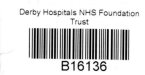
ANAESTHESIA
DATABOOK

A Perioperative and Peripartum Manual

3RD EDITION

ANAESTHESIA DATABOOK

A Perioperative and Peripartum Manual

3RD EDITION

Rosemary Mason MB ChB DObst RCOG FRCA

Consultant Anaesthetist
Swansea NHS Trust
Singleton Hospital
Swansea SA2 8QA
UK

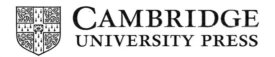

CAMBRIDGE
UNIVERSITY PRESS

CAMBRIDGE UNIVERSITY PRESS
Cambridge, New York, Melbourne, Madrid, Cape Town, Singapore, São Paulo, Delhi

Cambridge University Press
The Edinburgh Building, Cambridge CB2 8RU, UK

Published in the United States of America by Cambridge University Press, New York

www.cambridge.org
Information on this title: www.cambridge.org/9780521114196

First published 2001
Digitally reprinted by Cambridge University Press 2009

A catalogue record for this publication is available from the British Library

ISBN 978-0-521-11419-6 paperback

Contents

SECTION 1
Medical disorders and anaesthetic problems

A

Achalasia of the oesophagus 3
Achondroplasia 5
Acromegaly 8
Addiction 12
Addison's disease; adrenocortical
    insufficiency 14
AIDS; acquired immunodeficiency
    syndrome 17
Air embolism; see section 2 525
Alcoholism 23
Aldosteronism, Primary 26
Alkaptonuria 26
Alveolar proteinosis, pulmonary 27
Amniotic fluid embolism 29
Amphetamine abuse 29
Amyloidosis 32
Amyotrophic lateral sclerosis 36
Ankylosing spondylitis 36
Antiphospholipid syndrome (Hughes'
    syndrome) 40
Aortic regurgitation 43
Aortic stenosis 46
Arnold Chiari (and other Chiari)
    malformations 49
Arthrogryposis multiplex congenita 51
Asthma 54
Athletic heart syndrome 59
Automatic implantable cardioverter
    defibrillators 62
Autonomic failure 66

B

Becker muscular dystrophy 70

Beckwith-Wiedmann syndrome 71
Budd-Chiari syndrome 73
Buerger's disease 74

C

Carcinoid syndrome 76
Cardiac tamponade 79
Cardiomyopathies; dilated, hypertrophic,
    restrictive 82
Carnitine palmitoyl transferase deficiency 88
Carotid body tumour 90
Central core disease 91
C1 esterase inhibitor deficiency; acquired 93
Charcot-Marie-Tooth disease (peroneal
    muscular atrophy) 95
Charge association 96
Cherubism 98
Christmas disease (haemophilia B) 99
Churg-Strauss syndrome 99
Coarctation of the aorta, adult 100
Cocaine abuse 102
Cockayne syndrome 106
Conn's syndrome (primary aldosteronism) 107
Creutzfeldt-Jakob disease 109
Cri du Chat syndrome 111
Cushing's syndrome & Cushing's disease 112
Cystic fibrosis 114
Cystic hygroma (lymphangioma) 119

D

Dandy-Walker syndrome 122
Demyelinating diseases 123
Dermatomyositis/polymyositis complex 125
Diabetes insipidus 127
Diabetes mellitus 129
Diffuse idiopathic skeletal hyperostosis 134
Down's syndrome 136
Drowning and near drowning 139
Duchenne muscular dystrophy 142

v

Dystrophica myotonica; and other
   myotonic syndromes 147

E

Eaton-Lambert syndrome (Lambert-Eaton
   or myasthenic syndrome) 153
Ebstein's anomaly 155
Eclampsia and severe preeclampsia 156
Ehlers-Danlos syndrome 162
Eisenmenger's syndrome 166
Emery-Dreifuss muscular dystrophy 169
Epidermolysis bullosa (recessive dystrophic) 170
Epiglottitis 172
Epilepsy 176

F

Fabry's disease 182
Fallot's tetralogy 183
Familial dysautonomia (Riley-Day
   syndrome) 186
Familial periodic paralyses 188
Fat embolism syndrome 193
Fibrodysplasia (myositis) ossificans
   progressiva 196
Fraser syndrome 198
Freeman-Sheldon syndrome 199
Friedreich's ataxia 200

G

Gaucher's disease 203
Giant axonal neuropathy 204
Gilbert's disease (idiopathic unconjugated
   hyperbilirubinaemia) 205
Glomus jugulare tumour 205
Glucagonoma 207
Glucose-6-phosphate dehydrogenase
   deficiency 208
Glycogen storage diseases 209
Goldenhar's syndrome 210
Goodpasture's syndrome 212
Gorham's syndrome 213
Guillain-Barre syndrome 214

H

Haemoglobinopathies (sickle cell disease) 218
Haemophilias A; and haemophilia B 224
Hallervorden-Spatz disease (neuroaxonal
   dystrophy) 228

Heart block 229
HELLP syndrome 235
Hereditary angioneurotic oedema 238
Hereditary haemorrhagic telangiectasia
   (Osler-Weber-Rendu disease) 241
Hereditary spherocytosis 245
Hers' disease (Cori type VI glycogen
   storage disease) 246
Homocystinuria 247
Hunter's syndrome; see Hurler's and
   mucopolysaccharidoses 249
Huntington's disease 249
Hurler, Hurler-Schie, Schie, and Hunter's
   syndromes 250
Hydatid disease 255
Hypercalcaemia 256
Hyponatraemia 258
Hypothyroidism 262

I

Infectious mononucleosis 267
Insulinoma 269

J

Jehovah's Witnesses; management for
   surgery 272
Juvenile hyaline fibromatosis 277

K

Kawasaki disease (mucocutaneous lymph
   node syndrome) 279
Kearns-Sayre syndrome 280
Klippel-Feil syndrome 282
Klippel-Trenaunay-Weber syndrome 284

L

Lambert-Eaton syndrome 287
Laryngeal papillomatosis 287
Latex allergy 290
Lesch-Nyan disease 291
Ludwig's angina 292
Lysergic acid diethylamide (LSD) abuse 294

M

Malignant hyperthermia 296
Marcus-Gunn jaw winking syndrome 303
Marfan syndrome 303
Maroteaux-Lamy syndrome 307

Mastocytoses 308

McArdle's syndrome (myophosphorylase deficiency) 311

Mediastinal masses 313

Miller's syndrome 317

Mitochondrial encephalomyopathies 318

Mitral valve disease 321

Morquio's syndrome (mucopolysaccharidosis type IV) 328

Motor neurone disease (amyotrophic lateral sclerosis) 330

Moyamoya disease 332

Mucopolysaccharidoses 335

Multiple endocrine neoplasia 336

Multiple system atrophy (Shy-Drager syndrome) 337

Muscular dystrophies 339

Myasthenia gravis 340

Myasthenic syndrome 344

Myeloma, multiple 344

Myoglobinuria 345

Myotubular (centronuclear) myopathy 345

Myxoedema 346

Myxoma, cardiac 346

N

Nemaline myopathy 350

Neurofibromatosis (types 1 & 2; von Recklinghausen's disease) 351

Neurogenic pulmonary oedema 354

Neuroleptic malignant syndrome 354

Noonan's syndrome 357

O

Obesity 360

Obstructive sleep apnoea 363

Opiate addiction 368

Opitz-Frias syndrome 370

Osler-Weber-Rendu syndrome 370

Osteogenesis imperfecta 370

P

Pacemakers 375

Paget's disease 375

Papillomatosis 356

Parkinson's disease 356

Paroxsysmal nocturnal haemoglobinuria 380

Pemphigus vulgaris and foliaceous 382

Pericardial disease 384

Phaeochromocytoma 384

Phenylketonuria 391

Pierre-Robin syndrome and the Robin sequence 393

Pituitary apoplexy 397

Plasma cholinesterase abnormalities 399

Polycythaemia vera and secondary polycythaemias 402

Pompe's disease; and adult-onset acid maltase deficiency 405

Porphyria 407

Prader-Willi syndrome 413

Protein C deficiency 415

Protein S deficiency 418

Pulmonary hypertension 419

Pulmonary oedema 423

Q

QT interval syndromes, prolonged 433

R

Relapsing polychondritis 439

Rett syndrome 441

Rhabdomyolysis 442

Rheumatoid arthritis 447

S

Sarcoidosis 452

Schwartz-Jampel syndrome 454

Scleroderma 455

Scoliosis 458

Shy-Drager syndrome 461

Sick sinus syndrome (bradycardia/tachycardia syndrome) 461

Sipple's syndrome (MEN 2a) 463

Sjogren's syndrome 464

Solvent and volatile substance abuse 465

Spinal muscular atrophy 469

Spondyloepiphyseal dysplasia 470

Sturge-Weber syndrome 472

Systemic lupus erythematosus 473

T

Takaysu's arteritis 477

Tetanus 480

Thalassaemia 484

vii

Thalidomide-related deformities and
    other phocomelias 486
Thyrotoxicosis 487
Torsade de pointes (atypical ventricular
    tachycardia) 491
Tracheobronchomegaly 493
Treacher Collins syndrome 494
Tuberous sclerosis 496
Turner syndrome 497

V
Varicella 499
Vipoma 500
Von Gierke's disease and type 1b
    glycogenolysis 502
Von Hippel-Lindau disease 504
Von Recklinghausen's disease 506
Von Willebrand's disease 506

W
Wegener's granulomatosis 510
Werdnig-Hoffman disease 513
Williams syndrome 513
Wolff-Parkinson-White syndrome 516

Z
Zenker's diverticulum 520

SECTION 2
Emergency conditions arising during anaesthesia or in the immediate perioperative period

A
Addisonian crisis 523
Air embolism 525
Amniotic fluid embolism 531

Anaphylactoid/anaphylactic reactions to
    intravenous agents 534
Angioneurotic oedema 542
Aortocaval fistula 543
Arrhythmias 545

B
Bronchospasm 548

C
Carcinoid syndrome 549
Cardiac tamponade 551
Central anticholinergic syndrome 553

D
Glycine absorption syndrome 555

L
Latex allergy 555
Local anaesthetic toxicity 557

M
Malignant hyperthermia 563
Masseter muscle rigidity 566
Methaemoglobinaemia 569

P
Phaeochromocytoma 572
Pituitary apoplexy 576
Pulmonary oedema 577

S
Subdural block, accidental 577
Suxamethonium apnoea 580

T
Thyrotoxic crisis or storm 581
Torsade de pointes 584
Total spinal anaesthesia, accidental 586
TURP syndrome 588

Appendix 594

List of abbreviations

A

ACE	Angiotensin-converting enzyme
AChE	Acetylcholinesterase
ACLA	Anticardiolipin antibody
ACTH	Adrenocorticotrophic hormone
ADH	Antidiuretic hormone
AF	Atrial fibrillation
AFE	Amniotic fluid embolism
AIDS	Acquired immune deficiency syndrome
AIP	Acute intermittent porphyria
ALA	d-Aminolaevulinic acid (synthase)
AMP	Adenosine monophosphate
APA	Antiphospholipid antibody
APLS	Antiphospholipid antibody syndrome
APTT	Activated partial thromboplastin time
APUD	Amine precursor uptake and decarboxylation
ARDS	Adult respiratory distress syndrome
ASD	Atrial septal defect
AV	Atrioventricular
A-V	Arteriovenous
AVP	Arginine vasopressin
AZT	Zidovudine ('Retrovir')

B

BAL	Bronchoalveolar lavage
BBB	Bundle branch block
bd	Twice per day
BG	Blood glucose
BMR	Basal metabolic rate
BP	Blood pressure

C

C1	First component of complement
C2	Second component of complement
C4	Fourth component of complement
CABG	Coronary artery bypass graft
cAMP	Cyclical adenosine monophosphate
CAPD	Continuous ambulatory peritoneal dialysis
ChE	Cholinesterase
C1EI	C1 esterase inhibitor
CMV	Cytomegalic virus
CNS	Central nervous system
CPAP	Continuous positive airway pressure
CPB	Cardiopulmonary bypass
CK	Creatine kinase
CPR	Cardiopulmonary resuscitation
CRF	Corticotrophin-releasing factor
CSF	Cerebrospinal fluid
CT	Computerised tomography
CVP	Central venous pressure
CXR	Chest X-ray

D

DDC	3,5-Dicarbethoxy-1,4-dihydrocolidine
DDAVP	Desmopressin (1-desamino-8-D-arginine vasopressin)
DMD	Duchenne muscular dystrophy
DNA	Desoxyribose nucleic acid
DVI	Digital vascular imaging
DVT	Deep venous thrombosis

E

EBV	Epstein-Barr virus
ECF	Extracellular fluid
ECG	Electrocardiogram
ECM	External cardiac massage
ECMO	Extracorporeal membranous oxygenation

EEC	European Economic Community		HC	Hereditary coproporphyria
EMG	Electromyogram		HCM	Hypertrophic cardiomyopathy
EMLA	Eutectic mixture of local anaesthetics (cream)		HELLP	Haemolysis Elevated Liver enzymes and Low Platelet count (syndrome)
ENT	Ear nose and throat		HGPRT	Hypoxanthine guanine phosphoribosyl transferase
ESWL	Extracorporeal shock wave lithotripsy		HHT	Hereditary haemorrhagic telangiectasia
ETCO2	End tidal carbon dioxide		HIV	Human immunodeficiency virus
E_1f	Fluoride-resistant gene		HPA	Hypothalamic-pituitary-adrenal axis
EUA	Examination under anaesthesia			

F

FBG	Fasting blood glucose
FDA	Food and Drugs Administration (USA)
FDP	Fibrin degradation products
FEV1	Forced expiratory volume in the first second of expiration
FFP	Fresh frozen plasma
FGF	Fresh gas flow
FIO_2	Fractional inspired oxygen
FRC	Functional residual capacity
FSH	Follicle stimulating hormone

I

ICP	Intracranial pressure
IDD	Insulin-dependent diabetes
IgE	Immunoglobulin E
IGF-1	Insulin-like growth factor-1
IgG	Immunoglobulin G
IgM	Immunoglobulin M
ILMA	Intubating laryngeal mask airway
im	Intramuscular
INR	International normalized ratio
IPPV	Intermittent positive-pressure ventilation
IQ	Intelligence quotient
ISI	International sensitivity index
ITU	Intensive therapy unit
iu	International units
iv	Intravenous

G

G	Gauge
GABA	Gamma amino butyric acid
GFR	Glomerular filtration rate
GH	Growth hormone
GIK	Glucose, insulin, potassium (infusion)
GTT	Glucose tolerance test
G6PD	Glucose-6-phosphate dehydrogenase

J

J	Joule
JVP	Jugular venous pulse

K

kPa	Kilopascal
KCCT	Kaolin cephalin clotting time

H

Hb	Haemoglobin
HbA	Normal adult haemoglobin
HbAS	Sickle cell trait
HbA2	Haemoglobin A2
HbC	Haemoglobin C
HbCO	Carboxyhaemoglobin
HbF	Fetal haemoglobin
HbS	Sickle cell haemoglobin
HbSC	Sickle cell C disease
HbSS	Homozygous sickle cell anaemia
HbThal	Thalassaemia haemoglobin

L

l	Litre
L	Length
LA	Local anaesthesia
LAP	Left atrial pressure
LBBB	Left bundle branch block
LFTs	Liver function tests
LMA	Laryngeal mask airway
LMWH	Low molecular weight heparin

LSCS	Lower segment Caesarean section		OSA	Obstructive sleep apnoea
LSD	Lysergic acid diethylamide			
LT	Leukotrienes		**P**	
LVEDP	Left ventricular end diastolic pressure		$PaCO_2$	Arterial partial pressure of carbon dioxide
LVF	Left ventricular failure		PAN	Polyarteritis nodosa
			PaO_2	Arterial partial pressure of oxygen
M			PAP	Pulmonary artery pressure
MAC	Minimal alveolar concentration		PAVM	Pulmonary arteriovenous malformation
MAO	Monoamine oxidase		PAWP	Pulmonary artery wedge pressure
MAOI	Monoamine oxidase inhibitor		PCP	Pulmonary capillary pressure
MAP	Mean arterial pressure		PCV	Packed cell volume
MCV	Mean corpuscular volume		PV	Polycythaemia vera
MEN	Multiple endocrine neoplasia		PCWP	Pulmonary capillary wedge pressure
MH	Malignant hyperthermia			
MHE	Malignant hyperthermia equivocal result, consider as MHS		PDA	Patent ductus arteriosus
			PE	Pulmonary embolism
MHN	Malignant hyperthermia non-susceptible from proven MH pedigree		PEEP	Positive end expiratory pressure
			PEFR	Peak expiratory flow rate
			PH	Pulmonary hypertension
MHS	Malignant hyperthermia susceptible		P mitrale	A prolonged bifid P wave on ECG indicating left atrial enlargement
mIBG	*Meta*-iodobenzylguanidine			
mmHg	Millimetres of mercury		PP	Pancreatic polypeptide
MMR	Masseter muscle rigidity		P pulmonale	A taller than normal P wave on ECG indicating right atrial hypertrophy
MPS	Mucopolysaccharidosis			
MRI	Magnetic resonance imaging			
MS	Multiple sclerosis		PPF	Plasma protein fraction
MSA	Multiple system atrophy		PPH	Primary pulmonary hypertension
MSH	Melanocyte-stimulating hormone			
MV	Minute volume		PT	Prothrombin time
MVP	Mitral valve prolapse		PTH	Parathormone
MVV	Minute volume ventilation		PVC	Polyvinyl chloride
			PVR	Pulmonary vascular resistance
N				
N	Normal		**Q**	
NAB	Nasally assisted breathing		qds	Four times per day
NANBV	Non-A non-B virus (hepatitis)		QTc	Corrected QT interval
Nd:YAG	Neodynium: yttrium-aluminium-garnet (laser)			
			R	
NIDD	Non-insulin-dependent diabetes		RAP	Right atrial pressure
NMS	Neuroleptic malignant syndrome		RBBB	Right bundle branch block
NPO	Neurogenic pulmonary oedema		RBC	Red blood corpuscle
NSAID	Non-steroidal anti-inflammatory drug		RDS	Respiratory distress syndrome
			RF	Radio frequency
			RR	Respiratory rate
O			R-R variation	Variations in the intervals between two consecutive R waves (ECG)
OD	Outside diameter			

xi

RSR1	An initial upward deflection (R) is followed by a downward deflection (S) followed by a second upward deflection (R1) on ECG lead VI		TCT	Thrombin clotting time
			tds	Three times per day
			TIA	Transient ischaemic attack
			TRH	Thyrotrophin-releasing hormone
			TSH	Thyroid-stimulating hormone
RVEDP	Right ventricular end diastolic pressure		TURP	Transurethral resection of the prostate
			TV	Tidal volume

S

SAP	Systemic arterial pressure		**U**	
SBE	Subacute bacterial endocarditis		u	Unit
SIADH	Syndrome of inappropriate antidiuretic hormone		UK	United Kingdom
SIDS	Sudden infant death syndrome		**V**	
SLE	Systemic lupus erythematosus		VC	Vital capacity
SVC	Superior vena cava		VF	Ventricular fibrillation
SVR	Systemic vascular resistance		VIP	Vasoactive intestinal peptide
SVT	Supraventricular tachycardia		VP	Variegate porphyria
			VSD	Ventricular septal defect

T

t	Tesla (10 000 gauss)		VT	Ventricular tachycardia
T_3	Tri-iodothyronine		vWd	von Willebrand's disease
T_4	Thyroxine		vWF:Ag	von Willebrand factor
TCAD	Tricyclic antidepressant		**W**	
TCRE	Transcervical resection of the endometrium		WCC	White cell count
			WPW	Wolff-Parkinson-White syndrome

xii

Preface to the third edition

Fourteen years have elapsed since I began to write the first edition of Anaesthesia Databook. The original intention was to produce a medical text specifically for the experienced anaesthetist facing unusual conditions or difficult problems. The responses to both the first and second editions were gratifying.

Anaesthetists require an unusual skew of medical knowledge. In addition to common conditions that might require treatment before surgery, they need to be familiar with a variety of rare diseases which, in a standard medical textbook, would merit few lines. Certain genetic conditions, such as malignant hyperthermia, central core disease, the dystrophinopathies, periodic paralyses, phaeochromocytoma, hereditary angioneurotic oedema, long QT syndromes – to name but a few – have produced serious, or even fatal complications in association with anaesthesia.

This third edition reflects the many medical developments that have taken place in the last seven years. Four main changes have occurred that are particularly relevant to anaesthetists.

First, the quality of case reports has improved. A higher standard of preoperative assessment has resulted in a greater understanding of disease processes, and the potential negative effects of surgery and anaesthesia. Advice about management can be more firmly based on knowledge of the pathophysiology of an individual medical condition, and the likely effects of drugs and other invasive processes. In the sick patient, the use of continuous monitoring is essential to assist in the early diagnosis of complications.

Secondly, increasing numbers of evidence-based studies are being published about perioperative management, and the risks of anaesthesia and surgery, in uncommon conditions. Unfortunately, many of these studies, for example those of the Sickle Cell Disease Study Groups, appear in non-anaesthetic journals. One purpose of this book is to collate information from a wide variety of sources.

Thirdly, medical advances have increased, rather than decreased, anaesthetic difficulties. For example, development of new antiarrhythmic devices, such as automatic implantable cardioverter defibrillators, has implications for surgery and anaesthesia. Individuals with severely disabling genetic disorders, such as cystic fibrosis, now survive long enough to require incidental surgery, or to become pregnant. In either circumstance, it is assumed that the anaesthetist will provide safe anaesthesia or analgesia.

Since many anaesthetists now have obstetric sessions, this edition contains more information about the management of the pregnant patient. There have been many new developments in the understanding of medical disease in pregnancy, as well as some of the pregnancy-associated diseases. It is particularly important to educate obstetricians and midwives to refer patients to the anaesthetist sufficiently early, so that should the risks of continuing the pregnancy be considered to be too great, termination may be offered. I am grateful to my colleague, Dr Sue Catling, for her constructive criticisms of the sections on pregnancy-associated conditions. However, the responsibility for their content is mine alone.

Finally, in the year 2000, the first draft of the Human Genome Project was unveiled. Whilst the immediate clinical implications are uncertain, the contribution of genetic factors to disease processes has become increasingly apparent. The concept of one gene mutation causing a single defined clinical syndrome is being replaced. For example, in the long QT syndromes, genetic studies have shown at least five distinct mutations in genes influencing cardiac ionic channel function, each associated with different T wave patterns on ECG, and varying risks of ventricular arrhythmias and death. Deletions and mutations of mitochondrial DNA are responsible for the mitochondrial encephalomyopathies, a heterogenous group of multisystem diseases involving mitochondrial metabolic pathways. Mutations of tumour suppressor genes can result in a variety of conditions with an increased incidence of tumours, such as the multiple endocrine neoplasias, Beckwith–Wiedemann syndrome, and von Hippel Lindau disease.

In order to make room for new material, the book has been reduced to two sections; medical disorders and anaesthetic problems, and emergency conditions arising during anaesthesia or in the immediate perioperative period.

Once again, I hope that this book can ward off some problems and ease the predicament in others.

R.A.M.
Swansea 2001

SECTION 1

MEDICAL DISORDERS AND ANAESTHETIC PROBLEMS

Achalasia of the oesophagus

A chronic, progressive motor disorder of the oesophagus that is associated with degenerative changes in the myenteric ganglia and vagal nuclei. There are three components: a failure of the lower oesophageal sphincter to relax, with an increased resting sphincter pressure, which together result in a functional obstruction; an absence of sequential peristalsis in response to a bolus of food; a dilated, contorted oesophagus. Degeneration of the myenteric plexus and decreased nitric oxide synthesis may underly the problem. Overspill may produce bronchopulmonary complications, and 5–10% of patients ultimately develop carcinoma of the oesophagus. Nitrates and calcium channel blockers given before meals sometimes produce symptomatic improvement, but the mainstays of treatment are oesophageal dilatation and surgical myotomy. Open surgery has been mostly replaced by laparoscopic myotomy and fundoplication (Hunter & Richardson 1997). For elderly patients, endoscopic injection of botulinum toxin can give relief for several months without the risk of surgery.

Preoperative abnormalities

1. Symptoms include dysphagia, retrosternal pain, regurgitation, and weight loss. In young people the condition may be misdiagnosed as anorexia nervosa or asthma. Respiratory complications, which may be attributed to asthma or chronic bronchitis, are secondary to overspill of undigested material. Nocturnal coughing occurs in 30%, and bronchopulmonary complications in 10% of patients. The aspiration of larger volumes may result in lobar collapse, bronchiectasis, or lung abscess.

2. Rarely, it may present with a cervical mass and acute upper respiratory tract obstruction, necessitating urgent intervention (Dunlop & Travis 1997).

3. There is an increased risk of oesophageal carcinoma.

4. Diagnosis can be made on barium swallow, manometric studies and endoscopy. Occasionally, acute dilatation may be seen on CXR, in which case, abnormal flow volume curves will indicate variable intrathoracic tracheal obstruction.

Anaesthetic problems

1. A predisposition to regurgitation and pulmonary aspiration in the perioperative period.

2. Acute thoracic inlet obstruction with stridor, deep cyanosis of the face, and hypotension occurred during recovery from anaesthesia after gynaecological surgery (McLean et al 1976). Passage of the tracheal tube past the dilated oesophagus was achieved with difficulty. In a second, less severe case, neck swelling and venous engorgement was precipitated by coughing or straining (King & Strickland 1979).

3. Upper airway obstruction or respiratory failure, particularly in the elderly. Rarely, an acute dilatation of the oesophagus results in total airway obstruction (Travis et al 1981, Westbrook 1992). CXR shows a hugely dilated, air-filled upper oesophagus (Requena et al 1999). One patient developed acute respiratory failure 8 days after surgery for fractured neck of femur. The diagnosis was made on CXR, which showed an air-containing cavity along the right upper heart border (Kendall & Lin 1991). The opening pressure of the cricopharyngeus muscle from above is much lower than that from below, therefore progressive dilatation of the upper oesophagus may occur, particularly in association with air swallowing or IPPV. An increased intrathoracic pressure produced by a Valsalva manoeuvre forces air from the thoracic into the cervical oesophagus. Occasionally, death may occur.

4. If acute airway obstruction is present, sudden decompression of the oesophagus may cause the pharynx to flood with food and fluid, resulting in aspiration.

Management

1. If anaesthesia is required, precautions must be taken to reduce the risk of aspiration of gastric contents. The dilated oesophagus must be emptied and decompressed. This needs a period of prolonged starvation, possibly with washouts of the oesophagus, although the need for this has been challenged. A rapid sequence induction should be undertaken. Tracheal tube removal is performed in the awake patient, who should be nursed in the lateral position during recovery.

2. Sublingual nifedipine 10–20 mg has been shown to reduce the basal sphincter pressure after 10 min and the effect lasts for up to 40 min.

3. Management of acute upper airway obstruction secondary to tracheal compression has been reported using the following methods:

   a) Sublingual glyceryl nitrate (Westbrook 1992).

   b) Passage of a naso-oesophageal tube (Zikk et al 1989).

   c) Transcutaneous needle puncture (Evans et al 1982).

   d) Tracheal intubation (Becker & Castell 1989).

   e) Rigid oesophagoscopy (Carlsson-Norlander 1987).

   f) Emergency tracheostomy (Barr & MacDonald 1989).

   g) Cricopharyngeus myotomy (Ali et al 1995, Campbell et al 1995).

4. Treatment can be either surgical or medical. For the elderly and less fit patient, pneumatic dilatation, or endoscopic injection of botulinum toxin (Requena et al 1999), may be appropriate. Heller myotomy and partial fundoplication can be performed either as an open or a laparoscopic procedure.

Bibliography

Ali GN, Hunt DR, Jorgensen JO et al 1995 Esophageal achalasia and coexistent upper esophageal sphincter relaxation disorder presenting with airway obstruction. Gastroenterology 109: 1328–32.

Barr GD, MacDonald I 1989 Management of achalasia and laryngo-tracheal compression. Journal of Laryngology & Otology 103: 713–14.

Becker DJ, Castell DO 1989 Acute airway obstruction in achalasia. Possible role of defective belch reflex. Gastroenterology 97: 1323–6.

Campbell KL, Logie JR, Munro A 1995 Cricopharyngeus myotomy for upper airway obstruction in achalasia. British Journal of Surgery 82: 1668–9.

Carlsson-Norlander B 1987 Acute upper airway obstruction in a patient with achalasia. Archives of Otolaryngology & Head & Neck Surgery 113: 885–7.

Dunlop SP, Travis SP 1997 Achalasia presenting as acute stridor. European Journal of Gastroenterology & Hepatology 9: 1125–8.

Evans CR, Cawood R, Dronfield MW et al 1982 Achalasia: presentation with stridor and a new form of treatment. British Medical Journal 285: 1704.

Hunter JG, Richardson WS 1997 Surgical management of achalasia. Surgical Clinics of North America 77: 993–1015

Kendall AP, Lin E 1991 Respiratory failure as a presentation of achalasia of the oesophagus. Anaesthesia 46: 1039–40.

King DM, Strickland B 1979 An unusual cause of thoracic inlet obstruction. British Journal of Radiology 52: 910–13.

McLean RDW, Stewart CJ, Whyte DGC 1976 Acute thoracic inlet obstruction in achalasia of the oesophagus. Thorax 31: 456–9.

Requena R, Hart AK, Kuhn JJ 1999 Acute upper airway obstruction in achalasia. Otolaryngology—Head & Neck Surgery 120: 105–8.

Travis KW, Saini VK, O'Sullivan PT 1981 Upper-airway obstruction and achalasia of the oesophagus. Anesthesiology 54: 87–8.

Westbrook JL 1992 Oesophageal achalasia causing respiratory obstruction. Anaesthesia 47: 38–40.

Zikk D, Rapoport Y, Halperin D et al 1989 Acute airway obstruction and achalasia of the esophagus. Annals of Otology, Rhinology & Laryngology 98: 641–3.

Achondroplasia

A type of skeletal dysplasia inherited as autosomal dominant, and associated with mutations in the fibroblast growth factor receptor-3 gene. Cartilage formation at the epiphyses is defective. Bones dependent on cartilage proliferation are thus shortened, whereas periosteal and membraneous bones are unaffected. Head and trunk size are normal, but the extremities are undersized. Anaesthesia may be required for suboccipital craniectomy, laminectomy, ventriculoperitoneal shunts, limb lengthening, midface advancement, and Caesarean section. The incidence of sleep-related respiratory disturbances resulting in hypoxaemia is high. Mortality is increased at all ages, and infants are at particular risk of sudden death from brainstem compression or sleep apnoea.

Preoperative abnormalities

1.   Individuals are less than 1.4 m tall and of normal intelligence. Hands and feet are short, and the fingers are of equal length. The forehead protrudes, the nose is flattened, the mandible and tongue are large, but the maxilla is short. Hypoplasia of the midface and abnormalities of the skull base lead to obstructive sleep apnoea. There is severe lumbar lordosis, a reduced symphysis pubis to xiphoid distance, and often thoracic kyphoscoliosis with reduced anteroposterior diameter of the thorax. The pelvis is small.

2.   Spinal canal stenosis, craniocervical junction abnormalities and hydrocephalus are common; spinal cord compression may occur at any level and result in neurological symptoms. The foramen magnum is small at birth and growth rate is impaired. Recent studies have shown neurological deficits in children to be more common than was previously thought, and the risk of sudden death in the first year is high. Chronic hydrocephalus and ventriculomegaly may be caused by intracranial venous hypertension secondary to jugular foramen stenosis (Steinbok et al 1989). Surgical

decompression of the jugular foramen may relieve the hydrocephalus (Lundar et al 1990).

3.   Sleep-related respiratory abnormalities, from both peripheral and central causes, are prevalent in the child and young adult (Waters et al 1993).

4.   Restrictive lung disease can present at a young age.

5.   Although fertility is low, pregnancy does occur. As a result of the skeletal problems, the fetus remains high, in an intra-abdominal position. This may result in severe respiratory embarrassment in the later stages of pregnancy. The baby is, however, of near normal size, making Caesarean section mandatory.

Anaesthetic problems

1.   The larynx is smaller than normal, and its size is related to patient weight, rather than to age (Mayhew et al 1986). Upper airway obstruction has been reported, in association with adenotonsillar hypertrophy and pharyngeal hypoplasia. Mask ventilation may be difficult because of the facial structure.

2.   Intubation problems have occurred as a result of premature fusion of the bones at the base of the skull, and limited mobility of the cervical vertebrae. However, in one series of 36 patients no intubation difficulty was experienced (Mayhew et al 1986), and in another report of 15 patients, the single failed intubation was solved by use of a laryngeal mask airway (Monedero et al 1997).

3.   Extreme hyperextension of the neck during airway manoeuvres may result in compression of the brainstem, if there is a small, anteriorly placed foramen magnum.

4.   Intravenous access may be difficult, particularly in the infant, because of lax, folded skin and excessive subcutaneous fat. During resuscitation of a patient from multiple trauma, peripheral venous and central venous cannulation needed multiple attempts (Dvorak

5

et al 1993). Eventually, an infraclavicular approach to the subclavian vein was successful.

5. Technical problems using automatic blood pressure monitoring may be encountered, since it can be difficult to match the cuff size to a short, fat arm. McArthur (1992) found that excessive arterial pressures were recorded by indirect methods, when compared with direct arterial monitoring.

6. Sleep apnoea and hypoxaemia are common. Abnormal respiratory function may be central or peripheral in origin, and several studies have demonstrated multiple aetiologies. Three groups of abnormalities were identified in 17 infants with respiratory difficulties. They were, in increasing order of seriousness: i) mid face hypoplasia, producing 'relative' adenotonsillar hypertrophy, ii) jugular foramen stenosis, which resulted in muscular upper airway obstruction and progressive hydrocephalus, and iii) hypoglossal foramen stenosis, which again produced muscular upper airway obstruction, with or without foramen magnum compression. In group iii), the most severely affected group, gastro-oesophageal reflux was common (Tasker et al 1998). In another study of 88 children, aged from 1 month to 12.6 years, sleep-disordered breathing occurred in almost 50%, and 20% were severely affected (Mogayzel et al 1998). In infants with foramen magnum stenosis, a significant risk of sudden death from medullary compression exists. This group of patients requires brainstem decompression. However, hypotonia of the upper airway muscles is common in the infant and may contribute to airway obstruction during sleep (Berkowitz et al 1990). Studies in older children (mean age 4.7 years) showed that upper airway obstruction was the most important sleep disorder, and the pattern recorded was similar to that seen in children with adenotonsillar hypertrophy (Zucconi et al 1996). This was confirmed by Waters et al (1995), who found that, in children, measures designed to relieve upper airway obstruction produced considerable improvement in sleep pattern, and a reduction in obstructive episodes.

In adults, studies of lung volumes have shown that vital capacity is reduced out of proportion to that expected had the limb sizes been normal, but that the lungs and airways are functionally normal (Stokes et al 1990).

7. Adenotonsillectomy. The complication rate from this is higher than in the general population (Sisk et al 1999).

8. Regional anaesthesia. Technical difficulties may be experienced during regional anaesthesia as a consequence of the skeletal defects (Nguyen et al 1997). A narrow spinal canal, and reduced width of the epidural space, increases the risk of both accidental dural puncture and an extensive epidural block. Identification of inadvertent dural puncture may be more difficult because of impairment of the free flow of CSF. Engorged epidural veins also increase the likelihood of dural puncture, either by the needle or the catheter. Since neurological problems can develop spontaneously during the third and fourth decades, regional blockade should be approached with circumspect. Initial clinical symptoms of thoracolumbar involvement are lower limb motor weakness and low back pain, with sensory and sphincter disturbances occurring less frequently.

9. Neurosurgery. Twenty-four patients with achondroplasia undergoing craniectomies were reviewed (Mayhew et al 1986). Out of 16 patients whose surgery was performed in the sitting position, nine had some degree of air embolism, whereas only one operated on in the prone position had such a problem. The air was usually successfully aspirated, and no patient died. Six other major complications occurred; two patients had C1 level spinal cord infarctions, two had brachial plexus palsies, and one was extubated accidentally. The sixth patient, after developing severe oedema of the tongue, required tracheostomy. This was thought to be due to extreme flexion of the neck producing venous thrombosis (Mayhew et al 1985). A 6-month-old baby in the prone position had torrential haemorrhage, followed by air embolism and cardiac arrest (Kelleher &

Mackersie 1995).Visual loss occurred after prolonged spinal fusion surgery, in which a hypotensive technique was used whilst the patient was positioned head down (Roth et al 1997).

10. Anaesthesia for Caesarean section may compound many of the problems identified above. In the later stages of pregnancy the supine position can be associated with severe aortocaval compression and respiratory embarrassment. Successful anaesthesia, using both general and epidural techniques, has been described. However, even if the technical difficulties of regional anaesthesia are overcome, it should be remembered that small doses of local anaesthetic given epidurally can produce extensive, and sometimes patchy, neural blockade. In one patient, bupivacaine 0.5% 12 ml produced a block from C5 to S4 (Brimacombe & Caunt 1990), and in a second, 5 ml only was required for Caesarean section (Wardall & Frame 1990). Problems were not encountered in all patients and Carstoniu et al (1992) emphasise that a woman must not be denied epidural anaesthesia, should the need for it arise.

11. Problems secondary to chronic hydrocephalus were reported in a patient after a head injury (Dvorak et al 1993).An unusually large epidural haematoma was thought to have been caused by displacement of CSF through an open fourth ventricle. Postoperative IPPV may have exacerbated the elevation of ICP.

Management

1. Since upper airway obstruction can be improved by a number of manoeuvres (adenotonsillectomy, nasal continuous positive airway pressure (NCPAP) and weight loss), these might be considered before embarking on major surgery (Waters et al 1995). Overnight admission for ENT procedures is mandatory, and some patients may require longer observation.

2. Possible intubation difficulties should be considered when the patient is assessed.A range of tracheal tubes, of sizes smaller than normal,

should be available (Sisk et al 1999). Mayhew et al (1986) believe that size in children should be based on age, according to the formula: tube size (internal diameter in mm) = [age (years) + 16]/4. Extreme care should be taken to avoid hyperextension of the neck, which could result in brainstem compression.

3. If venous access is required urgently, the posterior approach to the internal jugular vein has been recommended (Dvorak et al 1993).

4. Particular care is needed when positioning the patient for surgery. Upper limbs should be well supported, and extreme neck flexion avoided.

5. During neurosurgical procedures performed in the sitting position, great care should be taken to avoid air embolus (Katz & Mayhew 1985, Mayhew et al 1986). However, no patient died in the series presented. In addition, the prone position may be associated with heavy blood loss, and does not guarantee freedom from air embolism.Asystolic cardiac arrest occurred in a baby after a combination of torrential haemorrhage and air embolism during foramen magnum decompression. However, successful external cardiac massage was performed in the prone position and the baby survived without neurological deficit (Kelleher & Mackersie 1995).Whatever position is chosen for surgery, air embolism must be anticipated, diagnosed, and treated early. Care should be taken in positioning of the head to avoid ischaemic optic neuropathy.

6. In late pregnancy, if breathing is compromised, blood gases should be taken before Caesarean section, to assess respiratory function.

7. Despite technical difficulties, epidural anaesthesia can be used for Caesarean section or other surgery, although the doses of local anaesthetic should be titrated carefully to avoid extensive blockade (Brimacombe & Caunt 1990, Wardall & Frame 1990, Carstoniu et al 1992, Nguyen et al 1997, Morrow & Black 1998). Final volumes of local anaesthetic required to produce

surgical block have varied from 5 ml to 18 ml, and in one patient, fentanyl 37.5 μg was added at the end. A microspinal catheter technique has been reported for Caesarean section (Crawford & Dutton 1992). A single shot spinal technique with 1.3 ml hyperbaric bupivacaine and 10 μg fentanyl produced a bilateral block to T3 for an emergency Caesarean section (Ravenscroft et al 1998).

8. In labour, aortocaval compression must be prevented.

Bibliography

Berkowitz ID, Raja SN, Bender KS et al 1990 Dwarfs: pathophysiology and anesthetic implications. Anesthesiology 73: 739–59.

Brimacombe JR, Caunt JA 1990 Anaesthesia in an achondroplastic dwarf. Anaesthesia 45: 132–4.

Carstoniu J, Yee I, Halpern S 1992 Epidural anaesthesia for Caesarean section in an achondroplastic dwarf. Canadian Journal of Anaesthesia 39: 708–11.

Crawford M, Dutton DA 1992 Spinal anaesthesia for caesarean section in an achondroplastic dwarf. Anaesthesia 47: 1007.

Dvorak DM, Rusnak RA, Morcos JJ 1993 Multiple trauma in the achondroplastic dwarf: an emergency medicine physician perspective case report and literature review. American Journal of Emergency Medicine 11: 390–5.

Katz J, Mayhew JF 1985 Air embolism in the achondroplastic dwarf. Anesthesiology 63: 205–7.

Kelleher A, Mackersie A 1995 Cardiac arrest and resuscitation of a 6-month-old achondroplastic baby undergoing neurosurgery in the prone position. Anaesthesia 50: 348–50.

Lundar T, Bakke J, Nornes H 1990 Hydrocephalus in an achondroplastic child treated by venous decompression at the jugular foramen. Journal of Neurosurgery 73: 138–40.

Mayhew JF, Miner M, Katz J 1985 Macroglossia in a 16 month old child following a craniotomy. Anesthesiology 62: 683–4.

Mayhew JF, Katz J, Miner M et al 1986 Anaesthesia for the achondroplastic dwarf. Canadian Anaesthetists' Society Journal 33: 216–21.

McArthur RDA 1992 Obstetric anaesthesia in an achondroplastic dwarf at a regional hospital. Anaesthesia & Intensive Care 20: 376–8.

Mogayzel PJ Jr, Carroll JL, Loughlin GM et al 1998 Sleep-disordered breathing in children with achondroplasia. Journal of Pediatrics 132: 667–71.

Monedero P, Garcia-Pedrajas F, Coca I et al 1997 Is management of anesthesia in achondroplastic dwarfs really a challenge? Journal of Clinical Anesthesia 9: 208–12.

Morrow MJ, Black IH 1998 Epidural anaesthesia for Caesarean section in an achondroplastic dwarf. British Journal of Anaesthesia 81: 619–21.

Nguyen TT, Papadakos PJ, Sabnis LU 1997 Epidural anesthesia for extracorporeal shock wave lithotripsy in an achondroplastic dwarf. Regional Anesthesia 22: 102–4.

Ravenscroft AJ, Govendor T, Rout C 1998 Spinal anaesthesia for emergency Caesarean section in an achondroplastic dwarf. Anaesthesia 53: 1236–7.

Roth S, Nunez R, Schreider BD 1997 Unexplained visual loss after lumbar spinal fusion. Journal of Neurosurgical Anesthesiology 9: 346–8.

Sisk EA, Heatley DG, Borowski BJ et al 1999 Obstructive sleep apnoea in children with achondroplasia. Otolaryngology—Head & Neck Surgery 120: 248–54.

Steinbok P, Hall J, Flodmark O 1989 Hydrocephalus in achondroplasia: the possible role of intracranial venous hypertension. Journal of Neurosurgery 71: 42–8.

Stokes DC, Wohl ME, Wise RA et al 1990 The lungs and airways in achondroplasia. Do little people have little lungs? Chest 98: 145–52.

Tasker RC, Dundas I, Laverty A et al 1998 Distinct patterns of respiratory difficulty in young children with achondroplasia: a clinical, sleep, and lung function study. Archives of Disease in Childhood 79: 99–108.

Wardall GJ, Frame WT 1990 Extradural anaesthesia for Caesarean section in achondroplasia. British Journal of Anaesthesia 64: 367–70.

Waters KA, Everett F, Sillence DO et al 1995 Treatment of obstructive sleep apnea in achondroplasia: evaluation of sleep, breathing, and somatosensory-evoked potentials. American Journal of Medical Genetics 59: 460–6.

Zucconi M, Weber G, Castronovo V et al 1996 Sleep and upper airway obstruction in children with achondroplasia. Journal of Pediatrics 129: 743–9.

Acromegaly

A rare, chronic disease of insidious onset, which usually presents in middle life. An increased secretion of growth hormone (GH), associated with high insulin-like growth factor (somatomedin, IGF-1) levels, results in an overgrowth of bone, connective tissue, and viscera. It is most commonly caused by an adenoma of the eosinophil cells of the pituitary. Lifespan is considerably shortened, and deaths are primarily from cerebrovascular, respiratory and cardiovascular complications. Death from respiratory causes is three times more common than in the general population, probably secondary to airway obstruction, less often in association with CNS dysfunction (Murrant & Gatland 1990). There is also a threefold increase in deaths from neoplastic conditions, in particular colonic and breast cancer.

The treatment of choice is now transsphenoidal hypophysectomy, although radiotherapy, dopamine agonists, and somatostatin analogues may play a part. Despite successful surgery, hormone secretion fails to return to normal in about 50% of patients. If untreated, these individuals are still at risk from complications, so either radiotherapy or pharmacological therapy must be given (Frohman 1996).

Drugs that suppress hormonal output include bromocriptine and long acting somatostatin analogues, such as octreotide. The aim should be for symptomatic control, and a GH level of $<5\,\mathrm{mU\,l^{-1}}$ (Wass 1993). Patients most commonly require surgery for the pituitary adenoma, colonic or breast carcinoma, airway problems, and gallstones.

Preoperative abnormalities

1. The head, tongue, jaw, hands and feet are enlarged. Facial features are coarse, and the voice husky.

2. Kyphoscoliosis, muscular weakness, nerve entrapment syndromes, hypertension, acromegalic heart disease (10%), goitre, diabetes mellitus (10–20%), diabetes insipidus, hypercalcaemia, and visual field defects may be present.

3. There is evidence of a distinct acromegalic cardiomyopathy which is independent of

hypertensive heart disease (Lopez–Valasco et al 1997), and cardiac structure and function may improve after octreotide treatment.

4. Sleep apnoea can occur in up to 39% of patients. In comparison with a group of acromegalics without sleep apnoea, those with sleep apnoea had higher GH and IGF-1 levels, were older, and had greater neck circumference (Rosenow et al 1996). It has been suggested that OSA in acromegalics is different from other forms. Isono et al (1999) have shown extreme collapsibility of the pharynx, both at the tongue base and the soft palate edges, when patients are anaesthetised and paralysed. Sleep apnoea syndrome may resolve with hypophysectomy, but not always (Mickelson et al 1994).

5. Patients with active disease have large lungs (Harrison 1978). However, upper airway obstruction is common and may be secondary to pharyngeal soft tissue hypertrophy, thickening of the glottis and supraglottis, or reduced mobility of the vocal cords. Bilateral laryngocoeles have also been reported (Motta et al 1997).

6. There is an increased incidence of colonic cancer (8%), skin tags, and colonic polyps (46%) compared with the normal population (de Herder et al 1997).

7. Muscle weakness may occur.

8. Enlargement of the sella turcica may be evident on skull X-ray in 90% of cases.

9. Levels of GH are high and GH stimulates the output of insulin-like growth factor from the liver. Levels of both of these hormones may fail to return to normal after apparently successful treatment. Thus, the patient may be taking long-term bromocriptine.

10. Somatostatin may cause gall stones.

Anaesthetic problems

1. There are reports of a variety of airway problems, which can occur at any stage of the perioperative period. Some complications are more likely in patients who are known, before

surgery, to have airway obstruction and sleep apnoea. Extrathoracic airway obstruction occurs in 30–50% of acromegalics (Murrant & Gatland 1990, Trotman–Dickenson et al 1991), it is particularly common in men, and results in nocturnal hypoxaemia. Fibreoptic endoscopy has demonstrated that obstruction results from airway collapse at the level of the soft palate, rather than at the tongue base, and persistence of airway problems after surgery is common (Pelttari et al 1995).

At least six types of perioperative airway problem have been described:

a) Difficulty in mask ventilation because of inability to obtain an airtight fit with the mask. This results from both skeletal and soft tissue hypertrophy. Once the patient is anaesthetised and paralysed, the pharynx becomes more collapsible at both the tongue base and the soft palate edges (Isono et al 1999). In acromegalics, the exceedingly rare combination of impossible mask ventilation and impossible intubation may occur.

b) Difficulty in visualising the larynx with conventional laryngoscopes—often because of massive hypertrophy of the pharyngeal mucosa. In a study of 15 patients, using a size 5 Macintosh blade, five were classified as having a grade 3 or 4 view (Hakala et al 1998).

c) Difficulty in passing the tracheal tube because of mucosal thickening, laryngocoeles, cricoarytenoid and laryngeal chondrocalcification, glottic stenosis, and fixation or paralysis of the vocal cords. Resistance to passage of the tube has also been encountered during asleep fibreoptic intubation, when preformed, standard-tipped tubes were used (Hakala et al 1998).

d) Difficulties in fibreoptic intubation, performed under general anaesthesia, occurred in four out of 15 patients (Hakala et al 1998). However, this is not surprising, in view of the collapsibility of the pharynx and upper airway, during both sleep and anaesthesia.

e) Postintubation, or postoperative, obstruction. After transsphenoidal hypophysectomy, packing of the nose may predispose to upper airway obstruction and pulmonary oedema (Singelyn & Scholtes 1988).

2. Increased daytime somnolence and sleep apnoea are both common in active disease (Rosenow et al 1996), but surgery does not necessarily cure the problem. Obstructive sleep apnoea, combined with CNS depressant effects of drugs, may result in severe postoperative hypoxia, hypercarbia or respiratory arrest (Ovassapian et al 1981). Sudden deaths, which sometimes occur on return to the ward, may be explained by a combination of these factors, and respiratory obstruction.

3. The presence of hypertension, ischaemic heart disease, or cardiomyopathy will increase the perioperative risks. In a controlled study of cardiac arrhythmias, complex ventricular arrhythmias were found in 48% of acromegalics, compared with 12% in normal subjects (Kahaly et al 1992a). Left ventricular muscle mass was increased secondary to concentric ventricular hypertrophy and was related to the duration of the disease, rather than to its severity (Kahaly et al 1992b).

4. Acute pulmonary oedema has occurred secondary to upper airway obstruction (Goldhill et al 1982).

5. Impaired ulnar artery circulation was found in five out of ten acromegalic patients undergoing hypophysectomy (Campkin 1980), however this problem has not been confirmed by others. Losasso et al (1990) inserted 51 radial artery cannulae in acromegalics without performing Allen's test, and no patient developed ischaemic complications subsequently.

Management

1. Airway problems must be anticipated in advance and a careful history should be directed

towards this. Cervical X-rays may indicate overgrowth of pharyngeal tissue, glottic stenosis, or chondrocalcinosis. Nasoendoscopy or indirect laryngoscopy may be helpful. Airway abnormalities in acromegaly may be classified (Southwick & Katz 1979) as:

a) No involvement.

b) Hypertrophied nasal and pharyngeal mucosa, but normal vocal cords.

c) Glottic stenosis or vocal cord paresis.

d) Combination of both b) and c).

In the presence of either c) or d), and especially if there is sleep apnoea, elective tracheostomy should be considered (Murrant & Gatland 1990). Otherwise, awake fibreoptic intubation is probably the safest method of induction (Hakala et al 1998). If possible, an armoured tube, or a tube with a special tip, should be used. Fibreoptic intubation has been claimed to obviate the need for tracheostomy (Venus 1980, Ovassapian et al 1981, Messick et al 1982). However, one patient in whom tracheostomy was avoided required emergency reintubation on three occasions in the postoperative period—twice for airway obstruction and once for respiratory arrest (Ovassapian et al 1981). Fibreoptic techniques may have transformed the management of difficult intubation as such, but in acromegalics the airway problems are not restricted to the intraoperative period, nor are they solely of a technical nature. The use of an airway exchange catheter has also been described, when a nasal tube needed to be converted to an oral tube. The larynx was visualised with a Negus bronchoscope, the catheter was passed alongside the nasal tube and, once ventilation was confirmed, a flexometallic tube was railroaded over the top (Hulme & Blues 1999).

2. Postoperatively, acromegalics should be admitted to an area of high dependency, where respiration and cardiac rhythm can be carefully monitored. If nasal packing is required following hypophysectomy, it has been suggested that 18-gauge suction catheters, cut to sufficient length to pass beyond the base of the tongue, be inserted into each nostril before packing (Singelyn & Scholtes 1988). Postoperative CPAP, given via two nasal airways and a double lumen tube connector, avoided the use of tracheostomy in one patient (Young et al 1993).

3. Octreotide pretreatment for 3–4 months prior to removal of pituitary adenoma has been shown to be associated with remission of symptoms and tumour shrinkage (Stevenaert & Beckers 1996). Other benefits from long term octreotide include improvement in sleep apnoea, and in the structure and function of the heart (Lombardi et al 1996, Buyse et al 1997). In a controlled trial, it was found that 3–6 months' treatment with octreotide limited the anaesthetic risks associated with metabolic and cardiac impairment, improved surgical outcome, and reduced the duration of hospital stay after operation (Colao et al 1997).

4. Care must still be taken in treated acromegalics who have not had their GH levels checked, or who are not receiving bromocriptine. In these patients, sleep apnoea is unlikely if the patient is <60 years of age and has GH levels <2 mU l^{-1} (Rosenow et al 1996).

5. It has been suggested that surgery for pituitary adenoma be confined to selected centres in the UK (Clayton et al 1999).

Bibliography

Buyse B, Michiels E, Bouillon R et al 1997 Relief of sleep apnoea after treatment of acromegaly: report of three cases and review of the literature. European Respiratory Journal 10: 1401–4.

Campkin TV 1980 Radial artery cannulation. Potential hazards in patients with acromegaly. Anaesthesia 35: 1008–9.

Clayton RN, Stewart PM, Shalet SM et al 1999 Pituitary surgery for acromegaly. British Medical Journal 319: 588–9.

Colao A, Ferone D, Cappabianca P et al 1997 Effect of octreotide pretreatment on surgical outcome in acromegaly. Journal of Clinical Endocrinology & Metabolism 82: 3308–14.

de Herder WW, van der Lely AJ, Lamberts SW 1997 Colorectal screening in acromegaly. Still many unresolved questions. Clinical Endocrinology 47: 644–6.

Frohman LA 1996 Acromegaly: what constitutes optimal therapy? Journal of Clinical Endocrinology & Metabolism 81: 443–5.

Goldhill DR, Dalgleish JG, Lake RHN 1982 Respiratory problems and acromegaly. Anaesthesia 37: 1200–3.

Hakala P, Randell T, Valli H 1998 Laryngoscopy and fibreoptic intubation in acromegalic patients. British Journal of Anaesthesia 80: 345–7.

Harrison 1978 Lung function in acromegaly. Quarterly Journal of Medicine 47: 517–33.

Hulme GJ, Blues CM 1999 Acromegaly and papillomatosis: difficult intubation and the use of the airway exchange catheter. Anaesthesia 54: 787–9.

Isono S, Saeki N, Tanaka A et al 1999 Collapsibility of passive pharynx in patients with acromegaly. American Journal of Respiratory & Critical Care Medicine 160: 64–8.

Kahaly G, Olshausen KV, Mohr-Kahaly S et al 1992a Arrhythmia profile in acromegaly. European Heart Journal 13: 51–6.

Kahaly G, Stover C, Beyer J et al 1992b Relation of endocrine and cardiac findings in acromegalics. Journal of Endocrinological Investigation 15: 13–18.

Lombardi G, Colao A, Ferone D et al 1996 Cardiovascular aspects in acromegaly: effects of treatment. Metabolism: Clinical & Experimental 45: 57–60.

Lopez-Velasco R, Escobar-Morreale HF, Vega B et al 1997 Cardiac involvement in acromegaly: specific myocardiopathy or consequence of hypertension. Journal of Clinical Endocrinology & Metabolism 82: 1047–53.

Losasso T, Dietz NM, Muzzi DA 1990 Acromegaly and radial artery cannulation. Anesthesia & Analgesia 71: 204.

Messick JM, Cucchiara RF, Faust RJ 1982 Airway management in patients with acromegaly. Anesthesiology 56: 157.

Mickelson SA, Rosenthal LD, Rock JP et al 1994 Obstructive sleep apnea syndrome and acromegaly. Otolaryngology—Head & Neck Surgery 111: 25–30.

Motta S, Ferone D, Colao A et al 1997 Fixity of vocal cords and laryngocele in acromegaly. Journal of Endocrinological Investigation 20: 672–4.

Murrant NJ, Gatland DJ 1990 Respiratory problems in acromegaly. Journal of Laryngology & Otology 104: 52–5.

Ovassapian A, Doka JC, Romsa DE 1981 Acromegaly—use of fiberoptic laryngoscopy to avoid tracheostomy. Anesthesiology 54: 429–30.

Pelttari L, Polo O, Rauhala E et al 1995 Nocturnal breathing abnormalities in acromegaly after adenoidectomy. Clinical Endocrinology 43: 175–82.

Rosenow F, Reuter S, Deuss U et al 1996 Sleep apnoea in treated acromegaly: relative frequency and predisposing factors. Clinical Endocrinology 45: 563–9.

Singelyn FJ, Scholtes JL 1988 Airway obstruction in acromegaly. Anaesthesia & Intensive Care 16: 491–2.

Southwick JP, Katz J 1979 Unusual airway difficulty in the acromegalic patient-indications for tracheostomy. Anesthesiology 51: 72–3.

Stevenaert A, Beckers A 1996 Presurgical octreotide: treatment in acromegaly. Metabolism: Clinical & Experimental 45: 72–4.

Trotman-Dickenson B, Weetman AP, Hughes JMB 1991 Upper airflow obstruction and pulmonary function in acromegaly: relationship to disease activity. Quarterly Journal of Medicine 290: 527–38.

Venus B 1980 Acromegalic patient—indication for fiberoptic bronchoscopy but not tracheostomy. Anesthesiology 52: 100–1.

Wass JA 1993 Acromegaly: treatment after 100 years. British Medical Journal 307: 1505–6.

Young ML, Hanson CW 1993 An alternative to tracheostomy following transsphenoidal hypophysectomy in a patient with sleep apnea. Anesthesia & Analgesia 76: 446–9.

Addiction (see also Alcoholism, Amphetamine abuse, Cocaine abuse, LSD abuse, Opiate addiction, Solvent (volatile) abuse)

The incidence of drug addiction is increasing. New drugs are being used and hence new complications are being reported. Anaesthesia may be required for addicts in either an acute or a chronic state of intoxication (Larson et al 1997). Alternatively, the anaesthetist is increasingly involved in resuscitation and treatment of patients suffering toxic side effects of drugs or drug cocktails. Hazards exist not only for the patient, but also for staff in the hospital. Accidental rupture of drug packages concealed in body cavities may result in severe acute absorption or intestinal obstruction. Problems are encountered during pregnancy and labour (Gerada & Farrell 1990, Birnbach 1998, Birnbach & Stein 1998).

Terminology may vary geographically, but the following are commonly used terms:

Speedballs—heroin laced with cocaine.

Ecstasy—3,4-methylenedioxy-methamphetamine (MDMA).

Eve—3,4-methylenedioxyethamphetamine (MDEA).

Ice or blue ice—crystalline methamphetamine.

Individual drugs are dealt with separately in the text, but the following comments are generally applicable.

Anaesthetic problems

1. Difficulties in obtaining an accurate history.

2. Problems associated with chronic abuse.

3. Problems of withdrawal syndrome during a period of illness.

4. Difficulties with venepuncture.

5. Associated malnutrition and liver disease.

6. Problems of acute toxicity. The possibility exists that the patient may inject a drug into his/her infusion.

7. Increased risk of hepatitis B and HIV, septicaemia, bacterial endocarditis and tetanus in intravenous drug users.

8. Rhabdomyolysis, and occasionally acute renal failure, may be associated with the consumption of cocaine.

9. During pregnancy there is increased maternal and fetal morbidity and mortality.

10. Problems of resuscitation from overdose of drug or drug cocktails.

11. Problems of mixing drugs and contamination with other substances.

12. Ecstasy (MDMA) and Eve (MDEA), sometimes in combination with other substances, have been associated with a syndrome of convulsions, hyperthermia, hyperkalaemia, rhabdomyolysis, and disseminated intravascular coagulation.

General management

1. In general, drugs should not be withdrawn in the perioperative period.

2. Patients should be treated as if they were infected with hepatitis B virus or HIV.

3. An addiction centre may provide information and advice.

Bibliography

Birnbach DJ 1998 Anesthesia and the drug abusing parturient. Anesthesiology Clinics of North America 16: 385–95.

Birnbach DJ, Stein DJ 1998 The substance-abusing parturient: implications for analgesia and anesthesia management. Bailliere's Clinical Obstetrics & Gynaecology 12: 443–60.

Caldwell TB 1990 Anesthesia for patients with behavioral and environmental disorders. In: Katz J, Benumof J (eds) Anesthesia and uncommon diseases. WB Saunders, Philadelphia, pp 792–922.

DHSS 1991 Drug misuse and dependence. Guidelines on clinical management. HMSO, London.

Gerada C, Farrell M 1990 Management of the pregnant opiate user. British Journal of Hospital Medicine 43: 138–41.

Larson MJ, Samet JH, McCarty D 1997 Managed care of substance abuse disorders. Implications for generalist physicians. Medical Clinics of North America 81: 845–65.

McCammon RL 1987 Anesthesia for the chemically dependent patient. Anesthesia & Analgesia Review Course Lectures 47–55.

McGoldrick KE 1980 Anesthetic implications of drug abuse. Anesthesiology Review 7: 12–17.

Wood PR, Soni N 1989 Anaesthesia and substance abuse. Anaesthesia 44: 672–80.

Addison's disease (Adrenocortical insufficiency, see also Section 2)

Chronic adrenocortical insufficiency results from a variety of causes (Oelkers 1996). In the commonest form (idiopathic), adrenal autoantibodies are found, and other endocrine deficiencies may be demonstrated. Tuberculosis, secondary carcinoma, AIDS (Hilton et al 1988), and amyloidosis are other causes. In patients with adenocarcinoma, adrenal metastases are not uncommon (Ihde et al 1990), but clinically apparent disease occurs only after a 90% loss of adrenocortical tissue. In the majority of patients, Addison's disease will present in a chronic form, and may be difficult to diagnose. However, hyponatraemia and hyperkalaemia in the absence of renal failure should immediately suggest the diagnosis. Cardiovascular collapse from classical, acute adrenocortical failure is only rarely seen. However, since surgery and anaesthesia are both potent stress factors that require an increased steroid output, this deficiency may become apparent under these circumstances. A small number of patients develop adrenal insufficiency during critical illness on the ITU, and this may be masked by other causes of hypotension (Duggan et al 1998). However, there is controversy about what constitutes normal adrenal function in the critically ill, the accepted values for the ACTH stimulation tests, and the doses of steroids to be used if hypofunction is suspected or confirmed (Masterson & Mostafa 1998, McAllister 1998, Absalom & Scott 1999).

Acute adrenocortical insufficiency following sudden withdrawal of long term steroid therapy is a potential problem, but there is some dispute about the duration of hypothalamic–pituitary–adrenal axis (HPA) suppression. Recent studies suggest that the problem has been overexaggerated (Salem et al 1994, Levy 1996, Nicholson et al 1998). Current recommendations for treatment are given at the end of the management section.

Preoperative abnormalities

1. Addison's disease can present with weight loss, weakness, infertility, emotional instability, abdominal pain, diarrhoea, hyperpigmentation of skin and mucous membranes (particularly lips, skin creases, elbows, and knees), and intractable hiccups. It can present suddenly, or after a longer period of vague ill health. Two fatal cases in young people have been reported, which illustrated both modes of presentation (Brosnan & Gowing 1996). At postmortem, complete destruction of the adrenals was found.

2. It may mimic anorexia nervosa or chronic fatigue syndrome.

3. In mild cases there may be a normochromic, normocytic anaemia, leucocytosis, eosinophilia, and a low normal plasma cortisol.

4. In severe cases, steroid hormones may be undetectable in the blood. The characteristic metabolic changes of hyponatraemia, hyperkalaemia, hypoglycaemia, hypercalcaemia, and an elevated urea will be present. Hypotension, cardiovascular collapse, confusion, or even coma, may occur.

5. ECG may be of low voltage with flattening of ST segments. Echocardiographic changes have been found in untreated patients; all had smaller ventricular dimensions than controls, and four out of seven patients had signs of mitral valve prolapse. These abnormalities regressed 4–8 months after steroid treatment (Fallo et al 1999).

6. In the cancer patient, symptoms of anorexia, nausea, orthostatic hypotension, and confusion may be attributed to the cancer itself, or too its treatment. CT scan may show bilateral enlargement of the adrenal glands (Kung et al 1990).

7. Although infertility is usual, patients can present during pregnancy with apparent hyperemesis gravidarum. A patient was admitted at 8 weeks' gestation with severe vomiting and was found to have a plasma sodium level of $115\,\mathrm{mmol\,l^{-1}}$ (Abu et al 1997).

Anaesthetic problems

1. A previously undiagnosed Addisonian crisis may be a rare cause of cardiovascular

collapse in the perioperative period (Salam & Davies 1974, Smith & Byrne 1981, Hertzberg & Schulman 1985, Hardy et al 1992, Aono et al 1999), or pregnancy (Seaward et al 1989, Abu et al 1997). Resuscitation may be required in the accident and emergency department (Frederick et al 1991).

In the majority of these cases, the diagnosis was made only in retrospect, saline, glucose, and steroids having formed part of the general resuscitation of the collapsed patient. Subsequent confirmation of this diagnosis in such patients is potentially hazardous, since withdrawal of the exogenous steroids to test adrenocortical function may put the patient at risk. The author knows of a case in which collapse first occurred during anaesthesia for investigation of infertility. Resuscitation with steroids and antibiotics was successful but during the later investigation to exclude Addison's disease, steroids were withdrawn, and sudden death followed. Postmortem examination showed adrenal tuberculosis. This danger can be minimised by the administration of dexamethasone which does not interfere with plasma cortisol estimation (see below).

2. Problems can also occur in patients with known Addison's disease. A patient with chronic insufficiency developed a crisis following cardiac surgery despite adequate preoperative replacement (Serrano et al 2000).

3. Drugs given during anaesthesia may modify a patient's response to stress. Etomidate can adversely affect pituitary–adrenal function (Owen & Spence 1984). Increased death rates from infection were reported in patients having intravenous etomidate for sedation in intensive care. Prolonged infusions were shown to produce reversible suppression of adrenocortical response, as a result of mitochondrial enzyme inhibition. One patient with alveolar proteinosis, who had received two bolus doses of etomidate within 18 h, developed cardiovascular instability and was subsequently found to have low serum cortisol levels (McGrady & Wright 1989). The effect and clinical significance of a single dose of etomidate, or an infusion limited to the duration of anaesthesia alone, is subject to debate (Owen & Spence 1984, Yeoman et al 1984, Boidin 1986).

4. Respiratory muscle weakness, including that of the diaphragm, may occur. This improves on treatment of the condition (Mier et al 1988).

Management

1. If the diagnosis is suspected preoperatively, and some adrenal reserve remains, the plasma corticosteroids will tend to be in the low normal range. A value of $>600 \, nmol \, l^{-1}$ excludes Addison's disease, but a low normal does not prove it. Therefore, for confirmation, a stimulation test will be required. If there is time, ACTH levels should be done as well (ACTH $>200 \, pg \, ml^{-1}$, together with a plasma cortisol of $<275 \, nmol \, l^{-1}$ under stress situations, should establish the diagnosis).

Short tetracosactrin test

09.00 am: 10 ml heparinised blood for plasma cortisol estimation. Tetracosactrin $250 \, \mu g$ given im or iv.

09.30 am: Blood taken for plasma cortisol and aldosterone levels.

Results:

Normal: Baseline $>200 \, nmol \, l^{-1}$. At 30 min an increase of at least $300 \, nmol \, l^{-1}$ above this.

Addison's disease: Low baseline. At 30 min, a less than $160 \, nmol \, l^{-1}$ increase in response to stimulation.

Normally, no steroids should be administered for 3 days before this test. However, if steroids have been given under emergency circumstances, they should be changed to dexamethasone 0.5 mg bd 24 h before the test starts. Dexamethasone does not register in plasma cortisol assays. An ACTH assay will demonstrate an inappropriate high level ($200 \, pg \, ml^{-1}$) in primary adrenocortical insufficiency.

2. Treatment of an Addisonian crisis. This should precede confirmation of the diagnosis, since any delay may prove fatal.

   a) Infuse 0.9% saline 1 litre rapidly, then more slowly.

   b) Hydrocortisone (hemisuccinate or sodium phosphate) 100 mg iv immediately, then 6-hourly.

   c) Correct hypoglycaemia, if present.

3. Maintenance therapy for Addison's disease. Normal production of cortisol is 15–20 mg day^{-1} but hypoadrenal patients require twice this amount. Although replacement has traditionally been given twice daily, there is evidence that a thrice daily regimen gives better plasma cortisol levels and improvement in well-being (Groves et al 1988).

   Hydrocortisone 10 mg tds, or prednisolone 2.5 mg tds.

   Fludrocortisone acetate 0.1–0.2 mg daily is required for primary, but not for secondary hypoadrenalism.

Equivalent dosages for a given gluco-corticoid effect:

Hydrocortisone	100 mg
Cortisone	130 mg
Prednisolone	25 mg
Prednisone	25 mg
Methylprednisolone	20 mg
Betamethasone	4 mg
Triamcinolone	25 mg
Dexamethasone	4 mg

Drugs with mineralocorticoid effects:

Hydrocortisone	weak
Cortisone	weak
Fludrocortisone	strong

4. Patients should wear a 'Medi-alert' bracelet.

5. Increases in replacement therapy may be required to cope with minor or major stress. For minor stress 50–100 mg hydrocortisone daily should be tapered off after 5–10 days. Under conditions of major stress, 100–300 mg cortisol acetate iv daily, withdrawing over 2 weeks once the stress factors have been removed.

6. For non-Addisonian patients who are receiving steroids, or have received them recently (Nicholson et al 1998):

   a) Receiving <10 mg day^{-1}: assume a normal HPA response, therefore give no additional steroid cover.

   b) Receiving >10 mg day^{-1}: *minor surgery* give 25 mg at induction; *moderate surgery* give usual steroids preoperatively, hydrocortisone 25 mg at induction and 100 mg day^{-1} for 24 h; *major surgery*, give usual preoperative steroids, hydrocortisone 25 mg at induction and 100 mg day^{-1} for 48–72 h.

   c) Patients who have stopped taking steroids: >3 months, no perioperative steroids necessary; <3 months, treat as if receiving steroids.

Bibliography

Absalom AR, Scott NB 1999 Adrenocortical function and steroid therapy in critical illness. British Journal of Anaesthesia 82: 474–8.

Abu MAE, Sinha P, Totoe I 1997 Addison's disease in pregnancy presenting as hyperemesis gravidarum. Journal of Obstetrics & Gynaecology 17: 278–9.

Aono J, Mamiya K, Ueda W 1999 Abrupt onset of adrenal crisis during routine preoperative examination in a patient with unknown Addison's disease. Anesthesiology 90: 313–14.

Boidin MP 1986 Can etomidate cause an Addisonian crisis? Acta Anaesthesiologica Belgica 37: 165–70.

Brosnan CM, Gowing NFC 1996 Addison's disease. British Medical Journal 312: 1085–7.

Duggan M, Browne I, Flynn C 1998 Adrenal failure in the critically ill. British Journal of Anaesthesia 81: 468–70.

Fallo F, Betterle C, Budano S et al 1999 Regression of cardiac abnormalities after replacement therapy in Addison's disease. European Journal of Endocrinology 140: 425–8.

Frederick R, Brown C, Renusch J L et al 1991 Addisonian crisis: emergency presentation of primary adrenal insufficiency. Annals of Emergency Medicine 20: 802–6.

Groves RW, Toms GC, Houghton BJ et al 1988 Corticosteroid replacement therapy: twice or thrice daily? Journal of the Royal Society of Medicine 81: 514–16.

Hardy K, Mead B, Gill G 1992 Adrenal apoplexy after coronary artery bypass surgery leading to Addisonian crisis. Journal of the Royal Society of Medicine 85: 577–8.

Hertzberg LB, Schulman MS 1985 Acute adrenal insufficiency in a patient with appendicitis during anesthesia. Anesthesiology 62: 517–19.

Hilton CT, Harrington PT, Prasad C et al 1988 Adrenal insufficiency in the acquired immunodeficiency syndrome. Southern Medical Journal 81: 1493–5.

Ihde JK, Turnbull AD, Bajorunas DR 1990 Adrenal insufficiency in the cancer patient: implications for the surgeon. British Journal of Surgery 77: 1335–7.

Kung AWC, Pun KK, Lam K et al 1990 Addisonian crisis as presenting feature in malignancies. Cancer 65: 177–9.

Levy A 1996 Perioperative steroid cover. Lancet 347: 846–7.

McGrady EM, Wright IH 1989 Cardiovascular instability following bolus dose of etomidate. Anaesthesia 44: 404–5.

Masterson GR, Mostafa SM 1998 Adrenocortical function in critical illness. British Journal of Anaesthesia 81: 308–10.

Mier A, Laroche C, Wass J et al 1988 Respiratory weakness in Addison's disease. British Medical Journal 297: 457–8.

Nicholson G, Burrin JM, Hall GM 1998 Perioperative steroid supplementation. Anaesthesia 53: 1091–4.

Oelkers W 1996 Adrenal insufficiency. New England Journal of Medicine 335: 1206–12.

Owen H, Spence AA 1984 Etomidate. British Journal of Anaesthesia 56: 555–7.

Salam AA, Davies DM 1974 Acute adrenal insufficiency during surgery. British Journal of Anaesthesia 46: 619–22.

Salem M, Tainsh RE Jr, Bromberg J et al 1994 Perioperative glucocorticoid coverage. Annals of Surgery 219: 416–25.

Seaward PG, Guidozzi F, Sonnendecker EW 1989 Addisonian crisis in pregnancy. Case report. British Journal of Obstetrics & Gynaecology 96: 1348–50.

Serrano N, Jiminez JJ, Brouard MT et al 2000 Acute adrenal insufficiency after cardiac surgery. Critical Care Medicine 28: 569–70.

Smith MG, Byrne AJ 1981 An Addisonian crisis complicating anaesthesia. Anaesthesia 36: 681–4.

Yeoman PM, Fellows IW, Byrne AJ et al 1984 The effect of anaesthetic induction using etomidate upon pituitary-adrenocortical function. British Journal of Anaesthesia 56: 1291–2.

AIDS (Acquired immunodeficiency syndrome)

A spectrum of disease thought to be caused by infection with a human immunodeficiency virus, HIV. It is one of a family of retroviruses, and several types and subtypes are now known. There is a long latent period after infection, which may lead to a chronic condition of lymphadenopathy, fever, weight loss, and diarrhoea, or to a state of cellular immune deficiency and the development of unusual malignancies or opportunistic infections. It is most common in the homosexual and drug-taking communities, but is also found in haemophiliac patients who received infected blood products before antibody screening and heat treatment of Factor VIII concentrates. Some individuals may be carriers, but the full significance of this state and its natural history is not yet known.

The virus has been isolated from body fluids, particularly blood, CSF, pleural, peritoneal, semen, saliva, breast milk, tears, synovial and vaginal fluid, but it would appear that a breach in either skin or mucosa is necessary for infection to occur. However, perforation of gloves is common during surgical operations. Saliva or airborne transmission when the mucosa is intact has not yet been demonstrated, but neither has it been disproved. HIV is probably less infectious than hepatitis B, and present surveys indicate that the risks to health workers are low unless accidental inoculation has occurred.

However, the recent appearance of this potentially fatal disease has meant that epidemiological studies are, as yet, incomplete. The most recent literature should be consulted. In the period 1981–95, 49 healthcare workers had occupationally transmitted HIV virus, 86% of which were from percutaneous exposure (Layon et al 1997). The authors discuss the problems of loss of livelihood, lack of disability programmes, and the debate about routine testing of patients and staff. Guidelines for anaesthetists have been produced by the Association of Anaesthetists (1988), but these were written before the most recent recommendations for post-exposure prophylaxis (Department of Health 1997).

For the patient, the prognosis has greatly improved in the last 5 years (Avidan et al 2000), as a result of better understanding of the disease, the ability to monitor immune response and viral loads, more vigorous drug treatment using triple therapy (Lipsky 1996), and information from multicentre drug trials.

Preoperative abnormalities

1. The patient may either be HIV antibody positive only, or show signs of the immunodeficiency syndrome as well.

2. The neurological manifestations include peripheral neuropathy, radiculopathy, cranial nerve palsies, and dementia. Five AIDS patients, one of whom died, had vasovagal episodes associated with lung biopsy. Subsequent investigation suggested a diagnosis of autonomic dysfunction (Craddock et al 1987).

3. The commonest opportunistic infection is *Pneumocystis carinii* pneumonia, but candidal, tuberculous, and viral pneumonias occur. Up to 85% of patients will develop pneumocystis pneumonia (PCP) at some time, and acute infections carry a mortality of 9–35% (Thomas et al 1990). The treatment of choice is now co-trimoxazole (trimethoprim and sulfamethoxazole), and pentamidine is a second line drug. Corticosteroids may prevent the early deterioration of oxygenation in PCP and has been recommended at a $Pa_{O_2} <9.3\,kPa$. Addison's disease has been reported as a complication (Hilton et al 1988).

4. HIV-associated neoplasia (Schulz et al 1996).

5. Patients may present to the ENT surgeon with a variety of unusual laryngeal infections or neoplasms (Tami et al 1999).

6. Drug treatment (Lipsky 1996, Gazzard & Moyle 1998). There are three classes of antiretroviral agent: nucleoside reverse transcriptase inhibitors (NRTIs); protease inhibitors (PIs) ; non-nucleoside reverse transcriptase inhibitors (NNRTIs). Side effects of treatment with antiviral agents may be severe and include nausea and vomiting, hepatic disease, peripheral neuropathy, pancreatitis, and Stevens–Johnson syndrome. Zidovudine (Retrovir, AZT) may cause megaloblastic anaemia and neutropenia. It is theoretically possible that interaction with nitrous oxide could occur (Phillips & Spence 1987). Neurological complications of the drugs may be difficult to distinguish from those of the disease.

7. Increasing numbers of children are becoming infected and the pattern of disease is slightly different from that seen in adults (Schwartz et al 1991). Lung disease is the commonest cause of morbidity and mortality, and infection with *P. carinii* carries a worse prognosis. Lymphoid interstitial pneumonitis can develop with chronic lung disease. Cardiac abnormalities occur in 90% (Lipschultz et al 1989). Most children have neurological abnormalities, including autoimmune neuropathy. General problems comprise recurrent infections, anaemia, and lymphadenopathy. Interventional procedures may involve CVP insertion, gastrostomy, and lung and liver biopsies.

Anaesthetic problems

These can be divided into problems for the AIDS patient undergoing anaesthesia, admission to the ITU, care during pregnancy, or for pain control, and problems for healthcare workers potentially exposed to infected body fluids.

1. The problems of anaesthesia in the presence of lung disease.

2. A high proportion of patients with advanced disease have ECG and echocardiographic abnormalities, but information about the individual risk of anaesthesia is limited.

3. The potential effects of antiretroviral drugs on the metabolism of drugs given during anaesthesia must be considered. Protease inhibitors inhibit cytochrome P-450, thus decreasing the metabolism of a number of drugs, including certain opiates and benzodiazepines (Avidan et al 2000).

4. Immune function. Although anaesthesia is known to suppress immune function, the significance of this effect on the AIDS patient is not yet clear (Hughes et al 1995). The patient's overall prognosis is related to the CD4 T-lymphocyte count, and is poor in those in whom the count is <50 mm^{-3} (Shapiro et al 1994).

5. Autonomic neuropathy may cause cardiovascular instability.

6. Central and peripheral nervous system effects. In view of the relatively high incidence of AIDS patients developing spinal cord lesions or encephalitis, the advisability of spinal and epidural anaesthesia has been questioned. Polyneuropathy, myelopathy and muscle wasting may be a contraindication to the use of suxamethonium. The presence of AIDS dementia can lead to problems with consent, and these patients may be sensitive to the effects of CNS-depressant drugs (Shapiro et al 1994).

7. Pregnancy is now common in patients with HIV and AIDS but only 17% are thought to be identified before delivery. Elective Caesarean section decreases the risk of transmission to the child (The International Perinatal Group 1999). One patient presented at 28 weeks' gestation with genital herpes and AIDS-related dementia (Birnbach et al 1995). The safety or otherwise of treating an HIV-seropositive patient with an epidural blood patch, should postdural puncture headache occur, has caused debate.

8. Patients may require ITU admission. In a survey of 127 patients admitted between 1993 and 1997, 70.7% were known HIV before admission, and 27% were diagnosed for the first time (Gill et al 1999). The majority were not receiving combination antiretroviral therapy. Pneumonia with *P. carinii* was the commonest reason (36.1%) for admission. ITU mortality was 33% and in-hospital mortality 56%. A previous AIDS-defining illness, sepsis, and a CD4 cell count of <100 cells ml^{-1}, were associated with a poor prognosis.

9. An increasing number of children are presenting with HIV infection (Schwartz et al 1991). The pattern of disease differs from that in adults and they should not be segregated from other children. Appropriate consent for treatment may be difficult to obtain.

10. Pain is a common, underestimated, and poorly treated, problem. A multicentre study of 315 AIDS patients, at different stages of their disease, found that pain was present in 62%, but that physicians were reluctant to prescribe potent analgesics (Larue et al 1997). Penfold and Clark (1992) discussed the wide variety of manifestations of pain syndromes in AIDS and classified them into the following groups: chest, headache, oral cavity, peripheral nervous syndrome, abdominal, musculoskeletal, and anorectal.

11. The possibility of transmission of the virus to healthcare workers, which is most likely to occur as a result of needlestick injuries. Surgical gloves constitute the most likely route of infection. At the end of surgery, about 15% of gloves tested were perforated (Johanet et al 1996). Double gloving reduced this to 5%. Porosity of the latex increases with duration of use. The incidence of seroconversion following needle puncture from an HIV-positive patient is calculated to be 0.5%. Eight healthcare workers who had either received a needlestick injury, or who had suffered from dermatitis (Weiss 1985), and five surgeons in whom there was massive exposure of skin or mucous membranes to blood (Gazzard & Wastell 1990) were reported as being

HIV positive. In a review of literature, the risk of percutaneous injury during surgery was calculated as 5–6%, and the risk of virus transmission after percutaneous injury with an infected needle was 0.3% (Flum & Wallack 1997). Studies have also suggested that the risk to anaesthetists is not trivial (Editorial 1990, Greene et al 1998). Buergler et al (1992) identified the three factors that determined occupational risk for HIV: the risk of needlestick injury per year, the risk of seroconversion should injury occur, and the prevalence of HIV in the particular population served by the hospital. Their occupational risk calculations for US anaesthetists, based on existing figures, was 0.05% in a low prevalence area increasing to 4.5% in a high prevalence area. Calculations from a multicentre study of anaesthesia personnel suggested that in the USA there would be 17 HIV infections from percutaneous injuries in 30 years (Greene et al 1998).

12. Prophylaxis after accidental exposure. A recent survey has shown that many anaesthetists are ignorant of the procedures that should be followed after needlestick injuries in high-risk patients, potentially increasing the risk of seroconversion (Diprose et al 2000).

13. The problems of handling and disposal of contaminated material, and the sterilisation of equipment.

Management

Again, this section is divided into management of the AIDS patient undergoing surgery, ITU treatment, peripartum care and therapy for pain syndromes, and protection of healthcare worker against accidental infection from a patient.

1. Full assessment of the patient for organ involvement by the disease itself, or from complications of treatment. Pulmonary, central and peripheral nervous systems, and hepatic involvement are the most important.

2. In patients receiving protease inhibitors, care should be taken with doses of analgesics and sedatives whose metabolism is known to be impaired by these drugs (Avidan 2000).

3. Postoperative complications. A study of 343 AIDS patients matched with 26 control patients found that the presence of HIV did not increase the risk of postoperative complications in the first 30 days (Ayers et al 1993). However, a prospective study of 48 males (HIV-seropositive or AIDS) undergoing haemorrhoidectomy, showed considerably delayed wound healing compared with controls (Morandi et al 1999).

4. Since the previously poor prognosis of AIDS has improved, patients are more likely to be considered for ITU care than they were in the past. A study of 127 patients admitted to ITU on 133 occasions between 1993 and 1997 showed an overall ITU mortality of 33% and an in-hospital mortality of 56%. Survival was highest in the respiratory HIV-related disease or an illness that was HIV unrelated (Gill et al 1999). During this study, few were receiving combination antiretroviral therapy, so the changing pattern of disease and mortality is difficult to predict.

5. In pregnancy, elective Caesarean section should be undertaken to protect the child (Riley et al 1999). It may also protect it from genital herpes (Birnbach et al 1995). Before administering regional anaesthesia, a neurological assessment should be performed. Local anaesthetic techniques might be contraindicated if parapareses are already present. However, in a study of HIV-positive patients, there were no neurological or infectious complications related to the administration of regional anaesthesia (Hughes et al 1995). Subsequent retrospective studies have shown no differences in complication rates between parturients given regional or general anaesthetic techniques (Gershon & Manning-Williams 1997).

6. A follow-up of six patients 6–24 months after having been given autologous epidural blood patch following dural puncture headache did not show any CNS morbidity which could be attributed to the procedure (Tom et al 1992).

7. Management of pain syndromes. It has been suggested that pain syndromes could be managed better, in a similar way to cancer pain, using a multidisciplinary team (Penfold & Clark 1992, Wood et al 1997). A wide variety of drugs are available, including non-narcotics, narcotics, and adjuvant drugs such as antidepressants, carbamazepine, local anaesthetics, and steroids.

8. To reduce risks to laboratory personnel, only urgent laboratory investigations likely to influence management should be contemplated. Sterilisation of any instrument used for the analysis of contaminated blood is mandatory.

9. Laparoscopic techniques minimise the dangers for all theatre staff (Diettrich & Kaplan 1991). However, trauma and emergency surgery can be performed safely, provided full precautions are taken (Carrillo et al 1995).

10. For hospital staff, the same precautions should be taken as for hepatitis B. Gown, gloves, and mask and eye protection should be worn during anaesthesia. Blood spillage should be avoided. Disposal of needles in a tough disposal bin, without resheathing, is crucial. They should not be passed from one person to another. Care should be taken not to spread blood, sputum, or saliva, during tracheal intubation and extubation. In the UK, the wearing of gloves at least is being recommended for all anaesthetics (Association of Anaesthetists 1988), but in a survey of anaesthetists undertaken in the UK in 1991, less than 16% routinely wore gloves (O'Donnell & Asbury 1992a,b). The use of double gloves, with or without reinforcement of the distal phalanges by application of adhesive tape directly to the gloves, has been suggested (Paglia & Sommer 1991). Double gloving may reduce the occupational risk of HIV by an average of 80% (Buergler et al 1992, Johanet et al 1996). Needlestick injuries should be taken seriously and reported (Greene et al 1998).

11. Equipment should be disposable or sterilisable. The virus is destroyed by both heat and chemicals. Reusable equipment should be scrubbed with detergent solution and decontaminated by soaking in glutaraldehyde or sodium hypochlorite solution. Nursing staff should wear goggles during cleaning of equipment. Steam or gas sterilisation is also reported to be effective.

a) Ventilators. Although HIV infection is not airborne, the use of disposable circuitry and bacterial filters is advisable.

b) Blood gas machines. The introducer port should be syringed through with 1% sodium hypochlorite and left for 5 min. This is followed by two wash cycles and recalibration.

c) Surfaces. Should be cleaned with sodium hypochlorite.

12. Response to occupational exposure by health workers. Following a needlestick injury, active bleeding should be promoted, and the wound washed in soap and running water. In the case of exposure to blood from a patient with HIV, or known to be high risk, prophylaxis should be given as soon as possible, preferably within 1 h. The recommended regimen at present is zidovudine 250 mg bd, lamivudine 150 mg bd, and indinavar 800 mg tds, for a period of 4 weeks (Department of Health 1997). This should be organised through the occupational health department, since counselling and follow-up will be necessary.

Bibliography

Association of Anaesthetists 1988 AIDS and hepatitis B. Guidelines for anaesthetists. Association of Anaesthetists, London.

Avidan MS, Jones N, Pozniak AL 2000 The implications of HIV for the anaesthetist. Anaesthesia 55: 344–54.

Ayers J, Howton MJ, Layon AJ 1993 Postoperative complications in patients with human immunodeficiency virus disease. Clinical data and a literature review. Chest 103: 1800–7.

Birnbach DJ, Bourlier RA, Choi R et al 1995 Anaesthetic management of Caesarean section in a patient with active recurrent genital herpes and AIDS-related dementia. British Journal of Anaesthesia 75: 639–41.

Buergler JM, Kim R, Thisted RA et al 1992 Risk of Human Immunodeficiency Virus in surgeons, anesthesiologists and medical students. Anesthesia & Analgesia 75: 118–24.

Carillo EH, Carrillo LE, Byers PM et al 1995 Penetrating trauma and emergency surgery in patients with AIDS. American Journal of Surgery 170: 341–4.

Craddock C, Pasvol G, Bull R et al 1987 Cardiorespiratory arrest and autonomic neuropathy in AIDS. Lancet 2: 16–18.

Department of Health 1997 Guidelines on post-exposure prophylaxis for health care workers occupationally exposed to HIV. Department of Health, London.

Diettrich NA, Kaplan G 1991 Laparoscopic surgery for HIV-infected patients: minimizing dangers for all. Journal of Laparoscopic Surgery 1: 295–8.

Diprose P, Deakin CD, Smedley J 2000 Ignorance of post-exposure prophylaxis guidelines following HIV needlestick injury may increase the risk of seroconversion. British Journal of Anaesthesia 84: 767–70.

Editorial 1990 Occupational infection among anaesthetists. Lancet 336: 1103.

Flum DR, Wallack MK 1997 The surgeon's database for AIDS: a collective review. Journal of the American College of Surgeons 184: 403–12.

Gazzard B, Moyle G 1998 Revision to the British HIV Association guidelines for antiretroviral treatment of HIV seropositive individuals. Lancet 352: 314–16.

Gazzard BG, Wastell C 1990 HIV and surgeons. British Medical Journal 301: 1003–4.

Gershon RY, Manning-Williams D 1997 Anesthesia and the HIV-infected parturient. International Journal of Obstetric Anesthesia 6: 76–81.

Gill JK, Greene L, Miller R et al 1999 ICU admission in patients infected with the human immunodeficiency virus—a multicentre survey. Anaesthesia 54: 727–34.

Greene ES, Berry AJ, Jagger J et al 1998 Multicenter study of contaminated percutaneous injuries in anesthesia personnel. Anesthesiology 89: 1392–8.

Hilton CT, Harrington PT, Prasad C et al 1988 Adrenal insufficiency in the acquired immunodeficiency syndrome. Southern Medical Journal 81:1493–5.

Hughes SC, Daily PA, Landers D et al 1995 Parturients infected with the human immunodeficiency virus and regional anesthesia. Anesthesiology 82: 565–71.

The International Perinatal HIV Group. The mode of delivery and risk of vertical transmission of HIV-1.

A meta-analysis of 15 prospective cohort studies. New England Journal of Medicine 340: 1032–3.

Johanet H, Chosidow D, Marmuse JP et al 1996 [Perforations and porosity of surgical gloves. Frequency, mechanism, risk.] Annales de Chirugie 50: 352–5.

Larue F, Fontaine A, Colleau SM 1997 Underestimation and undertreatment of pain in HIV disease. British Medical Journal 314: 23–8.

Layon J, Rosenbaum SH, Dirk L 1997 Human immunodeficiency virus and health care workers. Canadian Journal of Anaesthesia 44: 689–95.

Lipschultz SE, Chanock S, Sanders SP et al 1989 Cardiovascular manifestations of human immunodeficiency virus infections in infants and children. Americal Journal of Cardiology 63: 1489–97.

Lipsky JJ 1996 Antiretroviral drugs for AIDS. Lancet 348: 800–3.

Morandi E, Merlini D, Salvaggio A et al 1999 Prospective study of healing time after hemorrhoidectomy: influence of HIV infection, acquired immunodeficiency syndrome, and anal wound infections. Diseases of the Colon & Rectum 42: 1140–4.

O'Donnell NG, Asbury AJ 1992a The occupational hazard of human immunodeficiency virus and hepatitis. I Perceived risks and preventive measures adopted by anaesthetists: a postal survey. Anaesthesia 47: 923–8.

O'Donnell NG, Asbury AJ 1992b The occupational hazard of human immunodeficiency virus and hepatitis B virus. II. Effect of grade, age, sex and region of employment on perceived risks and preventive measures adopted by anaesthetists. Anaesthesia 47: 929–35.

Paglia SL, Sommer RM 1989 AIDS infection protection—reinforced gloves. Anesthesia & Analgesia 69: 407.

Penfold J, Clark AJ 1992 Pain syndromes in HIV infection. Canadian Journal of Anaesthesia 39: 724–30.

Phillips AJ, Spence AA 1987 Zidovudine and the anaesthetist. Anaesthesia 42: 799–800.

Riley LE, Greene MF 1999 Elective cesarean delivery to reduce the transmission of HIV. New England Journal of Medicine 340: 1032.

Shapiro HM, Grant I, Woinger MB 1994 AIDS and the central nervous system: implications for the anesthesiologist. Anesthesiology 80: 187–200.

Schulz TF, Boshoff CH, Weiss RA 1996 HIV infections and neoplasia. Lancet 348: 587–91.

Schwartz D, Schwartz T, Cooper E et al 1991 Anaesthesia and the child with HIV infection. Canadian Journal of Anaesthesia 38: 626–33.

Tami TA, Ferlito A, Rinaldo A et al 1999 Laryngeal pathology in the acquired immunodeficiency syndrome: diagnostic and therapeutic dilemmas. Annals of Otology, Rhinology & Laryngology 108: 214–20.

Thomas S, O'Doherty M, Bateman N 1990 *Pneumocystis carinii* pneumonia. Aerosolised pentamidine gives effective prophylaxis. British Medical Journal 300: 211–12.

Tom DJ, Gulevich SJ, Shapiro HM et al 1992 Epidural blood patch in the HIV-positive patient: a review of clinical experience. Anesthesiology 76: 943–7.

Weiss SH 1985 HTLV-III infections among health care workers. Association with needle stick injuries. Journal of the American Medical Association 254: 2089–93.

Wood CG, Whittet S, Bradbeer CS 1997 ABC of palliative care. HIV infection and AIDS. British Medical Journal 315: 1433–6.

Air embolism (see Section 2)

Alcoholism

Alcoholism has been defined as excessive drinking that results in impairment of the subject's health and social activities. Alcohol has a wide range of effects on many organs and increases the risk of cancer. More patients present to surgical departments (particularly ENT) than to any other department in the hospital, and about 50% of patients who are injured sustain their injury whilst under the influence of alcohol (Spies & Rommelspacher 1999). If surgical treatment is required, three main problems must be considered:

1. The effects of the numerous metabolic and endocrine changes that occur in longstanding alcoholics.

2. Whether or not there is also acute alcohol toxicity.

3. The problems of alcohol withdrawal, which can occur at any time between 8 h and 5 days after abstention.

The pathophysiology of withdrawal is complex, but it involves imbalance in cerebral neurotransmitter systems (eg glutamate, GABA, dopamine, serotonin, and opioid). Alterations in the regulation of GABA and NDMA (N-methyl-D-aspartate) systems and the cAMP pathway during abuse may be the basis of physiological dependence and the state of withdrawal (Hall & Zador 1997). There may also be disturbances in the hypothalamic–pituitary–adrenal (HPA) axis.

In known alcohol abusers, treatment should be given to prevent withdrawal syndrome. It is even better to persuade them to undergo a 1-month period of abstinence before elective surgery, which significantly reduces postoperative complications (Tonnesen et al 1992). More often, however, the alcohol dependence is neither diagnosed, nor admitted, and unexpected withdrawal occurs in the perioperative period.

There are several excellent reviews on the perioperative management of alcoholic patients and alcohol withdrawal syndromes (Spies et al 1995, Spies & Rommelspacher 1999, Tonnesen & Kehlet 1999).

Preoperative abnormalities

1. The patient may be truthful about his/her alcohol intake, but rarely about his/her dependence on it. There are formal assessments of alcohol dependence (CAGE), and a withdrawal assessment scale (Spies & Rommelspacher 1999).

2. Laboratory markers. High levels of gamma-glutamyltransferase, MCV and carbohydate-deficient transferrin suggest a problem. The MCV exceeds 93 fl in 85% of heavy drinkers. Bone marrow depression can occur, and, if liver function is impaired, there may be coagulation defects.

3. Biochemical. Blood alcohol levels:

80 mg dl^{-1}—legal limit for driving.

200 mg dl^{-1}—severe intoxication.

>400 mg dl^{-1}—stupor.

>500 mg dl^{-1}—frequently fatal.

Electrolyte disturbances, particularly hypokalaemia, may exacerbate delirium tremens.

4. Liver function. Gamma-glutamyltransferase and the aminotransaminases may be abnormal and the albumin low. Plasma cholinesterase activity is normal, unless hepatic damage is severe. There may be impaired glucose tolerance after alcohol, followed by hypoglycaemia occurring between 6 and 24 h after acute ingestion. Induction of microsomal alcohol oxidising systems occurs, which affects a variety of other drugs. These systems can metabolise certain substances into highly toxic metabolites.

5. Cardiac disease. A dilated cardiomyopathy may occur, and can be associated with dyspnoea, heart failure, conduction defects, bifid T waves, digitalis-like ST segments, and arrhythmias.

6. Central nervous system effects. Wernicke's encephalopathy (Reuler et al 1985) includes ocular abnormalities (horizontal nystagmus, lateral rectus paralysis), ataxia and a global confusional state. Korsakoff's psychosis (retrograde and anterograde amnesia, confabulation) and epileptic fits can also occur.

7. A peripheral neuropathy may be produced by the combined effects of alcohol and malnutrition.

8. Increased carcinogenesis.

9. Alcohol affects the individual's immune response and leucocyte function, and should be considered to be an immunosuppressive drug (McGregor 1986). In acute alcoholism, there is interference with primary responses to a new antigen and poor control of bacterial infection.

Anaesthetic problems

1. Acute alcohol toxicity, electrolyte imbalance, and hypoglycaemia.

2. Coagulation abnormalities.

3. The possible presence of a full stomach and delayed gastric emptying.

4. Acute withdrawal syndrome. This occurs 6–24 h after the last drink, and effects have been divided into autonomic, neuronal excitation, and delirium tremens (Hall & Zador 1997). Increased epinephrine (adrenaline) and norepinephrine (noradrenaline) concentrations are found when long term drinking is stopped suddenly. Clinical features include tremors, sweating, nausea and vomiting, agitation, and cognitive disorders. These are followed by delirium tremens, hallucinations, confusion, and intense autonomic hyperactivity. Grand mal seizures can occur at 12–24 h.

5. Impaired liver metabolism and cirrhosis.

6. Decreased adrenocortical response to stress.

7. Malnutrition and vitamin deficiencies.

8. H_2 blockers inhibit gastric alcohol dehydrogenase, thus increasing blood alcohol levels (Lieber 1995).

9. Dilated cardiomyopathy and arrhythmias. Heavy drinking increases the risk of cardiac arrhythmias, particularly idiopathic atrial fibrillation, whether or not heart disease is present (Koskinen & Kupari 1992).

10. The presence of, or bleeding from, oesophageal varices (Cello et al 1986).

11. Peripheral or autonomic neuropathy.

12. There is an increased postoperative complication rate (Tonnesen et al 1992). After hysterectomy, the morbidity was increased, and the length of stay in hospital was doubled, when heavy drinkers were compared with moderate and light drinkers. Complications included wound infection, cystitis, pneumonia, and vaginal abscess (Fielding et al 1992). Other studies showed an increased risk of wound infections, cardiovascular complications, and bleeding disorders (Tonnesen & Kehlet 1999). These accord with similar studies on men undergoing colonic and prostatic surgery and may result from interference with the immune system. Individuals with trauma and evidence of chronic abuse had a two-fold incidence of

complications, in particular pneumonia and other infections (Jurkovich et al 1993). There is also an increase in length of stay on the ITU in men having upper gastrointestinal surgery (Spies et al 1996).

Management

1. If acute alcohol toxicity is present, surgery should be delayed if possible. Alcohol levels above 250 mg dl^{-1} increase surgical morbidity. Correction of dehydration should be tempered by the knowledge that diuresis occurs mainly while the blood alcohol level is rising. Beware of fluid overload. Hypokalaemia can precipitate delirium tremens. Hypoglycaemia may occur 6 to 24 h after intake. If iv glucose is required, thiamine should be given concurrently. Alcohol-related cardiac arrhythmias usually stop spontaneously within 24–48 h.

2. In the case of elective surgery, attempts should be made to persuade the patient of the benefits of a period of alcohol withdrawal. Tonnesen et al (1999), in a randomised trial of 42 alcoholics undergoing elective colorectal surgery, found that withdrawal from alcohol for 1 month reduced the postoperative morbidity. In addition to this, there was objective evidence of improved cardiac and immune responses.

3. Withdrawal assessment and prophylaxis. In known alcoholics, the following have been used for prevention or treatment of acute withdrawal syndrome on a standard surgical ward (Spies & Rommelspacher 1999):

a) Diazepam 2.5–10 mg 6 hrly, or

   chlormethiazole capsules (192 mg) or syrup (250 mg in 5 ml), 0.25–1 g 6 hrly (but causes bronchial hypersecretion), or

   ethanol 0.5–1 g kg^{-1} d^{-1}, or 0.5 g kg^{-1} d^{-1} iv.

b) For autonomic signs, use clonidine or beta blockers.

c) For hallucinations use haloperidol.

4. An iv preparation of vitamins B and C, such as Pabrinex high potency, is given 8 hrly by infusion. Prevention of hypoglycaemia has been stressed, and the use of thiamine 100 mg iv first, to prevent Wernicke's encephalopathy, has been suggested (Mayes 1989).

5. Coagulation abnormalities, if present, should be treated with vitamin K$_1$, fresh frozen plasma, or platelets.

6. Cardiomyopathy (see Cardiomyopathies; dilated). Thiopentone is avoided if a cardiomyopathy is present or there is hypoalbuminaemia. Atracurium is the neuromuscular blocker of choice if liver function is impaired. Postoperative jaundice frequently occurs several days after surgery, irrespective of the anaesthetic agent used, and results from defective processing of old red blood cells by an impaired liver. The use of halothane is therefore best avoided. Isoflurane or sevoflurane undergo less liver metabolism. Short-acting opiates, such as remifentanil, are beneficial for intraoperative maintenance.

7. Longer-acting analgesics should be used with caution, and only to treat pain. Dependence can occur readily.

8. Intravenous treatment for withdrawal, only on ITU. Start with a benzodiazepine, and later add either haloperidol or clonidine.

a) Clormethiazole edisylate 0.8% soln, 320–800 mg (40–100 ml) over 5–10 min, then the rate is maintained at 0.5–1 ml min^{-1}. *Note*: Chlormethiazole is dangerous in severe liver disease, or when a patient is acutely intoxicated with alcohol. Severe respiratory depression can result from the combination (McInnes 1987).

b) Delirium tremens can be treated with midazolam 2.5 mg, using additional increments up to a maximum of 10 mg. Diazepam is used in increments up to a total dose of 20 mg.

c) Clonidine bolus dose 0.15–0.3 mg, followed by an infusion of 0.88 μg kg^{-1} h^{-1}.

d) Haloperidol 10–20 mg

9. An existing peripheral neuropathy is a contraindication to regional anaesthesia.

10. In the presence of cirrhosis, gastrointestinal bleeding may precipitate hepatic failure. Nasogastric tubes should be inserted cautiously, in case oesophageal varices are present.

Bibliography

Cello JP, Crass RA, Grendell JH et al 1986 Management of the patient with hemorrhaging esophageal varices. Journal of the American Medical Association 256: 1480–4.

Fielding C, Jensen IM, Tonnesen H 1992 Influence of alcohol intake on postoperative morbidity after hysterectomy. American Journal of Obstetrics & Gynecology 166: 667–70.

Hall W, Zador D 1997 The alcohol withdrawal syndrome. Lancet 349: 1897–900.

Jurkovich G, Rivara FP, Gurney JG et al 1993 The effect of acute intoxication and chronic alcohol abuse on outcome from trauma. Journal of the American Medical Association 270: 51–6.

Koskinen P, Kupari M 1992 Alcohol and cardiac arrhythmias. British Medical Journal 304: 1394–5.

Lieber CS 1995 Medical disorders of alcoholism. New England Journal of Medicine 333: 1058–65.

McGregor RR 1986 Alcohol and immune defense. Journal of the American Medical Association 256: 1474–9.

McInnes GT 1987 Chlormethiazole and alcohol. British Medical Journal 294: 592.

Mayes GA 1989 Thiamine for prevention of Wernicke's encephalopathy: a reminder. Anesthesia & Analgesia 69: 407–8.

Reuler JB, Giraud DE, Cooney TG 1985 Wernicke's encephalopathy. New England Journal of Medicine 312: 1035–9.

Spies CD, Rommelspacher H 1999 Alcohol withdrawal and the surgical patient; prevention and treatment. Anesthesia & Analgesia 88: 946–54.

Spies C, Dubisz N, Funk W et al 1995 Prophylaxis of alcohol withdrawal syndrome in alcohol dependent patients admitted to the intensive care unit following tumour resection. British Journal of Anaesthesia 75: 734–9.

Spies C, Nordmann A, Brummer G et al 1996 Intensive care unit stay is prolonged in chronic alcoholic men following tumor resection of the upper digestive tract. Acta Anaesthesiologica Scandinavica 40: 649–56.

Tonnesen H, Kehlet H 1999 Preoperative alcoholism and postoperative morbidity. British Journal of Surgery 86: 869–74.

Tonnesen H, Petersen K, Hojgaard L et al 1992 Postoperative morbidity amongst symptom-free alcohol misusers. Lancet 340: 334–40.

Tonnesen H, Rosenberg J, Nielsen HJ et al 1999 Preoperative abstinence improves the poor postoperative outcome in alcohol abusers. British Medical Journal 318: 1311–16.

Aldosteronism, primary (see Conn's syndrome)

Alkaptonuria

An autosomal recessive disease, in which there is reduced activity of homogentisic acid oxidase, so that homogentisic acid cannot be metabolised. Ochronosis (the presence of brown/black pigment), which is caused by abnormal accumulation of oxidised homogentisic acid, occurs in skin, connective tissue, and cartilage, including the cardiac valves.

Preoperative abnormalities

1. The urine becomes dark, from homogentisic aciduria, after exposure to air or alkali. There is bluish discoloration of nails, auricles and axillae, and brown pigmentation of the sclerae.

2. Musculoskeletal. Ochronosis of connective tissue and cartilage results in a degenerative arthritis.

3. Cardiovascular disease. Aortic stenosis and coronary artery disease have been reported (Vavuranakis et al 1998).

4. Genitourinary complications.

5. Diagnosis is made after detection of increased levels of homogentisic acid in the urine and plasma (normally not detected).

6. Treatment is with dietary restriction of protein and ascorbic acid.

Anaesthetic problems

1. A degenerative arthritis develops, and bone is more prone to fracture; disc prolapse (Reddy & Prasas 1998), and compression of spinal cord secondary to atlanto-axial arthropathy (Kusakabe et al 1995), can occur.

2. Failed epidural anaesthesia has been reported (Itoh et al 1993).

Management

1. Assessment of cardiac disease.

2. Look for evidence of cervical myelopathy.

Bibliography

Itoh K, Itimata M, Matsumoto K et al 1993 Anesthesia for a patient with alkaptonuria. Hiroshima Journal of Anesthesia 29: 329–32.

Kragel AH, Lapa JA, Roberts WC 1990 Cardiovascular findings in alkaptonuric ochronosis. American Heart Journal 120: 1460–3.

Kusakabe N, Tsuzuki N, Sonada M 1995 Compression of the cervical cord due to alcaptonuric arthropathy of the atlanto-axial joint. A case report. Journal of Bone & Joint Surgery 77A: 274–7.

Millea TP, Segal LS, Liss RG et al 1992 Spine fracture in ochronosis. Clinical Orthopaedics & Related Research 281: 208–11.

Reddy DR, Prasas VSS 1998 Alkaptonuria presenting as lumbar disc prolapse: case report and review of the literature. Spinal Cord 36: 523–4.

Vavuranakis M, Triantafillidi H, Stefanadis C et al 1998 Aortic stenosis and coronary artery disease caused by alkaptonuria, a rare genetic metabolic syndrome. Cardiology 90: 312–14.

Alveolar proteinosis

A lung condition in which protein, phospholipid, cholesterol and free fatty acids accumulate within the alveolar spaces. It may be secondary to a failure of surfactant to be reprocessed by type II alveolar cells, or defective clearance of material by alveolar macrophages (Gaine & O'Marcaigh 1997). Clinically, it is difficult to distinguish from interstitial lung disease, therefore alveolar proteinosis must be diagnosed on lung biopsy or bronchoalveolar lavage (BAL). In severely affected patients, the only successful treatment is whole-lung lavage with saline, to wash out the intra-alveolar phospholipids; this results in symptomatic and functional improvement in about 80% of patients. However, the course is rather variable, and in a series of 24 patients, whole-lung lavage was only needed once in 13 patients (Goldstein et al 1998). The diagnosis is often made late, and if it is delayed until hypoxia ensues, the prognosis is poor. Infection may supervene and the situation is worsened by inappropriate treatment with corticosteroids.

Occasionally, lung transplantation has been performed, but recurrence of the disease can occur in the transplanted lung, and an underlying immune defect has been postulated (Gaine & O'Marcaigh 1997).

Preoperative abnormalities

1. Symptoms are nonspecific, and include a dry cough and breathlessness at rest, which is worse on exercise, haemoptysis, chest pain, fever, fatigue, and weight loss (Wang et al 1997). Wheezing is usually absent, but there are fine inspiratory crepitations. Finger clubbing may be present.

2. Patients are predominantly male, mostly aged 20–50. Although it is generally an adult disease, children may be affected (Mahut et al 1996).

3. Chest X-ray shows an ill-defined nodular pattern, worse in the bases and the perihilar regions of the lung field. It has a similar appearance to pulmonary oedema.

4. Lung function tests indicate a restrictive ventilatory defect. In a series of ten patients, before bronchial lavage, the VC varied between 33% and 86% predicted, total lung capacity 35–89% predicted and transfer factor 16–74% predicted (du Bois et al 1983). Arterial blood gases often showed hypoxia (in one patient as low as 3.7 kPa), and sometimes hypocapnoea.

5. Most often affects smokers or exsmokers.

6. Opportunistic infections, such as nocardiosis, may be superimposed (Pascual et al 1989).

7. The diagnosis may be delayed because the condition is mistaken for interstitial lung disease or sarcoidosis.

8. Definitive diagnosis is made on electron microscopy of sputum, bronchial washings, or transbronchial lung biopsy (Goldstein et al 1998).

Anaesthetic problems

1. Hypoxaemia. Anaesthesia is required for BAL, during which significant reductions in arterial oxygen saturation may be a problem (Bradfield & Maynard 1989). Gas exchange and haemodynamic parameters have been studied (Cohen & Eisenkraft 1990, Aguinaga et al 1991). When the lung is filled with saline, improvement in Pao_2 occurs. When the lung is emptied, the Pao_2 decreases, but increases in cardiac output result in the oxygen delivery being unchanged.

2. Cardiovascular changes. Since there are increases in intrathoracic pressure and large fluctuations in cardiac output, the bronchial lavage may be stressful to a patient whose myocardium is compromised. Transoesophageal echocardiography (TOE) during BAL, under propofol and alfentanil infusions, showed a reduction in left ventricular filling when the lung was fluid filled, and this was accompanied by hypotension (Swenson et al 1995). McMahon et al (1998) also used TOE, in order to assess the degree of right ventricular afterload, to decide when to terminate the filling phase of the cycle, and whether or not to proceed to lavage of the other lung during the same anaesthetic.

3. The procedure is lengthy (up to 2 h), and hypoxaemia is sometimes severe.

4. Some of the technical problems that may occur have been described by Busque (1977). These include malposition of the double lumen tube, underinflation of the cuff resulting in overspill of fluid into the inflated lung, and overinflation of the cuff such that it is difficult to drain the fluid.

5. One patient with alveolar proteinosis who had received two bolus doses of etomidate within 18 h developed cardiovascular instability and was subsequently found to have low serum cortisol levels (McGrady & Wright 1989).

Management

1. BAL is now the treatment of choice and usually results in considerable improvement in oxygenation (Selecky et al 1977, Du Bois et al 1983). About 60% of patients have a good response within two lung washouts (Shah et al 2000). In a third of the patients in one series, alveolar proteinosis did not recur during a follow-up period of 8.8 years (Prakash et al 1987). BAL is performed after isolation of one lung with a double lumen tube. This side is filled with isotonic saline at 37°C until a volume equal to the FRC has been introduced. The lung is then washed with 0.5–1 l at a time, until washings are clear, or until 40 l has been used. Vigorous manual or mechanical chest percussion during lavage increases the efficiency of the technique (McKenzie et al 1989). Bronchial suction and manual ventilation are performed, and finally a standard tracheal tube is inserted and IPPV is instituted for 2–4 h. Lavage may need to be repeated at 2–3-day intervals. A technique in children, using a bronchoscopically positioned bronchial tube, whilst maintaining ventilation of the opposite lung via a modified nasal airway, has been described (McKenzie et al 1989). The addition of trypsin to the BAL fluid resulted in clinical improvement in two patients (Nagasaka et al 1996).

2. General anaesthesia using propofol/alfentanil (Swenson et al 1995) and propofol/fentanyl (McMahon et al 1998) have been described.

3. Monitor oxygenation with pulse oximeter or arterial blood gases.

4. Cardiopulmonary bypass has been used occasionally, when severe hypoxia exists (Lippman et al 1977, Freedman et al 1981). Venovenous ECMO has supported oxygenation in severe cases (Sivitanidis et al 1999).

5. Successful pregnancy has been reported following spontaneous remission (Canto et al 1995).

Bibliography

Aguinaga MA, Santos P, Renes E et al 1991 Hemodynamic changes during whole broncho-alveolar lavage in two cases of pulmonary alveolar proteinosis. Intensive Care Medicine 17: 421–3.

Bradfield HGC, Maynard JP 1989 Pulmonary lavage in a case of alveolar proteinosis: the value of continuous display oxygen-haemoglobin saturation using ear-oximetry. Anaesthesia 34: 1032–4.

Busque L 1977 Pulmonary lavage in the treatment of alveolar proteinosis. Canadian Anaesthetists' Society Journal 24: 380–8.

Canto MJ, Vives MA, Carmona F et al 1995 Successful pregnancy after spontaneous remission of familial pulmonary alveolar proteinosis. European Journal of Obstetrics, Gynecology, & Reproductive Biology 63: 191–3.

Cohen E, Eisenkraft JB 1990 Bronchopulmonary lavage: effects on oxygenation and hemodynamics. Journal of Cardiothoracic Anesthesia 4: 609–15.

Du Bois RM, McAllister WAC, Branthwaite MA 1983 Alveolar proteinosis: diagnosis and treatment over a 10-year period. Thorax 38: 360–3.

Freedman AP, Pelias A, Johnston RF et al 1981 Alveolar proteinosis lung lavage using partial cardiopulmonary bypass. Thorax 36: 543–5.

Gaine SP, O'Marcaigh AS 1997 Pulmonary alveolar proteinosis: lung transplantation or bone marrow transplant? Chest 113: 563–4.

Goldstein LS, Kavuru MS, Curtis-McCarthy P et al 1998 Pulmonary alveolar proteinosis: clinical features and outcome. Chest 114: 1357–62.

Lippman M, Mok MS, Wasserman K 1977 Anesthetic management for children with alveolar proteinosis using extracorporeal circulation. British Journal of Anaesthesia 49: 173–6.

McGrady EM, Wright IH 1989 Cardiovascular instability following bolus dose of etomidate. Anaesthesia 44: 404–5.

McKenzie B, Wood RE, Bailey A 1989 Airway management for unilateral lung lavage in children. Anesthesiology 70: 550–3.

McMahon CC, Irvine T, Conacher ID 1998 Transoesophageal echocardiography in the management of whole lung lavage. British Journal of Anaesthesia 81: 262–4.

Mahut B, Delacourt C, Scheinmann P et al 1996 Pulmonary alveolar proteinosis: experience with eight pediatric cases and a review. Pediatrics 97: 117–22.

Nagasaka Y, Takahashi M, Ueshima H et al 1996 Broncheolar lavage with trypsin in pulmonary alveolar proteinosis. Thorax 51: 769–70.

Pascual J, Aguinaga G, Vidal R et al 1989 Alveolar proteinosis and nocardiosis: a patient treated by bronchopulmonary lavage. Postgraduate Medical Journal 65: 674–7.

Prakash UBS, Bahram SS, Carpenter HA et al 1987 Pulmonary alveolar phospholipoproteinosis: experience with 34 cases and a review. Mayo Clinic Proceedings 62: 499–518.

Selecky PA, Wasserman K, Benfield JR et al 1977 The clinical and physiological effect of whole-lung lavage in pulmonary alveolar proteinosis: a ten-year experience. Annals of Thoracic Surgery 24: 451–61.

Shah PL, Hansell D, Lawson PR et al 2000 Pulmonary alveolar proteinosis: clinical aspects and current concepts on pathogenesis. Thorax 55: 67–77.

Sivitanidis E, Tosson R, Wiebalck A et al 1999 Combination of extracorporeal membrane oxygenation (ECMO) and pulmonary lavage in a patient with pulmonary alveolar proteinosis. European Journal of Cardio-Thoracic Surgery 15: 370–2.

Swenson JD, Astle KL, Bailey PL 1995 Reduction in left ventricular filling during bronchopulmonary lavage demonstrated by transesophageal echocardiography. Anesthesia & Analgesia 81: 634–7.

Wang BM, Stern EJ, Schmidt RA et al 1997 Diagnosing pulmonary alveolar proteinosis. A review and an update. Chest 111: 460–6.

Amniotic fluid embolism

(see Section 2)

Amphetamine abuse

Amphetamines are sympathomimetic amines, which, in the initial stages of intoxication, elevate the mood and increase alertness, thus reducing the need for sleep. They act both directly and indirectly on the sympathetic nervous system, via the peripheral nerve endings. Catecholamines are released within the CNS, and catecholamine re-uptake by adrenoceptor nerve endings is prevented. Tolerance readily occurs. A number of synthetic amines, which share structural similarities to methamphetamine, are used for their ability to produce euphoria and sociability. These include methylenedioxy-methamphetamine (MDMA, 'Ecstasy', 'E', 'XTC', 'Adam') and 3,4-methylenedioxy-ethamphetamine (MDEA, 'Eve'), 'Ice' or 'Blue ice' (crystalline methamphetamine). The use of these has been associated with deaths (Dowling et al 1987), and with a syndrome of convulsions, hyperthermia, hyperkalaemia and rhabdomyolysis, resembling MH, but unrelated to it (Brown & Osterloh 1987, Singarajah & Lavies 1992, Tehan et al 1993). There is evidence that serotoninergic mechanisms cause an increased heat production that is exacerbated by high ambient temperatures; this may account for the occurrence of the syndrome at 'rave' parties, where it is used as a 'dance drug' (Henry 1992). Amphetamine abusers often misuse other drugs, and street preparations frequently contain contaminants.

Maternal amphetamine use in pregnancy is associated with a high risk of prematurity and low birth weight (Furara et al 1999). Symptoms may be mistaken for preeclampsia, and fetal distress may be precipitated (Birnbach 1998).

The anaesthetist may be involved in anaesthesia for the acute or chronic abuser, for patients acutely intoxicated who injure themselves, or for resuscitation and intensive care of patients who present with convulsions, hyperthermia and rhabdomyolysis following synthetic amine abuse.

Preoperative abnormalities

1. The patient may be suffering from acute toxicity. Initially, signs of irritability, with tremor, dilated pupils and sweating may be displayed. Increasing doses cause tachycardia, fever, mild

hypertension and systemic vasoconstriction, with agitation and confusion. Delirium, increasing blood pressure, hyperthermia and the onset of arrhythmias, precede convulsions, coma and death.

2. Recreational use. There have been several reports of reactions to MDMA, in which rhabdomyolysis and hyperkalaemia are associated with convulsions and hyperthermia, producing a syndrome that resembles MH (Singarajah & Lavies 1992). Similar complications occur with MDEA (Tehan et al 1993). Coagulopathy (Chadwick et al 1991) and renal failure have also been reported (Fahal et al 1992).

3. Acute pulmonary oedema occurred 2 h following amphetamine ingestion, but the patient removed her tracheal tube 2 h later (Maury et al 1999).

4. In chronic abuse there may be significant tolerance.

5. The long term effects of MDMA are not yet fully known but may include psychiatric disturbances and hepatic damage.

6. In pregnancy, there is an increased risk of fetal distress and requirement for Caesarean section (Birnbach & Stein 1998).

Anaesthetic problems

1. Chronic amphetamine abusers or those who have acute toxicity may require anaesthesia. Intracranial hypertension was reported in a young girl who required elevation of a skull fracture (Michel & Adams 1979). Individuals who smuggle drugs by 'body-packing' may need urgent surgical intervention because of the risk of fatal toxicity (Watson et al 1991).

2. Studies on dogs have shown that MAC values for halothane were altered by both acute and chronic amphetamine intake. Acute intoxication resulted in an increased MAC for halothane (Johnston et al 1972), and duration of anaesthesia and time to ambulation was reduced. By contrast, chronic abuse for 7 days decreased

the MAC for halothane and dogs subjected to chronic abuse had a poor response to indirectly acting sympathetic agents.

3. Hazards during pregnancy, particularly during Caesarean section in chronic amphetamine abusers. In one patient, a longstanding heroin and amphetamine abuser, epidural anaesthesia was established with lidocaine 2% 10 ml (Samuels et al 1979). After transfer to the operating theatre, two successive doses of 12 ml and 6 ml of chloroprocaine 3% did not extend the block, and it was assumed that the catheter had become displaced. General anaesthesia was induced with thiopentone 200 mg and suxamethonium. Cardiac arrest occurred soon after surgery began. Resuscitation with epinephrine (adrenaline), bicarbonate, and isoprenaline proved successful. On recovery, the patient admitted to taking amphetamines just prior to admission. The authors postulated that chronic users of amphetamines do not respond to stress and may develop a type of autonomic dysfunction. Another patient, also a chronic amphetamine abuser, developed hypotension, tachycardia and vasoconstriction intraoperatively, for which 500 ml colloid and 1300 ml crystalloid was given (Smith & Gutsche 1980). After extubation, pulmonary oedema developed, and IPPV, with PEEP, was required for 8 h. Her rapid recovery was felt to be consistent with the diagnosis of hydrostatic pulmonary oedema, rather than gastric inhalation or septicaemia. A third patient, who had taken amphetamine in late pregnancy, presented with convulsions, agitation, hypertension and proteinuria which was misdiagnosed as eclampsia, for which a Caesarean section was performed (Elliott & Rees 1990).

4. An extensive consumptive coagulopathy has been reported in a 24-week-pregnant patient with abdominal pain who took iv amphetamine 3.5 h before admission (Hahn 1995).

5. Arrhythmias may occur, particularly in the presence of agents which sensitise the heart to the effects of catecholamines. The response to pressor agents is unpredictable (Birnbach 1998).

6. There may be delayed recovery from anaesthesia.

7. Overdoses of ecstasy produce hyperthermia, coagulopathy, rhabdomyolysis, rigidity, dilated pupils, cardiac arrest convulsions, coma, liver failure, and pulmonary oedema. Progressive muscle damage has been reported with maximum CK levels of 122 341 U l^{-1}, which, unusually, did not occur until the 10th day (Murphy et al 1997).

8. Low-dose MDMA induces plasma arginine vasopressin secretion, with a maximal pharmacological effect at 1–2 h following ingestion (Henry et al 1998).

Management

1. A careful history should be taken in an attempt to establish the presence of acute or chronic abuse. Denial or concealment is common (Michel & Adams 1979, Samuels et al 1979). Urinary estimations of amphetamines and their metabolites can be performed, but this facility is not usually available in the acute situation; in addition, samples may not be taken early enough because the diagnosis has not been considered.

2. ECG, core temperature and blood pressure should be monitored from the induction of anaesthesia. Benzodiazepines are reported as being suitable for the chronic abuser (Caldwell 1990).

3. Acute intoxication. Rehydration and mannitol may be required when toxicity is present, particularly in those who are pyrexial. In cases of acute intoxication, chlorpromazine has been recommended. The use of dantrolene sodium in the treatment of rhabdomyolysis and hyperthermia has been reported (Singarajah & Lavies 1992, Tehan et al 1993), but there are no definite scientific data to support its use. However, Hall (1997) believes that for the patient *in extremis*, there is some weight of clinical evidence in favour of dantrolene, to control dangerous hyperthermia.

4. The management of hypertension may require the use of alpha blockers. Because of its longer action, diazoxide 300 mg (or 5 mg kg^{-1}) may be more appropriate than phentolamine.

5. Halothane should be avoided in the presence of amphetamines.

6. Regional anaesthesia has been used for patients in labour, but hypotension can occur and the response to pressor agents is unpredictable (Birnbach 1998). Direct-acting vasopressors are recommended to treat hypotension in the chronic abuser (Johnston et al 1972).

Bibliography

Birnbach DJ 1998 Anesthesia and the drug-abusing parturient. Anesthesiology Clinics of North America 16: 385–95.

Birnbach DJ, Stein DJ 1998 The substance-abusing parturient: implications for analgesia and anaesthesia management. Baillieres Clinical Obstetrics & Gynaecology 12: 433–60.

Brown C, Osterloh J 1987 Multiple severe complications from recreational ingestion of MDMA ('Ecstasy'). Journal of the American Medical Association 258: 780–1.

Caldwell TB 1990 Anesthesia for patients with behavioral and environmental disorders. In: Katz J, Benumof J (eds) Anesthesia and uncommon diseases. WB Saunders, Philadelphia, pp 792–922.

Chadwick IS, Curry PD, Linsley A et al 1991 3–4 Methylenedioxymethamphetamine (MDMA), a fatality associated with hyperthermia and coagulopathy. Journal of the Royal Society of Medicine 84: 371.

Dowling GP, McDonough ET, Bost RO 1987 'Eve' and 'Ecstasy'. A report of five deaths associated with the use of MDEA and MDMA. Journal of the American Medical Association 257: 1615–17.

Elliott RH, Rees GB 1990 Amphetamine ingestion presenting as eclampsia. Canadian Journal of Anaesthesia 37: 130–3.

Fahal IH, Sallomi DF, Yaqoob M et al 1992 Acute renal failure after ecstasy. British Medical Journal 305: 29.

Furara SA, Carrick P, Armstrong D et al 1999 The outcome of pregnancy associated with amphetamine abuse. Journal of Obstetrics & Gynaecology 19: 377–80.

Hahn L 1995 Consumption coagulopathy after amphetamine abuse in pregnancy. Acta Obstetrica et Gynecologica Scandinavica 74: 652–4.

Hall AP 1997 'Ecstasy' and the anaesthetist. British Journal of Anaesthesia 79: 697–8.

Henry JA 1992 Ecstasy and the dance of death. Severe reactions are unpredictable. British Medical Journal 305: 5–6.

Henry JA, Fallon JK, Kieman AT et al 1998 Low-dose MDMA ('ecstasy') induces vasopressin secretion. Lancet 351: 1784.

Johnston RR, Way WL, Miller RD 1972 Alteration of anaesthetic requirements by amphetamine. Anesthesiology 36: 357–63.

Maury E, Darondel JM, Buisinne A et al 1999 Acute pulmonary edema following amphetamine ingestion. Intensive Care Medicine 25: 332–3.

Michel R, Adams AP 1979 Acute amphetamine abuse. Problems during general anaesthesia for neurosurgery. Anaesthesia 34: 1016–19.

Murphy BCS, Wilkes RG, Roberts NB 1997 Creatine kinase isoform changes following ecstasy overdose. Anaesthesia & Intensive Care 25: 156–9.

Samuels SI, Maze A, Albright G 1979 Cardiac arrest during Cesarean section in a chronic amphetamine abuser. Anesthesia & Analgesia 58: 528–30.

Singarajah C, Lavies N G 1992 An overdose of ecstasy. A role for dantrolene. Anaesthesia 47: 686–7.

Smith DS, Gutsche BB 1980 Amphetamine abuse and obstetrical anesthesia. Anesthesia & Analgesia 59: 710–11.

Tehan B, Hardern R, Bodenham A 1993 Hyperthermia associated with 3,4-methylenedioxyethamphetamine (Eve). Anaesthesia 48: 507–10.

Watson CJE, Johnston PS, Thomson HJ 1991 Body-packing with amphetamines—an indication for surgery. Journal of the Royal Society of Medicine 84: 311–12.

Amyloidosis

Amyloidosis is a general term for a variety of different disease processes involving the deposition of fibrillary material in tissues. This is formed of protein subunits sharing a common beta-pleated sheet structure, but derived from proteins of great chemical diversity. These fibrils are resistant to normal proteolytic digestion and share a common histochemical staining property to Congo red. In the light of advances in the understanding of the structural chemistry of amyloid, the disease is now classified according to the amyloid protein that makes up the deposit. The main forms are AL amyloid (primary, myeloma, or macroglobinaemia-related) and AA amyloid (reactive, secondary). Heart transplantation may be undertaken for cardiac amyloid, although the long term survival may be reduced because of progression of systemic disease and recurrence of the disease in the new heart (Hosenpud et al 1991).

1. AL amyloidosis predominantly involves mesenchymal tissue. This results in neuropathies, carpal tunnel syndrome, macroglossia, a restrictive cardiomyopathy, skin, gut, and kidney lesions.

2. AA amyloidosis can occur in association with chronic infective, inflammatory, and neoplastic disorders. In a survey of patients, the frequency of underlying disorder was rheumatoid arthritis (56%), recurrent pulmonary infections (11%), Crohn's disease (5%), ankylosing spondylitis (5%), and tuberculosis (3%) (Hazenberg & Van Rijswijk 1994). Parenchymal tissue tends to be involved primarily, particularly in the kidneys, liver, spleen, and thyroid. Cardiomyopathy occurs in less than 10%, compared with AL amyloid, in which involvement of the heart is almost universal. Amyloid deposition, particularly involving joints, bones, and tendons, may occur in patients on long term dialysis (Editorial 1991).

Preoperative abnormalities

1. Cardiac amyloidosis may present with a digoxin-resistant heart failure, arrhythmias, and conduction defects. In the AL form, heart involvement is almost universal, whereas in the AA form significant disease only occurs in less than 10% of patients. The classical restrictive cardiomyopathy carries a poor prognosis, with a median survival from diagnosis of about 1 year (Dubrey et al 1998). It is the main cause of death in about 65% of patients. Those with severe diastolic dysfunction may have atrial thrombi that can produce thromboembolism. Features

include ventricular, ventricular septal, and valvular thickening, and reduced chamber size. ECG may be of low voltage, particularly in the limb leads.

2. Unusual skin lesions, ecchymoses, nonthrombocytopenic purpura, or bullae feature in 40% of cases with AL amyloid, and macroglossia is common. Neurological lesions may affect any type of nerve including those of the autonomic system, resulting in an autonomic neuropathy.

3. AA amyloid may present with the nephrotic syndrome, renal failure, hepatosplenomegaly, adrenal failure, or lung disease. It is the main cause of death in 35% of patients with this form of disease.

4. Bleeding occurs frequently, although coagulation studies may be normal. Three types of abnormalities have been described (Mizutani & Ward 1990): abnormalities of platelet function, increased vessel fragility secondary to amyloid infiltration of the blood vessels (Yood et al 1983), and defects in coagulation and fibrinolysis. Qualitative and quantitative defects in Factors IX and X have been described, and there may be defects in the interactions between platelets and the vessel walls. In a series of 100 patients, 41 had one or more bleeding episodes, three of which resulted in death.

5. Amyloidosis should be suspected when a patient presents with multiple organ involvement. Confirmation is by biopsy of an affected organ, but rectal biopsy is diagnostic in 90% of cases of systemic amyloid.

6. Anaesthesia may be required for biopsies, for cardiac transplantation, or for incidental surgery.

7. Patients may be receiving long term immunosuppressive, cytotoxic, or steroid therapy.

Anaesthetic problems

1. Fatal arrhythmias have been described in the perioperative period. Intraoperative deaths occurred in two patients with AL amyloid

undergoing renal, and renal and liver transplantation, respectively. In the first, cardiac involvement was not anticipated, and in the second the diagnosis was known, but the severity of the cardiac disease was not appreciated at the time of surgery (Tallgren et al 1995). The QT dispersion was subsequently measured from preoperative ECGs, and in both it was found to be increased (125–128 ms, N 20–50 ms). Another patient developed VT followed by VF in the recovery room after laminectomy. Resuscitation failed and at postmortem, extensive cardiac amyloid was found (Wang & Pollard 2000).

2. Four patients had fatal perioperative myocardial infarctions. In retrospect, the only common features were low voltage QRS complexes and bundle branch block. As a result of diastolic dysfunction, the amyloid heart is resistant to cardiosupportive measures, and calcium channel blockers may worsen the condition (Kotani et al 2000). Resistant heart failure developed after general anaesthesia for cystoscopy, in a patient who had unusual skin petechiae. The diagnosis of amyloidosis was made subsequently, and death occurred on the 15th postoperative day (Welch 1982).

3. Macroglossia, common in the AL form, may cause difficulties with intubation and potential postoperative airway obstruction.

4. Extreme fragility of the skin, and ecchymoses of the mucosae, eyelids, face, neck, and axillary folds may be seen. In one patient, haemorrhagic rashes and frank bleeding occurred at all the sites where ECG electrodes and adhesive tape had been placed (Dixon 1987). In another, the appearance of two rectangular haemorrhagic, purpuric lesions on the cheekbones where the tracheal tube had been fastened, led to the diagnosis of amyloid first being made (Camposi 1999).

5. There have been several reports of bleeding during surgery, or bleeding that resulted in surgical investigation being required. A patient with small bowel obstruction, in whom there was mild prolongation of the bleeding time, rapidly developed large haematomas and

required 10 units of platelets and 4 units of FFP. Subsequently, Factor IX and X levels were found to be 70% of normal (Mizutani & Ward 1990). Routine coagulation studies are unreliable predictors of the likelihood of bleeding. Of 41 patients with amyloid who had bled, only 20% had an abnormal prothrombin time. Bleeding can follow mild trauma and may require surgical intervention. The gastrointestinal tract was the source in 18, a further eight bled after diagnostic procedures, and three had haematuria. Coagulation tests were normal in all eight who bled after diagnostic procedures (Yood et al 1983). An additional factor contributing to bleeding is amyloid infiltration of the blood vessels (Chow et al 1993).

6. In the reactive form, the additional problems are those of the primary associated disease, eg rheumatoid arthritis.

7. The larynx is the most common site for localised amyloidosis. Hoarseness was the commonest symptom and the false vocal cords were the most likely site to be affected (Lewis et al 1992). Laryngofissure and temporary tracheostomy were required in a 9-year-old child, in spite of which recurrence occurred 18 months later (O'Halloran & Lusk 1994). Urgent tracheal intubation, followed by tracheostomy, was needed for laser resection of subglottic amyloidosis (Woo et al 1990). A fatality occurred in a patient with undiagnosed localised laryngeal amyloidosis. The 38-year-old man had a 3-week history of hoarseness and coughing. Massive haemorrhage and suffocation took place in the middle of the night. At autopsy, a typical amyloid ulcer was found in the subglottis, and the airway was filled with blood (Chow et al 1993). Tracheal involvement can occur concurrently. In a patient with primary amyloid, massive cervical lymphadenopathy resulted in severe airway obstruction (Leach et al 1999).

Management

1. The diagnosis should be suspected in the patient with multiple organ involvement,

especially in the presence of a disease known to be associated with the AA form.

2. Careful assessment of the heart, lungs, and liver for impairment of function. Surgical decisions, and anaesthetic management, should be in the light of this information. Cardiac involvement should be suspected in all patients with heart failure who have chamber wall and valve leaflet thickening on echocardiography, normal chamber size, and low ECG voltages (Dubrey et al 1998). Such patients have a poor prognosis. Measurement of QT dispersion has been suggested as a method to predict patients in whom the likelihood of arrhythmias is high (Kirvela et al 1994). From a 12-lead ECG, the QT_c should be calculated manually from the onset of the QRS to the end of the T wave, defined as a return to the TP baseline. On three consecutive cycles, the mean QT_c is calculated, and the QT dispersion is measured as the difference between the maximum and minimum QT_c. An increase in the QT dispersion reflects variations in ventricular recovery of excitability, and therefore an increased risk of arrhythmias. If bradycardias develop, atropine may be ineffective, and isoprenaline and pacing may be required (Tallgren et al 1995).

3. If severe diastolic dysfunction is present, atrial thrombi should be sought on echocardiography and the appropriate prophylaxis given.

4. In the presence of macroglossia, difficulties in intubation may be experienced. Postoperatively, the patient should be nursed in an intensive recovery area. Treatment of laryngeal amyloid should be as for any upper airway lesion causing obstructive symptoms.

5. Coagulation studies should be performed, but even when these are normal the possibility of haemorrhage should be anticipated. A normal result does not guarantee that haemorrhage will not occur.

6. Epidural anaesthesia was given to a patient with secondary amyloidosis undergoing Caesarean section. She had been admitted at 34 weeks' gestation with hypertension and deteriorating renal function in a transplanted kidney (Weir & McLoughlin 1998).

Bibliography

Camposi JH 1999 A reaction to tape after tracheal extubation in a patient with systemic amyloidosis. Journal of Clinical Anesthesia 11: 126–8.

Chow LT-C, Chow HW, Shum BS 1993 Fatal upper respiratory tract haemorrhage: an unusual complication of localized amyloidosis of the larynx. Journal of Laryngology & Otology 107: 51–3.

Dixon J 1987 Primary amyloidosis and skin damage. Anaesthesia 42: 218.

Dubrey SW, Cha K, Anderson J et al 1998 The clinical features of immunoglobulin light-chain (AL) amyloidosis with heart involvement. Quarterly Journal of Medicine 91: 141–7.

Editorial 1991 Dialysis amyloidosis. Lancet 338: 349–50.

Gertz MA, Kyle RA 1991 Secondary systemic amyloidosis: response and survival in 64 patients. Medicine 70: 246–56.

Hazenberg BPC, Van Rijswijk MH 1994 Clinical and therapeutic aspects of AA amyloidosis. Baillieres Clinical Rheumatology 8: 627–34.

Hosenpud JD, DeMarco T, Frazier OH et al 1991 Progression of systemic disease and reduced long term survival in patients with cardiac amyloidosis undergoing heart transplantation. Circulation 84: 338–43.

Kirvela M, Yli-Hankala A, Lindgren L 1994 QT dispersion and autonomic function in diabetic and non-diabetic patients with renal failure. British Journal of Anaesthesia 73: 801–4.

Kotani N, Hashimoto H, Muraoka M et al 2000 Fatal perioperative myocardial infarction in four patients with cardiac amyloid. Anesthesiology 92: 873–5.

Leach DB, Hester TO, Farrell HA et al 1999 Primary amyloidosis presenting as massive cervical lymphadenopathy with severe dyspnoea: a case report and review of the literature. Otolaryngology—Head & Neck Surgery 120: 560–4.

Lewis JE, Olsen KD, Kurtin PJ et al 1992 Laryngeal amyloidosis: a clinicopathologic and immunohistochemical review. Otolaryngology—Head & Neck Surgery 106: 372–7.

Mizutani AR, Ward CF 1990 Amyloidosis-associated bleeding diathesis in the surgical patient. Canadian Journal of Anaesthesia 37: 910–12.

O'Halloran LR, Lusk RP 1994 Amyloidosis of the

larynx in a child. Annals of Otology, Rhinology & Laryngology 103: 590–4.

Tallgren M, Hockerstedt K, Isoniemi H et al 1995 Intraoperative death in cardiac amyloidosis with increased QT dispersion in the electrocardiogram. Anesthesia & Analgesia 80: 1233–5.

Wang MMJ, Pollard JB 2000 Postoperative ventricular fibrillation and undiagnosed primary amyloidosis. Anesthesiology 92: 871–2.

Weir PS, McLoughlin CC 1998 Anaesthesia for caesarean section in a patient with systemic amyloidosis secondary to familial Mediterranean fever. International Journal of Obstetric Anesthesia 7: 271–4.

Welch DB 1982 Anaesthesia and amyloidosis. Anaesthesia 37: 63–6.

Woo KS, Van Hasselt CA, Waldron J 1990 Laser resection of localized subglottic amyloidosis. Journal of Otolaryngology 19: 337–8.

Yood RA, Skinner M, Rubinow A et al 1983 Bleeding manifestations in 100 patients with amyloidosis. Journal of the American Medical Association 249: 1322–4.

Amyotrophic lateral sclerosis

(see Motor neurone disease)

Ankylosing spondylitis

An inflammatory arthropathy of insidious onset with systemic involvement. Granulation tissue infiltrates the bony insertions of ligaments and joint capsules, and the disease progresses variably to fibrosis, ossification, and ankylosis. The primary sites of involvement are the sacroiliac joints and the spine, but 50% of patients will have extraspinal joint involvement at some time. Since it is a systemic disorder, a proportion of the patients will develop nonarticular manifestations of the inflammatory process.

Preoperative abnormalities

1. *Bone and joints*

a) The inflammatory process usually begins at the sacroiliac joints and spreads upwards to involve the spine and costovertebral joints. A limitation of chest expansion to 2.5 cm or less is one of the criteria contributing to the clinical diagnosis. Ossification of interspinous ligaments, and the formation of bony bridges between vertebrae, occur in the lumbar spine, whilst cervical spine involvement varies from a degree of limitation of movement of the neck, to complete ankylosis. Those with advanced disease have an increased risk of sustaining a cervical fracture, often after minor trauma or hyperextension (Tico et al 1998), and 36% of this group have evidence of a previous occult cervical spine fracture. The majority of lesions involve the disc spaces of C5–C7, although sometimes a vertebral body is involved. A high proportion of the patients with spinal fractures have neurological damage.

b) Temporomandibular joint involvement causes limited mouth opening in 10% of patients, but in longstanding disease the incidence may be as high as 30–40%. Sometimes this progresses to complete ankylosis.

c) Cricoarytenoid arthritis occurs rarely. Dyspnoea, hoarseness, and vocal cord fixation may be present.

2. *Non-articular disease*

a) Systemic effects include fatigue, weight loss, fever, a high ESR, and hypochromic anaemia.

b) Thirty-five per cent of patients have uveitis, and 85% of male patients have prostatitis at some stage of the disease.

c) Cardiovascular complications have been reported in 3.5% of patients with a 15-year history, and in 10% of patients who have had the disease for 30 years. Scarring of the adventitia and fibrous proliferation of the intima of the aorta and the valve cusps produce aortitis and aortic regurgitation, and occasionally mitral valve disease. Purkinje tissue involvement may result in conduction defects. Occasionally patients present with complete heart block, yet have minimal skeletal symptoms (Bergfeldt et al 1982). Transoesophageal echocardiography may allow an earlier diagnosis of cardiac involvement than transthoracic, because there is better detection of fibrosis of the aortic root and intraventricular septum (Arnason et al 1996).

d) Pulmonary disease may occur. Upper lobe fibrosis is a well-recognised complication. The seriousness of any pulmonary complication will be accentuated by the limited chest expansion.

e) Neurological effects are protean. Spinal cord compression, cauda equina syndrome, focal epilepsy, vertebrobasilar insufficiency and peripheral nerve lesions have all been described. In addition there is an increased risk of trivial trauma causing cervical fractures (Murray & Persellin 1981), and the incidence of cervical fracture is 3.5 times greater than in the normal population. Fracture not infrequently leads to acute epidural haematoma formation, giving a picture of incomplete cord injury followed by rapid deterioration of neurological status (Wu & Lee 1998).

Anaesthetic problems

1. Difficult intubation. If the cervical spine is involved, intubation may be difficult or impossible, particularly since patients are young and often have full dentition. Repeated attempts under general anaesthesia may be hazardous. Death from a retropharyngeal abscess, which developed following several attempts at blind intubation, has been recorded (Hill 1980).

2. Bony fragility. The diseased bones are fragile. Forcible neck movements in the presence of neuromuscular blockade should therefore be avoided because of the possible risk of cervical fracture, or vertebrobasilar insufficiency.

Quadriparesis and dislocation of C6 vertebra became apparent after emergency tracheal intubation of a patient who had collapsed at work (Salathe & Johr 1989). The role of resuscitation manoeuvres in the generation of the lesion was unclear, but tracheal intubation was thought to have contributed. In a series of 33 patients requiring surgical intervention, three became quadriplegic after emergency intubation, and one, with an unrecognised L1 fracture, as a result of transfer from his bed (Fox et al 1993). Particular care should also be taken if ECT is required (Snyder et al 1992).

3. Cervical fixation. The position in which the neck becomes fixed in longstanding disease may preclude tracheostomy. As a result of flexion deformity, no structure below the thyroid cartilage may be palpable.

4. It is known that insertion of a laryngeal mask airway may be impossible in patients with extreme flexion deformities, because of the abnormal angle of the oropharyngeal axes (Ishimura et al 1995). In normal patients, the angle between the oral and pharyngeal axes at the back of the tongue is 105°. If this angle is less than 90°, the leading edge of the laryngeal mask airway becomes kinked at the angle and cannot be advanced. The authors demonstrated the problem with an aluminium plate. Although the patient described had rheumatoid arthritis, similar deformities occur in ankylosing spondylitis.

5. Difficulty in positioning and spinal deformity were thought to have contributed to the massive bleeding encountered during surgery to stabilise a traumatic lumbar spinal fracture (Tetzlaff et al 1998).

6. Patients with vertebrobasilar insufficiency should be treated with caution. The author encountered a patient who had syncope during cervical spine screening whenever extension of the neck was attempted. Presumably, bony encroachment into the vertebral canal had compromised blood flow in the artery. The radiologist considered general anaesthesia inadvisable, and limited abdominal surgery was

performed after difficult spinal anaesthesia. However, the patient had a respiratory arrest on the ward 1 week later and died after unsuccessful CPR.

7. Temporomandibular joint involvement may compound the intubation difficulties. Ankylosis of this joint, further complicated by massive haematemesis, has been described (Sinclair & Mason 1984). Cricoarytenoid arthritis, though rare, can occur (Miller et al 1994).

8. Respiratory problems and limited chest wall expansion increase the pulmonary complication rate, and hence the need for postoperative IPPV.

9. Aortic valve disease and conduction defects can occur. Early preclinical changes in the aortic root and intraventricular septum have been shown using transoesophageal echocardiography (Arnason et al 1996).

10. Although spinal anaesthesia can be technically difficult because of joint ankylosis, spinal anaesthesia may be a satisfactory alternative to general anaesthesia. In a series of 13 patients in which it was attempted, ten were successful (Schelew & Vaghadia 1996). The spinal needles, 22–27 G Sprotte, were inserted through introducers.

11. If intubation is predicted to be difficult, lumbar and caudal epidural anaesthesia should be undertaken with caution, and local anaesthetic doses carefully fractionated, to avoid total spinal anaesthesia. Technical difficulties may increase the risk of complications. Convulsions secondary to accidental intraosseous injection of bupivacaine 20 ml during an attempted caudal block (Weber 1985), and a spinal haematoma following epidural analgesia (Gustafsson et al 1988), are recorded. In a recent review of 51 confirmed spinal haematomas following epidural anaesthesia, ankylosing spondylitis was identified as a previously unreported risk factor (Wulf 1996). Possible predisposing factors include technical difficulties, treatment with NSAIDs, and the narrowness of the epidural space.

12. Difficulty in removing the epidural catheter has been reported in two patients who were in a flexed sitting position (Trikha 1996). Both catheters had been inserted in the left lateral position and return of the patient to that position enabled removal to be achieved without problem.

13. There is a high incidence of gastrointestinal bleeding following treatment with NSAIDs.

14. External cardiac massage is ineffective in patients with a rigid chest wall.

Management

1. Neck movements should be assessed with radiological screening in flexion and extension. If there is limitation of movement, and the patient has full dentition, intubation difficulties should be anticipated. Wittmann and Ring (1986), who reported hip replacement in eight spondylitics, emphasised the value of indirect laryngoscopy in advance, to predict difficult intubation. Conventional intubation failed in both patients in whom preoperative indirect laryngoscopy using a spatula and a dental mirror could not demonstrate the larynx. In such patients, awake fibreoptic intubation is the safest course of action. However, technical problems may sometimes arise and difficulty occurred as a result of distortion of the airway by a large anterior osteophyte (Ranasinghe & Calder 1994). A fibreoptic bronchoscope was used to perform nasal intubation in a patient whose upper lip was pressed against her chest wall (Ovassapian et al 1983). In this particular case, tracheostomy would have been impossible. However, in some circumstances, for example surgery for active haematemesis, preliminary tracheostomy under local anaesthesia may be the technique of choice (Sinclair & Mason 1984). A retrograde wire technique has been used in a patient who required endobronchial intubation (Alfery 1993). A modification of a retrograde technique was described, in which the final positioning of the tube is performed under

fibreoptic guidance (Roberts & Solgonick 1996).

2. The use of the laryngeal mask airway is controversial. Although anaesthetists have come to rely on it as a fallback in cases of intubation failure (Alexander et al 1988), laryngeal mask airway placement is not guaranteed to be satisfactory (Kumar & Mehta 1995), or may actually fail (Ishimura et al 1995), in patients with advanced ankylosing spondylitis.

3. A preoperative ECG is mandatory in longstanding disease, because of the risk of conduction defects; cardiovascular complications should be treated. Echocardiography will demonstrate valvular disease.

4. A cervical support should be used during anaesthesia, especially if there are signs of vertebrobasilar insufficiency. If vertebrobasilar insufficiency is severe, general anaesthesia may be contraindicated.

5. If general anaesthesia is contraindicated, spinal anaesthesia may be possible, if necessary using radiological control, a 19-G needle, and the assistance of an orthopaedic drill or hammer. In patients in whom a midline approach proves difficult, a lateral approach to spinal anaesthesia may be possible (Kumar & Mehta 1995). Epidural anaesthesia is technically more difficult, and carries increased risk of epidural haematoma. Local anaesthetics should be given gradually, in small doses, in patients known to be difficult to intubate.

6. Pregnancy sometimes occurs in severe disease. Awake fibreoptic intubation in the left lateral position was reported in a parturient with a history of failed intubation at previous surgery (Broomhead et al 1995).

7. Patients undergoing spinal surgery require particularly careful management, including aggressive postoperative mobilisation.

8. After major surgery, a short period of postoperative IPPV may be required to anticipate possible lung problems. Even without this, admission to an HDU may be advisable.

Bibliography

Alexander CA, Leach AB, Thompson AR et al 1988 Use your Brain! Anaesthesia 43: 893–4.

Alfery DD 1993 Double-lumen endobronchial tube intubation using a retrograde wire technique. Anesthesia & Analgesia 76: 1374–5.

Arnason JA, Patel AK, Rahko PS et al 1996 Transthoracic and transesophageal echocardiographic evaluation of the aortic root and subvalvular structures in ankylosing spondylitis. Journal of Rheumatology 23: 120–3.

Bergfeldt L, Edhag O, Vedin L et al 1982 Ankylosing spondylitis. An important cause of severe disturbances of the cardiac conduction system. American Journal of Medicine 73: 187–91.

Broomhead CJ, Davies W, Higgins D 1995 Awake fibreoptic intubation for caesarean section. International Journal of Obstetric Anesthesia 4: 172–4.

Fox MW, Onofrio BM, Kilgore JE 1993 Neurological complications of ankylosing spondylitis. Journal of Neurosurgery 78: 871–8.

Gustafsson H, Rutberg H, Bengtsson M 1988 Spinal haematoma following epidural analgesia. Anaesthesia 43: 220–2.

Hill CM 1980 Death following dental clearance in a patient suffering from ankylosing spondylitis. British Journal of Oral Surgery 18: 73–6.

Ishimura H, Minami K, Sata T et al 1995 Impossible insertion of the laryngeal mask airway and oropharyngeal axes. Anesthesiology 83: 867–9.

Kumar CM, Mehta M 1995 Ankylosing spondylitis: lateral approach to spinal anaesthesia for lower limb surgery. Canadian Journal of Anaesthesia 42: 73–6.

Miller FR, Wanamaker JR, Hicks DM et al 1994 Cricoarytenoid arthritis and ankylosing spondylitis. Otolaryngology—Head & Neck Surgery 120: 214–16.

Murray GC, Persellin RH 1981 Cervical fracture complicating ankylosing spondylitis. American Journal of Medicine 70: 1033–41.

Ovassapian A, Land P, Schafer MF et al 1983 Anesthetic management for surgical corrections of severe flexion deformity of the cervical spine. Anesthesiology 58: 370–2.

Ranasinghe DN, Calder I 1994 Large cervical osteophyte—another cause of difficult flexible fibreoptic intubation. Anaesthesia 49: 512–14.

Roberts KW, Solgonick RM 1996 A modification of retrograde wire-guided, fiberoptic-assisted endotracheal intubation in a patient with ankylosing spondylitis. Anesthesia & Analgesia 82: 1290–1.

Salathe M, Johr M 1989 Unexpected cervical fractures: a common problem in ankylosing spondylitis. Anesthesiology 70: 869–70.

Schelew BL, Vaghadia H 1996 Ankylosing spondylitis and neuraxial anaesthesia—a 10 year review. Canadian Journal of Anaesthesia 43: 65–8.

Sinclair JR, Mason RA 1984 Ankylosing spondylitis. The case for awake intubation. Anaesthesia 39: 3–11.

Snyder DS, Lipsey JR, McPherson RW 1992 Management for electroconvulsive therapy of a patient with inoperable coronary artery disease and ankylosing spondylitis. Journal of Clinical Anesthesia 3: 226–8.

Tetzlaff JE, Yoon HJ, Bell G 1998 Massive bleeding during spine surgery in a patient with ankylosing spondylitis. Canadian Journal of Anaesthesia 45: 903–6.

Tico N, Ramon S, Garcia-Ortun F et al 1998 Traumatic spinal cord injury complicating ankylosing spondylitis. Spinal Cord 36: 349–52.

Trikha A 1996 Removal of extradural catheters. British Journal of Anaesthesia 77: 295.

Weber S 1985 Caudal anaesthesia complicated by intraosseous injection in a patient with ankylosing spondylitis. Anesthesiology 63: 716–17.

Wittmann FW, Ring PA 1986 Anaesthesia in hip replacement in ankylosing spondylitis. Journal of the Royal Society of Medicine 79: 457–9.

Wu CT, Lee ST 1998 Spinal epidural hematoma and ankylosing spondylitis: case report and review of the literature. Journal of Trauma 44: 558–61.

Wulf H 1996 Epidural anaesthesia and spinal haematoma. Canadian Journal of Anaesthesia 43: 1260–71.

Antiphospholipid antibody syndrome (Hughes' syndrome)

This recently described syndrome of hypercoagulability associated with specific antibodies against phospholipids is the most common cause of acquired thrombophilia. It affects young patients, median age 35–45 years, and the main clinical features result from recurrent arterial and venous thromboses. There is a high incidence of pregnancy loss, often in the second trimester, and intrauterine growth retardation (Khamashta & Mackworth-Young 1997).

The disease can be either primary, or secondary to a variety of systemic diseases (Vianna et al 1994). These include SLE, lupus syndrome, and systemic sclerosis. The criteria for diagnosis are based on both clinical features and laboratory tests (Greaves 1999).

The condition encompasses a wide spectrum. At one end, individuals may have antibodies, but without any evidence of disease. At the other end, catastrophic antiphospholipid antibody (APLS) syndrome, the severest form, is associated with a high mortality (Asherson et al 1998). In between, there are a variety of manifestations, which include recurrent fetal loss, with or without thromboembolic phenomena, and valvular disease.

Preoperative abnormalities

1. Presence of antiphospholipid antibodies (APA) (positive IgG or IgM anticardiolipin antibodies or positive lupus anticoagulant tests), prolongation of activated thromboplastin time, and mild thrombocytopenia. However, the mere presence of antibodies is not necessarily associated with a disease process (Devine & Brigden 1996).

2. A history of thromboembolic disease with arterial and venous thromboses in an incidence of 2:1. Strokes, ocular ischaemia, leg ulcers, chorea, and recurrent cerebral ischaemia can occur.

3. There is an increased risk of fetal loss and maternal morbidity during pregnancy. The presence of lupus anticoagulant and anticardiolipin antibodies is associated with slow, progressive thrombosis and infarction in the placenta. The incidence of the antibody varies in different patient populations; normal obstetric patients (5.3%), women with recurrent pregnancy loss (20%), women with SLE (37%), and women undergoing IVF (24%) (Kutteh 1997).

4. Valvular disease occurs in 33–50% of patients with primary APLS and treatment does

not reverse the valvular lesions (Espinola–Zavaleta et al 1999).Verrucous endocarditis, especially of the mitral valve, and intracardiac thrombosis may occur (Ducceschi et al 1995).

5. Livedo reticularis, particularly on thighs, shins, or forearms, occurs in 15–20%.

6. Cerebral involvement and neuropsychiatric disturbances.

7. Catastrophic antiphospholipid syndrome lies at the extreme end of the spectrum and can be life-threatening. In an analysis of 50 patients from the literature, there was a mortality of about 60%. A variety of precipitating factors included surgical procedures, infections, and anticoagulant withdrawal. Death was mainly secondary to cardiac disease, although respiratory failure was often present as well (Asherson et al 1998). A patient with scleroderma presented with digital gangrene and multiorgan failure and died within 19 h (Kane et al 1998).

8. The disease is best controlled using warfarin at high doses, to keep the INR >3.0.

Anaesthetic problems

1. The perioperative course may be complicated, either by thromboses, or by coagulation problems. One 36-year-old female, admitted acutely with a pelvic mass, developed a coagulopathy and ARDS following laparoscopy. Initially, the patient's previous history of thromboses and SLE was not known, because the notes were unavailable and she did not speak English. Subsequent laparotomy led to cardiorespiratory and renal failure, with death at 10 days (Menon & Allt-Graham 1993). A second patient with primary APLS had a pulmonary embolus from a popliteal vein thrombosis on the third day after surgery for stenosis of the common bile duct, despite receiving low dose heparin (Madan et al 1997).

2. Catastrophic APLS (see above) may occasionally be precipitated by surgical procedures (Asherson et al 1998).

3. Obstetric problems. Patients may present for anaesthesia for miscarriages, intrauterine death, or delivery. Budd–Chiari syndrome from complete thrombosis of the right hepatic veins has also been described (Segal et al 1996).Three patients with severe preeclampsia and HELLP syndrome before 20 weeks' gestation, a time at which preeclampsia is rare, were all found to have antiphospholipid antibodies, and two had hepatic infarction (Alsulyman et al 1996). A higher than normal incidence of operative delivery is reported (Ringrose 1997), and decisions have to be made as to whether or not regional anaesthesia can be used safely (Ralph 1999).

4. A high incidence venous thromboses in the peripartum period, and in patients taking oral contraceptives (Krnic-Barrie et al 1997). A retrospective study of 61 patients showed recurrent arterial/venous thromboses in about 50% patients and that warfarin treatment was most effective in preventing it. In a series of 20 parturients with APLS, five had thrombotic episodes, two of whom were receiving sc heparin in addition to aspirin (Ringrose 1997).

5. Difficulty may be experienced in balancing anticoagulant therapy. In a 27-year-old with APLS, warfarin was stopped 2 days before debridement of an ankle ulcer. One day after surgery the patient developed a right hemiparesis and dysarthria. Investigation showed bleeding into a brainstem cavernous haemangioma, which was subsequently resected (Kiyama 1997). Bleeding may be particularly common in elderly patients receiving anticoagulants (Piette & Cacoub 1998).

Management

1. A full systematic history, for evidence of primary disease, or for previous thrombotic events.

2. Clinical examination for signs of cardiovascular disease. In patients with antibodies and arterial thrombosis, especially with cerebral or ocular involvement, echocardiography may be advisable.

3. Haematological assessment and advice. The patient or parturient may need high dose warfarin (INR >3). For surgery, a perioperative heparin infusion should be substituted, followed by a return to warfarin afterwards.

4. A difficult balance exists between prevention of bleeding at surgery and prophylaxis for postoperative thromboses.

5. Keep the patient warm and hydrated intraoperatively.

6. Anticipate a stormy postoperative course.

7. Initial trials on pregnant patients, although not randomised, suggested that subcutaneous heparin and aspirin might reduce fetal loss (Rai et al 1997). Subsequently, this was confirmed, and for recurrent miscarriages associated with the presence of APA, lupus antibodies and anticardiolipin antibodies, low dose aspirin, followed by heparin 5000 u bd when the fetal heart was heard, resulted in a live birth rate of 71% (Backos et al 1999). The addition of intravenous immunoglobulin during pregnancy was reported to increase the live birth rate to 84% (Clark et al 1999). However, in a small (16 women) pilot study of aspirin/low dose heparin/iv immunoglobulin, versus aspirin/low dose heparin/placebo, no statistical difference was found in fetal or maternal outcome between the two groups, although there was a nonsignificant decrease in fetal growth restriction and ITU admission in the iv immune globulin group (Branch et al 2000).

8. For those already anticoagulated. In early pregnancy, warfarin should be changed to heparin and aspirin, and only restarted after labour is completed.

9. Although some authors suggest that regional anaesthesia is contraindicated, this is not necessarily the case, and depends on the treatment being given. Ralph (1999) reported regional anaesthesia in which unfractionated heparin was stopped 4 h in advance and LMWH stopped 12 h in advance. When higher than standard doses are being given, a longer time and blood monitoring may be required. Fahy and

Malinow (1996) stopped heparin, monitored the whole blood heparin concentrations, and sited the epidural once the concentration decreased to zero. Single-shot techniques may be indicated if LMWH needs to be restarted rapidly.

Bibliography

Alsulyman OM, Castro MA, Zuckerman E et al 1996 Preeclampsia and liver infarction in early pregnancy associated with the antiphospholipid syndrome. Obstetrics & Gynecology 88: 644–6.

Asherson RA, Khamashta MA, Ordi Ros J et al 1989 The primary antiphospholipid syndrome: major clinical and serological features. Medicine 68: 366–74.

Asherson RA, Cervera R, Piett J-C et al 1998 Catastrophic antiphospholipid syndrome: clinical and laboratory features of 50 patients. Medicine 77: 195–207.

Backos M, Rai R, Baxter N et al 1999 Pregnancy complications in women with recurrent miscarriage associated with antiphospholipid antibodies treated with low dose aspirin and heparin. British Journal of Obstetrics & Gynaecology 106: 102–7.

Branch DW, Peaceman AM, Druzin M et al 2000 A multicenter, placebo-controlled pilot study of intravenous immune globulin treatment of antiphospholipid syndrome during pregnancy. The Pregnancy Loss Study Group. American Journal of Obstetrics & Gynecology 182: 122–7.

Clark AL, Branch DW, Silver RM et al 1999 Pregnancy complicated by the antiphospholipid syndrome: outcomes with intravenous immunoglobulin therapy. Obstetrics & Gynecology 93: 437–41.

Devine DV, Brigden ML 1996 The antiphospholipid syndrome: when does the presence of antiphospholipid antibodies require therapy? Postgraduate Medicine 99: 105–8.

Ducceschi V, Sarubbi B, Iacono A 1995 Primary antiphospholipid syndrome and cardiovascular disease. European Heart Journal 16: 441–5.

Espinola-Zavaleta N, Vargas-Barron J, Colmenares-Galvis T et al 1999 Echocardiographic evaluation of patients with primary antiphospholipid syndrome. American Heart Journal 137: 973–8.

Fahy BG, Malinow AM 1996 Anesthesia with antiphospholipid antibodies; anesthetic management of a parturient with lupus anticoagulant and anticardiolipin antibodies. Journal of Clinical Anesthesia 8: 49–53.

Greaves M 1999 Antiphospholipid antibodies and thrombosis. Lancet 353: 1348–53.

Kane D, McSweeney F, Swan N et al 1998 Catastrophic antiphospholipid syndrome in primary systemic sclerosis. Journal of Rheumatology 25: 810–12.

Khamashta MA, Mackworth-Young C 1997 Antiphospholipid (Hughes') syndrome. British Medical Journal 314: 253–7.

Khamashta MA, Cuadrado MJ, Mujic F et al 1995 The management of thrombosis in the antiphospholipid-antibody syndrome. New England Journal of Medicine 332: 993–7.

Kiyama S 1997 Antiphospholipid syndrome and neurosurgery. Anaesthesia 52: 612.

Krnic-Barrie S, O'Connor CR, Looney SW et al 1997 A retrospective review of 61 patients with antiphospholipid syndrome. Analysis of factors influencing recurrent thrombosis. Archives of Internal Medicine 157: 2101–8.

Kutteh WH 1997 Antiphospholipid antibodies and reproduction. Journal of Reproductive Immunology 35: 151–71.

Madan R, Khoursheed M, Kukla R et al 1997 The anaesthetist and the antiphospholipid syndrome. Anaesthesia 52: 71–4.

Menon G, Allt-Graham J 1993 Anaesthetic implications of the anticardiolipin syndrome. British Journal of Anaesthesia 70: 587–90.

Piette JC, Cacoub P 1998 Antiphospholipid syndrome in the elderly: caution. Circulation 97: 2196–6.

Rai R, Cohen H, Dave M et al 1997 Randomised controlled trial of aspirin and aspirin plus heparin in pregnant women with recurrent miscarriages associated with phospholipid antibodies (or antiphospholipid antibodies). British Medical Journal 314: 253–7.

Ralph CJ 1999 Anaesthetic management of parturients with antiphospholipid syndrome: a review of 27 cases. International Journal of Obstetric Anesthesia 8: 249–52.

Ringrose DK 1997 Anaesthesia and the antiphospholipid syndrome: a review of 20 obstetric patients. International Journal of Obstetric Anesthesia 6: 107–11.

Segal S, Shenhav S, Segal O et al 1996 Budd–Chiari syndrome complicating severe preeclampsia in a parturient with primary antiphospholipid syndrome. European Journal of Obstetrics, Gynecology, & Reproductive Biology 68: 227–9.

Vianna JL, Khamashta M, Ordi Ros J et al 1994 Comparison of primary and secondary antiphospholipid syndrome. A European multicenter study of 114 patients. American Journal of Medicine 96: 3–9.

Aortic regurgitation (incompetence)

Regurgitation of blood from the aorta into the left ventricle during diastole may result from aortic cusp distortion (rheumatic heart disease), cusp perforation (bacterial endocarditis), or dilatation of the aortic ring (Marfan's syndrome, aortic dissection, connective tissue diseases, etc.).

The volume of blood regurgitated depends on the extent of the incompetence, the aortic/left ventricular pressure gradient during diastole, and the diastolic filling time. The regurgitated volume is added to that entering from the left atrium, so that both left ventricular hypertrophy and dilatation occur. Left ventricular volume overload occurs in a ventricle that is initially distensible, and in some cases the stroke volume may be increased to more than $20 \, l \, min^{-1}$. Later the myocardium becomes stiffer, the LVEDP rises, premature mitral valve closure may occur, and cardiac failure finally supervenes. Symptoms may appear late in the disease, and do not correlate well with the severity of regurgitation, or the degree of myocardial depression. Severe aortic regurgitation carries a poor prognosis with conservative management, with excess mortality and high morbidity (Turina et al 1987, Dujardin et al 1999). Even those with moderate disease have an increased risk. Additional risk factors are an ejection fraction of <55%, and atrial fibrillation (Dujardin et al 1999). Surgery should be considered promptly, both to improve the quality of life and to prevent catastrophe (Cheitlin 1998). Once contractility has decreased, it will remain impaired after valve replacement.

Acute lesions, usually in association with endocarditis (but sometimes associated with aortic dissection, such as in Marfan's, Turner's or Ehlers–Danlos syndrome), may occasionally occur. In these cases of rapid onset, the haemodynamic situation is very different from that in the chronic disease, and many of the signs associated with the chronic lesion are absent. Hence, the presentation and treatment of the two forms is different. Acute severe aortic regurgitation is usually a surgical emergency.

Preoperative abnormalities

1. In chronic aortic regurgitation, symptoms do not correlate well with signs. Initially, reduced exercise tolerance and dyspnoea appear. Later, there are signs of congestive cardiac failure. Chest pain may occur in advanced disease, when diastolic coronary artery flow is impaired and coronary flow may be limited to systole.

2. The signs are a large volume, rapid upstroke, collapsing pulse (high systolic, low diastolic), a precordial left ventricular impulse, and an early diastolic blowing murmur, maximum on expiration, at the left sternal edge. The intensity of the murmur is correlated with the magnitude of the regurgitant fraction and volume (Desjardins et al 1996).

3. Increasing left ventricular hypertrophy and cavity dilatation can lead to gross cardiomegaly on CXR, and increased left ventricular voltages with repolarisation abnormalities on ECG.

4. The left ventricle is initially compliant, with a large stroke volume and a low LVEDP. Finally, when structural myocardial changes take place, the ejection fraction decreases and failure occurs, with signs of increased pulmonary venous pressure, a third heart sound, and pulmonary inspiratory crackles.

5. In acute aortic regurgitation, there is a normal sized left ventricle into which a large regurgitant volume suddenly enters. Acute pulmonary oedema is usually the presenting feature. Forward cardiac output is impaired, organ perfusion reduced, and myocardial ischaemia may occur.

6. In asymptomatic patients, treatment is with long term vasodilators, such as nifedipine (Gaasch et al 1997).

Anaesthetic problems

These largely depend upon the severity of the regurgitation, and the presence or absence of myocardial failure. In mild or moderate regurgitation there are usually no problems. In the severe case, risks may be high. Anaesthesia can acutely disturb compensatory mechanisms. Factors that oppose these compensatory mechanisms may produce pulmonary oedema, reduced forward cardiac output, and myocardial ischaemia.

1. There are significant pathophysiological differences between acute and chronic aortic regurgitation.

In *chronic* disease, compensation is accomplished by hypertrophy and dilatation of the left ventricle, and a reduction in systemic resistance. A tachycardia prevents overdistension of the ventricle in diastole. Initially, the left ventricle is compliant, and left ventricular filling pressures alter relatively little with volume changes. In these cases, systemic vasoconstriction is likely to increase the regurgitant volume.

In *acute* lesions however, the normal-sized left ventricle has only a limited capacity for distension, and life threatening pulmonary oedema occurs early. Indeed, severe, acute disease is a surgical emergency (Carabello & Crawford 1997). Forward cardiac output is impaired and organ perfusion reduced. Compensation for the decrease in stroke volume and cardiac output is in part achieved by systemic vasoconstriction and tachycardia. In such cases, the effect of anaesthetic techniques that produce systemic vasodilatation is potentially disastrous. A death occurred during epidural anaesthesia for Caesarean section, in a patient who presented with previously undiagnosed aortic regurgitation, systolic and diastolic hypertension, and increasing cardiac failure (Alderson 1987). Aortic dissection occurred at 24 weeks' gestation in a patient with Turner syndrome, producing pulmonary oedema secondary to severe aortic regurgitation, and myocardial infarction (Garvey et al 1998). In a pregnant patient with Marfan syndrome, the aortic root diameter increased from 8.1 cm to 8.9 cm at 38 weeks, by which stage she had developed severe aortic regurgitation. She had refused surgery, but accepted beta blockers and epidural analgesia, and survived (Mayet et al 1998).

2. A bradycardia is disadvantageous. It allows overdistension of the ventricles, an increase in left atrial pressure, and pulmonary congestion.

3. Inhalation agents may worsen myocardial depression.

Management

1. Mild or moderate chronic aortic regurgitation requires a careful anaesthetic, avoiding volume depletion, myocardial depression, and bradycardia. Antibiotic prophylaxis should be given. Both regional and general anaesthesia are well tolerated.

2. If there is evidence of decompensation, a detailed cardiological assessment is required. In addition, the differentiation between acute and chronic aortic regurgitation is crucial for the management of the severe case. In either case there may be sensitivity to changes in systemic vascular resistance.

3. Agents that depress myocardial contractility are avoided.

4. Bradycardia is prevented and a fairly fast heart rate maintained. Pancuronium has been suggested as a suitable agent for producing a mild tachycardia.

5. With severe disease, haemodynamic monitoring is essential. This will enable the effects of drug and fluid therapy to be monitored closely. The response to acute events cannot always be predicted. In the case of chronic aortic regurgitation, vasodilators and sometimes inotropic agents, may be required. The use of epidural anaesthesia, or a drug with mild alpha adrenoceptor blocking effects, such as droperidol, has been recommended to reduce afterload. However, adequate preload must first be achieved. In acute aortic regurgitation, however, techniques that produce an uncontrolled decrease in systemic vascular resistance must be avoided.

6. Catastrophic pulmonary oedema requires intensive therapy. A dilating inotrope such as dobutamine, a reduction of left atrial pressure with diuretics, and vasodilators such as glyceryl trinitrate or nitroprusside, and IPPV, may all be required (Stone et al 1980). Depending on the cause, urgent surgery may be needed.

Bibliography

Alderson JD 1987 Cardiovascular collapse following epidural anaesthesia for Caesarean section in a patient with aortic incompetence. Anaesthesia 42: 643–5.

Carabello BA, Crawford FA 1997 Valvular heart disease. New England Journal of Medicine 337: 32–41.

Cheitlin MD 1998 Finding 'just the right moment' for operative intervention in the asymptomatic patient with moderate to severe aortic regurgitation. Circulation 97: 518–20.

Desjardins VA, Enriquez-Sarano M, Tajik AJ et al 1996 Intensity of murmurs correlates with severity of valvular regurgitation. American Journal of Medicine 100: 149–56.

Dujardin KS, Enriquez-Sarano M, Schaff HV et al 1999 Mortality and morbidity of aortic regurgitation in clinical practice. A long term follow-up study. Circulation 99: 1851–7.

Gaasch WH, Sundaram M, Meyer TE 1997 Managing asymptomatic patients with chronic aortic regurgitation. Chest 111: 1702–9.

Garvey P, Elovitz M, Landsberger EJ 1998 Aortic dissection and myocardial infarction in a pregnant patient with Turner syndrome. Obstetrics & Gynecology 91: 864.

Lazar JM, Scott WC 1996 An unusual case of aortic insufficiency. Journal of Cardiothoracic & Vascular Anesthesia 10: 963–4.

Mayet J, Steer P, Somerville J 1998 Marfan syndrome, aortic dilatation, and pregnancy. Obstetrics & Gynecology 92: 713.

Sheikh F, Rangwala S, DeSimone C et al 1995 Management of the parturient with severe aortic incompetence. Journal of Cardiothoracic & Vascular Anesthesia 9: 575–7.

Stone JG, Hoar PF, Calabro JR et al 1980 Afterload reduction and preload augmentation improve the anaesthetic management of patients with cardiac failure and valvular regurgitation. Anesthesia & Analgesia 59: 737–42.

Turina J, Hess O, Sepulchri F et al 1987 Spontaneous course of aortic valve disease. European Heart Journal 8: 471–83.

Aortic stenosis (see also William's syndrome)

Aortic stenosis may be valvular, subaortic, or supravalvular. The normal area of the valve is $3 \, cm^2$. Symptoms and signs appear when the area is reduced to about $0.8 \, cm^2$. The long term prognosis depends upon the degree of stenosis; $\leq 0.7 \, cm^2$ is classified as severe, $0.8–1.5 \, cm^2$ moderate, and $>1.5 \, cm^2$ mild. Acquired disease results from degeneration and calcification of the valve leaflets, and is more likely to occur in congenitally bicuspid valves (Carabello & Crawford 1997). Unlike hypertension, in which the resistance to left ventricular function is variable, and depends upon the state of the systemic vasculature, the resistance to ejection of blood by the left ventricle in aortic stenosis is fixed. A pressure gradient across the valve of >50 mmHg is considered severe, and <20 mmHg mild. These gradients are increased by tachycardia and exercise. In order to overcome the obstruction, left ventricular hypertrophy occurs and this is associated with a loss of compliance, and without an increase in cavity size. Stroke volume is therefore limited. Ventricular dilatation occurs only in the late stages, or when the valve becomes incompetent.

The dangerous feature of this condition is that signs and symptoms appear late in the disease. Once symptoms occur, the prognosis is poor. However, even those with moderate disease are at risk, and those with valve areas from $0.7–1.2 \, cm^2$ are at significant risk of developing complications, particularly if there is a subnormal ejection fraction (Kennedy et al 1991). In a study of the natural history of aortic stenosis, 21% (66 patients) in the moderate group died in the short term from causes attributed to aortic stenosis (Kennedy et al 1991). In another longitudinal study, half of a group of patients with initially mild to moderate stenosis showed a progression of greater than, or equal to, 10 mmHg per year (Peter et al 1993). This group represented older patients, and in such patients, coronary artery disease may contribute to symptoms and cardiac dysfunction. Supravalvular stenosis is associated with William's syndrome (Larson & Warner 1989).

In the past, in patients with moderate to severe aortic stenosis, surgery and pregnancy were associated with considerable morbidity and mortality. With modern monitoring and anaesthesia, the risks of noncardiac surgery and parturition have decreased (Lao et al 1993, Raymer & Yang 1998). Traditionally, regional anaesthesia was said to be contraindicated, but in the presence of invasive monitoring, combined with techniques that allow gradual induction of regional blocks, some anaesthetists believe that this view should be modified.

Once symptoms develop, usually at a gradient of 50 mmHg (area $<0.8 \, cm^2$), surgery becomes urgent. In some units minimally invasive aortic surgery is being undertaken (Hearn et al 1996).

Preoperative abnormalities

1. The onset of symptoms occurs relatively late in the disease and includes dyspnoea, intolerance of exercise, angina, and syncope. LVEDP is increased and the occurrence of pulmonary oedema on exertion may be the first sign of decompensation. Even in haemodynamically severe disease, patients may be asymptomatic, or only mildly symptomatic.

2. The pulse is slow rising and of decreased amplitude. A pulse pressure of <30 mmHg reflects severe disease. Conversely, if the systolic blood pressure is >180 mmHg, the disease is not significant.

3. An ejection systolic murmur, maximal at the base and radiating into the right side of the neck. The intensity of the murmur correlates well with the Doppler aortic jet velocity (Munt et al 1999), although echocardiography is still needed to reliably exclude severe obstruction.

4. Chest X-ray initially shows normal cardiac size. Left atrial enlargement and dilatation of the aortic root may be seen later.

5. In the presence of significant stenosis, the ECG usually shows left ventricular hypertrophy, but not always. The diagnosis should be considered in elderly patients with LVF. In cardiac failure, when the output is low, the murmur is soft or absent.

6. Sudden death may occur.

7. The diagnosis and valve areas can be assessed rapidly by echocardiography, and Doppler studies give the transvalvular pressure gradients.

8. In severe aortic stenosis, pregnancy may be associated with decompensation of the disease, and occasionally death.

Anaesthetic problems

Significant aortic stenosis (a systolic ejection murmur of at least grade II–VI) in patients more than 40 years old was identified as a risk factor for life threatening and fatal cardiac complications in noncardiac surgical procedures (Goldman & Caldera 1977). However, more recent analyses suggest that the risks have improved with modern monitoring, drugs, and management techniques (Raymer & Yang 1998). In symptomatic aortic stenosis, a number of factors will alter the haemodynamic state and disturb compensatory mechanisms. One or more of the following problems may result:

1. Myocardial ischaemia. The hypertrophied myocardium is vulnerable to ischaemia. Tachycardia reduces the time available for coronary filling, and hypotension or hypovolaemia may produce myocardial ischaemia. At low heart rates, there is an inability to increase stroke volume.

2. Decreases in cardiac output or cardiovascular collapse. These can be precipitated by hypovolaemia, myocardial depressants, bradycardias, systemic vasodilatation, and atrial arrhythmias.

3. Pulmonary oedema. Interference with atrial function by arrhythmias or fluid overload causes cardiac decompensation.

4. Decreased cerebral blood flow.

5. Resuscitation from a state of asystole is extremely difficult. Following asystolic cardiac arrest, the prognosis is poor.

6. During pregnancy, cardiac failure may be precipitated by the physiological increase in blood volume. Angina, secondary to myocardial ischaemia, occurred during uterine contractions in a patient with a valve area of $0.7\,cm^2$ (Colclough et al 1995). Pregnancy has previously been discouraged because of decompensation and a high maternal mortality. However, a recent summary of the available literature on congenital aortic stenosis showed a maternal mortality of 11% (Lao et al 1993), which is significantly less than that previously quoted.

Management

Management of the symptomatic patient requires careful monitoring with the insertion of an arterial line and CVP. Some authors recommend PAP in addition. All anaesthetic drugs must be given with caution, and therapeutic manoeuvres, such as fluid loading and treatment of adverse heart rates, must be performed with particular care, to avoid wide swings in cardiovascular pressures and myocardial oxygen supply. There is division between those who recommend general anaesthesia and those who feel that a careful regional block is not contraindicated, provided invasive monitoring is used. For Caesarean section, the proponents of each technique produce convincing arguments in sequential editorials (Brighouse 1998, Whitfield & Holdcroft 1998).

1. If the condition is symptomatic, echocardiography should be performed and cardiological advice obtained. Aortic valve replacement or a balloon valvuloplasty may be more important than the proposed surgery. In

young patients, particularly those with congenital aortic stenosis, balloon valvuloplasty may be preferable because it delays the necessity for long-term anticoagulation (Hall & Kirk 1992). In older patients, any improvement produced by valvuloplasty is usually short lived and the complication rates, in particular the incidence of aortic regurgitation, are high.

2. Control of heart rate. Slow rhythms are treated with atropine, and atrial arrhythmias are prevented. Atrial fibrillation with decompensation may be an indication for cardioversion.

3. Prevention of hypotension. Whatever technique is used, the induction of anaesthesia, or establishment of a regional block, must be gradual. High concentrations of myocardial depressants, such as halothane and enflurane, are avoided, and the vascular volume maintained. The exact method of anaesthesia is probably less important than the care with which it is administered and the patient monitored. A Swan–Ganz catheter has been used to monitor absorption of irrigating fluid (Toft & Knudsen 1991). In the presence of severe outflow obstruction, a regional technique is probably less controllable than a general anaesthetic. However, opinions vary. Continuous spinal anaesthesia with invasive haemodynamic monitoring has been described in two patients for hip replacement (Collard et al 1995). Spinal anaesthesia with sufentanil alone, and without invasive monitoring, was reported in three patients for ESWL (Eaton 1998).

4. Precordial ECG lead is observed for evidence of myocardial ischaemia.

5. Prophylaxis against bacterial endocarditis.

6. Should cardiac arrest occur, effective cardiac massage can only be obtained after opening the chest.

7. Pregnant patients should be seen and assessed early, initially to decide about continuation of pregnancy, since, in severe disease, termination may be the safest option. Echocardiographic estimations of aortic valve

area are more reliable than gradients during pregnancy (Hustead et al 1989), and Doppler flow velocity should increase during pregnancy if the ventricle is coping. Oakley (1997) suggests that previously asymptomatic women, with a normal ECG, good ventricular function and satisfactory treadmill testing, should have no problems. Danger signs are tachycardia, dyspnoea, angina or a decrease in Doppler velocity, any of which warrant hospital admission and treatment with beta blockers. Balloon valvuloplasty may buy time, although regurgitation is a risk. Management plans should be documented, dated and, when necessary, revised. The conduct of labour is controversial. A variety of techniques have been recommended for Caesarean section. These include general anaesthesia (Oakley 1997), continuous spinal anesthesia using a microcatheter technique (Pittard & Vucevic 1998), epidural anaesthesia, with full invasive monitoring and fractional doses of lidocaine (lignocaine) (Brian et al 1993), and epidural anaesthesia using sufentanil (Colclough et al 1995).

8. If pressors are required, phenylephrine may be better than ephedrine (Goertz et al 1994). Inotropes may be needed.

Bibliography

Brian JE, Seifen AB, Clark RB et al 1993 Aortic stenosis, cesarean section, and epidural anesthesia. Journal of Clinical Anesthesia 5: 154–7.

Brighouse D 1998 Anaesthesia for Caesarean section in patients with aortic stenosis: the case for regional anaesthesia. Anaesthesia 53: 107–8.

Carabello BA, Crawford FA 1997 Valvular heart disease. New England Journal of Medicine 337: 32–41.

Colclough GW, Ackerman WE, Walmsley PM et al 1995 Epidural anesthesia for a parturient with critical aortic stenosis. Journal of Clinical Anesthesia 7: 264–5.

Collard C, Eappen S, Lynch E et al 1995 Continuous spinal anesthesia with invasive hemodynamic monitoring for surgical repair of the hip in two patients with aortic stenosis. Anesthesia & Analgesia 81: 195–8.

Eaton MP 1998 Intrathecal sufentanil analgesia for extracorporeal shock wave lithotripsy in three patients with aortic stenosis. Anesthesia & Analgesia 86: 943–4.

Goertz AW, Lindner KH, Schutz W et al 1994 Influence of phenylephrine bolus administration of left ventricular filling dynamics in patients with coronary artery disease and patients with valvular aortic stenosis. Anesthesiology 81: 49–58.

Goldman L, Caldera DL 1977 Multifactorial index of cardiac risk in non cardiac surgical procedures. New England Journal of Medicine 297: 845–50.

Hall R, Kirk R 1992 Balloon dilatation of heart valves. British Medical Journal 305: 487–8.

Hearn CJ, Kraenzler EJ, Wallace LK et al 1996 Minimally invasive aortic valve surgery: anesthetic considerations. Anesthesia & Analgesia 83: 1342–4.

Hustead ST, Quick A, Gibbs HR et al 1989 'Pseudocritical' aortic stenosis during pregnancy: role for Doppler assessment of aortic valve area. American Heart Journal 117: 1383–5.

Kennedy KD, Nishimura RA, Holmes DR et al 1991 Natural history of moderate aortic stenosis. Journal of the American College of Cardiology 17: 313–19.

Lao TT, Sermer M, MaGee L et al 1993 Congenital aortic stenosis and pregnancy—a reappraisal. American Journal of Obstetrics & Gynecology 169: 540–5.

Larson JS, Warner MA 1989 Williams syndrome: an uncommon cause of supravalvular aortic stenosis in a child. Journal of Cardiovascular Anesthesia 3: 337–40.

Munt B, Legget ME, Kraft CD et al 1999 Physical examination in valvular aortic stenosis: correlation with stenosis severity and prediction of clinical outcome. American Heart Journal 137: 298–306.

Oakley CM 1997 Pregnancy and congenital heart disease. Heart 78: 12–14.

Peter M, Hoffman A, Parker C et al 1993 Progression of aortic stenosis. Role of age and concomitant coronary artery disease. Chest 103: 1715–19.

Pittard A, Vucevic M 1998 Regional anaesthesia with subarachnoid microcatheter for Caesarean section in a parturient with aortic stenosis. Anaesthesia 53: 169–73.

Raymer K, Yang H 1998 Patients with aortic stenosis: cardiac complications in non-cardiac surgery. Canadian Journal of Anaesthesia 45: 855–9.

Toft P, Knudsen F 1991 [Prevention of the TURP syndrome by using the Swan–Ganz catheter in a patient with severe aortic stenosis. English abstract.] Ugeskr-Laeger 153: 3487–94.

Whitfield A, Holdcroft A 1998 Anaesthesia for Caesarean section in patients with aortic stenosis:
the case for general anaesthesia. Anaesthesia 53: 109–12.

Arnold–Chiari (and other Chiari) malformations

The Chiari malformation is a term encompassing a range of hindbrain maldevelopments. Problems include underdevelopment of the cranial fossa and overcrowding of normally developed hindbrain, the risks of descent of hindbrain structures below the foramen magnum and intermittent obstruction to CSF outflow from the fourth ventricle. There may be a relatively high CSF pressure in the head, and a relatively lower one in the spine. Arnold–Chiari actually refers to type 2 malformations, and in this type a myelomeningocoele (and sometimes syringomyelia) is present.

Preoperative abnormalities

1. There are four types.

    Type 1, downward herniation of cerebellar tonsils of at least 3–5 mm below the foramen magnum. A study of posterior cranial fossa and CSF volumes showed them to be reduced compared with normal patients, and hindbrain overcrowding results in direct compression of tissue (Milhorat et al 1999). Clinical symptoms thus relate to CSF disturbances and direct compression of nervous tissue; they include headaches, pseudotumour-like episodes, a syndrome resembling Menieres disease, lower cranial nerve signs and spinal cord disturbances without syringomyelia. It is mostly seen in young adults.

    Type 2 (Arnold–Chiari) is the most important and includes; thoracolumbar myelomeningocoele, hypoplasia of posterior fossa, and displacement of cerebellar vermis, brainstem and fourth ventricle. It presents in infancy or early childhood.

Type 3, dilated fourth ventricle with cervical meningomyelocoele.

Type 4, cerebellar hypoplasia.

Types 3 and 4 are rare.

2. May be associated with syringomyelia or syringobulbia, other skeletal abnormalities of skull base and cervical vertebrae, or myelomeningocoele. Syringomyelia is the term for an expanding, longitudinal cystic cavity within the spinal cord. In the communicating variety, there is continuity between the syrinx and the CSF in the central canal.

3. May need decompression of foramen magnum or cervical spine.

4. Progressive hydrocephalus may occur which needs shunt surgery.

5. Obstructive sleep apnoea (Doherty et al 1995).

6. Patients may present with respiratory arrest. Two adults with sudden respiratory arrest were found on MRI to have Chiari type 1 malformations (Omer et al 1996).

7. Sudden unexpected death may occur. A 27 year old presented to the emergency room with headache for which he was given a variety of sedatives and analgesics; 4 h later he was drowsy, and at 5 h he developed pulmonary oedema, VF and died. Postmortem showed severe cerebral oedema and herniation of the cerebellar tonsils (Rocker et al 1995). Two fatal cases of unexpected respiratory arrest occurred in two children with previously undiagnosed Chiari type 1 malformation (Martinot et al 1995).

8. Recurrent pulmonary aspiration (Nathadwarawala et al 1992).

9. May exhibit abnormal autonomic control.

Anaesthetic problems

1. Increased ICP may lead to coning. A 17 year old with spina bifida aperta coned and died after sevoflurane induction and anaesthesia for cystoscopy. She had had a VP shunt in infancy and at postmortem the CSF was under high pressure, there was an Arnold–Chiari malformation, the posterior cranial fossa was small, and the brain had herniated through a large foramen magnum. The ventricular end of the shunt was outside the brain tissue and there was no pumping chamber. Despite the nonfunctioning shunt she was apparently asymptomatic (Radhakrishna 2000).

2. Symptoms may start after dural puncture. In one patient, recurrent postdural puncture headaches occurred after spinal anaesthesia for Caesarean section (Hullander et al 1992). In another, signs and symptoms began after diagnostic lumbar puncture (Barton & Sharpe 1993).

3. Bolus injections into the epidural space may lead to ICP increases in susceptible individuals (Hilt & Gramm 1986).

4. Sleep apnoea may occur in Chiari type 1. Bilateral abductor vocal cord paralysis and sleep apnoea developed suddenly following general anaesthesia in a 13-year-old boy. Further investigation showed Chiari type 1 with syringomyelia (Ruff et al 1987).

5. Acute cardiovascular collapse secondary to inadvertent brainstem compression in an infant (Tanaka et al 1997).

6. A 33-year-old pregnant woman with a history of Chiari type 1, who had undergone a cadaver dural graft 5 years before, developed a rapidly progressive brain disorder. She died 18 months later and postmortem showed a spongiform encephalopathy. Her child was unaffected (Lane et al 1994).

Management

1. A careful history should be taken in a patient with a ventriculoperitoneal shunt, to check for any signs that it is nonfunctioning. If there is doubt, referral to a neurosurgeon is indicated. This is particularly important if the

notes are absent, there is a poor history, or lack of follow-up (Radhakrishna 2000).

2. Try to prevent anything that is likely to increase ICP, such as coughing, or hypercarbia from heavy sedation or analgesia (Rocker et al 1995).

3. Avoid straining in labour. Epidural anaesthesia for Caesarean section was performed in a patient with type 1 Chiari who had a previous difficult tracheal intubation (Semple et al 1996), and in another who had refused foramen magnum decompression for symptomatic Chiari type 1 malformation and syringomyelia (Nel et al 1998). Small doses of local anaesthetic should be titrated gradually, to avoid sudden decreases in arterial pressure or distension of the epidural space.

4. Spinal anaesthesia should be avoided.

Bibliography

Barton JJS, Sharpe JA 1993 Oscillopsia and horizontal nystagmus with accelerating slow phases following lumbar puncture in the Arnold–Chiari malformation. Annals of Neurology 33: 418–21.

Doherty MJ, Spence DP, Young C et al 1995 Obstructive sleep apnoea with Arnold–Chiari malformation. Thorax 50: 690–1.

Hilt H, Gramm H-J 1986 Changes in intracranial pressure associated with extradural anaesthesia. British Journal of Anaesthesia 58: 676–80.

Hullander RM, Bogard TD, Lievers D et al 1992 Chiari 1 malformation presenting as recurrent spinal headache. Anesthesia & Analgesia 75: 1025–6.

Lane KL, Brown P, Howells DN et al 1994 Creutzfeldt–Jakob disease in a pregnant woman with an implanted dura mater graft. Neurosurgery 34: 737–9.

Martinot A, Hue V, Leclerc F et al 1995 Sudden death revealing Chiari type 1 malformation in two children. Intensive Care Medicine 19: 73–4.

Milhorat TH, Chou MW, Trinidad EM et al 1999 Chiari I malformation redefined: clinical and radiographic findings for 364 symptomatic patients. Neurosurgery 44: 1005–17.

Nathadwarawala KM, Richards CA, Lawrie B et al 1992 Recurrent aspiration due to Arnold–Chiari type 1 malformation. British Medical Journal 304: 565–6.

Nel MR, Robson V, Robinson PN 1998 Extradural anaesthesia for Caesarean section in a patient with syringomyelia and Chiari type I anomaly. British Journal of Anaesthesia 80: 512–15.

Omer S, al-Kawi MZ, Bohlega S et al 1996 Respiratory arrest: a complication of Arnold–Chiari malformation in adults. European Neurology 36: 36–8.

Radhakrishna S 2000 Coning in a patient with spina bifida following general anaesthesia for cystoscopy. Anaesthesia 55: 295–6.

Rocker GM, MacAulay MA, Sangalang V 1995 Sudden deaths and Chiari malformations. Intensive Care Medicine 21: 621.

Ruff ME, Oakes WJ, Fisher SR et al 1987 Sleep apnea and vocal cord paralysis secondary to type 1 Chiari malformation. Pediatrics 80: 231–4.

Semple DA, McClure JH, Wallace EM 1996 Arnold–Chiari malformation in pregnancy. Anaesthesia 51: 580–2.

Tanaka M, Harukuni I, Naito H 1997 Intraoperative cardiovascular collapse in an infant with Arnold–Chiari malformation. Paediatric Anaesthesia 7: 163–6.

Arthrogryposis multiplex congenita (AMC)

Not a distinct entity, but rather a symptom complex, in which there is congenital but nonprogressive stiffness and deformity of joints, most probably associated with immobility of limbs in utero. More than 150 conditions are known to have congenital contractures (Steinberg et al 1996). The primary cause may be neurogenic, myopathic, an abnormality of joints or connective tissue, or restrictive, secondary to oligohydramnios. In a pathological study of 21 fatal cases, 11 were myogenic (10 congenital muscular dystrophy) in origin (Quinn et al 1991). One case occurred after the mother had received tubocurarine in the tenth week of pregnancy for the treatment of tetanus. It is suggested that those cases of neurogenic origin may be associated with degeneration of anterior horn cell columns. Those in the neurogenic group have a number of congenital abnormalities in association. Infants at birth who are ventilator dependent have a poor prognosis, unless myasthenia gravis is the basis of the arthrogryposis. Birth fractures are common (Thompson & Bilenker 1985), and patients may present for orthopaedic, ENT, and oral surgical procedures.

Preoperative abnormalities

1. The joint rigidity is fibrous, not bony, and most marked in distal joints. Frequently the arms are rotated internally and the hips externally, sometimes with dislocation. Talipes and flexion deformities of the wrists are common. Both contractures and muscle atrophy occur secondary to immobility. Although the postural deformities are similar, the underlying lesion, and hence the individual prognoses, are very different.

2. The face is expressionless, with drooling of saliva. More than 20% have involvement of the craniomaxillofacial area (Steinberg et al 1996). Problems include micrognathia, cleft or high arched palate, temporomandibular joint involvement, and trismus.

3. A number of other congenital abnormalities, including those of the cardiovascular, respiratory, nervous and genitourinary systems, have been reported.

4. About 20% of patients have ENT complications (Cohen & Isaacs 1976). It has been postulated that the primary CNS pathology results in dysfunction of the tongue, palate, pharynx, and larynx. Dysphagia, aspiration, and airway obstruction may occur.

5. EMG and muscle biopsy will distinguish neuropathic from myopathic and dystrophic conditions, and also from the congenital fibre type disproportion.

Anaesthetic problems

1. Patients are prone to recurrent aspiration pneumonitis (Laureano & Rybak 1990) secondary to dysphagia and poor control of pharyngeal and laryngeal reflexes. An 18-month-old child was managed with a propofol infusion at 6 mg kg^{-1} h^{-1} on a laryngeal mask airway for an 5-h orthopaedic operation. Postoperatively she developed hypoxia and a severe metabolic acidosis and needed IPPV. CXR was consistent with acute lung injury and pulmonary aspiration of gastric contents (Mehta et al 1999). Muscle biopsy suggested a possible mitochondrial respiratory chain deficiency and the question of an idiosyncratic reaction to propofol was raised. However, the possibility that pulmonary aspiration could have been the major contributory factor was not mentioned.

2. Severe deformities may cause difficulties in tracheal intubation. Temporomandibular joint involvement (Heffez et al 1985), micrognathia, high arched palate, and trismus have been reported.

3. Difficult venous access.

4. Hypermetabolic responses to anaesthesia have occurred. As a result of this, some authors suggested that AMC was associated with an increased incidence of MH, but the evidence has been largely anecdotal. In only one case were the MH criteria convincing (Baudendistel et al 1984). The likelihood of this association was also challenged in a review of 67 patients with arthrogryposis who had undergone a total of 398 anaesthetics (Baines et al 1986). No evidence could be found that an MH episode had occurred in any of them, although the temperature was not always recorded. A 7-year-old child developed a pyrexia of 38.5°C on sevoflurane, but no hypercapnoea (Kanaya et al 1996). Hopkins et al (1991) reported two cases of hypermetabolic reactions in AMC that were distinct from MH and independent of the anaesthetic agents used. However, they did observe that it could be possible for two rare conditions such as AMC and MH to be present coincidentally in the same patient. Intraoperative convulsions occurred in a 15-month-old infant, but without pyrexia (Ferris 1997).

5. Regional anaesthetics may be technically difficult.

6. Rarely, pregnancy has been reported. Quance (1988) described the management of Caesarean section in which failed epidural

anaesthesia was followed by moderate difficulty in tracheal intubation.

Management

1. Elucidation of the cause of the condition may be helpful, if only for the future resolution of anaesthetic risk factors. Conduction studies and EMG may assist in this.

2. If dysphagia and recurrent aspiration pneumonitis are features, gastrostomy and tracheostomy may be required (Cohen & Isaacs 1976).

3. If there are maxillofacial abnormalities, the possibility of difficult tracheal intubation should be borne in mind and appropriate precautions taken. An adaptation of a paediatric mask is described, with a side port to maintain anaesthesia, and a rubber cap through which to perform fibreoptic intubation (Kitamura et al 1999). This was successfully used for an 11 month old with AMC who was known to be difficult to intubate.

4. During general anaesthesia the patient should be observed and specifically monitored for signs of a hypermetabolic response. Should this occur, it will respond to active cooling (Hopkins et al 1991). Since the risk of MH is unproven, it is suggested that the use of volatile agents in these patients is justified, particularly if alternative agents may place the child at an even greater risk (Baines et al 1986). The only exception might be those in whom the AMC is secondary to a myopathy. A child with an arthrogryposis of myopathic origin requiring a pyelolithotomy, and whose CK was 880 iu l^{-1}, had an uneventful anaesthetic when ketamine and pancuronium were used (Oberoi et al 1987).

5. Regional techniques may be successful, despite problems having been encountered. Standl and Wappler (1996) inserted a caudal catheter for intra- and postoperative analgesia during extensive orthopaedic surgery. Rozkowski et al (1996) described continuous spinal bupivacaine through a 22-G catheter for

Caesarean section. They found that the vertebrae did not coincide with the anatomical midline.

Bibliography

Baines DB, Douglas ID, Overton JH 1986 Anaesthesia for patients with arthrogryposis multiplex congenita. What is the risk of malignant hyperpyrexia? Anaesthesia & Intensive Care 14: 370–2.

Baudendistel L, Goudsouzian N, Cote C et al 1984 End-tidal CO_2 monitoring. Its use in the diagnosis and management of malignant hyperthermia. Anaesthesia 39: 1000–3.

Cohen SR, Isaacs H 1976 Otolaryngological manifestations of arthrogryposis multiplex congenita. Annals of Otology, Rhinology & Laryngology 85: 484–90.

Ferris PE 1997 Intraoperative convulsions in a child with arthrogryposis. Anaesthesia & Intensive Care 25: 546–9.

Heffez L, Doku HC, O'Donnell JP 1985 Arthrogryposis multiplex congenita involving the temporomandibular joint. Journal of Oral & Maxillofacial Surgery 43: 539–42.

Hopkins PM, Ellis FR, Halsall PJ 1991 Hypermetabolism in arthrogryposis multiplex congenita. Anaesthesia 46: 374–5.

Kanaya N, Nakayama M, Nakae Y et al 1996 Hyperthermia during sevoflurane anaesthesia in arthrogryposis multiplex congenita with central nervous system dysfunction. Paediatric Anaesthesia 6: 428–9.

Kitamura S, Fukumitsu K, Kinouchi K et al 1999 A new modification of anaesthesia mask for fibreoptic intubation. Paediatric Anaesthesia 9: 119–22.

Laureano AN, Rybak LP 1990 Severe otolaryngologic manifestations of arthrogryposis multiplex congenita. Annals of Otology, Rhinology & Laryngology 99: 94–7.

Mehta N, DeMunter C, Habibi P et al 1999 Short-term propofol infusion. Lancet 354: 866–7.

Oberoi GS, Kaul HL, Gill IS et al 1987 Anaesthesia in arthrogryposis multiplex congenita: case report. Canadian Journal of Anaesthesia 34: 288–90.

Quance DR 1988 Anaesthetic management of an obstetrical patient with arthrogryposis multiplex congenita. Canadian Journal of Anaesthesia 35: 612–14.

Quinn CM, Wigglesworth JS, Heckmatt J 1991 Lethal arthrogryposis multiplex congenita: a pathological study of 21 cases. Histopathology 19: 155–62.

Rozkowski A, Smyczek D, Birnbach DJ 1996
Continuous spinal anesthesia for cesarean delivery
in a patient with arthrogryposis multiplex.
Regional Anesthesia 21: 477–9.

Standl T, Wappler F 1996 [Arthrogryposis multiplex
congenita: special anesthesiological aspects.
German.] Anasthesiologie, Intensivmedizin,
Notfellmedizin, Schmertherapie 31: 53–7.

Steinberg B, Nelson VS, Feinberg SE et al 1996
Incidence of maxillofacial involvement in
arthrogryposis multiplex congenita. Journal of Oral
& Maxillofacial Surgery 54: 956–9.

Thompson GH, Bilenker RM 1985 Comprehensive
management of arthrogryposis multiplex congenita.
Clinical Orthopedics 194: 6–14.

Asthma

A condition of hyperreactivity of the tracheobronchial tree, in which a number of exogenous and endogenous stimuli can produce reversible airway obstruction. Histamine and the leukotrienes (LT) are thought to be the most active chemical mediators, whilst acetylcholine may contribute via a disturbance in autonomic balance. As obstruction worsens, increasingly smaller airways are affected. Expiration is prolonged, residual volume and functional residual capacity are increased, whilst vital capacity, inspiratory capacity and expiratory reserve volume are reduced. Widespread ventilation perfusion inequalities may occur to produce hypoxia, at a time when the work of breathing is considerably increased. In addition to bronchospasm, the pathological changes include oedema of the bronchial mucosa, secretion of mucus, and epithelial desquamation.

The leukotrienes, which are arachidonic acid derivatives, are proinflammatory agents with actions that include airway smooth muscle contraction and bronchoconstriction, increased mucus secretion and inflammatory cell infiltrates, increased vascular permeability and oedema formation. Leukotriene antagonists have recently been introduced. They reduce the requirement for beta agonists and steroids, but their place in the overall management of asthma has yet to be defined (Drazen 1998, Drazen et al 1999).

New asthma guidelines have been produced to be read in conjunction with the 1993 guidelines (Guidelines for the Management of Asthma 1997, Keeley & Rees 1997). Available drugs are ranked in a series of steps (1–5), and 16% asthmatics are on step 3 (which is the most controversial area), or above (Tattersfield & Harrison 1999).

Preoperative abnormalities

1. There may be a history of wheezing, dyspnoea, cough, and sputum production. The chest may be hyperresonant and the breath sounds diminished, with prolonged expiration and an audible wheeze. In very severe cases the wheeze disappears.

2. Therapy in asthma can be aimed at blocking airway reflexes, relaxing smooth muscle, inhibiting the release of inflammatory mediators, and increasing beta adrenoceptor tone. An increasing appreciation of the role of the inflammatory component led to a change of emphasis in drug therapy for long term treatment (Barnes 1989, Guidelines for the Management of Asthma in Adults 1990, Guidelines for the Management of Asthma 1997). Bronchodilators are primarily indicated for short term relief of bronchospasm, acute asthma attacks, and the prevention of exercise-induced asthma. The main bronchodilators are, in decreasing order of effectiveness, $beta_2$ adrenoceptor agonists, theophylline derivatives, and anticholinergics. For the chronic state, emphasis is now placed on the early introduction of regular inhaled anti-inflammatory drugs such as corticosteroids (beclometasone dipropionate or budesonide), sodium cromoglycate, and nedocromil sodium. Since their onset of action is slow, long term therapy is required. The use of the aerosol form of bronchoactive drugs reduces systemic side effects. In addition, bronchodilators given by inhalation act more rapidly than oral ones, and equally as fast as intravenous preparations. The recently introduced

leukotriene receptor antagonists may replace inhaled steroids.

3. Chest X-ray may show an increase in bronchovascular markings and hyperinflation, and in the later stages, some degree of emphysema. In an acute asthma attack, a CXR is essential to exclude pneumothorax.

4. An FEV_1 of less than 1 litre, or an FEV_1/VC ratio of less than 40% and an increased $Paco_2$, may all indicate the need for postoperative IPPV. A PEFR of less than $120 \, l \, min^{-1}$ and an MVV of less than 50% of the predicted level also indicate severe obstruction.

5. There may be an improvement in pulmonary function tests and blood gases after administration of bronchodilators.

6. Studies of near fatal episodes of asthma on arrival in hospital suggest that they were secondary to asphyxia as a consequence of undertreatment, rather than overtreatment, of asthma by beta adrenoceptor agonists, as had been previously suggested (Molfino et al 1991).

7. Treatment is with inhaled short-acting beta agonists, long-acting beta agonists (salmeterol), or inhaled anti-inflammatory agents (beclometasone, budesonide, fluticasone, cromoglycate or nedocromil). The recent introduction of leukotriene antagonists, montelukast, pranlukast and zafirlukast (Drazen et al 1999), may decrease the need for rescue therapy with beta adrenoceptor agonist drugs and corticosteroids.

Anaesthetic problems

1. The inflammatory component is particularly significant for the patient needing anaesthesia (Hirshman & Bergman 1990). The effect of reflex increases in airway tone depends upon the initial calibre of the airway. If inflammation causing mucosal oedema and secretion of mucus is present, then reflex bronchospasm may have profound effects on airway resistance. An apparently asymptomatic patient who has inflamed airways may thus develop complete airway closure after tracheal intubation, despite having had no audible wheeze on preoperative examination.

2. There is an increased sensitivity to airway manipulations during light anaesthesia. Kim and Bishop (1999) showed that reversible bronchoconstriction occurs with tracheal tube insertion, but not with a laryngeal mask airway. Tracheal intubation may precipitate acute bronchospasm. In a computer-aided incidence study of 136 929 anaesthetics, it was found that bronchospasm was usually triggered by mechanical stimuli (Olsson 1987).

3. Cardiac arrhythmias can occur more frequently in the presence of hypoxia and acidosis, or following the overuse of sympathomimetic agents. Sudden spontaneous deaths in asthmatics have been attributed to the combination of nebulised high dose $beta_2$ sympathomimetics and long-acting theophylline derivatives, although doubt has been cast on this theory (Molfino et al 1991).

4. Halothane can interact with aminophylline to produce serious arrhythmias, even when theophylline levels are within the therapeutic range. This combination was suggested to have been the cause of ventricular fibrillation (Stirt & Sternick 1982) and ventricular tachycardia (Roizen & Stevens 1978). The xanthines are beta adrenoceptor stimulators that release norepinephrine (noradrenaline) and inhibit the breakdown of cyclic AMP.

5. Inhalational agents may worsen ventilation perfusion inequalities and increase hypoxia, by reducing hypoxic pulmonary vasoconstriction.

6. Perioperative steroid cover is advisable if steroids have been used within the previous 3 months.

7. In severe cases, postoperative IPPV may be required. It does, however, carry a high risk of complications such as pneumothorax, cardiac arrhythmias, pneumonia, and heart failure.

8. An increased incidence of postoperative pulmonary complications

9. The Churg–Strauss syndrome, a systemic vasculitis with eosinophilia, has been reported to occur following the start of treatment with leukotriene antagonists. It is suggested that the condition is associated with the withdrawal of steroids. The condition up until then had been masked by steroid treatment (Stirling & Chung 1999).

Management

1. Elective surgery should not take place in the presence of infection or untreated bronchospasm. Preoperative preparation will include physiotherapy, bronchodilators, antibiotics and corticosteroid cover, if steroids have been used within the previous 3 months. A short course of steroids is also indicated before surgery if inflammation is present (Hirshman & Bergman 1990). A study of 71 asthmatics undergoing 89 surgical procedures who were treated with steroids showed minimal complications (Kabalin et al 1995). In severe cases it is important to assess the likelihood of the need for IPPV in the postoperative period.

2. Anxiety may be a significant feature in the asthmatic patient. Care and understanding should be shown at the preoperative visit, and a sedative premedication, such as an antihistamine or benzodiazepine, is advantageous. The potential seriousness of this disease cannot be underestimated.

3. Despite having a drying effect on secretions, atropine may be desirable for a smooth induction. It can also improve dilatation in the larger bronchi by blocking vagal constrictor effects. Although pethidine has been promoted as a bronchodilator, it has recently been shown to be a more common cause of histamine release than morphine. Even when bronchospasm is absent, some form of preoperative bronchodilator therapy is advisable.

Beta blockers are contraindicated, since even those with a primarily cardiac action can aggravate airway obstruction.

4. Induction agent. Bronchoconstriction can arise from the drug itself, or directly from tracheal intubation (Kim & Bishop 1999). Even when attacks are infrequent, tracheal intubation is one of the commonest causes of intraoperative bronchospasm in patients who have any history of asthma. The carina is particularly sensitive to stimulation. However, in a controlled trial of asthmatics undergoing induction of anaesthesia, whilst 45% of patients who received thiopentone wheezed after intubation, none who received propofol did so (Pizov et al 1995). A study on the effect of either propofol or halothane on the respiratory mechanics of children found no difference between them (Habre et al 1996). There are no particular contraindications to the use of benzodiazepines or etomidate.

5. There is experimental evidence that reflex bronchospasm is prevented by iv lidocaine $(1 \, mg \, kg^{-1})$, but not that resulting from the release of allergic mediators (Downes et al 1980). In humans, the cough reflex in response to tracheal instillation of sterile water was suppressed by lidocaine $1.5 \, mg \, kg^{-1}$ (Nishino et al 1990). Thus the use of iv lidocaine $(1–1.5 \, mg \, kg^{-1})$ before induction has been recommended. However, topical lidocaine (lignocaine) spray is not effective, and may actually induce bronchoconstriction in asthmatic patients (McAlpine & Thomson 1989).

6. Use of a laryngeal mask airway has been shown to avoid the reversible bronchoconstriction associated with tracheal intubation (Kim & Bishop 1999).

7. Ketamine has been suggested to be a suitable induction agent for emergency anaesthesia in asthmatics, when a rapid sequence induction is required (Hirshman et al 1979). A comparison with thiopentone in dogs showed it to have a protective effect against bronchospasm, which was abolished by beta adrenoceptor blockers.

8. Halothane, enflurane and isoflurane are all effective at reversing antigen-induced bronchospasm (Hirshman et al 1982). The effect of halothane has been shown to be secondary to

blocking of baseline vagal tone (Brown et al 1993). However, halothane sensitises the heart to the effect of exogenous and endogenous catecholamines. It also interacts with aminophylline to produce arrhythmias, even when theophylline levels are within the therapeutic range. The choice of isoflurane, enflurane or sevoflurane may therefore be more appropriate. An inhalational induction with sevoflurane was given for emergency Caesarean section in a patient with status asthmaticus (Que & Lusaya 1999). However, in severe asthma, inhalational agents may worsen ventilation perfusion inequalities and increase hypoxia, by reducing hypoxic pulmonary vasoconstriction.

9. Neuromuscular blockers. Atracurium constricts peripheral airways in doses that produce significant cardiovascular effects, and this probably results from the release of histamine acting on H_2 receptors (Mehr et al 1992). The peak effects occur 3 min after a dose of $0.5 \, mg \, kg^{-1}$. However, in a controlled trial in asthmatics between atracurium and vecuronium, atracurium had more adverse cardiovascular events, but there were no differences in airway pressures between the two (Caldwell et al 1995).

10. Regional anaesthesia may be used for surgery or during labour. A retrospective study of asthmatic parturients (Ramanathan et al 1990), and a prospective study of suitable patients undergoing surgery (Tanaka et al 1991), showed that epidural anaesthesia could be safely administered, even during acute exacerbations of asthma.

11. Treatment of acute bronchospasm:

a) If this occurs following tracheal intubation, the easiest initial manoeuvre is to try and deepen the anaesthetic using a volatile agent.

b) Give salbutamol $250 \, \mu g$ in 20 ml saline over 10 min or aminophylline 250 mg over 20 min.

c) If there is complete airway closure, epinephrine 1 in 10 000 should be given in divided doses, 1–10 ml. This may need to be repeated.

d) For continued problems, a salbutamol infusion, $5 \, \mu g \, min^{-1}$ (5 ml of $1 \, mg \, ml^{-1}$ solution added to 500 ml 0.9% saline to give a final concentration of $10 \, \mu g \, ml^{-1}$).

e) The use of ketamine in subanaesthetic doses (bolus dose $0.75 \, mg \, kg^{-1}$, infusion of $0.15 \, mg \, kg^{-1} \, h^{-1}$) has been used to treat intractable bronchospasm in two patients (Sarma 1992).

f) Residual bronchospasm can be treated with aminophylline, as an infusion of $0.5 \, mg \, kg^{-1} \, h^{-1}$. In a small patient 750 mg in 24 h or in a large patient 1500 mg in 24 h. However, the narrow margin between therapeutic and toxic levels of theophylline means that the drug is being used less frequently. If aminophylline is used, plasma theophylline levels must be measured if treatment is prolonged for more than 24 h. The therapeutic range is $10–20 \, mg \, l^{-1}$ but toxic effects such as fits, arrhythmias and cardiac arrest have been described with plasma levels as low as $25 \, mg \, l^{-1}$. Extreme caution is necessary if the patient has already been taking sustained-release theophylline preparations.

g) Avoidance of IPPV in a severe asthmatic was achieved by administration of a subanaesthetic dose of halothane in 100% oxygen using a close fitting mask (Padkin et al 1997).

12. Indications for IPPV in asthmatics:

a) Distress and exhaustion.

b) Deterioration in arterial blood gases. $Pa_{O_2} < 6.7 \, kPa$ or $Pa_{CO_2} > 6.7 \, kPa$, and increasing metabolic acidosis.

c) Cardiac arrhythmias or hypotension.

d) Acute crises such as cardiorespiratory arrest, decreased conscious level due to sedatives, or a collapsed lung.

e) Technique of IPPV in asthmatics. Inotropes should be available at intubation. Patients should be underventilated and therefore neuromuscular blockers may be required. Provided that life-threatening hypoxia is avoided, it is unnecessary to aim for normal blood gases. Care should be taken to prevent hyperinflation.

13. Refractory asthma has been treated on the ITU with propofol (Pedersen 1992), magnesium sulphate (Mills et al 1997), and halothane (Padkin et al 1997).

Bibliography

Barnes PJ 1989 A new approach to the treatment of asthma. New England Journal of Medicine 321: 1517–27.

Brown RH, Mitzner W, Zerhouni E et al 1993 Direct in vivo visualization of bronchodilatation induced by inhalational anesthesia using high-resolution computed tomography. Anesthesiology 78: 295–300.

Caldwell JE, Lau M, Fisher DM 1995 Atracurium versus vecuronium in asthmatic patients. A blinded, randomized comparison of adverse events. Anesthesiology 83: 986–91.

Downes H, Gerber N, Hirshman CA 1980 Iv lignocaine in reflex and allergic bronchoconstriction. British Journal of Anaesthesia 52: 873–8.

Drazen J 1998 Clinical pharmacology of leukotriene receptor antagonists and 5-lipoxygenase inhibitors. American Journal of Respiratory & Critical Care Medicine 157: S233–7.

Drazen JM, Israel E, O'Byrne PM 1999 Treatment of asthma with drugs modifying the leukotriene pathway. New England Journal of Medicine 340: 197–206.

Guidelines for the Management of Asthma in Adults 1990 Statement by the British Thoracic Society, Research Unit of the Royal College of Physicians, King's Fund Centre, National Asthma Campaign. I—chronic persistent asthma in adults. British Medical Journal 301: 651–3; II—acute severe asthma in adults. British Medical Journal 301: 797–800.

Guidelines for the Management of Asthma 1997 Thorax: 52(suppl 1): S1–20.

Habre W, Matsumoto I, Sly PD 1996 Propofol or halothane anaesthesia for children with asthma: effects on respiratory mechanics. British Journal of Anaesthesia 77: 739–43.

Hirshman CA 1991 Perioperative management of the asthmatic patient. Canadian Journal of Anaesthesia 38: R26–38.

Hirshman CA, Bergman NA 1990 Factors influencing intrapulmonary airway calibre during anaesthesia. British Journal of Anaesthesia 65: 30–42.

Hirshman CA, Downes H, Farbood A et al 1979 Ketamine block of bronchospasm in experimental canine asthma. British Journal of Anaesthesia 51: 713–18.

Hirshman C, Edelstein G, Peetz S et al 1982 Mechanisms of action of inhalational agents on airways. Anesthesiology 56: 107–11.

Kabalin CS, Yarnold PR, Grammer LC 1995 Low complication rate of corticosteroid-treated asthmatics undergoing surgical procedures. Archives of Internal Medicine 155: 1379–84.

Keeley D, Rees J 1997 New guidelines on asthma management. British Medical Journal 314: 315–16.

Kim ES, Bishop MI 1999 Endotracheal intubation, but not laryngeal mask airway insertion, produces reversible bronchoconstriction. Anesthesiology 90: 391–4.

McAlpine LG, Thomson NC 1989 Lidocaine-induced bronchoconstriction in asthmatic patients. Relation to histamine airway responsiveness and effect of preservatives. Chest 96: 1012–15.

Mehr EH, Hirshman CA, Lindeman KS 1992 Mechanism of action of atracurium in airway constriction. Anesthesiology 76: 448–54.

Mills R, Leadbeater M, Ravalia A 1997 Intravenous magnesium sulphate in the management of refractory bronchospasm in a ventilated asthmatic. Anaesthesia 52: 782–5.

Molfino NA, Nannini LJ, Martelli AN et al 1991 Respiratory arrest in near-fatal asthma. New England Journal of Medicine 324: 285–8.

Nishino T, Hiraga K, Sugimori K 1990 Effects of iv lignocaine on airway reflexes elicited by irritation of the tracheal mucosa in humans anaesthetised with enflurane. British Journal of Anaesthesia 64: 682–7.

Olsson GL 1987 Bronchospasm during anaesthesia. A computer-aided incidence study of 136 929 patients. Acta Anaesthesiologica Scandinavica 31: 244–52.

Padkin AJ, Baigel G, Morgan GA 1997 Halothane treatment of severe asthma to avoid mechanical ventilation. Anaesthesia 52: 994–7.

Pedersen CM 1992 The effect of sedation with propofol on postoperative bronchoconstriction in patients with hyperreactive airway disease. Intensive Care Medicine 18: 45–6.

Pizov R, Brown RH, Weiss YS et al 1995 Wheezing during induction of general anesthesia in patients with and without asthma. Anesthesiology 82: 1111–16.

Que JC, Lusaya VO 1999 Sevoflurane induction for emergency cesarean section in a parturient in status asthmaticus. Anesthesiology 90: 1475–6.

Ramanathan J, Osborne B, Sibai B 1990 Epidural anesthesia in asthmatic parturients. Anesthesia & Analgesia 70: S317.

Roizen MF, Stevens WC 1978 Multiform ventricular tachycardia due to the interaction of aminophylline and halothane. Anesthesia & Analgesia 57: 738–41.

Sarma VJ 1992 Use of ketamine in acute severe asthma. Acta Anaesthesiologica Scandinavica 36: 106–7.

Stirling RG, Chung KF 1999 Leukotriene antagonists and Churg–Strauss syndrome: the smoking gun. Thorax 54: 865–6.

Stirt JA, Sternick CS 1982 Aminophylline and anesthesia. Anesthesiology 57: 252–3.

Tanaka K, Shono S, Watnabe R, Dan K 1991 Epidural anesthesia and analgesia is safe for patients with asthma—a survey of 383 patients. Anesthesia & Analgesia 72: S292.

Tattersfield AE, Harrison TW 1999 Step 3 of the asthma guidelines. Thorax 54: 753–4.

Tobias JD, Kubos KL, Hirshman CA 1989 Aminophylline does not attenuate histamine-induced airway constriction during halothane anesthesia. Anesthesiology 71: 723–9.

Athletic heart syndrome

A term given to certain cardiac and ECG changes which occur in some high performance athletes, and that probably represent physiological adaptations of the heart and cardiovascular system to the demands of the sport. The changes depend upon the nature of the demand: endurance (isotonic or dynamic) athletes such as marathon runners have chronic volume overload because of sustained increases in cardiac output (as much as seven-fold), whereas weight lifters (isometric or static athletes) experience transient episodes of enormous pressure overload. Both have cardiac enlargement. Left ventricular mass is increased as a result of increases in left ventricular diastolic cavity dimensions, thickness of the ventricular wall, or both. However, endurance athletes have increases in LV end-diastolic volume (from 120 ml in an untrained person to 220 ml in a resting athlete) and stroke volume (up to 170 ml during exercise), with proportionate, but mild, increases in ventricular wall thickness. Although it was previously thought that pure power training considerably increased LV wall thickness, a recent study showed that although LV mass was increased, the increase in absolute wall thickness was modest and rarely exceeded the upper limits of normal (Pelliccia et al 1993). From an echocardiographic study of 100 weight-trained, young athletes, the authors found that increases in LV wall thickness above 12 mm were unusual, and concluded that, if it was uneven in distribution, and exceeded 16 mm, a pathological cause should be sought.

In either case, when cardiac abnormalities occur, the main problem is to differentiate these from pathological heart disease, in particular, hypertrophic cardiomyopathy (HCM). This is increasingly recognised as an important cause of sudden death in young people, a number of whom have a family history (Editorial 1992).

However, those with 'athlete's heart' are not immune from problems, since the cardiovascular changes which prepare athletes for exercise may be disadvantageous during anaesthesia and surgery. In a study of normotensive athletes with cardiac hypertrophy, impairment of cardiopulmonary receptor reflexes was found (Giannattasio et al 1990). This indicates a potential lack of appropriate response to haemorrhage or orthostatic stress by means of a tachycardia.

Preoperative abnormalities

1. Physical examination may show a resting bradycardia and displaced LV impulse. Midsystolic murmurs may be heard in up to 50% of dynamic athletes and third and fourth heart sounds are common.

2. Chest X-ray shows an increased cardiothoracic ratio, a globular heart, and increased pulmonary vascularity.

3. ECG changes. Certain rhythm disturbances are more frequent than in the general population, but the patients are usually of an age group, and a degree of fitness, that would not justify a routine preoperative ECG. However, an unduly slow, and sometimes irregular, pulse may lead an observant physician to perform one. The ECG may show large voltages, tall T waves and ST elevation, with signs of right and left ventricular hypertrophy. A sinus bradycardia will be found in the majority of athletes and there is a significant correlation between the heart rate and fitness. There may be a range of depolarisation abnormalities including wandering atrial pacemaker, first- and second-degree heart block, right bundle branch block, or ST-segment abnormalities. There is a close relationship between incomplete right bundle branch block and right ventricular hypertrophy (Bjornstad et al 1993). Occasionally, third-degree heart block has been reported (Hernandez-Madrid et al 1991).

4. Echocardiography can help to differentiate between the athletic heart and the pathological heart (Maron et al 1995). In most athletes, although the calculated left ventricular mass and the size of the ventricular end-diastolic cavity are both increased (the latter may be >55 mm), the absolute ventricular wall thickness is usually normal or only mildly increased (<13 mm). In HCM, however, there is usually markedly (and often unevenly) increased LV wall thickness, ranging from 16 mm up to 50 mm, but the cavity dimension is <45 mm (Pelliccia et al 1991).

5. Endurance athletes have poor tolerance to orthostatic stress. Echocardiographic studies suggest that the cause is mechanical rather than autonomic in origin (Levine et al 1991). In endurance athletes, a greater effective LV chamber compliance and distensibility was found compared with non-athletes. This resulted in a steeper slope to the Starling curve, which relates LV filling pressure to stroke volume.

6. Elderly male athletes with a lifelong history of regular, strenuous exercise were shown to have more complex arrhythmias and profound bradyarrhythmias than did healthy, elderly controls (Jensen-Urstad et al 1998).

Anaesthetic problems

1. General anaesthesia. There have been reports of fit young athletes presenting with unexpected episodes of arrhythmias or conduction defects during general anaesthesia (Bullock & Hall 1985, Abdulatif et al 1987). However, in these cases, events were not serious and the problem was one of awareness of the diagnosis.

2. Whilst reduced heart rate responses to baroreceptor stimulation may favour cardiovascular function during exercise, it may be disadvantageous during haemorrhagic or orthostatic stress, when the ability to develop a tachycardia is an important component in the maintenance of stable cardiovascular haemodynamics (Giannattasio et al 1990).

3. Regional anaesthesia. One athlete had two periods of asystole and unconsciousness, from which he was resuscitated with atropine, 25 min after induction of spinal anaesthesia (Kreutz & Mazuzan 1990). Subsequent ECG showed resting sinus bradycardia, LV hypertrophy, and ST segment abnormalities. This may have been related to the recognised intolerance to orthostatic stress.

4. In the first week after athletic competition, endurance athletes can have elevated heart-specific serum CK-MB enzyme levels. Thus, caution must be exercised in the interpretation of such investigations. However, athletes are not immune from heart disease and sudden deaths during exercise have been caused by previously undiagnosed cardiomyopathies (Editorial 1992, Committee on Sports Medicine and Fitness 1995).

Management

1. In general, a careful preoperative history will help to distinguish between patients with physiological and pathological cardiac

abnormalities. ECG and echocardiography may contribute if the diagnosis is in doubt. Although both athletic heart syndrome and HCM can produce a wide range of not dissimilar ECG changes, the presence of prominent Q waves, deep inverted T waves and strikingly increased voltages would suggest a cardiomyopathy. Exercise ECGs in patients with coronary artery disease often show progressive abnormalities, whereas when athletes exercise, arrhythmias usually disappear.

2. During anaesthesia, if unexpected arrhythmias occur in young, apparently fit patients, the first problem is to exclude causes such as hypercarbia, hypoxia, inhalational agents, the response to surgical stimuli, and the use of vasoconstrictors. The second is to be aware of rarer causes of arrhythmias such as MH, substance abuse, ankylosing spondylitis, sarcoidosis, mitral valve prolapse, and cardiomyopathies.

If the above pathological abnormalities have been excluded, treatment is not necessarily indicated. Earlier reports suggested that patients with 'athlete's heart' remain haemodynamically stable during anaesthesia, and that conduction defects respond to atropine. However, not all arrhythmias during anaesthesia are benign and if serious conduction defects occur they should be treated expeditiously.

3. Care should be taken not to subject athletes to sudden orthostatic stress, particularly when performing spinal or epidural anaesthesia. Hypotension, bradycardias and hypovolaemia should be anticipated and treated.

4. It is essential that individuals with athletic heart syndrome are not labelled as having a pathological cardiac condition. If doubt persists, referral to a cardiologist who is known to be aware of the condition is advised. Extensive invasive investigations will not usually be appropriate, but echocardiographic measurement of LV wall thickness and LV cavity size will usually discriminate between athlete's heart and HCM. Maron et al (1995) have charted the criteria for discrimination in the small number of individuals whose LV wall thickness lies in the overlap zone between athlete's heart and HCM.

Bibliography

Abdulatif M, Fahkry M, Naguib M et al 1987 Multiple electrocardiographic anomalies during anaesthesia in an athlete. Canadian Journal of Anaesthesia 34: 284–7.

Bjornstad H, Storstein L, Dyre Meen H et al 1993 Electrocardiographic findings of heart rate and conduction times in athletic students and sedentary control subjects. Cardiology 83: 258–67.

Bullock RE, Hall RJC 1985 Athletic dysrhythmias. A case report. Anaesthesia 40: 647–50.

Committee on Sports Medicine and Fitness 1995 Cardiac dysrhythmias and sports. Pediatrics 95: 786–7.

Editorial 1992 Sporting hearts. Lancet 340: 1132–3.

Giannattasio C, Seravalle G, Bolla GB et al 1990 Cardiopulmonary receptor reflexes in normotensive athletes with cardiac hypertrophy. Circulation 82: 1222–9.

Hernandez-Madrid A, Moro C, Marin Huerta E et al 1991 Third-degree atrioventricular block in an athlete. Journal of Internal Medicine 229: 375–6.

Jensen-Urstad K, Bouvier F, Saltin B et al 1998 High prevalence of arrhythmias in elderly male athletes with a lifelong history of regular strenuous exercise. Heart 79: 161–4.

Kreutz JM, Mazuzan JE 1990 Sudden asystole in a marathon runner: the athletic heart syndrome and its anesthetic implications. Anesthesiology 73: 1266–8.

Levine BD, Lane L, Buckey JC et al 1991 Left ventricular pressure–volume and Frank–Starling relations in endurance athletes. Circulation 84: 1016–23.

Link MS, Olshansky B, Estes III NAM 1999 Cardiac arrhythmias and the athlete. Current Opinion in Cardiology 14: 24–9.

Maron BJ, Pelliccia A, Spirito P 1995 Cardiac disease in young trained athletes. Insights into methods for distinguishing athlete's heart from structural disease, with particular emphasis on hypertrophic cardiomyopathy. Circulation 91: 1596–601

Pelliccia A, Maron BJ, Spataro A et al 1991 The upper limit of physiologic cardiac hypertrophy in highly trained elite athletes. New England Journal of Medicine 324: 295–301.

Pellicia A, Spataro A, Caselli G et al 1993 Absence of left ventricular wall thickening in athletes engaged in intense power training. American Journal of Cardiology 72: 1048–54.

Automatic implantable cardioverter defibrillator (AICD) in

patients requiring surgery and anaesthesia

A device used in the treatment of patients with recurrent tachyarrhythmias that are unresponsive to medical treatment. The automatic implantable cardioverter defibrillator (AICD) senses VT or VF and responds with countershocks to the heart. Although there are significant complications from the insertion of this device and its subsequent aftercare, in this high-risk group of patients the AICD has been found to be superior to antiarrhythmic drugs in prolonging survival (Anonymous 1999).

The newer generation devices will provide high-energy shocks for VF and rapid VT, and antitachycardia and antibradycardia pacing as required (Pinski & Fahy 1999).

In the early days, AICD implantation required a general anaesthetic, because of the need to expose the apex of the heart, and anaesthesia was usually required on at least two occasions. However, with the newer generation, lightweight devices, some centres are using local anaesthesia and sedation, as for pacemaker implantation.

Increasing numbers of these devices are being implanted, therefore there is a greater chance of a patient with an implanted AICD needing incidental surgery. For a detailed review of the AICD, see Zaidan (1999).

Description

Modern systems consist of a light weight pulse generator, a programmer/recorder/monitor (PRM), software and a telemetry wand (Cardiac Pacemakers Incorporated). The PRM device communicates with the AICD system via radio waves through a handheld wand. The pulse generator has leads for sensing cardiac rate and delivering either shocks or pacing pulses. The metal housing of the pulse generator acts as an active electrode. There is a single, insulated lead with two electrodes, proximal and distal. A dual

current pathway sends energy from the lead's distal electrode to both the proximal electrode and the metal pulse generator. The endocardial cardioversion/defibrillation and pacing lead is inserted transvenously, via the left subclavian vein, and positioned such that the tip of the lead lies against the inner wall of the right ventricular apex. The pulse generator box can be implanted in a subcutaneous pocket in the left pectoral region, or in the abdomen, with the label side facing towards the skin. Most pulse generators have an identifier that is visible on X-ray film, displaying the model and manufacturer's name. The leads are usually tunnelled subcutaneously to the implantation pocket. An AICD can be programmed for both VF, and tachycardia or bradycardia pacing. At implantation, the lowest successful shock is recorded. The pulse generator automatically records information about arrhythmia detection and therapy for each detected episode. An 'episode' is defined as the period from the initial detection of an arrhythmia to its termination and this information is stored in the pulse generator.

The device can be programmed to detect tachycardias in certain ranges, to charge and to deliver a shock, if and when the predetermined criteria are fulfilled. It can also recharge to a higher charge, giving, if necessary, up to five countershocks of 30 joules each. The device can only be deactivated and reactivated by the programmer wand. Patients are followed up at an implantation centre and, from time to time, pulse generators and electrodes will need replacement.

Surgical diathermy should not be used when an AICD is active, because the pulse generator may interpret it as an arrhythmia and deliver a shock to the patient.

Indications for insertion

1. Recurrent ventricular tachyarrhythmias that are not controlled by drugs, or in patients who do not tolerate the appropriate therapy.

2. Recently, the indications have been extended to certain patients who have one of the

congenital long QT syndromes (eg Romano–Ward and Jervell, Lange–Nielsen, etc.). AICDs are now used in the small number of individuals who cannot tolerate beta blockers. Alternatively, if this therapy is ineffective in controlling episodes of syncope, left thoracocervical sympathectomy, with or without implantation of AICDs, may be required (Groh et al 1996).

Anaesthetic problems

1. If anaesthesia is required, the patient may need two anaesthetics, the first for insertion, the second about 3 months later to test device function. However, this is not always necessary (Lee 1992), and local anaesthesia with sedation is increasingly being used (Stix et al 1999). Patients with malignant ventricular arrhythmias are high-risk candidates for anaesthesia and surgery (Kam 1997), and the average operative mortality is 3.5%. Those with long QT syndrome, however, rarely have significant structural heart disease.

2. Awareness under anaesthesia has been reported when propofol infusions were administered on the same side as implantation, because propofol was lost from the central venous access site (Moerman et al 1995).

3. Testing of the device. Repeated intraoperative induction of VF may be needed to test thresholds, during which haemodynamics may be compromised, and cerebral oxygen uptake may be depressed for some time, if two or more shocks are required (de Vries et al 1998). The amount of cognitive dysfunction found 5 days later was related to the duration of the reperfusion interval between shocks (Murkin et al 1997). Testing with the patient awake is also necessary, so that he/she can experience the sensation of a shock. However, if reversion to sinus rhythm does not occur, an anaesthetist will be required urgently, so that external defibrillation can be applied. Each time a test is performed there is a risk that normal rhythm will not be restored (Horrow & Pharo 1991).

4. The presence of the AICD patches may increase the energy requirements for external defibrillation, to a level higher than usual with the paddles in the standard position. In one case, failure to convert an induced episode of VF was finally solved by placing the internal paddles perpendicular to the plane of epicardial patches and delivering two near-simultaneous (orthogonal) shocks discharged 50 ms apart (Horrow & Pharo 1991).

5. Most patients are receiving antiarrhythmic therapy, usually amiodarone. This drug may increase the threshold for defibrillation. Possible amiodarone-induced pulmonary toxicity was reported in two patients undergoing one-lung anaesthesia with high oxygen concentrations for AICD insertion (Herndon et al 1992).

6. Anaesthetic agents, or antiarrhythmics such as lidocaine (lignocaine) and verapamil, may alter cardiac conduction or the thresholds for defibrillation.

7. The AICD can be triggered by any form of electromagnetic radiation, including electrocautery (Gaba et al 1985). In one patient the countershock sequence that precipitated VT was initiated by the diathermy.

8. The AICD may discharge at any time, therefore staff handling the patient are advised to wear gloves (Lee 1992).

9. Poor ventricular function is associated with an increased mortality at operation. Ventricular arrhythmias can occur at any time, with a resultant decrease in cardiac output.

10. Problems associated with certain procedures:

a) Extracorporeal shock wave lithotripsy (ESWL). In patients undergoing ESWL for fragmentation of calculi, there is a danger of the piezoelectric crystal being shattered by the shock wave (Horrow & Pharo 1991, Long & Venditti 1991).

b) ECT needs special precautions. If the patient is earthed, ECT current may pass through the heart via the AICD and cause VF.

c) Problems of using transcutaneous electrical nerve stimulation (TENS).

11. Complications of initial AICD insertion include wound infection, seroma of the pocket holding the device, pleural effusion, device failure, and inappropriate activation.

Management

1. Anaesthesia for implantation of AICD. In the past, general anaesthesia was usually employed. However, with the newer generation, lightweight devices, there is increasing use of local anaesthesia and sedation. In a controlled trial of 40 patients undergoing either local anaesthesia and sedation, or general anaesthesia, local techniques were found to be safe, acceptable, cheaper, and less time consuming (Stix et al 1999). In addition, the use of lidocaine (lignocaine) did not adversely affect defibrillation thresholds. When general anaesthesia was used initially, intra-arterial monitoring was recommended, because testing involved induction of VF (Gaba et al 1985). This can be associated with adverse cardiopulmonary effects, which sometimes require treatment with inotropic agents (Hachenberg et al 1991). However, others have suggested that $ETCO_2$ monitoring may be sufficient to indicate decreases in cardiac output (Cashman et al 1992). Central venous access is needed for passage of the pacing wires and for administration of vasoactive drugs. A comparison between intravenous anaesthesia with propofol and inhalational anaesthesia with isoflurane showed no significant changes in the defibrillation threshold (Moerman et al 1998). If propofol infusions are used, they should be administered on the contralateral side, so that propofol is not lost through the central venous access (Moerman et al 1995).

2. Patients are regularly followed up at implanting centres, for retrieval of data from memory about therapy episodes, and checking the integrity of the leads and the battery life of the pulse generator.

3. Anaesthesia for incidental surgery that requires surgical diathermy. If incidental surgery is required for which diathermy is essential, the AICD must be deactivated first. If a hospital has neither an implanting centre nor access to an experienced programmer, the manufacturer will usually provide a technical service. First of all the function and frequency of firing needs to be assessed. The AICD is interrogated by holding the telemetry wand over the pulse generator, to access the history and therapy data stored in memory. The wand is also used to program, or delivery therapy, as required. The technician must also be present in theatre, to deactivate the device, to reactivate it, and to check it at the end of surgery. Before deactivation, external adhesive defibrillator pads are applied to the patient's chest and attached to a defibrillator figured in the mode for delivery through the pads. Should ventricular arrhythmias occur during surgery, defibrillation can take place without delay.

4. Interaction with antiarrhythmic drugs. The minimum energy requirements to deliver an effective shock may be altered by certain drugs. This is more likely to be a problem shortly after insertion of the AICD. For this reason, the trigger threshold for defibrillation should be assessed each time antiarrhythmic medication is changed. It has been shown that verapamil significantly increases the defibrillation energy requirement and for this reason it is recommended that verapamil should be used with caution in patients with AICDs and a marginal defibrillation threshold (Jones et al 1991). For anaesthetists managing patients with AICDs, it is important to remember this fact when treating perioperative arrhythmias.

5. Anaesthesia for ECT. This frequently induces transient arrhythmias, therefore current recommendations are that the AICD should be deactivated before the administration of each treatment and reactivated on completion, in order to minimise the risk of an inappropriate shock (Tchou et al 1989). However, more recently, successful use of ECT without deactivation has been reported (Pornnoppadol et

al 1998). External defibrillator pads and full resuscitation equipment will again be required.

6. Radiotherapy. Ionising radiation, particularly in high dosage, may adversely affect pulse generator operation. The device should be inactivated, shielded, and checked afterwards (Cardiac Pacemakers Incorporated).

7. Magnetic resonance imaging. Direct current magnetic fields can exert significant mechanical forces on an AICD pulse generator because of its ferromagnetic components (Menon et al 1992). These can cause physical pain and injury, and can damage the pulse generator. Alternating magnetic fields can cause a pulse generator to: i) charge and deliver a high-voltage shock to the patient, ii) inhibit bradycardia pacing, iii) disable antitachycardia therapy, or iv) change programmed parameters (Cardiac Pacemakers Incorporated).

8. Staff handling these patients are advised to wear gloves, because a shock can occur at any time (Lee 1992).

9. Extracorporeal shock wave lithotripsy (ESWL). Previously, this was not recommended in patients with an AICD, because of the powerful mechanical and electrical forces generated during treatment, and the close proximity of the AICD to the focus of the shock waves (Vassolas et al 1993). However, recent studies conclude that ESWL can be performed safely in selected patients with modern AICDs, although the device should be shielded, and a complete test should be performed on it after treatment (Streem 1997, Chung et al 1999). In order to investigate methods of protecting the device from the shock wave, an AICD generator was strapped to a patient who was undergoing ESWL. It was protected from the shockwave with 1 inch (2.5 cm) thick, styrofoam board and was subsequently examined for damage; none was found (Long & Venditti 1991).

10. Investigations have shown that emergency, noninvasive transcutaneous pacing is possible in patients with AICD patches, despite the fact that there is insulation of the epicardial patch electrodes (Kemnitz et al 1992). No difference in thresholds was found when compared with patients without them who were undergoing routine CABG.

11. Access to extracorporeal circulation facilities may be life saving if refractory VF occurs (Horrow & Pharo 1991).

12. Further information can be obtained from:

> http://www.implantable.com
>
> http://www:guidant.com
>
> http://www.medtronic.com

Bibliography

Anonymous 1999 Causes of death in the Antiarrhythmics Versus Implantable Defibrillator (AVID) Trial. Journal of the American College of Cardiology 34: 1552–9.

Cardiac Pacemakers Incorporated. CPI. Physician's system manual. Ventak Mini II 1762 and Ventak Mini II+ 1763. Guidant Corporation. Cardiac Pacemakers Incorporated, Basingstoke, Hampshire.

Carr CME, Whiteley SM 1991 The automatic implantable cardioverter-defibrillator. Implications for anaesthetists. Anaesthesia 46: 737–40.

Cashman JN, Garcia-Rodriguez C, Lamond C 1992 Anaesthesia for transvenous insertion of an automatic implantable converter-defibrillator. Anaesthesia 47: 720–1.

Chung MK, Streem SB, Ching E et al 1999 Effects of extracorporeal shock wave lithotripsy on tiered therapy implantable defibrillators. Pacing and Clinical Electrophysiology 22: 738–42.

de Vries JW, Bakker PF, Visser GH et al 1998 Changes in cerebral oxygen uptake and cerebral electrical activity during defibrillation threshold testing. Anesthesia & Analgesia 87: 16–20.

Gaba DM, Wynder J, Fish KJ 1985 Anesthesia and the automatic implantable cardioverter defibrillator. Anesthesiology 62: 786–92.

Groh WJ, Silka MJ, Oliver RP et al 1996 Use of implantable cardioverter-defibrillators in the congenital long QT syndrome. American Journal of Cardiology 78: 703–6.

Hachenberg T, Hammel D, Mollhoff I et al 1991 Cardiopulmonary effects of internal cardioverter defibrillator implantation. Acta Anaesthesiologica Scandinavica 35: 626–30.

Herndon JC, Cook AO, Ramsay MAE et al 1992 Postoperative unilateral pulmonary edema: possible amiodarone toxicity. Anesthesiology 76: 308–11.

Horrow JC, Pharo G 1991 Successful defibrillation with near-simultaneous orthogonal discharges. Anesthesiology 75: 362–4.

Jones FD, Fahy BG 1999 Intraoperative use of automated external defibrillator. Journal of Clinical Anesthesia 11: 336–8.

Jones DL, Klein GJ, Guiraudon GM et al 1991 Effects of lidocaine and verapamil on defibrillation in humans. Journal of Electrocardiography 24: 299–305.

Kam PCA 1997 Anaesthetic management of a patient with an automatic implantable cardioverter defibrillator in situ. British Journal of Anaesthesia 78: 102–6.

Kemnitz J, Winter J, Vester EG et al 1992 Transcutaneous cardiac pacing in patients with automatic implantable cardioverter defibrillators. Anesthesiology 77: 258–62.

Lee EM 1992 More on automatic cardioverter-defibrillators. Anaesthesia 47: 637–8.

Lehmann A, Boldt J, Zeitler C et al 1999 Total intravenous anesthesia with remifentanil and propofol for implantation of cardioverter-defibrillators in patients with severely reduced left ventricular function. Journal of Cardiothoracic & Vascular Anesthesia 13: 15–19.

Long AL, Venditti FJ 1991 Lithotripsy in a patient with an automatic implantable cardioverter defibrillator. Anesthesiology 74: 937–8.

Menon DK, Peden CJ, Hall AS et al 1992 Magnetic resonance for the anaesthetist. Part I: physical principles, applications, safety aspects. Anaesthesia 47: 240–55.

Moerman A, Herregods L, Foubert L et al 1995 Awareness during anaesthesia for implantable cardioverter defibrillator implantation. Recall of defibrillation shocks. Anaesthesia 50: 733–5.

Moerman A, Herregods L, Tavernier R et al 1998 Influence of anaesthesia on defibrillation threshold. Anaesthesia 53: 1156–9.

Murkin JM, Baird DL, Martzke JS et al 1997 Cognitive dysfunction after ventricular fibrillation during implantable cardioverter/defibrillator procedures is related to duration of reperfusion interval. Anesthesia & Analgesia 84: 1186–92.

Pinski SL, Fahy GJ 1999 Implantable cardioverter defibrillators. American Journal of Medicine 106: 446–58.

Pornnoppadol C, Isenberg K 1998 ECT with implantable cardioverter defibrillator. Journal of Electroconvulsive Therapy 14: 124–6.

Stix G, Anvari A, Podesser B et al 1999 Local anaesthesia versus general anaesthesia for cardioverter-defibrillator implantation. Wiener Klinische Wochenschrift 111: 406–9.

Streem SB 1997 Contemporary clinical practice of shock wave lithotripsy: a reevaluation of contraindications. Journal of Urology 157: 1197–203.

Tchou PJ, Piasecki E, Gutmann M et al 1989 Psychological support and psychiatric management of patients with automatic implantable cardioverter defibrillators. International Journal of Psychiatry in Medicine 19: 393–407.

Vassolas G, Roth RA, Venditti FJ 1993 Effect of extracorporeal shock wave lithotripsy on implantable cardioverter defibrillator. Pacing & Clinical Electrophysiology 16: 1245–8.

Zaidan JR 1999 Implantable cardioverter-defibrillators. Journal of Cardiothoracic & Vascular Anesthesia 13: 475–83.

Autonomic failure

Failure, or dysfunction, of the autonomic nervous system is being increasingly recognised as a complication of a number of disease processes. In familial dysautonomia (Riley–Day syndrome), there is a decrease in all neuronal populations, as well as a decrease in synthesis of norepinephrine (noradrenaline). Through its sympathetic and parasympathetic pathways, the autonomic nervous system supplies and influences every organ in the body (Mathias 1997). It is therefore not surprising that autonomic failure can have such widespread effects. Dysfunction may be secondary to diabetes, Guillain–Barré syndrome, Parkinson's disease, multiple system atrophy (formerly Shy–Drager syndrome), tetanus, AIDS, postcerebrovascular states, alpha adrenoceptor blocking drugs, and the peripheral neuropathy of amyloid disease. A pure neuropathy can also occur, which is peripheral in origin (Goldstein et al 1997). Occasionally, an acute autonomic neuropathy, of sudden onset, can occur in young people (Hart & Kanter 1990). Sympathetic or parasympathetic systems, or the functions of both, may be affected. Gastroparesis and syncope are the commonest presenting signs, and the CSF protein level may be increased.

Autonomic dysfunction can be central or peripheral in origin, and may affect sympathetic or parasympathetic nerves. A recent consensus statement classifying the different types of disease involving autonomic failure has been made (Anonymous 1996). Whilst autonomic failure will produce widespread disturbances of organ function, it is the cardiovascular and respiratory effects that are of particular concern to the anaesthetist.

Preoperative abnormalities

1. *General features.* The clinical manifestations of primary, chronic autonomic failure include the following features: orthostatic hypotension, anhydrosis, heat intolerance, constipation, dysphagia, nocturia, frequency, urgency, incontinence, retention of urine, erectile or ejaculatory failure, Horner's syndrome, stridor, apnoea, Parkinson's disease, cerebellar and pyramidal features (Mathias 1997). Erythropoietin depletion may cause anaemia, particularly in diabetic neuropathy (Watkins 1998).

2. *Cardiovascular.* Orthostatic hypotension, peripheral vasodilatation and an inability, in response to stress, to produce the normal pressor response that depends on reflex vasoconstriction and tachycardia. There is reversal of the usual diurnal pattern of blood pressure, and also of that normally produced by postural changes. A number of clinical features of autonomic dysfunction have been described:

a) Postural hypotension. The blood pressure increases when in the supine position at night, and decreases on standing. A decrease in the systolic blood pressure of 30 mmHg on standing is significant.

b) Abnormal blood pressure response to the Valsalva manoeuvre. This manoeuvre involves taking a maximum inspiration, blowing into a tube connected to a

mercury manometer, and elevating the mercury level to 40 mmHg for 10 s. A slow blow-off valve in the system requires the subject to blow continuously to maintain the pressure. Four phases of response are described in normal individuals:

i) A rapid increase in arterial pressure immediately after the onset of straining, when the intrathoracic pressure is added to systemic arterial pressure.

ii) A decrease in blood pressure, with an associated tachycardia secondary to diminished venous return. Some restoration in pressure occurs later in this phase.

iii) Following the release in straining, there is a sudden brief reduction in pressure.

iv) Finally there is a terminal elevation of pressure above control values, associated with a bradycardia. The release of the Valsalva manoeuvre restores venous pressure and cardiac output at a time when the systemic vessels are still constricted. The arterial pressure increases above normal, the baroreceptors are stimulated, and a bradycardia occurs until the pressure returns to its normal value.

Since a patient with autonomic failure cannot respond with vasoconstriction, the blood pressure continues to decrease during the Valsalva manoeuvre. There is no overshoot in blood pressure when the straining is released, with a gradual return to normal. No tachycardia or bradycardia occurs. In clinical practice this has been difficult to demonstrate without direct arterial monitoring (Brown 1987); however, a technique in which a pulse oximeter is linked to a chart recorder has been described to show this (Broome & Mason 1988).

3. *ECG.* The R–R variation on the ECG is lost, and there are no heart rate changes on taking six deep breaths.

4. *Fluid and electrolyte homeostasis.* This is disturbed, resulting in a failure to concentrate urine at night. There is a nocturnal diuresis and sodium loss (Watson 1987).

5. *Central versus peripheral failure.* Differences exist between autonomic failure of central origin and that of peripheral origin. Central lesions, in which there is preservation of sympathetic ganglia, have normal basal serum norepinephrine (noradrenaline) levels, whereas those with pure autonomic failure often have low values (Goldstein et al 1997, Mathias 1997).

6. *Sudden death.* Sudden death can occur during sleep in patients with multiple system atrophy and vocal fold dysfunction. This may be associated with dyskinesia of the muscles of the larynx. Sudden death can also occur in young people with type 1 diabetes mellitus; nocturnal hypoglycaemia may be compounded by autonomic dysfunction (Weston & Gill 1999).

Anaesthetic problems

1. Hypotension. Blood pressure is extremely sensitive to changes in extracellular fluid volume, and hypotension may occur on induction of anaesthesia. In a prospective study of 17 diabetic patients having eye surgery, 35% required vasopressors, compared with 5% of nondiabetic controls. They were required more often in those with the poorest autonomic function (Burgos et al 1989). Tracheal intubation produces less of a pressor response than is seen in normal patients and, in fact, the first few minutes after tracheal intubation is the period of highest risk for hypotension and bradycardia.

2. Arrhythmias, bradycardias, and unexpected cardiac arrest have all been described. Atropine-induced heart rate increases were found to be significantly less in diabetics than in nondiabetics (Tsueda et al 1991).

3. Respiratory arrest and diminished sensitivity to hypoxia and hypercarbia have been reported (Page & Watkins 1978).

4. The response to catecholamines is variable

(Stirt et al 1982). In central dysfunction, the response to indirect-acting catecholamines is normal, and there is no sensitivity to those acting directly. With peripheral dysfunction, there may be lesser response to indirect-acting catecholamines, but an exaggerated (denervation hypersensitivity) response to those acting directly.

Management

For the problems of individual diseases, see Diabetes, Familial dysautonomia, Multiple system atrophy, Guillain–Barré syndrome, Parkinson's disease, Tetanus, AIDS, etc. It is important to realise that autonomic dysfunction exists to varying degrees. It is not an all or none phenomenon (Ewing & Clarke 1986).

1. Awareness of the possibility of localised or generalised dysfunction in association with another disease. A wide variety of tests have been described (Ravits 1997), but for anaesthetic purposes, screening tests are best directed towards cardiovascular involvement.

2. Good management lies in the anticipation of possible problems, close patient monitoring, and the minimisation of cardiovascular changes by judicious fluid and drug therapy.

3. ECG and blood pressure should be monitored from the outset of the anaesthetic.

4. All drugs should be given with caution. Hypotension may require a fluid load and intropic agents.

5. The patient's lungs should be ventilated, or respiration closely monitored, particularly in the postoperative period.

6. Patients with multiple system atrophy and vocal cord abductor paralysis probably require tracheostomy (Isozaki et al 1996).

Bibliography

Anonymous 1996 Consensus statement on the definition of orthostatic hypotension, pure autonomic failure, and multiple system atrophy. Neurology 46: 1470.

Autonomic failure

Broome IJ, Mason RA 1988 Use of a pulse oximeter for the identification of autonomic dysfunction. Anaesthesia 43: 833–6.

Brown MJ 1987 The measurement of autonomic function in clinical practice. Journal of the Royal College of Physicians 21: 206–9.

Burgos LG, Ebert TJ, Asiddao C et al 1989 Increased intraoperative cardiovascular lability in diabetics with autonomic neuropathy. Anesthesiology 70: 591–7.

Ewing DJ, Clarke BF 1986 Autonomic neuropathy: its diagnosis and prognosis. Clinics in Endocrinology & Metabolism 15: 855–88.

Goldstein DS, Holmes C, Cannon RO III 1997 Sympathetic cardioneuropathies in dysautonomias. New England Journal of Medicine 336: 696–702.

Hart RG, Kanter MC 1990 Acute autonomic neuropathy. Two cases and a clinical review. Archives of Internal Medicine 150: 2373–6.

Isozaki E, Naito A, Horiguchi S et al 1996 Early diagnosis and stage classification of vocal cord abductor paralysis in patients with multiple system atrophy. Journal of Neurology, Neurosurgery & Psychiatry 60: 399–402.

Mathias CJ 1997 Autonomic disorders and their recognition. New England Journal of Medicine 336: 721–4.

Page MMcB, Watkins PJ 1978 Cardiorespiratory arrest and diabetic autonomic neuropathy. Lancet i: 14–16.

Ravits JM 1997 AAEM minimonograph 48: autonomic nervous system testing. Muscle & Nerve 20: 919–37.

Stirt JA, Frantz RA, Gunz EF, Connolly ME 1982 Anesthesia, catecholamines and hemodynamics in autonomic dysfunction. Anesthesia & Analgesia 61: 701–4.

Tsueda K, Huang KC, Dumont SW et al 1991 Cardiac sympathetic tone in anaesthetised diabetics. Canadian Journal of Anaesthesia 38: 20–3.

Watkins PJ 1998 The enigma of autonomic failure in diabetes. Journal of the Royal Society of Physicians of London 32: 360–5.

Watson RDS 1987 Treating postural hypotension. British Medical Journal 294: 390–1.

Weston PJ, Gill GV 1999 Is undetected autonomic dysfuction responsible for sudden death in Type 1 diabetes mellitus? The 'dead in bed' syndrome revisited. Diabetic Medicine 16: 623–5.

Becker muscular dystrophy (BMD)

A muscle dystrophy which is less severe than Duchenne muscular dystrophy (DMD) and ten times rarer. The two dystrophies share the same locus, Xp21, and the protein product of the gene is dystrophin. DMD has an absence of dystrophin, whereas BMD has an alteration in the size or quantity of dystrophin (Dubowitz 1992). Dystrophin is located to the inner surface of the sarcolemmal membrane. It probably forms a complex with other proteins, and is important in maintaining the integrity of the sarcolemma (Ohlendieck et al 1993, Dubowitz 1997). As a result of these abnormalities, the muscle becomes extremely susceptible to necrosis.

Preoperative abnormalities

1. May present with muscle cramps on walking long distances, or episodes of red-coloured urine following exercise.

2. It is a progressive muscle dystrophy similar to DMD, but less severe. It runs a parallel clinical course, but at a slower rate, and is more variable. Whereas the majority of boys with DMD are wheelchair bound by the age of 12 years, BMD patients are usually mobile until 16 years, and some still ambulatory in their 60s (Dubowitz 1992).

3. Cardiac disease in mild cases is more frequent than previously thought. In 28 patients with only subclinical or 'benign' BMD, myocardial involvement occurred in 72% and 60% respectively. The right ventricle was affected early by the cardiomyopathic process, and the left ventricle later (Melacini et al 1996). Mechanical stress could occur if individuals, unaware of the cardiac disease, exercised strenuously. Life-threatening arrhythmias complicate the later stages of BMD. A recent study of BMD carriers has shown that more than 60% had abnormalities on echocardiography (Hoogerwaard et al 1999).

4. The presence of a hypercoagulable state in X-linked dystrophic patients has been suggested (Porreca et al 1999).

5. The diagnosis can usually be confirmed by a combination of clinical features, family history, tests that examine the dystrophin protein, and those that examine the gene.

Anaesthetic problems

1. Serious or fatal events in BMD patients may have been preceded by apparently normal anaesthetics, or ones that were followed by myoglobinuria, or other evidence of rhabdomyolysis. Hyperkalaemic cardiac arrest and death during dental anaesthesia, 80 min after halothane and suxamethonium, has been reported in a 6-year-old boy with known BMD. A previous anaesthetic with halothane alone had been followed by myoglobinuria (Bush & Dubowitz 1991). Cardiac arrest occurred 25 min after halothane and suxamethonium for post-tonsillectomy bleeding in an 11 year old. Postmortem showed myopathy and evidence of several preceding episodes of muscle necrosis. Retrospective questioning revealed a history of leg cramps on walking, a family history of BMD, and a probable episode of myoglobinuria after a previous anaesthetic (Farrell 1994).

2. The diagnosis may be unknown, and the event associated with anaesthesia can be the first sign of the disease. Hyperkalaemic cardiac arrest occurred after halothane induction followed by suxamethonium in a 3-month-old boy. Resuscitation was successful, and muscle biopsy showed BMD (Sullivan & Thompson 1994).

3. Evidence of rhabdomyolysis alone may occur (Shoji et al 1998). Myoglobinuria followed maxillofacial surgery using enflurane in a 22-year-old man with BMD. Further anaesthesia 35 days later, but without volatile agents, showed no evidence of rhabdomyolysis (Umino et al 1989).

4. Evidence of metabolic stimulation, similar to that seen in MH, has been described. Hyperthermia, masseter spasm, rhabdomyolysis, and heart failure occurred in a 17-year-old boy following a GA (Ohkoshi et al 1995).

Management

1. Examination for possible cardiac disease.

2. In a patient with known BMD, there should be careful questioning about red-coloured urine following previous anaesthetics.

3. Volatile agents and suxamethonium should probably be avoided.

4. If sudden cardiac arrest occurs when suxamethonium has been used, hyperkalaemia must be assumed to have occurred, and treatment directed towards reduction in serum potassium. ECG will show peaked T waves and wide QRS complexes.

For a 70-kg adult give glucose 50% 50 ml with insulin 10–20 u. Calcium chloride 10% 10–20 ml over 5–10 min and sodium bicarbonate 8.4% 50 ml.

For a child give glucose $0.5\,g\,kg^{-1}h^{-1}$ and insulin $0.05\,u\,kg^{-1}$. Calcium gluconate 10% $0.5\,ml\,kg^{-1}$ and repeat twice if necessary. Sodium bicarbonate 8.4% $2.5\,ml\,kg^{-1}$.

5. Calcium acts immediately and its effect lasts for 15–30 min. Sodium bicarbonate and insulin/glucose act in 15–30 min and their effects last for 3–6 h.

Bibliography

Bush A, Dubowitz V 1991 Fatal rhabdomyolysis complicating general anaesthesia in a child with Becker muscular dystrophy. Neuromuscular Disorders 1: 204–10.

Dubowitz V 1992 The muscular dystrophies. Postgraduate Medical Journal 68: 500–6.

Dubovitz V 1997 The muscular dystrophies—Clarity or chaos? New England Journal of Medicine 336: 650–1.

Farrell PT 1994 Anaesthesia-induced rhabdomyolysis causing cardiac arrest: case report and review of anaesthesia and the dystrophinopathies. Anaesthesia & Intensive Care 22: 597–601.

Hoogerwaard EM, Van der Wouw PA, Wilde AAM et al 1999 Cardiac involvement in carriers of Duchenne and Becker muscular dystrophy. Neuromuscular Disorders 9: 347–51.

Melacini P, Fanin M, Danieli GA et al 1996 Myocardial involvement is very frequent among patients affected with subclinical Becker's muscular dystrophy. Circulation 94: 3168–75.

Ohkoshi N, Yoshizawa T, Mizusawa H et al 1995 Malignant hyperthermia in a patient with Becker muscular dystrophy: dystrophin analysis and caffeine contracture study. Neuromuscular Disorders 5: 53–8.

Ohlendieck K, Matsumura K, Ionasescu VV et al 1993 Duchenne muscular dystrophy. Deficiency of dystrophin-associated proteins in the sarcolemma. Neurology 43: 795–800.

Porreca E, Guglielmo MD, Uncini A et al 1999 Haemostatic abnormalities, cardiac involvement and serum tumor necrosis factor levels in X-linked dystrophic patients. Thrombosis & Haemostasis 81: 543–6.

Shoji T, Nishikawa Y, Saito N et al 1998 A case of Becker muscular dystrophy and massive myoglobinuria with minimal renal manifestations. Nephrology, Dialysis & Transplantation 13: 759–60.

Sullivan M, Thompson WK 1994 Succinylcholine-induced cardiac arrest in children with undiagnosed myopathy. Canadian Journal of Anaesthesia 41: 497–501.

Umino M, Kurosa M, Masuda T et al 1989 Myoglobinuria and elevated serum enzymes associated with partial glossectomy under enflurane anesthesia in a patient with muscular dystrophy. Journal of Oral & Maxillofacial Surgery 47: 71–5.

Beckwith–Wiedemann syndrome

A congenital overgrowth syndrome. Anaesthesia may be required for closure of omphalocoele, tongue reduction, tracheostomy, embryonic cancers, adenotonsillectomy, or renal investigations.

Preoperative abnormalities

1. Macroglossia (97%), abdominal wall defects (80%), >90% percentile on the growth chart (88%), ear creases (76%), facial naevus flammeus (62%), nephromegaly (59%), hypoglycaemia (63%), hemihypertrophy, and visceromegaly were found in a study of 76 patients (Elliott et al 1994). Congenital heart disease may occur.

2. Associated with an increased risk of embryonal cancers such as Wilm's tumour, neuroblastoma, hepatoblastoma, adrenocortical carcinoma, and rhabdomyosarcoma (DeBaun & Tucker 1998).

3. A high incidence of nonmalignant renal abnormalities; renal cysts, hydronephrosis, and nephrolithiasis (Choyke et al 1998).

4. Monitoring is required for tumours (Beckwith 1998).

Anaesthetic problems

1. Upper airway obstruction can occur in the presence of macroglossia, particularly when the patient is supine. Anterior tongue reduction surgery may be needed (Menard et al 1995, Morgan et al 1996). However, this may not necessarily improve the airway problems if the predominant anatomical feature is tongue base enlargement, in which case tracheostomy may be required (Rimell et al 1995). In addition, regrowth has been reported (Kopriva & Classen 1998). Accidental trauma of the large tongue may produce problems (Thomas & McEwan 1998). Extubation difficulties occurred secondary to upper airway obstruction in a neonate who had undergone omphalocoele repair (Suan et al 1996).

2. Obstruction may also be associated with adenotonsillar hypertrophy, which is common in these children. In these patients, adenotonsillectomy will improve the situation (Rimell et al 1995).

3. Severe hypoglycaemia may occur. Hypoglycaemic fits have been reported in early life (Suan et al 1996). Subtotal pancreatectomy was performed in an infant whose blood sugar was difficult to control (Gurkowski & Rasch 1989).

4. Preoperative polycythaemia required partial exchange transfusion before closure of an omphalocoele (Tobias et al 1992).

Management

1. Assessment of potential airway or intubation difficulties.

2. Monitoring of blood sugar for hypoglycaemia. For hypoglycaemia, a bolus dose of 10% dextrose, $2\,\mathrm{ml\,kg^{-1}}$ is required.

3. Postoperative respiratory monitoring for obstruction and respiratory insufficiency.

4. Tracheostomy may be required in the presence of tongue base obstruction.

Bibliography

Beckwith JB 1998 Children at increased risk for Wilms tumor: monitoring issues. Journal of Pediatrics 132: 377–9.

Choyke PL, Siegel MJ, Sotelo-Avila C et al 1998 Nonmalignant disease in pediatric patients with Beckwith–Wiedemann syndrome. American Journal of Roentgenology 171: 733–7.

DeBaun MR, Tucker MA 1998 Risk of cancer during the first four years of life in children with The Beckwith–Wiedemann Syndrome Surgery Register. Journal of Pediatrics 132: 398–400.

Elliott M, Bayly R, Cole T et al 1994 Clinical features and natural history of Beckwith–Wiedemann syndrome: presentation of 74 new cases. Clinical Genetics 46: 168–74.

Gurkowski MA, Rasch D 1989 Anesthetic considerations for Beckwith–Wiedemann syndrome. Anesthesiology 70: 711–12.

Kopriva D, Classen DA 1998 Regrowth of tongue following Beckwith–Wiedemann macroglossia. Journal of Otolaryngology 27: 232–5.

Menard RM, Delaire J, Schendel SA 1995 Treatment of the craniofacial complications of Beckwith–Wiedemann syndrome. Plastic & Reconstructive Surgery 96: 27–33.

Morgan WE, Friedman EM, Duncan NO et al 1996 Surgical management of macroglossia in children. Archives of Otolaryngology—Head & Neck Surgery 122: 326–9.

Rimell FL, Shapiro AM, Shoemaker DL et al 1995 Head and neck manifestations of Beckwith–Wiedemann syndrome. Otolaryngology—Head & Neck Surgery 113: 262–5.

Suan C, Ojeda R, Garcia-Perla JL et al 1996 Anaesthesia and the Beckwith–Wiedemann syndrome. Paediatric Anaesthesia 6: 231–3.

Tobias JD, Lowe S, Holcomb GW 1992 Anaesthetic considerations of an infant with Beckwith–Wiedemann syndrome. Journal of Clinical Anesthesia 4: 484–6.

Thomas ML, McEwan A 1998 The anaesthetic management of a case of Kawasaki's disease (mucocutaneous lymph node syndrome) and Beckwith–Wiedemann syndrome presenting with a bleeding tongue. Paediatric Anaesthesia 8: 500–2.

Budd–Chiari syndrome

A syndrome caused by obstruction to the hepatic venous outflow and resulting in a clinical picture of hepatomegaly and portal hypertension. It may be secondary to haematological disorders, malignancy, oral contraceptives, heart failure, or constrictive pericarditis. The three main sites of obstruction are: i) inferior vena cava, ii) large hepatic veins, and iii) small intrahepatic venules. The condition may be acute or chronic. Acute Budd–Chiari syndrome with hepatocyte necrosis may require urgent portosystemic, decompressive, surgical or interventional radiological procedures. Untreated hepatic venous thrombosis usually results in progressive liver failure and death. Medical treatment is of little help, therefore shunt procedures or liver transplantation will be needed (Gupta et al 1986, Klein et al 1990).

Preoperative abnormalities

1. Abdominal pain and swelling were the commonest symptoms in a review of 44 patients (Mahmoud et al 1996). Ascites and hepatomegaly will be present in the majority. Vomiting, splenomegaly, jaundice, or bleeding from oesophageal varices may also occur. If the vena cava is involved there will be dependent oedema.

2. Liver function abnormalities depend on the site and severity of the obstruction. Liver biopsy may show outflow obstruction, hepatic necrosis, and fibrosis.

3. Aetiological factors include polycythaemia, paroxysmal nocturnal haemoglobinuria, antiphospholipid syndrome, protein C deficiency, factor V Leiden, myeloproliferative disorders, and mechanical factors, such as webs and tumours. Hepatic venous thrombosis has been reported in association with ulcerative colitis, but in the patient described, iron deficiency had concealed an underlying polycythaemia vera (Whiteford et al 1999).

4. Treatment is aimed at the preservation of liver function and includes thrombolysis, angioplasty, stent placement, portacaval shunt, mesoatrial shunt, and liver transplantation (Henderson et al 1990).

Anaesthetic problems

1. Hepatic function may be compromised.

2. Surgery may be required for portacaval or mesoatrial shunt, or liver transplantation. This has been described in a patient with paroxysmal nocturnal haemoglobinuria (Taylor et al 1987).

3. Patients may present during pregnancy, when the condition must be distinguished from HELLP syndrome and acute fatty necrosis of the liver. Antiphospholipid syndrome and preeclampsia in a primipara presented with Budd–Chiari syndrome from thrombosis of the right hepatic veins (Segal et al 1996). Caesarean section and liver transplantation took place in a patient at 32 weeks of pregnancy (Valentine et al 1995, Salha et al 1996). Factor V Leiden was the basis for the Budd–Chiari syndrome presenting at 20 weeks' gestation in another patient. Caesarean section at 31 weeks' gestation was followed by acute hepatic failure 6 weeks postpartum, and liver transplantation corrected the coagulopathy (Fickert et al 1996). Thrombotic thrombocytopenic purpura resulted in postpartum hepatic venous thrombosis (Hsu et al 1995). Paroxysmal nocturnal haemoglobinuria has been associated with haemolytic crises and Budd–Chiari syndrome during pregnancy (Bais et al 1994). Maternal deaths have been reported.

Management

1. Haematological examination is important because, in the absence of mechanical causes for hepatic vein thrombosis, there is a high incidence of underlying haematological abnormalities (Boughton 1991); these include myeloproliferative disorders, paroxysmal nocturnal haemoglobinuria, systemic lupus erythematosus, and antithrombin III deficiency.

2. Assessment of liver function, including coagulation.

3. Low-dose heparin infusion from the first postoperative day has been recommended (Henderson et al 1990), with subsequent low-dose aspirin and long-term anticoagulation to reduce the risks of graft thrombosis.

4. Liver transplantation will cure the inherited thrombophilias, for example factor V Leiden, protein C and S, etc. (Fickert et al 1996).

5. In a boy with paroxysmal nocturnal haemoglobinuria who developed Budd–Chiari syndrome, resolution was achieved following bone marrow transplantation (Graham et al 1996).

6. Pregnant patients with paroxysmal nocturnal haemoglobinuria should be carefully monitored for the onset of Budd–Chiari syndrome (see Paroxysmal nocturnal haemoglobinuria).

Bibliography

Bais J, Pel M, von dem Borne A et al 1994 Pregnancy and paroxysmal nocturnal haemoglobinuria. European Journal of Obstetrics, Gynaecology & Reproductive Biology 53: 211–14.

Boughton BJ 1991 Hepatic and portal vein thrombosis. Closely associated with chronic myeloproliferative disorder. British Medical Journal 302: 190–2.

Fickert P, Ramschak H, Kenner L et al 1996 Acute Budd–Chiari syndrome with fulminant hepatic failure in a pregnant woman with factor Leiden mutation. Gastroenterology 111: 1670–3.

Graham ML, Rosse WF, Halperin EC et al 1996 Resolution of Budd–Chiari syndrome following bone marrow transplantation for paroxysmal nocturnal haemoglobinuria. British Journal of Haematology 92: 707–10.

Gupta S, Blumgart LH, Hodgson HJF 1986 Budd–Chiari syndrome: long-term survival and factors affecting mortality. Quarterly Journal of Medicine 60: 781–91.

Henderson JM, Warren WD, Millikan WJ et al 1990 Surgical options, hematologic evaluation, and pathologic changes in Budd–Chiari syndrome. American Journal of Surgery 159: 41–8.

Hsu HW, Belfort MA, Vernino S et al 1995 Postpartum thrombotic thrombocytopenic purpura complicated by Budd–Chiari syndrome. Obstetrics & Gynecology 85: 839–43.

Klein AS, Sitzmann JV, Coleman J et al 1990 Current management of the Budd–Chiari syndrome. Annals of Surgery 212: 144–9.

Mahmoud AEA, Mendoza A, Meshikhes AN et al 1996 Clinical spectrum, investigations and treatment of Budd–Chiari syndrome. Quarterly Journal of Medicine 89: 37–43.

Salha O, Campbell DJ, Pollard S 1996 Budd–Chiari syndrome in pregnancy treated by caesarean section and liver transplant. British Journal of Obstetrics & Gynaecology 103: 1254–6.

Segal S, Shenhav S, Segal O et al 1996 Budd–Chiari syndrome complicating severe preeclampsia in a parturient with primary antiphospholipid syndrome. European Journal of Obstetrics, Gynaecology & Reproductive Biology 68: 227–9.

Taylor MB, Whitwam JG, Worsley A 1987 Paroxysmal nocturnal haemoglobinuria. Perioperative management of a patient with Budd–Chiari syndrome. Anaesthesia 1987; 42: 639–42.

Valentine JMJ, Parkin G, Pollard SG et al 1995 Combined orthotopic liver transplantation and Caesarean section for the Budd–Chiari syndrome. British Journal of Anaesthesia 75: 105–8.

Whiteford MH, Moritz MJ, Ferber A et al 1999 Budd–Chiari syndrome complicating restorative proctocolectomy for ulcerative colitis. Diseases of the Colon & Rectum 42: 1220–4.

Buerger's disease

A type of occlusive peripheral vascular disease which, until recently, predominantly affected young men. Some changes in the disease pattern have been observed (Olin et al 1990). An increasing number of women, more common involvement of the upper extremity, and its occurrence in older patients are being reported (Sasaki et al 1999). There is a strong association with smoking. The disease primarily affects small vessels of the feet, legs, and hands, and is exacerbated by vasospasm. The aetiology is not fully understood, but there may be an immunological component. Abnormal responses to type I and III collagen have been demonstrated. The intense inflammation of the early stages progresses to fibrous encasement of the whole neurovascular bundle.

Preoperative abnormalities

1. Clinical criteria are: i) a smoking history, ii) onset before the age of 50 years, iii) infrapopliteal arterial occlusions, iv) either upper limb involvement or phlebitis migrans, and v) absence of risk factors for atherosclerosis, other than smoking (Shionya 1998).

2. Raynaud's disease, nonhealing ulcers or gangrene of the feet may occur, even in the presence of femoral and popliteal pulses. The hands may be similarly affected. Frequently there is preceding or accompanying phlebitis.

3. Peripheral pulses are reduced or absent. Allen's test may show a poor collateral circulation to the hand.

4. Patients may be improved by stopping smoking, the use of iloprost LD injections, and sympathectomy.

Anaesthetic problem

1. Intra-arterial cannulation for blood pressure monitoring is not usually recommended, and indirect Doppler methods are advised. However, in major procedures there may be overriding indications for direct pressure measurements.

2. Analgesia may be needed for peripheral ischaemia.

Management

1. Axillary artery pressure monitoring in a patient with Buerger's disease and an intracranial aneurysm has been described (Yacoub et al 1987). A continuous axillary brachial plexus block was established before cannulation of the axillary artery with a 20-G catheter. Care was taken to maintain the patient's core temperature with a warming blanket, and there was minimal reduction in arterial pressure during clipping of the aneurysm.

2. Continuous local anaesthesia via a silastic catheter inserted in the region of the median nerve has been reported (Saddler & Crosse 1988).

Bibliography

Mills JL, Porter JM 1991 Buerger's disease (thromboangiitis obliterans). Annals of Vascular Surgery 5: 570–2.

Olin JW, Young JR, Graor RA et al 1990 The changing clinical spectrum of thromboangiitis obliterans. Circulation 82(suppl IV): 3–8.

Saddler JM, Crosse MM 1988 Ischaemic pain in Buerger's disease. Anaesthesia 43: 305–6.

Sasaki S, Sakuma M, Kunihara T et al 1999 Current trends in thromboangiitis obliterans. American Journal of Surgery 177: 316–20.

Shionoya S 1998 Diagnostic criteria of Buerger's disease. International Journal of Cardiology 66(suppl 1): S243–5.

Yacoub OF, Bacaling JH, Kelly M 1987 Monitoring of axillary arterial pressure in a patient with Buerger's disease requiring clipping of an intracerebral aneurysm. British Journal of Anaesthesia 59: 1059–62.

Carcinoid syndrome

Carcinoids are gastrointestinal tumours that arise from the fore-, mid- and hindgut (Kulke & Mayer 1999). Midgut tumours are the commonest, 36–46% occurring in the appendix. Less than 25% of tumours produce the carcinoid syndrome, and the symptoms are probably proportional to the amount of secreting tissue present. Serotonin and the bradykinins are the commonest hormones produced. More recently, the role of the tachykinins (neuropeptides, which include substance P, neurokinin A, and neuropeptide K) has become apparent. Elevated plasma tachykinin levels have been found in nearly 80% of carcinoid tumours.

The majority of patients with the carcinoid syndrome have liver metastases. Exceptions to this are tumours from which the venous blood passes directly into the systemic circulation (eg bronchial and ovarian). In most cases, the liver inactivates the hormones, and no symptoms are produced.

The advent of somatostatin analogues has dramatically improved the medical control of carcinoid symptoms, and the management of the perioperative period (Janmohamed & Bloom 1997). In general, patients treated with octreotide, and prepared for surgery or embolisation, showed decreased basal and provoked release of 5HT and had no intraoperative complications. Two patients who had not initially been given octreotide, developed severe crises on induction of anaesthesia, which responded to iv octreotide (Ahlman et al 1988). The crises correlated well with extremely high levels of 5-HT in the arterial blood. However, even with preoperative sc octreotide, complications can occur. Severe refractory bronchospasm occurred following tracheal intubation after fentanyl, etomidate, lidocaine (lignocaine), and suxamethonium. Octreotide $200\,\mu g$ resolved the crisis within 15 s (Quinlivan & Roberts 1994).

Carcinoid heart disease still carries a poor prognosis, and since the advent of successful symptomatic medical treatment, the heart disease has had more impact on mortality rates (Anderson et al 1997).

Preoperative abnormalities

1. Serotonin can cause diarrhoea, hypertension and tachycardia, mild hyperglycaemia, hypoproteinaemia, and possibly flushing.

2. Bradykinin, if secreted, causes flushing, hypotension, bronchospasm and increased capillary permeability. The latter results in oedema and loss of electrolytes from the vascular compartment. A careful history may help to indicate whether significant amounts of bradykinins are being secreted.

3. Tachykinins cause vasodilatation, and possibly play a role in bronchospasm and fibrosis of the cardiac valves.

4. Other vasoactive peptides such as histamine and prostaglandins may be involved, but their part in the syndrome has not, as yet, been elucidated.

5. Preoperative investigations should include urinary 5-hydroxyindole acetic acid levels, which will be increased, and blood glucose, which may be increased. Liver scan and LFTs may be abnormal, with elevated liver enzyme levels and hypoproteinaemia.

6. In some cases there may be tricuspid or pulmonary valve disease secondary to chronic serotonin secretion.

7. Severe intrapulmonary shunting has been described in a patient with metastatic carcinoid in the absence of liver involvement (Lee & Lepler 1999).

8. Pharmacological treatment may involve inhibitors of 5HT synthesis, peripheral 5HT antagonists, and inhibitors of 5HT release. Ondansetron may improve gastrointestinal symptoms and slow gastric emptying. The main therapeutic indications for octreotide are: failure to control symptoms with surgery or other drugs, unfitness of the patient for surgery, and as

prophylaxis before surgery or investigative procedures (Woods et al 1990). Newer, longer-acting somatostatin analogues are being investigated. Initial reports of lanreotide, which can be given im, once a fortnight, suggest that it may be effective in reducing symptoms (Ruszniewski et al 1996).

Anaesthetic problems

A small number of patients with carcinoid syndrome have developed serious cardiovascular and respiratory complications during anaesthesia, thought to be secondary to secretion of hormones by the tumour, and provoked by mechanical, biochemical, or pharmacological stimuli. Symptoms may be proportional to the amount and nature of the hormone produced, and certainly the prognosis has been found to be related to the level of 5-HIAA (5-hydroxyindoleacetic acid) excreted at the time of diagnosis. This is poor if excretion is greater than $1000 \mu g 24 h^{-1}$. General anaesthesia is not always implicated. A fatal acute crisis has occurred immediately after fine-needle liver biopsy of liver metastases (Bissonnette et al 1990), and a nonfatal one after bronchial biopsy (Sukamaran et al 1982). Both of these procedures were performed under local anaesthesia.

1. Serotonin is invariably produced, and if secreted in excess during anaesthesia, is thought to cause hyperkinetic states of hypertension and tachycardia (Casthely et al 1986, Hughes & Hodkinson 1989), certain types of flushing, and prolonged recovery.

2. Bradykinins may or may not be secreted. Their possible effects include hypotension (Marsh et al 1987), secondary to both vasodilatation and increased capillary permeability, flushing, and bronchospasm (Miller et al 1980, Quinlivan & Roberts 1994). The bradykinin effects seem to be the most life threatening.

3. Tachykinins (substance P, neurokinin A, and neuropeptide K). These primarily cause vasodilatation, but in some cases they may be associated with flushing. However, the flush may occur in the absence of a detectable increase in circulating tachykinins.

4. Other vasoactive substances such as prostaglandins and histamine may be secreted, but their significance is still unknown.

Management

1. Treatment of heart failure, hypoproteinaemia, or electrolyte imbalance, if present.

2. Drugs used to block the release of mediators from the tumour, or to block the actions of the mediators. The mainstay of treatment is now the somatostatin analogue, octreotide. However, most authors still report the supplementary use of other drugs with antiserotonin and antihistamine properties.

   a) Somatostatin analogues have been found to inhibit the release of active mediators from carcinoid tumours. Octreotide (Sandostatin, Sandoz SMS 201–995) has been used both prophylactically as a preparation for surgery, and for emergency treatment of a carcinoid crisis (Marsh et al 1987, Quinlivan & Roberts 1994, Veall et al 1994).

      i) *Preoperative*: octreotide $100 \mu g$ sc bd or tds prior to surgery.

      ii) *Intraoperative*: octreotide $50–100 \mu g$ iv, diluted to $10 \mu g ml^{-1}$, to treat a carcinoid crisis.

   b) Specific antiserotonin or antihistamine therapy. Cyproheptadine is a nonspecific antihistamine. Ketanserin is a selective antagonist at $5HT_2$ receptors, alpha$_1$ adrenoceptors, and H_1 histamine receptors.

      i) *Preoperative*: EITHER cyproheptadine 4 mg tds for 3 days and 4 mg with the premedication OR ketanserin 40 mg bd for 3 days (if available). Recent studies have shown that ondansetron improves gastrointestinal symptoms in carcinoid by slowing gastric emptying (Wymenga et al 1998).

ii) *Intraoperative*: In attempts to treat hypertension and tachycardia arising during anaesthesia, a variety of antiserotoninergic drugs have been used. These have included levomepromazine (methotrimeprazine) 2.5 mg iv, cyproheptadine 1 mg iv (Solares et al 1987), ketanserin 10 mg given over a period of 3 min and then an infusion of 3 mg h^{-1} (Fischler et al 1983, Hughes & Hodkinson 1989). The choice is often governed by the availability of the drug.

3. Anaesthetic drugs. Etomidate and propofol have both been used (Veall et al 1994). Suxamethonium fasciculations may increase intra-abdominal pressure and release tumour hormones. Vecuronium or pancuronium are probably the most appropriate muscle relaxants.

4. Vasopressors of the catecholamine type, or those that act by the release of catecholamines, may activate tumour kallikrein which is the inactive precursor of bradykinin. However, the successful use of epinephrine (adrenaline) has been reported following cardiopulmonary bypass, when the hypotension was thought not to have been related to the carcinoid tumour (Hamid & Harris 1992).

5. Regional anaesthesia does not block the effects of the hormones on the receptors, and hypotension may precipitate a bradykininergic crisis. However, uneventful epidural anaesthesia for transurethral resection of the prostate has been reported in a patient treated with octreotide and other antihormonal drugs (Monteith & Roaseg 1990).

6. For postoperative pain, Veall et al (1994) have used both PCA systems and low-dose epidural fentanyl and bupivacaine infusions.

Bibliography

Ahlman H, Ahlund L, Dahlstrom A et al 1988 SMS 201–995 and provocation tests in preparation of patients with carcinoids for surgery or hepatic arterial embolization. Anesthesia & Analgesia 67: 1142–8.

Anderson AS, Krauss D, Lang R 1997 Cardiovascular complications of malignant carcinoid disease. American Heart Journal 134: 693–702.

Bissonnette RT, Gibney RG, Berry BR et al 1990 Fatal carcinoid crisis after percutaneous fine-needle biopsy of hepatic metastasis: case report and review of the literature. Radiology 174: 751–2.

Casthely PA, Jablons M, Griepp RB et al 1986 Ketanserin in the preoperative and intraoperative management of a patient with carcinoid tumour undergoing tricuspid valve replacement. Anesthesia & Analgesia 65: 809–11.

Fischler M, Dentan M, Westerman MN et al 1983 Prophylactic use of ketanserin in a patient with carcinoid syndrome. British Journal of Anaesthesia 55: 920.

Hamid SK, Harris DNF 1992 Hypotension following valve replacement surgery in carcinoid heart disease. Anaesthesia 47: 490–2.

Hughes EW, Hodkinson BP 1989 Carcinoid syndrome: the combined use of ketanserin and octreotide in the management of an acute crisis during anaesthesia. Anaesthesia & Intensive Care 17: 367–70.

Janmohamed S, Bloom SR 1997 Carcinoid tumours. Postgraduate Medical Journal 73: 207–14.

Kulke MH, Mayer RJ 1999 Carcinoid tumors. New England Journal of Medicine 340: 858–68.

Lee DF, Lepler LS 1999 Severe intrapulmonary shunting associated with metastatic carcinoid. Chest 115: 1203–7.

Lundin L, Hansson H-E, Landelius J et al 1990 Surgical treatment of carcinoid heart disease. Journal of Thoracic & Cardiovascular Surgery 100: 552–61.

Marsh HM, Martin JK, Kvols LK et al 1987 Carcinoid crisis during anesthesia: successful treatment with a somatostatin analogue. Anesthesiology 66: 89–91.

Miller R, Boulukos PA, Warner RRP 1980 Failure of halothane and ketamine to alleviate carcinoid syndrome-induced bronchospasm during anaesthesia. Anesthesia & Analgesia 59: 621–3.

Monteith K, Roaseg OP 1990 Epidural anaesthesia for transurethral resection of the prostate in a patient with the carcinoid syndrome. Canadian Journal of Anaesthesia 37: 349–52.

Quinlivan JK, Roberts WA 1994 Intraoperative octreotide for refractory carcinoid-induced bronchospasm. Anesthesia & Analgesia 78: 400–2.

Roberts LJ II, Marney SR Jr, Oates JA 1979 Blockade

of the flush associated with metastatic gastric carcinoid by combined histamine H_1 and H_2 receptor antagonists. New England Journal of Medicine 300: 236–8.

Ruszniewski P, Ducreux M, Chayvialle JA et al 1996 Treatment of the carcinoid syndrome with the longacting somatostatin analogue lanreotide: a prospective study in 39 patients. Gut 39: 279–83.

Solares G, Blanco E, Pulgar S et al 1987 Carcinoid syndrome and intravenous cyproheptadine. Anaesthesia 42: 989–92.

Sukamaran M, Wilkinson ZS, Christianson L 1982 Acute carcinoid syndrome: a complication of flexible fibreoptic bronchoscopy. Annals of Thoracic Surgery 34: 702–5.

Veall GRQ, Peacock JE, Bax NDS et al 1994 Review of the anaesthetic management of 21 patients undergoing laparotomy for carcinoid syndrome. British Journal of Anaesthesia 72: 335–41.

Woods HF, Bax ND, Ainsworth I 1990 Abdominal carcinoid tumours in Sheffield. Digestion 45: 17–22.

Wymenga AN, de Vries EG, Leijsma MK et al 1998 Effects of ondansetron on gastrointestinal symptoms in carcinoid syndrome. European Journal of Cancer 34: 1293–4.

Cardiac tamponade (see also Section 2)

This can occur when a pericardial effusion (or a collection of blood within the pericardial cavity), restricts, by the effect of external pressure, cardiac filling during diastole. When the pericardium can be distended no further, small volume increases produce a rapid increase in pericardial pressure. There is a fixed, decreased diastolic volume of both ventricles. In inspiration, the right ventricle fills at the expense of the left, and the left ventricular stroke volume decreases, producing pulsus paradoxicus, a cardinal sign. A tachycardia and systemic vasoconstriction will compensate initially for the decrease in cardiac output. Signs of respiratory distress supervene, and sudden cardiac arrest may occur. The mortality rate is 100% when the volume of pericardial fluid is >500 ml. As the tamponade develops, it is the right, rather than the left ventricle, that is compressed. On release of tamponade, there is sudden overload of the left ventricle, while the PVR (pulmonary vascular resistance) remains high.

Malignant disease is the commest cause; infection, trauma, postcardiac surgery, pacemaker or CVP line insertion, intracardiac injection, and anticoagulants are others. The long-term prognosis is related to the cause, irrespective of treatment (Markiewicz et al 1986).

Preoperative abnormalities

1. An elevated CVP, rapid, low-volume pulse, hypotension, and reflex systemic arterial and venous vasoconstriction. The fixed, low cardiac output may be aggravated by straining at stool, or on the assumption of the supine position. Straining may cause syncope (Keon 1981). In a study of 36 patients, the majority had respiratory distress, jugular venous distension, heart rate >90 beat min^{-1}, cardiomegaly, and pulsus paradoxicus (Markiewicz et al 1986). The combination of tachycardia, increased CVP, and hypotension is known as Beck's triad. Infants with pericardial tamponade may not show Beck's classical signs (Musumeci & Hickey 1994).

2. Pulsus paradoxicus. Normally on inspiration there is a slight decrease in systolic blood pressure. In cardiac tamponade this decrease is accentuated, usually to >10 mmHg, and sometimes to >20 mmHg. Pulsus paradoxicus is easily detected by palpation, but may be measured by an auscultation method (Lake 1983). With a sphygmomanometer, the cuff pressure should first be reduced until the sound is intermittent, then deflation continued until all the beats are heard. The difference between the two pressures is then measured.

3. Respiratory distress occurs, especially when lying down.

4. If the collection of fluid is greater than 250 ml, the CXR may show an enlarged, globular cardiac outline, the left border of which may be straight or even convex. The right cardiophrenic angle will be less than 90 degrees. The lung fields are clear. The diagnosis can be confirmed by echocardiography.

Anaesthetic problems

1. Induction of anaesthesia in the presence of cardiac tamponade may be fatal. Abolition of the vasoconstrictor compensation will cause cardiovascular collapse. Cardiac arrest and death during a halothane induction has been reported in a 9-year-old boy, who was about to have a cervical node biopsy (Keon 1981). The child had had a mild degree of respiratory distress, worse in the supine position. Before admission, an episode of loss of consciousness with cyanosis had occurred while straining at stool. Postmortem examination showed a large malignant lymphoma that enveloped the heart and infiltrated the pericardium. Profound hypotension following induction was the first sign of tamponade in a patient involved in a mountaineering accident (Cyna et al 1990). Immediate restoration of arterial pressure occurred after incision of the pericardium. An asymptomatic pericardial effusion in a young woman with seropositive rheumatoid arthritis presented with cardiovascular collapse after induction of anaesthesia for abdominal surgery (Bellamy et al 1990). Fenestration of the pericardium decreased the CVP from 24 mmHg to 10 mmHg.

2. Tamponade may result from central venous cannulation. This occurred in a 7 month old who presented with Beck's triad of tachycardia, hypotension, and increased CVP (Leech et al 1999). However, Beck's triad may not always occur in an infant (Musumeci & Hickey 1994). In a 3-day-old child following surgery for Hirschsprung's disease, parenteral nutrition was given via a right internal jugular catheter. Three hours later, the infant deteriorated abruptly, with cardiac arrest and severe metabolic acidosis. The infusion was stopped, the CVP measured as 22 cmH$_2$O and 12 ml milky fluid was aspirated from the pericardium (Cherng et al 1994). Perforation occurs most commonly in the right atrium, followed by the right ventricle, and finally the superior vena cava (Jiha et al 1996).

3. Sudden drainage of a chronic cardiac tamponade may cause acute haemodynamic changes and pulmonary oedema (Vandyke et al 1983, Downey et al 1991, Hamaya et al 1993). This gradually resolves over 24 h. In one patient, a volume of 500 ml had been removed. Full haemodynamic monitoring was being undertaken, and there was a sudden increase in pulmonary artery pressure after pericardiocentesis. In cardiac tamponade, it is the right rather than the left ventricle that is compressed. After release of the tamponade there is sudden overload of the left ventricle while the PVR is still high. Acute dilatation of the thinner walled right ventricle, and a temporary mismatch between the outputs of the two ventricles were thought to have been responsible for the pulmonary oedema in these patients. Other complications of drainage include laceration of the ventricular wall or a coronary artery, a pneumothorax, or perforation of a viscus (John & Treasure 1990).

4. Occasionally, isolated right atrial compression, which may be difficult to diagnose, can occur following cardiac surgery (Skacel et al 1990). A pulmonary artery catheter was in use and normal pressures were found in all chambers, except the right atrium. There was also a CVP to right ventricular end-diastolic gradient. The chest was reexplored and right atrial compression from bleeding was found. In this case, the pulmonary artery catheter helped to exclude other causes.

Management

1. Monitor direct arterial and central venous pressures.

2. Minimise any factors that can worsen the haemodynamic situation.

3. These are:

a) An increase in intrathoracic pressure. If IPPV is already being undertaken, for example after cardiac surgery, then PEEP should be avoided. This further reduces cardiac output, especially at slow rates of ventilation (Mattila et al 1984). Otherwise, the maintenance of spontaneous respiration, until relief of the tamponade is imminent, has been recommended (Moller et al 1979). High-frequency jet ventilation (HFJV) was found to produce less decrease in stroke volume in experimentally induced cardiac tamponade than continuous mandatory ventilation (CMV) (Goto et al 1990).

b) Low intravascular volume. The blood volume must be maintained with iv fluids, given according to the haemodynamic responses.

c) Decreased myocardial contractility. Dopamine is thought to have a favourable effect on haemodynamics, even in the presence of severe tamponade (Mattila et al 1984). Awake tracheal intubation was used for a patient with blunt chest trauma, followed by a gentle induction with isoflurane and fentanyl (Breen & MacVay 1996). If general anaesthesia is essential, diazepam has been recommended to prevent the reduction in ventricular filling pressure caused by other induction agents (Jain 1998).

4. Urgent relief of tamponade. If possible, needle pericardiocentesis, with or without catheter insertion should be performed under local anaesthesia. ECG and radiological screening should be used, with facilities for emergency thoracotomy available. A subxiphoid approach can be used. Local anaesthesia is infiltrated between the xiphisternum and the left costal margin. With the patient 30–45 degrees head up, a long, 16- or 18-G needle is directed towards the left shoulder. Safety may be increased by the use of a sterile ECG lead attached to the needle. When the epicardium is located, there is elevation of the ST segment. A Seldinger technique with insertion of a soft catheter should be used. Continuous gentle aspiration assists identification of the pericardial sac. A sample of blood is injected onto a gauze swab; defibrinated

pericardial blood does not clot. More recently a technique of percutaneous balloon periocardiotomy has been described. This involves passage of a guidewire into the pericardium via a subxiphoid approach, draining the effusion with a pigtail catheter, then dilating the pericardium with a balloon dilating catheter. The pigtail catheter can be left in place for 24 h. This technique may have a place in the management of malignant pericardial effusions, since it carries less risk than open surgery (Keane & Jackson 1992). It has been suggested that in chronic tamponade, fluid be removed gradually, with close monitoring of haemodynamics to prevent the occurrence of pulmonary oedema (Vandyke et al 1983). A maximum rate of 50 ml min^{-1} has been suggested (Hamaya et al 1993). Symptomatic improvement occurs with the removal of the first 50–200 ml of fluid withdrawn, so there is no urgency to fully decompress the heart.

5. Prevention of pericardial tamponade in association with central venous catheter insertion. The two risk factors are catheter tip location and the angle of incidence made by the catheter against the wall (Jiha et al 1996). It has been suggested that the tip of the catheter should not be more than 2 cm inferior to a line drawn between the lower borders of the medial ends of the clavicles on an upright CXR.

Bibliography

Bellamy MC, Natarajan V, Lenz RJ 1990 An unusual presentation of cardiac tamponade. Anaesthesia 45: 135–6.

Breen PH, MacVay MA 1996 Pericardial tamponade: a case for awake endotracheal intubation. Anesthesia & Analgesia 83: 658.

Brooker RF, Testa LD, Butterworth J et al 1998 Diagnosis and management of acute hypovolaemia after drainage of massive pericardial effusion. Journal of Cardiothoracic & Vascular Anesthesia 12: 690–71.

Cherng Y-G, Cheng Y-J, Chen T-G 1994 Cardiac tamponade in an infant. A rare complication of central venous catheterisation. Anaesthesia 49: 1052–4.

Cobbe SM 1980 Pericardial effusions. British Journal of Hospital Medicine 23: 250–5.

Cyna AM, Rodgers RC, McFarlane H 1990 Hypotension due to unexpected cardiac tamponade. Anaesthesia 45: 140–2.

Downey RJ, Bessler M, Weissman C 1991 Acute pulmonary oedema following pericardiocentesis for chronic cardiac tamponade secondary to trauma. Critical Care Medicine 19: 1323–5.

Goto K, Goto H, Benson KT et al 1990 Efficacy of high-frequency jet ventilation in cardiac tamponade. Anesthesia & Analgesia 70: 375–81.

Hamaya Y, Dohi S, Ueda N et al 1993 Severe circulatory collapse immediately after pericardiocentesis in a patient with chronic cardiac tamponade. Anesthesia & Analgesia 78: 169–71.

Jain AK 1998 Survival after cardiac tamponade and arrest in a paediatric patient with penetrating trauma to pulmonary artery. Paediatric Anaesthesia 8: 345–8.

Jiha JG, Weinberg GL, Laurito CE 1996 Intraoperative cardiac tamponade after central venous cannulation. Anesthesia & Analgesia 82: 664–5.

John RM, Treasure P 1990 How to aspirate the pericardium. British Journal of Hospital Medicine 43: 221–3.

Keane D, Jackson G 1992 Managing recurrent malignant pericardial effusions. Percutaneous balloon pericardiotomy may have a role. British Medical Journal 305: 729–30.

Keon TP 1981 Death on induction of anesthesia for cervical node biopsy. Anesthesiology 55: 471–2.

Lake CL 1983 Anesthesia and pericardial disease. Anesthesia & Analgesia 62: 431–43.

Leech RC, Watts ADJ, Heaton ND et al 1999 Intraoperative cardiac tamponade after central venous cannulation in an infant during orthotopic liver transplantation. Anesthesia & Analgesia 89: 342–3.

Markiewicz W, Borovik R, Ecker S 1986 Cardiac tamponade in medical patients; treatment and prognosis in the echocardiographic era. American Heart Journal 111: 1138–42.

Mattila I, Takkunen O, Mattila P et al 1984 Cardiac tamponade and different modes of ventilation. Acta Anaesthesiologica Scandinavica 28: 236–40.

Moller CT, Schoonbee CG, Rosendorff C 1979 Haemodynamics of cardiac tamponade during various modes of ventilation. British Journal of Anaesthesia 51: 409–15.

Musumeci R, Hickey PR 1994 Anaesthesia in a neonate with tamponade due to massive pericardial effusion. Anesthesia & Analgesia 78: 169–71.

Skacel M, Harrison GA, Verdi IS 1991 A case of isolated right atrial compression following cardiac surgery. The value of pulmonary artery catheterisation. Anaesthesia & Intensive Care 19: 114–15.

Susini G, Pepi M, Sisillo E et al 1993 Percutaneous pericardiocentesis versus subxiphoid pericardiotomy in cardiac tamponade due to postoperative pericardial effusion. Journal of Cardiothoracic & Vascular Anesthesia 7: 178–83.

Vandyke WH, Cure J, Chakko CS et al 1983 Pulmonary oedema after pericardiocentesis for cardiac tamponade. New England Journal of Medicine 309: 595–6.

Cardiomyopathies

A group of diseases of unknown aetiology, affecting cardiac muscle. There are three main pathophysiological groups, diagnosed by echocardiography:

1. *Dilated (congestive) cardiomyopathy*, in which there is a decrease in contractile force in the left or right ventricle, resulting in systolic failure. It may be associated with a number of conditions including those of toxic (eg alcohol), metabolic, neurological, and inflammatory origins. Peripartum cardiomyopathy is a dilated form specifically associated with late pregnancy or the first 5 months of the puerperium. A small group remain who have idiopathic dilated cardiomyopathy, and in whom no obvious cause can be found (Caforio et al 1990).

2. *Hypertrophic cardiomyopathy* (HCM) is an autosomal dominant, inherited condition involving a variety of mutations of genes that encode proteins of the sarcomere. The term 'obstructive' is now omitted because many cases are nonobstructive. Left ventricular hypertrophy is asymmetrical, and the left ventricle is nondilated. Ventricular wall thicknesses vary from mild (13–15 mm) to massive (>30 mm up

to 60 mm). Impaired left ventricular diastolic function may be associated with increased filling pressures and outflow obstruction (Maron 1997). Intermittent arrhythmias are common. It is a dynamic disease and progression occurs.

3. *Restrictive cardiomyopathy* is characterised by a loss of ventricular distensibility, secondary to either endocardial or myocardial problems. There is restriction to diastolic filling, resembling constrictive pericarditis, but systolic function is usually normal. Heart failure occurs in the absence of cardiomegaly or systolic function. This is a rare form (Wilmshurst & Katritsis 1990, Kushawa et al 1997).

Preoperative abnormalities

1. *Dilated cardiomyopathy*. There is significant reduction in ejection fraction (often <0.4 when heart failure supervenes). The heart becomes dilated and there is often increased systemic resistance to compensate. Vasodilators and ACE inhibitors therefore form part of the treatment, with the aim of reducing myocardial work. Systemic embolism can occur, and when arrhythmias (chronic AF or nonsustained ventricular tachycardia) supervene, the patient should be anticoagulated indefinitely. In idiopathic dilated cardiomyopathy there is a high incidence of sudden deaths, which suggests an arrhythmic cause (Caforio et al 1990).

2. *Hypertrophic cardiomyopathy* (HCM, idiopathic hypertrophic subaortic stenosis). The hypertrophy and fibrosis mostly affects the septum, but may involve the whole of the left ventricle. There is resistance to inflow, therefore in advanced disease, diastolic failure is the main problem. The patient may present with dyspnoea, dizziness, syncope or near-syncope, angina, or palpitations. Sudden death can occur, particularly during physical exercise. The strongest risk factors are previous cardiac arrest, multiple sudden deaths in the family, recurrent syncope, massive LVH, and repetitive nonsustained VT (Maron 1997). Whilst sinus rhythm is usual, the late onset of atrial

fibrillation is ominous. An apical and left sternal edge systolic murmur may occur. The patient may be taking beta blockers to prevent tachycardias, or calcium channel blockers to improve myocardial relaxation, and hence pressure/volume relationships (Lorell et al 1982). Once again, the risks of systemic embolism may necessitate anticoagulation. The ECG shows left ventricular hypertrophy, and often Q waves and ST and T wave changes. Chest X-ray usually shows slight cardiomegaly. It may occur as part of Noonan's syndrome. Treatment includes beta blockers, verapamil, diuretics, disopyramide, diltiazem, DDD pacing, septal myectomy, or heart transplantation. Those with risk factors for sudden death may need an AICD.

3. *Restrictive cardiomyopathy*. The individual features of this rare condition are very variable, and depend on the underlying cause. The main feature is the loss of ventricular distensibility secondary to rigidity imposed by endocardial or myocardial disease. One type is associated with marked eosinophilia. In this, there is a reduction in the ventricular cavity size and distortion of the AV valves. Again, there are diastolic filling problems, with a picture resembling that of constrictive pericarditis. It may be associated with Noonan's syndrome, Fabry's disease, sarcoid, and amyloid. The endocardial disease may produce thromboembolic problems, and patients may need anticoagulants. Treatment is with diuretics and amiodarone, and possibly a pacemaker. Vasodilators may be deleterious, and digitalis and beta blockers should only be used cautiously.

The table below provides a summary.

Anaesthetic problems

In advanced cases of these three disease types, the pathophysiology is extremely variable, and the effect of anaesthesia unpredictable. If the diagnosis is known in advance, expert cardiological assessment is essential. However, in many cases, the condition mimics ischaemic or hypertensive heart disease, or may be

	Dilated	**Hypertrophic**	**Restrictive**
Primary problem	systolic	diastolic	diastolic
Presents with	heart failure arrhythmias systemic embolism	dyspnoea syncope angina arrhythmias	eosinophilia heart failure
Principle treatment	diuretics anticoagulants vasodilators ACE inhibitors	amiodarone anticoagulants beta blockers Ca antagonists	steroids cytotoxics
Avoid	myocardial depressants	digoxin beta stimulators vasodilators hypotensives	morphine vasodilators diuretics

unrecognised until an anaesthetic causes decompensation. More detailed advice should be obtained from the references, but a broad outline is given.

1. *Dilated cardiomyopathy.*

a) Myocardial depressants may precipitate acute cardiac failure.

b) Arrhythmias are common, and sudden death can occur. Cardiac arrest followed SVT after induction of anaesthesia in a young man having day case surgery (Hanson 1989). A mild tachycardia and infrequent ventricular ectopics had been present on induction, and anaesthesia was induced with thiopentone 600 mg, atropine 1 mg and lidocaine 400 mg. Subsequent investigation showed a dilated cardiomyopathy. Cardiac arrest on induction for Caesarean section for fetal distress was also the first sign in a 32-year-old woman. Pulmonary oedema occurred on recovery and she was found to have a dilated, poorly contractile left ventricle. Anaphylaxis was excluded (McIndoe et al 1995).

c) Peripartum cardiomyopathy. Although this is associated with pregnancy, it is difficult to know whether or not it is a distinct disease entity, or an unmasking of a pre-

existing condition by the haemodynamic stresses of pregnancy (Witlin et al 1996). In a study of 28 patients, the prognosis was guarded, and recurrence at an early stage in subsequent pregnancies was common. In women presenting for the first time, decompensation usually occurs in association with the periods of maximum haemodynamic change. The peak increases in blood volume (35–40%), and cardiac output (30–40%), occur in the third trimester. In labour and immediately postpartum, there is a further increase in venous return and cardiac output. Thus, peripartum cardiac failure may occur, either in late pregnancy (Lavies & Turner 1989, Dodds et al 1991, Brown et al 1992), or at delivery. Three patients with unexpected peripartum cardiomyopathy presented with acute pulmonary oedema at Caesarean section (Malinow et al 1985, Brown et al 1992). One occurred during spinal anaesthesia, and two after a general anaesthetic. Postoperative echocardiography showed dilated, hypokinetic ventricles, that subsequently returned to normal. In general, the prognosis in the dilated form is poor, but that in the peripartum disease is variable. Some patients die in the acute phase, some have chronic cardiac problems, while others will make a complete recovery, but may relapse in subsequent pregnancies (O'Connell et al 1986, Witlin et al 1996). If cardiomegaly persists at the onset of the next pregnancy, the mortality may be as high as 60%. In a study of myocardial function, at a mean of 10.5 months after delivery, in apparently 'recovered' patients who had regained normal resting left ventricular size, dobutamine challenge testing revealed decreased contractile reserve (Lampert et al 1997).

2. *Hypertrophic cardiomyopathy (HCM).*

a) Patients with HCM undergoing noncardiac surgery have an increased risk of perioperative cardiac events, often manifested as cardiac failure. However, in a review of 77 patients, there were no perioperative deaths (Haering et al 1996).

b) Tachycardias from emotion, exercise and pain, and drugs such as digoxin and beta stimulators, will all increase the outflow tract gradients and may considerably reduce the cardiac output to essential organs, such as the myocardium and brain. Patients are often already taking beta blockers to prevent tachycardias.

c) Pulmonary oedema was reported in a patient during recovery after immersion in a bath for ESWL. Transient dynamic obstruction was thought to have occurred, secondary to a reduction in CVP and decrease in preload (Wulfson & LaPorta 1993).

d) Hypotension from blood loss, regional anaesthesia, or vasodilator drugs, cause similar reductions in cardiac output and can worsen obstruction. A series of 52 general and four spinal anaesthetics in patients with HCM was reviewed (Thompson et al 1985). One of the patients having a spinal anaesthetic sustained a myocardial infarction and subsequently died. Severe bradycardia and hypotension has been reported in patients

with hypertrophic cardiomyopathy during spinal anaesthesia (Baraka et al 1987), and epidural anaesthesia (Loubser et al 1984).

e) Pregnancy may be associated with increasing shortness of breath which responds to diuretics, and occasionally with angina.

f) A systolic murmur may be present, which increases in intensity when blood loss occurs, and decreases when intravascular volume is increased (Lanier & Prough 1984). These authors thought that HCM should be considered in any elderly patient who developed a systolic murmur during longstanding hypertension.

g) Arrhythmias. The patient may already be taking amiodarone for these.

h) Anticoagulant therapy.

3. *Restrictive cardiomyopathy.*

a) A reduction in intravascular volume will decrease the ventricular filling pressure and accentuate the existing restriction to diastolic filling.

b) Changes in heart rate in either direction will impair diastolic filling.

c) Frequently the systolic function is normal. In some cases there is an additional impairment of ventricular function. In these, myocardial depressants may cause cardiovascular collapse.

Management

In advanced cases, careful cardiological assessment is required. The presence of cardiac failure will necessitate the monitoring of direct arterial blood pressure and ventricular filling pressures. Facilities for temporary pacing should be immediately available. The anaesthetist should understand the pathophysiology of the condition and the cardiovascular effects of the drugs and anaesthetic agents used.

1. *Dilated cardiomyopathy.*

a) Myocardial depressants such as thiopentone, halothane, and enflurane should be avoided. A nitrous oxide, oxygen, narcotic, benzodiazepine, muscle relaxant technique is preferred.

b) The ECG should be carefully observed for ventricular arrhythmias and heart block, so that treatment can be instituted rapidly.

c) Regional anaesthesia may be considered for appropriate surgical procedures, provided the filling pressures are well controlled, and there is no myocardial ischaemia. An epidural anaesthetic was given for hip replacement, to a patient with severe dilated cardiomyopathy caused by alcohol (Amaranath et al 1986). PAP was measured, and the only complication was an episode of pulmonary hypertension after insertion of the femoral prosthesis. Epidural anaesthesia has also been used for Caesarean section using an impedance cardiograph for haemodynamic monitoring (Gambling et al 1987). Two episodes of hypotension were treated with ephedrine. If epidural anaesthesia is to be used in labour, it should be induced slowly, with time to make adjustments to fluid and inotrope therapy (George et al 1997).

d) Caesarean section was performed under infiltration anaesthesia in a 30-week-pregnant woman who presented with gross pulmonary oedema and an enlarged heart. Initial dramatic improvement after delivery was not sustained. Her echocardiograms showed deteriorating left ventricular function and she died at 72 h, despite intra-aortic balloon pumping (Mellor & Bodenham 1996).

e) Patients in heart failure require diuretics, and may need dobutamine or dopamine if there is a low cardiac output state. Occasionally isoprenaline may be necessary. Sodium nitroprusside can improve cardiac output by reducing the ventricular afterload. The use of continuous arteriovenous haemofiltration has been described to urgently treat refractory congestive heart failure, in preparation for Caesarean section under epidural anaesthesia (Dodds et al 1991).

2. *Hypertrophic cardiomyopathy.* The obstruction is dynamic (Maron et al 1997). Management should aim to decrease the obstruction, by reducing myocardial contractility, and increasing preload and afterload.

a) A tachycardia from premedication, intubation, too light anaesthesia, ketamine, or cardiac stimulants must be avoided. Preoperative beta blockers should be maintained. An infusion of esmolol was used for the management of cerebral aneurysm surgery (Freilich & Jacobs 1991), for postbypass treatment (Ooi et al 1993), and for vaginal delivery under epidural anaesthesia (Fairley & Clarke 1995).

b) Drugs and techniques that cause vasodilatation and hypotension must be avoided, therefore regional anaesthesia is generally contraindicated. However, with the greater ability to control the onset of epidural and spinal blocks by the use of continuous infusions and opiates, it has been suggested that regional blocks are no longer contraindicated. Ho et al (1997) describe the use of a fentanyl and 0.1% bupivacaine infusion and invasive monitoring for vaginal delivery.

c) An adequate preload should be given and blood loss should be replaced promptly. An intraoperative diagnosis of HCM was made during hip replacement in a patient with a history of hypertension (Lanier & Prough 1984). Blood loss was associated with a sudden increase in intensity of her systolic murmur and the appearance of a systolic click. Subsequent echocardiography confirmed the diagnosis.

d) Since isoflurane and morphine produce veno-dilatation, halothane or enflurane, and opiates such as fentanyl, alfentanil or remifentanil, should be used in preference (Campbell & Bousfield 1992). Harley et al (1996) used fentanyl and isoflurane in two patients undergoing orthotopic liver transplant. Intraoperative transoesophageal echocardiography was used to assist the management of haemodynamics and fluid therapy. A propofol infusion was used for clipping of a cerebral aneurysm, and phenylephrine was given whenever the systolic and pulmonary artery pressures decreased below 100 mmHg and 24/12 mmHg respectively (Edmends & Ghosh 1994).

Isoflurane, despite apparent contraindications, was used for a neurosurgical procedure (Freilich & Jacobs 1990), and again, in their patient, phenylephrine was used to control hypotension. Provided the pulse is slow, and the vascular volume maintained, halothane will minimise the severity of the obstruction by decreasing the force of ventricular contraction. A propofol infusion has been described for cardiac surgery (Bell & Goodchild 1989).

e) Caesarean section should be managed with general anaesthesia rather than epidural anaesthesia (Oakley et al 1979). The routine use of ergometrine has been recommended (Oakley et al 1979), although an infusion of syntocinon produces less vasodilatation than a bolus dose.

f) Hypotension should be treated by restoring vascular volume. If vasopressors are required, an alpha$_1$ agonist, such as phenylephrine (Freilich & Jacobs 1990), or methoxamine, is the most suitable.

3. *Restrictive cardiomyopathy.* Maintenance of the compensatory mechanisms for the impaired diastolic filling are essential.

a) Adequate ventricular filling. Blood volume is maintained, and morphine and isoflurane avoided because of venous dilatation.

b) Adequate heart rate. Pancuronium may be advantageous.

c) Myocardial contractility. In severe disease, fentanyl, ketamine, and benzodiazepines should be used rather than thiopentone or halothane.

d) Avoid the use of vasodilators and diuretics.

4. Some patients with end-stage cardiac failure require cardiac transplantation or dynamic cardiomyoplasty (Lehmann et al 1999), and these patients may subsequently appear for surgery.

Bibliography

Amaranath L, Esfandiari S, Lockrem J et al 1986 Epidural analgesia for total hip replacement in a patient with dilated cardiomyopathy. Canadian Anaesthetists' Society Journal 33: 84–8.

Baraka A, Jabbour S, Itani I 1987 Severe bradycardia following epidural anesthesia in a patient with idiopathic hypertrophic subaortic stenosis. Anesthesia & Analgesia 66: 1337–8.

Bell MD, Goodchild CS 1989 Hypertrophic obstructive cardiomyopathy in combination with prolapsing mitral valve. Anaesthesia for surgical correction with propofol. Anaesthesia 44: 409–11.

Brown G, O'Leary M, Douglas I et al R 1992 Perioperative management of a severe peripartum cardiomyopathy. Anaesthesia & Intensive Care 20: 80–3.

Caforio APL, Stewart JT, McKenna WJ 1990 Idiopathic dilated cardiomyopathy. Rational treatment awaits better understanding of pathogenesis. British Medical Journal 300: 890–1.

Campbell AM, Bousfield JD 1992 Anaesthesia in a patient with Noonan's syndrome and cardiomyopathy. Anaesthesia 47: 131–3.

Dodds TM, Haney MF, Appleton FM 1991 Management of peripartum congestive heart failure using continuous arteriovenous haemofiltration in a patient with myotonic dystrophy. Anesthesiology 75: 907–11.

Edmends S, Ghosh S 1994 Hypertrophic obstructive cardiomyopathy complicating surgery for cerebral artery aneurysm clipping. Anaesthesia 49: 608–9.

Fairley CJ, Clarke JT 1995 Use of esmolol in a parturient with hypertrophic obstructive cardiomyopathy. British Journal of Anaesthesia 75: 801–4.

Freilich JD, Jacobs BR 1990 Anesthetic management of cerebral aneurysm resection in a patient with idiopathic hypertrophic subaortic stenosis. Anesthesia & Analgesia 71: 558–60.

Gambling DR, Flanagan ML, Huckell VE et al 1987 Anaesthetic management and non-invasive monitoring for Caesarean section in a patient with cardiomyopathy. Canadian Journal of Anaesthesia 34: 505–8.

George LM, Gatt SP, Lowe S 1997 Peripartum cardiomyopathy: four case histories and a commentary on anaesthetic management. Anaesthesia & Intensive Care 25: 292–6.

Haering JM, Comunale ME, Parker RA et al 1996 Cardiac risk of noncardiac surgery in patients with asymmetric septal hypertrophy. Anesthesiology 85: 254–9.

Hanson CW 1989 Asymptomatic cardiomyopathy presenting as cardiac arrest in the day surgical unit. Anesthesiology 71: 982–4.

Harley ID, Jones EF, Liu G et al 1996 Orthotopic liver transplantation in two patients with hypertrophic obstructive cardiomyopathy. British Journal of Anaesthesia 77: 675–7.

Ho KM, Kee WDN, Poon MCM 1997 Combined spinal and epidural anesthesia in a parturient with idiopathic hypertrophic subaortic stenosis. Anesthesiology 87: 168–9.

Kushwaha SS, Fallon JT, Fuster V 1997 Restrictive cardiomyopathy. New England Journal of Medicine 336: 267–76.

Lampert MB, Weinert L, Hibbard J et al 1997 Contractile reserve in patients with peripartum cardiomyopathy and recovered left ventricular function. American Journal of Obstetrics & Gynecology 176: 189–95.

Lanier W, Prough DS 1984 Intraoperative diagnosis of hypertrophic obstructive cardiomyopathy. Anesthesiology 60: 61–3.

Lavies NG, Turner DAB 1989 Peripartum cardiomyopathy. A rare cause of pulmonary oedema in late pregnancy. Anaesthesia 44: 770–2.

Lehmann A, Faust K, Boldt J et al 1999 Dynamic cardioplasty in patients with end-stage heart failure; anaesthetic considerations. British Journal of Anaesthesia 82: 140–3.

Lorell BH, Paulus WJ, Grossman W et al 1982 Modification of abnormal left ventricular diastolic

properties by nifedipine in patients with hypertrophic cardiomyopathy. Circulation 65: 499–507.

Loubser P, Suh K, Cohen S 1984 Adverse affects of spinal anesthesia in a patient with idiopathic hypertrophic subaortic stenosis. Anesthesiology 60: 228–30.

McIndoe AK, Hammond EJ, Babington PCB 1995 Peripartum cardiomyopathy presenting as a cardiac arrest at induction of anaesthesia for Caesarean section. British Journal of Anaesthesia 75: 97–101.

Malinow AM, Butterworth JF, Johnson MD 1985 Peripartum cardiomyopathy presenting at Cesarean delivery. Anesthesiology 63: 545–7.

Maron BJ 1997 Hypertrophic cardiomyopathy. Lancet 350: 127–33.

Oakley GDG, McGarry K, Limb DG et al 1979 Management of pregnancy in patients with hypertrophic cardiomyopathy. British Medical Journal 1: 1749–50.

O'Connell JB, Constanzo-Nordin MR, Subramanian R et al 1986 Peripartum cardiomyopathy: clinical hemodynamic, histologic and prognostic characteristics. Journal of the American College of Cardiology 8: 52–6.

Ooi LG, O'Shea PJ, Wood AJ 1993 Use of esmolol in the postbypass management of hypertrophic obstructive cardiomyopathy. British Journal of Anaesthesia 70: 104–6.

Wilmshurst PT, Katritsis D 1990 Restrictive cardiomyopathy. British Journal of Cardiology 63: 323–4.

Witlin AG, Mabie WC, Sibai BM 1996 Peripartum cardiomyopathy: an ominous diagnosis. American Journal of Obstetrics & Gynecology 176: 182–8.

Wulfson HD, LaPorta RF 1993 Pulmonary oedema after lithotripsy in a patient with hypertrophic subaortic stenosis. Canadian Journal of Anaesthesia 40: 465–7.

Carnitine palmitoyl transferase deficiency (CPTD)

An autosomal recessive, metabolic myopathy involving an inability to use fatty acids for energy production in muscle. It is secondary to deficencies of CPT1 or CPT2, enzymes involved mitochondrial fatty acid oxidation (Schaefer et al 1997). It is thought to be an underdiagnosed condition, because episodes of muscle cramps and red urine following intense exercise may be ignored (Katzir et al 1996). It is characterised by episodes of rhabdomyolysis, myoglobinuria, and lipid accumulation. Carnitine palmitoyl transferase (CPT) is present on both sides of the mitochondrial membrane, CPT1 on the outer, and CPT2 on the inner (Schaefer et al 1997). It converts acyl-CoA to acylcarnitine, to enable it to cross the membrane, and on the inner side converts it back again. Thus, CPT deficiency impairs the entry of long chain acyl-CoA compounds from the cytosol into mitochondria, with the result that mitochondria are unable to utilise long chain fatty acids for energy production. Muscle requires 50% of its energy from fatty acids and ketone bodies, even at rest. During fasting or exercise, glucose becomes depleted and if fatty acids cannot be used, energy production is reduced, the ATP which is needed to maintain the integrity of the sarcoplasm is depleted, and rhabdomyolysis ensues (Kelly et al 1989). A high fat diet may also cause problems by overloading the system.

An alternative theory is that the disease involves alteration in the regulatory properties of CPT rather than a deficiency (Zierz & Schmitt 1989), and these authors have shown that CPT is abnormally inhibited by malonyl Co-A or by increasing the substrate/product concentration. The enzyme is vulnerable if lipid metabolism is stressed, and they suggest that general anaesthetics may initiate rhabdomyolysis by interfering with the lipid matrix.

Preoperative abnormalities

1. There are different forms of the disease. Infantile forms are usually associated with early death and will not be considered further here.

2. The adult 'benign' form involves CPT2 deficiency and the patient may be totally asymptomatic, or episodes of muscle pains, weakness, and rhabdomyolysis, may occur after exercise, with asymptomatic periods between (Faigel 1995, Katzir et al 1996).

3. A fatal attack of rhabdomyolysis and renal failure occurred in a child in association with a severe viral infection (Kelly et al 1989). Investigation of the child and her sister showed the unsuspected abnormality.

4. During an attack, patients are advised to rest, and maintain fluid intake and a suitable diet.

Anaesthetic problems

1. An adult male, given suxamethonium for gastrectomy, passed dark brown urine postoperatively, became oliguric, and subsequently developed renal failure (Katsuya et al 1988).

2. Starvation and dehydration may precipitate acute rhabdomyolysis and myoglobinuria.

3. A few patients have been described during pregnancy. In one, Caesarean section was performed because of failure to progress. Biopsy of uterine and abdominal wall showed an absence of CPT enzyme activity. However, glucose was given during her second labour and delivery was normal (Dreval et al 1994). Spinal anaesthesia has been used for vaginal delivery (Madirosoff et al 1997).

Management

1. Give glucose and fluids during periods of starvation. Avoid overloading with triglycerides.

2. Avoid the use of suxamethonium, in case it precipitates rhabdomyolysis.

Bibliography
Dreval D, Bernstein D, Zakut H 1994 Carnitine palmitoyl transferase deficiency in pregnancy—a case report. American Journal of Obstetrics & Gynecology 170: 1390–2.
Faigel HC 1995 Carnitine palmitoyl transferase deficiency in a college athlete: a case report and literature review. Journal of American College Health 44: 51–4.
Katsuya H, Misumi M, Ohtani Y et al 1988 Postanesthetic acute renal failure due to carnitine palmityl transferase deficiency. Anesthesiology 68: 945–8.

Katzir Z, Hochman B, Biro A et al 1996 Carnitine palmitoyltransferase deficiency: an underdiagnosed condition? American Journal of Nephrology 16: 162–6.

Kelly K, Garland JS, Tang TT et al 1989 Fatal rhabdomyolysis following influenza infection in a girl with familial carnitine palmityl transferase deficiency. Pediatrics 84: 312–16.

Mardirosoff C, Dumont L, Cobin L et al 1997 Labour analgesia in a patient with carnitine palmityl transferase deficiency and idiopathic thrombocytopenic purpura. International Journal of Obstetric Anesthesia 7: 134–6.

Schaefer J, Jackson S, Taroni F et al 1997 Characterisation of carnitine palmitoyltransferases in patient with carnitine palmitoyltransferase deficiency: implications for diagnosis and therapy. Journal of Neurology, Neurosurgery & Psychiatry 62: 169–76.

Zierz S, Schmitt U 1989 Inhibition of carnitine palmitoyl transferase by maloyl-CoA in human muscle is influenced by anesthesia. Anesthesiology 70: 373.

Carotid body tumour

A tumour of ectodermal origin. One of a group known as the paragangliomas, which are associated with the sympathetic nervous system. The cells of the carotid body normally act as chemoreceptors, but in common with other APUD cells, can secrete a variety of amines and peptides. Most carotid body tumours are nonfunctional, but occasionally they secrete norepinephrine (noradrenaline), dopamine, calcitonin, or ACTH. They may be malignant, may enlarge and invade locally, and can produce metastases. Surgery is, therefore, the treatment of choice (Bernard 1992, Bastounis et al 1999).

Preoperative abnormalities

1. The tumour usually presents as a mass in the neck.

2. Arteriography or DVI is essential to delineate the blood supply.

3. Radioisotope scans may show tumours elsewhere.

4. Clinical signs of catecholamine secretion should be sought, and if these are suggestive, biochemical tests may be required. However, endocrine activity is rare, except in the case of familial carotid body tumours, when the incidence has been shown to be 31.8% (Grufferman et al 1980, Netterville et al 1995).

Anaesthetic problems

1. Those of catecholamine secretion, if the tumour is functional. Patients with multiple carotid body tumours, or a family history, often have associated phaeochromocytomas (Campeau & Graves 1991), and these are detectable by mIBG scan. A patient with a previous resection of carotid body tumour, and a father with the same diagnosis, had severe hypertension during excision of the second tumour. He had a stormy perioperative period and was later found to have an adrenal mass secreting norepinephrine (noradrenaline) (Connelly & Baker 1995). Episodes of severe hypertension and tachycardia during anaesthesia for biopsy of undiagnosed neck masses have also been recorded (Clarke et al 1976, Newland & Hurlbert 1980). Both patients were found to have increased catecholamine levels, and were treated as for phaeochromocytoma during their subsequent tumour resection.

2. Blood loss may be brisk and heavy. In one operation, 11 litres were lost (Connolly & Baker 1995).

3. Heparinisation is occasionally required.

4. Reflex bradycardia, and occasionally cardiovascular collapse, secondary to carotid sinus stimulation (Kraayenbrink & Steven 1985).

5. Postoperative complications are not uncommon and include cranial nerve palsy, cerebrovascular accident (Wright et al 1979), severe hypertension, and aspiration pneumonia.

6. Postoperative baroreceptor failure. Patients with bilateral resection have had large fluctuations in blood pressure and sustained increases in heart rate (Netterville et al 1995).

On occasions, serious hypertensive events occurred, one of which resulted in a massive stroke. Baroreflex failure is recognised as a labile blood pressure associated with plasma catecholamine fluctuations, and clonidine attenuates the pressure surges and tachycardias (Robertson et al 1993).

7. It has been suggested that those patients who undergo resection on both carotid bodies may also lose their reflex respiratory stimulation to hypoxia. This was thought to have contributed to respiratory arrest in one patient receiving PCA morphine on return to the ward from ITU, although in his case, obstructive sleep apnoea may have contributed (Connolly & Baker 1995).

Management

1. Look for evidence of phaeochromo-cytoma. If present, see management of phaeochromocytoma.

2. Embolisation of the tumour before surgery has been reported to reduce intraoperative blood loss (LaMuraglia et al 1992).

3. The use of nasotracheal intubation improves surgical access (Bernard 1992).

4. Atropine may be required for bradycardias, although this may not protect the patient from cardiovascular collapse, even when the carotid sinus is only lightly stimulated. A technique has been proposed in which the dissection to expose the carotid bifurcation is performed so that it avoids pressure on the sinus. Lidocaine is irrigated locally, before infiltration with further lidocaine (Boyd 1980).

5. The surgeon may require to use a nerve stimulator to reduce the risk of nerve injury, in which case, only partial neuromuscular blockade should be employed.

6. In patients who have had resections to both sides, careful monitoring of postoperative blood pressure is required because of baroreceptor failure. Netterville et al (1995)

suggested that in those patients who have undergone vascular repair, sodium nitroprusside should be used initially, whilst waiting for the effects of an oral agent, such as clonidine or phenoxybenzamine, to take effect.

Bibliography

Bastounis E, Maltezos C, Pikoulis E et al 1999 Surgical treatment of carotid body tumours. European Journal of Surgery 165: 198–200.

Bernard RP 1992 Carotid body tumors. American Journal of Surgery 163: 494–6.

Boyd CH 1980 Anaesthesia for carotid body tumour resection. Anaesthesia 35: 720.

Campeau RJ, Graves C 1991 Pheochromocytoma associated with prior carotid body tumors (chemodectomas). Detection with I-131 mIBG. Clinical Nuclear Medicine 17: 511–12.

Clarke AD, Matheson H, Boddie HG 1976 Removal of catecholamine-secreting chemodectoma. Anaesthesia 31: 1225–30.

Connolly RA, Baker AB 1995 Excision of bilateral carotid body tumours. Anaesthesia & Intensive Care 23: 342–5.

Grufferman S, Gillman MW, Pasternak LR et al 1980 Familial carotid body tumours: case report and epidemiological review. Cancer 46: 2116–22.

Kraayenbrink MA, Steven CM 1985 Anaesthesia for carotid body tumour resection in a patient with the Eisenmenger syndrome. Anaesthesia 40: 1194–7.

LaMuraglia GM, Fabian RL, Brewster DC et al 1992 The current surgical management of carotid body paragangliomas. Journal of Vascular Surgery 15: 1038–44.

Netterville JL, Reilly KM, Robertson D et al 1995 Carotid body tumors: a review of 30 patients with 46 tumours. Laryngoscope 105: 115–26.

Newland MC, Hurlbert BJ 1980 Chemodectoma diagnosed hypertension and tachycardia during anesthesia. Anesthesia & Analgesia 59: 388–90.

Robertson D, Hollister AS, Biaggioni I et al 1993 The diagnosis and treatment of baroreflex failure. New England Journal of Medicine 329: 1449–55.

Wright DJ, Pandya A, Noel F 1979 Anaesthesia for carotid body tumour resection. Anaesthesia 34: 806–8.

Central core disease (CCD)

A nonprogressive, congenital myopathy, usually inherited as autosomal dominant. Pathological abnormalities of the sarcoplasmic reticulum and the t-tubules have been shown. There is a strong association with malignant hyperthermia (MH), although the conditions are not the same. Genetic studies suggest that the gene responsible is situated on chromosome 19 close to one of the MH genes (Haan et al 1990). However, not all individuals are susceptible to MH. Halsall et al (1996) studied six families; three were screened for MH because of they were known to have CCD, and three were diagnosed as having CCD as a result of investigation for a malignant hyperthermia reaction. Out of 19 patients, eight were MH susceptible, nine were negative and two were equivocal. Surgery may be required for correction of hip or other orthopaedic deformities.

Preoperative abnormalities

1. Can present with infantile or childhood hypotonia (floppy infant), motor delay, and proximal muscle weakness. However, in general the myopathy is mild and nonprogressive, and there is a broad range of clinical expression. In some the myopathy is clinically undetectable, whereas in a small number of patients it is severe (Halsall et al 1996).

2. Deep tendon reflexes may be reduced or absent.

3. Orthopaedic abnormalities included congenital dislocation or subluxation of the hip (probably secondary to muscle weakness), pes planus, and joint hypermobility (Gamble et al 1988). Scoliosis and patellar dislocation were also seen. Patients are prone to develop joint contractures.

4. An increased incidence of mitral valve prolapse has been reported (Shuaib et al 1987).

5. The diagnosis is made on muscle biopsy; type 1 fibres show 'cores' within the fibres, amorphous-looking areas, that have a deficiency of mitochondria and lack of oxidative enzyme activity (Loke & MacLennan 1998).

Anaesthetic problems

1. Some patients with central core disease are susceptible to malignant hyperthermia, a condition with which it is closely associated (Frank et al 1980, Halsall et al 1996), and death has occurred. Status epilepticus, a temperature of 42°C, and a pH of 7.1 developed in a patient 4 h after meningioma resection. Suxamethonium was given for subsequent evacuation of blood clot and the next day he developed myoglobinuria and renal failure from which he died (Prescott et al 1992). Histological examination of muscle showed central core disease. Sevoflurane was the triggering agent in one patient who had a nonfatal episode of MH that responded to dantrolene (Otsuka et al 1991). Harriman (1986) showed that seven out of eight patients with central core disease were susceptible to malignant hyperthermia on *in vitro* contracture testing. Another study confirmed that 11 patients from four families were found to be susceptible (Shuaib et al 1987). Halsall et al (1996) found that eight out of 19 individuals in three families with central core disease were susceptible to MH.

2. One 19-year-old patient developed an increase in $ETCO_2$, 30 min after suxamethonium and desflurane anaesthesia. Subsequent investigation showed a congenital myopathy and central core disease (Garrido et al 1999).

3. A patient with a psychiatric disorder given haloperidol developed hyperthermia, rigidity and hypertension. Muscle biopsy suggested central core disease (Calore et al 1994).

Management

1. Assessment of severity of myopathy.

2. It had been suggested that all patients with central core disease should be considered to be at risk for malignant hyperthermia unless *in vitro* contracture tests show that the particular patient is free from the trait (Shuaib et al 1987). Not all patients with central core disease are susceptible

to MH, and the disease is genetically heterogeneous (Curran et al 1999).The importance of all individuals with CCD being screened, regardless of the MH status of their relatives, has therefore been stressed (Halsall et al 1996, Curran et al 1999). If testing is not undertaken, individuals and their families will have to be treated as for MH, with all its implications.

3. Examination for mitral valve prolapse.

4. Avoidance of suxamethonium.

Bibliography

Allen GC, Brubaker CL 1998 Human malignant hyperthermia associated with desflurane anesthesia. Anesthesia & Analgesia 86: 1328–31.

Calore EE, Cavaliere MJ, Perez NM et al 1994 Hyperthermic reaction to haloperidol with rigidity, associated to central core disease. Acta Neurologica 16: 157–61.

Curran JL, Hall WJ, Halsall PJ et al 1999 Segregration of malignant hyperthermia, central core disease and chromosome 19 markers. British Journal of Anaesthesia 83: 217–22.

Frank JP, Harati Y, Butler IJ et al 1980 Central core disease and malignant hyperthermia syndrome. Annals of Neurology 7: 11–17.

Gamble JG, Rinsky LA, Lee JH 1988 Orthopedic aspects of central core disease. Journal of Bone & Joint Surgery 70A: 1061–6.

Garrido S, Fraga M, Martin MJ et al 1999 Malignant hyperthermia during desflurane-succinylcholine anesthesia for orthopedic surgery. Anesthesiology 90: 1208–9.

Haan EA, Freemantle CJ, Mccure JA et al 1990 Assignment of the gene for central core disease to chromosome 19. Human Genetics 86: 187–90.

Halsall PJ, Bridges LR, Ellis FR et al 1996 Should patients with central core disease be screened for malignant hyperthermia? Journal of Neurology, Neurosurgery & Psychiatry 61: 119–21.

Harriman DGF 1986 The definition of normal muscle and of malignant hyperthermia and the association of myopathies with the malignant hyperthermia trait. Muscle & Nerve 9 (suppl 1) 222.

Loke J, MacLennan DH 1998 Malignant hyperthermia and central core disease: disorders of Ca^{2+} release channels. American Journal of Medicine 104: 470–86.

Otsuka H, Komura Y, Mayumi T et al 1991 Malignant hyperthermia during sevoflurane anesthesia in a child with central core disease. Anesthesiology 75: 699–701.

Prescott RJ, Roberts SP, Williams G 1992 Malignant hyperpyrexia: a rare cause of postoperative death. Journal of Clinical Pathology 45: 361–3.

Shuaib A, Paasuke RT, Brownell KW 1987 Central core disease. Clinical features in 13 patients. Medicine 66: 389–96.

C1 esterase inhibitor deficiency (acquired)

This may be a familial (see Hereditary angioneurotic oedema) or, more rarely, an acquired disorder involving the complement system. The acquired form is mostly associated with a B-lymphocyte malignancy, and antibodies have been detected against abnormal immunoglobulins present on the malignant B-cells. Reaction between the two cause C1 activation, which in turn produces a secondary reduction in the concentrations of C1, C2 and C4 and a reduced functional activity of C1 esterase inhibitor (Geha et al 1985). This form must be distinguished from the physical forms of angioedema that occur in response to food, drugs or insect bites, or in association with connective tissue disorders. Recently, a number of patients have developed angioedema in response to treatment with ACE inhibitors, particularly enalapril and captopril (Barna & Frable 1990). Substantial increases in plasma bradykinin have been demonstrated during attacks of hereditary, acquired, and captopril-induced angioneurotic oedema (Nussberger et al 1998).

Preoperative abnormalities

1. Intermittent attacks of angioneurotic oedema that can involve any part of the body, and result from extravasation of intravascular fluid and protein into subcutaneous and mucosal structures (Gelfand et al 1979).

2. As with hereditary angioneurotic oedema,

there is a low level of C1 esterase inhibitor, and sometimes life threatening episodes of oedema of the upper airway may develop in response to stress or local trauma, particularly dental treatment (Frigas 1989). However, attacks of oedema may occur without any obvious reason, and recurrent abdominal pain may be a presenting feature.

3. As with the hereditary form, epinephrine (adrenaline), antihistamines, and steroids are ineffective for prophylaxis, and for treatment of these attacks.

4. The two conditions may be distinguished by the fact that in the acquired form the onset is late, no family history is elicited, no complement abnormalities are found in the patient's blood relatives, and the underlying malignancy may already have been diagnosed.

5. Differentiation may now be made on measurement of the C1q subunit of C1; patients with acquired deficiency have a decreased level of C1q, compared with those with the hereditary form, in whom the C1 level is normal (Alsenz et al 1987).

Anaesthetic problems

1. Tracheal intubation and manipulation of the upper airway may precipitate local angioneurotic oedema, for which treatment with epinephrine (adrenaline), steroids, and antihistamines is ineffective. Oedema may also occur after dental extractions.

2. Although tranexamic acid has been recommended to prevent attacks in both forms, venous thrombosis has been reported after its prophylactic use during surgery in the acquired disease (Razis et al 1986).

3. A patient with acquired C1 esterase inhibitor deficiency undergoing cardiopulmonary bypass had massive activation of the common pathway, coagulation problems, pulmonary oedema, and circulatory collapse (Bonser et al 1991).

Management

1. Danazol is a progestogen derivative that probably increases the hepatic synthesis of C1 esterase inhibitor. Its prophylactic value in the acquired and hereditary disorders has been reported (Razis et al 1986). Danazol 200 mg tds should be given preoperatively, but may take several days to become effective. Alternatively, stanozolol $0.5–8$ mg day^{-1} can also be used (Frigas 1989). The lower levels will be required for maintenance, whilst higher levels may be needed in the initial stages. A patient with autoimmune C1 EI, who was known to be carrying a male fetus, was given short-term therapy at 40 weeks' gestation (Marescal et al 1999).

2. Tranexamic acid should probably be avoided in the acquired form, especially in the presence of a thrombocytosis.

3. The preoperative prophylactic use of fresh frozen plasma, and C1 esterase inhibitor concentrate has been reported (Plenderleith et al 1988). Purified C1 esterase inhibitor can be obtained from Immuno Limited (Rye Lane, Dunton Green, Sevenoaks, Kent TN14 5HB, UK).

Bibliography

Alsenz J, Bork K, Loos M 1987 Autoantibody-mediated acquired deficiency of C1 inhibitor. New England Journal of Medicine 316: 1360–6.

Barna JS, Frable MA 1990 Life-threatening angioedema. Otolaryngology—Head & Neck Surgery 103: 795–8.

Bonser RS, Dave J, Morgan J et al 1991 Complement activation during bypass in acquired C1 esterase inhibitor deficiency. Annals of Thoracic Surgery 52: 541–3.

Frigas E 1989 Angioedema with acquired deficiency of the C1 inhibitor: a constellation of syndromes. Mayo Clinic Proceedings 64: 1269–75.

Ishoo E, Shah UK, Grillone GA et al 1999 Predicting airway risk in angioedema: staging system based on presentation. Otolaryngology—Head & Neck Surgery 121: 263–8.

Geha RS, Quinti I, Austen KF et al 1985 Acquired C1 inhibitor deficiency associated with anti-idiotypic antibody to monoclonal immunoglobulins. New England Journal of Medicine 312: 534–40.

Gelfand JA, Boss GR, Conley CL et al 1979 Acquired C1 esterase inhibitor deficiency and angioedema: a review. Medicine 58: 321–8.

Marescal C, Ducloy-Bouthors AS, Laurent J et al 1999 Parturition and angioneurotic oedema. International Journal of Obstetric Anesthesia 8: 135–7.

Nussberger J, Cugno M, Amstutz C et al 1998 Plasma bradykinin in angio-oedema. Lancet 351: 1693–7.

Plenderleith JL, Algie T, Whaley K 1988 Acquired C1 esterase inhibitor deficiency. Anaesthesia 43: 246–7.

Razis PA Coulson IH, Gould TR et al 1986 Acquired C1 esterase inhibitor deficiency. Anaesthesia 41: 838–40.

Charcot–Marie–Tooth disease

(Peroneal muscular atrophy)

An autosomal dominant, chronic peripheral motor and sensory neuropathy starting in childhood. Anaesthesia is most commonly required for orthopaedic procedures, muscle or nerve biopsies.

Preoperative abnormalities

1. Distal muscle weakness and wasting with a sensory ataxia, initially producing walking difficulties in the second decade. Later there may be involvement of the hand and forearm, with distal muscle atrophy.

2. A mild glove and stocking sensory loss.

3. Orthopaedic abnormalities include high pedal arches, club feet, and foot drop.

4. Respiratory problems may be more common than previously thought. In a study of patients with respiratory symptoms a correlation was found between proximal upper limb involvement and respiratory muscle dysfunction (Nathanson et al 1989). Diaphragmatic weakness has been reported (Laroche et al 1988). If respiratory insufficiency occurs, it is usually secondary to restrictive lung disease, and only appears late in the disease.

5. Although cardiac involvement has been suggested, a study of 12 patients with CMT disease showed that cardiomyopathy was no more frequent than in unaffected relatives (Dyck et al 1987).

6. The kidney is sometimes involved (Paul et al 1990).

7. Diagnosis on abnormal nerve conduction velocities and sural nerve biopsy.

Anaesthetic problems

1. In patients with upper limb involvement, there may be respiratory impairment. Those with diaphragmatic weakness may be unable to lie down, therefore regional anaesthesia is not always feasible (Hardie et al 1990).

2. A study of dose requirements of thiopentone found that patients with serious impairment of motor and sensory function required significantly lower doses for induction of anaesthesia (Kotani et al 1996).

3. The possibility of suxamethonium precipitating hyperkalaemia has been raised, but its uneventful use has been reported in 41 patients in one series (Antognini 1992), and seven in another (Greenberg 1992).

4. Although postoperative respiratory complications are rare, a perioperative death after spinal fusion secondary to restrictive lung disease and pneumonia has been reported (Antognini 1992).

5. Exacerbations of the disease may occur in pregnancy. In a study of 21 patients, 81% noticed increasing weakness, and the neurological disabilities persisted in 65% (Rudnik-Schoneborn et al 1993). In patients with respiratory complications, increasing support may be required in the third trimester. A 26 year old with a tracheostomy, who was receiving IPPV at night, had to increase her periods of ventilatory support towards term (Byrne et al 1992). Respiratory failure after Caesarean section necessitated prolonged IPPV (Brian et al 1987).

Management

1. Assessment of respiratory function, particularly in those patients with upper limb involvement.

2. Cautious use of neuromuscular blockers, especially in the more affected patients. However, Naguib & Samarkandi (1998) found normal responses to both atracurium and mivacurium in a 17-year-old man.

3. Epidural anaesthesia was used for vaginal delivery with no untoward sequelae (Scull & Weeks 1996). A continuous spinal technique has been described for elective Caesarean section at 35 weeks' gestation, in a patient with decreasing respiratory function (Reah et al 1998).

Bibliography

Antognini JF 1992 Anaesthesia for Charcot–Marie–Tooth disease: a review of 86 cases. Canadian Journal of Anaesthesia 39: 398–400.

Brian JE, Boyles GD, Quirk JG et al 1987 Anesthetic management for Cesarean section of a patient with Charcot–Marie–Tooth disease. Anesthesiology 66: 410–12.

Byrne DL, Chappatte OA, Spencer GT et al 1992 Pregnancy complicated by Charcot–Marie–Tooth disease, requiring intermittent ventilation. British Journal of Obstetrics & Gynaecology 99: 79–80.

Dyck PJ, Swanson CJ, Nishimura RA et al 1987 Cardiomyopathy in patients with hereditary motor and sensory neuropathy. Mayo Clinic Proceedings 62: 672–5.

Greenberg RS, Parker SD 1992 Anesthetic management for the child with Charcot–Marie–Tooth disease. Anesthesia & Analgesia 74: 305–7.

Hardie R, Harding AE, Hirsch NP et al 1990 Diaphragmatic weakness in hereditary motor and sensory neuropathy. Journal of Neurology, Neurosurgery & Psychiatry 53: 348–50.

Kotani N, Hirota K, Anzawa N 1996 Motor and sensory disability has a strong relationship to induction dose of thiopental in patients with the hypertrophic variety of Charcot–Marie–Tooth disease. Anesthesia & Analgesia 82: 182–6.

Laroche CM, Carroll N, Moxham J et al 1988 Diaphragmatic weakness in Charcot–Marie–Tooth disease. Thorax 43: 478–9.

Nathanson BN, Yu D-G, Chan CK 1989 Respiratory muscle weakness in Charcot–Marie–Tooth disease. A field study. Archives of Internal Medicine 149: 1389–91.

Naguib M, Samarkandi AH 1998 Response to atracurium and mivacurium in a patient with Charcot–Marie–Tooth disease. Canadian Journal of Anaesthesia 45: 56–9.

Paul MD, Fernandez D, Pryse-Phillips W et al 1990 Charcot–Marie–Tooth disease and nephropathy in a mother and daughter, with a review of the literature. Nephron 54: 80–5.

Reah G, Lyons GR, Wilson RC 1998 Anaesthesia for Caesarean section in a patient with Charcot–Marie–Tooth disease. Anaesthesia 53: 586–8.

Rudnik-Schoneborn S, Rohrig D, Nicholson G et al 1993 Pregnancy and delivery in Charcot–Marie–Tooth disease type 1. Neurology 43: 2011–16.

Scull T, Weeks S 1996 Epidural analgesia for labour in a patient with Charcot–Marie–Tooth disease. Canadian Journal of Anaesthesia 43: 1150–2.

CHARGE association

An association of congenital abnormalities characterised by **C**oloboma of the eye, **H**eart disease, **A**tresia of the choanae, **R**etarded growth development and/or central nervous system abnormalities, **G**enital hypoplasia in males, **E**ar anomalies and/or deafness. Diagnosis is made on the presence of at least four of the criteria. A retrospective study of 50 patients showed that, apart from choanal atresia and cleft lip and palate, 56% of patients had some other upper airway abnormality (Stack & Wyse 1991). Muscular hypotonia is common. Anaesthesia may be required for choanal atresia repair, cardiac surgery, tracheo-oesophageal fistula, ear surgery, Nissen's fundoplication, and tracheostomy. Treatment requires a multidisciplinary approach.

Preoperative abnormalities

1. In an analysis of 50 patients, more than 90% had colobomata, 56% had choanal atresia, 84% had congenital heart disease, 96% males had

external genital abnormalities, and 100% had ear abnormalities. Of those who were old enough to be assessed, 76% had developmental delay (Blake et al 1990). Similar figures were found in 45 patients described by Roger et al (1999), and in 47 cases by Tellier et al (1998). Severe sensorineural visual and vestibular deficits are suggested as the cause of delay in walking development, rather than retardation (Guyot & Vibert 1999).

2. Other abnormalities include facial palsy, tracheo-oesophageal fistula, and laryngeal malformations. Sixty-nine percent of 32 patients studied had genitourinary anomalies (Ragan et al 1999).

3. There is a high incidence of abnormal blood gas levels and sleep problems. Cardiorespiratory arrest is common in this group of patients (Roger et al 1999).

4. Gastro-oesophageal reflux has been reported in 80%.

Anaesthetic problems

1. An increased risk of airway obstruction, so that tracheal intubation or tracheostomy may be required in early life (Coniglio et al 1988). Fifty six percent had choanal atresia or stenosis, 40% micrognathia, 8% laryngomalacia, 6% subglottic stenosis, and 8% had other upper airway abnormalities.

2. Upper airway collapse. Stack & Wyse (1991) attributed the tendency for the airway to collapse during light anaesthesia to laryngomalacia. However, Roger et al (1999) felt that the inability to maintain the patency of the pharyngolaryngeal passage that could be seen on endoscopy would be better termed 'pharyngolaryngeal hypotonia', rather than laryngomalacia. The obstruction is variable, and becomes more pronounced during sleep and during inspiration. Oedematous arytenoids may result from gastro-oesophageal reflux.

3. Tracheal intubation difficulties have been recorded in 25–40%, and intubation problems

appeared to increase with increasing age (Stack & Wyse 1991, Roger et al 1999).

4. Patients require multiple anaesthetics, and in one series there was a significant postoperative mortality.

5. Feeding difficulties and a high incidence of gastro-oesophageal reflux (50–80%). Postoperative deaths were frequently associated with pulmonary aspiration.

6. Congenital heart disease, predominantly conotruncal abnormalities or patent ductus arteriosus. About 60% of these will require surgery.

Management

1. Careful preoperative assessment for upper airway abnormalities and cardiac disease.

2. A range of sizes of tracheal tube should be available.

3. If micrognathia present, a gaseous induction may be advisable.

4. Tracheostomy may be required for long-term management. In a review of 45 patients, 13 required tracheostomy, and the authors felt that early tracheostomy helped to avoid hypoxaemic events in infancy (Roger et al 1999).

5. Precautions should be taken against aspiration of gastric contents.

6. Careful postoperative observation for apnoea.

Bibliography

Blake KD, Russell-Eggitt IM, Morgan DW et al 1990 Who's in CHARGE? Multidisciplinary management of patients with CHARGE association. Archives of Disease in Childhood 65: 217–23.

Coniglio JU, Manzione JV, Hengerer AS 1988 Anatomic findings and management of choanal atresia and the CHARGE association. Annals of Otology, Rhinology & Laryngology 97: 448–53.

Guyot JP, Vibert D 1999 Patients with CHARGE association: a model to study saccular function in the human. Annals of Otolaryngology—Head & Neck Surgery 108: 151–9.

Ragan DC, Casale AJ, Rink RC et al 1999 Genitourinary anomalies in the CHARGE association. Journal of Urology 161: 622–5.

Roger G, Morisseau-Durand M-P, Van Den Abbeele T et al 1999 The CHARGE Association. The role of tracheostomy. Archives of Otolaryngology—Head & Neck Surgery 125: 33–8.

Stack CG, Wyse RKH 1991 Incidence and management of airway problems in the CHARGE association. Anaesthesia 46: 582–4.

Tellier AL, Cormier-Daire V, Abadie V et al 1998 CHARGE syndrome: report of 47 cases and review. American Journal of Medical Genetics 76: 402–9.

Cherubism

A benign, familial condition, transmitted as autosomal dominant, which may present during childhood with progressive mandibular, and sometimes maxillary, enlargement. It is named after renaissance cherubs, who gazed heavenwards (Kalantar Motamedi 1998). It usually regresses spontaneously during adolescence (Katz et al 1992), but sometimes facial or incidental surgery is required before regression.

Preoperative abnormalities

1. Bilateral swelling involves the mandible and sometimes the maxilla, usually starting at the age of 2–4 years. Skull X-ray shows multilocular cysts, expanding the bone, and leaving only a thin layer of cortex. Progression of the lesions slows down towards puberty, and sometimes they regress.

2. Speech, deglutition and mastication may be affected in gross cases.

3. There may be dental abnormalities and premature loss of teeth.

Anaesthetic problems

1. Intubation difficulties have been encountered. In one patient, visualisation of the vocal cords was made impossible by enlargement of the mandible, such that it displaced the area of soft tissue bounded by the lower jaw (Maydew & Berry 1985).

2. A limited range of jaw movements may contribute to intubation difficulties (Faircloth et al 1991).

3. Surgery for gross deformities may be associated with considerable blood loss and postoperative IPPV may be required (Kaugers et al 1992).

Management

1. Difficult intubation should be anticipated. An awake intubation technique is the safest but, if the patient refuses, a spontaneously breathing induction should be used. Facilities must be available for an immediate tracheostomy, should it be required.

2. Postoperative IPPV may be required and occasionally tracheostomy.

Bibliography

Faircloth WJ Jr, Edwards RC, Farhood VW 1991 Cherubism involving a mother and daughter: case reports and review of the literature. Journal of Oral & Maxillofacial Surgery 49: 535–42.

Kalantar Motamedi MH 1998 Treatment of cherubism with locally aggressive behavior presenting in adulthood: report of four cases and a proposed new grading system. Journal of Oral & Maxillofacial Surgery 56: 1336–42.

Katz JO, Dunlap CL, Ennis RL 1992 Cherubism: report of a case showing regression without treatment. Journal of Oral & Maxillofacial Surgery 50: 301–3.

Kaugars GE, Niamtu J, Svirsky JA 1992 Cherubism: diagnosis, treatment, and comparison with central giant cell granulomas and giant cell tumors. Oral Surgery, Oral Medicine, Oral Pathology 73: 369–74.

Maydew RP, Berry FA. Cherubism with difficult laryngoscopy and tracheal intubation. Anesthesiology 1985; 62: 810–12.

Pierce AM, Sampson WJ, Wilson DF et al 1996 Fifteen-year follow-up of a family with inherited craniofacial fibrous dysplasia. Journal of Oral & Maxillofacial Surgery 54: 780–8.

Christmas disease (haemophilia B)

(see Haemophilia A)

Churg–Strauss syndrome

A syndrome of asthma, allergic rhinitis, pulmonary and systemic small-vessel vasculitis and extravascular granulomas. Reid et al (1999) reported organ systems involvement as follows: lungs (48%), heart (44%), kidney (48%), nervous system (78%), skin (48%), bowel (30%), joints (57%), and muscle (57%). The presence of severe gastrointestinal disease or myocardial involvement is associated with a poor prognosis (Guillevin et al 1999). It has sometimes been associated with the new leukotriene antagonists used for asthma. However, it is thought that the disease is unmasked when these drugs replace corticosteroids for treatment, rather than being the cause of it (Churg & Churg 1998, Stirling & Chung 1999).

Preoperative abnormalities

1. Asthma, hypereosinophilia ($>1.5 \times 10^9 l^{-1}$), necrotising vasculitis, extravascular granulomas, and allergic rhinitis. The vasculitis involves two or more extrapulmonary organs. The combination of late onset asthma with severe, recurrent sinusitis that requires surgery, particularly if there are abnormal paranasal sinus X-rays, may give a clue to the presence of the disease (D'Cruz et al 1999).

2. Lung. Pulmonary infiltrates, alveolar haemorrhage, and pleural effusions.

3. Renal. Proteinuria, haematuria, impaired renal function.

4. Gastrointestinal tract. Diarrhoea and bleeding.

5. Myocardial involvement. Pericarditis, myocardial infarction, and cardiomyopathy.

6. Neurological involvement is common, and usually presents as mononeuritis multiplex or a polyneuropathy (Sehgal et al 1995).

7. Bronchoalveolar lavage in severe cases shows involvement of neutrophils as well as eosinophils (Schnabel et al 1999).

8. Treatment is with corticosteroids, alone or in combination with cyclophosphamide or plasma exchange (Guillevin et al 1999).

Anaesthetic problems

1. The problems of the management of asthma.

2. In one asthmatic patient, sudden withdrawal of steroid therapy in pregnancy was associated with development of bilateral pulmonary infiltrates, pleural infusion and eosinophilia (Priori et al 1998).

3. Rarely, a dilated cardiomyopathy may be present.

4. Two patients have been reported with decreased plasma cholinesterase levels (Taylor et al 1990). However, both were receiving immunosuppressive agents and had multiple organ involvement.

Management

1. Treatment of asthma.

2. Look for organ involvement and treat appropriately.

Bibliography

Churg A, Churg J 1998 Steroids and Churg–Strauss syndrome. Lancet 352: 32–3.

D'Cruz DP, Barnes NC, Lockwood CM 1999 Difficult asthma or Churg–Strauss syndrome. British Medical Journal 318: 175–6.

Guillevin L, Cohen P, Gayraud M et al 1999 Churg–Strauss syndrome: clinical study and long-term follow-up of 96 patients. Medicine 78: 26–37.

Priori R, Tomassini M, Magrini L et al 1998 Churg–Strauss syndrome during pregnancy after steroid withdrawal. Lancet 352: 1599–600.

Reid AJ, Harrison BD, Watts RA et al 1998 Churg–Strauss syndrome in a district hospital. Quarterly Journal of Medicine 91: 219–29.

Schnabel A, Csernok E, Braun J et al 1999

Inflammatory cells and cellular activation in the lower respiratory tract in Churg–Strauss syndrome. Thorax 54: 771–8.

Sehgal M, Swanson JW, DeRemee RA et al 1995 Neurologic manifestations of Churg–Strauss syndrome. Mayo Clinic Proceedings 70: 337–41.

Stirling RG, Churg KF 1999 Leukotriene antagonists and Churg–Strauss syndrome: the smoking gun. Thorax 54: 865–6.

Taylor BL, Whittaker M, Van Heerden CD et al 1990 Cholinesterase deficiency and the Churg–Strauss syndrome. Anaesthesia 45: 649–52.

Coarctation of the aorta, adult

A congenital narrowing of the aorta that may be pre- or post-ductal. The preductal form is usually a long, narrow segment, and is associated with other cardiac defects. This type generally presents with heart failure before the age of 1 year and requires treatment in a paediatric cardiac surgical unit. It will not be considered further here. The postductal form, however, is often asymptomatic, and the patient may present in later life for surgery of some other condition, or for correction of the coarctation itself. Even after correction of coarctation, abnormalities can continue (Moskowitz et al 1990). Those who have undergone repair show persistent alterations in left ventricular function and left ventricular mass, together with resting gradients between the arm and leg. There is a higher incidence than normal of ischaemic heart disease and sudden death. The optimal time for repair is disputed (Brouwer et al 1994). Hypertension is more common in late correction, but repair at a young age is associated with a higher risk of recoarctation. In addition, persistent abnormalities in aortic stiffness have been found (Ong et al 1992). Adult repairs are associated with a higher incidence of significant aortic valve disease (58%), compared with 37% of those repaired in childhood (Findlow & Doyle 1997).

Preoperative abnormalities

1. There may be moderate hypertension, the arm blood pressure being higher than that in the leg. If the left subclavian arises at or below the constriction there may be an absent or reduced left radial pulse. If both radial and femoral pulses are felt together, the small volume and delay of the femoral pulse will be obvious.

2. Collateral circulation develops in the internal mammary, intercostal, and subscapular arteries. The latter may be seen if the scapula is illuminated from the side.

3. A systolic murmur is usually heard along the left sternal edge radiating up into the neck.

4. Chest X-ray may show notching of the undersides of the ribs, secondary to intercostal artery dilatation. There may be pre- and poststenotic dilatation of the aorta.

5. Occasionally, cerebral berry aneurysms coexist with coarctation. In such cases, the high arterial pressure increases the risk of subarachnoid haemorrhage.

6. There is a 25–50% incidence of bicuspid aortic valve, and some aortic regurgitation.

7. Unusually, angina or left ventricular failure may present late in untreated adult coarctation. Other factors are often contributary.

8. Patients may require surgical resection or balloon dilatation. There is evidence that balloon angioplasty should be undertaken initially in discrete aortic coarctation in adolescents and adults (Fawzy et al 1999).

Anaesthetic problems

If, before elective surgery, a previously undiagnosed coarctation is found, treatment of the coarctation may be considered to be the priority. Even if coarctation has been treated, the possibility of residual cardiovascular abnormalities should be considered, since there is an increased risk of premature death compared with the normal population (Bobby et al 1991). Causes include aneurysms (cerebral, at the operative site, other parts of the aorta and intercostal arteries), hypertension, myocardial infarction, and cardiac failure (Editorial 1991). Balloon angioplasty may carry less risk.

1. Patients may present with hypertension-related complications. A 30-year-old man, who had been rejected for army service because of hypertension, presented with severe epistaxis and a blood pressure of 210/110. He had prominent rib notching on CXR, LVH on ECG, and decreased femoral pulses (Pulli 1999).

2. Any operation in the area of the dilated collateral vessels may result in heavy bleeding, especially when the chest is opened.

3. Hypoperfusion of the spinal cord. This may cause paraplegia, and is more likely in those patients with few collaterals. Induced hypotension for clipping of cerebral aneurysm may compromise spinal cord perfusion (Goodie & Rigg 1991).

4. Susceptibility to bacterial endocarditis.

5. If there are left subclavian abnormalities, the left arm cannot be used for blood pressure monitoring.

6. Patients may present during pregnancy with hypertension, which may be confused with preeclampsia. Three patients were described whose clinical signs (ejection systolic murmur and delayed or absent leg pulses) had gone unnoticed. Two required balloon dilatation and the third resection and aortoplasty (Lip et al 1998). A rare case of abdominal coarctation was diagnosed by MRI in a 26 year old with a 15-year history of hypertension (Dizon-Townson et al 1995). The patient had a Caesarean section under general anaesthesia at 36 weeks' gestation because of failure to control the hypertension with labetalol. One patient was noted to have a systolic murmur at 28 weeks' gestation. Cardiac assessment showed severe pulmonary hypertension and coarctation. Decompensation occurred at 35 weeks and Caesarean section under general anaesthesia was performed. Intensive care management included the use of glyceryl trinitrate and prostacyclin (O'Hare et al 1998). A patient with recurrent coarctation, with 50% narrowing of the aortic arch, developed chest pain, dyspnoea and claudication during late pregnancy. Caesarean section under general anaesthesia was performed using a remifentanil infusion and isoflurane (Manullang et al 2000).

Management

1. Antihypertensive therapy should be used until the day of operation. Beta adrenoceptor blockers may reduce the hypertensive response to intubation.

2. Appropriate prophylaxis for endocarditis should be given.

3. During clipping of an intracranial aneurysm, monitoring of the femoral artery pressure was undertaken to assess spinal cord perfusion during induced hypotension. A mean distal aortic pressure in excess of 50 mmHg has been suggested as adequate for spinal cord perfusion.

Bibliography

Bobby JJ, Emami JM, Farmer RDT et al 1991 Operative survival and 40 year follow-up of surgical repair of aortic coarctation. British Heart Journal 65: 271–6.

Brouwer RMHJ, Erasmus ME, Ebels T et al 1994 Influence of age on survival, late hypertension, and recoarctation in elective aortic coarctation repair. Journal of Thoracic & Cardiovascular Surgery 108: 525–31.

Dizon-Townson D, Magee KP, Twickler DM et al 1995 Coarctation of the abdominal aorta in pregnancy: diagnosis by magnetic resonance imaging. Obstetrics & Gynecology 85 (5II suppl) 817–19.

Fawzy ME, Sivanandam V, Pieters F et al 1999 Long-term effects of balloon angioplasty on systemic hypertension in adolescent and adult patients with coarctation of the aorta. European Heart Journal 20: 827–32.

Findlow D, Doyle E 1997 Congenital heart disease in adults. British Journal of Anaesthesia 78: 416–30.

Goodie DB, Rigg DL 1991 Controlled hypotension for cerebral aneurysm surgery in the presence of severe aortic coarctation. British Journal of Anaesthesia 67: 329–31.

Lip GYH, Singh SP, Beevers DG 1998 Aortic coarctation diagnosed after hypertension in pregnancy. American Journal of Obstetrics and Gynecology 179: 814–15.

C

Coarctation of the aorta, adult

Manullang TR, Chun K, Egan TD 2000 The use of remifentanil for Cesarean section in a parturient with recurrent aortic coarctation. Canadian Journal of Anaesthesia 47: 454–9.

Moskowitz WB, Schieken RM, Mosteller M et al 1990 Altered systolic and diastolic function in children after 'successful' repair of coarction of the aorta. American Heart Journal 120: 103–9.

O'Hare R, McLoughlin C, Milligan K et al 1998 Anaesthesia for Caesarean section in the presence of severe primary pulmonary hypertension. British Journal of Anaesthesia 81: 790–2.

Ong CM, Canter CE, Gutierrez FR et al 1992 Increased stiffness and persistent narrowing of the aorta after successful repair of coarctation of the aorta: relationship to left ventricular mass and blood pressure at rest and with exercise. American Heart Journal 123: 1594–600.

Pulli RS 1999 Management of epistaxis complicated by a previously undiagnosed aortic coarctation. Otolaryngology—Head & Neck Surgery 120: 584–7.

Cocaine abuse

Cocaine is an alkaloid present in the shrub, *Erythroxylon coca*. It has an onset of action of about 11 min and a half-life of 78 min, and produces CNS stimulation, euphoria and hallucinations. As a sympathetic stimulant, it acts by preventing the uptake of catecholamines into sympathetic nerve endings. In addition, it may release catecholamines from body stores. Whilst there is evidence that it has been used as a euphoriant in the Central Amazon from as early as the ninth century, the last 30 years has seen a notable increase in its use. It has been said to produce emotional, but not physical dependence. However, more recently, the use of chemically modified forms (paste, crack and freebase) for inhalation or smoking, has resulted in higher blood concentrations. These forms appear to be producing dependence. The consumption of cocaine for recreational purposes has been more prevalent in the USA than in the UK. The greatly increased production and illicit trade from South America is changing this.

Cocaine is a toxic drug. A series of 68 deaths were associated with its illicit use in Florida (Wetli & Wright 1979). Analysis of the cases showed that the effects after intravenous use included immediate respiratory collapse and death, or death after up to 3 h in coma. After nasal or oral ingestion a delay of up to an hour occurred before convulsions and death. Average blood levels were highest in those with oral intake (average 0.92 mg dl^{-1}), lowest in those after iv (0.3 mg dl^{-1}), and intermediate after use of the nasal route (0.44 mg dl^{-1}). Oral ingestion is an uncommon route for those seeking euphoria. The majority of deaths were deliberate, or accidental when packages of cocaine which were swallowed for concealment (body packing), burst in the gut. That cocaine is potentially dangerous even when given nonintravenously, has been confirmed (Isner et al 1986). Seven patients had acute cardiac events that bore a temporal relationship to intranasal cocaine use. These included myocardial infarction, ventricular tachycardia and fibrillation, myocarditis, and two sudden deaths. Existing heart disease was not a prerequisite. Large doses of cocaine were not essential, and seizures did not necessarily occur before cardiac toxicity. A further 19 case reports were analysed.

Cocaine is frequently taken in combination with other drugs (Birnbach 1998). Drug mixtures include speedballs (a combination of heroin laced with cocaine). Patients often do not admit to drug use, but may present with a variety of cardiopulmonary (40%), psychiatric (22%), and neurological (13%) symptoms (Brody et al 1990). Anaesthetists may be involved, often unknowingly, with anaesthesia for chronic users, or in the resuscitation of those with acute toxicity. Cocaine causes central and peripheral adrenoceptor stimulation, by blocking presynaptic uptake of norepinephrine (noradrenaline) and dopamine, and increasing postsynaptic concentrations. Cocaine is hydrolised by plasma cholinesterase into two major metabolites, which can be detected in urine for 14–60 h after administration.

Cocaine abuse

Presenting problems

1. The cardiovascular effects of cocaine are biphasic. An initial increase in blood pressure and a tachycardia, secondary to sympathetic stimulation, precedes the pronounced depression of the CNS. Sweating, vomiting and restlessness may occur. Sympathetic vasoconstriction can be intense, with increased metabolism, hyperthermia, hypoxia, and convulsions. Ventricular fibrillation or asystole has occurred with doses as low as 30 mg. Tachycardia and hypertension occurred during anaesthesia, when a patient injected two speedballs into his infusion just before surgery (Samuels et al 1991).

2. ECG abnormalities may be misinterpreted. Tachycardia, chest pain and large inferior Q waves on ECG in a young cocaine user led to the incorrect diagnosis of myocardial infarction (Lustik et al 1999). In the event she had WPW syndrome and successful ablation of the accessory pathway was accompanied by return to normal of the short PR interval and disappearance of the Q wave.

3. Toxic doses produce an initial tachypnoea and increased depth of respiration. This may be rapidly followed by central respiratory depression.

4. When taken nasally, the vasoconstrictor effects on the mucosa may eventually lead to nasal ulceration and septal perforation.

5. Anaesthetics may interact with cocaine when toxic levels exist. An animal study of a cocaine infusion in the presence of 0.75–1.5 MAC isoflurane showed reduction in cerebral and spinal cord blood flow and increased systemic vascular resistance, diastolic pressure, and coronary perfusion pressure (Boylan et al 1996). Arrhythmias and altered ventricular conduction also occurred. Ketamine potentiates strongly the cardiovascular toxicity of cocaine.

6. Vasoconstrictors, such as phenylephrine and felypressin, can precipitate hypertensive crises, ventricular tachycardia, and myocardial ischaemia during acute cocaine toxicity.

7. Intraoperative pulmonary oedema occurred after instillation of phenylephrine (0.5 ml 0.25%) into the nose of a 24-year-old man (Singh et al 1994). Echocardiography, whilst he received IPPV, showed right ventricular hypokinesia and an ejection fraction of 30%. When he had recovered, his echocardiogram became normal. Pulmonary oedema has also being reported after ketamine 50 mg, given for traction pain during tubal ligation under spinal anaesthesia (Murphy 1993). In both of these cases, a history of cocaine use was later obtained. The mechanism of the oedema is unclear. Contributing factors may be damaged pulmonary endothelium, or transient left ventricular dysfunction secondary to myocardial ischaemia or pulmonary vasocontriction.

8. There have been a number of reports of chronic rhabdomyolysis in association with cocaine abuse, and acute renal failure has occurred (Singhal et al 1989). In a study of cocaine users presenting to an emergency department, 24% had evidence of rhabdomyolysis (Welch et al 1991). One developed multiorgan failure and died.

9. A greatly increased risk of endocarditis in iv cocaine users (Chambers et al 1987).

10. Intravenous users are at risk of contracting hepatitis B, sexually transmitted diseases, and AIDS.

11. Hot cocaine fumes, when smoked or inhaled, may cause pulmonary damage, as may the chemicals used in the processing (Gossop 1987). Two patients presented with acute respiratory distress for which they eventually required tracheal intubation and IPPV. In both patients, superficial white plaques, mucosal ulceration, and severe supraglottic oedema had been found on fibreoptic laryngoscopy. Each patient finally admitted to aspirating hot fragments while smoking crack (Reino & Lawson 1993). A third patient had sudden airway obstruction whilst smoking crack. Following a CT scan for a confusional state, he developed stridor and upper airway obstruction. Numerous polyps, oedema, and a narrowed aperture were

found. Tracheostomy was required until the polyps healed at the end of 6 days (White & Reynolds 1999).

12. Plasma cholinesterase is essential for the metabolism of cocaine. Individuals with enzyme abnormality or deficiency are therefore at risk from sudden death (Cregler & Mark 1986). There is now definite evidence that those with cocaine-induced complications have a significantly lower level of plasma cholinesterase than those without complications (Om et al 1993).

13. Thrombocytopenia is associated with cocaine abuse (Orse 1991). It may be autoimmune in origin. Antibodies to platelets may be common in drug addicts.

14. Organophosphate insecticides have been used to prolong the action of cocaine by inhibiting plasma cholinesterase (Herschman & Aaron 1991). Under these circumstances the recovery from suxamethonium may be delayed.

15. In late pregnancy, some of the effects of cocaine may be mistaken for preeclampsia or eclampsia (Birnbach 1998). Eleven women were reported with signs typical of preeclampsia and a positive urine drug screen for cocaine. However, there was no laboratory evidence of preeclampsia, and, as the drug wore off, the symptoms resolved (Towers et al 1993). Another patient, admitted with haemolytic anaemia, thrombocytopenia, renal impairment, and intermittent episodes of pulmonary oedema, was found to have been smoking crack cocaine on the ward (Campbell et al 1996).

16. Cocaine crosses the placenta and has a direct effect on fetal vasculature. Experimentally, there is evidence that pregnancy increases the cardiovascular toxicity caused by cocaine. Cocaine-induced hypertension in gravid ewes was modified by hydralazine, but caused profound maternal tachycardia and failed to restore the cocaine-induced reduction in uterine blood flow (Vertommen et al 1992). It causes uterine contractility and an increased incidence of preterm labour. In the USA, where cocaine

abuse is said to be common among parturients, myocardial infarction and cardiovascular instability, which was temporally related to 'crack' use prior to delivery, has been reported (Liu et al 1992). Maternal death has occurred, and prematurity and perinatal mortality are increased (Neerhof et al 1989). The incidence of abruptio placenta is almost doubled and uterine rupture, hepatic rupture, and cardiac arrest, have all been reported. A patient had an abruptio placenta at 34 weeks' gestation, 18 h after using cocaine. She was oliguric on admission and this persisted after Caesarean section, despite hydration, dopamine, and frusemide. She developed myoglobinuria and required haemodialysis (Lampley et al 1996). Birnbach et al (1993) studied 25 cocaine users who required Caesarean section and found that general anaesthesia was associated with a greater number of complications than regional anaesthesia. Another study of Caesarean section showed that parturients are at a higher than normal risk for hypertension, hypotension, and wheezing (Kain et al 1996).

17. Medical complications include myocardial infarction, ventricular arrhythmias, aortic rupture, seizure, stroke, hyperthermia, bowel ischaemia, and malnutrition.

Management

1. Resuscitation may involve airway protection, and control of haemodynamic abnormalities, seizures, or hyperthermia (Cheng 1994).

2. Beta adrenoceptor blockers have been used to counteract the sympathetic effects of cocaine, but an alpha adrenoceptor blocker, such as phentolamine, should be available in case of severe hypertension. Regimens have included propranolol (1 mg iv each min up to a total of 8 mg) to obtain a decrease in heart rate within 1–3 min (Gay et al 1976). However, it has been suggested that beta blockade alone may worsen hypertension by unopposed alpha stimulation (Gay & Loper 1988). Labetalol (20 mg iv bolus,

followed by an infusion of 60 mg h^{-1}), may be more appropriate. That the beta effects of labetalol arc much greater than the alpha effects, must not be overlooked. A bolus of esmolol 20 mg followed by an esmolol infusion (1%) was used to treat toxicity from epinephrine (adrenaline) and cocaine given before nasal polypectomy (Pollan & Tadjziechy 1989).

3. Calcium channel blockers have been used for arrhythmias (Cregler & Mark 1986), and may be more effective than adrenoceptor blockers in the management of cocaine cardiovascular toxicity (Nahas 1991). However, it has been suggested that for protection, nifedipine needs to be given before cocaine use.

4. For the treatment of convulsions, either a benzodiazepine or incremental doses of thiopentone are indicated. Immediate attention should be paid to oxygenation and control of the airway. A profound metabolic acidosis occurs in association with convulsions, and their immediate control might decrease the cardiac effects of cocaine (Jonsson et al 1983). Treatment with sodium bicarbonate may be required for metabolic acidosis.

5. Restlessness or agitation in the chronic cocaine abuser can be treated with benzodiazepines. Increasing the usual dosage by 50% has been recommended (Gay et al 1976).

6. Phenothiazines are contraindicated because they potentiate cerebral depressant drugs.

7. The platelet count returns to normal 1–6 weeks after termination of drug exposure. Bleeding time is the best indicator of platelet function. If this is normal, no treatment is required.

8. The possibility that rhabdomyolysis might occur should be remembered. Since clinical symptoms do not predict rhabdomyolysis, laboratory evaluation may be necessary. Treatment with mannitol, intravenous fluids and, occasionally, dialysis may be required.

9. In the pregnant patient, regional anaesthesia produced fewer serious complications than general anaesthesia.

However, platelets and coagulation status should be checked first. Phenylephrine was found to be superior to ephedrine for treatment of hypotension after spinal anaesthesia (Birnbach et al 1993).

10. Avoid using direct-acting sympathomimetics and vasoconstrictors, because they may precipitate hypertension and arrhythmias.

Bibliography

Anonymous 1998 Cocaine and the brain. Journal of the American Medical Association 280: 594.

Birnbach DJ, Stein DJ, Thomas K et al 1993 Cocaine abuse in the parturient. What are the anesthetic implications? Anesthesiology 79: A988.

Birnbach DJ 1998 Anesthesia and the drug abusing parturient. Anesthesiology Clinics of North America 16: 385–95.

Birnbach DJ, Stein DJ 1998 The substance-abusing parturient: implications for analgesia and anesthesia management. Bailliere's Clinical Obstetrics & Gynaecology 12: 443–60.

Boylan J, Cheng D, Feindel C et al 1992 Cocaine toxicity and isoflurane anaesthesia–haemodynamics and myocardial metabolism. Canadian Journal of Anaesthesia 39: A27.

Boylan JFM, Cheng DC, Sandler AN et al 1996 Cocaine toxicity and isoflurane anesthesia— hemodynamic, myocardial metabolic, and regional blood flow in swine. Journal of Cardiothoracic & Vascular Anesthesia 10: 772–7.

Burkett Chambers HF, Morris DL, Tauber MG et al 1987 Cocaine use and the risk for endocarditis in intravenous drug users. Annals of Internal Medicine 106: 833–6.

Campbell D, Parr MJA, Shutt LE 1996 Unrecognised 'crack' cocaine abuse in pregnancy. British Journal of Anaesthesia 77: 553–5.

Cheng D 1994 Perioperative care of the cocaine abusing patient. Canadian Journal of Anaesthesia 41: 883–7.

Cregler LL, Mark H 1986 Medical complications of cocaine abuse. New England Journal of Medicine 315: 1495–500.

Fleming JA, Byck R, Barash PG 1990 Pharmacology and therapeutic applications of cocaine. Anesthesia & Analgesia 73: 518–31.

Gay GR, Inaba DS, Rappolt RT et al 1976 Cocaine in current perspective. Anesthesia & Analgesia 55: 582–7.

Gay GR, Loper KA 1988 Control of cocaine induced hypertension with labetalol. Anesthesia & Analgesia 67: 92.

Gossop M 1987 Beware cocaine. British Medical Journal 295: 945.

Herschman Z, Aaron C 1991 Prolongation of cocaine effect. Anesthesiology 74: 631–2.

Isner JM, Estes NA, Thompson PD et al 1986 Acute cardiac events temporally related to cocaine abuse. New England Journal of Medicine 315: 1438–43.

Jonsson S, O'Meara M, Young JB 1983 Acute cocaine poisoning. Importance of treating seizures and acidosis. American Journal of Medicine 75: 1061–4.

Kain ZN, Mayes LC, Ferris CA et al 1996 Cocaine-abusing parturients undergoing cesarean section. A cohort study. Anesthesiology 85: 1028–35.

Karch SB, Stephens B, Ho CH 1998 Relating cocaine blood concentrations to toxicity—an autopsy study. Journal of Forensic Sciences 43: 41–5.

Lampley EC, Williams S, Myers SA 1996 Cocaine-associated rhabdomyolysis causing renal failure in pregnancy. Obstetrics & Gynecology 87: 804–6.

Liu SS, Forrester RM, Murphy GS et al 1992 Anaesthetic management of a parturient with myocardial infarction related to cocaine use. Canadian Journal of Anaesthesia 39: 858–61.

Lustik SJ, Wotjczak J, Chhibber AK 1999 Wolff-Parkinson-White syndrome simulating inferior myocardial infarction in a cocaine abuser for urgent dilation and evacuation of the uterus. Anesthesia & Analgesia 89: 609–12.

Murphy JL 1993 Hypertension and pulmonary oedema in a patient with a history of substance abuse. Canadian Journal of Anaesthesia 40: 160–4.

Nahas GG 1991 Treatment of cocaine-induced cardiovascular toxicity. Anesthesiology 75: 544.

Neerhof MG, Macgregor SN, Retzky SS et al 1989 Cocaine abuse during pregnancy: peripartum prevalence and perinatal outcome. American Journal of Obstetrics & Gynecology 161: 633–8.

O'Brien TP, Pane MA, Traystman RJ et al 1999 Propranolol blocks cocaine-induced cerebral vasodilation in newborn sheep. Critical Care Medicine 27: 784–9.

Om A, Ellahham S, Ornato JP et al 1993 Medical complications of cocaine: possible relationship to low plasma cholinesterase enzyme. American Journal of Cardiology 125: 1114–17.

Orser B 1991 Thrombocytopenia and cocaine abuse. Anesthesiology 74: 195–6.

Pollan S, Tadjziechy M 1989 Esmolol in the management of epinephrine (adrenaline)- and cocaine-induced cardiovascular toxicity. Anesthesia & Analgesia 69: 663–4.

Reino AJ, Lawson W 1993 Upper airway distress in crack-cocaine users. Otolaryngology—Head & Neck Surgery 109: 937–40.

Samuels J, Schwalbe SS, Marx GF 1991 Speedballs: a new cause of intraoperative tachycardia and hypertension. Anesthesia & Analgesia 72: 397–8.

Singh PP, Dimich I, Shamsi A 1994 Intraoperative pulmonary oedema in a young cocaine smoker. Canadian Journal of Anaesthesia 41: 961–4.

Singhal P, Horowitz B, Quinones MC et al 1989 Acute renal failure following cocaine abuse. Nephron 52: 76–8.

Towers CV, Pircon RA, Nageotte MP et al 1993 Cocaine intoxication presenting as preeclampsia and eclampsia. Obstetrics & Gynecology 81: 545–7.

Vertommen JD, Hughes SC, Rosen MA et al 1992 Hydralazine does not restore uterine blood flow during cocaine-induced hypertension in the pregnant ewe. Anesthesiology 76: 580–7.

Welch RD, Todd K, Krause GS 1991 Incidence of cocaine-associated rhabdomyolysis. Annals of Emergency Medicine 20: 154–7.

Wetli CV, Wright RK 1979 Death caused by recreational cocaine use. Journal of the American Medical Association 241: 2519–22.

White MC, Reynolds F 1999 Sudden airway obstruction following inhalation drug abuse. British Journal of Anaesthesia 82: 808.

Cockayne syndrome

An autosomal recessive condition in which there is a defect in the repair of oxidative DNA damage in nuclear DNA. Sensitivity to ultraviolet light leads to premature aging and neurological abnormalities. It is associated with patchy demyelination in the cortex and cerebellum, with calcium deposition in basal ganglia and white matter (Woods 1998). Patients may need anaesthesia for cataract extraction, feeding gastrostomy, and Nissen's fundoplication.

Preoperative abnormalities

1. In a study of 25 patients there was dwarfism, microcephaly and mental retardation,

photosensitivity (84%), gait disturbance (84%), progeroid appearance (84%), and eye abnormalities (Ozdirim et al 1996). Facial features are dysmorphic, and limb contractures occur.

2. Eyes. Retinal dystrophy, enophthalmos, squint, cataract, and nystagmus.

3. Neurological abnormalities. Include sensorineural deafness, progressive arteriosclerosis, slowed neural conduction, and abnormal brainstem evoked responses (Nance et al 1992).

4. Patients may be receiving H_2 receptor antagonists, proton pump inhibitors, and cisapride, a gastrointestinal stimulant.

Anaesthetic problems

1. Difficult tracheal intubation is reported (Cook 1982, Wooldridge et al 1996). Attempted intubation under light inhalational anaesthesia produced coughing and laryngospasm. A patient may require a smaller sized tube than would be anticipated. A 3.0-mm tube was used in a 13-year-old girl, and a 4.5-mm one in a 19 year old weighing 12.9 kg.

2. Gastro-oesophageal reflux and aspiration pneumonia.

3. Postoperative treatment of systolic hypertension with sublingual nifedipine caused a pressure decrease to 138 mmHg and the patient became unconscious and developed convulsive-like involuntary movements in extremities (Sasaki et al 1997). Nifedipine was thought to have produced cerebral ischaemia.

Management

1. Assessment of potential intubation problems.

2. A range of tube sizes is necessary. In one patient, the laryngeal mask airway helped to deepen anaesthesia before intubation. In another who had a failed intubation, a laryngeal mask airway was used as a conduit for the passage of a guidewire (Wooldridge et al 1996).

3. Precautions against gastro-oesophageal reflux, if present.

Bibliography

Cook S 1982 Cockayne syndrome. Another cause of difficult intubation. Anaesthesia 37: 1104–7.

Sasaki R, Hirota K, Masuda A 1997 Nifedipine-induced transient cerebral ischaemia in a child with Cockayne syndrome. Anaesthesia 52: 1236.

Nance MA, Berry SA 1992 Cockayne syndrome. Review of 140 cases. American Journal of Medical Genetics 42: 68–84.

Ozdirim E, Topcu M, Ozon A et al 1996 Cockayne syndrome: review of 25 cases. Pediatric Neurology 15: 312–16.

Woods CG 1998 DNA repair disorders. Archives of Disease in Childhood 78: 178–84.

Wooldridge WJ, Dearlove OR, Khan AA 1996 Anaesthesia for Cockayne syndrome. Anaesthesia 51: 478–81.

Conn's syndrome (primary aldosteronism)

Excess aldosterone production may be caused by an adrenal adenoma, adrenal hyperplasia, or a carcinoma. For a differential diagnosis of the different features, see Ganguly (1998). Aldosterone is a mineralocorticoid secreted by the zona glomerulosa of the adrenal cortex. It promotes sodium reabsorption and potassium exchange, mainly in the renal tubules, but to a lesser extent in the intestine, and salivary and sweat glands. The final stage of aldosterone secretion is controlled by the renin-angiotensin system. Activation of this system occurs in response to sodium or water depletion. Primary aldosteronism should be suspected if spontaneous hypokalaemia occurs in association with untreated hypertension (Young 1997, Stewart 1999).

Preoperative abnormalities

1. The main features are hypertension, hypokalaemia, and alkalosis. Symptoms, should

they occur, are usually secondary to hypokalaemia, and may include muscle weakness, polyuria, polydipsia, and tetany. A patient who presented with a flaccid quadriparesis, had the condition reversed by a potassium infusion (Gangat et al 1976). In contrast to the original belief that serious hypertension was not a problem in Conn's syndrome, malignant hypertension may sometimes occur (Sunman et al 1992, Winship et al 1999). That it is not a benign condition is shown by the fact that cardiovascular complications, especially stroke and proteinuria, are relatively common (Nishimura et al 1999).

2. Urinary potassium is high, despite a low total body potassium, and the serum sodium may be in the upper range of normal or be slightly elevated. Plasma renin levels are low and plasma aldosterone is elevated. Conn's syndrome should be suspected if a hypertensive patient has a serum sodium >140 mmol l^{-1} and a plasma potassium below the normal range for the laboratory. The diagnosis can be confirmed by an elevated aldosterone:renin ratio in excess of 800 (Brown & Hopper 1999).

3. Tumours must be distinguished from bilateral adrenal hyperplasia, with radionuclide imaging, or occasionally by adrenal vein sampling. In adrenal hyperplasia, surgery is inappropriate.

4. The ECG may show mild left ventricular hypertrophy, prolonged ST segment, T-wave flattening, and U waves.

5. Glucose tolerance may be abnormal in up to 50% of patients.

6. The diagnosis of Conn's syndrome may be masked in patients receiving calcium channel blockers, because they can suppress the increased aldosterone secretion and consequent hypokalaemia (Brown & Hopper 1999).

7. Treatment is either medical or surgical. Adrenalectomy is increasingly being performed by the laparoscopic route, which has been associated with fewer complications (Shen et al 1999).

Anaesthetic problems

1. Hypertension and sodium retention. Hypertensive peaks may occur at intubation. Patients may be receiving multiple antihypertensives, with potential for drug interactions.

2. Low total body and plasma potassium levels cause muscle weakness and increased sensitivity to nondepolarising muscle relaxants. A pregnant woman presented at 29 weeks' gestation with muscle weakness, hypertension, and severe hypokalaemia (Fujiyama et al 1999). Intraoperative arrhythmias may also be produced. A patient in whom tonic muscle contractions occurred during induction, and whose subsequent potassium balance studies suggested that the potassium stores had been depleted by 30–40%, has been described (Gangat et al 1976). Sudden ventricular fibrillation was reported in a 37-year-old, otherwise healthy, woman. A serum potassium of 1.4 mmol l^{-1} and a right sided adrenal tumour were found (Abdo et al 1999).

3. Pregnancy occurred in a patient being investigated for probable Conn's syndrome. During the first trimester, blood pressure and serum potassium were so difficult to control that adrenalectomy was performed at 15 weeks' gestation (Solomon et al 1996). Another patient presented with weakness, hypertension and severe hypokalaemia at 29 weeks' gestation (Fujiyama et al 1999). There is dispute about the appropriate time to perform resection in the pregnant patient. Since the condition is difficult to treat at this time, and medical therapy is probably more risky than surgery, it has been suggested that surgery should be performed early in the second trimester (Baron et al 1995, Harrington et al 1999). Two patients who had been normotensive during their pregnancies developed severe postpartum hypertension, one at at 18 days, the other at 1 month. Both patients had mild hypokalaemia, and adrenal tumours were demonstrated and subsequently resected (Nezu et al 2000).

Management

1. Hypertension must be controlled preoperatively. An aldosterone antagonist, such as spironolactone 100 mg tds, should be given for 3–4 weeks before surgery, since both the hypertension and potassium loss will be improved (Ganguly 1998).

2. A potassium infusion is required both pre- and intra-operatively. Total body potassium is depleted, and ECG and plasma potassium levels are both unreliable guides (Gangat et al 1976).

3. Preoperative beta blockers may reduce the hypertensive peaks on intubation.

4. Normocapnoea should be maintained to prevent potassium returning to the cells. An initial period of IPPV may be required after surgery, to counteract the compensatory respiratory acidosis.

5. Following removal of the tumour, the reversal of the electrolyte abnormalities occurs earlier than the correction of hypertension.

6. Glucocorticoid replacement should not be required, provided the other adrenal is intact.

7. If a patient presents in the first two trimesters of pregnancy, consideration should be given to the risks of surgery versus those of medical treatment (Baron et al 1995).

Bibliography

Abdo A, Bebb RA, Wilkins GE 1999 Ventricular fibrillation: an extreme presentation of primary hyperaldosteronism. Canadian Journal of Cardiology 15: 347–8.

Baron F, Sprauve ME, Huddleston JF et al 1995 Diagnosis and surgical treatment of primary aldosteronism in pregnancy. Obstetrics & Gynecology 86: 644–5.

Brown MJ, Hopper RV 1999 Calcium-channel blockade can mask the diagnosis of Conn's syndrome. Postgraduate Medical Journal 75: 235–6.

Fujiyama S, Mori Y, Matsubara H et al 1999 Primary aldosteronism with aldosterone-producing adrenal adenoma in a pregnant woman. Internal Medicine 38: 36–9.

Gangat Y, Triner L, Baer L et al 1976 Primary aldosteronism with uncommon complications. Anesthesiology 45: 542–4.

Ganguly A 1998 Primary aldosteronism. New England Journal of Medicine 339: 1828–34.

Harrington JL, Farley DR, Van Heerden JA et al 1999 Adrenal tumors and pregnancy. World Journal of Surgery 23: 182–6.

Nezu M, Miura Y, Noshiro T et al 2000 Primary aldosteronism as a cause of severe postpartum hypertension in two women. American Journal of Obstetrics & Gynecology 182: 745–6.

Nishimura M, Uzu T, Fujii T et al 1999 Cardiovascular complications in patients with primary aldosteronism. American Journal of Kidney Diseases 33: 261–6.

Shen WT, Lim RC, Siperstein AE et al 1999 Laparoscopic vs open adrenalectomy for the treatment of primary hyperaldosteronism. Archives of Surgery 134: 628–32.

Solomon CG, Thiet M, Moore F et al 1996 Primary hyperaldosteronism in pregnancy. A case report. Journal of Reproductive Medicine 41: 255–8.

Stewart PM 1999 Mineralocorticoid hypertension. Lancet 353: 1341–7.

Sunman W, Rothwell M, Sever PS 1992 Conn's syndrome can cause malignant hypertension. Journal of Human Hypertension 6: 72–5.

Winship SM, Winstanley JHR, Hunter JM 1999 Anaesthesia for Conn's syndrome. Anaesthesia 54: 569–74.

Young WF Jr 1997 Pheochromocytoma and primary aldosteronism: diagnostic approaches. Endocrinology & Metabolism Clinics of North America 26: 801–27.

Creutzfeldt–Jakob disease (CJD)

A rare spongiform encephalopathy, classified as a prion (proteinaceous infective particle) disease. Kuru, linked with ritual cannibalism in Papua New Guinea, Gerstmann-Straussler-Schenker disease, usually inherited, and new variant CJD, are the other three human prion diseases. Four such diseases have been defined as occurring in animals, bovine spongiform encephalopathy having achieved substantial notoriety in the UK (Hughes 1993). All are widespread degenerative diseases of the CNS with long incubation periods, but, once manifested, there is rapid progression to death. Treatment is to no avail. Patients of late middle age are usually affected and death typically occurs within 6 months. The infective agent can be isolated from the brain, spinal cord, and many other tissues, and can be experimentally transmitted to animals. There is no detectable immune reaction. It is difficult to destroy by either physical or chemical methods (Johnson & Gibbs 1998).

Iatrogenic transmission of prions can occur in neurosurgical procedures, corneal grafts (MacMurdo et al 1984), and when growth hormone from cadaveric pituitaries is used (Buchanan et al 1991). In the latter, it usually follows an incubation period of about 18 months. Patients who have received human growth hormone are now excluded from being blood donors.

Variant CJD is associated with a distinct prion type 4 PrP^{sc}. At present, the risks of transmitting prions causing variant CJD are not yet known. It is known, however, that they can be found in the lymphoreticular system and can be diagnosed by tonsillar biopsy (Collinge 1999, Petersen 1999). Studies on tonsillar material are in progress, and the results could have implications for the reuse of surgical instruments.

Preoperative abnormalities

1. With classical CJD, there is dementia of rapid onset, and mutism in the 50–70 age group. However, variant CJD may appear in young people and have an unusual neurological profile. Cerebellar dysfunction with ataxia, increased tone and sometimes myoclonus, is common. Cortical blindness may occur. Deterioration to decerebrate or decorticate states is usually rapid. Epilepsy can occur.

2. The EEG has nonspecific changes, but there are often periodic discharges of slow waves and spikes.

3. Diagnosis is usually made on clinical grounds. It can only be confirmed by brain biopsy, but this is now not advised because of the risks of accidental transmission.

4. Treatment is symptomatic and the patient may be taking anticonvulsants.

Anaesthetic problems

1. Any tissue or body fluid should be considered as potentially infectious, although in reality the main danger probably lies in accidental inoculation. However, there is nothing to suggest that routine nursing care carries a risk, therefore barrier nursing is unnecessary. Accidental transmission has occurred by contaminated instruments, and a cadaveric dural graft (Lane et al 1994), or by pituitary hormones from cadavers before the use of recombinant growth hormone (Holmes et al 1996). Martinez-Lage et al (1994) have described four patients who developed CJD from lyophilised dura mater grafts.

2. Occasionally patients may have autonomic dysfunction.

3. Rarely, there are abnormalities of liver function.

Management

1. Particular care should be taken during brain biopsies in undiagnosed cases of presenile dementia (du Moulin & Hedley-Whyte 1983), although if Creutzfeldt–Jakob disease or its variant are suspected, biopsy is inadvisable. The anaesthetist should wear gown, gloves and mask. These should all be waterproof (Hernandez-Palazon et al 1998). Patients with dementia should not be used as organ donors.

2. Equipment, in particular surgical instruments, should preferably be disposable and should be incinerated at the end. Linen and instruments should be soaked in 1% sodium hypochlorite before being bagged (du Moulin & Hedley-Whyte 1983, Hernandez-Palacon et al 1998).

3. The virus is difficult to destroy by physical and chemical means. Experiments have shown that soaking in 5% sodium hypochlorite for 1 h, autoclaving for 1 h at 132°C (103.4 kPa), or a combination of these, will inactivate it (Brown et al 1982). Hands should be washed (not scrubbed) with aqueous povidone iodine, if

penetration of the skin has occurred. Equipment surfaces should be washed with 0.5% sodium hypochlorite.

Bibliography

Brown P, Gibbs CJ, Amyx HL et al 1982 Chemical disinfection of Creutzfeldt–Jakob disease virus. New England Journal of Medicine 306: 1279–82.

Buchanan CR, Preece MA, Milner RDG 1991 Mortality, neoplasia, and Creutzfeldt–Jakob disease in patients treated with pituitary growth hormone in the United Kingdom. British Medical Journal 302: 824–8.

Collinge J 1999 Variant Creutzfeldt–Jakob disease. Lancet 354: 317–23.

du Moulin GC, Hedley-Whyte J 1983 Hospital-associated viral infection and the anesthesiologist. Anesthesiology 59: 51–65.

Hernandez-Palazon J, Martinez-Lage JF, Tortosa JA 1998 Anaesthetic management in patients suspected of, or at risk of, having Creutzfeldt–Jakob disease. British Journal of Anaesthesia 80: 516–18.

Holmes SJ, Ironside JW, Shalet SM 1996 Neurosurgery in a patient with Creutzfeldt–Jakob disease after pituitary derived growth hormone in childhood. Journal of Neurology, Neurosurgery & Psychiatry 60: 333–5.

Hughes JT 1993 Prion diseases. British Medical Journal 306: 288.

Johnson RT, Gibbs CJ Jr 1998 Creutzfeldt–Jakob disease and related transmissible spongiform encephalopathies. New England Journal of Medicine 339: 1994–2004.

Lane KL, Brown P, Howell DN et al 1994 Creutzfeldt–Jakob disease in a pregnant woman with an implanted dura mater graft. Neurosurgery 34: 737–9.

MacMurdo SD, Jakymec AJ, Bleyaert AL 1984 Precautions in the anesthetic management of a patient with Creutzfeldt–Jakob disease. Anesthesiology 60: 590–2.

Martinez-Lage JF, Poza M, Sola J et al 1994 Accidental transmission of Creutzfeldt–Jakob disease by dural cadaveric grafts. Journal of Neurology, Neurosurgery & Psychiatry 57: 1091–4.

Petersen RB 1999 Antemortem diagnosis of variant Creutzfeldt–Jakob disease. Lancet 353: 163–4.

Cri du chat syndrome

A chromosomal abnormality secondary to short arm deletion on chromosome 5. It is associated with a number of characteristic features. Malformations have been observed in the sella turcica, the clivus, the cerebellum, and the larynx. Most patients die in childhood. Anaesthesia may be required for Nissen's fundoplication, or correction of congenital heart disease.

Preoperative abnormalities

1. The infant has microcephaly, micrognathia, hypertelorism, severe mental retardation, epicanthic folds, strabismus, hypotonia, and a cat-like cry.

2. There may be a number of other abnormalities, including congenital heart disease.

3. Obstructive sleep apnoea may occur.

Anaesthetic problems

1. Difficulties in intubation have been reported (Yamashita et al 1985). There are thought to be structural differences in the larynx from normal, and the epiglottis is long, curved and floppy. Failed intubation, in a 15 month old having Nissen's fundoplication, was followed by failed fibreoptic intubation. Eventually an ILMA was placed (Castresana et al 1994). Although the characteristic cry may be partially neurogenic in origin, a number of upper airway abnormalities have been described. These include a small, narrow larynx, a long floppy epiglottis, and retrognathia.

2. The babies are hypotonic and may be sensitive to non-depolarising muscle relaxants.

3. Gastro-oesophageal reflux and a tendency to pulmonary aspiration may lead to chronic respiratory infections.

4. Obstructive apnoea has followed surgery (Brislin et al 1995).

Management

1. Investigation for the presence of congenital heart disease. Antibiotic prophylaxis, if appropriate.

2. Awake intubation or inhalation induction has been suggested, although a laryngeal mask airway may be of assistance. Examination of the laryngeal view can sometimes be performed first, with mild sedation. In a 33-month-old child, fentanyl $4\,\mu g\,kg^{-1}$ was administered in increments, after which gentle laryngoscopy revealed a grade 2 laryngeal view. Rapid sequence induction was then performed with confidence (Brislin et al 1995).

3. Minimal doses of relaxants, or controlled ventilation without relaxation, may be advisable.

4. Care with nursing and feeding may reduce aspiration problems. Observation for obstructive sleep apnoea.

Bibliography

Brislin RP, Stayer SA, Schwartz RE 1995 Anaesthetic considerations for the patient with cri du chat syndrome. Paediatric Anaesthesia 5: 139–41.
Castresana MR, Stefansson S, Cancel AR et al 1994 Use of the laryngeal mask airway during thoracotomy in a pediatric patient with cri-du-chat syndrome. Anesthesia & Analgesia 78: 817.
Yamashita M, Tanioka F, Taniguchi K et al 1985 Anesthetic consideration in Cri du Chat syndrome. A report of three cases. Anesthesiology 63: 201–2.

Cushing's syndrome and Cushing's disease

Cushing's syndrome is the general term used for a disorder caused by excess circulating glucocorticoid. Cushing's disease specifies one of its causes; that of pituitary-dependent adrenal hyperplasia, secondary to ACTH secretion. This accounts for about 70–80% of cases of Cushing's syndrome. Other important causes are adrenal cortical tumour (5–10%), and ectopic ACTH producing tumour (5–10%). The diagnosis and treatment of Cushing's syndrome, particularly during pregnancy, is more complex than previously thought. For further details, see Invitti et al (1999) and Newell-Price & Grossman (1999). The complications following surgery are higher than those with other endocrine diseases, and surgery does not necessarily reverse the cardiovascular complications.

Preoperative abnormalities

1. A review of 31 patients with Cushing's disease showed that the commonest clinical features, in order of frequency, were: weakness, thin skin, obesity, easy bruising, hypertension, menstrual disorders, hirsutism, impotence, striae, proximal muscle weakness, oedema, osteoporosis, mental disorders, diabetic GTT, backache, acne, hypokalaemia and fasting hyperglycaemia (Urbanic & George 1981). Fractures occur, and wound healing is poor.

2. Biochemical abnormalities include hypokalaemic alkalosis, sodium and water retention, hyperglycaemia, lack of diurnal variation in plasma cortisol with failure to decrease at night, and increased urinary free cortisol.

3. Cushing's syndrome is associated with severe left ventricular hypertrophy, with disproportionate hypertrophy of the interventricular septum (Sugihara et al 1992). The cause is unknown.

4. Patients have an increased incidence of infections.

5. Screening by overnight dexamethasone test and 24-h urinary excretion of cortisol (Klibanski & Zervas 1991).

6. Occasionally patients become pregnant, in which case the commonest complications are hypertension and diabetes (Aron et al 1990, Prihoda & Davis 1991). A patient with Cushing's syndrome and a phaeochromocytoma underwent laparoscopic adrenalectomy at 17 weeks' gestation (Finkenstedt et al 1999).

7. Cushing's disease is more difficult to diagnose during pregnancy because of gestational changes in the HPA axis.

8. Patients with treated Cushing's disease who are considered 'cured' still have an increased risk of cardiovascular disease and atherosclerosis, despite having normal cortisol levels (Colao et al 1999).

9. Treatment of Cushing's syndrome may unmask other diseases. A patient treated with

adrenalectomy developed sarcoidosis 6 weeks later (Walmsley & Bevan 1995).

Anaesthetic problems

1. Venous access may be difficult because the veins are extremely fragile.

2. Hypertension, with or without heart failure, may be present. Left ventricular hypertrophy, particularly of the interventricular septum, has been reported (Sugihara et al 1992). Acute left ventricular failure was the initial presentation of Cushings in a 22-year-old woman (Younge et al 1995).

3. Hypokalaemia. There may be severe depletion of potassium stores.

4. Diabetes mellitus. In pregnancy, this may be difficult to control, and in one patient, a mid-trimester trans-sphenoidal pituitary adenomectomy was performed because high levels of insulin were required (Mellor et al 1998). Another patient presented with acute heart failure, hypertension, and glucose intolerance, and adrenalectomy was performed at 24 weeks' gestation. Emergency Caesarean section was required at 31 weeks' for severe preeclampsia and HELLP syndrome (Lo & Lau 1998). Another patient, who had experienced a 2-year history of weakness, was only diagnosed during pregnancy from routine glucose screening (MacGibbon & Brieger 1995).

5. Anatomical changes and obesity may contribute to either difficult intubation or difficult mask ventilation. A 30-year-old woman developed severe iatrogenic Cushing's syndrome from steroid treatment of autoimmune idiopathic thrombocytopenic purpura during pregnancy. Superimposed preeclampsia at 33 weeks resulted in massive oedema of the face, lips and neck. She was unable to tolerate lying supine, therefore awake blind nasal intubation was performed in the sitting position before GA for Caesarean section (Rosenberg & Gross 1993).

6. Muscle weakness may contribute to postoperative respiratory failure.

7. There is an increased risk of deep vein thrombosis, infection, and postoperative pneumonia. In a series of 105 patients undergoing transsphenoidal surgery, four patients developed deep venous thrombosis, and one pneumonia (Semple & Laws 1999).

Management

1. Hypertension and heart failure, if present, must be treated.

2. Diabetes must be controlled.

3. Hypokalaemia requires identification and correction.

4. In florid cases, drug control of adrenocortical function with metyrapone, an 11-beta-hydroxylase inhibitor, may be advisable before operation (Lo & Lau 1998). However, this is only available in oral form. A patient who developed severe peritonitis and underwent IPPV on ITU whilst waiting for adrenalectomy was unresponsive to octreotide. However, a low dose infusion of etomidate reduced the serum cortisol from 2500 to 500 mmol l^{-1}. Dexamethasone was given im so as not to interfere with the serum cortisol monitoring (Drake et al 1998).

5. To avoid fractures of osteoporotic bone, careful positioning of the patient is required.

6. Steroids should be maintained during and after surgery.

7. Awake fibreoptic intubation (Mellor et al 1998), and awake blind nasal intubation (Rosenberg & Gross 1993), have been described in obese patients.

8. Presentation during pregnancy may necessitate surgery.

9. Thromboprophylaxis should be given in the perioperative period.

Bibliography
Aron DC, Schnall AM, Sheeler LR 1990 Cushing's syndrome and pregnancy. American Journal of Obstetrics & Gynecology 162: 244–52.

Colao A, Pivonello R, Spiezia S et al 1999 Persistence of increased cardiovascular risk in patients with Cushing's disease after 5 years of successful care. Journal of Clinical Endocrinology & Metabolism 84: 2664–72.

Drake WM, Perry LA, Hinds CJ et al 1998 Emergency and prolonged use of intravenous etomidate to control hypercortisolemia in a patient with Cushing's syndrome and peritonitis. Journal of Clinical Endocrinology & Metabolism 83: 3542–4.

Finkenstedt G, Gasser RW, Hofle G et al 1999 Pheochromocytoma and sub-clinical Cushing's syndrome during pregnancy: diagnosis, medical pre-treatment and cure by laparoscopic unilateral adrenalectomy. Journal of Clinical Investigation 22: 551–7.

Invitti C, Giraldi FP, de Martin M et al 1999 Diagnosis and management of Cushing's syndrome: results of an Italian multicentre study. Journal of Clinical Endocrinology & Metabolism 84: 440–8.

Klibanski A, Zervas NT 1991 Diagnosis and management of hormone secreting pituitary adenomas. New England Journal of Medicine 324: 822–31.

Lo KW, Lau TK 1998 Cushing's syndrome in pregnancy secondary to adrenal adenoma. A case report and literature review. Gynecologic & Obstetric Investigation 45: 209–12.

MacGibbon AL, Brieger GM 1995 Cushing syndrome in pregnancy secondary to an adrenal cortical adenoma. Australian & New Zealand Journal of Obstetrics & Gynaecology 35: 217–19.

Mellor A, Harvey RD, Pobereskin LH et al 1998 Cushing's disease treated by trans-sphenoidal selective adenomectomy in mid-pregnancy. British Journal of Anaesthesia 80: 850–2.

Newell-Price J, Grossman A 1999 Diagnosis and management of Cushing's syndrome. Lancet 353–8.

Prihoda JS, Davis LE 1991 Metabolic emergencies in obstetrics. Obstetrics & Gynecology Clinics of North America 18: 301–18.

Rosenberg DB, Gross JB 1993 Awake, blind nasotracheal intubation for cesarean section in a patient with autoimmune thrombocytopenic purpura and iatrogenic Cushing's syndrome. Anesthesia & Analgesia 77: 853–5.

Semple PL, Laws ER Jr 1999 Complications in a contemporary series of patients who underwent transsphenoidal surgery for Cushing's disease. Journal of Neurosurgery 91: 175–9.

Sugihara N, Shimizu M, Kita Y et al 1992 Cardiac characteristics and postoperative courses in Cushing's syndrome. American Journal of Cardiology 69: 1475–80.

Urbanic RC, George JM 1981 Cushing's disease—18 years' experience. Medicine 60: 14–24.

Walmsley D, Bevan JS 1995 Suppression of medical conditions by Cushing's syndrome. British Medical Journal 310: 1537.

Younge PA, Schidt D, Wiles PG 1995 Cushing's syndrome: still a potential killing disease. Journal of the Royal Society of Medicine 88: 174–5P.

Cystic fibrosis

An autosomal recessive syndrome primarily involving the exocrine glands, and producing a variable pattern of the disease. Glandular secretions are relatively concentrated, with excess electrolytes and altered mucus glycoproteins. Faulty regulation of the movement of salt and water across cell membranes results in excessive sodium absorption and deficient chloride secretion. This leads to abnormal mucociliary transport, although ciliary function is normal. As a result, gland ducts become blocked. This predisposes to infection, hyperplasia, and hypertrophy.

The patient may develop progressive chronic respiratory problems in childhood, malabsorption, and cirrhosis of the liver. Progressive lung damage can lead to pulmonary hypertension and right heart failure. Death is usually caused by widespread pulmonary infection leading to respiratory failure. Advances in the management of the disease have extended life-expectancy, therefore more patients are likely to present for surgery, and pregnancy now occurs. Provided there is not severe disease, pregnancy does not have adverse effects (Frangolias et al 1997). Increasing numbers of patients are undergoing heart-lung and lung transplantion for advanced disease (Shale 1996). However, even after surgery, patients still have cystic fibrosis in other organs. Operative mortality has decreased dramatically during the last 20 years. In a review of 77 patients undergoing 126 procedures, of which 86% were operations directly related to the disease itself, no evidence was produced that anaesthesia had any deleterious effect on lung function (Lamberty & Rubin 1985). In a more recent review of 144 anaesthetics for 74 patients, only one patient died. This was secondary to respiratory failure 10 days after laparoscopic cholecystectomy (Weeks & Buckland 1995).

Some improvement in sputum viscosity and elasticity has been shown using aerosolised amiloride, a potassium-sparing diuretic, which blocks sodium uptake and increases the water content of sputum (Knowles et al 1990). Nebulised recombinant DNase reduces sputum viscoelasticity *in vitro*, by lysis of neutrophil DNA, but there are wide variations in clinical response (Ramsey 1996, Innes 1998). The effect of extracellular nucleotides on induction of chloride secretion in nasal mucosa is also being assessed (Knowles et al 1991). Recently, the gene responsible for cystic fibrosis has been identified and sequenced. It is located on chromosome 7 and encodes for a chloride channel. The abnormal protein is the cystic fibrosis transmembrane conductance regulator (CFTR). There is evidence that care in a specialist unit improves outcome (Mahadeva et al 1998). Clinical guidelines for cystic fibrosis care have been produced by the British Paediatric Association and the British Thoracic Society (see Jackson 1996).

For detailed reviews of anaesthesia and cystic fibrosis, see Walsh & Young (1995), Weeks & Buckland (1995).

Preoperative abnormalities

1. Sweat test. High sodium (>60 mmol l^{-1} in infants; >65 mmol l^{-1} suggestive, and >90 mmol l^{-1} diagnostic in children), and high chloride levels.

2. Abnormal viscoelastic properties of sputum, defective mucociliary transport and altered lung mechanics produce severe chest infections. The main organisms responsible are *Haemophilus influenzae*, *Staphylococcus aureus*, *pseudomonas aeruginosa* and *Burkholderia cepacia*.

Bronchiectasis, pulmonary fibrosis, and emphysema follow. Bronchopulmonary aspergillosis, aspergilloma, and haemoptysis are other complications. Bronchial reactivity is greater than in normal individuals.

3. Pneumothorax, which is difficult to treat, is common in adults (Spector & Stern 1989). A study of 243 adults showed that 46 (18.9%) had at least one pneumothorax, from which seven had died (Penketh et al 1982). This complication is much less frequent in children (2–7%).

4. Nasal polyps and sinusitis occur in 10–15% of cases. Surgery improves the symptoms, but has no effect on pulmonary function (Madonna et al 1997).

5. Pulmonary hypertension, secondary to hypoxia, may develop in advanced lung disease. Cor pulmonale finally supervenes.

6. A certain number of adults develop abnormal liver function, proceeding to portal hypertension, oesophageal varices, and cirrhosis.

7. Pancreatic insufficiency occurs in 80–90% of patients. Malabsorption, hypoproteinaemia, and low body weight result. The incidence of diabetes is high and increases with age. Prothrombin time may be prolonged as a result of loss of fat soluble vitamins.

8. Distal intestinal obstruction syndrome is the commonest gastrointestinal complication. This can usually be managed medically (Smith & Stableforth 1992). It may be associated with the use of concentrated pancreatic enzymes. Gallstones, peptic ulceration, and oesophageal reflux occur more commonly than in normal people.

9. Superior vena cava syndrome can occur, secondary to the use of long-term indwelling catheters (Chow et al 1998).

10. Osteoporosis is universal in adults with late stage cystic fibrosis and its complications include increased fracture rates and severe kyphoscoliosis (Aris et al 1998).

Anaesthetic problems

1. Despite the improvement in prognosis, when lung disease is severe, mortality is increased.

2. Gaseous induction is both slow, because of low ventilation perfusion ratios, and stormy.

3. Gastro-oesophageal reflux is a feature of both the childhood and adult disease, and there is an association between asthma and gastro-oesophageal reflux (Ledson et al 1998). In 60% of patients studied, the lower oesophageal sphincter pressure was subnormal. This factor may predispose to respiratory complications.

4. The tracheal tube is easily blocked by secretions.

5. There is a high incidence of perioperative respiratory complications. These include pneumothorax, pneumonia, airway obstruction, atelectasis, respiratory failure, and arrest.

6. Bronchoscopy and lung washout is associated with episodes of profound hypoxia (Harnik et al 1983).

7. Periods of oxygen desaturation during sleep may occur postoperatively.

8. Nasal polyps can cause airway obstruction.

9. There is a high sodium loss, especially when hot.

10. With aggressive treatment, more patients are surviving to become pregnant (Canney et al 1991). In a survey of 38 pregnancies in 25 patients, pregnancy was found to be well tolerated by most. However, the patients in this study had less severe disease, since half were pancreatic sufficient. In other series, mother and fetus fared less well. Maternal complications included pulmonary, liver, cardiac, and pancreatic insufficiency. There was poor fetal nutrition and oxygen delivery, and an increased perinatal mortality. Edenborough et al (1995) reported that an FEV_1 of <60% predicted was associated with an increased risk of premature delivery, Caesarean section, loss of lung function, and early maternal death. Recurrent infections may require continuous antibiotics and oxygen therapy. Parenteral nutrition may be necessary. In an older study, 12% of patients died within 6 months, and 18% within 2 years, of pregnancy, but this death rate was no more than that expected in nonpregnant patients (Cohen et al 1980). Death was reported 10 days postpartum in a patient in respiratory failure whose chest was colonised with *Burkholderia cepacia* (Bose et al 1997).

Management

1. Patients and/or their parents are usually knowledgeable about their disease and will need to be closely involved in discussions on management, to which they can contribute useful information. It is most important to listen to them, and to gain their confidence.

2. Respiratory and cardiovascular function must be carefully assessed. Active infection should be excluded when elective surgery is taking place. FEV_1 and arterial blood gases appear to have the best predictive value. An FEV_1 <30%, a decreased Pao_2, or an increased $PaCO_2$, are all ominous signs. Diabetes, hyponatraemia, and hypokalaemia should also be excluded. In the presence of hepatic involvement, a coagulation screen is necessary.

3. Regular, intensive physiotherapy is mandatory. This includes percussion and forced expiration, and encouragement to exercise. Positive expiratory pressure, with a mask, one way valve and resistor, was found to be superior to conventional postural drainage with percussion (Coates 1997). Some parents are taught to do physiotherapy at home, which minimises the necessity for admitting the child early for surgery. The use of head down tilt for postural drainage is now controversial. There is evidence that gastro-oesophageal reflux may cause aspiration and bronchospasm (Coates 1997). It has been suggested that surgery be timed to take place mid-morning, so that overnight secretions can be cleared.

4. Infections, especially those with

Pseudomonas aeruginosa, require iv treatment with an aminoglycoside, such as tobramycin and a beta lactam (azlocillin) combination. However, the drugs required depend on the culture and sensitivity. There is increasing use of regular nebulised antibiotics given via high powered air compressors (Mukhopadhya et al 1998, Campbell & Saiman 1999). However, it is difficult to know how much is delivered, or to which parts of the lung. In addition, many patients now have implantable venous access devices and are managed at home for as long as possible to reduce exposure to hospital infection (Yung et al 1996).

5. Continue nebulised steroid and bronchodilator drugs, which reduce bronchial hyperreactivity.

6. Parenteral vitamin K will be needed if the prothrombin time is prolonged.

7. Local or regional anaesthesia should be employed if possible. Recently, laparoscopic cholecystectomy under continuous epidural anaesthesia in a 30–40 degrees sitting position, has been reported (Edelman 1991).

8. Sedative premedication should be avoided. Anti-sialogogues may be used if essential, but preferably immediately before induction. An H_2 antagonist may be used in the presence of reflux.

9. Since gaseous inductions are slow and stormy, they should be avoided. Total intravenous anaesthesia, with propofol and remifentanil, is an ideal technique.

10. All patients require tracheal intubation to facilitate intermittent of aspiration of secretions, oxygenation, and ventilation, and to avoid gastro–oesophageal reflux.

11. Anaesthetic gases must be humidified and tracheal secretions aspirated regularly during surgery. The viscidity of secretions is reduced by keeping the patient well hydrated, but not overloaded.

12. Care must be taken to provide adequate pain relief after surgery, so as to minimise pulmonary complications. For abdominal surgery, postoperative epidural analgesia allows coughing and physiotherapy. A patient with pleuritic pain and pneumonia had excellent pain relief from an infusion of fentanyl via an epidural catheter sited at a T7–8 level (Cain et al 1994).

13. The role of bronchial washouts in the management of cystic fibrosis is controversial. Its benefit in some patients has been supported (Harnik et al 1983). Repeated aliquots of up to 20 ml 5% acetylcysteine in saline were instilled into the main divisions of the bronchial tree, to a total volume of 200–300 ml, over a period of 20–30 min. Concomitant monitoring with a transcutaneous oxygen analyser enabled oxygenation to be restored before dangerous hypoxia occurred.

14. Pneumothorax in the adult, treated by simple drainage, is associated with a high incidence of recurrence (Penketh et al 1982). A persistent leak for 7 days was suggested as an indication for surgical intervention, and recurrence of a pneumothorax within 6 months of surgery was found to denote a very poor prognosis (Robinson & Branthwaite 1984). However, in decisions about treatment now, the possibility of future lung transplantation must be considered. Pleurectomy results in surgical problems, therefore suture of the bleb alone has been suggested (Noyes & Orenstein 1992). Difficulties may also occur in locating the site for drainage, because of the complex appearance of the lungs, and partial adherence to the chest wall. The benefit of a CT scan for diagnosis and the selection of the optimum site for drainage has been shown (Phillips et al 1997).

15. Haemoptysis requires location of the bleeding point with fibreoptic or rigid bronchoscopy. Life-threatening haemoptysis has been treated using desmopressin 4 μg followed by vasopressin 20 u over 15 min then an infusion of 0.2 u min^{-1} for 36 h (Bilton et al 1991). More invasive therapy includes embolisation of the bronchial artery, bronchial artery ligation, or lobectomy. However, many adults are not fit enough for major surgery.

16. Lung transplantation may be considered

in patients with progressive disease (Smyth et al 1991). After an analysis of serial investigations to study prediction of mortality in 673 patients, Kerem et al (1992) concluded that patients should be considered as candidates for lung transplantation when the FEV_1 decreased below 30% of the predicted value.

17. If pregnancy occurs, and the patient does not accept its termination, a multidisciplinary team must be assembled at an early stage. Assessment of activity, physical findings, nutrition, and CXR should be undertaken. Patient-controlled epidural analgesia has been used for labour (Howell et al 1993), and in another patient who had undergone double lung transplantation, epidural anaesthesia was described for vaginal delivery and tubal ligation (Deshpande 1998).

Bibliography

Aris RM, Renner JB, Winders AD et al 1998 Increased rate of fractures and severe kyphosis: sequelae of living into adulthood with cystic fibrosis. Annals of Internal Medicine 128: 186–93.

Bilton D, Webb AK, Foster H et al 1990 Life threatening haemoptysis in cystic fibrosis: an alternative therapeutic approach. Thorax 45: 975–6.

Bose D, Yentis SM, Fauvel NJ 1997 Caesarean section in a parturient with respiratory failure caused by cystic fibrosis. Anaesthesia 52: 578–82.

Cain JC, Lish MC, Passannante AN 1994 Epidural fentanyl in a cystic fibrosis patient with pleuritic chest pain. Anesthesia & Analgesia 78: 793–4.

Campbell PW 3rd, Saiman L 1999 Use of aerosolised antibiotics in patients with cystic fibrosis. Chest 116: 775–88.

Canny GJ, Corey M, Livingstone RA et al 1991 Pregnancy and cystic fibrosis. Obstetrics & Gynecology 77: 850–3.

Coates AL 1997 Chest physiotherapy in cystic fibrosis: spare the hand and spoil the cough? Journal of Pediatrics 131: 506–8.

Chow BJ, McKim DA, Shennib H et al 1998 Superior vena cava obstruction secondary to mediastinal lymphadenopathy in a patient with cystic fibrosis. Chest 113: 1732–3.

Cohen LF, Sant'Agnese PA, Friedlander J 1990 Cystic fibrosis and pregnancy. A national survey. Lancet 2: 842–4.

Deshpande S 1998 Epidural analgesia for vaginal delivery in a patient with cystic fibrosis following double lung transplantation. International Journal of Obstetric Anesthesia 7: 42–5.

Edelman DS 1991 Laparoscopic cholecystectomy under continuous epidural anesthesia in patients with cystic fibrosis. American Journal of Diseases of Children 145: 723–34.

Edenburgh FP, Stableforth DE, Mackenzie WE 1995 Pregnancy in women with cystic fibrosis. British Medical Journal 311: 822–3.

Elborn JS, Shale DJ 1990 Lung injury in cystic fibrosis. Thorax 45: 970–3.

Frangolias DD, Nakielna EM, Wilcox PG 1997 Pregnancy and cystic fibrosis: a case controlled study. Chest 111: 963–9.

Harnik E, Kulczycki L, Gomes MN 1983 Transcutaneous oxygen monitoring during bronchoscopy and washout for cystic fibrosis. Anesthesia & Analgesia 62: 357–62.

Jackson A 1996 Clinical guidelines for cystic fibrosis care. Summary of guidelines prepared by a working group of the Cystic Fibrosis Trust, the British Paediatric Association and the British Thoracic Society. Journal of the Royal College of Physicians of London 30: 305–8.

Howell PR, Kent N, Douglas MJ 1993 Anaesthesia for the parturient with cystic fibrosis. International Journal of Obstetric Anesthesia 2: 152–8.

Innes JA 1998 Dnase in cystic fibrosis: the challenge of assessing response and maximising benefit. Thorax 53: 1003–4.

Kerem E, Reisman J, Corey M et al 1992 Prediction of mortality in patients with cystic fibrosis. New England Journal of Medicine 326: 1187–91.

Knowles MR, Church NL, Waltner WE et al 1990 A pilot study of aerosolized amiloride for the treatment of lung disease in cystic fibrosis. New England Journal of Medicine 322: 1189–94.

Knowles MR, Clarke LL, Boucher RC 1991 Activation by extracellular nucleotides of chloride secretion in the airway epithelia of patients with cystic fibrosis. New England Journal of Medicine 325: 533–8.

Lamberty JM, Rubin BK 1985 The management of anaesthesia for patients with cystic fibrosis. Anaesthesia 40: 448–59.

Ledson MJ, Tran J, Walshaw MJ 1998 Prevalence and mechanism of gastro-oesophageal reflux in adult cystic fibrosis. Journal of the Royal Society of Medicine 91: 7–9.

Ledson MJ, Wilson GE, Tran J et al 1998 Tracheal

microaspiration in adult cystic fibrosis. Journal of the Royal Society of Medicine 91: 10–12.

Madonna D, Isaacson G, Rosenfeld RM et al 1997 Effect of sinus surgery on pulmonary fuction in patients with cystic fibrosis. Laryngoscope 107: 328–31.

Mahadeva R, Webb K, Westerbeek RC et al 1998 Clinical outcome in relation to care in centres specialising in cystic fibrosis: cross sectional study. British Medical Journal 316: 1771–5.

Noyes BE, Orenstein DM 1992 Treatment of pneumothorax in cystic fibrosis in the era of lung transplantation. Chest 101: 1187–8.

Penketh A, Knight RK, Hodson ME et al 1982 Management of pneumothorax in adults with cystic fibrosis. Thorax 37: 850–3.

Phillips GD, Trotman-Dickenson B, Hodson ME et al 1997 Role of CT in the management of pneumothorax in patients with complex cystic lung disease. Chest 112: 275–8.

Ramsey BW 1996 Management of pulmonary disease in patients with cystic fibrosis. New England Journal of Medicine 335: 179–88.

Robinson DA, Branthwaite MA 1984 Pleural surgery in patients with cystic fibrosis. Anaesthesia 39: 655–9.

Shale DJ 1996 Predicting survival in cystic fibrosis. Thorax 52: 309.

Smyth RL, Higginbottam T, Scott J et al 1991 The current state of lung transplantation for cystic fibrosis. Thorax 46: 213–16.

Spector ML, Stern RC 1989 Pneumothorax in cystic fibrosis: a 26-year experience. Annals of Thoracic Surgery 47: 204–7.

Taylor CJ, Threlfall D 1997 Postural drainage techniques and gastro-oesophageal reflux in cystic fibrosis. Lancet 349: 1567–8.

Walsh TS, Young CH 1995 Anaesthesia and cystic fibrosis. Anaesthesia 50: 614–22.

Weeks AM, Buckland MR 1995 Anaesthesia for adults with cystic fibrosis. Anaesthesia & Intensive Care 23: 332–8.

Yankaskas JR, Mallory GB Jr 1998 Lung transplantation in cystic fibrosis: consensus conference statement. Chest 113: 217–26.

Yung B, Campbell IA, Elborn JS et al 1996 Totally implantable venous access devices in adult patients with cyctic fibrosis. Respiratory Medicine 90: 353–6.

Cystic hygroma or lymphangioma

A spectrum of rare developmental anomalies of the lymphatic system, consisting of sequestrations of lymphatic tissue that fail to join up with the venous system. Endothelially-lined, thin walled, lymphatic cysts penetrate and canalise, their spread being dependent on the space available for expansion. Fifty percent are present at birth, and 80% appear before the age of 2 years. Surgery is the treatment of choice but carries a high morbidity from the disease itself, and from surgery. Recurrence is common, even after apparently total resection, and it usually occurs within the first postoperative year. Mortalities of 2–6%, and permanent nerve palsies in 12–33%, have been quoted. The postoperative complication rate is high and varies from 19–33% (Hancock et al 1992). Surface CO_2 laser photocoagulation has been used for suitable cases. Rarely, the condition may present in adult life (Scally & Black 1990, Wiggs & Sismanis 1994). Recently, the use of suction and injection of fibrin sealant has been assessed (Castanon et al 1999).

119

Preoperative abnormalities

1. Lymphangiomas are mostly sited in the head and neck, including the larynx. The shoulder, axilla, arm, chest wall, mediastinum, abdomen, inguinal region, and leg can also be involved. In a study of 193 cases, the distribution was as follows: cervical 31.4%, craniofacial 18.9%, extremity 18.9%, intra-abdominal 9.2%, cervico-axillothoracic 4.9%, multiple 3.8%, cervicomediastinal 2.2%, and intrathoracic 1.6% (Hancock et al 1992).

2. They transilluminate, are multilocular, and can range from 1 mm to 20 cm in size. There is no skin attachment, but fixation to deep tissues occurs.

3. Those in the head and neck may cause airway obstruction, dysphagia, feeding difficulties, and speech problems. If the tongue is involved there may be protrusion beyond the lip margin (Balakrishnan & Bailey 1992). Recurrent enlargement may occur secondary to infection, trauma, or bleeding. Suprahyoid lesions are more of a problem than infrahyoid ones, and more

likely to recur. Any child with tongue or floor of mouth lesions is at risk from sudden airway compromise.

4. Infiltrates vessels and nerves.

5. The lesion may rapidly expand as a result of haemorrhage or infection, particularly in association with either trauma or respiratory tract infection.

6. Recurrence is common, particularly with the suprahyoid lesions.

Anaesthetic problems

1. Airway problems. In a survey of 37 cases, 41% suffered airway obstruction at some stage. Tracheostomy may be required. Lymphangiomas may also involve the larynx (Cohen & Thompson 1986) and the epiglottis (Weller 1974). Out of a series of lymphatic malformations of the head and neck, 17 patients had extensive involvement of the lower face, tongue, floor of mouth, and mandible. Of these, 11 (65%) patients required tracheostomy for a threatened airway (Padwa et al 1995).

Airway problems may sometimes become evident in utero. Prenatal diagnosis of a cystic hygroma involving the chin, neck and anterior thoracic wall posed a challenge for delivery (Tanaka et al 1994). Airway control had to be achieved as soon as possible after uterine incision, but before interruption of maternal-fetal circulation. One fetus had a neck mass aspirated in utero, followed by surgery at 2 days. On day 5, the infant developed stridor, and the lymphangioma was found to extend from the skull base into the mediastinum (Chen 1999).

2. Lymphangiomas of the tongue may suddenly increase in size secondary to bleeding, trauma, or infection. Recurrent infection is a common problem.

3. Induction, airway maintenance, or intubation problems (MacDonald 1966, Scally & Black 1990).

4. Surgery is often prolonged and difficult

because the tumour infiltrates and destroys normal dissection planes.

5. Lingual oedema can occur after resection of submandibular lesions. Postoperative swelling of the tongue and floor of mouth may be alarming in the rapidity of its development.

6. Obstructive sleep apnoea and hypoxaemia may occur.

7. Infection is a danger because of impaired lymphatic drainage.

Management

1. Accurate diagnosis and anatomical localisation is essential to safe surgery and prediction of airway problems. MRI scans produce the best pictures (Fung et al 1998).

2. The patient may need a tracheostomy either pre- or postoperatively. Forty-one percent of children with cystic hygroma involving the neck suffered significant upper airway or feeding problems, and two-thirds of those with airway problems required tracheostomy (Emery et al 1984). Thus, it is essential to perform surgery where there are adequate facilities for paediatric intensive care.

3. May need a feeding gastrotomy.

4. Intralaryngeal tumours may require laser treatment (Cohen & Thompson 1986).

5. Infections will need prompt antibiotic therapy.

6. Sudden swelling in an adult cystic hygroma recurrence responded to emergency tracheostomy and corticosteroids (Scally & Black 1990).

7. In the case of prenatal diagnosis of potential airway obstruction in the fetus, a multidisciplinary approach must be planned.

Bibliography
Balakrishnan A, Bailey CM 1991 Lymphangioma of the tongue. A review of pathogenesis, treatment and the use of surface laser coagulation. Journal of Laryngology & Otology 105: 924–9.

Castanon M, Margarit J, Carrasco R et al 1999 Long-term follow-up of nineteen cystic lymphangiomas with fibrin sealant. Journal of Pediatric Surgery 34: 1276–9.

Chen C-P 1999 Congenital cervical cystic hygroma causing an airway emergency. American Journal of Emergency Medicine 17: 622–4.

Cohen SR, Thompson JW 1986 Lymphangiomas of the larynx in infants and children. A survey of pediatric lymphangioma. Annals of Otology, Rhinology & Laryngology 95 (suppl) 1–20.

Editorial 1990 Cystic hygroma. Lancet 335: 511–12.

Emery PJ, Bailey CM, Evans JNG 1984 Cystic hygroma of the head and neck. A review of 37 cases. Journal of Laryngology & Otology 98: 613–19.

Fung K, Poenaru D, Soboleski DA et al 1998 Impact of magnetic resonance imaging on the surgical management of cystic hygromas. Journal of Pediatric Surgery 33: 839–41.

Goodman P, Yeung CS, Batsakis JG 1990 Retropharyngeal lymphangioma presenting in an adult. Otolaryngology, Head & Neck Surgery 103: 476–9.

Hancock BJ, St-Vil D, Luks FI et al 1992 Complications of lymphangiomas in children. Journal of Pediatric Surgery 27: 220–4.

MacDonald DJF 1966 Cystic hygroma. An anaesthetic and surgical problem. Anaesthesia 21: 66–71.

Padwa BL, Hayward PG, Ferraro NF et al JB 1995 Cervicofacial lymphatic malformation: clinical course, surgical intervention, and pathogenesis of skeletal hypertrophy. Plastic & Reconstructive Surgery 95: 951–60.

Ricciardelli EJ, Richardson MA 1991 Cervicofacial cystic hygroma. Patterns of recurrence and management of the difficult case. Archives of Otolaryngology & Head & Neck Surgery 117: 546–53.

Scally CM, Black JHA 1990 Cystic hygroma: massive recurrence in adult life. Journal of Otology & Laryngology 104: 908–10.

Tanaka M, Sato S, Naito H et al 1994 Anaesthetic management of a neonate with prenatally diagnosed cervical tumour and upper airway obstruction. Canadian Journal of Anaesthesia 41: 236–40.

Weller RM 1974 Anaesthesia for cystic hygroma in a neonate. Anaesthesia 29: 588–94.

Wiggs WJ Jr, Sismanis A 1994 Cystic hygroma in the adult: two case reports. Otolaryngology—Head & Neck Surgery 110: 239–41.

Dandy–Walker syndrome

Dandy–Walker syndrome

The Dandy–Walker syndrome or complex describes abnormalities of the posterior fossa that usually present in infancy with hydrocephalus. Occasionally it is found incidentally in adult life. Anaesthesia may be required for CT or MRI scan, ventriculoperitoneal shunts, cystoperitoneal shunts, or resection of cyst membranes.

Preoperative abnormalities

1. Hypoplasia or absence of the cerebellar vermis, and a posterior fossa cyst in continuity with the fourth ventricle. Obstructive hydrocephalus develops in about 90% of infants. There is a gradual increase in intracranial pressure until a shunt is required. Other CNS anomalies may occur and patients are often of low IQ.

2. A large head may result from the hydrocephalus, or from the cyst. Other craniofacial abnormalities can include cleft palate, macroglossia, and micrognathia.

3. An association has been described between facial haemangiomas and posterior fossa anomalies. Four out of the nine infants described also had haemangiomas involving the larynx or pharynx (Reese et al 1993).

4. Cardiac defects, such as PDA and septal defects.

5. Renal and skeletal abnormalities.

6. An MRI scan will delineate the abnormalities.

Anaesthetic problems

1. Central ventilatory abnormalities occur, possibly involving the brainstem, with apnoeic episodes.

2. Potential difficult intubation. A 5-month-old infant with cleft lip and palate, micrognathia, and hydrocephalus had a failed intubation (Selim et al 1999).

3. A child with a blocked shunt developed hypertension, tachycardia and pulmonary oedema on induction of anaesthesia (Ashley 1998). Aspiration of CSF from the Holter valve relieved the tachycardia, but IPPV was required for 24 h.

4. Presentation may be delayed until adulthood. The abnormality was found incidentally in a 39 year old who had sustained a head injury (Cone 1995).

5. Multiple anaesthetics may be required for shunt surgery (Ewart & Oh 1990). Complications of posterior fossa shunts may occur, in particular the development of cranial nerve damage (Lee et al 1995). Brainstem tethering and formation of a posterior fossa cyst caused cranial nerve deficits in a 5-year-old child, who had undergone multiple shunt revisions for Dandy–Walker syndrome from the age of 2 months (Liu et al 1995).

Management

1. Assess intubation problems. MRI was used to view the relationship between the tongue and glottic opening in a 3-kg child with partial upper airway obstruction and a large Dandy–Walker cyst. A laryngeal mask airway was inserted under local anaesthesia (Abouleish & Mayhew 1998). Use of a laryngeal mask airway was reported in a 5 month old with failed intubation (Selim et al 1999). Fibreoptic bronchoscopy ascertained the position of the vocal cords and a 2.5-mm tube was used to railroad a 3-mm tube through the vocal cords.

2. Upper airway obstruction may be relieved by nasal CPAP (Abouleish & Mayhew 1998).

3. Close respiratory monitoring in the perioperative period.

Bibliography
Abouleish AE, Mayhew JF 1998 Magnetic resonance imaging of the airway in an infant with micrognathia. Anesthesia & Analgesia 86: 964–6.
Ashley EMC 1998 Acute arrhythmias on induction of anaesthesia in a child with a blocked shunt. Anaesthesia 53: 930–1.

Cone AM 1995 Head injury in an adult with previously undiagnosed Dandy–Walker syndrome: a review of the condition and discussion of its anaesthetic implications. Anaesthesia & Intensive Care 23: 613–15.

Ewart MC, Oh TE 1990 The Dandy–Walker syndrome. Relevance to anaesthesia and intensive care. Anaesthesia 45: 646–8.

Lee M, Leahu D, Weiner HL et al 1995 Complications of fourth-ventricular shunts. Paediatric Neurosurgery 22: 309–14.

Liu JC, Ciacci JD, George TM 1995 Brainstem tethering in Dandy–Walker syndrome: a complication of cystoperitoneal shunting. Journal of Neurosurgery 83: 1072–4.

Mayhew JF, Miner ME, Denneny J 1985 Upper airway obstruction following cyst-to-peritoneal shunt in a child with a Dandy–Walker cyst. Anesthesiology 62: 183–4.

Reese V, Frieden IJ, Paller AS et al 1993 Associations of facial haemangiomas with Dandy–Walker and other posterior fossa malformations. Journal of Pediatrics 122: 379–84.

Selim M, Mowafi H, Al-Ghamdi A et al 1999 Intubation via laryngeal mask airway in pediatric patients with difficult airways. Canadian Journal of Anaesthesia 46: 575–7.

Demyelinating diseases

A general name for a group of neurological diseases involving myelin sheath abnormalities, of which multiple sclerosis (MS) is the most common. The myelin surrounding an axon may develop normally and be lost later, but leaving the axon preserved. Alternatively, there may be some defect in the original formation of myelin as a result of an error of metabolism. Multiple sclerosis is thought to be autoimmune in nature.

Susceptibility to MS may be genetically determined. Viral and immune factors are possibly involved. It is characterised by a combination of inflammation, demyelination, and axonal damage in the CNS (Whitaker 1998). Disruption of the blood–brain barrier is an early event (McFarland 1998). Plaques of demyelination are scattered throughout the nervous system, usually in the optic nerve, brainstem, and spinal cord. The peripheral nerves are not involved. Only the problems of MS will be discussed further.

Preoperative abnormalities

1. The diagnosis is made on clinical grounds, when neurological lesions are disseminated both in time and space. Consequently the clinical picture is highly variable.

2. The commonest presenting symptoms, in order of frequency, are limb weakness, visual disturbances, paraesthesiae, and incoordination. Legs are more commonly involved before the arms, with signs of spasticity and hyperreflexia. Urinary symptoms may occur.

3. Progression, with remissions and relapses, is very variable. Infection, trauma, and stress may be associated with relapses. A small increase in body temperature can cause a definite deterioration in neural function. The third trimester of pregnancy is associated with a 70% decrease in relapse rate, but this is followed by an increase of about 70% in the first 3 months postpartum (Confavreux et al 1998). This may impair the ability of a mother to care for her child.

4. Pain may be a prominent feature, occurring at any one time in 45% of patients.

5. Mild dementia and dysarthria may appear as the disease progresses.

6. In advanced disease, and sometimes earlier during acute relapses, respiratory complications may occur secondary to a variety of causes; they were, in decreasing order of importance, respiratory muscle weakness, bulbar weakness, and central control of breathing (Howard et al 1992).

7. MRI now plays an important part in the diagnosis, and abnormalities in the white matter can be seen in 99% of cases. Gadolinium enhancement seems to reflect areas of inflammation where the blood–brain barrier has broken down. However, there appears to be little relationship between the extent of the lesions seen on MRI and the clinical picture.

8.   Patients may be receiving baclofen, gabapentin, or beta interferon.

Anaesthetic problems

Reports of anaesthetics given to patients with MS are both numerous and conflicting. Advice regarding the avoidance of particular drugs or techniques is inconsistent, and is often based on small numbers of patients. In the event of a relapse, major difficulty exists in the separation of the effects of drugs, surgery, pyrexia, or stress. An analysis of 88 general anaesthetics given to 42 patients did not show a relapse rate greater than that which would have been expected to have occurred spontaneously (Bamford et al 1978).

1.   Both experimentally and clinically, an increase in body temperature has been shown to cause a deterioration in nerve conduction and neurological signs.

2.   Spinal anaesthesia. A review of the medical literature, and a limited personal experience, led one group to the conclusion that spinal anaesthesia was associated with an increased incidence of neurological complications (Bamford et al 1978).

3.   Epidural anaesthesia. A recent study of 256 pregnancies in 241 women with MS showed that there was no difference between those who had been given an epidural and those who had not (Confavreux et al 1998). This confirms previous experiences of uncomplicated epidural anaesthetics in pregnant MS patients (Crawford et al 1981). Another study showed that epidural anaesthesia for delivery was not associated with a significantly higher incidence of relapses than local infiltration (Bader et al 1988). Temporary neurological deficits have, however, been reported. One patient developed localised paraesthesiae lasting 7 h and 7 weeks respectively following two epidurals, in consecutive labours (Warren et al 1982). The longer deficit followed a total dose of bupivacaine of 562.5 mg during a 15-h period. It was postulated that neurotoxicity might have resulted from the diffusion of the anaesthetic into the dural space. There is no

reason to deny a patient the benefits of an epidural anaesthetic, should it be considered necessary. However, it has been suggested that concentrations of bupivacaine of not greater than 0.25% should be used, since postpartum relapse has been reported with those in excess of this (Bader et al 1988).

4.   Local anaesthesia. One thousand procedures performed under local anaesthesia in 98 patients did not significantly increase the relapse rate (Bamford et al 1978). However, early disruption of the blood–brain barrier in MS means that local anaesthetics can cross more readily, and toxicity is more likely to occur.

5.   Neuromuscular blockers. Resistance to atracurium, in association with an abnormally high concentration of skeletal muscle acetylcholine receptors, has been reported in a patient with MS and spastic paraparesis (Brett et al 1987).

6.   There is an increased incidence of epilepsy in MS patients.

Management

1.   It is vital to know, either from the notes or from staff, whether or not the patient is aware of the precise diagnosis. Appropriate discussions can take place with the patient in the light of this knowledge.

2.   Elective surgery should not be undertaken in the presence of fever.

3.   Spinal anaesthesia should probably be avoided (Bamford et al 1978), although the use of local anaesthetic and diamorphine given through an intrathecal catheter has been used for sigmoid colectomy, in a patient with advanced disease involving paralysis of his intercostal muscles (Leigh et al 1990).

4.   If a regional block is required, epidural anaesthesia is preferable, and should not be denied. It is essential to document existing signs and symptoms accurately, and have a full discussion with the patient. Epidural anaesthesia

has been performed for Caesarean section in a patient with MS and von Hippel–Lindau disease associated with a small haemangioblastoma of the spine (Wang & Sinatra 1999). Following MRI of the spine, the needle was sited distal to the lesion.

5. Fourteen patients were given intravenous gamma globulin immediately after delivery, and none relapsed in the first 6 months postpartum (Orvieto et al 1999).

6. The maximum dose of local anaesthetic should be reduced below that normally recommended. Techniques that require large doses should be avoided.

7. Patients may require treatment for pain and spasticity. Kim and Ferrante (1998) describe relief of adductor spasticity for 5 months after a cryoprobe was applied to the obturator nerve under fluoroscopic control.

Bibliography

Bader AM, Hunt CO, Datta S et al 1988 Anaesthesia for the obstetric patient with multiple sclerosis. Journal of Clinical Anesthesia 1: 21–4.

Bamford C, Sibley W, Laguna J 1978 Anesthesia in multiple sclerosis. Le Journal Canadien des Sciences Neurologiques 5: 41–4.

Brett RS, Schmidt JH, Gage JS et al 1987 Measurement of acetylcholine receptor concentration in skeletal muscle from a patient with multiple sclerosis and resistance to atracurium. Anesthesiology 66: 837–9.

Confavreux C, Hutchinson M, Hours MM et al 1998 Rate of pregnancy-related relapse in multiple sclerosis. New England Journal of Medicine 339: 285–91.

Crawford JS, James FM, Nolte H et al 1981 Regional analgesia for patients with chronic neurological disease and similar conditions. Anaesthesia 36: 821.

Howard RS, Wiles CM, Hirsch NP et al 1992 Respiratory involvement in multiple sclerosis. Brain 115: 479–94.

Kim PS, Ferrante FM 1998 Cryoanalgesia: a novel treatment for hip adductor spasticity and obturator neuralgia. Anesthesiology 89: 534–6.

Leigh J, Fearnley SJ, Lupprian KG 1990 Intrathecal diamorphine during laparotomy in a patient with advanced multiple sclerosis. Anaesthesia 45: 640–2.

McFarland HF 1998 The lesion in multiple sclerosis: clinical, pathological, and magnetic resonance imaging considerations. Journal of Neurology, Neurosurgery & Psychiatry 64 (suppl 1): S26–30.

Orvieto R, Achiron R, Rotstein Z et al 1999 Pregnancy and multiple sclerosis: a 2-year experience. European Journal of Obstetrics, Gynecology, & Reproductive Biology 82: 191–4.

Wang A, Sinatra RS 1999 Epidural anesthesia for cesarean section in a patient with von Hippel–Lindau disease and multiple sclerosis. Anesthesia & Analgesia 88: 1083–4.

Warren TM, Datta S, Ostheimer GW 1982 Lumbar epidural anesthesia in a patient with multiple sclerosis. Anesthesia & Analgesia 61: 1022–3.

Whitaker JN 1998 Effects of pregnancy and delivery on disease activity in multiple sclerosis. New England Journal of Medicine 339: 339–40.

Dermatomyosititis/polymyositis complex

A group of autoimmune chronic inflammatory disorders primarily affecting muscle and skin, although there may be multisystem involvement. The related diseases include primary idiopathic polymyositis, primary idiopathic dermatomyositis, dermatomyositis associated with malignancy, a childhood form of dermatomyositis, and a form of the complex which is associated with other collagen diseases.

Preoperative abnormalities

1. A rash is a presenting feature in 100% of cases. A violaceous appearance of the eyelids and upper part of the face is caused by the cutaneous lesions. The rash may also be seen on the knees, knuckles, elbows, and periungually.

2. The inflammatory myopathy may present with muscle aches, tenderness, and weakness, involving proximal and distal muscles and the limb-girdle muscles. Contractures and muscle atrophy may occur later. Respiratory muscle weakness can occur simultaneously.

3. There is an increased risk of malignancy, in particular nasopharyngeal (Peng et al 1995) and

colonic cancer, and both carry a higher mortality rate than normal.

4. There may be patchy infiltration of the lungs with interstitial fibrosis, peripheral oedema, alveolitis, and soft-tissue calcification. A restrictive ventilatory pattern is seen and 40% of patients develop lung disease within a mean of 17 months of onset (Marie et al 1998).

5. Although all muscle enzymes may be elevated, the CK is said to be the most sensitive indicator of disease activity. Serum myoglobin may be better, but is not routinely measured. The patient may be anaemic.

6. Attendance at an ENT department is a common mode of presentation (Metheny 1978). Voice changes and upper oesophageal dysphagia were found to be the most frequent problems. Laryngo-oesophageal tone is reduced, with dysfunction of the tongue and soft palate. Saliva pools in the pyriform fossa, and regurgitation and aspiration leading to pneumonia, may occur. Aspiration pneumonia is a frequent cause of death. Nasopharyngeal carcinoma is also common.

7. Up to 40% of patients have cardiac problems; these include ECG changes and congestive heart failure. The presence of cardiac involvement is associated with a less good prognosis. Necrotising vasculitis and cardiac involvement may sometimes appear in the childhood form.

8. The patient may be taking steroids or immunosuppressives.

9. Pregnancy may be associated with fetal loss, particularly in active disease, but reports are contradictory (King & Chow 1985).

10. An abnormal EMG and evidence of a necrotising inflammatory process on muscle biopsy.

Anaesthetic problems

1. Dermatomyositis is associated with an increased incidence of malignancy (Richardson & Callen 1989, Sigurgeirsson et al 1992).

2. Prolonged neuromuscular blockade after vecuronium has been reported (Flusche et al 1987), but the reason for this is obscure since an inflammatory myopathy should not affect the neuromuscular junction. However, neuromuscular monitoring in two patients receiving atracurium (Ganta et al 1988), one having vecuronium (Saarnivaara 1988), and another having both suxamethonium and atracurium (Brown et al 1992), did not suggest sensitivity. However, one child had an abnormal response to suxamethonium. Before muscle relaxation occurred, fasciculations were followed by a short period of muscle contraction (Johns et al 1986). Nevertheless, marked increases in muscle tone following suxamethonium may occur in some normal patients, so the significance of this is uncertain (Leary & Ellis 1990).

3. Swallowing and vocal cord dysfunction may cause pooling of secretions and aspiration of gastric contents (Metheny 1978).

4. Aspiration pneumonia is the commonest pulmonary problem and postoperative respiratory insufficiency may occur.

5. Dermatomyositis presented in the first trimester with a painful, inflammatory myopathy, rhabdomyolysis (CK 3974 u l^{-1}), and fetal loss (Kofteridis et al 1999).

Management

1. A careful assessment of the systems involved in the disease, and in particular for signs of malignancy.

2. Monitoring of neuromuscular function is essential.

3. In view of the problems with swallowing and pooling of secretions, tracheal intubation may be advisable.

Bibliography
Brown S, Shupak RC, Patel C et al 1992 Neuromuscular blockade in a patient with active dermatomyositis. Anesthesiology 77: 1031–3.
Flusche G, Unger-Sargon J, Lambert DH 1987 Prolonged neuromuscular paralysis with

vecuronium in a patient with polymyositis. Anesthesia & Analgesia 66: 188–90.

Ganta R, Campbell IT, Mostafa SM 1988 Anaesthesia and acute dermatomyositis/polymyositis. British Journal of Anaesthesia 60: 854–8.

Johns RA, Finholt DA, Stirt JA 1986 Anaesthetic management of a child with dermatomyositis. Canadian Anaesthetists' Society Journal 33: 71–4.

King CR, Chow S 1985 Dermatomyositis and pregnancy. Obstetrics & Gynecology 66: 589–92.

Kofteridis DP, Malliotatis PI, Sotsiou F et al 1999 Acute onset dermatomyositis presenting in pregnancy with rhabdomyolysis and fetal loss. Scandinavian Journal of Rheumatology 28: 192–4.

Leary NP, Ellis FR 1990 Masseteric muscle spasm as a normal response to suxamethonium. British Journal of Anaesthesia 64: 488–92.

Lie JT 1995 Cardiac manifestations in polymyositis/dermatomyositis: how to get to the heart of the problem. Journal of Rheumatology 22: 809–11.

Marie I, Hatron PY, Hachulla E et al 1998 Pulmonary involvement in polymyositis and in dermatomyositis. Journal of Rheumatology 25: 1336–43.

Metheny JA 1978 Dermatomyositis: a vocal and swallowing disease entity. Laryngoscope 88: 147–61.

Peng JC, Sheen TS, Hsu MM 1995 Nasopharyngeal carcinoma with dermatomyositis. Analysis of 12 cases. Archives of Otolaryngology—Head & Neck Surgery 121: 1298–301.

Richardson JB, Callen JP 1989 Dermatomyositis and malignancy. Medical Clinics of North America 73: 1121–30.

Saarnivaara LHM 1988 Anesthesia for a patient with polymyositis undergoing myomectomy of the cricopharyngeal muscle. Anesthesia & Analgesia 67: 701–2.

Sigurgeirsson B, Lindelof B, Edhag O et al 1992 Risk of cancer in patients with dermatomyositis or polymyositis. A population based study. New England Journal of Medicine 326: 363–7.

Strauss KW, Gonzalez-Buritica H, Khamashta MA et al 1989 Polymyositis–dermatomyositis: a clinical review. Postgraduate Medical Journal 65: 437–43.

Diabetes insipidus

The result of a failure of arginine vasopressin secretion by the posterior part of the pituitary. In the presence of low levels of ADH, the kidney is unable to conserve water, and large volumes of dilute urine are excreted. It may be secondary to pituitary or hypothalamic surgery, head injury, tumour, multiple sclerosis, or in pregnancy. Diabetes insipidus (DI) is also common in brain dead patients. Lithium treatment may rarely be associated with a mild DI-like syndrome (Anonymous 1995). Diabetes insipidus appeared 2 days after chemical meningitis following spinal anaesthesia, and was thought to be caused by detergent used for washing a reusable glass syringe (Garfield et al 1986).

Preoperative abnormalities

1. Results from one of four different defects; impaired secretion by the neurohypophysis, impaired renal response (nephrogenic DI), excessive fluid intake, and increased metabolism of the hormone (gestational DI) (Robertson 1995).

2. Polyuria and polydipsia. The urine volume may reach $24 \, day^{-1}$.

3. Hypovolaemia and hypernatraemia.

4. Urinary osmolality is low, $50–100 \, mOsm \, kg^{-1}$, (median range=$50–1400 \, mosm \, kg^{-1}$), and there is an increased plasma osmolality (median range=$275–295 \, mosm \, kg^{-1}$).

5. Treatment will depend on the cause (Singer et al 1997).

Anaesthetic problems

1. Dehydration. If the patient does not increase his/her fluid intake, there will be dehydration, hypernatraemia, and plasma hyperosmolality. Untreated, the condition may lead to permanent brain damage (Vin-Christian & Arieff 1993).

2. Electrolyte imbalance.

3. Postoperative diabetes insipidus may occur following surgery to the pituitary or adrenal

gland (Lehrnbecher et al 1998). However, other causes may be less clear cut. In one patient after lung surgery, polyuria was suggested to be secondary to central causes (Otsuka et al 1997). MRI changes were seen in the hypophysis and its stalk, and these had disappeared 2 months later.

4. Diabetes insipidus can occur as a complication of pregnancy, without any previous history. This may be secondary to vasopressinase secreted by the placenta, or to latent central or nephrogenic DI. A patient with a twin pregnancy presented at 32 weeks, with a seizure, dry mucous membranes, extreme thirst, and a urinary output of 5 l in 6 h. DDAVP was given intranasally bd. Since epidural anaesthesia was requested, a central venous catheter was inserted first, so that fluid balance could be assessed. By the fourth day postpartum, there were no signs of DI. The abrupt onset, and immediate cessation following delivery, was suggestive of placental secretion of vasopressinase. The thirst stimulus for nonpregnant individuals is 298 mosm kg^{-1}, whereas in pregnancy it is reduced to 287 mosm kg^{-1} and the normal serum osmolality decreases from 280–270 mosm kg^{-1} (Passannante et al 1995). A 14-year-old girl was admitted at 33 weeks' gestation with abdominal pain and oligohydramnios. On day 2, her intake was 8 l and her output 13.6 l, her serum sodium 153 mmol l^{-1}, and her plasma osmolality 312 mmol l^{-1}. Desmopressin resolved both the oligohydramnios and her fluid output (Hanson et al 1997). Two convulsions occurred 20 min postpartum in a healthy woman. Her serum sodium was found to be 118 mmol l^{-1} and she admitted to drinking several litres of a commercial drink, promoted for use during physical exertion, which contained water, glucose, sodium 8 mmol l^{-1}, and potassium 4 mmol l^{-1}. Synocinon 5 u im was given after delivery (Paech 1998). Permanent central DI developed during pregnancy when a VP shunt was functionally occluded by the expanding uterus. The patient was admitted unconscious, at 26 weeks' gestation, with a plasma sodium of 158 mmol l^{-1} and a osmolality of 332 mosm kg^{-1} (Goolsby & Harlass 1996).

5. Severe hypovolaemia associated with diabetes insipidus in cadaveric organ donors will require treatment. If vasopressin is used, and its administration continued until the kidneys are removed, there is an increase in the incidence of tubular necrosis and graft failure in the recipient. Its analogue, desmopressin, has no vasoconstrictor effects.

6. Hypothermia has been reported in a patient with idiopathic diabetes insipidus following thoracic surgery. There was delayed recovery from anaesthesia and his temperature had decreased to below 32°C. A hypothalamic mechanism was postulated (Johnston & Vaughan 1988).

Management

1. Desmopressin nasally 10–20 μg bd, or 0.5–2 μg iv, increases water reabsorption from the renal tubules.

2. The urine output and serum osmolality is monitored. If the serum osmolality is >290 mmol kg^{-1}, iv fluids and desmopressin are required. In pregnancy, the threshold for treatment is lower.

3. In pregnancy, CVP monitoring may be needed, and fluid boluses given, if an epidural is required. Free water is needed in DI, and this may be a problem if fluids are restricted during labour (Passannante et al 1995).

Bibliography

Anonymous 1995 Hyperosmolar coma due to lithium-induced diabetes insipidus. Lancet 346: 413–17.

Garfield JM, Andriole GL, Vetto JT et al 1986 Prolonged diabetes insipidus subsequent to an episode of chemical meningitis. Anesthesiology 64: 253–4.

Goolsby L, Harlass F 1996 Central diabetes insipidus: a complication of ventriculoperitoneal shunt malfunction. American Journal of Obstetrics and Gynecology 174: 1655–7.

Hanson RS, Powrie PO, Larson L 1997 Diabetes insipidus in pregnancy: a treatable cause of oligohydramnios. Obstetrics & Gynecology 89: 816–17.

Johnston KR, Vaughan RS 1988 Delayed recovery from general anaesthesia. Anaesthesia 43: 1024–5.

Lehrnbecher T, Muller-Scholden J, Danhauser-Leistner I et al 1998 Perioperative fluid and electrolyte management in children undergoing surgery for craniopharyngioma. A 10-year experience in a single institution. Childs Nervous System 14: 276–9.

Otsuka F, Mizobuchi S, Morita K et al 1997 Postanesthetic polyuria attributable to central diabetes insipidus. Anesthesia & Analgesia 85: 940–3.

Paech MJ 1998 Convulsions in a healthy parturient due to intrapartum water intoxication. International Journal of Obstetric Anesthesia 7: 59–61.

Passannante AN, Kopp VJ, Mayer DC 1995 Diabetes insipidus and epidural analgesia for labor. Anesthesia & Analgesia 80: 837–8.

Robertson GL 1995 Diabetes insipidus. Endocrine & Metabolism Clinics of North America 24: 549–72.

Singer I, Oster JR, Fishman LM 1997 The management of diabetes insipidus in adults. Archives of Internal Medicine 157: 1293–301.

Vin-Christian K, Arieff AI 1993 Diabetes insipidus, massive polyuria, and hypernatremia leading to permanent brain damage. American Journal of Medicine 94: 341–2.

Diabetes mellitus

In insulin-dependent diabetes (IDD, type I), the insulin deficiency means that catabolism exceeds anabolism, and in the absence of treatment, a state of hyperosmolar ketoacidosis will progress to hypokalaemia, dehydration, coma, and death.

In noninsulin-dependent diabetes (NIDD, type II) the pancreas still secretes insulin, but supply may not meet demand, so that under certain circumstances, such as surgical stress, there is insulin resistance and gluconeogenesis. The metabolic changes produced by surgery will worsen the state of diabetes.

Surgery should not be undertaken in diabetics who are out of control. Conversely, hypoglycaemia is undetectable, and hence dangerous, during anaesthesia. The increased insulin requirements must therefore be monitored closely and balanced with a supply of glucose and potassium.

Preoperative abnormalities

1. *Diagnosis.* A fasting venous or capillary whole blood glucose of >6.7 mmol l^{-1}, or a venous plasma level of >7.8 mmol l^{-1}. This can then be confirmed with a second FBG or a value after a glucose load. In symptomatic patients a random glucose of 11.1 mmol l^{-1} or more is usually diagnostic.

2. *Metabolic.* In the absence of insulin there is increased lipid metabolism with fatty acid release, increased ketone production such that the supply exceeds utilisation, and increased gluconeogenesis and glycogenolysis. The net result is acidaemia, ketoacidosis, and hyperglycaemia. This hyperosmolar state leads to polyuria that in turn causes urinary loss of sodium, potassium, calcium, phosphate, and magnesium. The acidosis results in loss of cellular potassium and the deficiency of insulin prevents cellular uptake of potassium. Sodium is also lost with the urinary excretion of ketoacids.

3. *Cardiovascular disease.* Large vessel disease leads to atherosclerosis and myocardial disease. The microangiopathy, which affects particularly renal, retinal and digital vessels, appears to be related to the increased levels of blood glucose. There is a high mortality from myocardial and peripheral vascular disease.

4. *Infection.* Resistance to infection and wound healing are both impaired.

5. *Renal failure.* A common complication of diabetes, and the mortality from renal transplantation is two to four times greater than in nondiabetic patients.

6. *Neuropathy.* Peripheral and autonomic neuropathies, which may be related to high levels of sorbitol, are common.

7. *'Stiff joint syndrome'.* Limited joint mobility, in which patients are unable to approximate their palms (the prayer sign), is said

to occur in 30–40% of insulin-dependent diabetics. The joints of the hands are usually involved early, and the skin becomes thick and waxy. There is a positive correlation with microvascular disease and the condition is progressive, ultimately involving all joints. It may be related to abnormal collagen cross-linkages. Lung elasticity may also be reduced.

8. *Mortality.* In a study of type 1 diabetics diagnosed under the age of 30 years the relative risks for death was 4.0 for females and 2.7 for males (Laing et al 1999). However, there was a peak of 5.7 for females aged 20–29 and of 4.0 in males age 40–49.

Anaesthetic problems

1. There is a higher perioperative morbidity and mortality in diabetic than in nondiabetic patients. Myocardial disease and infection are chiefly responsible for this.

2. Surgery and stress aggravate diabetes and may be accompanied by some degree of insulin resistance. In addition, insulin resistance occurs in association with severe infection, obesity, liver disease, steroid therapy, and cardiopulmonary bypass.

3. There is an increased incidence of infections. Multiple epidural abscesses have been reported following spinal anaesthesia (Mahendru et al 1994). A trial of aggressive insulin therapy versus standard insulin therapy during cardiac surgery showed an improvement in neutrophil function in those in whom continuous insulin was given. Whilst the aim was not to look at infection, there were two major infections and one minor in the standard insulin group, whilst none occurred in the continuous infusion group (Rassias et al 1999).

4. Hypoglycaemia can occur suddenly during anaesthesia. The clinical signs are undetectable and brain damage can ensue.

5. Whilst a mild elevation of blood glucose is acceptable during surgery, it should be maintained between 6 and 13 mmol l^{-1}. The renal threshold for glucose is 10 mmol l^{-1}. At levels above this, glycosuria causes an osmotic diuresis, with loss of water and electrolytes. In addition, hyperglycaemia is associated with impaired wound healing and disordered phagocyte function.

6. Administration of lactate-containing solutions may increase blood glucose, or may exacerbate lactic acidosis when this occurs in hyperglycaemic states.

7. Ketosis may produce insulin resistance and alter the metabolism of anaesthetic agents. It also increases potassium loss from the body. Hypokalaemia may induce cardiac arrhythmias during anaesthesia.

8. Ketoacidosis is associated with gastric atony and ileus, which increase the risk of inhalation of gastric contents.

9. Autonomic neuropathy may be responsible for cardiovascular and respiratory complications during anaesthesia. Five diabetics were reported in whom episodes of cardiorespiratory arrest occurred in association with anaesthesia (Page & Watkins 1978). Episodes of respiratory arrest and loss of consciousness may continue into the second postoperative day (Thomas & Pollard 1989). It was suggested that autonomic neuropathy could reduce the respiratory responses to hypoxia and hypercarbia. Certainly, the diabetic heart is more susceptible to hypoxia in the absence of sympathetic drive. In some patients, prolongation of the QT interval has been associated with arrest or sudden death. Ventricular fibrillation occurred following renal transplant in a 31-year-old man and the QT$_c$ was 503 ms (Reissell et al 1994). A 39-year-old with a QT$_c$ of 447 ms developed asystole at the end of surgery (but before neostigmine), and he required epinephrine (adrenaline) followed by cardioversion for resuscitation (Usher & Shaw 1999). There is also an impaired ability to respond to stress by vasoconstriction and tachycardia (see Autonomic failure). In a prospective study of 17 diabetic patients having eye surgery, 35% required vasopressors compared with 5% of nondiabetic controls, and

those with worse autonomic function required them more often (Burgos et al 1989). However, no relationship was found between cardiac autonomic function and haemodynamic behaviour during anaesthetic induction in diabetic and nondiabetic patients scheduled for CABG (Keyl et al 1999). Atropine-induced heart rate was found to be significantly lower in diabetics than nondiabetics (Tsueda et al 1991).

10. Local anaesthetic procedures are not without problems. Twenty minutes after brachial plexus block for the creation of an arteriovenous fistula, two patients suffered progressive bradycardia and hypotension that responded to external cardiac massage and epinephrine (adrenaline) (Lucas & Tsueda 1990). Although in one patient the combined local anaesthetic blood level approached the seizure threshold, it was considerably less than that likely to produce cardiovascular collapse.

11. Difficult intubation is more likely in patients with type 1 diabetes (Salzarulo & Taylor 1986, Reissell et al 1990). This may be related to involvement of the atlanto-occipital joint in 'stiff joint syndrome'. A group of type 1 diabetics have joint contractures and a thick waxy skin, associated with rapidly progressive microvascular disease. This accounts for the higher than normal incidence of difficult laryngoscopy found in diabetics undergoing renal and pancreatic transplantation. However, series vary in the percentage and degree of difficulty reported. Out of 115 diabetics having renal or pancreas transplants, difficult laryngoscopy was found in about 40%, whereas in 112 nondiabetic patients having renal transplants, the incidence was only about 2–3% (Hogan et al 1988). Most of the difficult patients had blind intubation after several attempts, but three were woken up for fibreoptic intubation, and two had emergency tracheostomies. Laryngeal structures tended to be anterior to the line of vision, with only the posterior part of the arytenoids or epiglottis seen. However, Warner et al (1998) reported a much lower incidence than this. Only 15 out of 725 (2.1%) were identified as difficult, and none required special techniques.

12. Severe lactic acidosis was associated with the use of the biguanide, metformin, in a patient who underwent repair of abdominal wall hernia. Metformin was omitted on the day of surgery but continued daily thereafter, even though the patient's calorie intake was low. On day 4 he developed cardiorespiratory failure, with a base deficit of 12.5 and a serum lactate concentration of 95 mg dl^{-1}. Despite respiratory and renal support he died on day 10 (Mercker et al 1997).

Management

1. *General assessment.* A thorough assessment of the degree of multiorgan involvement by the diabetic process is required. In particular, the presence of cardiovascular and renal diseases, or autonomic neuropathy (see Autonomic failure) must be determined. If there is autonomic failure, then there should be close respiratory and cardiovascular monitoring throughout the perioperative period. After major surgery, oxygen supplements, ECG and oxygen saturation monitoring should be continued for 48 h (Thomas & Pollard 1989).

2. *Assessment of intubation problems.* If there is physical evidence of 'stiff joint syndrome', flexion-extension views of the cervical spine may be helpful. The presence of limited atlanto-occipital extension indicates the possible need for awake tracheal intubation. Examination of the ability of the patient to approximate his fingers may reveal the 'palm sign'. In addition, a palm print, obtained by inking the dominant hand and placing it, with fingers spread, on white paper, has also been used to predict difficult laryngoscopy (Reissell et al 1990). If only the finger tips were visible, laryngoscopy was likely to be difficult.

3. *Assessment of diabetic control.* This includes estimations of FBG levels, glucose test strips, and urinalysis. Variations in the level occur, dependent on the method of sampling. Whole blood glucose values are 10–15% less than plasma values, and fasting capillary is 7% greater than venous values.

4. *Management of diabetes during elective surgery.* Traditionally, it was recommended that diabetics be admitted 2–3 days in advance of surgery and appear first on a morning operating list, and that long-acting oral hypoglycaemic agents be discontinued 2 days in advance, or changed to short-acting ones. Similarly, long-acting insulins should be changed to either actrapid or other short-acting insulin. In practice, the anaesthetist is often presented with diabetic patients the evening before operation—none of these conditions having been met! Practical approaches are:

a) *Diet-controlled diabetics and patients with NIDD*:

   i) Minor surgery. May need no treatment, but the latter should be monitored closely for hypoglycaemia. There is certainly no evidence that insulin is necessary, unless the fasting blood glucose is >13 mmol l^{-1}, in which case an insulin regimen should be established.

   ii) Major surgery (or in NIDD patients with a FBG >10 mmol l^{-1} on the morning of operation). Treat with an insulin infusion as for IDD.

b) *Insulin-dependent diabetics.*

   Various methods of administering insulin have been described. These include short-acting insulin given iv 4 hrly, continuously iv by syringe pump, or mixed in an infusion with glucose and potassium. Subcutaneous insulin is absorbed erratically in the perioperative period and should not be used.

   Management is divided between separate insulin and glucose infusions and the glucose/insulin/potassium (GIK) infusion as described by Alberti.

   i) *Separate iv infusion of glucose and insulin.* With improvement in infusion pumps, and in glucosimetry, the separate infusion regimen seems now to be more in favour (Eldridge & Sear 1996). Actrapid 50 u is mixed in a syringe with 50 ml saline (1 u ml^{-1})

and infused according to a sliding scale:

Blood sugar 3–5 mmol l^{-1}: actrapid 1 ml h^{-1}.

Blood sugar 6–9 mmol l^{-1}: actrapid 1.5 ml h^{-1}.

Blood sugar 10–12 mmol l^{-1}: actrapid 2 ml h^{-1}.

Blood sugar 13–16 mmol l^{-1}: actrapid 4 ml h^{-1}.

Blood sugar >16 mmol l^{-1}: actrapid 6 ml h^{-1}.

Glucose 10% 500 ml, (with or without 10 mmol potassium chloride) is infused at 100 ml h^{-1}. Obviously, care must be taken not to stop one without the other being stopped.

   ii) *GIK technique* (Alberti 1991). Preoperative FBG should be <13 mmol l^{-1}. Postponement of the proposed surgery should be considered if levels are higher than this. The aim should be to maintain a BG of 5–10 mmol l^{-1}. Infuse actrapid 15 u + KCl 10 mmol + 10% glucose 500 ml, at a rate of 100 ml h^{-1}. Repeat BG in 2–3 h. If BG >10 mmol l^{-1} increase insulin to 15 u and check BG in further 2 h. If BG <5 mmol l^{-1} then no insulin should be given. BG should be measured 2-hrly, and serum potassium twice on the day of infusion.

   Despite past fears of insulin absorption into the container and tubes, if the first 50 ml are washed through, 75–90% of the insulin is delivered. Should the infusion run too fast or stop, all the constituents are similarly affected. In addition, if the infusion is started when the morning insulin would have been due, the need for early morning surgery is less urgent. The main disadvantage is the wasted solutions if the insulin dose has to be altered frequently.

5. *The ketoacidotic diabetic*

a) In young diabetics, severe ketoacidosis may cause abdominal pain. If the vomiting starts before the pain, the cause is more likely to be ketoacidosis, whereas pain preceding vomiting is more likely to be surgical.

b) If severe ketoacidosis is present and conditions permit, surgery should be delayed for 4–5 h. Without prior control of the diabetes, mortality is high.

c) Treatment of severe diabetic ketoacidosis (adult).

   i) Investigations: glucose, sodium, potassium, urea, serum osmolality, blood gases.

   ii) Monitoring: BP, pulse, respiration, urine output, CVP measurement.

   iii) Rehydration 0.9% saline 1 l is given in 30 min, then 1 l per hour for 2 h, followed by 500 ml hrly until a total of 5–7 l has been given. 500 ml is then infused 2–4 hrly. When a BG of 10–14 mmol l^{-1} has been achieved, change to 5% glucose 4 hrly. If sodium >146 mmol l^{-1} then, after the second litre of 0.9% saline, substitute sodium chloride 0.18% and glucose 4%.

   iv) Insulin therapy. Give 6 u iv stat, then using hourly glucose test strips, regulate the rate on a sliding scale.

   v) Potassium. Immediately following the first dose of insulin, give potassium chloride 13 mmol h^{-1} in the saline. Monitor serum potassium:

     K$^+$ 3 mmol l^{-1} give 39 mmol h^{-1}.

     K$^+$ 3–4 mmol l^{-1} give 26 mmol h^{-1}.

     K$^+$ 4–6 mmol l^{-1} give 13 mmol h^{-1}.

     K$^+$ >6 mmol l^{-1} stop potassium.

   vi) Acidosis. pH≤7.0, give sodium bicarbonate 100 mmol and KCl 20 mmol in the first 30 min.

pH = 7.0–7.1, give sodium bicarbonate 50 mmol and KCl 10 mmol.

6. *Insulin resistance.* Insulin resistance occurs in a number of circumstances. Normally the ratio of insulin to glucose required is 15 u insulin to 500 ml 10% dextrose. In patients with severe infection, obesity, liver disease, steroid therapy, or undergoing cardiopulmonary bypass, the dose of insulin may have to be increased by up to four times the normal ratio.

7. *Impaired conscious level in diabetics.* Causes include hypoglycaemia, diabetic ketoacidosis, hyperglycaemic hyperosmolar nonketotic coma, and lactic acidosis.

Typical laboratory findings are:

a) *Hypoglycaemia*: BG <2 mmol l^{-1}.

b) *Severe diabetic ketoacidosis*: BG >15 mmol l^{-1}, ketones + to +++, dehydration +++, hyperventilation +++.

c) *Hyperglycaemic, hyperosmolar, nonketotic coma*: BG >15 mmol l^{-1}, ketones 0 to +, dehydration ++++, no hyperventilation.

d) *Lactic acidosis*: BG variable, ketones 0 to +, dehydration 0 to +, hyperventilation +++.

Other nondiabetic causes should not be forgotten.

8. *Diabetic gastroparesis.* The use of erythromycin, which may act as a motilin agonist, has been shown to improve gastric emptying in gastroparesis (Janssens et al 1990).

Bibliography

Alberti KGMM 1991 Diabetes and surgery. Anesthesiology 74: 209–11.

Burgos LG, Ebert TJ, Asiddao C et al 1989 Increased intraoperative cardiovascular morbidity in diabetics with autonomic neuropathy. Anesthesiology 70: 591–7.

Eldridge AJ, Sear JW 1996 Peri-operative management of diabetic patients. Any changes for the better since 1985? Anaesthesia 51: 45–51.

Hall GM 1994 Insulin administration in diabetic patients—return of the bolus. British Journal of Anaesthesia 72: 1–2.

Hogan K, Rusy D, Springman SR 1988 Difficult laryngoscopy and diabetes mellitus. Anesthesia & Analgesia 67: 1162–5.

Janssens J, Peeters TL, Vantrappen G et al 1990 Improvement of gastric emptying in diabetic gastroparesis by erythromycin. New England Journal of Medicine 322: 1028–30.

Keyl C, Lemberger P, Palitzsch K-D et al 1999 Cardiovascular autonomic dysfunction and hemodynamic response to anesthetic induction in patients with coronary artery disease and diabetes mellitus. Anesthesia & Analgesia 88: 985–91.

Laing SP, Swerdlow AJ, Slater SD et al 1999 The British Diabetic Association Cohort Study 1: all-cause mortality in patients with insulin-treated diabetes mellitus. Diabetic Medicine 16: 459–65.

Lucas LF, Tsueda K 1990 Cardiovascular depression following brachial plexus block in two diabetic patients with renal failure. Anesthesiology 73: 1032–5.

Mahendru V, Bacon DR, Lema MJ 1994 Multiple epidural abscesses and spinal anesthesia in a diabetic patient. Case report. Regional Anesthesia 19: 66–8.

Mercker SK, Maier C, Neumann G et al 1997 Lactic acidosis as a serious perioperative complication of antidiabetic biguanide medication with metformin. Anesthesiology 87: 1003–5.

Milaskiewicz RM, Hall GM 1992 Diabetes and anaesthesia: the past decade. British Journal of Anaesthesia 68: 198–206.

Page MMcB, Watkins PJ 1978 Cardiorespiratory arrest and diabetic autonomic neuropathy. Lancet i: 14–16.

Ralley FE 1996 The diabetic patient: a challenge or just routine. Canadian Journal of Anaesthesia 43: R14–18.

Rassias AJ, Marrin CA, Arruda J et al 1999 Insulin infusion improves neutrophil function in diabetic cardiac surgery patients. Anesthesia & Analgesia 88: 1011–16.

Reissell E, Orko R, Maunuksela E-L et al 1990 Predictability of difficult laryngoscopy in patients with long-term diabetes mellitus. Anaesthesia 45: 1024–7.

Reissell E, Yli-Hankala A, Orko R et al 1994 Sudden cardiorespiratory arrest after renal transplantation in a patient with diabetic autonomic neuropathy and prolonged QT interval. Acta Anaesthesiologica Scandinavica 38: 406–8.

Salzarulo HH, Taylor LA 1986 Diabetic 'stiff joint syndrome' as a cause of difficult endotracheal intubation. Anesthesiology 64: 366–8.

Thomas AN, Pollard BJ 1989 Renal transplantation and diabetic autonomic neuropathy. Canadian Journal of Anaesthesia 36: 590–2.

Tsueda K, Huang KC, Dumont SW et al 1991 Cardiac sympathetic tone in anaesthetised diabetics. Canadian Journal of Anaesthesia 38: 20–3.

Usher S, Shaw A 1999 Peri-operative asystole in a patient with diabetic autonomic neuropathy. Anaesthesia 54: 1125.

Warner ME, Contreras MG, Warner MA et al 1998 Diabetes mellitus and difficult laryngoscopy in renal and transplant patients. Anesthesia & Analgesia 86: 516–19.

Diffuse idiopathic skeletal hyperostosis (DISH)

A disease in which spinal rigidity of varying degrees is associated with the formation of anterior and anterolateral osteophytes. Flowing ossification results in bridges between several vertebrae. These hyperostotic complexes occur particularly in the thoracic and cervical regions, but there may be normal areas in between. The condition can resemble ankylosing spondylitis, but differs from it in the absence of sacroiliac disease, lack of involvement of the posterior apophyseal joints, and relative preservation of spinal function. The X-ray features have been reported in 2.4–5.4% of those over 40 years of age (Rotes-Querol 1996). Problems can result from compression of adjacent structures, or increased fragility of the diseased spine.

Preoperative abnormalities

1. Varying degrees of spinal rigidity, which may be asymptomatic or produce morning stiffness. Anterior or anterolateral calcification and ossification occurs between several vertebral bodies, with relative preservation of disc spaces. Areas of hyperostosis can coexist with unaffected segments, which in turn may become stressed.

2. The hyperostotic lesions may cause compression of the oesophagus, the pharynx or the medulla, producing dysphagia, the sensation

of a foreign body, aspiration, snoring, sleep apnoea, or signs of a cervical myopathy.

3. Although rare, atlantoaxial subluxation has been reported (Chiba et al 1992, Oostveen et al 1996).

Anaesthetic problems

1. Several cases of either difficult, or impossible, intubation have been described. Most were not predicted using standard bedside tests, but subsequent lateral cervical X-rays revealed the characteristic anterior osteophytes and flowing ossification (Yamamoto et al 1992, Crosby & Grahovac 1993, Togashi et al 1993, Broadway 1994).

2. Obstruction to the passage of a laryngeal mask airway by a large posterior pharyngeal swelling, which was subsequently found to be a large cervical osteophyte (Aziz et al 1995). A giant cervical osteophyte was also responsible for dysphagia and aspiration pneumonia in an 80 year old (Barbores & Finnerty 1998).

3. Ulceration of the posterior plate of the cricoid cartilage, inflammatory oedema, and secondary bilateral vocal cord paralysis with airway obstruction, have been reported in two patients (Hassard 1984). In another patient, oedema of the larynx necessitated emergency tracheostomy (Marks et al 1998).

4. The affected segments may be fragile and more prone to fracture. Paraplegia from fracture-dislocation of the T9–10 interspace occurred after surgery for a retroperitoneal tumour, during which the patient had been positioned in hyperextension and rotation (Israel et al 1994). Although fractures usually occur through the vertebral body, in this patient it involved the disc space.

5. Potential for aspiration pneumonia (Babores & Finnerty 1998).

6. Acute respiratory failure occurred 10 min after interscalene block, using 40 ml 0.375% bupivacaine, for carpal tunnel surgery in a patient with an 8-year history of DISH. Phrenic nerve paralysis was the cause (Tortosa & Hernandez-Palazon 1998).

Management

1. Assessment of possible intubation difficulties. If DISH is suspected, lateral X-rays of the cervical spine will show osteophytes and areas of hyperostosis.

2. Techniques described include awake intubation through the ILMA using a fibrescope (Palmer & Ball 2000), although in another patient a laryngeal mask airway could not be passed because of the pharyngeal mass (Aziz et al 1995). In cases of severe laryngeal oedema, tracheostomy may be required.

3. Care with surgical positioning or manipulation.

Bibliography

Aziz ES, Thompson AR, Baer S 1995 Difficult laryngeal mask insertion in a patient with Forestier's disease. Anaesthesia 50: 370.

Babores M, Finnerty JP 1998 Aspiration pneumonia secondary to giant cervical osteophyte formation (diffuse idiopathic skeletal hyperostosis or Forestier's disease): a case report. Chest 114: 1481–2.

Broadway JW 1994 Forestier's disease (ankylosing hyperostosis): a cause for difficult intubation. Anaesthesia 49: 912–20.

Chiba H, Annen S, Shimada T et al 1992 Atlantoaxial subluxation complicated by diffuse idiopathic skeletal hyperostosis. A case report. Spine 17: 1414–17.

Crosby ET, Grahovac S 1993 Diffuse idiopathic hyperostosis: an unusual cause of difficult intubation. Canadian Journal of Anaesthesia 40: 54–8.

Hassard AD 1984 Cervical ankylosing hyperostosis and airway obstruction. Laryngoscope 94: 966–8.

Israel Z, Mosheiff R, Gross E et al 1994 Hyperextension fracture-dislocation of the thoracic spine with paraplegia in a patient with diffuse idiopathic skeletal hyperostosis. Journal of Spinal Disorders 7: 455–7.

Marks B, Schober E, Swoboda H 1998 Diffuse idiopathic skeletal hyperostosis causing obstructing laryngeal edema. European Archives of Oto-Rhino-Laryngology 255: 256–8.

Oostveen JC, van de Laar MA, Tuynman FH 1996 Anterior atlantoaxial subluxation in a patient with diffuse idiopathic skeletal hyperostosis. Journal of Rheumatology 23: 1441–4.

Palmer HMcG, Ball DR 2000 Awake tracheal intubation with the intubating laryngeal mask airway in a patient with diffuse idiopathic skeletal hyperostosis. Anaesthesia 55: 70–3.

Rotes-Querol J 1996 Clinical manifestations of diffuse idiopathic skeletal hyperostosis (DISH). British Journal of Rheumatology 35: 1193–6.

Togashi H, Hirabayashi Y, Mitsuhata H et al 1993 The beveled tracheal tube orifice abutted on the tracheal wall in a patient with Forestier's disease. Anesthesiology 79: 1452–3.

Tortosa JA, Hernandez-Palazon J 1998 Forestier disease and interscalene brachial plexus block. European Journal of Anaesthesiology 15: 805–6.

Yamamoto T, Katoh H, Wakamatsu M 1992 [Anesthetic problems with Forestier's disease. Japanese.] Masui—Japanese Journal of Anesthesiology 41: 1008–10.

Down's syndrome

This well-known syndrome, with characteristic morphological features and mental retardation, results from the chromosomal abnormality, trisomy 21. Anaesthetic risk is increased in these children (Mitchell et al 1995). Indeed, the mortality is increased at any stage of life, but improved medical and nursing care means that many more individuals are surviving into adulthood and may present for surgery. Between 60 and 70% of patients now survive beyond 10 years of age.

Preoperative abnormalities

1. Cardiac abnormalities occur in 50–60% of patients and are usually responsible for the initial mortality in infancy. The commonest lesions are septal defects, Fallot's tetralogy, and patent ductus arteriosus. In adults, there is an increased risk of mitral valve prolapse, and mitral and aortic valve regurgitation.

2. A defect in the immune system results in an increased incidence of infection. Granulocyte abnormalities, decreased adrenal responses, and defects in cell-mediated immunity have all been identified. There is an increased incidence of lymphomas and leukaemias.

3. Skeletal abnormalities occur. Atlantoaxial instability was recognised as being a problem, at a time when these children were encouraged to participate in gymnastics! In one survey, 18% of 85 Down's children had C1–C2 articulation abnormalities; 12% had subluxation alone, and 6% were associated with odontoid peg abnormalities (Semine et al 1978). Four cases occurred in association with either medical procedures or physical activity (Msall et al 1990). The cause of instability is still uncertain, but poor muscle tone, ligamentous laxity and abnormal development of the odontoid peg may act in concert.

4. Biochemical abnormalities have been found and may involve metabolism of serotonin, catecholamines, and amino acids.

5. Thyroid hypofunction is common in both adults and children, although hyperthyroidism can sometimes occur. A child with Down's syndrome had a thyrotoxic crisis which mimicked malignant hyperthermia (Peters et al 1981).

6. Sleep-induced ventilatory dysfunction has been reported.

7. Institutionalised Down's patients have an increased incidence of hepatitis B antigen.

8. Autonomic dysfunction, in particular increased sympathetic function and decreased vagal activity, results from brainstem abnormalities.

Anaesthetic problems

The incidence of significant abnormalities is high. In a review, 100 cases of Down's syndrome requiring surgery, 44 patients had lesions requiring cardiac surgery, and 41 others had abnormalities or diseases with anaesthetic implications (Kobel et al 1982).

1.   Cervical spine abnormalities increase the risk of dislocation of certain cervical vertebrae on intubation, or when the patient is paralysed with muscle relaxants. Atlantoaxial subluxation and spinal cord compression were discovered in two children, after anaesthesia for surgical procedures. In neither case had cervical spine screening been carried out, nor had precautions been taken during intubation (Moore et al 1987, Williams et al 1987). An adult, admitted to the ITU for treatment of acute respiratory failure attributed to postoperative pneumonia, was subsequently found to have atlantoaxial subluxation with a sagittal canal diameter in extension of only 2.5 mm (Powell et al 1990). By this stage, irreversible neurological damage had occurred. Acute symptomatic atlantoaxial instability followed ENT surgery in a child who had previously had a normal neck X-ray (Morton et al 1995), and after middle ear surgery (Litman & Perkins 1994).

2.   The larynx is often underdeveloped and a smaller tracheal tube size is required than would be anticipated for the age of the patient (Kobel et al 1982). The adult larynx may only accept a size 6-mm tube.

3.   Airway and intubation difficulties sometimes occur, from a combination of anatomical features. These include a large tongue, a small mandible and maxilla, a narrow nasopharynx, and irregular teeth. Even in the absence of teeth, intubation is made more difficult by excessive pharyngeal tissue.

4.   Postoperative stridor after prolonged nasal intubation. Congenital subglottic stenosis occurs occasionally.

5.   Obstructive sleep apnoea is common in Down's syndrome (Silverman 1988). Compared with normal children they had an increased incidence of stridor and chest wall recession, lower baseline oxygen saturations, and a greater number of episodes of desaturation to 90% or less (Stebbens et al 1991). Chronic episodes of hypoxia and hypercarbia may lead to pulmonary hypertension and congestive heart failure (Ayeni & Roper 1998). Airway patency depends upon both the anatomical structure of the upper respiratory tract, and the normal functioning of the pharyngeal muscles. Abnormalities of either or both may occur.

6.   Upper airway obstruction, because it has multiple causes, is not necessarily resolved with surgical treatment. In a retrospective analysis of 71 Down's syndrome patients with upper airway obstruction, over a 5-year period, one-third of the patients with mild OSA improved with adenotonsillectomy. The younger group with more severe symptoms often had multiple sites of obstruction, and a high incidence of cardiac disease. Five deaths occurred during the study period; three were attributable to upper airway obstruction, two to cardiac causes, and one to obstruction of a tracheostomy (Jacobs et al 1996).

7.   Problems of the associated cardiac disease, which in later life may lead to pulmonary hypertension (Riley & McBride 1991).

8.   A high incidence of atelectasis and pulmonary oedema after surgery for congenital heart disease (Morray et al 1986). Those with Down's syndrome and ventricular septal defects were predisposed to pulmonary vascular obstruction.

9.   Posterior arthrodesis of the upper cervical spine carries a high complication rate (Segal et al 1991). Problems included infection and wound dehiscence, instability at a lower level, neurological sequelae, and postoperative death.

Management

1.   Lateral cervical X-rays are required, in full flexion and extension positions, to detect atlantoaxial instability. This may show as an increase in the distance between the posterior surface of the anterior arch of the atlas, and the anterior surface of the odontoid process (Hungerford et al 1981). Patients with an atlanto-odontoid interval of 4.5–6.0 mm were asymptomatic, but those in whom the distance exceeded 7 mm had neurological signs. If

instability is present, great care should be taken to immobilise the neck during intubation and muscle relaxation. These changes do not appear to progress with time. A longitudinal study of 141 patients having serial X-ray examinations showed that significant changes of the atlanto–dens interval did not take place (Pueschal et al 1992), therefore the authors suggested that the necessity for regular screening is removed. In a questionnaire to members of a paediatric anaesthesia society, only 18% said they would obtain X-rays in an asymptomatic child (Litman et al 1995). However, the fact that instability can occur in the absence of symptoms (Hartley et al 1998) and that symptomatic atlantoaxial instability followed ENT surgery in a child whose neck X-ray was previously reported as normal, suggests that extreme care should be taken when these patients undergo surgery. However, plain X-rays may be unreliable, and Selby et al (1991) found no reliable clinical predictors of subluxation.

2. If significant cardiac disease is present, management must be appropriate to the lesion and endocarditis prophylaxis given as recommended.

3. A tracheal tube should be used that is 1–2 sizes smaller than would be expected from the patient's age.

4. If prolonged nasotracheal intubation is required, steroids should be given before extubation. The child should receive humidification and be observed carefully for signs of stridor.

5. Close observation is required in the perioperative period, to detect episodes of obstructive apnoea. A pulse oximeter is useful.

6. Loss of locomotor skills or disturbances of gait after surgery or acute trauma should alert staff to the possibility of subluxation and cord compression (Powell et al 1990, Morton et al 1995). In the event of this, an urgent neurological opinion should be sought. However, in the absence of neurological signs, nonoperative management has been advised,

because of the high complication rate after surgery (Segal et al 1991).

7. In patients with adenotonsillar hypertrophy, surgery may improve obstruction. However, close monitoring and oxygen therapy is important for the first postoperative night (Bower & Richmond 1995).

Bibliography

Ayeni TI, Roper HP 1998 Pulmonary hypertension resulting from upper airways obstruction in Down's syndrome. Journal of the Royal Society of Medicine 91: 321–2.

Bower CM, Richmond D 1995 Tonsillectomy and adenoidectomy in patients with Down syndrome. International Journal of Pediatric Otorhinolaryngology 33: 141–8.

Hartley B, Newton M, Albert A 1998 Down's syndrome and anaesthesia. Paediatric Anaesthesia 8: 182–3.

Hungerford GD, Akkaraju V, Rawe SE et al 1981 Atlanto-occipital and atlanto-axial dislocations with spinal cord compression in Down's syndrome: a case report and review of the literature. British Journal of Radiology 54: 758–61.

Jacobs IN, Gray RF, Todd NW 1996 Upper airway obstruction in children with Down syndrome. Otolaryngology—Head & Neck Surgery 122: 945–50.

Kobel M, Creighton RE, Steward DJ 1982 Anaesthetic considerations in Down's syndrome. Canadian Anaesthetists' Society Journal 29: 593–9.

Litman RS, Perkins FM 1994 Atlantoaxial subluxation after tympanomastoidectomy in a child with trisomy 21. Otolaryngology—Head & Neck Surgery 110: 584–6.

Litman RS, Zerngast BA, Perkins FM 1995 Preoperative evaluation of the cervical spine in children with trisomy-21: results of questionnaire study. Paediatric Anaesthesia 5: 355–61.

Mitchell V, Howard R, Facer E 1995 Down's syndrome and anaesthesia. Paediatric Anaesthesia 5: 379–84.

Moore RA, McNicholas KW, Warran SP 1987 Atlantoaxial subluxation with symptomatic spinal cord compression in a child with Down's syndrome. Anesthesia & Analgesia 66: 89–90.

Morray JP, MacGillivray R, Duker G 1986 Increased perioperative risk following repair of congenital heart disease in Down's syndrome. Anesthesiology 65: 221–4.

Morton RE, Khan MA, Murrary-Leslie C et al 1995 Atlantoaxial instability in Down's syndrome: a five year follow up study. Archives of Disease in Childhood 72: 115–18.

Msall ME, Reese ME, DiGaudio K et al 1990 Symptomatic atlantoaxial instability associated with medical and rehabilitation procedures in children with Down syndrome. Pediatrics 85: 447–9.

Peters KR, Nance P, Wingard DW 1981 Malignant hyperthyroidism or malignant hyperthermia? Anesthesia & Analgesia 60: 613–15.

Powell JF, Woodcock T, Luscombe FE 1990 Atlanto-axial subluxation in Down's syndrome. Anaesthesia 45: 1049–51.

Pueschel SM, Scola FH, Pezzullo JC 1992 A longitudinal study of atlanto–dens relationships in asymptomatic individuals with Down syndrome. Pediatrics 89: 1194–8.

Riley DP, McBride LJ 1991 Ketamine, midazolam and vecuronium infusion. Anaesthesia for Down's syndrome and congenital heart disease. Anaesthesia 46: 122–3.

Ruggieri M, Pavone V, Polizzi A et al 1998 Life-threatening neurological syndrome in Down's syndrome. Postgraduate Medical Journal 74: 257–9.

Segal LS, Drummond DS, Zanotti RM et al 1991 Complications of posterior arthrodesis of the cervical spine in patients who have Down syndrome. Journal of Bone & Joint Surgery 73: 1547–54.

Selby KA, Newton RW, Gupta S et al 1991 Clinical predictors and radiological reliability in atlantoaxial subluxation in Down's syndrome. Archives of Disease in Childhood 66: 876–8.

Semine AA, Ertel AN, Goldberg MJ et al 1978 Cervical spine instability in children with Down's syndrome. Journal of Bone & Joint Surgery 60A: 649–52.

Silverman M 1988 Airway obstruction and sleep apnoea in Down's syndrome. British Medical Journal 296: 1618–19.

Stebbens VA, Dennis J, Samuels MP et al 1991 Sleep related upper airway obstruction in a cohort with Down's syndrome. Archives of Disease in Childhood 66: 1333–8.

Williams JP, Somerville GM, Miner ME et al 1987 Atlanto-axial subluxation and trisomy-21: another perioperative complication. Anesthesiology 67: 253–4.

Drowning and near drowning

Drowning is one of the commonest causes of accidental death in young people, but is potentially remediable if appropriate treatment is instituted without delay. Early animal studies led to undue emphasis being placed on the differences between immersion in salt or fresh water, the accompanying osmotic changes, and, in fresh water, the possibility of massive haemolysis. In practice, the inhaled volumes are much less than those induced experimentally, the haemolysis is not significant, and, in large series of patients reaching hospital, electrolyte and blood values showed no significant difference between the two (Golden et al 1997). The management of drowning depends, therefore, on the clinical state, not the medium. Of more importance is the diagnosis of incidents possibly contributing to the clinical state, such as alcohol or other drug intoxication, head and neck injury, abdominal injury, epilepsy, or myocardial infarction. One of the crucial factors affecting survival from near drowning is the institution of prompt, effective CPR at the site of the incident, and before hospital admission. In general, patients who arrive in hospital with fixed, dilated pupils have a poor prognosis. The only exception to this is the patient in whom hypothermia is a feature, when resuscitation should be continued and judgement delayed until rewarming has occurred (Kemp & Sibert 1991). In these cases, a rapid decrease in temperature on immersion probably protects the brain, rather than the so-called 'diving' reflex. This probably accounts for the greater protection in children, who have a higher surface area to body weight ratio. The major problem nowadays is to prevent brain injury in the patients who survive the immediate near-drowning event, and to decide on the management of those who have signs of a bad prognosis. There is no evidence that measures specifically aimed at brain preservation improve outcome (Modell 1993).

At the site of the accident, the immediate initiation of artificial ventilation and circulation is imperative, but there is no evidence that the Heimlich abdominal thrust manoeuvre should be used routinely, unless there is obstruction to the airway by a foreign body. A recent on-site classification has been proposed on the basis of an analysis of 1831 cases (Szpilman 1997):

Grade 1—cough but normal sounds on auscultation.

Grade 2—crepitations in the lung fields.

Grade 3—evidence of pulmonary oedema without hypotension.

Grade 4—pulmonary oedema with hypotension.

Grade 5—isolated respiratory arrest.

Grade 6—cardiopulmonary arrest.

In the cases grades 1–6 the respective mortalities were 0%, 0.6%, 5.2%, 19.4%, 44%, and 93%.

Presentation

1. Nearly all near-drowning victims are hypoxic, acidotic, and hypothermic. Pulmonary surfactant properties are altered and the alveoli become unstable, affecting the ventilation–perfusion ratios. In addition, pulmonary oedema occurs, worsening oxygenation. However, signs of inhalation may not be immediately evident, but can appear some hours later. Aspiration of gastric contents may also occur in up to 25% of victims, and secondary infection in up to 40%.

2. Respiration may be adequate, inadequate, or absent. In a review of 130 cases, those with adequate respiration on arrival in hospital had an excellent prognosis (Simcock 1986). However, in hypothermic children, the absence of respiration did not necessarily predict a poor outcome (Kemp & Sibert 1991).

3. Circulatory changes are complex and are associated with hypoxia, hypothermia, pH, volume, and electrolyte changes. In the most serious group, asystole or VF may be present. Severe vasoconstriction may make it difficult to determine whether or not there is cardiac output (Modell 1993). In less severe cases there may be hypovolaemia and poor peripheral perfusion.

4. Hypothermia is common. At 26–28°C it may be difficult to reverse VF or asystole. Above 30°C the problem is less urgent. A moderate degree of hypothermia has a cerebral protectant effect.

5. A number of features are associated with a poor prognosis. These include: immersion incidents of duration exceeding 5–9 min; delay in initiating effective CPR; arrival in hospital pulseless; in VT or VF; fixed dilated pupils; fits; and a poor Glasgow coma score (Russell 1992). Fits continuing 24 h after admission also predicted a poor outcome (Kemp & Sibert 1991). Most children with reactive pupils did survive, whereas if the return of pupil reactivity was delayed for 6 h or more, this was associated with neurological deficit or death. The prognosis also depended on the conditions of the incident; in cold water, even if the patient has dilated pupils, resuscitation should be continued until rewarming occurs. However, when the incident was associated with warm water swimming pools, fixed dilated pupils and coma accurately predicted patients with a bad prognosis (Orlowski 1988). Secondary drowning, in which pulmonary oedema may develop at any time up to 3 days after the event, can occur. In children, secondary drowning in salt water has a worse prognosis than that after fresh-water incidents (Pearn 1980).

6. Other complications include pulmonary oedema, infection, hypoxic encephalopathy and cerebral oedema, coagulopathy, and rhabdomyolysis.

Investigations

1. After the initial resuscitation, monitoring of blood gases, CXR, and base deficit will indicate whether there is further development, or resolution, of any respiratory complications.

2. ECG may show arrhythmias, especially on rewarming. CVP indicates hypovolaemia, and urine output guides therapy.

3. Core temperature monitoring.

4. Determinations of haemoglobin, haematocrit, electrolytes and urea, coagulation,

blood and tracheal aspirate for cultures are required. These will give baseline values in case of subsequent complications, but changes are usually small and rarely need therapy. If the possibility of drug or alcohol overdose exists, a drug screen should be performed.

Management

1. If there is still no cardiac output on admission to hospital, full resuscitation should be continued until the nature of the cardiac rhythm is established on ECG (Harries 1995). If the temperature is <33°C, attempts should be made to rewarm the patient.

2. An attempt is made to maintain the Pa_{O_2} above 8 kPa with up to 50% oxygen. If this is impossible, and there is significant intrapulmonary shunting, CPAP is effective, either with spontaneous breathing, or with IPPV. In fresh-water drowning, IPPV and PEEP are probably superior to spontaneous respiration. Should hypotension result, expansion of the vascular volume will be required.

3. Treatment of circulatory failure should be monitored with a CVP. Hypovolaemia occurs commonly, particularly in salt-water drowning. Colloids may be required. In salt-water drowning, dextrose 5% may be needed, and in fresh water, saline. If the pH is <7.2, partial correction of the acidosis is advisable.

4. Unless the temperature is less than 30–32°C, in which case serious cardiac arrhythmias may occur, rapid treatment of hypothermia is unnecessary and possibly dangerous. Sudden vasodilatation may cause hypotension, and increases the hazard of cold acidotic blood returning to the heart. Moderate hypothermia is of positive benefit in reducing hypoxic brain damage, especially in children. Successful resuscitation has been achieved after total immersion for 25 min at 4°C in a child (Theilade 1977). However, if the temperature is below 30°C, then warmed peritoneal dialysis should be considered.

5. Antibiotic therapy depends on the likely water pollution. In the absence of gross contamination, antibiotics should be withheld.

6. More recent techniques include the use of emergency cardiopulmonary bypass in severe hypothermia (Bolte et al 1988, Ireland et al 1997), and artificial surfactant installation for persistent respiratory distress (McBrien et al 1993).

7. In the presence of the features associated with a poor prognosis, overenthusiastic treatment should be avoided.

8. Treatment of late complications, such as cerebral oedema, pulmonary infection, and renal failure.

Bibliography

Bolte BG, Black PG, Bowers RS 1988 The use of extracorporeal warming in a child submerged for 66 minutes. Journal of the American Medical Association 260: 377–9.

Golden FS, Tipton MJ, Scott RC 1997 Immersion, near-drowning and drowning. British Journal of Anaesthesia 79: 214–25.

Harries MG 1995 Near drowning. In: Colquhoun MC, Handley AJ, Evans T (eds) ABC of resuscitation. BMJ, London, pp 50–4.

Ireland AJ, Pathi VL, Crawford R et al 1997 Back from the dead: extracorporeal warming of severe accidental hypothermia victims in accident and emergency. Journal of Accident & Emergency Medicine 14: 255–7.

Kemp AM, Sibert JR 1991 Outcome in children who nearly drown: a British Isles study. British Medical Journal 302: 931–3.

McBrien M, Katumba JJ, Mukhtar AI 1993 Artificial surfactant in the treatment of drowning. Lancet 342: 1485–6.

Modell JH 1993 Drowning. New England Journal of Medicine 328: 253–6.

Orlowski JP 1988 Drowning, near drowning and ice water drowning. Journal of the American Medical Association 260: 390–1.

Pearn JH 1980 Secondary drowning in children. British Medical Journal 281: 1103–5.

Russell RIR 1992 Drowning and near-drowning in children. British Journal of Intensive Care 2: 135–44.

Simcock AD 1986 Treatment of near drowning—a review of 130 cases. Anaesthesia 41: 643–8.

Szpilman D 1997 Near-drowning and drowning classification: a proposal to stratify mortality based on an analysis of 1831 cases. Chest 112: 660–5.

Theilade D 1977 The danger of fatal misjudgement in hypothermia after immersion. Anaesthesia 32: 889–92.

Duchenne muscular dystrophy (DMD)

An X-linked recessive, severe muscular dystrophy, that usually presents with proximal lower limb and pelvic muscle weakness. The weakness, which is progressive and varies between muscles, results from a decrease in the total number of muscle fibres. The young child, on attempting to rise, will use its arms to 'climb' up its own legs. Cardiac muscle disease occurs, with characteristic ECG changes and a hypertrophic cardiomyopathy. The condition steadily progresses to involve other muscles until finally death, from respiratory failure (75% of cases), pneumonia, or cardiac disease, occurs between the ages of 10 and 20. The commonest genetic muscular dystrophy, it shares the same locus at Xp21 as Becker muscular dystrophy (BMD), but is more severe and ten times more common. The protein product of the gene is dystrophin. Most patients with DMD have an absence of dystrophin, whereas in BMD there is an alteration in size or quantity of dystrophin (Dubowitz 1992). Dystrophin is located to the inner surface of sarcolemmal membrane. It probably forms a complex with other proteins, and is important in maintaining the integrity of the sarcolemma (Ohlendieck et al 1993). As a result of these abnormalities, the muscle becomes extremely susceptible to breakdown and necrosis.

Anaesthesia in patients with this condition may be hazardous, particularly in the early stages of the disease, before the diagnosis has been made. The occurrence of cardiac arrest during anaesthesia, secondary to hyperkalaemia, has sometimes been the first indication that the child had a muscle dystrophy (Seay et al 1978, Benton & Wolgat 1993).

Preoperative abnormalities

1. Varying degrees of muscle weakness are present, with initial involvement of the thighs and pelvis. The calf muscles are enlarged by fatty tissue (pseudohypertrophy) and, if the shoulder girdle is affected, there is winging of the scapulae. Relentlessly progressive scoliosis, which may require spinal fusion to improve stability and comfort, usually occurs after this (Shapiro et al 1992). The child is often obese and eventually becomes confined to a wheelchair.

2. Vital capacity decreases progressively, and when it falls below 700 ml, the risk of death is high. Diaphragmatic weakness occurs and blood gases may show hypoventilation and hypoxia in the later stages of the disease. Once diurnal hypercapnoea develops, life expectancy is less than 1 year (Simonds et al 1998).

3. Sleep hypoxaemia is frequent once individuals are no longer mobile, and it worsens with age. Initially, apnoeas are obstructive in nature (Khan & Heckmatt 1995). Nocturnal hypoxaemia leads to diurnal ventilatory failure and cor pulmonale.

4. Serum CK levels can be grossly elevated, the highest levels often occurring in the early stages of the disease, before loss of muscle tissue. An EMG will confirm the presence of a myopathy.

5. Clinical signs of a hypertrophic cardiomyopathy, with diastolic failure secondary to left ventricular inflow obstruction, may exist. The ECG shows abnormalities in over 90% of patients. Characteristic changes are a tall R wave and an RSR1 in lead V1, a deep Q wave in leads V3–6, a prolonged PR interval, and a sinus tachycardia. Echocardiography will demonstrate mitral valve prolapse in 25% of patients. Sudden death can occur.

6. The diagnosis can usually be confirmed by a combination of clinical features, family history, tests that examine the dystrophin protein, and those that study the gene.

Anaesthetic problems

Although many apparently uneventful anaesthetics have been given to patients with DMD, a substantial number of individual cases have been reported in which serious complications have occurred. Some have resulted in death. Attempts have been made to quantify the risks of anaesthesia in DMD (Sethna et al 1988, Larsen et al 1989). Most studies have been retrospective. Problems occurred in 16–27% of patients having general anaesthesia, whereas surgery performed under local anaesthesia was uneventful.

Complications have been associated with suxamethonium and all of the volatile agents. The exact aetiology of the anaesthetic complications has not always been clear, but they can be broadly divided into respiratory problems, abnormal metabolic responses, and cardiac events. The metabolic complications share many of the features of MH, but they are entirely separate diseases. Occasionally the two conditions have been noted to coexist, but both traits may occur independently.

Whilst the respiratory complications usually occur with advanced disease, secondary to progressive muscle weakness, this is not necessarily the case with acute cardiac and metabolic events, which are more likely to happen early in the disease. It is in this period that the greatest muscle bulk is present and the highest CK levels are recorded.

1. Tachycardia, ventricular fibrillation, and cardiac arrest have all been reported during induction of anaesthesia (Genever 1971, Linter et al 1982, Smith & Bush 1985, Buzello & Huttarsch 1988, Chalkiadis & Branch 1990, Shapiro et al 1992, Sullivan et al 1994). Most reports have involved the use of suxamethonium, and, when biochemical evidence was available, the acute cardiac events seemed mostly to be associated with hyperkalaemia. Cardiac arrest is usually precipitated by suxamethonium, but may occur at any stage, even during the recovery period.

Presumably this is because suxamethonium-induced hyperkalaemia persists for longer in patients with DMD. In normal individuals given suxamethonium, the increase in plasma potassium usually lasts for less than 10 min, whereas in DMD it may be significantly prolonged. Serum potassium concentration increased from $3.6\,mmol\,l^{-1}$ to $4.6\,mmol\,l^{-1}$ in a patient given suxamethonium before undergoing tracheal intubation for IPPV (Stephens 1990). Hyperkalaemia may also be precipitated by volatile agents alone. In one particular patient, who had cardiac arrest during recovery from anaesthesia with isoflurane, the serum potassium did not return to normal levels until 5 h after the initial event, despite active treatment (Chalkiadis & Branch 1990). Hyperthermia and cardiac arrest after 11 min of a gaseous induction (assisted ventilation) with halothane alone, was reported in a child with a CK of $14\,000\,iu\,l^{-1}$, who was to undergo muscle biopsy (Sethna & Rockoff 1986). Ventricular fibrillation and prolonged cardiac arrest occurred in a 15-year-old boy, 6 h into scoliosis surgery using isoflurane and IPPV (Reid & Appleton 1999). The prone position and instability of the spinal column at the time of arrest hampered resuscitation and open cardiac massage had to be performed with the patient still prone. A left ventricular blood gas sample taken 40 min later showed a metabolic acidosis with a pH of 6.95, but a potassium level of $4.6\,mmol\,l^{-1}$. Preoperative ECG had shown the characteristic signs of cardiomyopathy, therefore this was assumed to be the cause.

2. Perioperative pyrexia is common and in the past an association with MH was suggested. This is incorrect. Although cases have been reported that have some, and occasionally all, of the clinical features of MH, few papers present *in vitro* or electron microscopic evidence of MH (Gronert et al 1992). Muscle from a 4-year-old boy with DMD showed abnormal contraction to halothane, but not to caffeine (Rosenberg & Heiman-Patterson 1983). Another had abnormal responses to both tests in a 5-year-old child, who had suffered cardiac arrest, metabolic acidosis

and acute rhabdomyolysis following suxamethonium (Brownell et al 1983). A 7-week-old infant with suxamethonium-induced rhabdomyolysis was claimed to be the youngest child with MH (Wilhout et al 1989). However, since muscle biopsy was diagnostic for DMD and the parents declined MH testing, this claim must be viewed with scepticism.

Most authors believe that the two conditions are unrelated, but are both capable of producing common features under anaesthesia. Contracture testing was negative in two children, one with Becker muscle dystrophy, and the other with DMD (Gronert et al 1992), and these authors considered that the MH-like features seen during anaesthesia were the result of alterations in the muscle membrane secondary to the dystrophy itself. Exposure to volatile agents and suxamethonium might increase membrane permeability, and compensatory hypermetabolism is suggested to result from attempts to re-establish membrane stability and prevent calcium flux.

Whatever the initiating mechanisms, in DMD, as in MH, suxamethonium or volatile agents can trigger a variety of nonspecific complications that are associated with acute disruption of muscle. These include pyrexia, tachycardia, acidosis, hyperkalaemia, asystole, VF, muscle spasm, acute rhabdomyolysis, and a high CK. All of these complications have been reported, either singly, or in various combinations, in some patients with DMD.

3. Adverse cardiac events have been reported, even in the absence of suxamethonium and volatile agents. Intraoperative cardiac arrest occurred during a total intravenous technique with propofol and alfentanil. Seven hours into scoliosis surgery, a broad complex bradycardia developed, followed by asystole, from which the 14 year old was resuscitated (Irwin & Henderson 1995). Serum potassium and blood gases had been within the normal range and postoperatively there was no evidence of rhabdomyolysis.

4. If asystole or VF should occur, then the cardiomyopathic heart may be resistant to resuscitation measures (Sethna et al 1988).

5. Central venous catheter insertion initiated atrial fibrillation in a 13 year old. Neither removal of the guidewire, nor of the catheter itself, resolved the problem, which responded to cardioversion (Keohane & Allen 1999).

6. Problems with scoliosis surgery. When a patient was turned prone for spinal surgery there was complete tracheal obstruction. Bronchoscopy confirmed a slit-like narrowing of the lower trachea, distal to the tube, thought to be caused by compression against the vertebral bodies (Rittoo & Morris 1995). Blood loss during scoliosis surgery is greater in DMD than in other conditions, and is related to the length of surgery (Noordeen et al 1999). It has been attributed to a poor vascular smooth muscle vasoconstrictive response. Should cardiac arrest occur in the prone position, resuscitation is hampered (Irwin & Henderson 1995, Reid & Appleton 1999).

7. The response to nondepolarising agents may be abnormal. This cannot be predicted in advance. The stage of the disease, and the muscles monitored, will presumably have some bearing on this. Cumulative 50% and 90% blocking doses of vecuronium were determined in two 4-year-old boys (Buzello & Huttarsch 1988). Although the authors found no increase in sensitivity to vecuronium, the recovery time from 75% to 25% block of twitch tension was three to nearly six times that of normal.

8. Postoperative respiratory insufficiency. There are a number of reports of 'uneventful' anaesthetics using a barbiturate, suxamethonium, and halothane, but in which delayed respiratory insufficiency occurred from 5 to 36 h postoperatively (Smith & Bush 1985). Difficulty in swallowing, breathing, and clearing secretions all featured in the pattern of deterioration. Despite intubation and IPPV, a number of the children later developed cardiac arrest from which resuscitation failed.

9. Rhabdomyolysis with myoglobinuria has usually been associated with the administration

of suxamethonium (Boltshauser et al 1980, Jerusalem 1980, Larsen et al 1989). However, isolated myoglobinuria following adenoidectomy was the first indication of DMD in a 5-year-old boy (Rubiano et al 1987). Myoglobinuria was also observed 3 h after a sevoflurane anaesthetic for squint surgery. The CK at that time was 55 700 iu l⁻¹ (Obata et al 1999).

Management

1. Assessment of respiratory function is helpful, provided the child is old enough to cooperate. Diaphragmatic involvement suggests serious impairment. A difference in vital capacity of more than 25% between the erect and supine positions is indicative of diaphragmatic weakness (Heckmatt 1987). In the later stages of DMD, arterial blood gases will show impending respiratory failure. Assessment is particularly important when major elective surgery, such as scoliosis correction, is contemplated (Milne & Rosales 1982, Shapiro et al 1992). It has been suggested that, for scoliosis surgery, the patient should have a VC of at least 20 ml kg⁻¹ (or 30% of predicted), and an inspiratory capacity of 15 ml kg⁻¹.

2. Evidence of cardiac involvement should be sought. This may vary from ECG changes alone to diastolic failure.

3. If scoliosis surgery is performed in the prone position, precordial defibrillator pads should be sited at induction (Reid & Appleton 1999).

4. If advanced disease is present, the wisdom and possible benefits of surgery should be weighed against the risks. If the assessment is misjudged, elective surgery may hasten death, or commit a patient with progressive and ultimately fatal disease to a period of prolonged artificial ventilation.

5. Noninvasive nasal ventilation increases the survival time when ventilatory failure develops (Simonds et al 1998).

6. A local anaesthetic technique should be considered. Larsen et al (1989), in a retrospective review, found that no complications occurred in 19 operations under local anaesthesia, whereas in 65 general anaesthetics, 18 were complicated.

7. Suxamethonium is absolutely contraindicated in patients with DMD since, at present, it does not appear possible to predict which patients might develop hyperkalaemia, cardiac arrest, rigidity, rhabdomyolysis or postoperative respiratory failure, all of which complications have been attributed to its use. Larsen et al (1989) found that nine out of ten patients given suxamethonium in their series developed complications. Should cardiac arrest occur in association with suxamethonium, hyperkalaemia should be assumed. Treatment in an adult is with calcium chloride (0.5–1 g), sodium bicarbonate (50 mmol), insulin and dextrose (actrapid 10–15 units with 25 g dextrose). Calcium acts immediately and lasts for 15–30 min. Sodium bicarbonate and insulin/glucose act in 15–30 min and last for 3–6 h. In a patient with hyperkalaemia resistant to these treatments, peritoneal dialysis reduced the serum potassium to 4.3 mmol l⁻¹ (Jackson et al 1996).

8. In view of the variability of response, neuromuscular monitoring and incremental dosages should be employed for nondepolarising muscle relaxants, since there may be a prolonged duration of action. Responses in the peripheral muscles do not always reflect those in respiratory muscles, and the evoked EMG may recover faster than the actual mechanical response (Buzello & Huttarsch 1988).

9. Although many patients have been safely anaesthetised with volatile agents, their use is controversial, particularly when the CK is very high (Morris 1997, Goresky & Cox 1999). The report of cardiac arrest occurring during a gaseous induction with halothane is of concern (Sethna & Rockoff 1986), so also is the critical review condemning the use of halothane in patients with DMD and a high CK (Roizen 1987). The causes of the arrest cannot be

accurately determined, but it is easy to visualise how a serious arrhythmia might occur in a myopathic heart with a combination of even mild respiratory obstruction, light anaesthesia, and halothane. That halothane, isoflurane, and sevoflurane given alone are all capable of producing muscle breakdown is demonstrated by the reports of myoglobinuria following anaesthetics in which suxamethonium was not used (Rubiano et al 1987, Obata et al 1999). Avoidance of suxamethonium and volatile agents has been reported in 27 patients undergoing spinal fusion (Shapiro et al 1992).

10. Whichever technique is chosen, ECG, temperature and ETCO$_2$ should be monitored from the start of the anaesthetic. Urine should be observed for the presence of myoglobin. If there is evidence of rhabdomyolysis, intravenous fluids and mannitol should be given early.

11. Observation in a high dependency area for the first 24–48 h after surgery will assist in the early detection of pulmonary insufficiency. If doubt arises, it is safer to support respiration until all drugs have been eliminated.

Bibliography

Benton NC, Wolgat RA 1993 Sudden cardiac arrest during adenotonsillectomy in a patient with subclinical Duchenne's muscular dystrophy. Ear, Nose, & Throat Journal 72: 130–1.

Boltshauser E, Steinmann B, Meyer A et al 1980 Anaesthesia-induced rhabdomyolysis in Duchenne's muscular dystrophy. British Journal of Anaesthesia 52: 559.

Brownell AKW, Paasuke RT, Elash A et al 1983 Malignant hyperthermia in Duchenne muscular dystrophy. Anesthesiology 58: 180–2.

Buzello W, Huttarsch H 1988 Muscle relaxation in patients with Duchenne's muscular dystrophy. British Journal of Anaesthesia 60: 228–31.

Chalkiadis GA, Branch KG 1990 Cardiac arrest after isoflurane anaesthesia in a patient with Duchenne's muscular dystrophy. Anaesthesia 45: 22–5.

Dubowitz 1992 The muscular dystrophies. Postgraduate Medical Journal 68: 500–6.

Genever EE 1971 Suxamethonium induced cardiac arrest in unsuspected pseudohypertrophic muscular dystrophy. British Journal of Anaesthesia 43: 984–6.

Goresky GV, Cox RG 1999 Inhalation agents and Duchenne's muscular dystrophy. Canadian Journal of Anaesthesia 46: 525–8.

Gronert GA, Fowler W, Cardinet GH et al 1992 Absence of malignant hyperthermia contractures in Becker–Duchenne dystrophy at age 2. Muscle & Nerve 15: 52–6.

Heckmatt JZ 1987 Respiratory care in muscular dystrophy. British Medical Journal 295: 1014–15.

Irwin MG, Henderson M 1995 Cardiac arrest during major spinal surgery in a patient with Duchenne's muscular dystrophy undergoing intravenous anaesthesia. Anaesthesia & Intensive Care 23: 626–9.

Jackson MA, Lodwick R, Hutchinson SG 1996 Hyperkalaemic cardiac arrest successfully treated with peritoneal dialysis. British Medical Journal 312: 1289–90.

Jerusalem F 1980 Anaesthesia-induced rhabdomyolysis in Duchenne's muscular dystrophy. British Journal of Anaesthesia 52: 559.

Keohane M, Allen R 1999 Persistent atrial fibrillation following central venous cannulation. Paediatric Anaesthesia 9: 178–9.

Khan Y, Heckmatt JZ 1995 Obstructive apnoeas in Duchenne muscular dystrophy. Thorax 49: 157–61.

Larsen UT, Juhl B, Hein-Sorensen O et al 1989 Complications during anaesthesia in patients with Duchenne's muscular dystrophy (a retrospective study). Canadian Journal of Anaesthesia 36: 418–22.

Linter SPK, Thomas PR, Withington PS et al 1982 Suxamethonium associated hypertonicity and cardiac arrest in unsuspected pseudohypertrophic muscular dystrophy. British Journal of Anaesthesia 54: 1331–3.

Milne B, Rosales JK 1982 Anaesthetic considerations in patients with muscular dystrophy undergoing spinal fusion and Harrington rod insertion. Canadian Anaesthetists' Society Journal 29: 250–4.

Morris P 1997 Duchenne muscular dystrophy: a challenge for the anaesthetist. Paediatric Anaesthesia 7: 1–4.

Noordeen MH, Haddad FS, Muntoni F et al 1999 Blood loss in Duchenne muscular dystrophy: vascular smooth muscle dysfunction. Journal of Pediatric Orthopedics 8: 212–15.

Obata R, Yasumi Y, Suzuki A et al 1999 Rhabdomyolysis in association with Duchenne's muscular dystrophy. Canadian Journal of Anaesthesia 46: 564–6.

Ohlendieck K, Matsumura K, Ionasescu VV et al 1993 Duchenne muscular dystrophy. Deficiency of dystrophin-associated proteins in the sarcolemma. Neurology 43: 795–800.

Reid JM, Appleton PJ 1999 A case of ventricular fibrillation in the prone position during back stabilisation surgery in a boy with Duchenne's muscular dystrophy. Anaesthesia 54: 364–7.

Rittoo DB, Morris P 1995 Tracheal occlusion in the prone position in an intubated patient with Duchenne muscular dystrophy. Anaesthesia 50: 719–21.

Roizen MF 1987 Comment. Survey of Anesthesiology 31: 232–3.

Rosenberg H, Heiman-Patterson T 1983 Duchenne's muscular dystrophy and malignant hyperthermia: another warning. Anesthesiology 59: 362.

Rubiano R, Chang J-L, Carroll J et al 1987 Acute rhabdomyolysis following halothane anesthesia without succinylcholine. Anesthesiology 67: 856–7.

Seay AR, Ziter FA, Thompson JA 1978 Cardiac arrest during induction of anaesthesia in Duchenne muscular dystrophy. Journal of Pediatrics 93: 88–90.

Sethna NF, Rockoff MA 1986 Cardiac arrest following inhalation induction of anesthesia in a child with Duchenne's muscular dystrophy. Canadian Anaesthetists' Society Journal 33: 799–802.

Sethna NF, Rockoff MA, Worthen HM et al 1988 Anesthesia related complications in children with Duchenne muscular dystrophy. Anesthesiology 68: 462–5.

Shapiro F, Sethna N, Colan S et al 1992 Spinal fusion in Duchenne muscular dystrophy: a multidisciplinary approach. Muscle & Nerve 15: 604–14.

Simonds AK, Muntoni F, Heather S et al 1998 Impact of nasal ventilation on survival in hypercapnic Duchenne muscular dystrophy. Thorax 53: 949–52.

Smith CL, Bush GH 1985 Anaesthesia and progressive muscular dystrophy. British Journal of Anaesthesia 57: 1113–18.

Sullivan M, Thompson WK, Hill GD 1994 Succinylcholine-induced cardiac arrest in children with undiagnosed myopathy. Canadian Journal of Anaesthesia 41: 456–8.

Stephens ID 1990 Succinylcholine and Duchenne's muscular dystrophy. Canadian Journal of Anaesthesia 37: 274.

Wilhoit RD, Brown RE, Bauman LA 1989 Possible malignant hyperthermia in a 7-week-old infant. Anesthesia & Analgesia 68: 688–91.

Dystrophia myotonica (and other myotonic syndromes)

Dystrophia myotonica, myotonia congenita (see below), paramyotonia, and the periodic paralyses are a group of diseases known as the ion channelopathies, in which myotonia occurs. They are caused by abnormalities in the muscle membrane voltage-gated channels. Minor changes in resting potential can produce either hyperexcitability or paralysis. The term 'myotonia' means persistence of muscle contraction beyond the duration of the voluntary effort or stimulation. In *myotonia congenita* (Thomsen's disease), the generalised myotonia is enhanced by cold and resting, but may be improved by exercise. Subjects with *paramyotonia* have attacks of muscle weakness resembling those in periodic paralysis, to which it is probably closely related. Again, the myotonia is provoked by cold (see under Familial periodic paralysis).

Dystrophia myotonica is a multisystem disease in which myotonia and dystrophic changes occur in certain muscles, in association with other clinical features. The site of the abnormality is the muscle fibre, since myotonia persists after the administration of neuromuscular blocking agents and local anaesthetics, and neural section.

Preoperative abnormalities

1.   Dystrophia myotonica usually presents in the third and fourth decades. Myotonia is associated with weakness and muscle wasting. Unlike most other myopathies, it predominantly involves the distal and cranial muscles. Handshake is weak and reduced in maximum grip strength, and there is prolonged onset to maximum grip strength, but once this is achieved, the patient cannot relax. Percussion myotonia may be demonstrated, particularly in the tongue or thenar eminence. Ocular movements, eye closure, swallowing, and chewing may also be affected.

2.   Dystrophic features dominate the clinical picture as the patient ages, and the weakness is progressive.

3. Cardiac conduction is impaired, arrhythmias are common, and there is an increased incidence of sudden death (Merino et al 1998). In an electrophysiological study of 83 patients, both atrial and ventricular arrhythmias could be induced easily, particularly in the young. Patients had AV conduction defects and ventricular tachyarrhythmias. The most common abnormalities were distal conduction defects, which can only be detected by special testing (Lazarus et al 1999).

4. Frontal baldness, ptosis and facial weakness, cataracts, hypogonadism, and a low IQ, are other features of the condition. There is an increase in serum CK levels.

5. EMG shows electrical after-discharge and molecular genetic studies will confirm the diagnosis.

6. The myotonia may be improved by keeping warm and the use of class I antiarrhythmics, such as phenytoin and procainamide.

7. In pregnancy, if the neonate carries the disease, there is polyhydramnios.

8. Life expectancy is greatly reduced. In a study of 367 patients over a 10-year period, 20% died; 43% from respiratory problems, 20% from cardiovascular disease, 11% from malignancy, and 11% had sudden death (Mathieu et al 1999).

Anaesthetic problems

1. There may be chronic underventilation and respiratory muscle weakness. Vital capacity, expiratory reserve volume, maximum breathing capacity, and maximal inspiratory pressure are all markedly reduced, secondary to abnormalities in the respiratory muscles. CNS disease may contribute to the poor respiratory reserve. Somnolence and prolonged apnoea can occur, and respiration is readily depressed by barbiturates, volatile agents, benzodiazepines, and opiates (Aldridge 1985, Harper 1989). However, there may be a wide variation in a patient's response to drugs. This may reflect the state of

his/her disease, as is suggested by two contrasting reports of the use of propofol; one patient showed extreme sensitivity to propofol (Speedy 1990), the other did not (White & Smyth 1989, 1990).

2. In common with other diseases in which there is chest wall restriction, hypoventilation may occur during sleep, (Branthwaite 1990). Accessory muscle function is lost, and, during rapid eye movement sleep so is that of the intercostal muscles. The additional presence of diaphragmatic weakness results in hypoventilation, therefore analgesics and sedatives will depress the arousal response to hypoxia and hypercarbia. Such a mechanism was suggested to account for the death of a child after tendon transfer (Brahams 1989, Branthwaite 1990). In a study of 130 patients, respiratory insufficiency was associated with proximal weakness and daytime sleepiness (Begin et al 1997).

3. It may be difficult to prevent myotonia from occurring during surgical manipulation and diathermy, since it is not necessarily abolished by muscle relaxants, local or regional anaesthesia. Depolarising relaxants can produce a prolonged contraction that outlasts the duration of effect. Nondepolarising relaxants may or may not produce relaxation. In one case, masseter spasm and shivering occurred for 4 min after the administration of fentanyl (Paterson et al 1985). Hypothermia, shivering and potassium may all cause generalised myotonia.

4. Cardiovascular disease. Arrhythmias, including AF and conduction defects, cardiomyopathy, mitral valve prolapse, and heart failure, may occur.

5. Disordered oesophageal contraction and delayed gastric emptying predispose to pulmonary aspiration.

6. There is an increased incidence of postoperative problems (Moore & Moore 1987, Blumgart et al 1990, Mathieu et al 1997). In a study of 219 cases undergoing their first operation, 8.2% had complications. The majority were pulmonary; five patients required

ventilatory support and the remainder had either atelectasis or pneumonia (Mathieu et al 1997). This is lower than previously reported, but in 28.6% of cases, surgery was performed before the onset of symptoms, and 90% involved the periphery or lower abdomen. A 32-year-old man had a stormy course after thymectomy (Mudge et al 1980). Other complications have included pulmonary emboli and cardiac arrhythmias.

7. Although pregnancy is rare, it may be associated with an increase in myotonic symptoms (Paterson et al 1985). Hypotonia can also occur, and there is an increased risk of postpartum haemorrhage which may not respond to oxytocics and has sometimes necessitated hysterectomy (Blumgart et al 1990). Patients occasionally present for emergency Caesarean section, therefore anaesthesia must be planned in advance (Walpole & Ross 1992).

8. Hypermetabolic events similar to those in patients with MH have occasionally been reported in dystrophia myotonica and myotonia congenita. A group of 44 patients with either myotonias or periodic paralyses underwent *in vitro* testing for MH (Lehmann–Horn & Iaizzo 1990). Four with myotonic dystrophy had positive results, although two had increased resting myoplasmic calcium levels. Suxamethonium also produced muscle contracture in some individuals. It was concluded not that these patients had a susceptibility to MH (and indeed, neither they, nor their families had ever experienced any untoward effects from anaesthesia), but that the standard MH testing lacks specificity.

9. The problem is not always known because adults may conceal their symptoms (Russell & Hirsch 1994).

Management

1. A detailed clinical examination for the distribution of muscle weakness and myotonia.

2. If respiratory muscles are involved, lung function tests and blood gases will give some

indication of the severity of the restrictive lung defect.

3. Arrhythmias should be diagnosed and treated. Occasionally a temporary or permanent pacemaker (Tanaka & Tanaka 1991) may be required. Catheter ablation has been suggested for persistent ventricular re-entrant tachycardias.

4. Induction agents should be given in small doses because apnoea often follows.

5. Suxamethonium should be avoided. Tracheal intubation is possible using an induction and a volatile agent alone.

6. Nondepolarising neuromuscular blockers can be used, but they do not guarantee muscle relaxation. Reports about the reliability of neostigmine as an antagonist are conflicting. Incomplete reversal of neuromuscular blockade is common and a second dose of neostigmine has aggravated the paralysis. Uneventful anaesthetics using atracurium and propofol infusions (White & Smyth 1989), vecuronium (Castano & Pares 1987), and atracurium (Nightingale et al 1985), have been described, although myoclonus was seen after propofol induction (Bouly et al 1991). Neuromuscular monitoring must be undertaken. If there is any doubt about the return of function, IPPV should be provided until all drugs have been excreted, and respiration is adequate.

7. Local or regional techniques will avoid some of the problems associated with drugs used for general anaesthesia (Wheeler & James 1979). Successful spinal anaesthesia (Boyle 1999), epidural anaesthesia (Paterson et al 1985), and a combination of spinal and local anaesthesia (Cope & Miller 1986), were used in patients for Caesarean section. Abdominal hysterectomy was performed under combined spinal and epidural anaesthesia (Cherng et al 1994). A caudal epidural was used in a 2-year-old child (Alexander et al 1981), and epidural anaesthesia and sedation in a 11-year-old child (Tobias 1995). However, once again, these techniques do not guarantee surgical muscle relaxation.

8. Several measures have been used in

attempts to reduce myotonia. Severe uterine spasm, occurring during Caesarean section under spinal anaesthesia, was relieved by the application of bupivacaine 30 ml 0.5% to the cut surface of the myometrium (Cope & Miller 1986). However, administration of dantrolene failed to produce muscle relaxation in a patient undergoing cholecystectomy (Phillips et al 1984).

9. Measures to prevent pulmonary aspiration, prompt attention to respiratory inadequacy, and antibiotics, may all help to prevent pneumonia and lung abscess.

10. The operating theatre should be kept warm and measures taken to avoid shivering.

11. Although there is no evidence that there is any direct relationship between myotonic dystrophy and MH, close monitoring of $ETCO_2$ and temperature are advisable.

Bibliography

Aldridge M 1985 Anaesthetic problems in myotonic dystrophy. British Journal of Anaesthesia 57: 1119–30.

Alexander C, Wolf S, Ghia JN 1981 Caudal anesthesia for early onset myotonic dystrophy. Anesthesiology 55: 597–8.

Begin P, Mathieu J, Almirall J et al A 1997 Relationship between chronic hypercapnia and inspiratory muscle weakness. American Journal of Respiratory & Critical Care Medicine 156: 133–9.

Blumgart CH, Hughes DG, Redfern N 1990 Obstetric anaesthesia in dystrophia myotonica. Anaesthesia 45: 26–9.

Bouly A, Nathan N, Feiss P 1991 Propofol in myotonic dystrophy. Anaesthesia 46: 705.

Boyle R 1999 Antenatal and preoperative genetic and clinical assessment in myotonic dystrophy. Anaesthesia & Intensive Care 27: 301–6.

Brahams D 1989 Postoperative monitoring in a patient with muscular dystrophy. Lancet ii: 1053–4.

Branthwaite MA 1990 Myotonic dystrophy and respiratory function. Anaesthesia 45: 250.

Castano J, Pares N 1987 Anaesthesia for major abdominal surgery in a patient with myotonia dystrophica. British Journal of Anaesthesia 59: 1629–31.

Cherng YG, Wang YP, Liu CC et al 1994 Combined spinal and epidural anesthesia for abdominal hysterectomy in a patient with myotonic dystrophy. Regional Anesthesia 19: 69–72.

Cope DK, Miller JN 1986 Local and spinal anesthesia for Cesarean section in a patient with myotonic dystrophy. Anesthesia & Analgesia 65: 687–90.

Harper PS 1989 Postoperative complications in myotonia dystrophica. Lancet ii: 1269.

Lazarus A, Varin J, Ounnoughene Z et al 1999 Relationships among electrophysiological findings and clinical status, heart function and extent of DNA mutation in myotonic dystrophy. Circulation 99: 1041–6.

Lehmann-Horn F, Iaizzo PA 1990 Are myotonias and periodic paralyses associated with susceptibility to malignant hyperthermia? British Journal of Anaesthesia 65: 692–7.

Mathieu J, Allard P, Gobeil G et al 1997 Anesthetic and surgical complications in 219 cases of myotonic dystrophy. Neurology 49: 1646–50.

Mathieu J, Allard P, Potvin L et al 1999 A 10-year study of mortality in a cohort of patients with myotonic dystrophy. Neurology 52: 1658–62.

Merino JL, Carmona JR, Fernandez-Lozano I et al 1998 Mechanisms of sustained tachycardia in myotonic dystrophy: implications for catheter ablation. Circulation 98: 541–6.

Moore JK, Moore AP 1987 Postoperative complications of dystrophia myotonica. Anaesthesia 42: 529–33.

Mudge BJ, Taylor PB, Vanderspek AFL 1980 Perioperative hazards of myotonic dystrophy. Anaesthesia 35: 492–5.

Nightingale P, Healy TEJ, McGuiness K 1985 Dystrophia myotonia and atracurium. British Journal of Anaesthesia 57: 1131–5.

Paterson RA, Tousignant M, Skene DS 1985 Caesarean section for twins in a patient with myotonic dystrophy. Canadian Anaesthetists' Society Journal 32: 418–21.

Phillips DC, Ellis FR, Exley KA et al 1984 Dantrolene sodium and dystrophia myotonica. Anaesthesia 39: 568–73.

Russell SH, Hirsch NP 1994 Anaesthesia and myotonia. British Journal of Anaesthesia 72: 210–16.

Speedy H 1990 Exaggerated physiological response to propofol in myotonic dystrophy. British Journal of Anaesthesia 64: 110–12.

Tanaka M, Tanaka Y 1991 Cardiac anaesthesia in a patient with myotonic dystrophy. Anaesthesia 46: 462–5.

Tobias JD 1995 Anaesthetic management of a child with myotonic dystrophy; epidural as an alternative to general anaesthesia. Paediatric Anaesthesia 5: 335–8.

Walpole AR, Ross AW 1992 Acute cord prolapse in an obstetric patient with myotonia dystrophica. Anaesthesia & Intensive Care 20: 526–8.

Wheeler AS, James MFM 1979 Local anesthesia for laparoscopy in cases of myotonia dystrophica. Anesthesiology 50: 169.

White DA, Smyth DG 1989 Continuous infusion of propofol in dystrophia myotonica. Canadian Journal of Anaesthesia 36: 200–3.

White DA, Smyth DG 1990 Exaggerated physiological responses to propofol in myotonic dystrophy. British Journal of Anaesthesia 64: 758.

Myotonia congenita (Thompsen's disease and Becker's myotonia)

This includes an autosomal dominant form (Thomsen's disease), and an autosomal recessive form (Becker's myotonia), both of which are caused by mutations in the skeletal muscle voltage-gated chloride channel gene (CLCN1) (Zhang et al 1996). In the past, the term myotonia congenita has been used rather loosely in the literature, sometimes to refer to the myotonic dystrophy occurring in infants of mothers with the disease. Recent genetic and electrophysiological advances have allowed the diagnosis to be made more accurately. In view of this, past anaesthetic reports of infants with 'congenital myotonic dystrophy' have been excluded.

Preoperative abnormalities

1. In both diseases, there is painless myotonia, that is improved, or totally abolished, by exercise. Sportsmen may complain of stiffness, but only when starting after a period of rest.

2. Transient weakness that can also be 'warmed up' occurs in Becker's myotonia. It is not cold induced, nor potassium induced, nor is it progressive. However, in Thomsen's disease weakness is not a feature.

3. Muscle may be normal in size, or hypertrophied. Atrophy does not occur.

4. EMG shows myotonic discharges. Type 2B fibre is usually absent on muscle biopsy (Ptacek et al 1993).

5. Unlike myotonic dystrophy, other systems are not involved.

6. In Becker's, symptoms may be improved with acetazolamide, mexilitene, or tocainide. Thompsen's is not improved by acetazolamide, but may respond to quinine, procainamide, or phenytoin (Ptacek 1998).

Anaesthetic problems

1. Sustained contractions lasting 45 s following suxamethonium (Anderson & Brown 1989), and hypertonus in two sisters (Heiman-Patterson et al 1988). Sensitivity to nondepolarising agents has also been reported.

2. Hypermetabolic events resembling those in patients with MH have occasionally been reported in myotonia congenita and a fatality has occurred. Leg spasms developed 7 h after an uneventful anaesthetic (in which no trigger agents for MH were used) had been given to a child with a clinical diagnosis of myotonia congenita (Haberer et al 1989). The clinical condition deteriorated over the next 5 h, with severe, diffuse rigidity, notably of the thorax, slowly increasing pyrexia, and metabolic acidosis. A serum CK level of >11 500 iu l^{-1} was recorded. Cardiac arrest occurred in the 14th hour, despite treatment with dantrolene, and resuscitation was hampered by the thoracic rigidity.

3. A group of 44 patients with either myotonias or periodic paralyses underwent *in vitro* testing for MH (Lehmann-Horn & Iaizzo 1990). None of the six patients with congenital myotonia had positive results, although suxamethonium produced muscle contractures in three, and most showed a small response and slow relaxation after caffeine and halothane. None had family histories of anaesthetic problems. However, muscle rigidity with

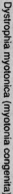

suxamethonium has been reported in myotonia congenita, and two sisters developed contractures on exposure to halothane whilst the third did not (Heiman–Patterson et al 1988).

Management

1. Assessment and monitoring of neuromuscular function.

2. $ETCO_2$ and temperature should be monitored.

Bibliography

Anderson BJ, Brown TCK 1989 Anaesthesia for a child with congenital myotonic dystrophy. Anaesthesia & Intensive Care 17: 351–4.

Haberer J-P, Fabre F, Rose E 1989 Malignant hyperthermia and myotonia congenita (Thomsen's disease). Anaesthesia 44: 166.

Heiman-Patterson T, Martino C, Rosenberg H et al 1988 Malignant hyperthermia in myotonia congenita. Neurology 38: 810–12.

Lehmann-Horn F, Iaizzo PA 1990 Are myotonias and periodic paralyses associated with susceptibility to malignant hyperthermia? British Journal of Anaesthesia 65: 692–7.

Ptacek L 1998 The familial periodic paralyses and nondystrophic myotonias. American Journal of Medicine 104: 58–70.

Ptacek LJ, Johnson KJ, Griggs RC 1993 Genetics and physiology of the muscle disorders. New England Journal of Medicine 328: 482–9.

Zhang J, George AL Jr, Griggs RC et al 1996 Mutations in human skeletal muscle chloride channel gene (CLCN1) associated with dominant and recessive myotonia congenita. Neurology 47: 993–8.

Eaton–Lambert syndrome (Lambert–Eaton or myasthenic syndrome)

A myasthenia-like disorder secondary to an abnormality of neuromuscular transmission in which weakness and fatiguability often primarily involve the thigh and pelvic muscles. It was orginally described in association with carcinoma of the lung, but patients were subsequently reported in whom no carcinoma was found. There is now evidence that both types of Eaton–Lambert syndrome are autoimmune in origin, and autoantibodies to P/Q-type voltage-gated calcium channels are thought to be involved (Voltz et al 1999). There is a presynaptic abnormalitiy that results in a decrease in the quanta of acetylcholine released by the passage of the nerve impulse, although each quantum released is normal. This contrasts with myasthenia gravis in which the abnormality involves the postganglionic receptors. The tumour-associated cases are almost exclusively found in association with small cell carcinoma of the lung, and the syndrome sometimes precedes the tumour by as long as 2 years. Tumour therapy may result in improvement of the neurological problems.

Preoperative abnormalities

1. Muscles are fatiguable, as in myasthenia gravis, but the proximal limbs and trunk are initially affected, and the external ocular muscles tend to be spared. By contrast with myasthenia, although the patient complains of fatiguability, the muscle power may actually increase after brief exercise. Lower limb reflexes are reduced or absent, but may be enhanced by prior voluntary contraction, whereas in true myasthenia, reflexes are preserved. Neostigmine produces little or no improvement in the weakness. In a review of 50 cases (O'Neill et al 1988), the main neurological features were proximal lower limb weakness (100%), reduced or absent tendon reflexes (92%), post-tetanic facilitation (78%), autonomic dysfunction, in particular dryness of the mouth (74%), and mild to moderate ptosis (54%). Recent work shows that, despite the proximal distribution of the weakness, the most sensitive muscles for demonstrating abnormalities are abductor digiti minimi and abductor pollicis brevis (Maddison et al 1998).

2. Electrophysiological criteria for diagnosis include a decrease in amplitude of EMG muscle potentials and further decline at low rates of stimulation. By contrast, there is an increase in amplitude of the action potential in response to stimulation at high rates, or following muscle contraction.

3. Patients tend to be older than those with myasthenia.

4. Associated lung carcinomas are usually oat cell in type, and are often small and less aggressive than normal. In O'Neill's review, half of the patients had a malignancy (O'Neill et al 1988).

5. Some improvement has been reported with guanidine and 4-aminopyridine, which enhance release of acetylcholine. However, the allowable dose is limited by CNS excitation. More recently, 3,4-diaminopyridine, an oral preparation with less CNS effects, has been used (McEvoy et al 1989). It is thought to have an effect on the efflux of calcium ions from the presynaptic nerve terminal. Low-dose guanidine ($<1000\,\mathrm{mg\,d^{-1}}$) and pyridostigmine, as required, may help in long-term treatment (Oh et al 1997). Corticosteroids, plasma exchange, and iv immunoglobulin may result in short-term improvement (Chapel 1996).

6. Diagnosis may be confirmed by an assay for antibodies (Voltz et al 1999).

Anaesthetic problems

1. Prolonged paralysis can occur after the use of depolarising or nondepolarising neuromuscular blockers. In one patient, this occurred several months in advance of clinical symptoms, although postoperative EMG and serological testing confirmed Eaton–Lambert

syndrome (Small et al 1992). Respiratory failure following anaesthesia may be a presenting feature (O'Neill et al 1988), and reversal with anticholinesterases may be incomplete (Telford & Hollway 1990). An improvement in evoked action potential occurred after treatment with both 4-aminopyridine (Agoston et al 1978) and 3,4-diaminopyridine, which prolong the activation of the voltage-gated calcium channel at the nerve terminal.

2. Autonomic dysfunction may be a prominent feature and is most severe in older men with cancer (O'Suilleabhain et al 1998). Symptoms include mouth dryness (77%), impotence (45% of men), constipation, and urinary retention. Orthostatic hypotension and decreased R–R intervals on ECG may be noted. In such patients, there may be impairment of cardiovascular responses to hypotension.

Management

1. Neuromuscular blockers should, if possible, be avoided. If essential, small doses should be given and monitored. A local anaesthetic technique may be appropriate.

2. Intravenous immunoglobulin, $2\,g\,kg^{-1}$ given over 2 days, resulted in a short-term improvement in muscle strength, peaking at 2–4 weeks and declining by 8 weeks (Bain et al 1996). In a dose of $400\,mg\,kg^{-1}day^{-1}$ for 5 days, it improved the weakness in a patient scheduled for open lung biopsy (Biarnes & Rochera 1996), so that the response to atracurium was within the normal range.

3. Respiratory insuffiency should be treated with postoperative IPPV. Sakura et al (1991) used postoperative epidural analgesia in a patient undergoing thoracotomy and biopsy for lung carcinoma, and studied its effects on pulmonary function.

4. If there is evidence of autonomic dysfunction, drugs producing myocardial depression or systemic vasodilatation should be used with caution.

Bibliography

Agoston S, van Weerden T, Westra P et al 1978 Effects of 4-aminopyridine in Eaton–Lambert syndrome. British Journal of Anaesthesia 50: 383–5.

Bain PG, Motomura M, Newsom-Davis J et al 1996 Effects of intravenous immunoglobulin on muscle weakness and calcium-channel autoantibodies in the Lambert–Eaton myasthenic syndrome. Neurology 47: 678–83.

Biarnes A, Rochera MI 1996 Lambert–Eaton (myasthenic) syndrome: pre-anaesthetic treatment with intravenous immunoglobulins. Anaesthesia 51: 797.

Chapel H 1996 Intravenous immunoglobulin therapy. Quarterly Journal of Medicine 89: 641–3.

McEvoy KM, Windebank AJ, Daube JR et al 1989 3,4-diaminopyridine in the treatment of Lambert–Eaton myasthenic syndrome. New England Journal of Medicine 321: 1567–71.

Maddison P, Newsom-Davis J, Mills KR 1998 Distribution of electrophysiological abnormality in Lambert–Eaton myasthenic syndrome. Journal of Neurology, Neurosurgery & Psychiatry 65: 213–17.

Oh SJ, Kim DS, Head TC et al 1997 Low-dose guanidine and pyridostigmine: relatively safe and effective long-term symptomatic therapy in Lambert–Eaton myasthenic syndrome. Muscle & Nerve 20: 1146–52.

O'Neill JH, Murray NM, Newsom-Davies J 1988 The Lambert–Eaton myasthenic syndrome: a review of 50 cases. Brain 111: 577–96.

O'Suilleabhain P, Low PA, Lennon VA 1998 Autonomic dysfunction in the Lambert–Eaton myasthenic syndrome: serologic and clinical correlates. Neurology 50: 88–93.

Sakura S, Saito Y, Maeda M et al 1991 Epidural analgesia in Eaton–Lambert myasthenic syndrome. Effects on respiratory function. Anaesthesia 46: 560–2.

Small S, Ali HH, Lennon VA et al 1992 Anesthesia for an unsuspected Lambert–Eaton myasthenic syndrome with autoantibodies and occult small cell lung carcinoma. Anesthesiology 76: 142–4.

Telford RJ, Hollway TE 1990 The myasthenic syndrome: anaesthesia in a patient treated with 3,4-diaminopyridine. British Journal of Anaesthesia 64: 363–6.

Voltz R, Carpentier AF, Rosenfeld MR et al 1999 P/Q-type voltage-gated calcium channel antibodies in paraneoplastic disorders of the central nervous system. Muscle & Nerve 22: 119–22.

Ebstein's anomaly

A rare congenital cardiac abnormality. The septal and posterior cusps of the tricuspid valve are displaced downwards and are elongated, such that a varying amount of the right ventricle effectively forms part of the atrium. Its wall is thin and it contracts poorly. The remaining functional part of the right ventricle is therefore small. The foramen ovale is patent, or defective, in 80% of cases.

The degree of abnormality of right ventricular function, and the size of the ASD, are probably the main determinants of the severity of the condition, which varies considerably. The right ventricular systolic pressure is low, and the RVEDP is elevated. Tricuspid incompetence can occur. There may be a right to left shunt, with cyanosis, on effort, and pulmonary hypertension and right heart failure may supervene. However, the natural history of the disease is very variable. Fifty percent of cases present in infancy with cyanosis, and 42% die in the first 6 weeks of life. In those who survive to adulthood, symptoms may be precipitated by the onset of arrhythmias, or by pregnancy. A few patients remain asymptomatic, even as adults, although once symptoms develop, the disability can increase rapidly (Mair 1992).

Factors predicting death were examined in a long-term study of survival (Gentles et al 1992). A cardiothoracic ratio of greater than, or equal to, 0.65 was a better predictor of sudden death than the symptomatic state, and those who developed atrial fibrillation died within 5 years. It has therefore been suggested that tricuspid surgery should be undertaken before the cardiothoracic ratio reaches 0.65.

Preoperative abnormalities

1. There may be a right to left shunt, with dyspnoea and cyanosis at rest, or on moderate exertion. Alternatively, the patient may be asymptomatic.

2. Episodes of tachyarrhythmias occur in 25% of patients. Some provoke syncopal attacks.

3. The ECG may show varying abnormalities, including large peaked P waves, a long P–R interval, Wolff–Parkinson–White syndrome, RBBB, and right heart strain. Paroxysmal supraventricular tachycardia occurs in 15%, usually because of the presence of WPW syndrome.

4. Chest X-ray may show cardiomegaly, with a prominent right heart border, and poorly perfused lung fields.

5. Paradoxical systemic embolism and bacterial endocarditis may occur.

6. A number of other lesions of the tricuspid valve or right ventricle may mimic Ebstein's anomaly, therefore the discriminating clinical and echocardiographic features for correct diagnosis have been enumerated (Ammash et al 1997).

Anaesthetic problems

These will depend upon the anatomical abnormality, the degree of right to left shunt, and the presence or absence of right heart failure.

1. Induction times are prolonged, because of pooling of drugs in the large atrial chamber (Elsten et al 1981, Halpern et al 1985).

2. Intracardiac catheter insertion may be hazardous, because it can provoke serious cardiac arrhythmias.

3. Air entering peripheral venous lines or any open veins at subatmospheric pressure may cause paradoxical air emboli.

4. Tachycardia is poorly tolerated because of impaired filling of the functionally small right ventricle.

5. Hypotension may increase the right to left shunt, if present.

6. Hypoxia causes pulmonary vasoconstriction, which also increases a right to left shunt.

7. There is a risk of bacterial endocarditis, especially if a CVP line is in place.

8. Deterioration may occur in pregnancy because of a decrease in right ventricular function, and an increase in blood volume and cardiac output (Linter & Clarke 1984, Groves & Groves 1995), or with the onset of arrhythmias. However, a review of 42 pregnancies in 12 women showed that, in the absence of cyanosis or arrhythmias, pregnancy was well tolerated (Donnelly et al 1991). Presumably, those who survive to child bearing age represent a less severely affected group.

Management

1. The severity of the lesion must be assessed. In the presence of maternal cyanosis or arrhythmias during pregnancy, there should be close monitoring of both mother and fetus. Deterioration may occur, despite previous successful pregnancies (Groves & Groves 1995).

2. Heart failure and arrhythmias require treatment.

3. Antibiotic prophylaxis against bacterial endocarditis.

4. If a CVP is used for monitoring, its tip should be kept within the superior vena cava. The use of intracardiac catheters should probably be avoided.

5. Techniques should aim to minimise tachycardia and hypotension.

6. Oxygen therapy increases pulmonary vasodilatation. Long-term maternal therapy was required during pregnancy from 14 weeks, to treat fetal hypoxia that was demonstrated by umbilical venous blood gases (Negishi et al 1995).

7. A number of anaesthetic techniques have been described. A two-catheter epidural technique was used for vaginal delivery to minimise hypotension (Linter & Clarke 1984). Bupivacaine doses must be fractionated and saline rather than air used to site the epidural, to avoid paradoxical air emboli (Groves & Groves 1995). Caesarean section under general anaesthesia, preceded by fentanyl (Halpern et al 1985), and a neurolept analgesic technique for hysterectomy (Bengtsson et al 1977), have been described.

Bibliography

Ammash NM, Warnes CA, Connolly HM et al 1997 Mimics of Ebstein's anomaly. American Heart Journal 134: 508–13.

Bengtsson IM, Magno R, Wickstrom 1977 Ebstein's anomaly—anaesthetic problems. British Journal of Anaesthesia 49: 501–3.

Donnelly JE, Brown JM, Radford DJ 1991 Pregnancy outcome and Ebstein's anomaly. British Heart Journal 66: 368–71.

Elsten JL, Kim YD, Hanowell ST et al 1981 Prolonged induction with exaggerated chamber enlargement in Ebstein's anomaly. Anesthesia & Analgesia 60: 909–10.

Gentles TL, Calder AL, Clarkson PM et al 1992 Predictors of long-term survival with Ebstein's anomaly of the tricuspid valve. American Journal of Cardiology 69: 377–81.

Groves ER, Groves JB 1995 Epidural analgesia for labour in a patient with Ebstein's anomaly. Canadian Journal of Anaesthesia 42: 77–9.

Halpern S, Gidwaney A, Gates B 1985 Anaesthesia for Caesarean section in a preeclamptic patient with Ebstein's anomaly. Canadian Anaesthetists' Society Journal 32: 244–7.

Linter SPK, Clarke K 1984 Caesarean section under extradural analgesia in a patient with Ebstein's anomaly. British Journal of Anaesthesia 56: 203–5.

Mair DD 1992 Ebstein's anomaly: natural history and management. Journal of the American College of Cardiology 19: 1047–8.

Negishi H, Yamada H, Okuyama K et al 1995 Pregnancy complicated by Ebstein's anomaly: oxygen administration to mother for chronic fetal hypoxemia. A therapeutic case report. Fetal Diagnosis & Therapy 10: 22–5.

Eclampsia and severe preeclampsia (see also HELLP syndrome)

Preeclampsia is a syndrome of unknown aetiology which is associated with pregnancy. It affects a wide variety of organs and therefore produces diverse manifestations. The main presenting feature is hypertension, with either proteinuria or oedema, or both. Maternal complications include eclampsia, cerebral haemorrhage, cerebral oedema, left ventricular failure, and renal failure.

Eclampsia, a cerebral complication, is marked by the onset of convulsions. Cerebral haemorrhage and cerebral oedema are the most frequent causes of death in preeclampsia. Hypertensive disease is still the second most important cause of maternal mortality in the UK and accounts for almost 15% of direct maternal deaths (Department of Health 1998).

Occasionally, an intracranial aneurysm can rupture, or a cerebral AV malformation may bleed, during pregnancy. The presentation will share some of the features of eclampsia and severe preeclampsia, an acute severe headache and neurological signs, with or without a period of unconsciousness. It is crucial that it is distinguished from preeclampsia. Early diagnosis and surgery will improve morbidity and mortality.

A small group of patients have been described with the HELLP syndrome, which comprises preeclampsia, in association with Haemolysis, Elevated Liver enzymes, and a Low Platelet count.

The use of iv magnesium sulphate as the anticonvulsant of choice for patients with eclampsia is now well established (The Eclampsia Trial Collaborative Group 1995). This study of 1680 women showed a lower risk of recurrent convulsions in those receiving magnesium sulphate compared with the groups receiving diazepam or phenytoin. The use of magnesium sulphate for prophylaxis in severe preeclampsia is now being examined. At present, a multicentre study (the MAGPIE trial) is being undertaken to determine whether or not prophylactic administration of magnesium sulphate to women with severe preeclampsia reduces the incidence of eclampsia, and if it does, the safety of giving it routinely. In the interim period, a South African study of 699 women, randomised to receive either placebo or magnesium sulphate, has been published. The authors found an incidence of

eclampsia of 0.3% in those receiving magnesium sulphate and 3.2% in those having the placebo (Coetzee et al 1998). Following this paper there have been arguments for and against the continuation of the MAGPIE trial (Anthony & Rush 1998, Duley 1998, Moodley 1998).

Presentation

1. The definition of preeclampsia includes diastolic hypertension of ≥90 mmHg (Cunningham & Lindheimer 1992). It has also been recommended that the disappearance of the Korotkoff sound (phase V), rather than the muffling (phase IV), be used in its determination. Severe preeclampsia is associated with a BP of 160/110 or more on at least two occasions 6 h apart, and proteinuria of >5 g in 24 h.

2. Whilst preeclampsia is common in the young primiparous patient, there appears to be a subgroup for whom the maternal and fetal risks are particularly high. The patient with preeclampsia at special risk, is the older (>25 years), multiparous patient, and particularly the one who develops an impairment in her level of consciousness.

3. The onset of convulsions denotes eclampsia. It may be associated with cerebral haemorrhage or diffuse oedema.

4. The HELLP syndrome may present with bleeding as a result of thrombocytopenia, a decrease in haemoglobin secondary to haemolysis, and abnormal LFTs.

Problems

1. Hypertension, which may be complicated by cerebral oedema, haemorrhage, or heart failure. Both preeclampsia and existing hypertension are associated with exaggerated pressor responses to accelerated labour, or to noxious stimuli such as tracheal intubation or extubation. In normotensive patients, mean arterial pressures exceeding 130–150 mmHg

may be associated with a loss of protective cerebral autoregulation, and the hypertensive response to intubation has provoked cerebral haemorrhage.

2. Impaired renal function which may progress to anuria. Even in mild preeclampsia, the GFR is decreased by 25%. Renal failure accounts for about 10% of deaths from eclampsia, and long-term renal problems are now being seen in ITU survivors (Umo-Etuk et al 1996).

3. Plasma volume may be decreased by up to 40% in severe cases. Despite sodium and water retention, the CVP is low or normal. This is in part due to an increased vascular permeability causing loss of fluid and protein from the circulation. In a study of patients who had pulmonary artery pressure monitoring, variable results were obtained (Mabie et al 1989). However, the general impression was of a high cardiac output state, with an inappropriately high systemic vascular resistance. The haemodynamic profile suggested that the intravascular volume in preeclampsia is centrally redistributed.

4. Maternal systemic blood flow is reduced secondary to increased systemic resistance, and increased blood viscosity. Diminished placental blood flow results in placental infarction and separation, which leads to decreased fetal growth and sometimes death. Maternal vessels become particularly sensitive to the effects of exogenous catecholamines.

5. A coagulopathy may occur, which is probably consumptive in origin. The number and quality of platelets commonly decrease and the thrombin time becomes prolonged. Prothrombin time, partial thromboplastin time, and fibrinogen abnormalities may occur. Significant thrombocytopenia and coagulation abnormalities are usually only encountered in severe preeclampsia (Barker & Callander 1991).

6. Pulmonary oedema, which can be vascular or neurogenic in origin, may produce cyanosis and respiratory distress.

7. Headache, epigastric pain, visual disturbances, hyperreflexia, or cerebral irritability may be warning signs of impending eclampsia. Delayed recovery of consciousness following an eclamptic fit may indicate the occurrence of cerebral oedema or intracranial haemorrhage. In a study of 175 women with eclampsia, almost 6% developed symptomatic cerebral oedema, and one died from transtentorial herniation (Cunningham & Twickler 2000). Patients with eclampsia have increases in cerebral perfusion pressure, but an accompanying decrease in cerebrovascular resistance resulting in loss of autoregulation and overperfusion of the brain (Williams & Wilson 1999). A patient who developed acute cortical blindness, preeclampsia and HELLP syndrome at 33 weeks' gestation had ischaemic lesions on CT scan which involved basal ganglia, posterior parietal and occipital regions (Crosby & Preston 1998). Vision returned fully by 72 h, and MRI confirmed the ischaemic lesions, and an absence of major vascular abnormalities.

8. Not all fits occurring during pregnancy and labour are the result of eclampsia. Eclamptic fits must be distinguished from those secondary to hyponatraemia associated with the concomitant administration of oxytocics and dextrose-containing fluids, epilepsy, phaeochromocytoma, a ruptured intracranial aneurysm or AV malformation, or other intracranial pathology (Cheng & Kwan 1997).

9. Pulmonary aspiration and airway obstruction are both more likely to occur in oversedated or unconscious patients.

10. Rarely, severe preeclampsia is associated with haemolysis, abnormal liver function, hepatic damage and thrombocytopenia (see HELLP syndrome), which carries a mortality of up to 24%.

11. Occasionally, pharyngeal or laryngeal oedema may occur unexpectedly, and cause intubation problems (Seager & MacDonald 1980, Brimacombe 1992). One patient developed breathing difficulties after extubation. At laryngoscopy, severe laryngeal oedema was found, despite the vocal cords having been

normal at induction of anaesthesia (Rocke & Scoones 1992).

12. Phaeochromocytoma occasionally presents during pregnancy and is associated with a high mortality (Harper et al 1989). The majority of patients have hypertension, and one presented with convulsions (see Phaeochromocytoma).

Management of severe preeclampsia

This is a potentially lethal condition which should be managed in a high dependency area. Monitoring and treatment requires close cooperation between obstetrician, anaesthetist, and paediatrician, whether or not operative delivery is required. All labour wards should have local guidelines for the management of severe preeclampsia and eclampsia. General anaesthesia may be particularly hazardous in some patients, and additional precautions should be taken to prevent hypertensive peaks during intubation and extubation.

Management of severe preeclampsia, throughout the peripartum period, should be directed towards:

1. Monitoring. CVP, ECG, arterial pressure and urine output is monitored, as is neuromuscular function if general anaesthesia is required.

2. Control of maternal blood pressure by arteriolar dilatation. A number of different methods of controlling blood pressure prior to delivery have been described. The care with which blood pressure is monitored and regulated is probably of more importance to maternal and fetal welfare than the precise method of control. The majority of patients will already be receiving oral methyldopa from the obstetrician.

a) Epidural analgesia. This has the dual therapeutic advantages of providing both vasodilatation and analgesia in preeclampsia, provided that no coagulation defect is present. Platelet count should be $>100 \times 10^9 l^{-1}$, and the prothrombin time and partial thromboplastin time normal.

b) Hydralazine, in 5–10 mg increments iv, or by infusion, has been used traditionally for emergency treatment of hypertension in late pregnancy. However, an analysis of available data has suggested that it may not be the most appropriate choice in pregnancy (Magee et al 1999).

c) Labetalol is a non-selective beta adrenergic blocker, with beta effects predominating over alpha, in a ratio of seven to one. Intravenously it is given as an initial bolus of 5–10 mg, repeated at 5-min intervals up to 1 mg kg^{-1}.

d) Nifedipine, a calcium channel blocker, can be given orally or sublingually. Although it has been used both orally (10 mg) and sublingually (5 mg) in acute hypertension, there have been no large controlled studies of severe hypertension in pregnancy (Smith et al 2000). In a small study comparing the haemodynamic effects of oral nifedipine and iv labetalol using thoracic electrical bioimpedance, nifedipine significantly increased cardiac index and reduced systemic vascular resistance, whilst labetalol affected neither, but significantly reduced heart rate (Scardo et al 1999).

e) Magnesium sulphate is both a vasodilator and a sedative. Magnesium sulphate 4 g stat and 2 g h^{-1}, via an infusion.

Magnesium (Mg) levels:

Normal serum	0.7–1.0 mmol l^{-1}.
Therapeutic anticonvulsant levels	2–3.5 mmol l^{-1}.
Loss of patellar reflex	5 mmol l^{-1}.
Skeletal muscle relaxation	6 mmol l^{-1}.
Respiratory paralysis	6–7.5 mmol l^{-1}.
Cardiac asystole	>12 mmol l^{-1}.
Accidental high levels can be treated by calcium gluconate 10%	10 ml slowly.

3. Restoration of vascular volume and vasodilatation. This should take place synchronously, preferably using plasma protein fraction or a colloid. The CVP should be maintained around 6–8 cmH$_2$O, with reference to the midaxillary line. Prevention of vasoconstriction and restoration of blood volume has the additional benefit of improving renal function and uteroplacental blood flow. Fluid administration must be carried out cautiously, since pulmonary oedema is not uncommon in severe preeclampsia, and some studies suggest that the CVP may be normal and there is redistribution of intravascular volume centrally (Mabie et al 1989).

4. Prevention of eclampsia. Currently, the MAGPIE trial is examining the effectiveness and safety of magnesium sulphate for prophylaxis against convulsions in severe preeclampsia.

5. Protection against acid aspiration syndrome. Patients with impaired conscious levels are particularly at risk, and this has, in part, influenced the decrease in the use of heavy sedation.

6. Operative intervention. For Caesarean section, there has been a move towards spinal anaesthesia as the technique of choice, because of the improvement in quality of anaesthesia and onset time (Sharwood-Smith et al 1999). However, this is a controversial area. Some feel that epidural anaesthesia permits an incremental technique; this carries less risk of the sudden haemodynamic changes that are produced by spinal anaesthesia (Howell 1998). Large controlled trials are now awaited.

In the very severe case, or if regional anaesthesia is contraindicated, general anaesthesia may be required, but carries additional risks. A careful technique should aim to modulate the hypertensive peaks provoked by intubation and extubation, and to prevent sudden uncontrolled reductions in blood pressure. The latter can, however, be produced by either general or regional anaesthesia. It has been suggested that drugs that will help modify the hypertensive response to intubation should be given before induction. These are administered in addition to the preoperative antihypertensive regimen. As yet, there appears to be no technique that guarantees protection in every patient. The following drugs have been used:

a) Lidocaine 1 mg kg^{-1} iv, prior to induction, to reduce haemodynamic responses. It prevented intracranial hypertension during tracheal suction in comatose head injury patients (Donegan & Bedford 1980).

b) A combination of an alfentanil and magnesium sulphate by bolus prior to induction (Allen et al 1991).

c) Alfentanil 10–25 μg kg^{-1} has been shown to modify the hypertensive response to intubation in the nonhypertensive pregnant patient.

7. Management of HELLP syndrome (see HELLP).

Management of eclampsia

1. Although magnesium sulphate is now recommended as the first line of treatment, the ABC management of a fitting patient may require initial control of convulsions with diazepam 2.5–5 mg, in order to secure the airway and maintain oxygenation whilst magnesium is being prepared. Magnesium therapy should be initiated without delay to prevent recurrence of fits (Brodie & Malinow 1999). Tracheal intubation, blood gas estimation and IPPV may be required at this stage.

2. Care should be taken to ensure that the diagnosis of eclampsia is correct. If a convulsion is not associated with hypertension and either oedema or proteinuria, or if the history and signs are atypical, then other causes must be eliminated. If an intracranial aneurysm is suspected, a CT scan should be performed.

3. For control of hypertension, see above.

4. The only ultimate control of eclampsia is termination of the pregnancy, either by rapid vaginal delivery or LSCS.

5. If an eclamptic patient remains unconscious 4–6 h postpartum, neurosurgical advice should be sought. A CT scan will distinguish cerebral oedema from intracranial haemorrhage. It has been suggested that the combination of diffuse white matter oedema and basal cisternal effacement is an indication for intracranial pressure monitoring (Richards et al 1986). A high intracranial pressure ($n = 10$–$15\,mmHg$) may require specific treatment.

Post-delivery care

In the UK, 44% of eclamptic fits occurred postpartum (Douglas & Redman 1994). In the severe case, intensive monitoring and treatment should continue for 24–72 h.

Bibliography

Allen RW, James MF, Uys PC 1991 Attenuation of the pressor response to tracheal intubation in hypertensive proteinuric pregnant patients by lignocaine, alfentanil and magnesium sulphate. British Journal of Anaesthesia 66: 216–23.

Anthony J, Rush R 1998 A randomised controlled trial of intravenous magnesium sulphate versus placebo. British Journal of Obstetrics and Gynaecology 105: 300–3.

Barker P, Callander CC 1991 Coagulation screening before epidural analgesia in pre-eclampsia. Anaesthesia 46: 64–7.

Brimacombe T 1992 Acute pharyngolaryngeal oedema and pre-eclamptic toxaemia. Anaesthesia & Intensive Care 20: 97–8.

Brodie H, Malinow AM 1999 Anesthetic management of preeclampsia/eclampsia. International Journal of Obstetric Anesthesia 8: 110–24.

Cheng AY, Kwan A 1997 Perioperative management of intrapartum seizure. Anaesthesia & Intensive Care 25: 535–8.

Coetzee EJ, Dommisse J, Anthony J 1998 A randomised controlled trial of intravenous magnesium sulphate versus placebo in the management of women with severe pre-eclampsia. British Journal of Obstetrics & Gynaecology 105: 300–3.

Crosby ET 1991 Obstetrical anaesthesia for patients with the syndrome of haemolysis, elevated liver enzymes and low platelets. Canadian Journal of Anaesthesia 38: 227–33.

Crosby ET, Preston R 1998 Obstetrical anaesthesia for a parturient with preeclampsia, HELLP syndrome and acute cortical blindness. Canadian Journal of Anaesthesia 45: 452–9.

Cunningham FG, Lindheimer MD 1992 Hypertension in pregnancy. New England Journal of Medicine 326: 927–32.

Cunningham FG, Twickler D 2000 Cerebral edema complicating eclampsia. American Journal of Obstetrics & Gynecology 182: 94–100.

Dann WL, Hutchinson A, Cartwright DP 1987 Maternal and neonatal responses to alfentanil administered before induction of general anaesthesia for Caesarean section. British Journal of Anaesthesia 59: 1392–6.

Department of Health 1998 Report on Confidential Enquiries into Maternal Deaths in the United Kingdom 1994–1996. HMSO, London.

Donegan MF, Bedford RF 1980 Intravenously administered lidocaine prevents intracranial hypertension during endotracheal suction. Anesthesiology 52: 516–18.

Douglas KA, Redman CWG 1994 Eclampsia in the United Kingdom. British Medical Journal 309: 1395–400.

Duley L 1998 Magnesium sulphate in eclampsia. Eclampsia Trial Collaborative Group. Lancet 352: 67–8.

Easterling TR, Benedetti TJ, Schmucker BC et al 1990 Maternal hemodynamics in normal and preeclamptic pregnancies: a longitudinal study. Obstetrics & Gynecology 76: 1061–9.

The Eclampsia Trial Collaborative Group 1995 Which anticonvulsant for women with eclampsia? Evidence from the Collaborative Eclampsia Trial. Lancet 345: 1455–63.

Fawcett WJ, Haxby EJ, Male DA 1999 Magnesium: physiology and pharmacology. British Journal of Anaesthesia 83: 302–20.

Giannotta SL, Daniels J, Golde SH et al 1986 Ruptured intracranial aneurysms during pregnancy. Journal of Reproductive Medicine 31: 139–47.

Hanretty KP 1989 Effect of nifedipine in severe preeclampsia. British Medical Journal 299: 1205.

Harper MA, Murnaghan GA, Kennedy L et al 1989 Phaeochromocytoma in pregnancy. British Journal of Obstetrics & Gynaecology 96: 594–606.

Howell P 1998 Spinal anaesthesia in severe preeclampsia: time for reappraisal, or time for caution. International Journal of Obstetric Anesthesia 7: 217–19.

James MFM 1998 Magnesium in obstetric anesthesia. International Journal of Obstetric Anesthesia 7: 115–23.

Mabie WC, Ratts TE, Sibai BM 1989 The central hemodynamics of severe preeclampsia. American Journal of Obstetrics & Gynecology 161: 1443–8.

Magee LA, Ornstein MP, Von Dadelszen P 1999 Management of hypertension in pregnancy. British Medical Journal 318: 1332–6.

Moodley J 1998 Magnesium sulphate in clinical practice: an obstetrician's viewpoint. International Journal of Obstetric Anesthesia 7: 73–5.

Mortl MG, Schneider MC 2000 Key issues in assessing, managing and treating patients presenting with severe preeclampsia. International Journal of Obstetric Anesthesia 9: 39–41.

Patterson KW, O'Toole DP 1991 HELLP syndrome: a case report with guidelines for management. British Journal of Anaesthesia 66: 513–15.

Ramanathan J, Sibai BM, Vu T, Chaudhan D 1989 Correlation between bleeding times and platelet counts in women with pre-eclampsia undergoing Cesarean section. Anesthesiology 71: 188–91.

Redman CWG 1988 Eclampsia still kills. British Medical Journal 296: 1209–10.

Richards AM, Moodley J, Graham DI et al 1986 Active management of the unconscious eclamptic patient. British Journal of Obstetrics & Gynaecology 93: 554–62.

Rocke DA, Scoones GP 1992 Rapidly progressive laryngeal oedema associated with pregnancy-aggravated hypertension. Anaesthesia 47: 141–3.

Rout CC, Rocke DA 1990 Effects of alfentanil and fentanyl on induction of anaesthesia in patients with severe pregnancy-induced hypertension. British Journal of Anaesthesia 65: 468–74.

Scardo JA, Vermillion ST, Newman RB et al 1999 A randomized, double-blind, hemodynamic evaluation of nifedipine and labetalol in preeclamptic hypertensive emergencies. American Journal of Obstetrics & Gynecology 181: 862–6.

Schindler M, Gatt S, Isert P et al 1990 Thrombocytopenia and platelet functional defects in pre-eclampsia: implications for regional anaesthesia. Anaesthesia & Intensive Care 18: 361–5.

Seager SJ, MacDonald R 1980 Laryngeal oedema and preeclampsia. Anaesthesia 35: 360–2.

Sharwood-Smith G, Clark V, Watson E 1999 Regional anaesthesia for caesarean section in severe preeclampsia: spinal anaesthesia is the preferred choice. International Journal of Obstetric Anesthesia 8: 85–9.

Smith P, Anthony J, Johanson R 2000 Nifedipine in pregnancy. British Journal of Obstetrics & Gynaecology 107: 299–307.

Umo-Etuk J, Lumley J, Holdcroft A 1996 Critically ill parturient women and admission to intensive care. International Journal of Obstetric Anesthesia 5: 79–84.

Williams KP, Wilson S 1999 Persistence of cerebral hemodynamic changes in patients with eclampsia: a report of three cases. American Journal of Obstetrics & Gynecology 181: 1162–5.

Ehlers–Danlos syndrome (EDS)

A group of conditions, of varying inheritance, in which there is a defect in collagen. Many different subtypes have been identified, each showing a wide spectrum of effects, from mild to severe. There have been recent advances in understanding of the genetic and molecular abnormalities of the variants (Pope 1991), and a new classification has recently been proposed (Beighton et al 1998). Detailed descriptions of each type are beyond the scope of this book; however, for further information, several references may be consulted (Pope et al 1988, Anstey et al 1991, Pope 1991). The clinical picture is one of multiple skin, connective tissue, and musculoskeletal abnormalities. Cardiac defects have also been described. Anaesthesia may be required for joint dislocations, vascular or visceral rupture, and surgery may be complicated by abnormal haemorrhage. Type IV disease is the most dangerous, and in this type, surgery and pregnancy carry a high mortality.

Preoperative abnormalities

1. The whole group is characterised by a hyperextensible and sometimes fragile, soft skin, hypermobile joints, and a tendency to bruise and bleed without definite coagulation abnormalities. Paper-tissue scars may occur over the knees, shins, forehead, and chin.

2. The ecchymotic form (type IV EDS), which involves abnormalities in type III collagen synthesis, is the most severe, although in this

form the loose-jointedness and skin hyperextensibility are uncommon. Type III collagen is the predominant collagen of blood vessels, uterus, fetal skin, and the gastrointestinal tract; complications therefore include aneurysmal dilatation, rupture of blood vessels, and visceral rupture. Aortic dissection, similar to that in Marfan's syndrome, may occur. Type III collagen also forms 10–15% of the collagen in adult skin. Pregnancy carries a 25% mortality, and the complications of surgery can be disastrous.

3. Valvular disease, in the form of either regurgitation or prolapse, congenital heart disease, and a variety of conduction defects, have been described in association with some forms of EDS.

4. Type VI disease can be associated with severe kyphoscoliosis, probably secondary to muscular hypotonia and ligamentous laxity (Heim et al 1998).

5. Orthostatic stress may occur in EDS, secondary to abnormal connective tissue in dependent blood vessels causing venous pooling (Rowe et al 1999).

Anaesthetic problems

1. The ecchymotic form (type IV) may present with uncontrollable haemorrhage, aneurysm formation, and arterial or venous rupture.

2. Spontaneous perforation of a viscus, particularly the colon, may be the first event leading to the diagnosis (Sparkman 1984). Surgery may be followed by wound dehiscence, infection, or recurrent perforation.

3. In types IV and VI EDS, arterial and central venous lines used for monitoring, or intravascular or radiological procedures, can cause severe bleeding. Perforation of the superior vena cava occurred during digital angiography (Driscoll et al 1984).

4. Vascular surgery carries a high mortality

because of the extreme fragility of the arterial wall (Memon et al 1996). In a review of published reports in 112 patients with type IV, 50% had actually died (Bergqvist 1996). The commonest causes were arterial aneurysms (50%), arterial rupture (38%), and carotidocavernous fistula (24%).

5. A variety of haemostatic defects were reported in a study of 51 patients (Anstey et al 1991). Although the majority gave a history of bruising, or a bleeding tendency, only 17.6% had significant abnormalities. These included platelet storage pool defects, factor XI deficiency, and factor XIII deficiency. The remainder had either mild abnormalities of doubtful significance, or no abnormality at all. Thus, the bleeding and bruising that occurs must be related to structural abnormalities in the collagen and blood vessels, rather than coagulation defects.

6. There is an increased incidence of radiological evidence of atlantoaxial subluxation in type IV disease (Halko et al 1995). Even in the absence of subluxation, overall hypermobility of the cervical spine was seen in ten patients.

7. Spinal or epidural anaesthesia may be complicated by an epidural haematoma. However, combined spinal and epidural anaesthesia for Caesarean section was undertaken in a patient with type IV disease who had refused general anaesthesia (Brighouse & Guard 1992).

8. Milder forms may have postoperative wound dehiscence.

9. Venous access can be technically difficult because of the hyperextensible skin. Displacement of the cannula from a vein, and consequent venous extravasation, may remain undetected. Ectasia of the internal jugular vein has been reported (Heim et al 1998).

10. If conduction defects such as RBBB and left anterior hemi-block are present, it is possible that the patient could progress to complete heart block under anaesthesia. Elective repair of an aortic aneurysm was complicated by acute myocardial ischaemia and ventricular tachycardia

in a 38-year-old man (Price et al 1996). Q waves had been observed on preoperative ECG, but had been attributed to previous repair of a patent ductus arteriosus.

11. There is an increased risk of pneumothorax in type IV disease.

12. Mandibular hypoplasia (type VI), periodontal disease (type VIII), and recurrent mandibular joint dislocation may complicate airway management (Sacks et al 1990). In one patient, the occurrence of repeated jaw dislocations with facial ecchymosis led to the diagnosis of EDS.

13. A variety of complications may occur during pregnancy. In type I disease (30–50% of cases), they were associated mainly with tissue laxity, and included vaginal lacerations, abdominal herniae, ante- and postpartum haemorrhage, joint subluxations, and bruising, but none of these complications was associated with death. In type IV disease, however, pregnancy carries a high mortality (Peaceman & Cruikshank 1987), and death may occur at any time. In a study of 26 women with type IV, undergoing 50 pregnancies, ten died during pregnancy or immediately postpartum (Lurie et al 1998). Spontaneous pulmonary artery rupture caused exsanguination during the seventh month of pregnancy (Pearl & Spicer 1981). Intrapartum deaths have resulted from aortic, uterine, and vena caval rupture (Rudd et al 1983). Death occurred secondary to a postpartum haemorrhage in a patient with normal coagulation tests (Dolan et al 1980). Widespread bleeding from fragile vessels and a ruptured splenic artery aneurysm were found at exploratory laparotomy. Postpartum deaths have resulted from spontaneous rupture of the aorta on day 1 (Rudd et al 1983), day 5 (Snyder et al 1983), and at an unspecified time (Barabas 1972), and renal artery rupture on day 6 (Peaceman & Cruikshank 1987). In a vaginal delivery in a patient with type II disease, a large central perineal rupture involved the posterior wall, through which the baby was delivered (Georgy et al 1997).

14. Local anaesthesia, either by intradermal infiltration or topical application (EMLA), was found not to be as effective in EDS type III, compared with controls (Arendt-Nielsen et al 1990). Reduced depth and duration of anaesthesia probably results from the looseness of the connective tissue.

Management

1. If the condition is suspected and time permits, genetic advice should be obtained to assess the type and severity.

2. Blood should be cross-matched and coagulation defects excluded.

3. Intramuscular injections must not be given in type IV, and regional anaesthesia is relatively contraindicated. However, a combined spinal and epidural technique was used for Caesarean section in a patient with type IV who refused general anaesthesia (Brighouse & Guard 1992), and spinal anaesthesia for type II (Goldstein & Miller 1997).

4. Good peripheral venous access or a venous cutdown should be established. Central venous monitoring via a large cannula, at a site where bleeding cannot be controlled by pressure, should be avoided in types IV and VI. If essential, a small needle should be used, in a peripheral site.

5. Particular care should be taken to avoid tissue trauma or jaw dislocation when tracheal or nasogastric tubes are inserted.

6. During artificial ventilation, low airway pressures should be used to reduce the risk of a pneumothorax.

7. If conduction defects are present, the temporary insertion of a pacemaker should be considered.

8. Antibiotic prophylaxis is required if there is mitral valve prolapse.

9. Patients with type IV disease should be counselled against pregnancy, and those who

become pregnant should be recommended to have termination before 16 weeks (Peaceman & Cruikshank 1987, Lurie et al 1998). If this is declined, delivery by elective Caesarean section at 32 weeks has been recommended (Lurie et al 1998), and close observation for signs of vascular or bowel rupture maintained in the postpartum period.

10. Analysis of literature reports of surgical complications over 20 years, associated with vascular or bowel surgery, showed a high incidence of reperforations, anastomotic leaks, haemorrhage, aneurysms, and vascular dissection. The authors suggest that colonic perforations should be treated with total colectomy and end ileostomy. If vascular surgery must be done, simple vessel ligation, rather than reconstruction, should be attempted (Bergqvist 1996, Freeman et al 1996).

Bibliography

Anstey A, Mayne K, Winter M et al 1991 Platelet and coagulation studies in Ehlers–Danlos syndrome. British Journal of Dermatology 125: 155–61.

Arendt-Nielsen L, Kaalund S, Bjerring P et al 1990 Insufficient effect of local analgesics in Ehlers–Danlos type III patients (connective tissue disorder). Acta Anaesthesiologica Scandinavica 34: 358–61.

Beighton P, De Paepe A, Steinmann B et al 1998 Ehlers–Danlos syndromes: revised nosology, Villefranche, 1997. American Journal of Medical Genetics 77: 31–7.

Bergqvist D 1996 Ehlers–Danlos type IV syndrome. A review from a vascular surgical point of view. European Journal of Surgery 162: 163–70.

Brighouse D, Guard B 1992 Anaesthesia for Caesarean section in a patient with Ehlers–Danlos syndrome type IV. British Journal of Anaesthesia 69: 517–20.

De Paepe A 1996 The Ehlers–Danlos syndrome: a heritable collagen disorder as a cause of bleeding. Thrombosis & Haemostasis 73: 379–86.

Dolan P, Sisko F, Riley E 1980 Anesthetic considerations for Ehlers–Danlos syndrome. Anesthesiology 52: 266–9.

Driscoll SHM, Gomes AS, Machleder HI 1984 Perforation of the superior vena cava: a complication of digital angiography in Ehlers–Danlos syndrome. American Journal of Roentgenology 142: 1021–2.

Freeman RK, Swegle J, Sise MJ 1996 The surgical complications of Ehlers–Danlos syndrome. American Surgeon 62: 869–73.

Georgy MS, Anwar K, Oates SE et al 1997 Perineal delivery in Ehlers–Danlos syndrome. British Journal of Obstetrics & Gynaecology 104: 505–6.

Giunta C, Superti-Furga A, Spranger S et al 1999 Ehlers–Danlos type VII: clinical features and molecular defects. Journal of Bone & Joint Surgery 81: 225–8.

Goldstein M, Miller R 1997 Anesthesia for cesarean delivery in a patient with Ehlers–Danlos syndrome. Regional Anesthesia 22: 280–3.

Halko GJ, Cobb R, Abeles M 1995 Patients with type IV Ehlers–Danlos syndrome may be predisposed to atlantoaxial subluxation. Journal of Rheumatology 22: 2152–5.

Heim P, Raghunath M, Meiss L et al 1998 Ehlers–Danlos syndrome type VI (EDS VI): problems of diagnosis and management. Acta Paediatrica 87: 708–10.

Lurie S, Manor M, Hagay ZJ 1998 The threat of type IV Ehlers–Danlos syndrome on maternal well-being during pregnancy: early delivery may make the difference. Journal of Obstetrics & Gynaecology 18: 245–8.

Memon MA, Nicholson CM, Clayton-Smith J 1996 Spontaneous aortic rupture in a 22-year-old. Postgraduate Medical Journal 72: 311–13.

Peaceman AM, Cruikshank DP 1987 Ehlers–Danlos syndrome and pregnancy: association of type IV disease with maternal death. Obstetrics & Gynecology 69: 428–31.

Pearl W, Spicer M 1981 Ehlers–Danlos syndrome. Southern Medical Journal 74: 80–1.

Pope FM 1991 Ehlers–Danlos syndrome. Baillière's Clinical Rheumatology 5(2): 321–49.

Pope FM, Narcisi P, Nicholls AC et al 1988 Clinical presentation of Ehlers–Danlos Syndrome. Archives of Disease in Childhood 63: 1016–25.

Price CM, Ford S, St John Jones L et al 1996 Myocardial ischaemia associated with Ehlers–Danlos syndrome. British Journal of Anaesthesia 76: 464–6.

Rowe PC, Barron DF, Calkins H et al 1999 Orthostatic intolerance and chronic fatigue syndrome associated with Ehlers–Danlos syndrome. Journal of Pediatrics 135: 494–9.

Rudd NL, Holbrook KA, Nimrod C et al 1983 Pregnancy complications in type IV Ehlers–Danlos syndrome. Lancet i: 50–3.

Sacks H, Zelig D, Schabes G 1990 Recurrent

temporomandibular joint subluxation and facial ecchymosis leading to diagnosis of Ehlers–Danlos syndrome. Journal of Oral & Maxillofacial Surgery 48: 641–7.

Snyder RR, Gilstrap LC, Hauth JC 1983 Ehlers–Danlos syndrome and pregnancy. Obstetrics & Gynecology 61: 649–51.

Sparkman RS 1984 Ehlers–Danlos syndrome type IV: dramatic, deceptive, and deadly. American Journal of Surgery 147: 703–4.

Eisenmenger's syndrome

A rare syndrome of pulmonary hypertension associated with a reversed or bidirectional cardiac shunt, occurring through a large communication between the left and right sides of the heart. The defect may be interventricular, interatrial, or aortopulmonary. The development of Eisenmenger's syndrome, from the initial left to right shunt, is usually a gradual process. Contributory factors to the pulmonary hypertension are hypoxia, high pulmonary blood flow, and high left atrial pressure. Irreversible structural changes take place in the small vessels, causing pulmonary vascular obstruction and a reduction in the size of the capillary bed. The pulmonary artery pressure is the same as, or sometimes exceeds, the systemic arterial pressure. The incidence of this syndrome is decreasing because of the more vigorous approach to diagnosis and treatment of congenital heart disease in childhood. In a long-term study of 188 patients over a median period of 31 years, noncardiac surgery with general anaesthesia carried risks of 23.5%, and pregnancy was associated with a deterioration in physical status and a maternal mortality of 27% (Daliento et al 1998). A lower mortality (10%) was quoted in a series of nonparturients, but only half involved general anaesthesia (Raines et al 1996). The mortality is also lower in children (Lyons et al 1995).

Preoperative abnormalities

1. Presenting symptoms include dyspnoea, tiredness, episodes of cyanosis, syncope, or chest pain. Haemoptysis may occur. A haemoglobin of $17.5\,\mathrm{g\,dl^{-1}}$ was noted at booking clinic with a community midwife at 17 weeks' gestation. Eisenmenger's syndrome was only diagnosed a month later when the patient was admitted to hospital with abdominal pain (Stoddart & O'Sullivan 1993).

2. The direction of the shunt, and hence the presence or absence of cyanosis, depends on a number of factors. These include hypoxaemia, the pulmonary and systemic pressure differences, and the intravascular volume. It can also be affected by certain drugs.

3. Sleep studies have shown that there is a nocturnal deterioration in arterial oxygen saturation, which seems to be related to ventilation/perfusion distribution abnormalities occurring in the supine position (Sandoval et al 1999).

4. Chest X-ray shows right ventricular hypertrophy, and ECG indicates varying degrees of right ventricular hypertrophy and strain.

5. Complications include thrombosis secondary to polycythaemia, air embolus, bacterial endocarditis, gout, cholelithiasis, and hypertrophic osteoarthropathy. Cerebral abscess may occur secondary to clot embolism.

Anaesthetic problems

1. Reductions in systemic arterial pressure by myocardial depression or loss of sympathetic tone are potentially dangerous. Reversal of the shunt may occur, and sudden death has been reported. A direct correlation between systemic pressure and oxygen saturation was found in a patient undergoing laparoscopic cholecystectomy (Sammut & Paes 1997). Hypovolaemia and dehydration are poorly tolerated. Syntocinon may cause a dramatic reduction in SpO_2 secondary to vasodilatation.

2. Sinus tachycardia results from exercise or emotion, and episodes of SVT are common after the age of 30. The onset of atrial fibrillation is

associated with a sudden deterioration in the condition of the patient.

3. The relative merits of general and regional anaesthesia are arguable. General anaesthesia tends to be favoured, since the reduction in systemic vascular resistance associated with regional blockade increases the shunt. However, successful use of epidural anaesthesia for bilateral inguinal herniorrhaphy (Selsby & Sugden 1989), and Caesarean section (Spinnato et al 1981), have been reported.

4. Pregnancy is contraindicated because it carries considerable risks. Recent maternal mortality rates of 40% have been reported (Yentis et al 1998). A Caesarean section may increase it to over 60%. Termination of pregnancy is usually recommended in the first trimester, but is still associated with a mortality of 7%. The diagnosis may be missed at booking clinic. An increased haemoglobin level in early pregnancy was the only abnormality in one patient, but the significance was not recognised. She died postpartum (Stoddart & O'Sullivan 1993). In another patient, unexplained cyanosis during Caesarean section for antepartum haemorrhage was the first sign. Postoperative cardiorespiratory failure and coagulopathy resulted in death, and autopsy showed persistent ductus arteriosus and pulmonary hypertension (Gilman 1991). Complications from the insertion of pulmonary artery catheters for monitoring have included systemic and pulmonary emboli, pulmonary artery rupture, and arrhythmias (Robinson 1983). Postpartum death is not uncommon. One patient deteriorated and died 66 h following Caesarean section under general anaesthesia (Stoddart & O'Sullivan 1993); one died during removal of a pulmonary artery catheter on the fourth day after Caesarean section (Devitt et al 1982); another died on the sixth day (Huytens & Alexander 1986). It has been argued that the risks of pulmonary artery catheters in Eisenmenger's syndrome outweigh the benefits (Robinson 1983), and that it is not always possible to obtain wedge pressures (Schwalbe et al 1990).

5. Patients are at risk from paradoxical air or clot embolism, and infective endocarditis.

Management

1. Since death can occur in association with relatively minor surgery, it has been suggested that these patients should be referred to centres with expertise (Ammash et al 1999). Understanding of the pathophysiology of the complex is essential, and both pregnancy and noncardiac surgery require a multidisciplinary approach.

2. Maintenance of an adequate circulating blood volume is important. Myocardial depressants and peripheral vasodilators should be used with caution. Bradycardia must be prevented. If regional anaesthesia is used, the block should be instituted with caution, and hypovolaemia avoided. High-dose spinal morphine for the first stage of labour, and pudendal block for the second, were used in a woman with a patent ductus arteriosus (Pollack et al 1990). Simultaneous monitoring of oxygen saturations in the right arm (predominantly preductal), and left arm, gave information about the right-to-left shunt.

3. It is unclear as to whether oxygen can cause pulmonary vasodilatation. Although the pulmonary vascular resistance was believed to be fixed in pulmonary hypertension, a high oxygen concentration has been shown to reduce it during Caesarean section (Spinnato et al 1981). A proportion of children with Eisenmenger's complex had reversible airway obstruction that responded to inhaled albuterol (O'Hagan et al 1999). Improved oxygenation occurred in labour with inhaled nitric oxide (Lust et al 1999), but the patient in question died 21 days later of pulmonary hypertension and heart failure.

4. Maintenance of systemic vascular resistance is critical. The use of a norepinephrine (noradrenaline) infusion before induction has been described (Sammut & Paes 1997). Alpha adrenergic vasopressors, such as methoxamine or phenylephrine, have also been used for the

treatment of hypotension on induction of anaesthesia (Foster & Jones 1984).

5. Pulmonary ventilation should be performed with low inflation pressures and early tracheal extubation is advised, because of the deleterious effects of IPPV.

6. Air must be completely eliminated from all intravenous lines and the epidural space should be located with loss of resistance to saline, not to air.

7. Appropriate antibiotics are given to prevent bacterial endocarditis.

8. Low-dose heparin may reduce the risk of emboli.

9. Patients are usually advised against pregnancy. If anaesthesia is required either for termination of pregnancy or operative delivery, intensive cardiac care is indicated. It has been suggested that those reaching the end of the second trimester should be admitted to hospital until delivery and given heparin 20–40 000 u daily and oxygen therapy (Avila et al 1995). Successful epidural anaesthesia has been reported for Caesarean section (Spinnato et al 1981).

Bibliography

Ammash NM, Connolly HM, Abel MD et al 1999 Noncardiac surgery in Eisenmenger's syndrome. Journal of the American College of Cardiology 33: 222–7.

Avila WS, Grinberg M, Snitcowsky R et al 1995 Maternal and fetal outcome in pregnant women with Eisenmenger's syndrome. European Heart Journal 16: 460–4.

Barzaghi N, Locatelli A, Minzioni G 1999 An unexpected intraoperative echocardiographic finding in a patient with Eisenmenger's syndrome. Journal of Cardiothoracic and Vascular Anesthesia 13: 363–4.

Daliento L, Somerville J, Presbitero P et al 1998 Eisenmenger syndrome. Factors relating to deterioration and death. European Heart Journal 19: 1845–55.

Devitt JH, Noble WH, Byrick RJ 1982 A Swan–Ganz catheter related complication in a patient with Eisenmenger's syndrome. Anesthesiology 57: 335–7.

Foster JMG, Jones RM 1984 The anaesthetic management of the Eisenmenger syndrome. Annals of the Royal College of Surgeons of England 66: 353–5.

Gilman DH 1991 Caesarean section in undiagnosed Eisenmenger's syndrome. Report of a fatal outcome. Anaesthesia 46: 371–3.

Huytens L, Alexander JP 1986 Maternal and neonatal death associated with Eisenmenger's syndrome. Acta Anaesthesiologica Belgica 37: 45–51.

Lust KM, Boots RJ, Dooris M et al 1999 Management of labor in Eisenmenger syndrome with inhaled nitric oxide. American Journal of Obstetrics & Gynecology 181: 419–23.

Lyons B, Motherway C, Casey W et al 1995 The anaesthetic management of a child with Eisenmenger's syndrome. Canadian Journal of Anaesthesia 42: 904–9.

O'Hagan AR, Stillwell PC, Arroliga A 1999 Airway responsiveness to inhaled albuterol in patients with pulmonary hypertension. Clinical Pediatrics 38: 27–33.

Pollack KL, Chestnut DH, Wenstrom KD 1990 Anesthetic management of a parturient with Eisenmenger's syndrome. Anesthesia & Analgesia 70: 212–15.

Raines DE, Liberthson RR, Murray JR 1996 Anesthetic management and outcome following noncardiac surgery in nonparturients with Eisenmenger's physiology. Journal of Clinical Anesthesia 8: 341–7.

Robinson S 1983 Pulmonary artery catheters in Eisenmenger's syndrome: many risks, few benefits. Anesthesiology 58: 588–9.

Sammut MS, Paes ML 1997 Anaesthesia for laparoscopic cholecystectomy in a patient with Eisenmenger's syndrome. British Journal of Anaesthesia 79: 810–12.

Sandoval J, Alvarado P, Martinez-Guerra ML et al 1999 Effect of body position changes on pulmonary gas exchange in Eisenmenger's syndrome. American Journal of Respiratory & Critical Care Medicine 159: 1070–3.

Schwalbe SS, Deshmukh SM, Marx GF 1990 Use of pulmonary artery catheterization in parturient with Eisenmenger's syndrome. Anesthesia & Analgesia 71: 442–3.

Selsby DS, Sugden JC 1989 Epidural anaesthesia for bilateral inguinal herniorrhaphy in Eisenmenger's syndrome. Anaesthesia 44: 130–2.

Spinnato JA, Kraynack BJ, Cooper MW 1981 Eisenmenger's syndrome in pregnancy: epidural anesthesia for elective Cesarean section. New England Journal of Medicine 304: 1215–17.

Stoddart P, O'Sullivan G 1993 Eisenmenger's
syndrome in pregnancy: a case report and review.
International Journal of Obstetric Anesthesia 2:
159–68.
Yentis SM, Steer PJ, Plaat F 1998 Eisenmenger's
syndrome in pregnancy: maternal and fetal
mortality in the 90s. British Journal of Obstetrics &
Gynaecology 105: 921–2.

Emery–Dreifuss muscular dystrophy (EDMD)

An X-linked muscular dystrophy with affected
males, and female carriers. Both patients and
female carriers can develop cardiac problems and
are at risk from sudden death. Atrial standstill is
said to be pathognomonic (Buckley et al 1999).
EDMD involves emerin gene deletion on the
long arm of the X chromosome, and an absence
of the protein emerin, which is localised to the
nuclear membrane of skeletal, cardiac, and
smooth muscle (Emery 1998, Funakoshi et al
1999).

Preoperative abnormalities

1. Early development of flexion contractures
in childhood, before the onset of muscle
weakness. Flexion of the elbows, shortening of
the Achilles tendon, with limitation of posterior
cervical and lower back flexion, may occur.

2. A slowly developing, mild muscular
weakness and wasting, of scapulo-humero-
peroneal distribution. The individual usually
remains mobile, but occasionally becomes
wheelchair bound.

3. Cardiac problems begin in the teenage
years and worsen with age (Funakoshi et al
1999). The myocardium becomes infiltrated by
fibrous and fatty tissue. The atria, which become
enlarged and thin walled, are involved first. The
first signs may be atrial tachy- and
bradyarrhythmias, or heart block.

4. Ventricular pacemakers are required.

5. Sudden death, from arrhythmias, CHF

(congestive heart failure), or thromboembolism
from atrial thrombi may occur.

6. A moderate increase in serum CK in the
early stages, with chronic rhabdomyolysis.

Anaesthetic problems

1. Problems of AV dissociation. After spinal
anaesthesia for testicular biopsy in a 26 year old
with atrial flutter, cardioversion was attempted.
Asystole occurred and a permanent pacemaker
had to be inserted (Jensen 1996).

2. Problems associated with flexion
contractures.

Management

1. Cardiac assessment may include
echocardiography, ECG, or 24-h Holter
monitor.

2. In the presence of conduction defects, a
pacemaker may be needed. Ventricular pacing
will usually be appropriate, in view of the
presence of atrial disease.

3. Care should be taken with positioning
because of flexion contractures.

4. Morrison and Jago (1991) used spinal
anaesthesia for lengthening of Achilles tendons
in a patient whose mother had died suddenly in
her early thirties.

5. Anticoagulants may be required.

Bibliography
Buckley AE, Dean J, Mahy IR 1999 Cardiac
involvement in Emery–Dreifuss muscular
dystrophy: a case series. Heart 82: 105–8.
Emery AE 1998 The muscular dystrophies. British
Medical Journal 317: 991–5.
Funakoshi M, Tsuchiya Y, Arahata K 1999 Emerin and
cardiomyopathy in Emery–Dreifuss muscular
dystrophy. Neuromuscular Disorders 9: 108–14.
Jensen V 1996 The anaesthetic management of a
patient with Emery–Dreifuss muscular dystrophy.
Canadian Journal of Anaesthesia 43: 768–71.

Miller RG, Layzer RB, Mellenthin MA et al 1985 Emery–Dreifuss muscular dystrophy with autosomal dominant transmission. Neurology 35: 1230–3.

Morrison P, Jago RH 1991 Emery–Dreifuss muscular dystrophy. Anaesthesia 46: 33–5.

Epidermolysis bullosa (EB)

(recessive dystrophic)

Epidermolysis bullosa (EB) refers to a spectrum of genetic diseases in which the primary feature is the formation of bullae in the skin or mucous membranes, either spontaneously, or in response to mechanical injury. The individual types can be distinguished by genetic, clinical, and pathological features. The three commonest types are EB simplex, junctional EB, and dystrophic EB. Recessive dystrophic epidermolysis bullosa, which presents at birth or in infancy, is one of the severest forms. The gene mutation for dystrophic EB codes for type VII collagen, and very low amounts of this collagen are present in this variant. Anaesthesia may be required for surgery for syndactyly, dressing changes, balloon or other dilatation of the oesophagus, skin grafting, excision of squamous cell carcinoma, and dental surgery.

Preoperative abnormalities

1. Frictional or other trauma causes the formation of bullae in the dermis and mucous membranes. When healing takes place, scarring occurs. There appears to be a decreased number, or an absence, of anchoring fibrils in the dermis, together with an increase in collagenase activity in the blistered skin.

2. The scarring may result in flexion contractures of the limbs, fusion of digits, contraction of the mouth, and fixation of the tongue.

3. Oesophageal strictures mainly involve the cervical oesophagus, and symptoms of dysphagia start in the first decade, even before pathological changes are obvious (Ergun et al 1992). Anal blistering and constipation are common.

4. Protein loss from the skin results in growth failure, anaemia, and malnutrition. Teeth are malformed and nails are shed; severe dental caries is common. Dehydration and sepsis are additional problems, particularly when hospital admission is required.

5. Drug treatment may include steroids, phenytoin, and vitamin E. A combination of iv iron and human recombinant erythropoietin may be required in patients with refractory anaemia.

6. There is an increased incidence of amyloidosis and porphyria.

Anaesthetic problems

1. The face mask may cause bullae on the chin, nose, and cheek. Poor eyelid retraction increases the risk of corneal damage, which in one audit was high (Griffin & Mayou 1993).

2. Tracheal intubation may produce oral bullae, which can bleed or rupture. Surprisingly, there are no reports of laryngeal or tracheal bullae forming as a result of tracheal intubation. In fact, involvement of the larynx and trachea is rare; in a recent review, only 18 cases of laryngeal involvement, and three of tracheolaryngeal, had been reported. Most of those described had junctional epidermolysis bullosa, as opposed to dystrophic. Lyos et al (1994) and Liu et al (1999) between them described four infants who required tracheostomy. The rarity of the problem has been attributed to the fact that the epithelium of the larynx and trachea is of the ciliated columnar type, which appears to be more resilient than the squamous. In a 3-month-old child, a spontaneous bulla sited above the vocal cords resulted in stridor (Fisher & Ray 1989). There have been two reports of laryngeal stenosis, but neither patient had ever had tracheal intubation.

3. Oral airways can produce massive bullae in the mouth, but, in a series of 57 uses of the laryngeal mask airway, only one new lingual bulla was reported (Ames et al 1999).

4. Microstomia from oropharyngeal scarring can cause problems with tracheal intubation.

5. Venepuncture may be difficult and venous occlusion can cause trauma.

6. Full monitoring may be difficult to apply. Bullae may occur at the sites of a BP cuff, ECG electrodes, or adhesive tape. From a mechanical point of view, shearing forces are the most damaging to the skin.

7. Poor handling of the patient whilst anaesthetised can cause damage. Extensive blistering occurred in one child, from being lifted under the arms to be comforted (Ames et al 1999).

8. There is increased risk of regurgitation and aspiration secondary to oesophageal strictures. Oesophageal dilatation carries the risk of perforation, which may be fatal.

Management

1. Direct pressure is less damaging than frictional or shearing forces. Thus, care should be taken to avoid shearing stresses to the skin when the patient is asleep. If feasible, the patient should be allowed to position him/herself on the operating table.

2. Adhesive tapes or dressings should not be applied.

3. The decision whether to use a mask, laryngeal mask airway or intubation technique is governed by factors such as the estimated duration of the operation, and the pressure required to maintain the mask in position. In a review of 131 patients who had tracheal intubation, there was no evidence that a careful technique caused laryngeal problems (James & Wark 1982). In one adult undergoing plastic surgery that lasted for 12 h, the tracheal tube was wired to a tooth without problems (Yonker-Sell & Connolly 1995). More commonly, bullae in the mouth have arisen from the trauma of an oral airway, the laryngoscope, or caused by the surgeon. In a review of 306 anaesthetics,

laryngeal mask airways were inserted on 57 occasions; in one case a new bulla formed on the tongue, but caused no airway problem (Ames et al 1999). Bullae have also occurred on the face as a result of pressure from the mask. If the patient is to undergo tracheal intubation, a well-lubricated, smaller than normal size of tube, should be used. Controlled ventilation and neuromuscular blockade is advisable under these circumstances, to reduce frictional damage from the patient coughing or straining against the tube. Fibreoptic intubation under general anaesthesia was performed in a patient with known intubation difficulties who refused to be awake for any procedure (Ishimura et al 1998).

4. Eye protection requires the use of simple eye ointments; taping of the eyelids must be avoided.

5. All instruments should be well lubricated. Petroleum jelly gauze is placed around the mask and at the sites where the anaesthetist's fingers support the chin.

6. Modifications have been made to monitoring attachments, in an attempt to reduce skin damage (Kelly et al 1987). Moist gauze was placed beneath the BP cuff, ECG pads had their adhesive trimmed, and gel electrodes were placed under the patient's back. Adhesive dots have been placed over suitable holes on an X-ray film, on which the patient is then placed (Ciccarelli et al 1995). Adhesive tape causes shearing stresses and should be avoided if possible. When invasive monitoring is necessary, adhesive attachments can be dispensed with. Central venous and arterial lines should be sutured into place.

7. Ketamine has been used, to avoid both mask anaesthesia and intubation.

8. Brachial plexus anaesthesia can be used for surgery of pseudosyndactyly (Kelly et al 1987, Hagen & Langenberg 1988), and in combination with ketamine supplements (Kaplan & Strauch 1987). Axillary blocks in 33 patients were performed without complications (Lin et al 1994).

9. Regional anaesthesia may be appropriate on occasions. Lumbar and caudal epidural and spinal anaesthesia have been reported (Spielman & Mann 1984, Broster et al 1987, Yee et al 1989, Farber et al 1995). The epidural catheters were not secured.

Bibliography

Ames WA, Mayou BJ, Williams K 1999 Anaesthetic management of epidermolysis bullosa. British Journal of Anaesthesia 82: 746–51.

Broster T, Placek R, Eggers GWN 1987 Epidermolysis bullosa: anesthetic management for Cesarean section. Anesthesia & Analgesia 66: 341–3.

Ciccarelli AO, Rothaus KO, Carter DM et al 1995 Plastic and reconstructive surgery in epidermolysis bullosa: clinical experience with 110 procedures in 25 patients. Annals of Plastic Surgery 35: 254–61.

Ergun GA, Lin AN, Dannenberg AJ et al 1992 Gastro-intestinal manifestations of epidermolysis bullosa. A study of 101 patients. Medicine 71: 121–7.

Farber NE, Troshynski TJ, Turco G 1995 Spinal anesthesia in an infant with epidermolysis bullosa. Anesthesiology 83: 1364–7.

Fisher GC, Ray DAA 1989 Airway obstruction in epidermolysis bullosa. Anaesthesia 44: 449.

Griffin RP, Mayou BJ 1993 The anaesthetic management of patients with dystrophic epidermolysis bullosa. A review of 44 patients over a 10 year period. Anaesthesia 48: 810–15.

Hagen R, Langenberg C 1988 Anaesthetic management in patients with epidermolysis bullosa dystrophica. Anaesthesia 43: 482–5.

Ishimura H, Minami K, Sata T 1998 Airway management for an uncooperative patient with recessive dystrophic epidermolysis bullosa. Anaesthesia & Intensive Care 26: 110–11.

James IG, Wark H 1982 Airway management during anesthesia in patients with epidermolysis bullosa dystrophia. Anesthesiology 56: 323–6.

Kaplan R, Strauch B 1987 Regional anesthesia in a child with epidermolysis bullosa. Anesthesiology 67: 262–4.

Kelly RE, Koff HD, Rothaus KO et al 1987 Brachial plexus anesthesia in eight patients with recessive dystrophic epidermolysis bullosa. Anesthesia & Analgesia 66: 1318–20.

Lin AN, Lateef F, Kelly R et al 1994 Anesthetic management in epidermolysis bullosa: review of 129 anesthetic episodes in 32 patients. Journal of the American Academy of Dermatology 30: 412–16.

Liu RM, Papsin BC, De Jong AL 1999 Epidermolysis bullosa of the head and neck: a case report of laryngotracheal involvement and 10-year review of cases at the Hospital for Sick Children. Journal of Otolaryngology 28: 76–82.

Lyos AT, Levy ML, Malpica A et al 1994 Laryngeal involvement in epidermolysis bullosa. Annals of Otology, Rhinology & Laryngology 103: 542–6.

Spielman FJ, Mann ES 1984 Subarachnoid and epidural anaesthesia for patients with epidermolysis bullosa. Canadian Anaesthetists' Society Journal 31: 549–51.

Yee LL, Gunter JB, Manley CB 1989 Caudal epidural anesthesia in an infant with epidermolysis bullosa. Anesthesiology 70: 149–51.

Yonker-Sell AE, Connolly LA 1995 Twelve hour anaesthesia in a patient with epidermolysis bullosa. Canadian Journal of Anaesthesia 42: 735–9.

Epiglottitis (acute)

An acute inflammation and swelling of the epiglottis, the aryepiglottic folds and the mucosa over the arytenoid cartilages, usually associated with *Haemophilus influenzae* type B, but increasingly with beta haemolytic streptococcus. It occasionally results in complete laryngeal obstruction, and death from hypoxia. Although epiglottitis was considered to be primarily a paediatric disorder, with a peak incidence between the ages of 1 and 4 years, there has been a dramatic decrease in its incidence in children. This is probably the result of the introduction of an effective vaccine against *H. influenzae* type B (Rhine & Roberts 1995, Park et al 1998). By contrast, the adult incidence is now increasing. The use of antibiotics during childhood may mean that adults have less immunity to *H. influenzae*; in addition, a significant percentage of adults with the disease are immunocompromised. However, children and adults present with slightly different clinical features. In children, the treatment of choice is short-term nasotracheal intubation, until the swelling has subsided. In adults, nasotracheal intubation may also be required, but the clinical course can be less severe than in children, so that an increasing number of clinicians are adopting a more conservative policy (Wolf et al 1990,

Crosby & Reid 1991). However, sudden death is still reported, even in adults, and such a change is not universally accepted.

Presentation

1. Although, since the Hib vaccine, epiglottitis in children has become rare, it is still worthwhile describing the clinical features. In children, the illness was usually of sudden onset (6–12 h), with high fever, marked constitutional symptoms, stridor, the development of a muffled voice, and the absence of a harsh cough. The child was agitated and often leaned forward, drooling saliva, because he/she was unable to swallow. Boys were more frequently affected than girls. Although before the introduction of the Hib vaccine the peak incidence was in the age group 2–4 years, some cases were reported in younger children, in whom the presentation could be atypical (Emmerson et al 1991).

2. In children, differentiation from laryngotracheobronchitis was sometimes difficult. In a prospective study, three findings on physical examination were associated with epiglottitis (Mauro et al 1988): drooling, agitation, and the absence of spontaneous cough.

3. The child sometimes presented with increasing respiratory distress and cyanosis. Total airway obstruction could be sudden and without warning. Occasionally, cardiorespiratory arrest occurred before hospital admission.

4. A high leucocyte count, and, in the past, *H. influenzae* type B was often grown from blood culture or swabs. However, since the introduction of Hib vaccine, a beta haemolytic streptococcus is now more commonly seen. A lateral X-ray of the neck may show a swollen epiglottis. However, if epiglottitis is suspected, the patient should only be sent to X-ray accompanied by an experienced member of staff, in case of sudden respiratory obstruction.

5. Adults are more likely to complain of dysphagia and painful swallowing, and one-third presented with shortness of breath (Hebert et al 1998). However, there is still the risk of sudden airway obstruction. The reported death rates vary, partly because of the small numbers in each study. Of 56 adult cases of epiglottitis, death occurred in four. Two of these were in hospital under observation, and both died before airway intervention had been undertaken (Mayosmith et al 1986). Overall death rates from an 813-patient cohort in Canada were 1.2%, whereas in the detailed review of 51 patients admitted to two tertiary care hospitals there were no deaths (Hebert et al 1998).

6. In adults, epiglottitis is increasingly associated with patients who are immunocompromised, with conditions such as HIV, drug and alcohol abuse. There is a high incidence in smokers (Hebert et al 1998).

Anaesthetic problems

1. Although the distinction between acute epiglottitis and acute laryngotracheobronchitis, the other more common cause of stridor, can frequently be made on clinical grounds, occasionally the diagnosis is difficult.

2. In children, examination of the mouth and throat, or even distress caused by insertion of an iv infusion, may precipitate complete upper airway obstruction.

3. Induction of anaesthesia may abolish accessory respiratory muscle movement, and also cause obstruction.

4. Perioperative complications include cardiorespiratory arrest, accidental extubation, tracheal tube blockage, pulmonary oedema, and pneumothorax. A report of 161 cases of epiglottitis revealed 45 complications in 34 patients and five deaths (Baines et al 1985). Complications included 18 episodes of cardiorespiratory arrest, ten incidents involving accidental extubation, three cases of pneumothorax, and three episodes of pulmonary oedema following relief of the obstruction.

5. Pulmonary oedema has occurred after intubation in 2% of children, usually those with

severe obstruction progressing to respiratory arrest (Bonadio & Losek 1992). In adults, the presence of a cardiac problem may increase the incidence of this complication. Postobstructive pulmonary oedema occurred in a 36 year old with severe coronary artery disease (Wiesel et al 1993).

6. The appearance of an ampicillin-resistant *H. influenzae* strain was reported in the early 1990s (Emmerson et al 1991), and the use of a cephalosporin is now more common.

7. In adults, elective intubation carries risks, therefore medical treatment is more often considered. However, this must only be carried out when there are staff at hand who are experienced at managing the emergency airway.

Management

1. Acute epiglottitis represents a serious emergency that should be attended by an experienced anaesthetist, whenever the diagnosis is suspected. In any child with stridor a high index of suspicion must be maintained. Investigation should not be allowed to delay the treatment of life-threatening obstruction.

2. In children, no examination of the throat should be made, except under an anaesthetic given by an experienced anaesthetist, and preferably with an ENT surgeon present.

3. In adults, in contrast, an accurate diagnosis of moderate to severe epiglottitis is important and a nasoendoscopic view of the larynx, without the application of local anaesthetic, may be obtained by an experienced endoscopist, without the risk of precipitating complete obstruction (Hebert et al 1998).

4. In adults, conservative management is increasingly used. In general, patients are divided into those who need immediate emergency intubation, those who have elective intubation because of a deterioration during observation, and those who require medical treatment only. However, it is still possible to precipitate complete airway obstruction, therefore should

this approach be used, the endoscopist should be experienced, and the facility for emergency tracheostomy immediately available.

5. Although there is no reliable method of predicting those who will obstruct (Park et al 1998), one study in adults found that dyspnoea at the time of admission predicted the need for intubation (Hebert et al 1998).

6. Traditionally, when intubation is required, inhalation anaesthesia with halothane and oxygen, with or without nitrous oxide, was used. Some authors now consider sevoflurane to be a superior agent (Milligan 1997, Spalding & Ala-Kokko 1998). However, at high concentrations, sevoflurane may cause respiratory depression and it can be difficult to achieve anaesthesia deep enough, or for a long enough period. Young (1999) described an uneventful induction in the sitting position, but when the patient was laid supine, apnoea and obstruction occurred. These controversies are now more difficult to resolve, because of the small number of patients requiring intervention.

7. Once the patient is sufficiently deep, the airway should be secured, first with an oral tube. This can be replaced at leisure with a suitably sized nasotracheal tube.

8. The tube must be firmly fixed and an intravenous infusion set up to prevent dehydration. However, it is amazing how rapidly a small child can remove a tracheal tube or cannula that is inadequately secured. Firm bandaging of the hands will reduce the risks of self-extubation. The emergency use of a Seldinger minitracheostomy kit has been reported in two adults (Ala-Kokko et al 1996).

9. In those patients with severe obstruction, pulmonary oedema may occur after intubation. Management requires airway patency, oxygen, and, in about 50% of cases IPPV and PEEP (Lang et al 1990).

10. One of the most difficult problems is to provide sufficient humidification to prevent crusting of the tube. Examination under anaesthesia at 24 h is advisable. Even if

extubation is not possible at this stage, the tube should be changed. In a small child, partial blockage of the tube by secretions is almost invariably found. The mean duration of intubation in one series was 36 h (Rothstein & Lister 1983). Direct observation of the epiglottis was found to be the only reliable way to determine the stage at which the tube was no longer necessary.

11. Anaesthetists are divided over the best method of managing the patient, once intubated. Increasingly, IPPV is used for the period of tracheal intubation, to allow adequate sedation, oxygenation, and humidification. However, in a study of 349 patients (Butt et al 1988), 83% received nasotracheal intubation and were allowed to breathe spontaneously through a condenser humidifier. No sedation was given but the patient was restrained. Criteria for extubation were: the resolution of fever to <37.5°C, the time of intubation (12–16 h), and general improvement in appearance. It was accepted that this scheme of management requires the invariable presence on the ITU of someone experienced in intubation. If the patient is allowed to breathe spontaneously, a sedative, but not a respiratory depressant, may be permitted. Accidental extubation and tracheal tube blockage are the most serious complications, and ones that can prove fatal if respiration is depressed. Whichever method is employed, facilities should be available for rapid reintubation.

12. Whereas ampicillin used to be the drug of choice, there is increasing evidence of ampicillin resistance. Cephalosporins are now more commonly used. Antibiotics should be given empirically; the insistence on having bacteriological specimens before antibiotics are given may be unnecessary and potentially hazardous.

13. Racemic epinephrine administered in a nebulizer (1 mg in 5 ml 0.9% saline) has been reported to improve symptoms in an adult with epiglottitis (MacDonnell et al 1995).

14. The use of steroids is debatable. A retrospective uncontrolled comparison between one area using them routinely and one only using them occasionally, showed no difference in outcome (Welch & Price 1983). However, in practice, steroids are often given. Those patients who fail the first attempt at extubation may benefit from a course of prednisolone $2\,mg\,kg^{-1}\,day^{-1}$ before the second attempt (Freezer et al 1990).

15. Short-lived pulmonary oedema occasionally occurs after relief of the obstruction, and should be treated with oxygen, or if necessary, IPPV (Lang et al 1990).

Bibliography

Ala-Kokko TI, Kyllonen M, Nuutinen L 1996 Management of upper airway obstruction using a Seldinger minitracheotomy kit. Acta Anaesthesiologica Scandinavica 40: 385–8.

Baines DB, Wark H, Overton JH 1985 Acute epiglottitis in children. Anaesthesia & Intensive Care 13: 25–8.

Bonadio WA, Losek JD 1992 The characteristics of children with epiglottitis who develop the complication of pulmonary edema. Archives of Otolaryngology & Head & Neck Surgery 117: 205–7.

Butt W, Shann F, Walker C et al 1988 Acute epiglottitis: a different approach to management. Critical Care Medicine 16: 43–7.

Crosby E, Ried D 1991 Acute epiglottitis in the adult: is intubation mandatory? Canadian Journal of Anaesthesia 38: 914–18.

Emmerson SG, Richman B, Spahn T 1991 Changing patterns of epiglottitis in children. Otolaryngology—Head and Neck Surgery 104: 287–92.

Freezer N, Butt W, Phelan P 1990 Steroids in croup: do they increase the incidence of successful extubation. Anaesthesia & Intensive Care 18: 224–8.

Hebert PC, Ducic Y, Boisvert D et al 1998 Acute epiglottitis in a Canadian setting. Laryngoscope 108: 64–9.

Lang SA, Duncan PG, Shephard DA et al 1990 Pulmonary oedema associated with airway obstruction. Canadian Journal of Anaesthesia 37: 210–18.

MacDonnell SPJ, Timmins AC, Watson JD 1995 Adrenaline administered via a nebulizer in adult patients with upper airway obstruction. Anaesthesia 50: 35–6.

Mauro RD, Poole SR, Lockhart CH 1988 Differentiation of epiglottitis from laryngotracheitis in the child with stridor. American Journal of Diseases in Childhood 142: 679–82.

Mayosmith MJ, Hirsch PJ, Wodzinski SF et al 1986 Acute epiglottitis in adults. New England Journal of Medicine 314: 1133–9.

Milligan K 1997 Sevoflurane induction and acute epiglottitis. Anaesthesia 52: 810.

Park KW, Darvish A, Lowenstein E 1998 Airway management for adult patients with acute epiglottitis: a 12-year experience at an academic medical center (1984–1995). Anesthesiology 88: 254–61.

Rhine EJ, Roberts D 1995 Acute epiglottitis— revisited. Paediatric Anaesthesia 5: 345–6.

Rothstein P, Lister G 1983 Epiglottitis—duration of intubation and fever. Anesthesia & Analgesia 62: 785–7.

Spalding MB, Ala-Kokko TI 1998 The use of inhaled sevoflurane for endotracheal intubation in epiglottitis. Anesthesiology 89: 1025–6.

Welch DB, Price DG 1983 Acute epiglottitis and severe croup. Experience in two English regions. Anaesthesia 38: 754–9.

Wiesel S, Gutman JB, Kleiman SJ 1993 Adult epiglottitis and postobstructive pulmonary edema in a patient with severe coronary artery disease. Journal of Clinical Anesthesia 5: 158–62.

Wolf M, Strauss B, Kronenberg J et al 1990 Conservative management of adult epiglottitis. Laryngoscope 100: 183–5.

Young PJ 1999 Sevoflurane induction and acute epiglottitis. Anaesthesia 54: 301.

Epilepsy

Epilepsy is a clinical diagnosis, based on the occurrence of at least two seizures. A seizure is an abnormal paroxysmal discharge from a group of neurones, resulting in a clinical manifestation or a sensory perception. It may occur with or without loss of consciousness. The incidence of epilepsy is 0.5–1%. It may be a symptom of an underlying pathology, in which case there is a focal cerebral lesion. Alternatively, it may be idiopathic. In the latter there is a constitutional and sometimes hereditary disposition to seizures,

and a focal lesion is not necessarily demonstrated. However, with the increasing use of MRI, focal lesions may be found even in apparent idiopathic epilepsy.

Determination of the type of epilepsy is usually made on the pattern of the fit, the age of onset, the timing, and the EEG changes. The international classification of seizure types is complex and detailed discussion is beyond the scope of this book. However, seizures can be divided broadly into 'partial' (that include the former terms Jacksonian, temporal lobe, and psychomotor epilepsy), and 'generalised' (previously described as grand mal or major convulsions). Partial seizures begin locally in the cortex and have an aura reflective of the origin of the discharge. This type of seizure can be further divided into simple, complex and those that become secondarily generalised. Generalised seizures are characterised by a sudden loss of consciousness without an aura, and bilateral manifestations. Further subdivisions include tonic-clonic, absence, and myoclonic seizures.

Status epilepticus is a recurrence of convulsions, without intervening periods when consciousness is recovered. At the start of status epilepticus there is a characteristic EEG sequence of events and changes in levels of neurotransmitters. Neuronal necrosis may occur secondary to the accumulation of neurotransmitters. The associated mortality is about 10%, and if seizures last for more than 2 h there may be permanent neurological sequelae (O'Brien 1991). Those who have recurrent episodes of status epilepticus are more prone to develop new lesions, or are more likely to die in an event. Diazemuls has been replaced by lorazepam in the first line treatment of status epilepticus. It has a higher success rate, less respiratory depression, and a longer duration of anticonvulsant effect (Bleck 1999).

Occasionally surgery is required for epilepsy, and this may be performed under light general anaesthesia using proconvulsant agents, or conscious analgesia (Kofke et al 1997).

There is continuing debate about the suitability

of propofol for epileptics, and conflicting clinical and experimental evidence surrounding the nature of excitatory events that are sometimes associated with its use. When selecting agents, it is important to know whether or not the patient holds a current driving licence or is seeking to become eligible for one (Sneyd 1999). Drugs that can produce perioperative events that could be interpreted as 'fits', and might precipitate licence withdrawal, should probably be avoided.

Preoperative abnormalities

1. The interictal EEG usually shows abnormal features, but if the epilepsy is mild, the EEG can be normal between fits. In addition, if the neuronal discharge originates from a medial temporal focus, a specialised lead may record an abnormality.

2. The nature of the lesions can now often be determined using MRI.

3. Side effects with anticonvulsants. Most cause enzyme induction and can interfere with the metabolism of other drugs. Patients receiving long-term therapy with phenytoin, phenobarbitone or primidone may develop folate deficiency and megaloblastic anaemia. Sodium valproate may interfere with haemostasis and excessive bleeding during surgery has been reported (Tetzlaff 1991). Thrombocytopenia is the commonest defect. Its incidence is dose related and it is more common in children than in adults. Platelet dysfunction, prolonged bleeding time and hypofibrinogenaemia have been reported. Phenytoin has a narrow therapeutic range and certain drugs (including sulfonamides, cimetidine, and halothane) have been known to precipitate acute phenytoin toxicity. Clinical signs of this may include ataxia, nystagmus, and respiratory depression.

Anaesthetic problems

1. Poor drug control, or noncompliance by the patient, increases the likelihood of seizures. A seizure is a highly undesirable event, since it is accompanied by systemic changes such as hypertension, tachycardia, respiratory and metabolic acidosis, hypoxia, and hyperthermia. Traumatic injury may occur. At a cellular level, focal increases in metabolism may cause local hypoxia or ischaemia. Rarely, recurrent postoperative fits have been reported: status epilepticus carries significant morbidity and occasionally death occurs.

2. Many anaesthetic drugs have both pro- and anticonvulsant activity. Confusion also exists in the terminology surrounding perioperative excitatory events. It is often difficult to distinguish between seizures resulting from cortical activity, and rigidity and myoclonus.

a) Methohexitone possesses excitatory activity and is used to provoke focal discharges in epileptics undergoing surgery for focal epilepsy. Several isolated reports of fits have occurred, and in one study of 48 epileptics in whom anticonvulsants had been withheld, five had fits in association with either the induction or cessation of methohexitone (Male & Allen 1977).

b) Etomidate may produce strong myoclonic movements on induction of anaesthesia. They are reputed not to be associated with epileptiform discharge on EEG. However, in some epileptics, increased epileptiform discharges on EEG have been seen (Opitz et al 1983, Ebrahim et al 1986). Generalised seizures have been associated with etomidate, often when given with fentanyl (Kreiger & Korner 1987). As with methohexitone, etomidate has been used to activate epileptic foci. Both generalised and focal seizures have occurred after etomidate infusions (Grant & Hutchinson 1983), and in rats, myoclonic movements have been accompanied by increases in brain glucose utilisation. There is powerful activation of beta activity on EEG and recording from scalp electrodes may be obscured. Several authors have suggested its avoidance in epilepsy. However, it has been successfully used as an anticonvulsant.

c) The effects of propofol on the brain are complex and there are conflicting reports with regard to excitatory activity. Propofol has been associated with a number of CNS effects, more than 30 of which have been recorded in the literature. These have included convulsions, opisthotonus, myoclonus, and prolonged unconsciousness. By October 1989, 101 similar events had been reported to the Committee on Safety of Medicine (Shearer 1990). Nearly one-third of 37 patients who had seizures were epileptics (Committee on Safety of Medicines 1989). In some cases, repeated fits have occurred, and in one patient, these continued for 7 days (Bredahl 1990). However, there has been little evidence of cortical epileptiform discharge on EEG. Conversely, decreased duration of fits during ECT has been documented (Simpson et al 1988), and propofol has been used for the treatment of status epilepticus. Smith et al (1996) found that small doses of propofol produced activation of the electrocorticogram in 17 out of 20 patients under anaesthesia for epilepsy surgery, whereas Hewitt et al (1999), in a crossover study with propofol and thiopentone, found no differences between the two drugs.

d) During enflurane anaesthesia, EEG studies have shown that an increase in depth of anaesthesia is accompanied by the appearance of high voltage spikes and spike waves with burst suppression. A reduction in Pa_{CO_2} increases the occurrence of these abnormalities (Neigh et al 1971). Enflurane has been used to activate epileptic foci during surgery for epilepsy. Convulsions have been reported at times, of durations varying from minutes to several hours, and in one case, several days (Grant 1986), after such anaesthesia. On another occasion, status

epilepticus occurred (Nicoll 1986). In all cases, enflurane was not the sole agent used and, in most patients, no seizures had occurred previously. Cerebral glucose utilisation studies in rats suggested activation of intercortical and corticothalamic pathways (Nakakimura et al 1988). However, in one study when enflurane was given to epileptics, EEG recordings could not demonstrate provocation of epileptic foci (Opitz et al 1977). Inhibition of seizure activity during enflurane anaesthesia has also been reported (Opitz et al 1983).

e) In contrast to enflurane, isoflurane has been reported to suppress spike activity during craniotomy (Ito et al 1988, Fiol et al 1993).

f) Sevoflurane. Epileptiform EEG patterns have been noted during gaseous induction with sevoflurane (Yli-Hankala et al 1999), and during 2 MAC sevoflurane anaesthesia in two healthy volunteers (Kaisti et al 1999).

g) Rigidity and epileptiform or myoclonic movements have been noted after high-dose opioids. Simultaneous cortical EEG recordings have not demonstrated abnormal activity in man, although animal studies have shown accompanying seizure activity on the EEG and activation of subcortical brain metabolism. High-dose pentazocine, used for cardiac surgery, has been associated with seizures. Grand mal convulsions have occurred during induction with fentanyl, but not necessarily at high dosage. In those in whom EEG recording was available, no cortical seizure activity was seen. During a study of alfentanil-induced rigidity in ten patients, the EEG showed no evidence of seizure activity, and a neurochemical mechanism has been suggested (Benthuysen et al 1986). A subsequent study of 127 patients with high-dose opioids produced similar conclusions (Ty

Smith et al 1989). Pethidine has been associated with seizures, particularly when used for a long period, and in patients with renal failure. Norpethidine, one of the metabolites, was probably responsible.

h) Ketamine, given to both epileptics and nonepileptics, did not show cortical or clinical seizure activity on EEG (Corssen et al 1974, Celisia et al 1975). However, ketamine is known to be excitatory to the thalamus and limbic system, in which it produces a seizure pattern that does not extend to the cerebral cortex (Ferrer-Allado et al 1973). Thus, cortical electrodes do not reflect seizure activity. Increases in cerebral blood flow and oxygen consumption have been shown, and activation of experimentally induced corticoreticular epilepsy in cats has been reported. However, ketamine also possesses anticonvulsant properties and has been used to treat status epilepticus.

3. Patients taking long-term anticonvulsant therapy may have altered responses to anaesthetic drugs. The recovery from atracurium in epileptics taking long-term phenytoin, valproic acid, and carbamazepine is two to three times shorter than those of nonepileptics (Tempelhoff et al 1990a). There can be similar resistance to metocurine, pancuronium, and vecuronium (Bulkey et al 1987), and an increased requirement for fentanyl during craniotomy (Tempelhoff et al 1990b).

4. Anaesthetists may be involved in the management of seizures in the emergency department, but these patients are not necessarily epileptics. Seizures have been reported in association with drug abuse. In one study of emergency hospital admissions, 32 were associated with cocaine, 11 with amphetamine, seven with heroin and four with phencyclidine (Alldredge et al 1989). In 11 patients, a combination of drugs was used. The seizures were usually short lived, and there were no neurological sequelae.

5. A number of cases of pseudostatus epilepticus, or psychogenic seizures, have been reported (Reuber et al 2000), and can occur in the perioperative period. Unless suspected, potentially harmful treatment can be given.

Management

1. Evaluation of haemostasis in patients on long-term sodium valproate undergoing major surgery.

2. Continuance of anticonvulsant medication.

3. The choice of anaesthetic agents must be left to the individual anaesthetist. However, it might be prudent to avoid the use of those drugs which are particularly implicated in the production of clinical excitatory events or EEG excitation. In view of the complex effects of propofol on epileptics, and the difficulty in interpreting excitatory events, it has been suggested that it should be avoided in those holding a driving licence, or who might wish to do so in the future (Sneyd 1999). However, should the use of a drug be indicated, particularly in those not eligible for a driving licence, then provided adequate anticonvulsant therapy is given in the perioperative period, the risk of precipitating seizures must be slight.

4. Treatment of status epilepticus. Prompt control is important.

   a) Remove false teeth, establish an airway, and give oxygen.

   b) Monitor.

   c) Gain iv access; give lorazepam 4 mg iv and repeat after 10 min if no response.

   d) Take bloods for FBC, U&E, calcium, glucose, alcohol, anticonvulsant levels, and arterial blood gases.

   e) If no response after 30 min give either:

      i) Phenobarbitone $10 \, mg \, kg^{-1}$ iv at a rate of $100 \, mg \, min^{-1}$ or,

      ii) Phenytoin $15 \, mg \, kg^{-1}$ iv at a rate of $50 \, mg \, min^{-1}$ or,

iii) Fosphenytoin 15 mg kg^{-1} iv at up to 150 mg min^{-1}.

f) If fits cannot be controlled, the patient must be transferred to an ITU for more specialist treatment. If still in status give thiopentone/atracurium or vecuronium, tracheal intubation, and IPPV.

g) If the patient is hypoglycaemic give 25 ml 50% glucose. If alcohol is likely to have been the precipitating factor, give thiamine 100 mg.

5. Psychogenic seizures can occasionally occur, but there are a number of features that can help to distinguish pseudostatus from genuine status epilepticus (Reuber et al 2000). Pseudostatus is characterised by closed eyes, resistance to opening them, and retention of pupillary reflexes during an attack. In addition, seizures usually take place in front of a doctor, last more than 90 s, but are not usually accompanied by cyanosis. If the arm is released above the head, the individual will avoid hitting themselves and they will respond to painful stimuli. The individuals are more likely to be young females, who volunteer a history of postoperative 'seizures', have had multiple hospital admissions, and often have a psychiatric history. It is important that these patients are not given powerful sedatives or anticonvulsants.

Bibliography

Alldredge BK, Lowenstein DH, Simon RP 1989 Seizures associated with recreational drug abuse. Neurology 39: 1037–9.

Benthuysen JL, Ty Smith N, Sanford TJ et al 1986 Physiology of alfentanil-induced rigidity. Anesthesiology 64: 440–6.

Bleck TP 1999 Management approaches to prolonged seizures and status epilepticus. Epilepsia 40(suppl 1): S59–63.

Borgeat A, Dessibourg C, Popovic V et al 1991 Propofol and spontaneous movements: an EEG study. Anesthesiology 74: 24–7.

Bredahl C 1990 Krampeanfald og opitotonus efter propofol-anaestesi. [Seizures and opisthotonos after propofol anesthesia. A possible connection.] Ugeskr Laeger 152: 748–9.

Bulkey R, Ebrahim Z, Roth S et al 1987 Resistance to vecuronium in patients receiving carbamazepine. Anesthesiology 67: A345.

Celisia C, Chen R, Bamforth B 1975 Effects of ketamine in epilepsy. Neurology 25: 169.

Committee on Safety of Medicines 1989 Current problems. No 26. Consumer's Association, London.

Corssen G, Little S, Tavakoli M 1974 Ketamine and epilepsy. Anesthesia & Analgesia 53: 319.

Ebrahim ZY, DeBoer GE, Luders H et al 1986 Effect of etomidate on the electroencephalogram of patients with epilepsy. Anesthesia & Analgesia 65: 1004–6.

Ferrer-Allado T, Brechner VL, Dymond A et al 1973 Ketamine-induced electroconvulsive phenomena in the human limbic and thalamic region. Anesthesiology 38: 333–4.

Fiol ME, Boening JA, Cruz-Rodriguez R et al 1993 Effect of isoflurane (Forane) on intraoperative electrocorticogram. Epilepsia 34: 897–900.

Grant IS 1986 Delayed convulsions following enflurane anaesthesia. Anaesthesia 41: 1024–5.

Grant IS, Hutchinson G 1983 Epileptiform seizures during prolonged etomidate sedation. Lancet ii: 511–12.

Hewitt PB, Chu DLK, Polkey CE et al 1999 Effect of propofol on the electrocorticogram in epileptic patients undergoing cortical resection. British Journal of Anaesthesia 82: 199–202.

Ito BM, Sato S, Kufta CV et al 1988 Effect of isoflurane and enflurane on the electrocorticogram of epileptic patients. Neurology 38: 924–8.

Kaisti KK, Jaaskelainen SK, Rinne JO et al 1999 Epileptiform discharges during 2 MAC sevoflurane anesthesia in two healthy volunteers. Anesthesiology 91: 1952–5.

Kofke WA, Young RSK, Davis P et al 1989 Isoflurane for refractory status epilepticus: a clinical series. Anesthesiology 71: 653–9.

Kofke WA, Tempelhoff R, Dasheiff RM 1997 Anesthetic implications of epilepsy, status epilepticus, and epilepsy surgery. Journal of Neurosurgical Anesthesiology 9: 349–72.

Kreiger W, Koerner M 1987 Generalized grand mal seizure after recovery from uncomplicated fentanyl-etomidate anesthesia. Anesthesia & Analgesia 66: 284–5.

Kumar A, Bleck TP 1992 Intravenous midazolam for the treatment of status epilepticus. Critical Care Medicine 20: 483–8.

Male CG, Allen EM 1977 Methohexitone-induced convulsions in epileptics. Anaesthesia & Intensive Care 5: 226–30.

Modica PA, Tempelhoff R, White PF 1990a Pro- and anticonvulsant effects of anesthetics (Part I). Anesthesia & Analgesia 70: 303–15.

Modica PA, Tempelhoff R, White PF 1990b Pro- and anticonvulsant effects of anesthetics (Part II). Anesthesia & Analgesia 70: 433–44.

Nakakimura K, Sakabe T, Funatsu N et al 1988 Metabolic activation of intercortical and corticothalamic pathways during enflurane anesthesia in rats. Anesthesiology 68: 777–82.

Neigh JL, Garman JK, Harp JR 1971 The electroencephalographic pattern during anesthesia with ethrane: effects of depth of anesthesia, Pa_{CO_2}, and nitrous oxide. Anesthesiology 35: 482–7.

Nicoll JMV 1986 Status epilepticus following enflurane anaesthesia. Anaesthesia 41: 927–30.

O'Brien MD 1991 Management of status epilepticus in adults. British Medical Journal 301: 918.

Opitz A, Brecht S, Stenzel E 1977 Enfran-Anestheseien bei epilptikem. [Enflurane anaesthesia for epileptic patients.] Anesthetist 26: 329–32.

Opitz A, Marschall M, Degen R et al 1983 General anaesthesia in patients with epilepsy and status epilepticus. Advances in Neurology 34: 531–5.

Paech MJ, Storey JM 1990 Propofol and seizures. Anaesthesia & Intensive Care 18: 585.

Reuber M, Enright SM, Goulding PJ 2000 Postoperative pseudostatus. Not everything that shakes is epilepsy. Anaesthesia 55: 74–8.

Shearer ES 1990 Convulsions and propofol. Anaesthesia 45: 255–6.

Simpson KH, Halsall PJ, Carr CME et al 1988 Propofol reduces seizure duration in patients having anaesthesia for electroconvulsive therapy. British Journal of Anaesthesia 61: 343–4.

Smith M, Smith SJ, Scott CA et al 1996 Activation of the electrocorticogram by propofol during surgery for epilepsy. British Journal of Anaesthesia 76: 499–502.

Sneyd JR 1999 Propofol and epilepsy. British Journal of Anaesthesia 82: 168–9.

Tempelhoff R, Modica PA, Jellish WS et al 1990a Resistance to atracurium-induced neuromuscular blockade in patients with intractable seizure disorders treated with anticonvulsants. Anesthesia & Analgesia 71: 665–9.

Tempelhoff R, Modica PA, Spitznagel EL 1990b Anticonvulsant therapy increases fentanyl requirements during anaesthesia for craniotomy. Canadian Journal of Anaesthesia 37: 327–32.

Tetzlaff JE 1991 Intraoperative defect of haemostasis in a child receiving valproic acid. Canadian Journal of Anaesthesia 38: 222–4.

Ty Smith N, Benthuysen JL, Bickford RG et al 1989 Seizures during opioid induction—are they opioid-induced rigidity? Anesthesiology 71: 852–62.

Walker MC, Smith SJM, Shorvon SD 1995 The intensive care treatment of convulsive status epilepticus. Results of a national survey and recommendations. Anaesthesia 50: 130–5.

Yli-Hankala A, Vakkuri A, Sarkela M et al 1999 Epileptiform electroencephalogram during mask induction of anesthesia with sevoflurane. Anesthesiology 91: 1596–603.

Fabry's disease

An X-linked disorder of glycolipid catabolism, in which a deficiency of alpha-galactosidase A results in accumulation of glycosphingolipid deposits within the lysosomes of vascular endothelial cells. Cardiac problems are common. There is also a high incidence of thrombotic events leading to myocardial infarction and strokes. Abnormalities involve the skin, nervous system, eyes, heart, and kidneys (Peters et al 1997). In addition to the classical form, there is an atypical group of individuals who have cardiac involvement alone. In an unselected group of men with left ventricular hypertrophy, 3% had low levels of alpha-galactosidase (Nakao et al 1995). Anaesthesia may be required for cardiac transplantation.

Preoperative abnormalities

1. Childhood angiokeratoma, corneal dystrophy, and decreased sweating. Cutaneous telangiectatic lesions around the lower half of the body. Painful, burning, tingling sensations in the extremities, known as acroparaesthesia. This results from damage to small myelinated and unmyelinated cutaneous fibres. Autonomic neuropathy may be present.

2. Cardiac lesions are common; problems include restrictive cardiomyopathy, valvular disease, and heart block (Cantor et al 1998).

3. There is a high incidence of thrombotic events, leading to premature myocardial infarcts and strokes. In a study of 60 patients, four out of 45 hemizygous males, and three out of 15 heterozygous females, had had thrombotic events (Utsumi et al 1997). Cerebrovascular complications occurred at a young age (average 33.8 years hemizygotes and 40.3 years heterozygotes) (Mitsias & Levine 1996). They mainly involve the vertebrobasilar circulation and denote a poor prognosis. Diffuse neuronal involvement occurred outside the areas of vascular abnormality.

4. There is an association with airway obstructive disease. In a study of 25 unselected men, 36% showed obstruction on spirometry and the majority responded to bronchodilators (Brown et al 1997).

5. In addition, there may be gastrointestinal, renal and ocular abnormalities (Peters et al 1997).

6. The diagnosis is confirmed by decreased leucoctye alpha-glucosidase activity in leucocytes and by skin biopsy.

7. Patients may be receiving carbamazepine or phenytoin for painful crises.

Anaesthetic problems

1. Cardiac disease; in particular the presence of a restrictive cardiomyopathy.

2. Delayed gastric emptying may increase the risk of pulmonary aspiration.

3. Intermittent painful crises, burning in hands and feet may require pain control (Gordon et al 1995).

Management

1. Assessment of cardiac involvement and appropriate management. Treatment of heart failure, arrhythmias, heart block, and valvular disease. For restrictive cardiomyopathy, see Cardiomyopathies.

2. If the patient has respiratory symptoms, spirometry with and without bronchodilators should be performed.

3. For painful peripheral crises, low-dose morphine infusion with amitryptiline has been tried. In seven crises, pain relief was immediate and the infusion could be gradually tapered over 24 h (Gordon et al 1995).

4. Multidisciplinary involvement may be required.

5. Metoclopramide may help delayed gastric emptying.

Bibliography

Brown LK, Miller A, Bhuptani A et al 1997 Pulmonary involvement in Fabry disease. American Journal of Respiratory & Critical Care Medicine 155: 1004–10.

Cantor WJ, Butany J, Iwanochko M et al 1998 Restrictive cardiomyopathy secondary to Fabry's disease. Circulation 98: 1457–9.

Gordon KE, Ludman MD, Finley GA 1995 Successful treatment of painful crises of Fabry disease with low dose morphine. Pediatric Neurology 12: 250–1.

Mitsias P, Levine SR 1996 Cerebrovascular complications of Fabry's disease. Annals of Neurology 40: 8–17.

Nakao S, Takenaka T, Maeda M et al 1995 An atypical variant of Fabry's disease in men with left ventricular hypertrophy. New England Journal of Medicine 333: 288–93.

Peters FP, Sommer A, Vermeulen A et al 1997 Fabry's disease: a multidisciplinary disorder. Postgraduate Medical Journal 73: 710–12.

Utsumi K, Yamamoto N, Kase R et al 1997 High incidence of thrombosis in Fabry's disease. Internal Medicine 36: 327–9.

Fallot's tetralogy (tetralogy of Fallot, TOF)

A congenital cardiac abnormality. The primary defects are pulmonary infundibular stenosis and VSD. The VSD is sufficiently large for the pressure in both ventricles to be equal to that of the aorta. The tetralogy is completed by two secondary features, a variable degree of overriding of the aorta, and right ventricular hypertrophy. Dynamic right ventricular outflow obstruction may occur (infundibular spasm), which is accentuated by sympathetic stimulation. The fraction of the right to left shunt depends primarily upon the relative resistances between the pulmonary (or right ventricular) and systemic outflows. The aim of surgery is to relieve the right ventricular outflow obstruction and to close the VSD. The traditional management by a two-stage repair has been replaced by definitive correction. Recent surgical advances include conduits to connect the RV to the PA, and transatrial repair of the VSD (Rosenthal 1993). There is evidence that early definitive correction reduces later complications that are related to right ventricular hypertrophy and dysfunction. The problems encountered during anaesthesia will depend upon whether or not corrective surgery has been undertaken, and the functional result.

Preoperative abnormalities

1. Dyspnoea may occur on exertion, and is hypoxia related. Cyanosis and finger clubbing are variable, depending on the degree of pulmonary stenosis and the size of the shunt. Polycythaemia (more correctly termed erythrocytosis) is common. There is a pulmonary stenotic murmur, but no murmur from the VSD because of the size of the defect. Squatting is thought to reduce the fraction of the shunt, since by kinking the large arteries it increases systemic vascular resistance. Squatting is commonly seen in children with uncorrected lesions.

2. ECG shows right atrial and right ventricular hypertrophy, right axis deviation, and right bundle branch block.

3. Chest X-ray shows right ventricular hypertrophy and oligaemic lungs. In the 2.6–6% of individuals who also have an absent pulmonary valve, aneurysmal dilatation of the pulmonary arteries may cause bronchial compression.

4. Initial surgery may have been undertaken to anastomose a systemic to a pulmonary artery, to improve the pulmonary blood flow, and reduce cyanosis. A definitive procedure is now more commonly undertaken in infancy.

5. In the occasional patient who has undergone shunt surgery without a definitive repair, there is chronic hypoxia and polycythaemia. These patients have a high mortality, and an increased risk of bacterial endocarditis, thrombotic stroke, emboli, and intracerebral abscess.

6. In adults who have undergone repair there is an increased risk of arrhythmias, conduction

defects, and sudden deaths, possibly related to mechanical events, such as ventricular dilatation and stretch, in the proximity of the conduction system (Bricker 1995, Gillette 1997). Although it is difficult to predict the population at risk, in an analysis of 178 adult survivors, Gatzoulis et al (1995) showed a relationship between QRS prolongation (>180 ms), right ventricular dilatation, sustained ventricular arrhythmias, and sudden cardiac death. Atrial brady- and tachyarrhythmias have also been observed. In a study of 53 patients who had surgery in the past two decades, sinus node dysfunction was observed in 36% and atrial tachyarrhythmias in 34% (Roos-Hesselink et al 1995). However, new approaches to surgery may result in a lower incidence of such problems in the future (Perloff & Natterson 1995).

Anaesthetic problems

1. In individuals with uncorrected lesions, the right to left shunt, and hence the cyanosis, is increased by a reduction in systemic vascular resistance produced by systemic vasodilatation. This may result from factors such as hypovolaemia, drugs effects, or pyrexia.

2. Cyanosis is also worsened by an increase in pulmonary vascular resistance, or spasm of the right ventricular infundibulum. Right ventricular outflow obstruction is produced by increases in catecholamine output, or the administration of drugs with positive inotropic effects. Anxiety, pain, hypercarbia, hypoxia and acidosis are all precipitating factors. These cyanotic attacks or 'tet' spells, which can occur when awake or under anaesthesia, may initiate a cycle of increasing hypoxia that can result in cerebral damage or death. Direct intraoperative observations of shunt direction and flow have been made with Doppler colour flow imaging using epicardial leads (Greeley et al 1989). These studies, made in an infant and a child before surgery, have confirmed that intracardiac right to left shunting is responsible for the sudden onset of cyanosis, and that this is corrected as soon as the shunt is reversed by treatment. Four patients

with severe life-threatening hypoxaemic spells, refractory to other treatment, responded to phenylephrine ($5\,\mu g\,kg^{-1}$ plus an infusion of 0.4–$2\,\mu g\,kg^{-1}min^{-1}$).

3. Dehydration in the presence of polycythaemia and high plasma viscosity may combine to increase the incidence of cerebral thrombosis. Polycythaemia may also be associated with coagulation defects.

4. In patients with an absent pulmonary valve, positional airway compromise occurred secondary to bronchial compression of dilated pulmonary arteries (Hosking & Beynen 1989).

5. A significant incidence of tracheal anomalies has been found. In 44 children undergoing cardiac surgery, five had undiagnosed tracheal problems and in four, these resulted in perioperative complications (Kazim et al 1996).

6. In adults who have undergone repair, ventricular and atrial arrhythmias are common, particularly during exercise. It has been suggested that patients scheduled for elective surgery should have Holter monitors, or undergo exercise testing, in case antiarrhythmic treatment is needed first (Findlow & Doyle 1997).

7. Cyanosed patients with Fallot's rarely become pregnant. However, adults who have undergone corrective surgery increasingly present during pregnancy. In a study of 19 patients who had had corrective surgery, the outcome was favourable (Zuber et al 1999).

Management

1. Antibiotic cover, as prophylaxis against bacterial endocarditis, when appropriate.

2. A good premedication to prevent excitement and anxiety.

3. In patients with cyanosis, measures aimed at reducing the right to left shunt. Specific treatment of cyanotic attacks include:

a) Oxygen 100% to decrease PVR.

b) Pressor agents, such as phenylephrine, to increase systemic vascular resistance (Shaddy et al 1989).

c) Fluids to correct hypovolaemia.

d) Propranolol to decrease outflow tract obstruction. Used iv it was successful for an attack occurring during cardiac catheterisation under local anaesthesia (Kam 1978).

e) Deepening of light anaesthesia to reduce tachycardia associated with catecholamine output (Greeley et al 1989).

f) Compression of the abdominal aorta. In four infants, the aorta was compressed against the vertebrae, sufficiently firmly to stop the femoral artery pulsations. This dramatically and immediately improved the arterial oxygen saturation (Baele et al 1991).

4. Techniques to avoid hypoxia and hypercarbia, and minimise vasodilatation and sudden increases in cardiac output. Ketamine or fentanyl, with or without N_2O, has been used (Shaddy et al 1989). Two children undergoing dental anaesthesia prior to repair had successful gaseous induction with sevoflurane (Chiu et al 1999).

5. Hydration is maintained in the perioperative period and, if there is severe polycythaemia, venesection may be necessary.

6. Metabolic acidosis should be prevented or treated.

7. In pregnancy, the outcome is satisfactory in patients whose ventricular function is good, and in whom no residual shunt occurs (Zuber et al 1999). However, close observation should be undertaken by an experienced team.

8. In general, the erythrocytosis that is associated with cyanotic congenital heart disease should not be treated. Thorne (1998) observed, that unlike the situation in polycythaemia vera, there is no evidence that routine venesection prevents stroke in these patients. In fact, since recurrent venesection causes iron deficiency anaemia, venesection in adults should only take place if there are symptoms of hyperviscosity with a haematocrit >65, and only provided volume replacement takes place at the same time.

Bibliography

Baele PL, Rennotte M-T E, Veyckemans FA 1991 External compression of the abdominal aorta reversing tetralogy of Fallot cyanotic crisis. Anesthesiology 75: 146–9.

Bricker JT 1995 Sudden death and tetralogy of Fallot. Risks, markers and causes. Circulation 92: 158–9.

Chiu CL, Wang CY 1999 Sevoflurane for dental extraction in children with tetralogy of Fallot. Paediatric Anaesthesia 9: 268–70.

Findlow D, Doyle E 1997 Congenital heart disease in adults. British Journal of Anaesthesia 78: 416–30.

Gatzoulis MA, Till JA, Somerville J et al 1995 Mechanoelectrical interaction in tetralogy of Fallot. QRS prolongation relates to right ventricular size and predicts malignant ventricular arrhythmias and sudden death. Circulation 92: 231–7.

Gillette PC 1997 Ventricular arrhythmia after repair of tetralogy of Fallot. Journal of the American College of Cardiology 30: 1384.

Greeley WJ, Stanley TE, Ungerleider RM et al 1989 Intraoperative hypoxaemic spells in tetralogy of Fallot. An echocardiographic analysis of diagnosis and treatment. Anesthesia & Analgesia 68: 815–19.

Hosking MP, Beynen F 1989 Anesthetic management of tetralogy of Fallot with absent pulmonary valve. Anesthesiology 70: 803–5.

Kam CA 1978 Infundibular spasm in Fallot's tetralogy. Anaesthesia & Intensive Care 6: 138–40.

Kazim R, Quaegebeur JM, Sun LS 1996 The association of tracheal abnormalities and tetralogy of Fallot. Journal of Cardiothoracic & Vascular Anesthesia 10: 589–92.

Mahoney MC, Hosking MP 1993 Anesthetic management for a palliative surgical procedure in a 72-year-old patient with tetralogy of Fallot. Journal of Cardiothoracic & Vascular Anesthesia 7: 724–6.

Perloff JK, Natterson PD 1995 Atrial arrhythmias in adults after repair of tetralogy of Fallot. Circulation 91: 2118–19.

Roos-Hesselink J, Perlroth MG, McGhie J et al 1995 Atrial arrhythmias in adults after repair of tetralogy of Fallot. Correlations with clinical, exercise and echocardiographic findings. Circulation 91: 2214–19.

Rosenthal A 1993 Adults with tetralogy of Fallot—repaired, yes; cured, no. New England Journal of Medicine 329: 655–6.

Shaddy RE, Viney J, Judd VE et al 1989 Continuous intravenous phenylephrine infusion for treatment of hypoxemic spells in tetralogy of Fallot. Journal of Pediatrics 114: 468–70.

Thorne SA 1998 Management of polycythaemia in adults with cyanotic congenital heart disease. Heart 79: 315–16.

Zuber M, Gautschi N, Oechslin E et al 1999 Outcome of pregnancy in women with congenital shunt lesions. Heart 81: 271–5.

Familial dysautonomia (Riley–Day syndrome)

A rare, autosomal recessive neurological disease associated with gastrointestinal dysfunction, presenting from birth, and usually occurring in Jewish children of Ashkenazi descent. Although most of the nervous system is involved, the autonomic and peripheral neuronal elements are of most concern to the anaesthetist. A decrease in sympathetic, parasympathetic and sensory neurones, a decrease in synthesis of norepinephrine (noradrenaline) (but with a normal adrenal medulla), and a sensitivity to exogenous catecholamines, have been shown. There is an increased risk of sudden death. Emotional lability is common but the IQ is normal. Patients may present for fundoplication, gastrostomy, or orthopaedic procedures.

Preoperative abnormalities

1. There is a decreased sensitivity to pain and temperature, muscle hypotonia, incoordination, and reduced tendon reflexes. About 90% of children develop curvature of the spine that results in kyphosis, scoliosis, or a combination of both, presumably secondary to inadequate muscle tone and impaired muscle proprioception. The kyphoscoliosis is progressive and may require correction (Rubery et al 1995).

2. Features include autonomic dysfunction with postural hypotension and lability of blood pressure, syncope, increased vagal reflexes, swallowing difficulties with excess salivation, gastric reflux, reduced gastrointestinal motility, absent sweating, and impaired temperature control.

3. Dysautonomic and emotional crises may be precipitated by stress, and can be associated with elevated plasma norepinephrine (noradrenaline) and dopamine levels. During these, there may be nausea, vomiting, hypertension, tachycardia, sweating, and the appearance of erythematous skin lesions.

4. Unexplained cardiac arrests and deaths have occurred. Prolonged QT_c intervals, which do not shorten during exercise, and unexpected heart rate and blood pressure responses, have been found (Glickstein et al 1993).

5. Crowded teeth, malocclusion, and a smooth tongue are characteristic.

6. Respiratory symptoms are common. In a study of 65 patients undergoing fundoplication and gastrostomy, 55% had severe lung disease, with increased markings or atelectasis, before operation (Axelrod et al 1991). Only nine had normal CXRs.

Anaesthetic problems

1. Emotion and fear may precipitate a dysautonomic crisis.

2. Disorders of swallowing are a major problem. In a study of 65 patients, gastro-oesophageal reflux was demonstrated in 95%, and disturbances of oropharyngeal function resulted in misdirected swallows with aspiration (Axelrod et al 1991). The development of lung disease secondary to recurrent pulmonary aspiration is a common feature.

3. Chronic dehydration occurs frequently, because of dysphagia for fluids.

4. Respiratory responses to hypercarbia and hypoxia are impaired.

5. Abnormal ventricular repolarisation

abnormalities may result in bradyarrhythmias, asystole, or sudden death (Glickstein et al 1999).

6. Autonomic nervous system dysfunction, apparently secondary to reduced endogenous catecholamine release, means that the patient is unable to respond to hypovolaemia and to drugs causing myocardial depression (Meridy & Creighton 1971, Foster 1983). Several cases have been reported in which either cardiac arrest, or severe hypotension, occurred during general anaesthesia (Kritchman et al 1959, Axelrod et al 1988).

7. Successful control of intraoperative hypotension has been achieved with both epinephrine (adrenaline) and dopamine infusions (Stenqvist & Sigurdsson 1982). However, exaggerated responses to norepinephrine (noradrenaline) have occurred, therefore any catecholamines should be administered with caution.

8. The use of atropine is controversial. Reports exist of sensitivity to anticholinergic agents, and, conversely, of pronounced reactions to vagal stimulation. Both its cautious use and its avoidance have been suggested.

9. Profound vomiting may occur in the perioperative period.

10. Core temperature variations may be a problem.

11. Major complications have occurred after surgery (Meridy & Creighton 1971, Albanese & Bobechko 1987, Axelrod et al 1988, 1991, Rubery et al 1995). These have included fever, pulmonary atelectasis or infection, aspiration, cardiovascular instability, and vomiting crises. An analysis of 127 procedures in 81 patients was reported (Axelrod et al 1988). A high incidence of postoperative atelectasis after gastric surgery prompted a policy of elective IPPV.

Management

1. Fundoplication with gastrostomy has been shown to improve nutrition and decrease respiratory problems (Axelrod et al 1991), but the patients require careful perioperative management. Intravenous fluid therapy should be started before surgery to prevent dehydration. Anxiety should be treated. Diazepam has been found to be effective in controlling dysautonomic crises. Cimetidine reduces gastric secretions. Premedication with both drugs has been suggested (Axelrod et al 1988), but the use of opiates and anticholinergics should be avoided. Laparoscopic-modified Nissen fundoplication has reduced the incidence of postoperative complications and removed the necessity for IPPV after surgery (Szold et al 1996).

2. Monitoring of arterial pressure and temperature should preferably be started before induction. Vascular access is facilitated by the relative sensory deficit.

3. The uneventful use of both depolarising and nondepolarising relaxants has been reported. However, the presence of hypotonia reduces the requirement for relaxants, and residual neuromuscular blockade may necessitate IPPV in the postoperative period.

4. Blood and fluid loss must be replaced promptly.

5. A dopamine or an epinephrine (adrenaline) infusion may be needed for intraoperative hypotension. However, catecholamines must be given with care, because sensitivity to their effects has been reported. Close monitoring is required, so that the blood pressure is increased, but an unacceptable tachycardia prevented.

6. Intraoperative IPPV is required, even for short operations, because of the impaired response to hypoxia and hypercarbia.

7. Local or regional techniques should be considered. Caesarean section for fetal growth retardation has been performed under local anaesthetic (Leiberman et al 1991).

8. Good postoperative analgesia is required for abdominal surgery. It has been suggested in

these cases that IPPV should be continued until analgesics are no longer required (Axelrod et al 1988). In three patients undergoing repeat Nissen's, the postoperative course was greatly improved by the use of epidural anaesthesia for pain relief (Challands & Facer 1998). This avoided the need for IPPV.

9. Vomiting crises should be treated with gastric decompression, diazepam, and cimetidine.

Bibliography

Albanese SA, Bobechko WP 1987 Spine deformity in familial dysautonomia (Riley Day syndrome). Journal of Pediatric Orthopedics 7: 179–83.

Axelrod FB, Donenfeld RF, Danziger F et al 1988 Anesthesia in familial dysautonomia. Anesthesiology 68: 631–5.

Axelrod FB, Gouge TH, Ginsburg HB et al 1991 Fundoplication and gastrostomy in familial dysautonomia. Journal of Pediatrics 118: 388–94.

Challands JF, Facer EK 1998 Epidural anaesthesia and familial dysautonomia (the Riley Day syndrome). Three case reports. Paediatric Anaesthesia 8: 83–8.

Foster JMG 1983 Anaesthesia for a patient with familial dysautonomia. Anaesthesia 38: 391.

Glickstein JS, Schwartzman D, Friedman D et al 1993 Abnormalities of the corrected QT interval in familial dysautonomia: an indicator of autonomic dysfunction. Journal of Pediatrics 122: 925–8.

Glickstein JS, Axelrod FB, Friedman D 1999 Electrocardiographic repolarization abnormalities in familial dysautonomia: an indicator of cardiac autonomic dysfunction. Clinical Autonomic Research 9: 109–12.

Kritchman MM, Schwartz H, Papper EM 1959 Experiences with general anesthesia in patients with familial dysautonomia. Journal of the American Medical Association 170: 529–33.

Leiberman JR, Cohen A, Wiznitzer A et al 1991 Cesarean section by local anesthesia in patients with familial dysautonomia. American Journal of Obstetrics & Gynecology 165: 110–11.

Meridy HW, Creighton RE 1971 General anaesthesia in eight patients with familial dysautonomia. Canadian Anaesthetists' Society Journal 18: 563–70.

Rubery PT, Spielman JH, Hester P et al 1995 Scoliosis in familial dysautonomia. Operative treatment. Journal of Bone & Joint Surgery 77A: 1362–9.

Stenqvist O, Sigurdsson J 1982 The anaesthetic management of a patient with familial dysautonomia. Anaesthesia 37: 929–32.

Szold A, Udassin R, Maayan C et al 1996 Laparoscopic-modified Nissen fundoplication in children with familial dysautonomia. Journal of Pediatric Surgery 31: 1560–2.

Familial periodic paralyses

1. Hypokalaemic periodic paralysis.

2. Hyperkalaemic and normokalaemic periodic paralysis.

3. Paramyotonia.

Genetic and electrophysiological studies have resulted in a better understanding of these complex conditions. They share similar clinical features; that is, periods of paralysis with apparently normal muscle function between, but they are associated with different genetic mutations of proteins involved in skeletal muscle membrane activity. Hypokalaemic periodic paralysis is a calcium channel disorder, in which periods of paralysis are associated with low, or decreasing, serum potassium levels. Hyperkalaemic periodic paralysis and paramyotonia are both sodium channel disorders, caused by a mutation of the voltage-gated sodium channel gene. In these, and in the so called 'normokalaemic' form, the administration of potassium worsens the paralysis.

It had been observed for some time that there was a close relationship between the clinical and electrophysiological features of hyperkalaemic periodic paralysis (hyperPP) and paramyotonia. In fact, they are allelic disorders, and genetic linkage studies showed the site of the defect to be the skeletal muscle sodium channel on chromosome 17. In view of this, hyperPP, paramyotonia and 'normokalaemic' paralysis will be considered together. An increasing number of similar diseases are being described that involve slightly different mutations. For a more detailed account of some of these rarer variants, see Ptacek (1998).

Thyrotoxic periodic paralysis (TPP), whose clinical features resemble those of hypoPP, is an acquired disease, in which paralysis is associated with a low serum potassium. Since TPP resolves with the treatment of the underlying thyrotoxicosis, it will be considered under thyrotoxicosis (section 1).

Hypokalaemic periodic paralysis (HypoPP)

A rare disease that usually starts in teenagers, but before the age of 30. Episodes of painless, flaccid paralysis are precipitated by a variety of stress factors. Attacks may last from several hours to 2 days. Certain muscle groups are more likely to be involved than others. It is usually associated with hypokalaemia, but the exact mechanism for its periodic nature, and its skeletal and cardiac effects, is not known. Increased potassium excretion from the body is not involved. There does, however, seem to be an increased uptake of potassium by the cells. The cell membrane potential has been found to be reduced during attacks, making the muscle inexcitable. Insulin and glucose, steroids, thyroxine, and beta stimulation can all increase cellular potassium uptake and intensify an existing hypokalaemia. HypoPP is a calcium channel disorder and about 66% of patients will have a family history.

Preoperative abnormalities

1. Attacks of paralysis are most likely to involve the arms, legs, trunk, and neck, but usually in an asymmetrical manner. They often occur at night, or during rest after exercise. Precipitating factors include stress, trauma, surgery, infections, and high-carbohydrate, high-sodium meals. Proximal muscles are mainly affected. Rarely, death may occur during an attack, from respiratory failure or pulmonary aspiration. Fortunately, however, the diaphragm and cranial muscles are not usually involved. Patients are more sensitive than normal to a reduction in serum potassium, such that muscle weakness may start at a level of $3 \, \text{mmol} \, l^{-1}$, and become profound when it is $<2.5 \, \text{mmol} \, l^{-1}$.

2. In between attacks, physical examination is normal, except that occasionally eyelid myotonia can be seen.

3. Patients are usually taking oral potassium. Symptoms may be improved by acetazolamide. This probably acts by producing a metabolic acidosis, thus reducing potassium uptake by the cells. Spironolactone or triamterene can also be used prophylactically, but these drugs cannot improve the paralysis once it has occurred. Intravenous potassium may cause problems because the solutions use vehicles that may worsen hypokalaemia (Ptacek 1998).

4. Hypokalaemia, which can be as low as $1.6 \, \text{mmol} \, l^{-1}$, may be accompanied by ECG changes such as T-wave flattening, U waves, arrhythmias, and bradycardias.

5. Muscle fibres in hypoPP are permanently depolarised. Experimentally, if a muscle fibre is exposed to a $1 \, \text{mM}$ potassium solution, depolarisation to $-50 \, \text{mV}$ occurs and muscle becomes inexcitable. During an attack, the EMG shows action potential lengthening, progressing into electrical silence.

6. HypoPP is a voltage-gated calcium channel disorder. Although the disease is not well understood, many cases involve mutations in the calcium channel (CACNL1A3) gene, the dihydropyridine-sensitive receptor in skeletal muscle fibres. There may also be abnormalities in the ATP-sensitive K^+ channel. Although CACNL1A3 is a calcium channel, its main role is to serve as a voltage sensor for the ryanodine receptor (Ptacek 1998).

Anaesthetic problems

1. Attacks of paralysis can be precipitated by administration of glucose and insulin, sodium bicarbonate, diuretics, a heavy carbohydrate meal, undue stress, hypothermia, or a salt load.

2. Although patients with spontaneous attacks rarely require respiratory support, this is not always so in the postoperative period. Most case reports have shown uneventful intraoperative courses using a wide range of

anaesthetic techniques. However, the incidence of postoperative paralysis, often developing some hours later, is about 25%. Most of these episodes have been associated with hypokalaemia (Siler & Discavage 1975, Rollman & Dickson 1985, Lema et al 1991). Emergency tonsillectomy in a 13 year old was followed by respiratory failure (Bunting & Allen 1997).

3. Hypokalaemia during surgery may be accompanied by ECG changes that are out of proportion to the measured serum potassium.

4. The effect of muscle relaxants may be difficult to distinguish from the paralysis itself. One family had a total of 21 anaesthetics. The three patients who received muscle relaxants were the only ones who had postoperative paralyses (Horton 1977).

5. Epidural, axillary, and intercostal blocks have all been reported to produce a decrease in serum potassium of 0.3–0.7 mmol l^{-1}. These changes are thought to have paralleled increases in plasma epinephrine (adrenaline) levels (Lofgren & Hahn 1994).

6. One patient was described in whom an MH-like reaction occurred. Hyperthermia, tachycardia, respiratory acidosis and a moderate increase in CK at 16 h (5740 IU l^{-1}) were seen in association with an anaesthetic that included suxamethonium, isoflurane, and halothane (Lambert et al 1994). Resolution occurred after cessation of halothane and administration of dantrolene sodium. However, subsequent testing showed the patient to be MH equivocal according to the European MH group protocol.

7. In another patient undergoing Caesarean section, severe trismus occurred after topical local anaesthesia to the upper airway, and again following induction of anaesthesia. Suxamethonium produced generalised muscle rigidity and the mechanomyograph showed a large increase in muscle tone lasting for 1 min (Neuman & Kopman 1993). The patient had a low serum potassium and generalised muscle weakness for 36 h. In this case, the exact form of periodic paralysis was not known.

8. Occasionally, the patient may be undiagnosed before surgery, or may fail to inform the medical staff. A young man developed weakness in his arms and legs in the recovery room following eye surgery (Melnick et al 1983). A family history was subsequently elicited and a serum potassium level of 3.1 mmol l^{-1} was treated with a potassium infusion. The weakness had improved by the following day.

Management

1. Stress and anxiety can be reduced by using adequate premedication. Treatment with beta blockers has been reported, but only during anaesthesia.

2. Core temperature should be monitored and the operating theatre warmed. Precautions should be taken against heat loss during prolonged surgery.

3. The ECG should be closely observed throughout the operation for changes associated with hypokalaemia.

4. Avoid a carbohydrate load and minimise glucose infusions. Large sodium loads, particularly bicarbonate, should be avoided. Serum potassium must be monitored and hypokalaemia treated. Ptacek (1998) suggests that iv potassium should be avoided if possible because the crystalloid vehicles may worsen the symptoms, but in the perioperative period, this may not be possible.

5. Muscle relaxants may not be required. If they are necessary, small increments can be given and the effects assessed with a nerve stimulator. The problems of distinguishing between the effects of relaxants and those of the disease itself may be reduced by stimulating the facial nerve, since it supplies muscles that are rarely affected. However, even this may be unreliable. Atracurium was used without complication in a patient with periodic paralysis and a cardiomyopathy (Rooney et al 1988).

6. The patient's pulmonary ventilation, and

his/her serum potassium, should be closely monitored postoperatively in a high dependency area. Avoid hyperventilation.

7.   Combined epidural/spinal has been described during labour, and for forceps delivery (Viscomi et al 1999). An arterial line allowed regular serum potassium and pH levels to be measured. An infusion of Ringer lactate with KCL 40 mmol was given at a rate of 200 ml h^{-1} during labour and postpartum. Glucose was avoided. Epidural anaesthesia was performed for vaginal delivery in a patient with hypoPP and WPW syndrome (Robinson et al 2000). Continuous spinal anaesthesia was used for vaginal hysterectomy in a patient in whom a long QT interval was present during attacks. Sudden death had occurred in her four brothers and a cousin (Hecht et al 1997).

Bibliography

Bunting HE, Allen RW 1997 Prolonged muscle weakness following emergency tonsillectomy in a patient with periodic paralysis and infectious mononucleosis. Paediatric Anaesthesia 7: 171–5.

Hecht ML, Valtysson B, Hogan K 1997 Spinal anesthesia for a patient with a calcium channel mutation causing hypokalemic periodic paralysis. Anesthesia & Analgesia 84: 461–4.

Horton B 1977 Anesthetic experiences in a family with hypokalaemic periodic paralysis. Anesthesiology 47: 308–10.

Lambert C, Blanoeil Y, Horber RK et al 1994 Malignant hyperthermia in a patient with hypokalaemic periodic paralysis. Anesthesia & Analgesia 79: 1012–14.

Lema G, Urzua J, Moran S et al 1991 Successful anesthetic management of a patient with hypokalemic familial periodic paralysis undergoing cardiac surgery. Anesthesiology 74: 373–5.

Lofgren A, Hahn RG 1994 Hypokalemia from intercostal nerve block. Regional Anesthesia 19: 247–54.

Melnick B, Chang J, Larson C et al 1983 Hypokalemic familial periodic paralysis. Anesthesiology 58: 263–5.

Neuman GG, Kopman AF 1993 Dyskalemic periodic paralysis and myotonia. Anesthesia & Analgesia 76: 426–8.

Ptacek L 1998 The familial periodic paralyses and nondystrophic myotonias. American Journal of Medicine 105: 58–70.

Robinson JE, Morin VI, Douglas MJ et al 2000 Familial hypokalemic periodic paralysis and Wolff–Parkinson–White syndrome in pregnancy. Canadian Journal of Anaesthesia 47: 160–4.

Rollman JE, Dickson CM 1985 Anesthetic management of a patient with hypokalaemic periodic paralysis for coronary bypass surgery. Anesthesiology 63: 526–7.

Rooney R, Shanahan E, Sun T et al 1988 Atracurium and hypokalemic familial paralysis. Anesthesia & Analgesia 67: 782–3.

Rosen CA, Thomas JP, Anderson D 1999 Bilateral vocal fold paralysis caused by familial hypokalemic periodic paralysis. Otolaryngology—Head & Neck Surgery 120: 785–6.

Siler JN, Discavage WJ 1975 Anesthetic management of hypokalemic periodic paralysis. Anesthesiology 43: 489–90.

Viscomi CM, Ptacek LJ, Dudley D 1999 Anesthetic management of familial hypokalemic periodic paralysis during parturition. Anesthesia & Analgesia 88: 1081–2.

Hyperkalaemic periodic paralysis and paramyotonia

A similar, but separate, inherited disease of which three clinical variants are recognised: hyperPP with myotonia, hyperPP without myotonia, and hyperPP with paramyotonia, the last of which is cold induced and worse on exercise. The serum potassium may increase by 20% during an attack, and paralysis may occur with serum levels no greater than 4 mmol l^{-1}. Both changes in membrane potential, and release of potassium from muscle, have been demonstrated. Administration of potassium can precipitate an attack, although the serum potassium levels may remain normal. Changes in potassium alone cannot account for the problem. An abnormality of sodium channel function causing spontaneous depolarisation is suggested, and genetic studies showed that mutations in the gene encoding the skeletal muscle sodium channel are responsible (Ptacek et al 1993).

In a study of muscle taken from patients with periodic paralyses, several were found to have equivocal results from the contracture tests for MH. It was not suggested that these patients were susceptible to MH, but rather that the tests lacked specificity. The significance of this is not known.

Preoperative abnormalities

1. HyperPP. Transient attacks of paralysis, which usually last for less than 3 h, start in early childhood. The distribution of paralysis is similar, but the facial and tongue muscles may be involved. They are shorter than in the hypokalaemic form, lasting 1–3 h, and may be precipitated by emotional stress, hunger, rest after exercise, certain foods, and the administration of potassium. Hyperkalaemia is not always present during an attack, but diagnosis is usually made by the patient's response to being given potassium (Ptacek 1998). Thus, paralysis defined as normokalaemic in the past may actually be the hyperPP form. Weakness is not induced by cold.

2. Percussion myotonia may be marked during an attack, which can be precipitated by giving an oral potassium load, and reversed with iv calcium gluconate. Myotonia may also be evident between attacks.

3. The EMG shows increased spontaneous activity and myotonic discharges. In paramyotonia these changes are augmented by cold.

4. The ECG may show peaking of the T waves, even before the episode of paralysis.

5. The serum CK may be increased and muscle biopsy often shows nonspecific myopathic changes.

6. Symptomatic treatment includes diuretics, and anti-arrhythmic drugs such as procainamide (which affects sodium influx during depolarisation) and mexilitene.

7. HyperPP and paramyotonia are genetic disorders linked to the sodium channel on chromosome 17. A mutation in a number of the sodium channels of skeletal muscle results in abnormal inactivation when subjected to increased extracellular potassium concentrations (Ptacek 1998).

Anaesthetic problems

1. Anaesthesia may precipitate paralysis, which can continue for some hours postoperatively (Egan & Klein 1959). Although avoidance of nondepolarising neuromuscular blockers has been suggested, there have been several cases in which they have been used without problems (Aarons et al 1989, Ashwood et al 1992).

2. Jaw rigidity following suxamethonium, with subsequent global weakness, has been reported in two patients with hyperPP with paramyotonia (Ashwood et al 1992). However, there is no evidence of an association between MH and hyperPP (Lehmann-Horn & Iaizzo 1990).

3. In paramyotonia, cold may trigger myotonia and weakness.

4. Epidural anaesthesia in a patient with paramyotonia and lupus anticoagulant has been described (Howell & Douglas 1992). Spinal anaesthesia for Caesarean section with bupivacaine 0.5% and fentanyl 20 μg was uneventful in a patient whose mother had a flaccid quadriparesis for several days following epidural anaesthesia (Grace & Roach 1999).

Management

1. Dextrose should be infused during the period of fasting before anaesthesia, to supply carbohydrate.

2. Thiazide diuretics should be given prophylactically before operation to deplete potassium. Hyperkalaemia occurring during surgery will respond to calcium gluconate, or dextrose and insulin, which act by moving potassium back into the cells.

3. Warmed, sodium-containing, potassium-free, intravenous fluids should be used.

4. As with the hypokalaemic form, it is essential to monitor serum potassium, ECG, and neuromuscular function.

5.   Core temperature should be monitored and attention paid to the maintenance of normothermia. A heat and moisture exchanger, heat-retaining fabrics, and a warming device should be used.

6.   Suxamethonium should be avoided, but nondepolarising blockers may be given, provided monitoring takes place.

7.   The possible need for postoperative ventilation should be anticipated.

Bibliography

Aarons JJ, Moon RE, Camporesi EM 1989 General anesthesia and hyperkalemic periodic paralysis. Anesthesiology 71: 303–4.

Ashwood EM, Russell WJ, Burrow DD 1992 Hyperkalaemic periodic paralysis and anaesthesia. Anaesthesia 47: 579–84.

Egan TJ, Klein R 1959 Hyperkalemic periodic paralysis. Pediatrics 24: 761–73.

Grace RF, Roach VJ 1999 Caesarean section in a patient with paramyotonia congenita. Anaesthesia & Intensive Care 27: 534–7.

Howell PR, Douglas MJ 1992 Lupus anticoagulant, paramyotonia congenita and pregnancy. Canadian Journal of Anaesthesia 39: 992–6.

Lehmann-Horn F, Iaizzo PA 1990 Are myotonias and periodic paralyses associated with susceptibility to malignant hyperthermia? British Journal of Anaesthesia 65: 692–7.

Ptacek L 1998 The familial periodic paralyses and nondystrophic myotonias. American Journal of Medicine 104: 58–70.

Ptacek LJ, Johnson KJ, Griggs RC 1993 Genetics and physiology of the myotonic muscle disorders. New England Journal of Medicine 328: 482–9.

Fat embolism

Fat embolism refers to the presence of fat globules in the lung and peripheral circulation after trauma, most commonly following fracture of long bones (Levy 1990). The fat embolism syndrome (FES) is a multisystem disorder that occurs when fat emboli produce serious clinical manifestations. The exact pathogenesis is unknown, but there are two main theories. The mechanical theory suggests that bone marrow fat enters the venous system as a result of high intramedullary pressures (up to 800–1600 mmHg) secondary to reaming, cement application, or prosthesis insertion, and embolises to the lungs (Hofmann et al 1998, Pitto et al 1998). It can sometimes reach the systemic circulation, either by traversing the pulmonary vascular bed as small droplets, or by passing through a patent foramen ovale. The passage of emboli has now been demonstrated, using transoesophageal echocardiography, by a sufficient number of authors to prove that this is a major cause of FES (Pell et al 1993, Christie et al 1995, Pitto et al 1998, 2000). The alternative theory is that mediators released at the time of the trauma may alter the lipid composition of the blood to generate free fatty acids that act on pneumocytes, and produce acute lung injury and impairment of gaseous exchange. It is probable that a number of mechanisms contribute.

The main clinical features involve the lungs, the brain, and the skin. Emboli to the pulmonary capillaries are of particular clinical significance. Local endothelial damage and small vessel obstruction occur, probably from a combination of interactions between marrow fat, free fatty acids, and platelets (Gossling & Donohue 1979). The resulting increase in capillary permeability produces ventilation/perfusion abnormalities and hypoxaemia. Whilst fat emboli probably pass to the pulmonary vessels in the majority of cases of long bone fracture, only a small proportion of patients develop the classical syndrome. The fat embolism syndrome has also been reported after joint replacement (Green 1992), bone marrow transplantation, and liposuction. In experimental animals, arachidonic acid metabolites, such as prostaglandins and thromboxane, are released during cemented arthroplasty and may be responsible for the haemodynamic and respiratory changes (Byrick et al 1991).

A prospective study of long bone or pelvic fractures showed that clinical fat embolism occurs in at least 11% of these patients and may be associated with a 10% mortality (Fabian et al 1990). Pulmonary shunting is an early feature, followed by mental changes, confusion, and lethargy. The authors selected an alveolar–arterial difference for O_2 of >100 mmHg as indicative of a pulmonary shunt, and this usually occurred within 24–48 h. Laboratory tests show that changes associated with coagulopathy (decreasing Hct, thrombocytopenia, and hypofibrinogenaemia) begin at the same time, or soon after, the shunt. The petechial rash appears relatively late.

At postmortem examination of fatal cases, severe systemic embolisation was shown, and sometimes a patent foramen ovale was demonstrated (Christie et al 1995).

Presenting problems

1. Signs and symptoms may occur immediately after injury or surgery, but more often there is a latent period of 24–48 h. FES occurs most commonly in association with long bone fractures, and hip and knee replacements. However, liposuction from the abdomen, hips, and trochanteric area resulted in hypoxia and bilateral pulmonary infiltrates 1 h after surgery in a young woman. Bronchoalveolar lavage showed large numbers of fat droplets (Fourme et al 1998).

2. Alveolar–arterial differences in oxygen (>100 mmHg) occur early, although other causes of lung injury must be excluded. An interstitial pneumonitis may present with tachycardia, dyspnoea, pyrexia, cyanosis, and frothy sputum. Chest X-ray may show bilateral pulmonary infiltrates. Florid pulmonary oedema has been reported and respiratory failure may ensue. ECG may suggest right ventricular strain. Burnstein et al (1998) used a gas exchange model to demonstrate the contribution of both shunt and V/Q abnormalities to the hypoxaemia of the FES.

3. Neurological signs include an altered conscious level, with confusion and restlessness, which are usually signs of cerebral hypoxia. Coma may follow (Jacobson et al 1986), occasionally without pulmonary signs. Neurological complications are frequently a cause of long-term morbidity.

4. A petechial rash, particularly over the nondependent parts (the skin folds of the upper half of the body, the conjunctivae, and mucous membranes of the mouth), appears in 50–60% of cases, usually within the first 36 h. This rash is diagnostic of the syndrome. The retina may show exudates and haemorrhages, and sometimes fat droplets can be seen in the retinal vessels.

5. A decrease in haemoglobin, hypoxia, acidosis, and thrombocytopenia can all occur. Three fatal cases were reported in which a coagulopathy was a prominent feature (Hagley 1983).

6. In fulminant cases the mortality may range from 10% to 45%. Pulmonary involvement is the predominant cause of death.

Diagnosis

1. Initially the diagnosis is made on clinical grounds, by the occurrence of some or all of the features, appearing within 48 h of a long bone fracture. The femoral shaft or neck, the pelvis, and the tibia, are the bones most commonly involved. Rarely, fatal fat embolism has been reported during total hip replacement (Green 1992, Heine et al 1998), and at closed manipulation of the hip (Van Miert et al 1991).

2. Alveolar–arterial oxygen pressure differences exceeding 100 mmHg, in the absence of other causes of lung damage. V/Q abnormalities are also demonstrated (Burnstein et al 1998). These may be accompanied by early changes of a coagulopathy.

3. Examination of the sputum and urine may show fat globules. If the patient is sufficiently cooperative during ophthalmic examination, fat may also be seen in the retinal vessels, together with exudates and haemorrhages.

4. The use of bronchoalveolar lavage has been recommended (Fourme et al 1998).

5. Pulmonary microvascular cytology has been used to analyse samples of capillary blood in a case of fat embolism (Castella et al 1992).

6. In a study of 42 patients following severe musculoskeletal injuries, levels of serum unionised calcium were significantly lower in the eight who developed the fat embolism syndrome than in those who did not (Henderson et al 1992).

7. Sequential examination of blood from the right atrium in five patients showed considerable activation of clotting cascades during reaming (Christie et al 1995).

Management

1. It is important to try and identify individuals who are at risk. It has been suggested that respiratory status is recorded before surgery for trauma using pulse oximetry and blood gas analysis (Burnstein et al 1998, Hofmann et al 1998). Any significant emboli that occur during surgery may be noted by a decrease in $ETCO_2$.

2. Patients who should be monitored closely are those with early, unexplained pulmonary shunt or V/Q abnormalities, in the absence of pulmonary injury. Care mainly involves regular monitoring and supportive treatment during the acute phase. Respiratory management is of prime importance, since death is most commonly secondary to respiratory complications. Continual assessment of the clinical situation, including blood gases, is essential. Hypoxia should be initially treated with oxygen and, if necessary, with CPAP, or IPPV, and PEEP.

3. Early stabilisation of fractures. It is a surgical responsibility to modify the surgical techniques so that intramedullary pressures are reduced, during reaming of the femur, application of cement, or insertion of the prosthesis. Pitto et al (1998, 2000) showed that if a vacuum is created in the medullary cavity of the femur during insertion of the stem during arthroplasty, there is a much lower incidence of transatrial embolic events, compared with patients having conventional cementation.

4. There are no specific prophylactic or therapeutic measures. Cardiovascular and respiratory support may be required. Crystalloid transfusion should be minimised, and volume maintained using colloid.

Bibliography

Burnstein RM, Newell JP, Jones JG 1998 Sequential changes in gas exchange following traumatic fat embolism. Anaesthesia 53: 373–8.

Byrick RJ, Mullen JB, Wong PY et al 1991 Prostanoid production and pulmonary hypertension after fat embolism are not modified by methylprednisolone. Canadian Journal of Anaesthesia 38: 660–7.

Castella X, Valles J, Cabezuela MA et al 1992 Fat embolism syndrome and pulmonary microvascular cytology. Chest 101: 1710–12.

Christie J, Robinson CM, Pell AC et al 1995 Transcardiac echocardiography during invasive intramedullary procedures. Journal of Bone & Joint Surgery 77B: 450–5.

Djejouah I, Lefevre G, Ozier Y et al 1997 Fat embolism in orthopedic surgery: role of bone marrow fatty acid. Anesthesia & Analgesia 85: 441–3.

Fabian TC 1993 Unravelling the fat embolism syndrome. New England Journal of Medicine 329: 961–3.

Fabian TC, Hoots AV, Stanford DS et al 1990 Fat embolism syndrome: prospective evaluation in 92 fractures. Critical Care Medicine 18: 42–6.

Fourme T, Vieillard-Baron A, Loubieres Y et al 1998 Early fat embolism after liposuction. Anesthesiology 89: 782–4.

Gossling HR, Donohue TA 1979 The fat embolism syndrome. Journal of the American Medical Association 241: 2740–2.

Gossling HR, Pellegrini VD 1982 Fat embolism syndrome. Clinical Orthopaedics & Related Research 165: 68–82.

Green CP 1992 Fatal intra-operative fat embolism. Anaesthesia 47: 168.

Hagley SR 1983 Fulminant fat embolism. Anaesthesia & Intensive Care 11: 162–6.

Heine TA, Halambeck BL, Mark JB 1998 Fatal pulmonary fat embolism in the early postoperative period. Anesthesiology 89: 1589–91.

Henderson SA, Graham HK, Mollan RA 1992 Serum and other calcium fractions in patients after severe musculoskeletal trauma. Clinical Orthopaedics & Related Research 275: 306–11.

Hofmann S, Huemer G, Salzer M 1998 Pathophysiology and management of the fat embolism syndrome. Anaesthesia 53 (suppl 2): 35–7.

Jacobson DM, Terrence CF, Reinmuth OM 1986 The neurologic manifestations of fat embolism. Neurology 36: 847–51.

Levy D 1990 The fat embolism syndrome. Clinical Orthopaedics & Related Research 261: 281–6.

Needham AP, McLean AS, Stewart DE 1996 Severe cerebral fat embolism. Anaesthesia & Intensive Care 24: 502–4.

Pell ACH, Hughes D, Christie J et al 1993 Fulminating fat embolism caused by paradoxical embolism through a patent foramen ovale. New England Journal of Medicine 329: 926–9.

Pitto RP, Koessler M, Draenert K 1998 The John Charnley Award. Prophylaxis of fat and bone marrow embolism in cemented total hip arthroplasty. Clinical Orthopaedics & Related Research 355: 23–4.

Pitto RP, Blunk J, Kossler M 2000 Transesophageal echocardiography and clinical features of fat embolism during cemented total hip arthroplasty. A randomized study in patients with femoral neck fracture. Archives of Orthopaedic and Trauma Surgery 120: 53–8.

Van Miert M, Thornington RE, Van Velzen D 1991 Cardiac arrest after massive acute fat embolism. British Medical Journal 303: 396–7.

Fibrodysplasia (myositis) ossificans progressiva

A disorder of connective tissue in which there is progressive heterotopic bone formation involving axial muscles, joints, tendon, and ligaments. It is chemically and histologically identical to normal bone, but present in soft tissue (Connor 1996). These changes are superimposed on a variety of skeletal defects that particularly affect the spine and jaw. Diagnosis may be delayed unless the significance of the hand or feet anomalies is recognised (Smith 1998). Eventually the patient develops a rigid spine, kyphoscoliosis, and ankylosis of costovertebral and temporomandibular joints, to produce a clinical picture similar to that of ankylosing spondylitis.

Presentation is at a mean age of 3–4 years. Patients are wheelchair bound in their early 20s, and death occurs in the third to fourth decade, usually secondary to pneumonia or poor nutrition. The terms 'Stone man' and 'dure comme du bois' are eloquent descriptions of the latter stages of the disease.

Surgery is usually required for skeletal problems, including trismus. Ectopic bone formation may be precipitated by trauma, surgical or anaesthetic procedures. Pregnancy has been reported, but is rare, therefore new cases usually arise from fresh mutations. In excess of 600 cases have been reported in the literature.

Preoperative abnormalities

1. The condition usually presents with a swelling in the neck at 4–5 years of age. Further localised swellings form in the muscles of the neck and back over succeeding weeks. These eventually become ossified and may ulcerate, discharging a chalky substance.

2. Neck movements become limited and sometimes cervical fusion occurs (Connor & Smith 1982).

3. There are characteristic anomalies in the skeleton of the feet; a short big toe with a single phalanx, sometimes with valgus deformity. Less commonly, the hands may have an incurving fifth digit and short first metacarpal.

4. Bony bridges form between the mandible and the zygoma to cause trismus and jaw problems.

5. Eventually the patient develops a rigid spine and kyphoscoliosis, with ankylosis of the costovertebral and temporomandibular joints. The resulting clinical picture is similar to that seen in ankylosing spondylitis.

6. Restrictive lung disease. In a study of 21 patients, the chest expansion was 1–3 cm (mean 1.4 cm), FEV_1 27–64% (mean 45%), and mean FVC 40% (Connor et al 1981). By the age of 15 years there is severe limitation of chest expansion. However, chronic respiratory failure and cor pulmonale are not evident, probably because diaphragmatic function remains

adequate for the restricted mobility permitted by the disease. Patients are prone to recurrent chest infections, and death from pneumonia is common.

7. A CT scan in the early stages shows that soft tissue swelling precedes ectopic ossification. The ossification becomes evident on tomography before it can be seen on plain X-ray (Reinig et al 1986).

8. Some patients show ECG changes of RBBB, or T-wave inversion in the inferior leads, but there is no evidence of cardiac failure. However, right ventricular abnormalities on ECG were associated with severely restricted chest wall disease (Kussmaul et al 1998).

9. There is often a low grade fever and increased ESR.

10. There is no specific treatment, but patients may be receiving calcitonin, steroids, disodium etidronate, and warfarin.

Anaesthetic problems

1. Difficult intubation.

a) Limited mouth opening as a result of bony bridges between the coronoid process of the mandible and the zygoma. Trismus cannot be overcome by neuromuscular blockers.

b) Restricted neck movement secondary to soft-tissue ossification in the neck, narrowing of the AP diameter (hypoplasia) of vertebral bodies, and fusion of the posterior elements. There has been one report of atlantoaxial subluxation.

2. If submandibular ossification from the condition is not diagnosed, airway problems may occur (Janoff et al 1996).

3. The presence of restrictive lung disease means that patients are susceptible to chest infections.

4. Any area of local trauma can form a focus for ectopic calcification, therefore the use of

invasive procedures should be considered carefully. This may occur at the site of biopsies, tracheostomy, and im or iv injections. Nineteen out of 20 operations to remove ectopic calcification in ten patients resulted in recurrence at the site of surgery (Connor & Evans 1982).

5. Routine injections of local anaesthetic for dental procedures have been associated with a flare-up of the condition and, in some patients, permanent jaw ankylosis (Luchetti et al 1996).

6. Problems of positioning patients with joint contractures.

7. Pregnancy has been reported (Thornton et al 1987), but is rare. The patient had cervical and temporomandibular ankylosis, joint contractures, and an inability to abduct her hips. Caesarean section was carried out under local anaesthesia with lidocaine (lignocaine).

Management

1. Assessment of respiratory function, and treatment for, or prophylaxis against, lung infection.

2. Airway assessment and management. Awake fibreoptic intubation may be required if there is trismus or neck fixation (Newton et al 1990). Otherwise, neuromuscular blockers should not be given until it can be established that tracheal intubation is possible (Stark et al 1990). Tracheostomy should only be undertaken after careful consideration, because of the risk of ectopic calcification. Ketamine infusions have been used for short procedures in order to avoid intubation in patients with trismus and partial fixation of the cervical vertebrae (Shipton et al 1985, Liniger et al 1989).

3. Careful positioning and padding of joints involved in contractures.

Bibliography
Connor JM 1996 Fibrodysplasia ossificans progressiva—lessons from rare maladies. New England Journal of Medicine 335: 591–3.

Connor JM, Evans DAP 1982 Fibrodysplasia ossificans progressiva: the clinical features and natural history of 34 patients. Journal of Bone & Joint Surgery 64B 64–76.

Connor JM, Smith R 1982 The cervical spine in fibrodysplasia ossificans progressiva. British Journal of Radiology 55: 492–6.

Connor JM, Evans CC, Evans DAP 1981 Cardiopulmonary function in fibrodysplasia ossificans progressiva. Thorax 36: 419–23.

Janoff HB, Zasloff MA, Kaplan FS 1996 Submandibular swelling in patients with fibrodysplasia ossificans progressiva. Otolaryngology—Head & Neck Surgery 114: 599–604.

Kussmaul WG, Esmail AN, Sagar Y et al 1998 Pulmonary and cardiac function in advanced fibrodysplasia ossificans progressiva. Clinical Orthopaedics & Related Research 346: 104–9.

Lininger TE, Brown EM, Brown M 1989 General anesthesia and fibrodysplasia ossificans progressiva. Anesthesia & Analgesia 68: 175–6.

Luchetti W, Cohen RB, Hahn GV et al 1996 Severe restriction in jaw movement after routine injection of local anesthetic in patients who have fibrodysplasia ossificans progressive. Oral Surgery, Oral Medicine, Oral Pathology, Oral Radiology & Endodontics 81: 21–5.

Newton MC, Allen PW, Ryan DC 1990 Fibrodysplasia ossificans progressiva. British Journal of Anaesthesia 64: 246–50.

Reinig JW, Hill SC, Fang M et al 1986 Fibrodysplasia ossificans progressiva. Radiology 159: 153–7.

Shipton EA, Retief LW, Theron HDuT et al 1985 Anaesthesia in myositis ossificans progressiva. A case report and clinical review. South African Medical Journal 67: 26–8.

Smith R 1998 Fibrodysplasia (myositis) ossificans progressive. Clinical lessons from a rare disease. Clinical Orthopaedics & Related Research 346: 7–14.

Smith R, Athanasou NA, Vipond SE 1996 Fibrodysplasia (myositis) ossificans progressiva: clinicopathological features and natural history. Quarterly Journal of Medicine 89: 445–6.

Stark WH, Krechel SW, Eggers GWN 1990 Anesthesia in 'stone man': myositis ossificans progressiva. Journal of Clinical Anesthesia 2: 332–5.

Thornton YS, Birnnbaum SJ, Lebowitz N 1987 A viable pregnancy in a patient with myositis ossificans progressiva. American Journal of Obstetrics & Gynecology 156: 577–8.

Fraser syndrome

An autosomal recessive syndrome in which cryptophthalmos is associated with a number of ear, nose, digit, and genital abnormalities.

Preoperative abnormalities

1. Cryptophthalmos, meatal stenosis, low-set ears, flattened nasal bridge, notching of nares, choanal atresia, cleft palate, high arched palate, and laryngeal or subglottic stenosis (Mina et al 1988).

2. Malformed genitalia and renal abnormalities.

3. Syndactyly of fingers and toes.

4. Cardiac lesions, including ASD and VSD.

5. Surgery may be required for ophthalmic, ENT, plastic, gynaecological, and orthopaedic procedures.

Anaesthetic problems

1. Difficult intubation, that was overcome by a retrograde catheter technique (Jagtap et al 1995).

2. Airway narrowing may produce respiratory difficulties (Ford et al 1992). A requirement for tracheal tube sizes smaller than predicted (Dakin & Bingham 1995). Stridor may be worsened after endoscopy and occasionally tracheostomy may be required (Dakin & Bingham 1995).

Management

1. Assessment of intubation difficulties in the possible presence of mental retardation.

2. A range of tube sizes should be available.

Bibliography

Dakin MJ, Bingham RM 1995 Anaesthetic considerations in patients with Fraser syndrome. Anaesthesia 50: 746.

Ford GR, Irving RM, Jones NS et al 1992 ENT manifestations of Fraser syndrome. Journal of Laryngology & Otology 106: 1–4.

Jagtap SR, Malde AD, Pantvaidya SH 1995 Anaesthetic considerations in a patient with Fraser syndrome. Anaesthesia 50: 38–41.

Mina MMF, Greenberg C, Levin B 1988 ENT abnormalities associated with Fraser syndrome: case report and review of the literature. Journal of Otolaryngology 17: 233–6.

Freeman–Sheldon syndrome (distal arthrogryposis type 2, craniocarpotarsal dysplasia)

One of the distal arthrogryposes, a congenital myopathy, usually of autosomal dominant inheritance, with facial and orthopaedic deformities. Anaesthesia may be required for inguinal hernia repair, orchidopexy, feeding gastrostomy, muscle biopsy, release of contractures around the mouth, or plastic surgery (Guyuron & Winkler 1988).

Preoperative abnormalities

1. A myopathy, with the development of contractures around the mouth, producing the characteristic 'whistling face' appearance. This feature contributes to microstomia and the formation of a small 'mound' on the chin. There may be hypertelorism, a small nose, a high arched palate, and an abnormal mandible with micrognathia. Limited neck flexion and extension may occur.

2. Kyphoscoliosis may develop as the myopathy progresses. Thoracic cage deformity and respiratory muscle myopathy can combine to produce restrictive lung disease.

3. Anatomical abnormalities and contractures may also affect the hands and feet. Camptodactyly occurs, with ulnar deviation of the fingers.

4. Diagnosis is made on EMG and muscle biopsy.

Anaesthetic problems

1. Intubation problems are common and may be secondary to micrognathia, microstomia, and a short neck (Munro et al 1997, Vas & Naregal 1998). Awake intubation was achieved with difficulty in an 11-week-old baby, and after inhalational anaesthesia in two children (Laishley & Roy 1986). Successful intubation was finally achieved using a stylet in a 7 month old, who was subsequently given caudal anaesthesia for surgery for club foot (Duggar et al 1989). Malkawi and Tarawneh (1983) reported impossible intubation in a child, and intubation achieved with great difficulty in the father. In one neonate, difficulties were experienced because of both nasal and oral narrowing and tracheostomy was performed at 3 weeks (Robinson 1997).

2. Muscle rigidity followed halothane anaesthesia in two patients (Jones & Delacourt 1992). In the first, this did not recede after pancuronium, but relaxation occurred 5 min after dantrolene 5 mg kg^{-1} was given. No hyperthermia, hyperkalaemia, or cardiac arrhythmias occurred, but the following day the serum CK was 9215 iu l^{-1}. In the second, masseter muscle spasm followed suxamethonium, and the maximum CK recorded was 1193 iu l^{-1}. The operation was allowed to continue but halothane was withdrawn.

3. Difficulty in obtaining venous access secondary to hand and foot deformities. Limbs may be encased in plaster.

4. Physical problems may make regional anaesthesia technically difficult. Dural puncture occurred at a depth of only 2.6 cm during epidural anaesthesia in a 12-year-old, 41-kg boy (Vas & Naregal 1998).

5. Patients are susceptible to pneumonia.

Management

1. Assessment of intubation difficulties and appropriate management. Difficult intubation

has been managed in a variety of ways, including intubation through an LMA blindly (Rabb et al 1996), with a fibrescope (Munro et al 1997), and with a stylet.

2. Although suxamethonium has been used, apparently uneventfully (Laishley & Roy 1986), it would seem prudent to avoid it in a myopathy, particularly in view of the evidence of muscle breakdown. Cruickshank et al (1999) used a propofol infusion and a laryngeal mask in a 2 year old for a hernia repair.

3. Observe for evidence of muscle rigidity, rhabdomyolysis, or hypermetabolism.

Bibliography

Cruikshank GF, Brown S, Chitayat D 1999 Anaesthesia for Freeman–Sheldon syndrome using a laryngeal mask airway. Canadian Journal of Anaesthesia 46: 783–7.

Duggar RG, DeMars PD, Bolton VE 1989 Whistling face syndrome: general anesthesia and early postoperative caudal analgesia. Anesthesiology 70: 545–7.

Guyuron B, Winkler PA 1988 Craniocarpotarsal dysplasia: the whistling face syndrome. Annals of Plastic Surgery 20: 86–8.

Jones R, Delacourt JL 1992 Muscle rigidity following halothane anesthesia in two patients with Freeman–Sheldon syndrome. Anesthesiology 77: 599–600.

Laishley RS, Roy WL 1986 Freeman–Sheldon syndrome: report of three cases and the anaesthetic implications. Canadian Anaesthetists' Society Journal 33: 388–93.

Malkawi H, Tarawneh M 1983 The whistling face syndrome, or craniocarpotarsal dysplasia. Report of two cases in a father and son and review of the literature. Journal of Pediatric Orthopedics 3: 364–9.

Munro HM, Butler PJ, Washington EJ 1997 Freeman–Sheldon (whistling face) syndrome. Anaesthetic and airway management. Paediatric Anaesthesia 7: 345–8.

Rabb MF, Minkowitz HS, Hagberg CA 1996 Blind intubation through the laryngeal mask airway for management of the difficult airway in infants. Anesthesiology 84: 1510–11.

Robinson PJ 1997 Freeman Sheldon syndrome: severe upper airway obstruction requiring neonatal tracheostomy. Pediatric Pulmonology 23: 457–9.

Vas L, Naregal P 1998 Anaesthetic management of a patient with Freeman Sheldon syndrome. Paediatric Anaesthesia 8: 175–7.

Friedreich's ataxia

An autosomal recessive, hereditary ataxia involving all four limbs. Degeneration of the pyramidal and spinocerebellar tracts, and atrophy of the dorsal root ganglia, result in ataxia and combined upper and lower motor neurone lesions. Asymptomatic ECG abnormalities occur in many patients. Disorders of cardiac muscle affect about 30% of individuals and are of two types; a hypertrophic form and a dystrophic form. The condition usually presents between the ages of 5 and 15 years, with a mean of 9 years. The disease is steadily progressive and sudden death may occur. It is associated with mutations in the frataxin gene on chromosome 9, and a broader spectrum of disease has been found than was previously thought (Rosenberg 1995, Durr et al 1996). Frataxin is a protein involved in regulation of mitochondrial iron content and its deficiency may cause iron-induced injury (Rustin et al 1999).

Preoperative abnormalities

1. Usually presents with gait ataxia. Later the upper limbs become clumsy, with intention tremor. The cerebellar lesion causes nystagmus and dysarthria. The dorsal root lesion is associated with sensory impairment and depressed or absent reflexes in the upper or lower limbs. The corticospinal tract degeneration causes progressive weakness and extensor plantar responses. Pes cavus is often present. Lower limbs and pelvic girdle are affected early, and upper limb and trunk muscles spared until late in the disease process (Beauchamp et al 1995).

2. Cardiac abnormalities are frequent, although these may simply consist of asymptomatic ECG or echocardiographic changes. In a study of 75 consecutive patients, 95% had one or more abnormalities (Child et al

1986). These consisted of ST/T-wave abnormalities (79%), right axis deviation (40%), a short PR interval (24%), an abnormal R wave in V1 (20%), abnormal inferolateral Q waves (14%), and left ventricular hypertrophy (11%). However, up to 50% of patients have clinical cardiac disease. Hypertrophic cardiomyopathy occurred in 20%, less frequently than previously thought, whilst 7% had nonhypertrophic cardiomyopathy, in which there was global hypofunction of the left ventricle. In a recent study of 55 patients, wide variations in cardiomyopathy were found and there was no relationship between it and the presence of ECG abnormalities (Dutka et al 1999). In affected patients, symptoms include palpitations and chest pain, and heart failure may supervene. Sudden death can occur.

3. The onset of symptoms is usually before the age of 25, and disability increases progressively. The development of scoliosis and loss of ambulation are closely associated. Scoliosis occurs in 80% of patients and surgery may be required for its correction. Chest infections are common and respiratory failure may occur.

4. Diabetes has been found in 18% of patients and a diabetic glucose tolerance curve in 40%. Insulin resistance is present in nondiabetic patients and alterations in the binding function of the insulin receptor have been shown (Fantus et al 1993).

5. The EMG is usually normal, but motor nerve conduction velocities are decreased.

Anaesthetic problems

1. Although sensitivity to nondepolarising relaxants has been reported, this is not always so. When nerve stimulators and train-of-four monitoring have been used, suggestions of a myasthenic-like response have not been confirmed (Bell et al 1986, Mouloudi et al 1998). However, since different muscles are affected to a variable degree, the response may depend both on the progression of the disease, and the muscle group being monitored.

2. If cardiac disease is present, there is a risk of arrhythmias and heart failure. A patient having scoliosis surgery developed heart failure on the 34th postoperative day, possibly from pulmonary emboli in addition to longstanding cardiomyopathy (Bell et al 1986). This subsequently proved fatal.

3. As the degree of scoliosis increases, or if diaphragmatic weakness develops, cardiopulmonary failure becomes a significant problem (see also Scoliosis). Chest infections occur readily.

4. Abnormal pharyngeal function may predispose to bronchopulmonary complications.

5. Obstructive sleep apnoea and periodic breathing may cause nocturnal desaturation (Botez et al 1997).

Management

1. Assessment of respiratory reserve, and vigorous treatment of chest infections with physiotherapy and antibiotics.

2. Assessment, monitoring, and treatment of cardiac lesions as appropriate.

3. Neuromuscular monitoring should be instituted, before induction of anaesthesia. The monitoring of more than one muscle group may be necessary.

4. Spinal anaesthesia has been used for Caesarean section (Kubal et al 1991), and epidural anaesthesia for laparoscopic tubal ligation (Alon & Waespe 1988). Combined spinal–epidural anaesthesia was performed with some difficulty for vaginal delivery in a patient with a cardiomyopathy who had undergone Harrington rod fixation for thoracic scoliosis (Wyatt & Brighouse 1998). However, in view of the incidence of cardiomyopathy, caution has been advised if regional anaesthesia is considered. If cardiomyopathy is present, full cardiac assessment is recommended (Finley & Campbell 1992).

5. Epidural narcotics were given for

postoperative pain relief in a 13-year-old girl who required colorectal surgery (Campbell & Finley 1989).

Bibliography

Alon E, Waespe W 1988 Epidura anaesthesie bei einer patient mit Friedreichscher ataxie. Regional Anaesthesia 11: 58–60.

Beauchamp M, Labelle H, Duhaime M et al 1995 Natural history of muscle weakness in Friedreich's ataxia and its relation to loss of ambulation. Clinical Orthopaedics & Related Research 311: 270–5.

Bell CF, Kelly JM, Jones RS 1986 Anaesthesia for Friedreich's ataxia. Anaesthesia 41: 296–301.

Botez MI, Mayer P, Bellemare F et al 1997 Can we treat respiratory failure in Friedreich's ataxia? Archives of Neurology 54: 1030–3.

Campbell AM, Finley GA 1989 Anaesthesia for a patient with Friedreich's ataxia and cardiomyopathy. Canadian Journal of Anaesthesia 36: 89–93.

Child JS, Perloff JK, Bach PM et al 1986 Cardiac involvement in Friedreich's ataxia. A study of 75 patients. Journal of the American College of Cardiology 7: 1370–8.

Durr A, Cossee M, Agid Y et al 1996 Clinical and genetic abnormalities in patients with Friedreich's ataxia. New England Journal of Medicine 335: 1169–75.

Dutka DP, Donnelly JE, Nihoyannopoulos P et al 1999 Marked variation in the cardiomyopathy associated with Friedreich's ataxia. Heart 81: 141–7.

Fantus IG, Seni MH, Andermann E 1993 Evidence for abnormal regulation of insulin receptors in Friedreich's ataxia. Journal of Clinical Endocrinology & Metabolism 76: 60–3.

Finley GA, Campbell AM 1992 Spinal anesthesia and Friedreich's ataxia. Anesthesia & Analgesia 74: 318.

Kubal K, Pasricha SK, Bhargava M 1991 Spinal anaesthesia in a patient with Friedreich's ataxia. Anesthesia & Analgesia 72: 257–8.

Mouloudi H, Katsanoulas C, Frantzeskos G 1998 Requirements for muscle relaxation in Friedreich's ataxia. Anaesthesia 53: 177–80.

Rosenberg RN 1995 Spinocerebellar ataxias and ataxins. New England Journal of Medicine 333: 1351–3.

Rustin P, von Kleist-Retzow JC, Chantreal-Groussard K et al 1999 Effect of idebenone on cardiomyopathy in Friedreich's ataxia: a preliminary study. Lancet 354: 477–9.

Wyatt S, Brighouse D 1998 Anaesthetic management of vaginal delivery in a woman with Friedreich's ataxia complicated by cardiomyopathy and scoliosis. International Journal of Obstetric Anesthesia 7: 185–8.

Gaucher's disease

An inherited sphingolipid storage disease in which there is a deficiency of a lysosomal enzyme, glucocerebrosidase, resulting in pathological storage of glycolipid in the macrophages of the reticuloendothelial system. There are three types, each with different features: type 1 (about 99% of cases), type 2 (infantile, results in early death), and type 3 (juvenile). There is a high incidence in Ashkenazi Jews (Zimran et al 1992). Enzyme therapy decreases the signs and symptoms, but is associated with other complications. Anaesthesia may be required for endoscopy, fundoplication, ENT, splenectomy, and orthopaedic surgery.

Preoperative abnormalities

1. In type 1 disease, the most common form, accumulation of glucocerebrosidase occurs in the spleen, liver, and bone marrow, producing hepatosplenomegaly, growth retardation and bone necrosis. Splenic infarcts are common. Type 2 (infantile) and type 3 (juvenile), are rare, but are complicated by CNS involvement, bone necrosis, and susceptibility to infection. Seizures, bulbar involvement and gastro-oesophageal reflux are also features.

2. There is X-ray evidence of skeletal involvement in 90% of cases, but not all patients are symptomatic. Avascular necrosis of the hip joint and bone crises can occur. Spinal involvement results in vertebral collapse with root compression.

3. In children, anaemia and thrombocytopenia are present in 80% and 60% respectively. A number of coagulation abnormalities have been reported, including factor IX deficiency and acquired von Willebrand's disease. In 32 patients with type 1 disease who did not have thrombocytopenia, 22% had abnormal platelet aggregation (Gillis et al 1999). It has been suggested that abnormal coagulation tests may be secondary to the presence of increased cerebroside levels interfering with assays (Billett al 1996).

4. Enzyme replacement with ceredase involves close monitoring of patients (Zevin et al 1993).

5. An unexpectedly high rate of pulmonary hypertension has been found in patients receiving enzyme replacement (Elstein et al 1998).

Anaesthetic problems

1. Bleeding manifestations are common, even in patients without thrombocytopenia, and may result from platelet dysfunction (Gillis et al 1999).

2. Difficult intubation has been reported secondary to trismus, opisthotonos, and a small mouth (Kita et al 1998, Kitamura et al 1999). Insertion of a laryngeal mask airway was difficult because of trismus. Infiltration of the airway with glycolipids may lead to airway obstruction (Tobias et al 1993). Pulmonary aspiration may be a problem in type 2 and 3 disease.

3. There is an increased risk of infection, especially in type 3 disease, possibly secondary to abnormalities of neutrophil chemotaxis. A splenic abscess, which was difficult to diagnose radiologically because of previous splenic infarcts, was eventually drained at laparotomy. The patient was receiving enzyme replacement therapy via a long-term catheter, although there was no proof that this was the source of the pus, from which *Streptococcus viridans* was grown (Maclean & Wilson 1999).

4. Pregnancy. In a study of 53 obstetric patients, seven developed bone crisis in the third trimester of pregnancy. There was an increased incidence of spontaneous abortions, postpartum haemorrhage, and fever, regardless of the mode of delivery (Granovsky-Grisaru et al 1995).

Management

1. Assessment of organ involvement and dysfunction.

2. Assessment of potential airway or intubation difficulties. The use of a mask and adapter has been described that allows placement of the tube using fibreoptic intubation (Kitamura et al 1999).

3. Enzyme replacement during pregnancy has reduced the spontaneous abortion rate (Elstein et al 1997).

Bibliography

Billett HH, Rizvi S, Sawitsky A 1996 Coagulation abnormalities in patients with Gaucher's disease: effect of therapy. American Journal of Hematology 51: 234–6.

Elstein D, Granovsky-Grisaru S, Rabinowitz R et al 1997 Use of enzyme replacement therapy for Gaucher disease during pregnancy. American Journal of Obstetrics & Gynecology 177: 1509–12.

Elstein D, Klutstein MW, Lahad A 1998 Echocardiographic assessment of pulmonary hypertension in Gaucher's disease. Lancet 351: 1544–6.

Gillis S, Hyam E, Abrahamov A et al 1999 Platelet function abnormalities in Gaucher disease patients. American Journal of Hematology 61: 103–6.

Granovsky-Grisaru S, Aboulafia Y, Diamant YZ et al 1995 Gynecologic and obstetric aspects of Gaucher's disease: a survey of 53 patients. American Journal of Obstetrics & Gynecology 172: 1284–90.

Kita T, Kitamura S, Takeda K et al 1998 [Anesthetic management involving difficult intubation in a child with Gaucher disease.] Masui-Japanese Journal of Anesthesiology 47: 69–73.

Kitamura S, Fukumitsu K, Kinouchi K et al 1999 A new modification of anaesthesia mask for fibreoptic intubation in children. Paediatric Anaesthesia 9: 119–22.

Maclean K, Wilson MJ 1999 Splenic abscess in a patient with type 3 Gaucher's disease receiving enzyme replacement therapy. Journal of Pediatrics 134: 245–7.

Tobias JD, Atwood R, Lowe S et al 1993 Anesthetic considerations in a child with Gaucher disease. Journal of Clinical Anesthesia 5: 150–3.

Zevin S, Abrahamov A, Hadas-Halpern I et al 1993 Adult type Gaucher disease in children: genetics, clinical features and enzyme replacement therapy. Quarterly Journal of Medicine 86: 565–73.

Zimran A, Kay A, Gelbart T et al 1992 Gaucher disease. Clinical, laboratory, radiologic, and genetic features of 53 patients. Medicine 71: 337–53.

Giant axonal neuropathy

An autosomal recessive neurological disorder of cytoplasmic intermediate filaments, in which there are swollen axons with accumulation of neurofilaments (Berg et al 1972). A mild sensory neuropathy is accompanied by severe CNS involvement, mental retardation, seizures, cerebellar dysfunction, and pyramidal signs. Occasionally the CNS abnormalities predominate (Lampl et al 1992). The condition develops in early childhood, with death occurring in adolescence, frequently secondary to muscle weakness and respiratory infection.

Preoperative abnormalities

1. Tightly kinked hair is characteristic.

2. There is profound limb weakness and wasting, usually accompanied by kyphoscoliosis.

3. Diffuse demyelination is evident on CT scan and MRI.

4. EMG shows decreased sensory nerve conduction.

5. Diagnosis is confirmed by sural nerve biopsy.

Anaesthetic problems

1. Respiratory problems may occur secondary to muscle weakness.

2. Profound weakness following diazepam was reported in one patient (Mitchell & Moskovits 1991).

Bibliography

Berg BO, Rosenberg SH, Asbury AK 1972 Giant axonal neuropathy. Pediatrics 49: 894–9.

Lampl Y, Eshel Y, Ben-David E et al 1992 Giant axonal neuropathy with predominant central nervous system manifestations. Developmental Medicine & Childhood Neurology 34: 164–9.

Maia M, Pires MM, Guimar ES 1988 Giant axonal disease: report of three cases and review of the literature. Neuropediatrics 19: 10–15.

Mitchell A, Moskovits PE 1991 Anaesthesia for a patient with giant axonal neuropathy. Anaesthesia 46: 469–70.

Gilbert's disease (idiopathic unconjugated hyperbilirubinaemia)

An autosomal dominant, benign condition, in which there is a mildly elevated unconjugated bilirubin, without either structural liver disease or haemolytic anaemia. It possibly results from an impaired uptake and conjugation of bilirubin, secondary to a deficiency of UDP-glucuronyltransferase. The diagnosis is made on a level of unconjugated bilirubin of $17–102 \mu$ mol l^{-1}. Alternatively, a serum total bilirubin of $25–50 \mu$ mol l^{-1} after a 24-h restricted diet.

Preoperative abnormalities

1. Serum unconjugated bilirubin is increased, but usually to a level $<50 \mu$ mol l^{-1}, and clinical jaundice is barely detectable. However, fluctuating mild jaundice may occur, particularly in the presence of stress, infection, starvation, or surgery.

2. Other liver function tests are normal, and there is no haemolytic anaemia.

Anaesthetic problems

1. The condition itself is of no significance. However, the appearance of jaundice postoperatively may suggest more serious problems, therefore the confirmation of Gilbert's syndrome as the cause is useful (Taylor 1984).

2. Starvation may elevate the bilirubin level and produce visible jaundice.

3. The metabolism of morphine (Nishimura et al 1973), and papaveretum (Danks & Jackson 1991), may be delayed. Two patients were reported in whom papaveretum 10 mg caused profound sedation and respiratory depression. A study on paracetamol elimination showed that in a subgroup of patients with Gilbert's syndrome, there was considerable reduction in glucuronidation (Esteban & Perez-Mateo 1999). It has been suggested that these individuals might be more susceptible to liver damage secondary to drug overdose. There are potential toxicological implications for any drug or chemical that is eliminated primarily via glucuronidation mechanisms (de Morais et al 1992).

Management

1. If Gilbert's disease is suspected, the administration of nicotinic acid 50 mg iv will double or treble the plasma unconjugated bilirubin within 3 h. In normal patients, or in those with other liver disease, the increase will be less.

2. Morphine, papaveretum, and paracetamol should be used with caution.

3. Early morning surgery and a dextrose infusion will reduce the increase in bilirubin provoked by starvation.

Bibliography

Danks JL, Jackson AFP 1991 Sensitivity to papaveretum in Gilbert's disease. Anaesthesia 46: 998–9.

de Morais SMF, Uetrecht JP, Welles PG 1992 Decreased glucuronidation and increased bioactivation of acetaminophen in Gilbert's syndrome. Gastroenterology 102: 577–86.

Esteban A, Perez-Mateo M 1999 Heterogeneity of paracetamol metabolism in Gilbert's syndrome. European Journal of Drug Metabolism & Pharmacokinetics 24: 9–13.

Nishimura TG, Jackson SH, Cohen SN 1973 Prolongation of morphine anaesthesia in a patient with Gilbert's disease. Canadian Anaesthetists' Society Journal 20: 709–12.

Taylor S 1984 Gilbert's syndrome as a cause of postoperative jaundice. Anaesthesia 39: 1222–4.

Glomus jugulare tumour

A rare, slow-growing, benign vascular tumour of the glomus bodies, usually arising from the dome of the jugular bulb. It is one of the paraganglionic tumours, related to the branchial arches. The symptoms, which vary, will depend in part on local extension, or invasion of structures by the tumour. The mode of presentation includes a swelling in the neck, middle ear disease, or symptoms indicative of involvement of the cerebellum, brainstem, or skull base. Although normally nonfunctional, it occasionally produces catecholamines. It must be distinguished from glomus tumours, which arise from the tympanic plexus. Surgical removal is either through the auditory canal or via a mastoid approach; in the presence of extensive spread, postoperative complications are significant, in which case radiotherapy may be a safer option (Larner et al 1992).

Preoperative abnormalities

1. Pulsatile tinnitus, hearing loss and facial paralysis can occur when the middle ear is involved. In a series of 52 patients, 98% had pulsatile tinnitus, 63% hearing loss, 94% middle ear masses, and 34% vocal cord paralyses (Green et al 1994).

2. Clinical signs of IX, X, XI and XII cranial nerve lesions denote extension of the tumour into the base of the skull.

3. Intracranial extension may give V and VI nerve lesions.

4. Invasion of the jugular vein or internal carotid may occur.

5. Occasionally, functioning tumours can produce catecholamines, including dopamine (Troughton et al 1998).

6. Ten percent of patients will have another paraganglionic tumour.

7. The tumours can be visualised using carotid angiography or digital vascular imaging. Vascularity and collateral circulation need to be assessed.

8. Treatment may be by surgery, radiation, or embolisation (Gjuric et al 1996).

Anaesthetic problems

1. The site and locally infiltrative behaviour makes them difficult to resect. Excision may require extensive surgery involving more than one surgical discipline. Combined or two-stage procedures may be necessary.

2. Blood loss can be heavy (Ghani et al 1983). The blood supply usually comes from the external carotid artery, but extensive tumours may also be supplied by collateral circulation from the internal carotid.

3. Occasionally the tumour may actually involve the internal carotid artery itself or invade the jugular vein to give tumour emboli.

4. Surgery has been reported as lasting for up to 17 h, therefore heat loss can be a problem.

5. The problems of any neurosurgical procedure, including that of air embolism.

6. Ligation of the internal carotid artery may be necessary (Braude et al 1986).

7. Patients with undiagnosed catecholamine secretion have cardiovascular instability during surgery (Anand et al 1993).

Management

1. A two-stage operation may be planned if the tumour is very extensive and involves two different surgical fields (Mather & Webster 1986).

2. Hypotensive anaesthesia may be required to reduce blood loss.

3. Prior radiological embolisation of the tumour may be required to reduce haemorrhage.

4. If carotid artery ligation is contemplated, adequacy of the collateral circulation must be assessed.

Hypothermia and cerebral protection may be required in tumours involving the carotid artery. A technique has been described in which moderate hypothermia, normocarbia, normotension and thiopentone infusion provided successful cerebral protection for resection of an extensive tumour which involved the internal carotid (Braude et al 1986).

Prolonged surgery has also been described using fentanyl and low-dose isoflurane (Jellish et al 1994).

Bibliography

Anand VK, Leonetti JP, al-Mefty O 1993 Neurovascular considerations in surgery of glomus tumors with intracranial extensions. Laryngoscope 103: 722–8.

Braude BM, Hockman R, McIntosh WA et al 1986 Management of a glomus jugulare tumour with internal carotid artery involvement. Anaesthesia 41: 861–5.

Ghani GA, Sung Y-F, Per-Lee JH 1983 Glomus jugulare tumours—origin, pathology and anesthetic considerations. Anesthesia & Analgesia 62: 686–91.

Gjuric M, Wigand ME, Wolf SR et al 1996 Cranial nerve and hearing function after combined-approach surgery for glomus jugulare tumors. Annals of Otology, Rhinology & Laryngology 105: 949–54.

Green JD Jr, Brackmann DE, Nguyen CD et al 1994 Surgical management of previously untreated glomus jugulare tumors. Laryngoscope 104: 917–21.

Jellish WS, Murdoch J, Leonetti J 1994 Intraoperative anesthetic management of patients undergoing glomus tumor resection using a low-dose isoflurane-fentanyl technique. Skull Base Surgery 4: 82–6.

Larner JM, Hahn SS, Spaulding CA et al 1992 Glomus jugulare tumors. Long-term control by radiation therapy. Cancer 69: 1813–17.

Mather SP, Webster NR 1986 Tumours of the glomus jugulare. Anaesthesia 41: 856–60.

Troughton RW, Fry D, Allison RS et al 1998 Depression, palpitations, and unilateral pulsatile tinnitus due to a dopamine-secreting glomus jugulare tumor. American Journal of Medicine 1–4: 310–11.

Glucagonoma

A rare glucagon-secreting tumour of the alpha cells of the pancreatic islets, the majority of which have metastasised at the time of presentation. One of the group of tumours classified as APUDomas. Glucagon causes glycogenolysis, release of insulin and catecholamines, protein breakdown, lipolysis, and ketogenesis. In addition, it has positive inotropic and chronotropic effects, which are not prevented by beta adrenoceptor blockers. In a series of 21 patients with glucagonoma syndrome, 71% had weight loss, 67% necrolytic migratory erythema, 38% diabetes mellitus, 29% diarrhoea, and 29% stomatitis (Wermers et al 1996). There have only been five cases reported in the anaesthetic literature.

Preoperative abnormalities

1. The patient, more frequently a woman, may present with a bullous skin condition, known as necrolytic migratory erythema (Price et al 1989).

2. There may be weight loss, anaemia, and diarrhoea.

3. Glucose tolerance tests may show mild or frank diabetes.

4. Basal plasma glucagon levels are increased.

5. Plasma pancreatic polypeptide levels are often increased.

6. Treatment includes surgical debulking, chemotherapy and hepatic artery embolisation. Somatostatin may provide symptomatic relief and palliation.

Anaesthetic problems

1. An increased incidence of venous thrombosis.

2. Wide fluctuations in plasma glucagon levels during handling of the tumour (Nicoll & Catling 1985). The levels recorded were, however, less than those needed to produce pharmacological effects, and no cardiovascular changes were seen.

3. Fluctuations of blood sugar also occurred in three cases reported by Boskovski et al (1991), but the levels were not clinically significant.

4. Other endocrinopathies may coexist, including insulinoma and phaeochromocytoma (see Multiple endocrine neoplasia).

Management

1. Evidence of secretion of other neuroendocrine hormones should be sought.

2. Careful monitoring of intraoperative cardiovascular function and blood glucose levels (Mercadal et al 1993).

3. Octreotide may be an effective treatment for the glucagonoma syndrome (Wynick & Bloom 1991). Doses of 150–500 μg tds sc may give symptomatic relief (Wermers et al 1996).

4. Prophylaxis against thromboembolism.

Bibliography

Boskovski NA, Chapin JW, Becker GL et al 1991 Anesthesia for glucagonoma resection. Journal of Clinical Anesthesia 3: 48–52.

Mercadal M, Suarez M, Cata C et al 1993 [Anesthesia in a case of glucagonoma.] Revista Espanola de Anestesiologia y Reanomation 40: 153–5.

Nicoll JMV, Catling SJ 1985 Anaesthetic management of glucagonoma. Anaesthesia 40: 152–7.

Price ML, Darley CR, Kirkham N 1989 The glucagonoma syndrome. Journal of the Royal Society of Medicine 82: 553–4.

Wermers RA, Fatourechi V, Wynne AG et al 1996 The glucagonoma syndrome. Clinical and pathologic features in 21 patients. Medicine 75: 53–63.

Wynick D, Bloom SR 1991 Clinical review 23. The use of long-acting somatostatin analog octreotide in the treatment of gut neuroendocrine tumours. Journal of Clinical Endocrinology & Metabolism 73: 1–3.

Glucose-6-phosphate dehydrogenase deficiency (G6PDD)

A sex-linked, hereditary abnormality in which the activity or stability of the enzyme glucose-6-phosphate dehydrogenase (G6PD) is severely decreased. It is most commonly found among blacks and people of Mediterranean origin. It is also found in North European and South East Asian populations. G6PD is an essential enzyme for glucose metabolism in the pentose phosphate pathway within the RBC. This pathway is ultimately involved in the production of reduced glutathione, and the reduction of methaemoglobin within the RBC. When G6PD activity is impaired, the accumulation of methaemoglobin, and a deficiency of reduced glutathione, alter cell integrity. Globin precipitates, known as Heinz bodies, are produced and the RBCs become more prone to haemolysis. Several variants of the A and B G6PD subtypes have been described, resulting in different clinical severity. Management is directed towards the avoidance of a variety of oxidant stimulants which initiate haemolysis (Martin & Casella 1991).

Preoperative abnormalities

1. With rare exceptions, the only clinical manifestation of G6PD deficiency is haemolytic anaemia. Usually the anaemia is episodic and is associated with stress, most notably drug administration, infection, the newborn period, and, in certain individuals, exposure to fava beans (favism). Drugs known to cause haemolysis in G6PD-deficient subjects include: acetanilid, primaquine, certain sulphonamides, tolbutamide, nitrofurantoin, the sulphones, methylene blue, nalidixic acid, high-dose aspirin, vitamin C in very high doses, vitamin K, phenacetin, and nitrates. Chloramphenicol, quinidine and quinine affect those with the Mediterranean form of the condition only. Two to 5 days after ingestion of one of these drugs, there may be abdominal or back pain and jaundice associated with a decrease in haemoglobin level. Heinz bodies appear in the blood during this period.

2. Chronic nonspherocytic haemolytic anaemia, with jaundice. Splenomegaly may be seen occasionally. The anaemia is not usually severe, but in some instances there is a need for frequent transfusions.

3. There is an increased incidence of cataracts and vitreous haemorrhage.

Anaesthetic problems

1. Drug-induced haemolysis can occur after administration of any of the above drugs.

However, haemolysis has occurred intraoperatively in the absence of these drugs (Sazama et al 1980), and the possibility that it was initiated by a stress reaction, or red cell damage during cardiopulmonary bypass, was considered.

2. Infection is another important precipitant of haemolytic anaemia (Beutler 1994).

3. Infants are more susceptible to oxidative stress than adults (Martin & Casella 1991).

4. The appearance of postoperative jaundice may cause confusion as to its origin (Shapley & Wilson 1973).

5. G6PD-deficient individuals may be sensitive to overdoses of prilocaine and sodium nitroprusside, not as a result of methaemoglobinaemia as sometimes stated, but because of the concurrent production of oxidising chemicals which can produce haemolysis (Smith & Snowden 1987). If clinically significant toxic methaemoglobinaemia occurs in a G6PDD patient, methylene blue is ineffective in treatment and may itself cause haemolysis (Rosen et al 1971, Smith & Snowden 1987). Cyanosis occurred in a young woman during laparoscopy, when tubal patency was being checked, 30 min after injection of methylene blue. The SpO$_2$ was 86%, but on blood gases oxygen levels were normal. Low levels of G6PD were found (Bilgin et al 1998).

6. Malignant hyperthermia was reported to have occurred in a patient with G6PD deficiency (Younker et al 1984). However, there was no mention of confirmation of the diagnosis of MH, with standard muscle tests.

Management

1. Elective surgery should not be undertaken during a haemolytic episode, or in the presence of an infection.

2. Agents known to produce haemolysis should be avoided. Particular care should be taken not to exceed the maximum safe doses of

sodium nitroprusside or prilocaine (Smith & Snowdon 1987, Martin & Casella 1991).

3. A folic acid supplement may be required.

4. Safe drugs include benzhexol, chloroquine, paracetamol, aspirin, l-Dopa, phenacetin, phenytoin, streptomycin, phenylbutazone, trimethoprim. For a complete safe list of drugs, see Beutler (1994).

Bibliography

Beutler E 1994 G6PD Deficiency. Blood 84: 3613–36.

Bilgin H, Ozcan B, Bilgin T 1998 Methemoglobinemia induced by methylene blue perturbation during laparoscopy. Acta Anaesthesiologica Scandinavica 42: 594–5.

Martin LD, Casella ES 1991 Anesthesia and glucose-6-phosphate dehydrogenase deficiency in a child with congenital heart disease. Journal of Cardiovascular & Vascular Anesthesia 5: 596–9.

Mason PJ 1996 New insights into G6PD deficiency. British Journal of Haematology 94: 585–91.

Mehta AB 1994 Glucose-6-phosphate dehydrogenase deficiency. Postgraduate Medical Journal 70: 871–7.

Rosen PJ, Johnson C, McGehee WG et al 1971 Failure of methylene blue treatment in toxic methemoglobinemia. Association with glucose-6-phosphate dehydrogenase deficiency. Annals of Internal Medicine 75: 83–6.

Sazama K, Klein HG, Davey RJ et al 1990 Intraoperative hemolysis: the initial manifestation of glucose-6-phosphate dehydrogenase deficiency. Archives of Internal Medicine 140: 845–6.

Shapley JM, Wilson JR 1973 Post-anaesthetic jaundice due to glucose-6-phosphate dehydrogenase deficiency. Canadian Anaesthetists' Society Journal 20: 390–2.

Smith CL, Snowdon SL 1987 Anaesthesia and glucose-6-phosphate dehydrogenase deficiency. Anaesthesia 42: 281–8.

Younker D, DeVore M, Hartlage P 1984 Malignant hyperthermia and glucose-6-phosphate dehydrogenase deficiency. Anesthesiology 60: 601–3.

Glycogen storage diseases

A group of genetic diseases in which there are defects in enzymes concerned with either the

Type	Enzyme deficiency	Affected organs
0	glycogen synthase deficiency	liver
I	glucose-6-phosphatase	liver and kidneys
II	alpha-1,4 glucosidase	skeletal and cardiac muscle
III	amylo-1,6 glucosidase	liver, skeletal and cardiac muscle and blood cells
IV	amylo-1,4 to 1,6-transglucosidase	liver, skeletal and cardiac muscle and blood cells
V	muscle phosphorylase	muscle
VI	liver phosphorylase	liver and white blood cells
VII	phosphoglucomutase	muscle
VIII	muscle fructokinase	muscle and red blood cells

breakdown or the branching of glycogen. The current classification is:

0— glycogen synthase deficiency

I—von Gierke's

II—Pompe's

III—Cori's, Forbes

IV—Andersen's

V—McArdle's

VI—Hers'

VII—Thompson

VIII—Tarin

The classifications are described in further detail in the table above.

The commonest of the diseases are dealt with under the individual names; see von Gierke's, Pompe's, McArdle's and Hers' diseases. Glycogen 0, which is not on the original Cori classification, is secondary to a deficiency of glycogen synthase activity in the liver. This produces fasting hypoglycaemia and hyperketonaemia, which alternates with postprandial hyperglycaemia and hyperlactic acidaemia (Wolfsdorf et al 1999).

Bibliography

Burchell A 1998 Glycogen storage diseases and the liver. Baillieres Clinical Gastroenterology 12: 337–54.

Casson H 1975 Anaesthesia for portacaval bypass in patients with metabolic disease. British Journal of Anaesthesia 47: 969–75.

Cox JM 1968 Anesthesia and glycogen-storage disease. Anesthesiology 29: 1221–5.

Edelstein G, Hirshman CA 1980 Hyperthermia and ketoacidosis during anesthesia in a child with glycogen storage disease. Anesthesiology 52: 90–2.

Ellis FR 1980 Inherited muscle disease. British Journal of Anaesthesia 52: 153–64.

Lee PJ, Leonard JV 1995 The hepatic glycogen storage diseases—problems beyond childhood. Journal of Inherited Metabolic Disease 18: 462–72.

Mendoza A, Fisher NC, Duckett J et al 1998 Successful pregnancy in a patient with type III glycogen storage disease managed with cornstarch supplements. British Journal of Obstetrics & Gynaecology 105: 677–80.

Wolfsdorf JI, Holm IA, Weinstein DA 1999 Glycogen storage diseases. Phenotypic, genetic, and biochemical characteristics, and therapy. Endocrine & Metabolism Clinics of North America 28: 801–23.

Goldenhar's syndrome

An inherited condition, the alternative name of which is oculo-auriculo-vertebral dysplasia. Two criteria are required for a diagnosis; an eye abnormality associated with any two of the three following: ear, mandibular, or vertebral anomalies (Feingold & Baum 1978). Anaesthesia is needed for ocular, cardiac or orthopaedic surgery.

Preoperative abnormalities

1. Ocular abnormalities include coloboma of the eyelid, epibulbar dermoid, subconjunctival lipoma, and defects of the extraocular muscles.

2. Micrognathia, maxillary hypoplasia, and cleft or high arched palate.

3. Orthopaedic abnormalities include vertebral anomalies (40%), club foot, congenital dislocation of the hip, Sprengel's deformity, and radial limb defects.

4. Cervical anomalies and basilar impression can occur (Gosain et al 1994, Manaligod et al 1999). Radiographic evidence of fusion of the cervical vertebrae was present in 11 out of 18 patients.

5. A range of cardiac defects (35%) have been reported: Fallot's tetralogy, ventricular septal defect, transposition of the great vessels, and total anomalous pulmonary venous drainage.

6. Mental retardation is usual.

7. There may be abnormalities of the immune system.

Anaesthetic problems

1. Mask ventilation may be difficult.

2. Problems with tracheal intubation have been reported (Stehling 1978, Cooper & Murray-Wilson 1987, Mohandas & Selvarajah 1988, Madan et al 1990), although only one patient out of 17 in Madan's series produced problems. These difficulties may be secondary to either facial or vertebral abnormalities.

3. Incidence of obstructive sleep apnoea.

4. Problems of associated congenital heart disease.

Management

1. Careful clinical assessment of upper airway problems. A child with a history of respiratory distress underwent respiratory inductance plethysmography and pulse oximetry before surgery, to assess the patency of the upper airway during sleep. Results did not suggest the presence of severe obstruction, therefore inhalation induction was undertaken (Aoe et al 1990).

2. Intubation problems may be resolved by tracheostomy (Stehling 1978), retrograde intubation (Cooper & Murray-Wilson 1987), a laryngeal mask airway (Bahk et al 1999), awake fibreoptic intubation via a laryngeal mask airway (Johnson & Sims 1994), or fibreoptic intubation using a guidewire or a mask adaptor (Okuyama et al 1994).

3. Management of associated abnormalities. Management of a neonate with transposition of the great vessels and hydrocephalus has been described (Scholtes et al 1987).

Bibliography

Aoe T, Kohchi T, Mizuguchi T 1990 Respiratory inductance plethysmography and pulse oximetry in the assessment of upper airway patency in a child with Goldenhar's syndrome. Canadian Journal of Anaesthesia 37: 369–71.

Bahk J-H, Han S-M, Kim S-D 1999 Management of difficult airways with a laryngeal mask airway under propofol anaesthesia. Paediatric Anaesthesia 9: 163–6.

Cooper CMS, Murray-Wilson A 1987 Retrograde intubation. Management of a 4.8 kg, 5-month infant. Anaesthesia 42: 1197–200.

Feingold M, Baum J 1978 Goldenhar's syndrome. American Journal of Diseases of Children 132: 136–8.

Gallagher DM, Hyler RL, Epker N 1990 Hemifacial microsomia: an anesthetic airway problem. Oral Surgery 49: 2–4.

Gosain AK, McCarthy JG, Pinto RS 1994 Cervicovertebral anomalies and basilar impression in Goldenhar syndrome. Plastic & Reconstructive Surgery 93: 498–506.

Johnson CM, Sims C 1994 Awake fibreoptic intubation via a laryngeal mask in an infant with Goldenhar's syndrome. Anaesthesia & Intensive Care 22: 194–7.

Madan R, Trikha A, Ventataraman RK et al 1990 Goldenhar's syndrome: an analysis of anaesthetic management. A retrospective study of seventeen cases. Anaesthesia 45: 49–52.

Manaligod JM, Bauman NM, Menezes AH et al 1999 Cervical vertebral anomalies in patients with anomalies of the head and neck. Annals of Otology, Rhinology & Laryngology 108: 925–33.

Mohandas K, Selvarajah S 1988 Failed intubation in a case of oculoauriculovertebral dysplasia (Goldenhar's syndrome). Medical Journal of Malaysia 43: 255–8.

Okuyama M, Imai M, Fujisawa E et al 1994 [Fiberscopic intubation under general anesthesia for children with Goldenhar syndrome. Japanese.] Masui—Japanese Journal of Anesthesiology 43: 1885–8.

Scholtes JL, Veyckemans F, Obbergh LV et al 1987 Neonatal anaesthetic management of a patient with Goldenhar's syndrome with hydrocephalus. Anaesthesia & Intensive Care 15: 338–40.

Stehling L 1978 Goldenhar's syndrome and airway management. American Journal of Diseases of Children 132: 818.

Goodpasture's syndrome

A rapidly progressive syndrome of glomerulonephritis and pulmonary haemorrhage, in association with antibodies to glomerular basement membrane (anti-GBM) type IV collagen, detectable in plasma by radioimmunoassay and by immunofluorescence techniques on muscle biopsy. These antibodies cross-react with alveolar basement membrane, although those individuals with lung haemorrhage are usually smokers, and those with isolated anti-GBM nephritis are nonsmokers. The term is often applied more loosely, to any disease with pulmonary haemorrhage and glomerulonephritis, whether or not anti-GBM antibodies are present (Holdsworth et al 1985, Lee & Marks 1999). Systemic vasculitides such as PAN and Wegener's granulomatosis cause lung haemorrhage and renal failure, but without the antibodies.

Preoperative abnormalities

1. Usually presents with cough, dyspnoea, haemoptysis (that can be massive), and anaemia.

2. The pulmonary lesions proceed to interstitial fibrosis, with haemosiderin deposits. Lung function tests show a restrictive type of abnormality (Ball & Young 1998).

3. Glomerulonephritis, which usually follows or coincides with pulmonary lesions, may produce proteinuria, haematuria, and casts. The end result is renal failure.

4. Treatment may be with corticosteroids for pulmonary haemorrhage, cytotoxic drugs to stop renal damage, and plasmapheresis to remove antibodies (Kelly & Haponik 1994).

Anaesthetic problems

1. Poor respiratory function with hypoxaemia and respiratory alkalosis.

2. Pulmonary haemorrhage that may, on occasions, be life-threatening (Klasa et al 1988).

3. Impaired renal function and sometimes renal failure.

4. Hypochromic anaemia and a high ESR.

5. Patients may be receiving immunosuppressives or steroids, or undergoing plasma exchange, with the aim of reducing the antibody titre. Plasma exchange may reduce levels of plasma cholinesterase.

Management

1. Preoperative assessment of lung function and, in particular, blood gases. Elective pulmonary surgery should not be undertaken during periods of active haemorrhage.

2. Assessment of renal function and appropriate management.

3. The management of a successful pregnancy has been described (Yankowitz et al 1992). It requires regular assessment of pulmonary and renal function. The use of steroids was associated with hyperglycaemia, which needed treatment with insulin. Plasmapheresis was required.

Bibliography

Ball JA, Young KR Jr 1998 Pulmonary manifestations of Goodpasture's syndrome. Antiglomerular basement membrane disease and related disorders. Clinics in Chest Medicine 19: 777–91.

Bolton WK 1996 Goodpasture's syndrome. Kidney International 50: 1753–66.

Holdsworth S, Boyce N, Thomson NM et al 1985 The clinical spectrum of acute glomerulonephritis and lung haemorrhage (Goodpasture's syndrome). Quarterly Journal of Medicine 55: 75–86.

Kalluri R 1999 Goodpasture syndrome. Kidney International 55: 1120–2.

Kelly PT, Haponik EF 1994 Goodpasture syndrome: molecular and clinical advances. Medicine 73: 171–85.

Klasa RJ, Abboud RT, Ballon HS et al 1988 Goodpasture's syndrome: recurrence after a five-year remission. American Journal of Medicine 84: 751–5.

Lee SM, Marks EA 1999 The emerging spectrum of IgA-mediated renal diseases: is there an IgA variant of Goodpasture's syndrome. American Journal of Kidney Diseases 34: 565–8.

Yankowitz J, Kuller JA, Thomas RL 1992 Pregnancy complicated by Goodpasture syndrome. Obstetrics & Gynecology 79: 806–8.

Gorham's syndrome

A nonmalignant, but sometimes fatal, syndrome of massive osteolysis complicated by lymphangiomatosis. Bone is replaced by fibrovascular tissue with capillary proliferation. A mass of proliferating, thin-walled vascular and lymphatic channels extend into adjacent bones, viscera, and soft tissues. The process often begins after minor trauma. It may result from enhanced osteoclastic activity, and interleukin-6 may have a role (Devlin et al 1996). It occurs predominantly in young people. Surgery may be required for ligation of the thoracic duct. Although grafting can be performed, resorption of the grafted bone may occur.

Preoperative abnormalities

1. Osteolysis; areas most commonly affected are the shoulder, upper arm, pelvis, jaw, thorax, and spine. Pain and discomfort may result from bone involvement and deformity, neural damage and chest problems may occur.

2. Pathological, thin-walled vascular or lymphatic channels develop in association with the osteolysis. These extend into bones, viscera, and soft tissues.

3. Pleural effusions or chylothorax may occur, and when the latter develops, it is associated with a high mortality. Malnutrition, lymphopenia and sepsis result from massive fluid and protein losses into the pleural cavity.

4. Treatment includes radiotherapy, bleomycin, ligation of thoracic duct, and bone grafts.

5. Deaths have occurred from chest wall involvement, spinal cord transection, sepsis, and pulmonary aspiration (Choma et al 1987).

Anaesthetic problems

1. Problems of reduction in lung function in the presence of an effusion or a chylothorax (McNeil et al 1996).

2. Complications associated with malnutrition from loss of protein from the chylothorax; one patient was draining 1500 ml day^{-1} (Riantawan et al 1996). Anaesthesia was reported for revision of pleurosubclavian shunt (Mangar et al 1994). Another patient developed bilateral pleural effusions following spinal decompression (Szabo & Habre 2000).

3. Vertebral destruction, vertebral collapse, and spinal cord compromise (Aoki et al 1996).

4. Mandibular and maxillary involvement (Ohya et al 1990). The disease can present with a pathological fracture after only minor trauma (Fisher & Pogrel 1990). In one patient, massive mandibular osteolysis resulted in obstructive sleep apnoea syndrome (Kayada et al 1995). Bone grafts may subsequently undergo resorption.

5. Potential difficult intubation.

6. Pregnancy has been reported in a young woman who had 70% destruction of the left hemipelvis with thigh involvement (Porter et al 1993). Severe preeclampsia and thrombocytopenia occurred, but a low forceps vaginal delivery was achieved.

Management

1. Assessment of respiratory function; blood gases, and spirometry.

2. Drainage of pleural effusion or chylothorax, if present.

3. Cervical spine screening if the cervical vertebrae are involved.

4. Calcitonin and pamidronate may reduce osteolysis.

5. CPAP device may be needed for OSA.

Bibliography

Aoki M, Kato F, Saito H et al 1996 Successful treatment of chylothorax by bleomycin for Gorham's disease. Clinical Orthopaedics & Related Research 330: 193–7.

Choma ND, Biscotti CV, Bauer TW et al 1987 Gorham's syndrome: a case report and review of the literature. American Journal of Medicine 83: 1151–16.

Devlin RD, Bone HG 3rd, Roodman GD 1996 Interleukin-6: a potential mediator of the massive osteolysis in patients with Gorham–Stout disease. Journal of Clinical Endocrinology & Metabolism 81: 1983–7.

Fisher KL, Pogrel MA 1990 Gorham's syndrome (massive osteolysis): a case report. Journal of Oral & Maxillofacial Surgery 48: 1222–5.

Freedy RM, Bell KA 1992 Massive osteolysis (Gorham's disease) of the temporomandibular joint. Annals of Otology, Rhinology & Laryngology 101: 1018–20.

Kayada Y, Yoshiga K, Takada K et al 1995 Massive osteolysis of the mandible with subsequent obstructive sleep apnea. Journal of Oral & Maxillofacial Surgery 53: 1463–5.

McNeil KD, Fong KM, Walker QJ et al 1996 Gorham's syndrome: a usually fatal cause of pleural effusion treated successfully with radiotherapy. Thorax 51: 1275–6.

Mangar D, Murtha PA, Aquilina TC et al 1994 Anesthesia for a patient with Gorham's syndrome: 'disappearing bone disease'. Anesthesiology 80: 466–8.

Ohya T, Shibata S, Takeda Y 1990 Massive osteolysis of the maxillofacial bones. Report of two cases. Oral Surgery, Oral Medicine, Oral Pathology 70: 698–703.

Porter KB, O'Brien WF, Towlsey G et al 1993 Pregnancy complicated by Gorham disease. Obstetrics & Gynecology 81: 808–10.

Riantawan P, Tansupasawasdikul S, Subhannachart P 1996 Bilateral chylothorax complicating massive osteolysis (Gorham's syndrome). Thorax 51: 1277–8.

Szabo C, Habre W 2000 Gorham syndrome. Anaesthesia 55: 157–9.

Guillain–Barré syndrome (GBS)

A collective name given to a group of acute ascending polyneuropathies in which motor involvement predominates. Some of these may have an autoimmune basis and antecedent infection, surgery and immunisations have all been implicated in their development. Two-thirds of patients have an URTI or a gastrointestinal infection 1–4 weeks before the onset of symptoms and *Campylobacter jejuni* is the most frequent antecedent pathogen, with CMV and EBV also being implicated (Hartung 1999). Almost exclusively, the target is myelin, although an axonal form may occur. The progress is variable, with advancement for 1–3 weeks, a plateau phase of several weeks, often followed by slow improvement (Ropper 1992). Diagnostic criteria have been agreed (Hahn 1998). Chronic inflammatory demyelinating neuropathy is now thought to be a continuum of GBS. Admission to an ITU is needed in about one-third of cases (Hahn 1998), and the anaesthetist may be involved in treatment of respiratory insufficiency, or for surgery. The mortality rate is 5–20%, whilst in 3% of patients the disease becomes chronic or relapsing. In a series of 79 patients admitted to the ITU (Ng et al 1995), significant complications included pulmonary infections (45.6%), hyponatraemia (25.3%), dysautonomia (19%), urinary tract infections (12.7%), and cognitive dysfunction (8.9%). Deaths can occur from sepsis, ARDS, pulmonary emboli, and unexplained cardiac arrest. Ventilator-associated pneumonia is the commonest cause, and those who died were older and more likely to have underlying pulmonary disease (Lawn & Wijdicks 1999a).

Preoperative abnormalities

1. Muscle weakness usually starts in the legs, is symmetrical, and progresses upwards at a variable rate. This progressive weakness, together with areflexia, are required for the diagnosis. Cranial nerve involvement, usually of the bulbar and facial nerves, may occur in up to 50% of cases, although involvement of other nerves has been described. One patient presented to hospital in coma, with absent brainstem reflexes (Coad & Byrne 1990), and the diagnosis was only made after CSF protein levels of $2\,gl^{-1}$ were found. In another patient, acute bilateral vocal cord paralysis was the first sign (Panosian & Quatela 1993). In some cases there is respiratory insufficiency and an inability to clear secretions. The requirement for IPPV in respiratory failure is 10–23%.

2. Mild paraesthesiae in the toes and fingertips may precede the muscle weakness.

3. Muscle pain or aching is common (50–76%). Two distinct types are reported; deep muscular pain with tenderness, and burning or hyperaesthesia in the extremities.

4. Autonomic dysfunction may produce cardiovascular instability and an impairment of normal compensatory vasoconstrictor responses. Changes of position can be accompanied by significant decreases in blood pressure. Attacks of sweating, tachycardia and hypertension may occur. Brady- and tachyarrhythmias may necessitate pacemaker insertion. Sudden deaths have occurred, probably secondary to arrhythmias. It has been suggested that the lack of respiratory variation in heart rate, which is

characteristic of autonomic dysfunction, occurs more often in the group of patients with respiratory muscle weakness who require IPPV (Oakley 1984). In those patients with autonomic complications, the mortality rate may be as high as 13%, although in specialist units a rate of only 1.3% has been quoted (Winer 1992).

5. The CSF protein content is elevated, with no increase in cell count.

6. Characteristic electrodiagnostic features may be present.

Anaesthetic problems

1. If the intercostal muscles are affected, respiration and sputum clearance may be compromised. Bulbar weakness may result in pulmonary aspiration and segmental collapse. One patient had such severe involvement of the cranial nerves that an initial, mistaken diagnosis of brainstem death was made (Coad & Byrne 1990). Subsequently, full recovery took place.

2. Autonomic dysfunction can produce postural variations in blood pressure and profound hypotension on induction of anaesthesia. Cardiovascular collapse has occurred immediately after the administration of a spinal anaesthetic (Perel et al 1977). This was thought to be caused by a combination of hypotension secondary to sympathetic blockade, and a 30 degrees head-up tilt.

3. Pain may be a troublesome feature and is difficult to treat.

4. Administration of suxamethonium may be associated with transient severe hyperkalaemia and cardiac arrest (Dalman & Verhagen 1994). In one patient, asystole after suxamethonium was subsequently followed by rhabdomyolytic renal failure (Hawker et al 1985).

5. Hyponatraemia may occur, as a result of inappropriate ADH secretion. In one series of 79 patients admitted to the ITU, about 25% had hyponatraemia (Ng et al 1995).

6. Guillain–Barré syndrome has been

described during pregnancy, under which circumstances decisions are required about the method of analgesia, anaesthesia, and delivery (McGrady 1987). A chronic demyelinating polyneuropathy presented suddenly at 25 weeks' pregnancy (Nwosu et al 1999). Cardiac arrest after suxamethonium was reported in a pregnant patient who had recently recovered from GBS (Feldman 1990).

7. Weakness following general anaesthesia occurred in a patient who failed to disclose a previous history of GBS (Sibert & Sladen 1994). In another patient, the onset of GBS began with leg weakness 48 h following major colorectal surgery. Morphine 2 mg in 10 ml had been given through an epidural catheter for postoperative pain relief. The subsequent clinical course, EMG and CSF findings supported the diagnosis of GBS (Collier 1994).

Management

1. In the presence of decreasing respiratory function, IPPV may be required. Vital capacity should be measured 4-hrly during the phase of deterioration. The use of accessory muscles of respiration, and the reduction of vital capacity to 1 litre (or 15 ml kg^{-1}), presages respiratory failure. Facial weakness is an ominous sign. The institution of IPPV may be accompanied by hypotension. Tracheostomy is required when prolonged ventilation is anticipated (Lawn & Wijdicks 1999b).

2. In patients who need IPPV, continuous cardiac monitoring is required. It has been suggested that regularity of the heart rate, measured by minimal R–R interval variation on deep breathing, may indicate autonomic failure and the possibility of sudden death as a result of arrhythmias (Oakley 1984) (see Autonomic failure). Pacemaker insertion may have to be considered. When tachycardia compromises cardiac output, beta adrenoceptor blockade may be considered. The use of esmolol has been described for this purpose (Calleja 1990).

3. Multicentre controlled trials of both

plasma exchange and high-dose intravenous immunoglobulin have showed benefit, if given early. Randomised trials of plasma exchange, immunoglobulin, or both, given in the first 2 weeks after onset of symptoms, showed no difference in outcome (van der Meche et al 1992, Winer 1992, Anonymous 1997). Plasma exchange is usually given about five times over 1–2 weeks and Sandoglobulin 0.4 g kg^{-1} for 5 days.

4. General care includes:

a) Physiotherapy for the chest, with passive movements for the limbs.

b) Nasogastric feeding. Constipation should be anticipated, with the use of stool softeners or enemas.

c) Psychological management. The patient may be very frightened, and constant reassurance is needed. Depression is a frequent problem in the later stages.

d) Prevention of thromboembolic complications.

5. Epidural opiates have been used for the treatment of intractable pain (Connelly et al 1990).

6. If general anaesthesia is required, suxamethonium should be avoided, even after recovery from GBS.

7. Epidural anaesthesia has been used both for Caesarean section and pain relief (McGrady 1987, Connelly et al 1990).

Bibliography

Anonymous 1997 Randomised trial of plasma exchange, intravenous immunoglobulin, and combined treatments in Guillain–Barré syndrome. Plasma Exchange/Sandoglobulin Guillain–Barré Syndrome Trial Group. Lancet 349: 225–30.

Calleja MA 1990 Autonomic dysfunction and Guillain–Barré syndrome. The use of esmolol in its management. Anaesthesia 45: 736–7.

Coad NR, Byrne AJ 1990 Guillain–Barré syndrome mimicking brainstem death. Anaesthesia 45: 456–7.

Collier CB 1994 Postoperative paraplegia: an unusual case. Anaesthesia & Intensive Care 22: 293–5.

Guillain–Barré syndrome (GBS)

Connelly M, Shagrin J, Warfield C 1990 Epidural opioids for the management of pain in a patient with the Guillain–Barré syndrome. Anesthesiology 72: 381–3.

Dalman JE, Verhagen WI 1994 Cardiac arrests in Guillain–Barré syndrome and the use of suxamethonium. Acta Neurologica Belgica 94: 259–61.

Feldman JM 1990 Cardiac arrest after succinylcholine administration in a pregnant patient recovered from Guillain–Barré syndrome. Anesthesiology 72: 942–4.

Hahn AF 1998 Guillain–Barré syndrome. Lancet 352: 635–41.

Hartung HP 1999 Infections and the Guillain–Barré syndrome. Journal of Neurology, Neurosurgery & Psychiatry 66: 277.

Hawker F, Pearson IY, Soni N et al 1985 Rhabdomyolytic renal failure and suxamethonium. Anaesthesia & Intensive Care 13: 208–9.

Lawn ND, Wijdicks EF 1999a Fatal Guillain–Barré syndrome. Neurology 52: 635–8.

Lawn ND, Wijdicks EFM 1999b Tracheostomy in Guillain–Barré syndrome. Muscle & Nerve 22: 1058–62.

McGrady EM 1987 Management of labour and delivery in a patient with Guillain–Barré syndrome. Anaesthesia 42: 899–900.

Ng KK, Howard RS, Fish DR et al 1995 Management and outcome of severe Guillain–Barré syndrome. Quarterly Journal of Medicine 88: 243–50.

Nwosu EC, Tandon S, Breeze C et al 1999 Chronic demyelinating polyneuropathy in pregnancy treated with intravenous immunoglobulin. British Journal of Obstetrics & Gynaecology 106: 174–6.

Oakley CM 1984 The heart in the Guillain–Barré syndrome. British Medical Journal 288: 94.

Panosian MS, Quatela VC 1993 Guillain–Barré syndrome presenting as acute bilateral vocal cord palsy. Otolaryngology—Head & Neck Surgery 108: 171–3.

Perel A, Reches A, Davidson JT 1977 Anaesthesia in the Guillain–Barré syndrome. Anaesthesia 32:257–60.

Rees JH 1998 Risk factors for treatment related clinical fluctuations in Guillain–Barré syndrome. Journal of Neurology, Neurosurgery & Psychiatry 64: 148–9.

Ropper AH 1992 The Guillain–Barré syndrome. New England Journal of Medicine 326: 1130–6.

Sibert KS, Sladen RN 1994 Impaired ventilatory capacity after recovery from Guillain–Barré syndrome. Journal of Clinical Anesthesia 6: 133–8.

Van der Meche FGA, Schmitz PIM and the Dutch Guillain Barre Study Group 1992 A randomized trial comparing intravenous immune globulin and plasma exchange in Guillain–Barré syndrome. New England Journal of Medicine 326: 1123–9.

Winer J 1992 Guillain–Barré syndrome revisited. British Medical Journal 304: 65–6.

Haemoglobinopathies (sickle cell disease) (see also Thalassaemia)

Normal haemoglobin (HbA) consists of a colourless protein, globin, which is made up from two alpha and two beta polypeptide chains, and four haem radicals. The haem radical is a porphyrin structure, at the centre of which is a hexavalent iron atom. Four of the valencies are occupied by the nitrogen atoms of pyrrole rings, and the fifth, by one of the globin polypeptide chains. The last one is therefore free, for haemoglobin to transport oxygen, in a reversible combination.

The haemoglobinopathies result from inherited structural alterations in one of the globin chains. The thalassaemias, on the other hand, result from inherited defects in the rate of synthesis of one or more of the globin chains.

Types of haemoglobinopathies

1. Sickle cell disease and allied disorders.

2. Haemoglobinopathies producing cyanosis.

3. Haemoglobinopathies associated with unstable haemoglobin.

4. Haemoglobinopathies producing polycythaemia.

Types of normal haemoglobin

HbA—Normal adult haemoglobin. Has two alpha and two beta chains. Ninety-eight per cent of adult molecule is in this form.

HbF—Fetal haemoglobin. Has two alpha and two gamma chains. Is gradually replaced during the first 6 months of life, but varying amounts may persist in the haemoglobinopathies and modify the disease severity.

HbA2—Forms 2.5% of adult haemoglobin. Has two alpha and two delta chains.

Sickle cell disease

A genetic abnormality of haemoglobin synthesis involving the substitution of valine for glutamic acid at the sixth amino acid position in the beta chain of the globin molecule. It occurs most frequently in blacks of African origin and in some Mediterranean races. Resistance to malaria occurs.

> Sickle cell disease—A general term encompassing all abnormal combinations in which HbS forms a part, for example HbSS, HbSC, HbSThal.
>
> Sickle cell anaemia—Refers to HbSS only.
>
> Sickle cell trait—Refers to HbAS.

The homozygous form (HbSS, sickle cell anaemia) affects 0.25% of the UK black population, while the heterozygous form (HbAS, sickle cell trait) affects up to 10%. In HbAS, the red blood cells contain 20–45% HbS, whereas in HbSS the content is 85–95% HbS.

The solubility of deoxygenated HbS is much lower than that of HbA and it has a tendency to gel. A decreased oxygen tension within the red cells is associated with stacking of the haemoglobin molecules into long crystals. The cell membrane is deformed by these molecular changes, and the red cell assumes a sickle shape. Dehydration promotes this tendency, and sickling increases the blood viscosity. Once initiated, the process can be self perpetuating. The process is complex and the precise mechanism of vaso-occlusion is not known (Steinberg 1999). However, sickle cells obstruct blood vessels, damage the endothelium, and cause vascular injury and tissue infarction. Oxygenation can reverse the sickling process in the initial stages, but repeated sickling episodes cause irreversible changes in the cell membrane. Haemolytic anaemia and jaundice occur as a result of premature destruction of these abnormal RBCs. The mean red cell life will depend on the percentage of abnormal haemoglobin within an individual cell. Cells with a majority of abnormal haemoglobin can have their life reduced from 120 days to less than 20 days.

In sickle cell anaemia, variable increases in fetal haemoglobin of up to 20% can occur. The levels may be genetically determined. High levels of HbF are advantageous, because its mixture with HbS will increase the solubility of the reduced haemoglobin and thus decrease the severity of the disease. A high level of fetal haemoglobin predicts improved survival (Platt et al 1994). Levels of HbF of 10% protect against stroke and avascular necrosis, whilst levels above 20% reduce painful crises and pulmonary complications.

A number of important observational and randomised studies have been undertaken by the Cooperative Study of Sickle Cell Disease and the Preoperative Transfusion in Sickle Cell Disease Study Group. These are prospective studies of a large number of patients, and they involve life expectancy and risk factors (Platt et al 1994), morbidity and mortality associated with surgery and anaesthesia (Koshy et al 1995), and a trial of preoperative aggressive transfusion versus conservative transfusion (Vichinksy et al 1995, Waldron et al 1999).

The median age for death in sickle cell anaemia (HbSS) was 42 years for males and 48 years for females. That for sickle cell HbC disease (HbSC) was considerably higher; 60 years for males and 68 years for females.

Acute pain teams are increasingly being involved in the management of painful sickle cell crises. Vijay et al (1998) have reviewed the anaesthetist's role in this, and in the management of acute chest syndrome.

Preoperative abnormalities

1. Sickle cell screening (Sickledex) is a rapid diagnostic test, which detects the presence of HbS, but does not distinguish HbSS from HbAS or HbSC. For elective procedures, the genotype should be determined by haemoglobin electrophoresis.

Sickle-cell trait (AS) has 55–70% HbA, 2–4% HbA_2, normal HbF, and 38–45% HbS.

Homozygous sickle-cell disease (SS) has no HbA, 2–5% HbA_2, 1–20% HbF, 75–95% HbS.

Sickle-cell HbC disease (HbSC) has no HbA, 30–50% HbC + HbA_2, 1–5% HbF, and 50–65% HbS.

2. Patients with HbSS have a severe haemolytic anaemia, whereas those with HbAS are asymptomatic and usually have a normal haemoglobin. The clinical severity of HbSC varies. Some individuals with HbSC are virtually asymptomatic, but half of them will develop symptoms during childhood and most others become symptomatic in adolescent or adult life.

3. Sickle cell disease is associated with small vessel occlusion and episodes of infarction in affected organs. These may involve bone, bone marrow, liver, spleen, brain, and lung. The episodes cause pain, pyrexia, and tachycardia. Reduced oxygen tension and acidosis cause sickling of red cells. The increased viscosity encourages stasis and sludging, which in turn produces occlusion, ischaemia, and infarction. Further hypoxia and acidosis will perpetuate the cycle.

4. Fever may denote either a crisis, or an infective focus, particularly in those who have defaulted on penicillin prophylaxis.

5. Renal problems may occur both in HbAS and HbSS. Papillary necrosis and haematuria can develop as a result of sickling in the juxtamedullary glomeruli. The concentrating capacity of the kidney is reduced and at least 2 l of fluid per day is required to excrete the normal osmolar load.

6. In HbSS, varying crises can occur.

a) The vaso-occlusive problems have been described.

b) Sequestration crises occur, particularly in infants and young children, and result from massive sudden pooling of red cells, especially in the spleen. It is the main cause of infant death in the first year of life.

c) An aplastic crisis results from sudden marrow depression, and is generally associated with infection, especially viral.

d) Haemolytic crises sometimes occur in association with glucose-6-phosphate dehydrogenase deficiency following drug therapy.

7. Infants less than 6 months old have high percentages of HbF, therefore may not require transfusion.

8. Chest syndrome is a term used for recurrent episodes of chest pain, fever, with the presence of pulmonary infiltrates on CXR. The aetiology is unclear, but multiple microinfarctions may contribute. An alternative theory is that rib infarction causes pleuritis and splinting of the ribs, leading to atelectasis (Rucknagel et al 1991).

9. Sickle cell lung disease, which comprises both perfusion and diffusion defects, results in progressive changes in blood gases and lung function. This complication contributes to the mortality in young people from pulmonary failure and cor pulmonale (Powars et al 1988). Recurrent episodes of intravascular sickling and acute chest syndrome appear to be two of the risk factors for the development of lung disease.

10. There is an increased morbidity and mortality associated with *Streptococcus pneumoniae* in the first 3 years of life. Penicillin prophylaxis, started at 2–3 months, and given twice daily up to the age of 5 years, reduces the incidence of pneumococcal sepsis.

11. Cardiovascular adaptations to sickle cell anaemia occur, even in the steady state. These consist of an increased cardiac output (70–100% higher for given Hb level), and a reduced systemic vascular resistance. Doppler ultrasound techniques showed that these changes are further accentuated in a sickle cell crisis, possibly as a result of shunting (Singer et al 1989).

12. Cerebral complications, including silent infarcts, have been reported in 17% of young patients with sickle cell disease (Kinney et al 1999).

13. Treatment in severe cases has included hydroxyurea, transfusion therapy, and bone marrow transplantation (Steinberg 1999). At present, the benefits have to be weighed against the possible complications (Cohen 1998).

Anaesthetic problems

1. Sickling of red blood cells may be precipitated by hypoxia, acidosis, cold, and hyperosmolality. Organ infarction, ischaemia, and further hypoxia, may result. The postoperative period is often the most hazardous time. Increased sickling of red blood cells occurs, with progressive decreases in the saturation of haemoglobin with oxygen.

2. In HbSS:

a) 100% oxygen saturation—some sickling occurs.

b) 65% saturation—75% of cells are sickled.

c) 50% saturation—all cells are sickled.

d) The critical Pao_2 for irreversible sickling is 5.5 kPa.

3. In HbAS:

a) If 40% HbS, sickling starts at 40% saturation.

b) The critical Pao_2 for irreversible sickling is 2.7 kPa.

4. Sickle cell trait does carry a small risk. Sudden deaths during exercise, and splenic infarcts at altitude, have been reported in the US forces literature. There appears to be an association between sickle cell trait and cerebral infarction that is more than coincidental (Radhakrishnan et al 1990). Despite statements to the contrary, anaesthetics in those with sickle cell trait have not been entirely free from complications. Adequate oxygenation cannot always be guaranteed in the perioperative period. Superior sagittal sinus thrombosis occurred in a child following eye surgery (Dalal et al 1974). Failure to detect airway obstruction and cyanosis in the recovery room, resulted in hypoxic fits, cerebral infarction, and subsequent death, in a patient with HbAS (personal

communication). In another case, cardiac arrest and subsequent maternal death occurred during Caesarean section (Anaesthetic Advisory Committee to the Chief Coroner of Ontario 1987). It was postulated that aortocaval compression had occurred, and its relief at Caesarean delivery allowed the sudden return of hypoxic, acidotic and sickled blood to the heart.

5. The recent Cooperative Studies of Sickle Cell Disease have shown that nowadays SCD carries a lower mortality from anaesthesia and surgery than was previously reported (Koshy et al 1995). In a study of 1079 procedures in 717 patients, the overall mortality within 30 days of a surgical procedure was 1.1%. Painful crisis was the commonest SCD complication and it was more common in those who had had regional anaesthesia compared with general anaesthesia. It is possible that the high incidence of pregnant patients in the regional anaesthesia group may have influenced this, since there is a relatively high complication rate in obstetric procedures. Fever was the commonest nonSCD complication. There was a beneficial effect of transfusion on painful crises.

6. Patients with sickle cell states who are shocked, hypoxic and acidotic are difficult to resuscitate.

7. The reduced concentrating capacity of the kidney, which tends to be progressive, means that the patient cannot compensate for dehydration. Renal manifestations of the disease may result in end-stage renal disease requiring chronic haemodialysis or renal transplantation (Gyasi et al 1990).

8. Some cases of von Willebrand's disease have been reported in association with HbSS and HbAS in patients presenting with haematuria.

9. Children less than 3 years old are at risk from sepsis, usually pneumococcal, and from acute splenic sequestration.

10. The anaesthetist or the pain team may become involved in problems of pain relief, either postoperatively, or following a sickle cell crisis (Vijay et al 1998).

11. Cholelithiasis is common, and reported incidences vary from 4% to 55%, depending on the method of diagnosis. Laparoscopic techniques are becoming common (Ware et al 1992). Nine patients had RBC transfusions to reduce HbS levels and increase the Hb to $10\,g\,dl^{-1}$. In one patient, conversion to open cholecystectomy was required because of intraoperative hypoxaemia and high pulmonary airway pressures (Cunningham & Schlanger 1992). The patient was only admitted on the morning of surgery and no formal assessment of lung disease had been made.

12. Problems of adenotonsillectomy (Derkay et al 1991).

13. Postoperative problems. Acute chest syndrome is the most common serious postoperative problem, and it has been reported in about 10% of patients (Delatte et al 1999). The average peak incidence is 72 h, and average duration is 8 days. The syndrome may be fatal, and those with existing lung disease are most at risk. Painful crises may prolong hospital stay. Pulmonary embolism can also occur.

14. Pregnancy carries a high risk of sickling complications, and had a higher rate of Caesarean section, anaemia, preeclampsia and preterm delivery than a comparable group (Howard et al 1995).

Management

1. Diagnosis. Sickle cell screening should be done in at-risk populations before anaesthesia, even when the Hb is normal. A normal haemoglobin can also occur in patients with HbSC disease, yet severe sickling can take place.

2. Generally, a multidisciplinary team is involved.

3. Preoperative transfusion therapy. A number of large studies have shown that for intermediate or high risk surgical procedures, a conservative transfusion regimen (correcting the anaemia to an Hb of $10\,g\,dl^{-1}$) produced no difference in postoperative SCD complications, compared

with an aggressive one (lowering the HbS level to less than 30%). In addition, the conservative approach (adults: average transfusion 2.5 u, median value HbS 59%) versus aggressive (5 u and HbS 31%), had only half as many transfusion-related complications. These included the appearance of new antibodies and haemolytic reactions (Vichinsky et al 1995). For elective gall bladder surgery (Haberkern et al 1997), and adenotonsillectomy (Waldron et al 1999), similar conservative transfusion regimens were supported, again after large studies. A laparoscopic approach to elective cholecystectomy and splenectomy is also suggested.

4. When surgery is required, admission to hospital 24 h in advance to allow optimal hydration with iv fluids.

5. Lung function should be assessed.

6. Manoeuvres to prevent sickling of red blood cells:

a) Hypoxia in both the arterial and venous sides of the circulation must be avoided. Monitoring of both arterial and central venous P_{O_2} may be useful.

b) Acidosis must not occur. A mild respiratory alkalosis can be maintained by IPPV.

c) Body temperature is monitored and maintained. Hypothermia increases sickling and blood viscosity, which result in stasis.

d) Local circulatory stasis is prevented. Increased oxygen extraction, possibly producing dangerously low venous P_{O_2} levels despite a normal Pa_{O_2}, is avoided. Vasopressors should preferably not be given. Although it has been recommended that tourniquets should not be used, two studies suggest that they are safe, provided oxygenation and acid–base status are normal (Stein & Urbaniak 1980, Abu-Gyamfi et al 1993). However, some of the patients had relative protection from high HbF levels. During labour, precautions against aortocaval compression are essential. Epidural anaesthesia was reported to have improved a sickle cell crisis involving the extremities, in a patient in active labour (Finer et al 1988).

e) Dehydration, which increases sickling, must be avoided. The decreased concentrating capacity of the kidney accentuates the problem.

f) In a patient undergoing femoropopliteal bypass for claudication, before arterial cross clamping, the leg was raised and the femoral artery compressed to reduce the amount of blood within the limb (Vipond & Caldicott 1998).

7. Elective surgery should not take place in the presence of infection, because a crisis may be precipitated.

8. Management of vaso–occlusive crisis.

a) General measures of rest, warmth, rehydration, and simple analgesics.

b) Treat infection promptly.

c) Pain relief. PCA with morphine was compared with iv morphine for sickle cell crises and found to be equally safe and effective (Gonzalez et al 1991).

d) Chemotherapeutic agents such as hydroxyurea (Davies 1991).

9. Management of acute chest syndrome. Intravenous dexamethasone $0.3 \, mg \, kg^{-1}$ every 12 h for four doses has been found to have a beneficial effect (Bernini et al 1998).

10. Penicillin prophylaxis.

11. Although the use of a cell saver has been proposed (Romanoff et al 1988), this has been questioned because of the 50% incidence of sickling that was observed when the processed blood was examined under the microscope (Brajtbord et al 1989). This was attributed to the cell-saver washing process.

12. Exchange transfusion from 28 weeks is

associated with a decreased risk of third trimester and peripartum complications (Howard et al 1995).

Bibliography

Abu-Gyamfi Y, Sankarankutty M, Marwa S 1993 Use of a tourniquet in patients with sickle-cell disease. Canadian Journal of Anaesthesia 40: 24–7.

Anaesthesia Advisory Committee to the Chief Coroner of Ontario 1987 Intraoperative death during Caesarean section in a patient with sickle cell trait. Canadian Journal of Anaesthesia 34: 67–70.

Bernini JC, Rogers ZR, Sandler ES et al 1998 Beneficial effects of intravenous dexamethasone in children with mild to moderately severe acute chest syndrome complicating sickle cell disease. Blood 92: 3082–9.

Brajtbord D, Johnson D, Ramsay M et al 1989 Use of the cell saver in patients with sickle cell trait. Anesthesiology 70: 878.

Cohen AR 1998 Sickle cell disease—new treatments, new questions. New England Journal of Medicine 339: 42–4.

Cunningham AJ, Schlanger M 1992 Intraoperative hypoxemia complicating laparoscopic cholecystectomy in a patient with sickle hemoglobinopathy. Anesthesia & Analgesia 75: 838–43.

Dalal FY, Schmidt GB, Bennett EJ et al 1974 Sickle-cell trait. A report of postoperative neurological complication. British Journal of Anaesthesia 46: 387–8.

Davies SC 1991 The vaso-occlusive crisis of sickle cell disease. Time for coordinated trials of new treatment. British Medical Journal 302: 1551–2.

Delatte SJ, Hebra A, Tagge EP et al 1999 Acute chest syndrome in the postoperative sickle cell patient. Journal of Pediatric Surgery 34: 188–91.

Derkay CS, Bray G, Milmoe GJ et al 1991 Adenotonsillectomy in children with sickle cell disease. Southern Medical Journal 84: 205–8.

Editorial 1991 The vaso-occlusive crisis of sickle cell disease. British Medical Journal 302: 1551–2.

Finer P, Blair J, Rowe P 1988 Epidural analgesia in the management of labour pain and sickle cell crisis. Anesthesiology 68: 799–800.

Goldberg MA, Brugnara C, Dover GJ et al 1990 Treatment of sickle cell anemia with hydroxyurea and erythropoietin. New England Journal of Medicine 323: 366–72.

Gonzalez ER, Bahal N, Hansen LA et al 1991 Intermittent injection vs patient-controlled analgesia for sickle cell crisis pain. Comparison in patients in the emergency department. Archives of Internal Medicine 151: 1373–8.

Gyasi HK, Zarroug AW, Matthew M et al 1990 Anaesthesia for renal transplantation in sickle cell disease. Canadian Journal of Anaesthesia 37: 778–85.

Haberkern CM, Neumayr LD, Orringer EP et al 1997 Cholecystectomy in sickle cell anemia patients: perioperative outcome of 364 cases from the National Preoperative Transfusion Study. Preoperative Transfusion in Sickle Cell Disease Study Group. Blood 89: 1533–42.

Howard RJ, Tuck SM, Pearson TC 1995 Pregnancy in sickle cell disease in the UK: results of a multicentre survey of the effect of prophylactic blood transfusion on maternal and fetal outcome. British Journal of Obstetrics & Gynaecology 102: 947–51.

Kinney TR, Sleeper LA, Wang WC et al 1999 Silent cerebral infarcts in sickle cell anemia: a risk factor analysis. The Cooperative Study of Sickle Cell Disease. Pediatrics 103: 640–5.

Koshy M, Chisum D, Burd L et al 1991 Management of sickle cell anemia and pregnancy. Journal of Clinical Apheresis 6: 230–3.

Koshy M, Weiner SJ, Miller ST et al 1995 Surgery and anesthesia in sickle cell disease. Blood 86: 3676–84.

Morris JS, Dunn DT, Poddar D et al 1994 Haematological risk factors for pregnancy outcome in Jamaican women with homozygous sickle disease. British Journal of Obstetrics & Gynaecology 101: 770–3.

Plante LA 1998 Transfusion issues in a gravida with sickle cell disease. Obstetrics & Gynecology 92 (4 II suppl): 712.

Platt OS, Brambilla DJ, Rosse WF 1994 Mortality in sickle cell disease. Life expectancy and risk factors for early death. New England Journal of Medicine 330: 1639–44.

Powars DP, Weidman JA, Odom-Maryon T et al 1988 Sickle cell chronic lung disease: prior morbidity and the risk of pulmonary failure. Medicine 67: 66–75.

Rahakrishnan K, Thacker AK, Maloo JC et al 1990 Sickle cell trait and stroke in the young adult. Postgraduate Medical Journal 66: 1078–80.

Rathmell JP, Viscomi CM, Ashburn MA 1997 Management of nonobstetric pain during pregnancy and lactation. Anesthesia & Analgesia 85: 1074–87.

Romanoff ME, Woodward DG, Bullard WG 1988
Autologous blood transfusion in patients with sickle
cell trait. Anesthesiology 68: 820–1.

Rucknagel DL, Kalinyak KA, Gelfand MJ 1991 Rib
infarcts and acute chest syndrome in sickle cell
diseases. Lancet 337: 831–3.

Singer M, Boghossian S, Bevan DH et al 1989
Hemodynamic changes during sickle cell crisis.
American Journal of Cardiology 64: 1211–13.

Stein RE, Urbaniak J 1980 Use of the tourniquet
during surgery in patients with sickle cell
haemoglobinopathies. Clinical Orthopaedics &
Related Research 151: 231–3.

Steinberg MH 1999 Management of sickle cell
disease. New England Journal of Medicine 340:
1021–30.

Vichinsky EP, Haberkern CM, Neumayr L et al 1995
A comparison of conservative and aggressive
transfusion regimens in the perioperative
management of sickle cell disease. New England
Journal of Medicine 333: 206–13.

Vijay V, Cavenagh JD, Yate P 1998 The anaesthetist's
role in acute sickle cell crisis. British Journal of
Anaesthesia 80: 820–8.

Vipond AJ, Caldicott LD 1998 Major vascular surgery
in a patient with sickle cell disease. Anaesthesia 53:
1204–6.

Waldron P, Pegelow C, Neumayr L et al 1999
Tonsillectomy, adenoidectomy, and myringotomy in
sickle cell disease: perioperative morbidity.
Preoperative Transfusion in Sickle Cell Disease
Study Group. Journal of Pediatric
Haematology/Oncology 21: 129–35.

Ware RE, Kinney TR, Casey JR et al 1992
Laparoscopic cholecystectomy in young patients
with sickle hemoglobinopathies. Journal of
Pediatrics 120: 58–61.

Yaster M, Tobin JR, Billett C et al 1994 Epidural
analgesia in the management of severe vaso-
occlusive sickle-cell crisis. Pediatrics 93: 310–15.

Haemophilia A (see also Haemophilia B)

Haemophilia A is a sex-linked, recessive
inherited coagulation disorder, associated with
reduced levels of Factor VIII. Males are affected,
whilst females are the carriers. For female
carriers, half of their sons will have haemophilia
and half of their daughters will be carriers. Most
female carriers are unaffected, but 10–20% will
have a substantial reduction in Factor VIII to
<40 u dl^{-1}. Rarely, instances of female deficiency
have been described, in which the mother is a
carrier and the father has haemophilia A. Under
these circumstances, the female will be at risk of
serious bleeding.

Haemophilia A is indistinguishable clinically
from haemophilia B (Christmas disease), which
is a rarer condition associated with a deficiency
of Factor IX. Haemophilia A will be dealt with
in detail, but the principles of the anaesthetic
management of haemophilia B are similar.

Recent advances in therapy include the
production of Factor VIII using recombinant
DNA technology, to reduce the risk of viral
transmission, and the use of regular or
continuous infusions as prophylaxis to prevent
orthopaedic complications.

Acquired haemophilia can occur secondary to
the development of Factor VIII inhibitors (Bossi
et al 1998). In a series of 34 patients, the mean
age was 61 (range 22–93 years), and more than
50% had an underlying cause, such as cancer or
an autoimmune disorder. A small number
presented with bleeding in the postpartum
period, and although it usually stops within 2
weeks of delivery when the antibodies disappear,
deaths have occurred during the haemorrhagic
stage.

Preoperative abnormalities

1. The clinical severity is related to Factor
VIII levels as measured by clotting assay. The
factor level can be expressed as iu ml^{-1}, or as a
percentage of normal. The normal range is
50–200 iu ml^{-1}, or 50–200%.

2. Spontaneous bleeding affects mainly joints
and muscles. Inadequately treated, recurrent joint
bleeds can lead to ankylosis and permanent joint
deformities (Rodriguez-Merchan 1998). There
is evidence that the use of prophylactic therapy,
rather than treatment of bleeding episodes only
when they occur, delays the joint problems in
those who are severely affected. However,

Factor level (%)	Clinical severity	Type of bleeding
<1	severe	frequent spontaneous bleeding
2–5	moderate	variable—some spontaneous bleeding; severe bleeding after trauma
6–15	mild	bleeding on trauma
>15	very mild	bleed only after severe trauma

prophylaxis has to start when the patient is 1–2 years old.

3. Coagulation tests detect the abnormality in intrinsic pathway with prolongation of partial thromboplastin generation. Whole blood clotting time is usually normal, except in the most severe cases. Bleeding time is normal. Definitive diagnosis is by Factor VIII:C assay.

4. Treatment is by replacement of deficient Factor VIII, either using intermediate or high purity products, or recombinant Factor VIII. For mild disease, desmopressin will release endogenous stores and increase the Factor VIII levels by two- or three-fold.

5. Complications of treatment include development of Factor VIII antibodies of varying strength in 10–20% of patients, allergic reactions, transmission of viruses, hepatitis A, B, and C, and HIV.

6. Implantable venous access devices may be used in haemophiliacs (Miller et al 1998).

7. At present, the main causes of death in severe haemophilia are AIDS and intracranial haemorrhage (Cahill & Colvin 1997). Those who received clotting factors before 1986 will also have hepatitis C.

8. Although the majority of female carriers have Factor VIII levels >50 iu dl⁻¹, in some, the activity is lower. However, there is an increase in Factor VIII levels during pregnancy.

Anaesthetic problems

1. High risk of hepatitis B, C, or AIDS in older patients.

2. The need to avoid im injections. Regional anaesthesia is contraindicated except in carriers who have Factor VIII levels >50 iu dl⁻¹. Special care is required during laryngoscopy and tracheal intubation.

3. Problems of venous access.

4. Although Factor VIII levels in female carriers are usually above 50%, there may be a wide range of Factor VIII:C activity. An 11-month-old girl who required adenoidectomy had a level of 22% and needed perioperative treatment (Harrison & Lammi 1991).

5. Desmopressin must be used with care, since hyponatraemic convulsions were associated with its use for bleeding after tonsillectomy in a 3-year-old child (Francis et al 1999).

6. Pregnancy in female carriers of haemophilia is associated with a high incidence of primary (22%) and secondary (11%) haemorrhage (Kadir et al 1997a). If mothers will not accept prenatal diagnosis of fetal gender, trauma to the infant may occur at delivery.

7. Peripartum acquired Factor VIII deficiency, secondary to the development of autoantibodies, can cause bleeding in the third trimester or postpartum. This is difficult to diagnose. A woman was admitted in labour at term, and 5 h after insertion of an epidural catheter, a large haematoma was noted at the site, with continual oozing of blood. At this stage, an increased APTT of 57 s (reference range 25–38 s) was the only abnormality. A presumptive diagnosis was made of lupus anticoagulant or a clotting factor deficiency. After delivery the epidural catheter accidentally fell out and the site continued to bleed at a rate

of 150 ml h^{-1}, although serial neurological examinations were normal. After extensive cryoprecipitate and blood transfusions, a diagnosis of acquired haemophilia, as a result of Factor VIII inhibitor, was made (Christie-Taylor & McAuliffe 1999). Readmission for bleeding occurred on day 15 and she was treated with Factor VIII, immunoglobulin and steroids. The inhibitor subsequently cleared. Another patient presented with postpartum bleeding at 1 week, and eventually developed a renal haematoma and intraperitoneal haemorrhage. Once again, the initial abnormality was an increased APTT (Kadir et al 1997b).

A nonparturient, admitted after a minor fall 5 days previously, developed extensive bruising, bleeding and neck swelling, which progressed to acute upper airway obstruction. Awake fibreoptic intubation was performed and subsequent haematological investigations revealed the presence of a Factor VIII inhibitor (Joynt et al 1996).

Management

1. Advice of a haematologist, or communication with a haemophilia centre, and knowledge of an individual patient's history, are essential.

2. Sources of Factor VIII concentrate.

a) Human freeze-dried Factor VIII. Both NHS and commercial preparations are available. All preparations are now heat treated to eliminate HIV infections.

b) Animal freeze-dried Factor VIII. Commercially produced bovine and porcine with high potency of animal Factor VIII. The material is highly antigenic and is indicated for patients with high titre Factor VIII antibodies.

c) Dose of Factor VIII (in units) = % rise needed × patient's weight in kg/1.5–2

3. Before major surgery, patients should be tested to exclude Factor VIII antibodies, and to assess the response to Factor VIII infusion.

4. During surgery, the infusion therapy should be controlled by specific factor assay. The amount and duration of treatment depends on the response to Factor VIII infusion, and its half-life (between 7 and 22 h, with an average of 12 h). It also depends on the nature of the operation and the time taken for the wound to heal. In severe haemophilia A, it is usual to give an immediate preoperative dose of 50 iu kg^{-1} of Factor VIII, and on the evening of operation a second dose of 25 iu kg^{-1}. The pre- and postinfusion Factor VIII level should be measured for the first dose. On the second day 25 iu kg^{-1} is given twice daily and continued for 7–10 days. A safe objective is to keep the post-infusion Factor VIII near 100% and the pre-infusion level near 50% for the first week postoperatively. Daily assays are thus needed for the first week, then less frequently. After 7–10 days, it is usually safe to reduce the frequency of doses from twice to once daily. If Factor VIII level is found to be particularly low in individual patients, then more frequent administration of Factor VIII is needed. Continuous infusions of concentrates during and after surgery are currently being assessed (Menart et al 1998, Rochat et al 1999).

5. In mild haemophiliacs undergoing minor surgery or dental extraction, the iv infusion of desmopressin in a dose of 0.3 μg kg^{-1} in 50 ml saline 0.9% will give a short-term increase in Factor VIII. Water retention may occur. Stimulation of the fibrinolytic system necessitates the simultaneous use of tranexamic acid.

6. Dental surgery may be carried out if covered by a single dose of Factor VIII, 25–30 iu kg^{-1}. Tranexamic acid 10 mg kg^{-1} iv is given initially, then 15 mg kg^{-1} tds orally is continued for 10 days. Postoperatively, infection predisposes to bleeding, so prophylactic antibiotics are needed.

7. Essential ENT surgery is possible, provided strict guidelines are adhered to (Conlon et al 1996). These include the use of Factor VIII (or Factor IX) 30 min before surgery, with

postinfusion levels checked at 20 min. Treatment needs to be continued 10 days after operation. Tranexamic acid 1 g iv and 500 mg qds may also be given. For myringotomies in mild cases with levels >10%, desmopressin $0.4 \mu g\,kg^{-1}$ is given in 100 ml saline over 15–30 min 1 h before surgery.

8. The presence of Factor VIII antibody is a contraindication to surgery, except when life-saving. Under such circumstances large doses have to be given.

9. Analgesia must be carefully managed. In the above series, persistence of bleeding was sometimes related to the inadvertent use of aspirin-containing compounds or NSAIDs. Mild pain should be treated with paracetamol, pentazocine, dihydrocodeine, or buprenorphine. Opiate analgesics should be used with caution to prevent addiction.

10. There are now guidelines for the management of pregnancy in female carriers, and a multidisciplinary approach is essential (Walker et al 1994, Kadir et al 1997a).

    a) Levels should be checked early in pregnancy and at 28 and 30 weeks.

    b) Knowledge of fetal gender will influence management. In an affected male, traumatic delivery should be avoided.

    c) Those with levels <50 iu dl⁻¹ will need prophylaxis for any surgical procedure and for delivery. In pregnant patients, recombinant Factor VIII should be used.

    d) During labour, a coagulation screen and factor assay are needed. If levels are <50 iu dl⁻¹, prophylaxis should be given.

    e) A vaginal delivery is preferable. Epidural anaesthesia for vaginal delivery, and spinal anaesthesia for Caesarean, have been suggested for women whose factor levels are >50 iu dl⁻¹ (Kadir et al 1997a).

    f) A cord blood sample should be taken into a citrated tube and sent to a haematologist within 2 h.

11. In the rare event of acquired haemophilia of pregnancy secondary to Factor VIII antibodies, suspect the diagnosis if there is unexplained bleeding postpartum and an abnormal APTT. Reduced Factor VIII activity and the identification of antibodies will confirm the diagnosis. Treatment will require blood, Factor VIII replacement (possibly with porcine Factor VIII), and immunosuppressive treatment with steroids and iv immunoglobulin. For details see Walker et al (1994) and Kadir et al (1997b).

Haemophilia B (Christmas disease) (see also Haemophilia A)

A sex-linked recessive inherited coagulation disorder associated with reduced levels of Factor IX.

Preoperative abnormalities

1. For clinical features and severity see Haemophilia A.

2. Coagulation tests detect the abnormality in intrinsic pathway and the definitive diagnosis is made on Factor IX assay.

Anaesthetic problems

See Haemophilia A.

Management

1. The principles of treatment for major surgery and dental extraction are the same as in haemophilia A. However, desmopressin is not effective in Factor IX deficiency.

2. Treatment is by replacement with Factor IX concentrates (both NHS and commercial). A combination of purified Factor IX and tranexamic acid for prophylaxis against bleeding during dental extraction is described (Djulbegovic et al 1996).

3. The recovery of Factor IX is less than in Factor VIII, so the dose required is greater:

Dose of Factor IX in units = % rise needed × patient's weight in kg/0.9

Bibliography

Bossi P, Cabang J, Ninet J et al 1998 Acquired hemophilia due to factor VIII inhibitors in 34 patients. American Journal of Medicine 105: 400–8.

Cahill MR, Colvin BT 1997 Haemophilia. Postgraduate Medical Journal 73: 201–6.

Christie-Taylor GA, McAuliffe GL 1999 Epidural placement in a patient with undiagnosed acquired haemophilia from Factor VIII inhibitor. Anaesthesia 54: 367–71.

Conlon B, Daly N, Temperely I et al 1996 ENT surgery in children with inherited bleeding disorders. Journal of Laryngology & Otology 110: 947–9.

Donahue BS, Emerson CW, Slaughter TF 1999 Case 1—1999. Elective and emergency cardiac surgery on a patient with hemophilia B. Journal of Cardiothoracic & Vascular Anesthesia 13: 92–7.

Djulbegovic B, Marasa M, Pesto A et al 1996 Safety and efficacy of purified Factor IX concentrate and antifibrinolytic agents for dental extractions in hemophilia B. American Journal of Hematology 51: 168–70.

Donmez A, Turker H, Sekerci S et al 1999 Dealing with a hemophilia-A patient undergoing cerebral aneurysm surgery. Journal of Neurosurgical Anesthesiology 11: 214–5.

Ehrenforth S, Kreuz W, Scharrer I et al 1992 Incidence of development of Factor VIII and Factor IX inhibitors in haemophiliacs. Lancet 339: 594–8.

Francis JD, Leary T, Niblett DJ 1999 Convulsions and respiratory arrest in association with desmopressin administration for the treatment of a bleeding tonsil in a child with borderline haemophilia. Acta Anaesthesiologica Scandinavica 43: 870–3.

Harrison HC, Lammi A 1991 Adenoidectomy in a girl with haemophilia. Journal of Otology & Laryngology 105: 957–8.

Joynt GM, Wickham NWR, Young RJ et al 1996 Upper airway obstruction caused by acquired inhibitor to Factor VIII. Anaesthesia 51: 687–8.

Kadir RA, Economides DL, Braithwaite J et al 1997a The obstetric experience of carriers of haemophilia. British Journal of Obstetrics & Gynaecology 104: 803–10.

Kadir RA, Koh MB, Lee CA et al 1997b Acquired haemophilia, an unusual cause of severe postpartum haemorrhage. British Journal of Obstetrics & Gynaecology 104: 854–6.

Menart C, Petit PY, Attali O et al 1998 Efficacy and safety of continuous infusion of Mononine during five surgical procedures in three hemophiliac patients. American Journal of Hematology 58: 110–16.

Miller K, Buchanan GR, Zappa S et al 1998 Implantable access devices in children with hemophilia: a report of low infection rates. Journal of Pediatrics 132: 934–8.

Rochat C, McFadyen ML, Schwyzer R et al 1999 Continuous infusion of intermediate-purity Factor VIII in haemophilia A patients undergoing elective surgery. Haemophilia 5: 181–6.

Rodriguez-Merchan EC 1998 Management of the orthopaedic complications of haemophilia. Journal of Bone & Joint Surgery 80B: 191–6.

Sultan Y, Algiman M 1990 Treatment of Factor VIII inhibitors. Blood Coagulation and Fibrinolysis 1: 193–9.

Walker ID, Walker JJ, Colvin BT et al 1994 Investigation and management of haemorrhagic disorders in pregnancy. Haemostasis and Thrombosis Task Force Journal of Clinical Pathology 47: 100–8.

Hallervorden–Spatz disease (neuraxonal dystrophy)

Now known as neuraxonal dystrophy, this rare autosomal recessive neurodegenerative disease of the basal ganglia involves abnormalities of iron and lipid metabolism. The clinical syndrome is one of childhood onset, progressive dementia, choreoathetosis, dystonia, and spasticity. Hallervorden–Spatz disease was technically considered to be a postmortem diagnosis because only after death could the histological features of massive iron deposition in the substantia nigra and pallidal nuclei, with gliosis, demyelination, and axonal swelling, be confirmed. However, recent MRI studies have shown features in the basal ganglia thought to be specific to the disease. There is no evidence of systemic overload. Iron levels in the plasma and cerebrospinal fluid are normal, as are those of the protein-bound ferritin, transferrin, and caeruloplasmin. Stereotactic pallidotomy has been reported recently for control of severe dystonia (Jussen et al 1999).

Preoperative abnormalities

1. Clinical features of dyskinesia, spasticity, torticollis, increasing scoliosis, and severe mental retardation. Pigmentary degeneration of the retina has been decribed. There has been recent suggestion of muscle involvement with increased serum CK and histological signs of a myopathy (Maladrini et al 1995).

2. The spontaneous appearance of an NMS-like syndrome has been reported; hyperthermia, rigidity, impaired conscious level, and autonomic imbalance (Hayashi et al 1993).

3. Occasionally, late onset disease may occur. One patient presented with Parkinsonian features in a family in which all the children died before the age of 25 (Jankovic et al 1985).

4. Sea-blue histiocytes are seen on bone marrow examination.

Anaesthetic problems

1. Oropharyngeal rigidity has been reported (Roy et al 1983).

2. Swallowing disorders are common and patients tend to choke on food and secretions.

3. Noxious stimuli may intensify the dystonia.

4. It has been suggested that these patients may present spontaneously with clinical features similar to those of neuroleptic malignant syndrome, but in the absence of precipitating neuroleptic drugs (Hayashi et al 1993).

Management

1. Increasing depth of anaesthesia caused relaxation of rigidity, torticollis, and some scoliosis (Roy et al 1983). The dystonia returned on emergence.

2. Suxamethonium should be avoided.

3. The use of dantrolene for hyperthermia and muscle rigidity has been described (Hayashi et al 1993).

Bibliography

Hayashi K, Chihara E, Sawa T et al 1993 Clinical features of neuroleptic syndrome in basal ganglia disease. Spontaneous presentation in a patient with Hallervorden–Spatz syndrome in the absence of neuroleptic drugs. Anaesthesia 48: 499–502.

Jankovic J, Kirkpatrick JB, Blomquist KA et al 1985 Late-onset Hallervorden–Spatz disease presenting as familial parkinsonism. Neurology 35: 227–34.

Jussen CR, Penn RD, Kroin JS et al 1999 Stereotactic surgery in a child with Hallervorden–Spatz disease: case report. Journal of Neurosurgery 90: 551–4.

Maladrini A, Bonuccelli U, Parrotta E et al 1995 Myopathic involvement in two cases of Hallervorden–Spatz disease. Brain & Development 17: 286–90.

Roy RC, McClain S, Wise A et al 1983 Anesthetic management of a patient with Hallervorden–Spatz disease. Anesthesiology 58: 382–4.

Heart block (see also Sick sinus syndrome)

A patient may present for surgery either with a permanent pacemaker implanted, or with a bradyarrhythmia that may require the insertion of a temporary transvenous pacemaker for the perioperative period. Increasing numbers of pacemakers are being implanted, and in many cases more complex electronic devices are being used.

Preoperative abnormalities

1. Heart block may be congenital or acquired, and the latter either acute or chronic.

a) Congenital heart block may occur alone, or in association with other cardiac abnormalities. As an isolated phenomenon it is relatively benign, since the block to conduction is at the level of the AV node. The ventricular pacemaker is proximal to the bifurcation of the bundle of His, so the

QRS complexes are narrow, and the ventricular conduction system intact. The rate is relatively high and can vary from 40–80 beat min^{-1}, and may increase with exercise. However, sudden death may occasionally occur.

b) In chronic, acquired heart block the defect is more distal in the conducting system. The AV junction or bundle branches are usually involved, the QRS complexes are wide, the heart rate is lower and is not increased by exercise. The prognosis is generally worse, but ultimately depends on the underlying cause.

2. Heart block can be divided into three types:

a) First-degree AV block: PR interval prolonged beyond 0.21 s.

b) Second-degree AV block:

 i) Type I: Progressive PR lengthening until a complete failure of conduction and a beat is dropped (Wenkebach phenomenon).

 ii) Type II: Intermittent failure of AV conduction without preceding prolongation of PR interval. This type is of more serious significance than type I, and often progresses to third-degree AV block.

c) Third-degree AV block. Complete dissociation of the atria and ventricles secondary to failure of atrial impulses to be transmitted.

3. Patients may present with syncopal (Stokes–Adams) attacks, fatigue, angina, or heart failure.

Anaesthetic problems

1. Patients with second-degree heart block, particularly type II, may progress to complete heart block under anaesthesia, since most volatile agents prolong cardiac conduction. Lesser degrees of block can also deteriorate. Although it has been suggested that the combination of bifascicular block and first-degree heart block rarely constitutes a significant perioperative risk (Gauss et al 1998), problems have been reported. After induction of anaesthesia, a patient with first-degree AV block and bifascicular block proceeded to complete AV dissociation. This was unresponsive to atropine, ephedrine, isoprenaline, and external transcutaneous pacing (Mamiya et al 1999). However, transoesophageal pacing restored the blood pressure.

2. Those with complete heart block may be unable to compensate for a decrease in cardiac output by increasing their ventricular rate. Organ blood flow may be dramatically reduced. When increases in stroke volume can no longer compensate for slow heart rates, cardiac failure occurs.

3. When patients with heart block are anaesthetised, there is no method of monitoring the adequacy of cerebral blood flow, therefore cerebral damage is a risk.

4. The problems of the underlying cause. The commonest cause of third-degree AV block in the elderly is idiopathic fibrosis. However, other causes include coronary artery disease, cardiomyopathy, drugs, and cardiac surgery.

5. The use of surgical diathermy in the presence of pacemakers may produce complications:

a) Ventricular fibrillation has been reported. This was a problem with older types of pacemaker (Titel & El Etr 1968). However, ventricular fibrillation has also occurred during use of cutting diathermy in a patient who had had a temporary transvenous pacemaker inserted that was in demand mode (Andrade & Grover 1997). Accidental stimulation of myocardial leads was probably responsible for the VF that occurred during pacemaker replacement (Aggarwal et al 1996).

b) Inhibition of demand pacemaker function (Wajszczuk et al 1969), or interference with AV sequential pacemaker (Dressner & Lebowitz 1988).

c) 'Phantom' reprogramming of a programmable pacemaker (Domino & Smith 1983).

d) Idiosyncratic responses in multiprogrammable pacemakers. In one case, interference with the quartz crystal clock was interpreted as impending battery failure and the pacemaker went into a slow backup mode aimed at preserving battery life (Shapiro et al 1985).

e) Asystole occurred as a result of the diathermy indirectly causing battery drainage and pacemaker failure (Mangar et al 1991).

f) Despite improved technology, diathermy can cause the pacemaker to fail, although the mechanism is not always clear (Nercessian et al 1998, Peters & Gold 1998).

6. In the past, the use of a strong magnet over the pulse generator to change a demand pacemaker to an asynchronous one was recommended. This should not be attempted with modern pacemakers, because it may allow the electromagnetic waves of the diathermy to reprogramme and change the firing rate of the pacemaker.

7. Pacemaker failure can occur during anaesthesia. The pulse generator failed on induction of anaesthesia after administration of suxamethonium (Finfer 1991). Myopotentials were thought to have inhibited pacemaker function. Generator failure may also occur if the stimulator threshold increases above the maximum output of the generator. This has been attributed to endocardial burns following defibrillation (Finfer 1991), and the use of unipolar diathermy during TURP (Kellow 1993).

8. Pacemaker failure occurred after a magnetic instrument mat was placed on the chest of a patient before surgery started (Purday & Towey 1992). In this particular pacemaker, the application of a magnet activated the test sequence for determining the stimulation threshold for capture. This was confirmed subsequently in the cardiology clinic using the surgical magnetic mat.

9. Special problems may occur with rate-responsive pacemakers (Andersen & Madsen 1990). Changes during surgery and anaesthesia can act as a stimulus to a rate increase and result in unphysiological pacing rates. For example, respiration-sensing pacemakers may respond to manual hyperventilation by producing a tachycardia. This was initially interpreted as a sign of light anaesthesia and later on as hypovolaemia, in a patient undergoing a TURP. The pulse rate only returned to normal when the anaesthetist stopped manual ventilation in order to set up a blood transfusion (Madsen & Andersen 1989). A movement-sensing pacemaker may respond to vigorous surgical stimulation.

10. Pacemaker failure may occur during surgery. This may be due to loose connections, battery failure, displacement of a lead, or a change in pacemaker threshold.

11. Ventricular demand pacemakers do not allow sequential AV contraction, therefore left ventricular systolic performance may be decreased when pacing takes over (Ducey et al 1991). Reprogramming of the pacemaker or therapeutic suppression may be required.

12. Halothane increases the pacing threshold and should be avoided.

13. Potential problems for patients undergoing extracorporeal shock wave lithotripsy (ESWL) (Celentano et al 1992). One episode of bradycardia that responded to isoprenaline was reported, but in general, cardiac pacemakers do not seem to be damaged. In a survey of 98 units undertaking ESWL, complications were minor and in only one patient was the pacemaker spontaneously deprogrammed by lithotripsy (Drach et al 1990).

14. Patients should not undergo MRI. The magnet may cause pacemaker failure, reprogramming, or microshock.

Management

1. The indications for insertion of a transvenous pacemaker before surgery are sometimes debatable, but may include:

   a) Sinoatrial node dysfunction producing a brady/tachyarrhythmia syndrome.

   b) Second- or third-degree AV block.

   c) LBBB and first-degree heart block.

   d) Bifascicular block. RBBB in combination with posterior fascicular block often progresses to third-degree heart block (Jordaens 1996). It has therefore been suggested that bifascicular block is an indication for a temporary pacemaker. However some authors believe this to be unnecessary (Rooney et al 1976, Gauss et al 1998). No complications occurred during epidural anaesthesia in patients with RBBB and left anterior fascicular block who were asymptomatic (Coriat et al 1981). It has also been suggested that a temporary pacemaker is unnecessary in congenital complete heart block, especially in children, since the rate is usually relatively high and the prognosis good (Bennie et al 1997). However, should problems occur, temporary transvenous cardiac pacing takes time to initiate. In a prospective survey of 153 insertions, the median time was found to be 20 min (Donovan & Lee 1984). The use of transoesophageal pacemakers may be safer in an emergency situation (Mamiya et al 1999).

2. If a permanent pacemaker is already in place, information on its mode of function should be sought. All patients with pacemakers are reviewed in a pacemaker clinic. Its markings, date of insertion, and battery life are regularly checked.

a) Pacemaker markings:

   I *Chamber paced*: V = ventricle; A = atrium; D = dual (A & V).

   II *Chamber sensed*: V = ventricle; A = atrium; D = dual (A & V); O = none.

   III *Mode of response*: T = triggered; I = inhibited; D = dual (T or I); O = none.

   IV *Programmable functions*: P = programmable (rate and/or output); M = multiprogrammable; C = communicating; O = none; R = rate-response; B = bursts of impulses; N = normal rate competition.

   V *Special antitachyarrhythmic functions*: S = scanning response; E = externally activated.

b) Pacemaker type and function. The most common type of pacemaker in use is VVI. The chamber paced is the ventricle, as is the chamber sensed, and the pacemaker is inhibited by spontaneous ventricular activity. A programmable pacemaker is one in which certain parameters such as rate, sensitivity, output, and refractory period, can be changed noninvasively. This is accomplished by the use of a programmer, which sends electromagnetic coded signals to the pacemaker. Some of the multiprogrammable ones have very complex functions to treat difficult arrhythmias, and to anticipate problems such as battery failure. Although VVI will be the most frequently encountered, other types of pacemaker may be needed on occasions, to cope with individual requirements or pacing problems (Andersen & Madsen 1990). Some of these are associated with particular individual problems during anaesthesia and if a complex rate-responsive pacemaker is in use, reference to Andersen and Madsen's article is suggested.

   i) Maintenance of atrial transport. Atrial demand pacemakers (AAI) are useful in sick sinus syndrome, when atrioventricular conduction is intact. It is haemodynamically advantageous if atrial synchrony is maintained, since an atrial contribution to ventricular filling may improve the cardiac output by up to 30%, as compared with that produced by VVI pacemakers. This may be important for patients with ventricular pacing, who are experiencing symptoms suggestive of the pacemaker syndrome. Dizziness or syncope may result from hypotension from loss of atrioventricular synchrony, or from retrograde ventriculoatrial conduction.

ii) Rate responsiveness to exercise. Dual-chamber pacemakers (eg DDD) can stimulate both chambers in sequence, and if atrial activity is normal they allow a 'physiological' response to exercise. Where there is sinus disease, other variables will have to be used to assess body activity. A new generation of rate-responsive pacemakers has been developed that are responsive to various physiological variables such as respiration, temperature, QT interval, myocardial contractility, oxygen saturations, and blood pH changes.

iii) Antitachycardia pacemakers. These have been designed to detect tachycardias, then terminate them by breaking the re-entrant circuit.

c) Pacemaker threshold. If a pacemaker has not been checked recently, a cardiologist should be asked to check the pacing threshold, which is the minimum voltage necessary for the pacing stimulus to capture the ventricles consistently. Pacemaker function depends on both electrical and nonelectrical factors. The threshold for capture is dependent upon cellular factors such as acid–base balance, hypoxia, serum potassium, and drug therapy. If the threshold increases, there may be intermittent failure of pacing. If

the threshold decreases, there is a risk of inducing ventricular fibrillation.

d) Detection of pacemaker dysfunction. The occurrence of syncope may suggest pacemaker dysfunction. A 10% decrease in heart rate in a fixed rate pacemaker may indicate impending battery failure. An irregular heart rate in a VVI pacemaker means that R waves are not being sensed.

3. The use of diathermy. Advice is still usually given that this should only be used if really necessary. Although many of the modern pacemakers are said to be safe with diathermy, problems have been encountered (Mangar et al 1991, Kellow 1993). As pacemakers have become more complex, with programmes both to detect and eliminate external electrical interference, and to provide back-up for programme or battery failure, so idiosyncratic complications may arise. Two cases of apparent pacemaker malfunction have been reported that were a direct result of the complex back-up functions of the pacemaker (Shapiro et al 1985). If diathermy is needed:

a) Place the indifferent electrode of the diathermy on the same side as the operating site and as far away from the pacemaker as possible.

b) Limit its frequency and duration of use, and keep the diathermy current as low as possible.

c) Use a bipolar rather than a unipolar diathermy.

d) Check the patient's pulse for inhibition of pacemaker function.

e) With a programmable pacemaker, it might be helpful to have the programmer itself available in theatre, so that the programming could be checked at the end of the operation. However, in many cases this is not feasible.

4. Pacemaker failure. Whenever a pacemaker is in place, atropine, epinephrine (adrenaline) and isoprenaline should be available, for use in the

event of pacemaker failure. If failure to pace occurs with a temporary pacemaker:

a) Try reversing the polarity.

b) Try increasing the output to maximum.

c) Change to V00 (asynchronous) mode.

d) Check that the connections are intact.

e) Change the whole unit, or the batteries.

f) If using a bipolar lead, try each as unipolar.

g) Turn the patient into the left lateral position to improve electrode contact.

h) Change the pacing lead.

5. If pacing with a ventricular demand pacemaker results in decreased cardiac output, pacemaker suppression may be required. The use of a peripheral nerve stimulator on the ipsilateral shoulder provided a stimulus which suppressed the pacemaker and allowed the patient's normal sinus rhythm to return the blood pressure and cardiac output to normal (Ducey et al 1991).

6. Monitoring of pulse and blood pressure. Blood pressure should be carefully monitored. If the ECG is susceptible to diathermy influence, then other methods of pulse observation, such as palpation or an oesophageal stethoscope, should be used to detect pacemaker inhibition. Direct arterial monitoring is advisable in all major cases.

7. In patients requiring ESWL, the presence of a cardiologist and equipment for emergency transvenous pacing has been recommended (Drach et al 1990, Celentano et al 1992).

8. Should defibrillation be required, the paddles should be positioned as far away from the generator as possible, preferably anterior/posterior positioning. Loss of capture may occur subsequently secondary to an endocardial burn, and an increase in stimulus output may be required.

Bibliography

Aggarwal A, Farber NE, Kotter GS et al 1996 Electrosurgery-induced ventricular fibrillation during pacemaker replacement. Journal of Clinical Monitoring 12: 339–42.

Andrade AJ, Grover ML 1997 Cardiac arrest from the use of diathermy during total hip arthroplasty in a patient with an external pacemaker. Annals of the Royal College of Surgeons of England 79: 69–70.

Andersen C, Madsen GM 1990 Rate-responsive pacemaker and anaesthesia. A consideration of possible implications. Anaesthesia 45: 472–6.

Bennie RE, Dierdorf SF, Hubbard JE 1997 Perioperative management of children with third degree heart block undergoing pacemaker placement: a ten year review. Paediatric Anaesthesia 7: 301–4.

Celentano WJ, Jahr JS, Nossaman BD 1992 Extracorporeal shockwave lithotripsy in a patient with a pacemaker. Anesthesia & Analgesia 74: 770–2.

Coriat P, Harari A, Ducardonet A et al 1981 Risk of advanced heart block during extradural anaesthesia in patients with right bundle branch block and left anterior hemiblock. British Journal of Anaesthesia 53: 545–8.

Domino KB, Smith TC 1983 Electrocautery-induced reprogramming of a pacemaker using a precordial magnet. Anesthesia & Analgesia 62: 609–12.

Donovan KD, Lee KY 1984 Indications for and complications of temporary transvenous cardiac pacing. Anaesthesia & Intensive Care 13: 63–70.

Drach GW, Weber C, Donovan JM 1990 Treatment of pacemaker patients with extracorporeal shock wave lithotripsy: experience from two continents. Journal of Urology 143: 895–6.

Dressner DL, Lebowitz PW 1988 Atrioventricular sequential pacemaker inhibition by transurethral electrosurgery. Anesthesiology 68: 599–601.

Ducey JP, Fincher CW, Baysinger CL 1991 Therapeutic suppression of a permanent ventricular pacemaker using a peripheral nerve stimulator. Anesthesiology 75: 533–6.

Finfer SR 1991 Pacemaker failure on induction of anaesthesia. British Journal of Anaesthesia 66: 509–12.

Gauss A, Hubner C, Radermacher P et al 1998 Perioperative risk of bradyarrhythmias in patients with asymptomatic chronic bifascicular block or left bundle branch block: does an additional first-degree atrioventricular block make any difference? Anesthesiology 88: 679–87.

Jordaens L 1996 Are there any useful investigations that predict which patients with bifascicular block will develop third degree atrioventricular block? Heart 75: 542–3.

Kellow NH 1993 Pacemaker failure during

transurethral resection of the prostate. Anaesthesia 48: 136–8.

Madsen GM, Andersen C 1989 Pacemaker-induced tachycardia during general anaesthesia: a case report. British Journal of Anaesthesia 63: 360–1.

Mamiya K, Aono J, Manabe M 1999 Complete atrioventricular block during anaesthesia. Canadian Journal of Anaesthesia 46: 265–7.

Mangar D, Atlas GM, Kane PB 1991 Electrocautery-induced pacemaker malfunction. Canadian Journal of Anaesthesia 38: 616–18.

Morley-Davies A, Cobbe SM 1997 Cardiac pacing. Lancet 349: 41–6.

Nercessian OA, Wu H, Nazarian D et al 1998 Intraoperative pacemaker dysfunction caused by the use of electrocautery during total hip arthroplasty. Journal of Arthroplasty 13: 599–602.

Peters RW, Gold MR 1998 Reversible prolonged pacemaker failure due to electrocautery. Journal of Interventional Cardiac Electrophysiology 2: 343–4.

Purday JP, Towey RM 1992 Apparent pacemaker failure caused by activation of ventricular threshold test by a magnetic instrument mat during general anaesthesia. British Journal of Anaesthesia 69: 645–6.

Rodriguez-Merchan EC 1998 Management of the orthopaedic complications of haemophilia. Journal of Bone and Joint Surgery 80B: 191–6.

Rooney S-M, Goldiner PL, Muss E 1976 Relationship of right bundle branch block and marked left axis deviation to complete heart block during general anesthesia. Anesthesiology 44: 64–6.

Shapiro WA, Roizen MF, Singleton MA et al 1985 Intraoperative pacemaker complications. Anesthesiology 63: 319–22.

Titel JH, El-Etr AA 1968 Fibrillation resulting from pacemaker electrodes and electrocautery during surgery. Anesthesiology 29: 845–6.

Wajszczuk WJ, Mowry FM, Dugan NL 1969 Deactivation of a demand pacemaker by transurethral electrocautery. New England Journal of Medicine 280: 34–5.

HELLP syndrome (see also Eclampsia)

A rare complication of preeclampsia, it is characterised by **H**aemolysis, **E**levated **L**iver enzyme activity, and **L**ow **P**latelet count. Reported to occur in 5–10% of patients with preeclampsia, it carries a maternal mortality of 2–24% and a perinatal mortality of 8–40%. Comparisons of severity have been attempted by grading the condition according to the level of the platelet count. Class 1 $\leq 50 \times 10^9 l^{-1}$, class 2 >50 but <100 $\times 10^9 l^{-1}$, class 3 >100 $\times 10^9 l^{-1}$ to $\leq 150 \times 10^9 l^{-1}$. Most deaths occurred in class 1 patients and factors that contributed to death were delay in diagnosis, haemorrhage into the liver or brain, vascular insult to the kidneys, or cardiopulmonary arrest (Isler et al 1999). Martin et al (1999) studied the three grades of HELLP syndrome and compared them with severe preclampsia without HELLP. They appeared to represent a spectrum of disease, with decreasing morbidity.

A high proportion of patients require operative delivery: in a series of 33 patients presenting over 5 years, 94% required Caesarean section (Crosby 1991). In another study of 112 cases, there were two maternal deaths, two patients had ruptured liver haematomas, and nine had renal failure (Sibai et al 1986). In a study of 442 pregnancies, 70% cases occurred antepartum and 30% postpartum, and those arising postpartum had a significantly higher incidence of pulmonary oedema and renal failure (Sibai et al 1993). Delivery should be expedited and treatment should be supportive. Measures include control of haemorrhage, hypertension, coagulation, renal, and liver complications. There is increasing evidence that corticosteroids are beneficial (Tompkins & Thiagarajah 1999), but that plasma exchange is not. In patients who develop HELLP in one pregnancy, the risk of recurrence in a subsequent one is 19–27% (Sullivan et al 1994).

Preoperative abnormalities

1. The presence of preeclampsia or eclampsia is 100%, although this is not always severe.

2. Upper abdominal pain (65%), nausea or vomiting (36%), headaches (31%), and visual disturbances (10%), are the commonest presenting complaints (Sibai et al 1993). Clinical signs include epigastric pain and tenderness, hypertension, oedema, proteinuria, and bleeding.

3. Thrombocytopenia is present and haemolytic anaemia is of the microangiopathic

type, with an increased reticulocyte count and a peripheral film showing burr cells and schistocytes. There is increased platelet consumption and a decreased lifespan. In a study of 132 patients divided into two classes according to the platelet count (class 1 $\leq 50 \times 10^9 l^{-1}$, class 2 > 50 but $< 100 \times 10^9 l^{-1}$), those with a count $< 40 \times 10^9 l^{-1}$ were at significant risk from postpartum bleeding, whereas those above that value were not (Roberts et al 1994).

4. Jaundice and disordered liver function. Rarely, subcapsular haematoma or liver rupture has been reported (Risseeuw et al 1999).

5. Hypovolaemia, decreasing urine output, and increasing creatinine levels.

6. Other complications have included ARDS, acute renal failure, and placental abruption. Abruption was strongly correlated with the development of DIC, acute renal failure, and pulmonary oedema (Sibai et al 1993). Death may occur from cardiorespiratory failure or intracerebral haemorrhage.

7. Abnormalities of coagulation (other than thrombocytopenia) are not commonly observed, and at one time, some authors concluded that coagulopathy was not a complication. However, it occurred in three out of 33 in one series (Crosby 1991). In addition, close observation suggests that many patients develop some coagulation activation. One study compared coagulation in 15 consecutive patients with HELLP syndrome with 12 who had preeclampsia alone. Sensitive and specific coagulation assays showed that the HELLP syndrome patients had a compensated coagulopathy. These abnormalities persisted over several days indicating that there was a continuing, but mild trigger to the coagulation system (de Boer et al 1991). It has been suggested that fibrin deposition may occur and may be responsible for the liver, kidney and placental dysfunction in these patients.

8. The differential diagnosis is from acute fatty liver of pregnancy or an infectious cause unrelated to pregnancy (Pereira et al 1997).

Anaesthetic problems

1. The diagnosis is often delayed because symptoms are often vague. There is an average delay of 8 days.

2. Care of the ill parturient with preeclampsia.

3. Possible bleeding problems secondary to thrombocytopenia. Patients with HELLP and an intrapartum platelet count of $\leq 40 \times 10^9 l^{-1}$ are at significant risk from postpartum bleeding, whereas in those with levels above this, significant bleeding is unlikely (Roberts et al 1994). Frequently, epidural catheters are in place before the syndrome is recognised, and persistent bleeding into the epidural space has been reported (Sibai et al 1986).

4. Problems of expediting delivery.

5. Management of complications such as renal failure, ARDS.

6. About 30% of patients present postpartum.

7. The management of liver rupture or subcapsular haematoma. A patient had a Caesarean section at 29 weeks' gestation for severe preeclampsia and HELLP syndrome. The liver was noted to be intact. Ten hours later she deteriorated, with a platelet count of $41 \times 10^9 l^{-1}$, at which stage laparotomy revealed liver rupture, which was treated with packing (Risseeuw et al 1999).

8. The differential diagnosis is from acute fatty liver of pregnancy, haemolytic uraemic syndrome, and thrombotic, thrombocytopenic purpura.

9. Laryngeal oedema may occur in severe cases of PIH. In a series of 442 pregnancies with HELLP, two patients out of five who died, did so as a result of failed intubation secondary to laryngeal oedema (Sibai et al 1993).

Management

1. Investigations include Hb, white cell, platelet and reticulocyte count, partial

thromboplastin time, fibrinogen concentration, FDP, liver function tests, and urea and electrolyte concentrations. Thromboelastography may be of help (Mallet & Cox 1992). In one patient undergoing haemodialysis for renal failure during which heparin had been given, the use of thromboelastography differentiated between two possible causes of haemorrhage. Once the heparin had been neutralised with protamine, the trace was characteristic of fibrinolysis, which was then treated with aprotinin (Whitta et al 1995).

2. The baby should be delivered expeditiously, preferably vaginally, if the gestation is beyond 34 weeks. However, Caesarean section is usually required, and unless an epidural catheter is already sited, general anaesthesia is necessary (Barton & Sibai 1991).

3. Ill patients may need transfer to an ITU where close monitoring of CVP and urinary output can take place. Hypovolaemia should be treated and a urine output of $0.5 \, ml \, kg^{-1} \, h^{-1}$ maintained. Patients should be monitored on the ITU for at least 48 h.

4. Haemorrhage may require surgical intervention. Bleeding from mucous membranes is not usually of clinical significance, but intrapartum bleeding from abruptio placentae should be managed aggressively.

5. FFP and platelets are required to increase the platelet count to $>50 \times 10^9 l^{-1}$ and the INR <1.5. Patterson and O'Toole (1991) described the management of Caesarean section for twins in a patient with a platelet count of $22 \times 10^9 l^{-1}$, haemolytic anaemia, and abnormal liver function tests. CVP and urinary output were monitored. Fresh frozen plasma and 6 u of platelets increased the platelet count to $50 \times 10^9 l^{-1}$, and a hydralazine infusion controlled the arterial blood pressure.

6. Control of hypertension with hydralazine infusion and, if general anaesthesia is required, treatment to attenuate the hypertensive response to tracheal intubation (see Eclampsia and preeclampsia).

7. There is evidence that the use of high-dose corticosteroids in women with HELLP syndrome improves the laboratory and clinical parameters, and hastens recovery. In the first study, antepartum patients with HELLP received either dexamethasone 10 mg iv 12-hrly until delivery or were untreated (Magann et al 1994a). In the second, postpartum patients with HELLP received four doses iv dexamethasone in 36 h (10 mg, 10 mg, 5 mg, 5 mg) or no treatment (Magann et al 1994b). In a later study of 93 patients, im betamethasone 12 mg two doses 12 h apart was thought to be the most effective (Tompkins & Thiagarajah 1999).

8. Should an epidural catheter be in place when thrombocytopenia develops, a neurological assessment must be carried out before each top up. It should be left in place until the coagulopathy has resolved. Otherwise, epidural anaesthesia should not be undertaken.

9. Radiological assistance may be required to diagnose the presence of spontaneous subcapsular, intrahepatic or renal haematomas. If complaints are of right upper quadrant, shoulder or neck pain, or relapsing hypotension, liver imaging should be performed (Barton & Sibai 1996). Abnormal liver scans correlated with the severity of the thrombocytopenia. Surgery may be needed.

10. In the event of liver failure, referral to a liver unit may be required. Transfer is suggested for patients who have deteriorating liver function despite early delivery, or for those who develop features of severe liver dysfunction, such as encephalopathy, coagulopathy, or hypoglycaemia. Treatment should include control of blood pressure, correction of INR to <1.5, maintenance of platelet count to $>50 \times 10^9 l^{-1}$, and acetylcysteine to maintain microcirculatory flow (Pereira et al 1997).

Bibliography
Barton JR, Sibai BM 1996 Hepatic imaging in HELLP syndrome (hemolysis, elevated liver enzymes, and low platelet count). American Journal of Obstetrics & Gynecology 174: 1820–7.

Crosby ET 1991 Obstetrical anaesthesia for patients

with the syndrome of haemolysis, elevated liver enzymes and low platelets. Canadian Journal of Anaesthesia 38: 227–33.

De Boer K, Buller HR, Ten Cate JW et al 1991 Coagulation studies in the syndrome of haemolysis, elevated liver enzymes and low platelets. British Journal of Obstetrics & Gynaecology 98: 42–7.

Geary M 1997 The HELLP syndrome. British Journal of Obstetrics & Gynaecology 104: 887–91.

Isler CM, Rinehart BK, Terrone DA et al 1999 Maternal mortality associated with HELLP (hemolysis, elevated liver enzymes, and low platelets) syndrome. American Journal of Obstetrics & Gynecology 181: 924–8.

Magann EF, Bass D, Chauhan SP et al 1994a Antepartum corticosteroids: disease stabilization in patients with the syndrome of hemolysis, elevated liver enzymes, and low platelets (HELLP). American Journal of Obstetrics & Gynecology 171: 1148–53.

Magann EF, Perry KG, Meydrech EF et al 1994b Postpartum corticosteroids: accelerated recovery from the syndrome of hemolysis, elevated liver enzymes, and low platelets (HELLP). American Journal of Obstetrics & Gynecology 171: 1154–8.

Mallet SV, Cox DJA 1992 Thromboelastography. British Journal of Anaesthesia 69: 307–13.

Martin JN Jr, Rinehart BK, May WL et al 1999 The spectrum of severe preeclampsia: comparative analysis by HELLP (hemolysis, elevated liver enzyme levels, and low platelet count) syndrome classification. American Journal of Obstetrics & Gynecology 180: 1373–84.

Mushambi MC, Halligan AW, Williamson K 1996 Recent developments in the pathophysiology and management of pre-eclampsia. British Journal of Anaesthesia 76: 133–48.

Patterson KW, O'Toole DP 1991 HELLP syndrome: a case report with guidelines for management. British Journal of Anaesthesia 66: 513–15.

Pereira SP, O'Donahue J, Wendon J et al 1997 Maternal and perinatal outcome in severe pregnancy-related liver disease. Hepatology 26: 1258–62.

Risseeuw JJ, de Vries JE, van Eyck J et al 1999 Liver rupture postpartum associated with preeclampsia and HELLP syndrome. Journal of Maternal-Fetal Medicine 8: 32–5.

Roberts WE, Perry KG Jr, Woods JB et al 1994 The intrapartum platelet count in patients with HELLP (hemolysis, elevated liver enzymes, and low platelets) syndrome: is it predictive of later hemorrhagic complications? American Journal of Obstetrics & Gynecology 171: 799–804.

Sibai BM, Taslimi MM, El-Nazer A et al 1986 Maternal-perinatal outcome associated with the syndrome of hemolysis, elevated liver enzymes, and low platelets in severe preeclampsia-eclampsia. American Journal of Obstetrics & Gynecology 155: 501–9.

Sibai BM, Ramadan MK, Usta I et al 1993 Maternal morbidity and mortality in 442 pregnancies with hemolysis, elevated liver enzymes and low platelets (HELLP syndrome). American Journal of Obstetrics & Gynecology 169: 1000–6.

Stone JH 1999 HELLP syndrome: hemolysis, elevated liver enzymes, and low platelets. Journal of the American Medical Association 280: 559–62.

Sullivan CA, Magann EF, Perry Jr KG et al 1994 The recurrence risk of the syndrome of hemolysis, elevated liver enzymes, and low platelets (HELLP) in subsequent gestations. American Journal of Obstetrics & Gynecology 171: 940–3.

Tompkins MJ, Thiagarajah S 1999 HELLP (hemolysis, elevated liver enzymes, and low platelet count) syndrome: the benefit of corticosteroids. American Journal of Obstetrics and Gynecology 181: 304–9.

Whitta RK, Cox DJ, Mallett SV 1995 Thromboelastography reveals two causes of haemorrhage in HELLP syndrome. British Journal of Anaesthesia 74: 464–8.

Hereditary angioneurotic oedema

(see also C1 esterase inhibitor deficiency)

A symptom complex of intermittent painless, nonitching, swelling of subcutaneous tissue, respiratory mucosa, and intestinal walls. Acute attacks are commonly precipitated by trauma or stress, and can last for a few hours up to 4 days. Often presenting in early childhood or adolescence, it is an autosomal dominant condition in which there is a deficiency, or abnormality, of the inhibitor of the activated first component of complement (C1 esterase inhibitor, C1 EI). Complement, whose major function is to eliminate antigen, is present in serum and a number of other body fluids, and is a mediator of immunological tissue damage. The complement system is a cascade resembling the clotting sequence, in which a series of normally inactive proteins sequentially activate each other. The complement cascade is initially activated by either the classical or alternate pathways. It is normally kept under control by inhibitors, or when activated, by the spontaneous decay of the active component. The kinin-generating and fibrinolytic systems are also involved, and the oedema appears to result from the generation of a peptide that causes increased capillary permeability. The C1 inhibitor gene has been mapped to chromosome 11, and many different mutations can be responsible. Two types have been identified. Type I has no C1 EI, whereas type II has normal levels of protein, but it is dysfunctional (Cicardi & Agostini 1996). The hereditary form is responsible for only a small proportion of cases of angioedema.

Until recently, severe attacks were treated with FFP, but this has probably been superseded by heat-treated C1 EI. In a double-blind, placebo-controlled study, prophylactic C1 EI produced nearly normal functional levels of C1 and C4 and resulted in significantly lower symptom scores. On average, the time from administration of the infusion to the beginning of the effect was 55 min (Waytes et al 1996). However, it is not licensed for general use because of concerns about viral infections, or the effects of long-term treatment, although it is used for emergency purposes on a named-patient basis.

Preoperative abnormalities

1. Attacks of angioneurotic oedema can be precipitated by minor trauma, mental or physical stress, pregnancy, or there may be no obvious cause. Cutaneous swellings are not red, itchy, or painful. However, serious effects occur if the oedema involves the upper airway or leads to intestinal obstruction. Shock may occur as a result of fluid sequestration into the peritoneal cavity and intestinal wall. The crisis does not respond to treatment with steroids, antihistamines, or epinephrine (adrenaline). The pulmonary vascular tree is spared because cells lining the pulmonary vessels have surface

enzymes that inactivate vasoactive peptides (Cicardi & Agostoni 1996).

2. A family history of the disease is usually elicited, sometimes with deaths at a young age. In the past, the development of acute laryngeal oedema carried a high mortality.

3. Plasma C1 EI levels are zero or below normal, or are normal but dysfunctional. A functional abnormality exists in about 15% of cases. During attacks there is a low C4 and often a low C2. Measurement of serum C4 titre is a good screening test during symptomatic periods. If the levels are normal, the condition is excluded. If the levels are low, then assay of C1 EI is warranted (Sim & Grant 1990).

4. Some patients with disabling symptoms may be on long-term therapy with stanozolol or danazol.

Anaesthetic problems

1. Patients may present with acute upper airway compromise from laryngeal oedema (Jensen & Weiler 1998). Emergency tracheostomy may be needed (Hamilton et al 1977). Severe postoperative angioedema occurred in a 61-year-old man after cervical surgery, performed because osteophytes were thought to be causing dysphagia and choking episodes (Krnacik & Heggeness 1997). Fatal obstruction occurred in a 27 year old on ITU, whilst preparations for tracheostomy were being made (Nielsen et al 1995).

2. Dental or surgical procedures, tracheal intubation or other trauma, all carry the risk of initiating an attack. Fatal laryngeal oedema has been reported after dental extraction (Wall et al 1989). Death, secondary to exaggerated complement common pathway activation, occurred during cardiopulmonary bypass in one patient whose C1 EI levels were 30% normal (Bonser et al 1991), whereas another patient in whom they were 75% had uneventful cardiac surgery (Haering & Communale 1993). It was suggested that haemodilution of existing low levels contributed to the fatality.

3. Attacks of abdominal pain may result from intestinal oedema. Unless the diagnosis is made, patients may be submitted to unnecessary surgery.

4. Although it has been suggested that pregnancy provides a protective effect against attacks, complications may still arise, and abdominal pain may become a diagnostic problem (Chappatte & de Swiet 1988, Galan et al 1996). A maternal death from hypovolaemia has also been reported, which was secondary to widespread oedema in the absence of serum C1 EI (Postnikoff & Pritzker 1979). The terminal episode started with perineal oedema, in association with episiotomy infection 48 h after delivery, and the immediate cause of death was pericardial effusion, and pulmonary and laryngeal oedema. One patient being given FFP for attacks during pregnancy developed a severe reaction (Boulos et al 1994).

5. The use of epsilon aminocaproic acid, a fibrinolytic inhibitor, as a prophylactic measure, has been associated with the development of deep venous thrombosis (Hamilton et al 1977). However, this drug is now unavailable in the UK.

Management

1. At present, the treatment of acute attacks and emergency surgery is controversial. There is some division in the profession between the use of FFP and C1 EI (Cox & Holdcroft 1995, Hawthorne & Gooi 1996). At present, although C1 EI is only licensed in a limited number of countries (Italy, France & Austria), increasing numbers of clinical trials from the USA and Canada show the heat-treated C1 EI to be effective and safe (Cicardi & Agostini 1996, Kunschak et al 1998, Visentin et al 1998). It also lacks the disadvantage of FFP, which contains C2 and C4 (that have the theoretical risk of worsening an attack), and it has not been shown to be associated with the transmission of virus diseases. It should be used mainly to treat attacks

of glottic oedema and abdominal pain. Clinical improvement has been seen within 40 min of administration. However, there should be close observation, even when appropriate treatment has been given. A young man who received both danazol and C1 EI concentrate for tonsillectomy developed facial swelling and difficulty in swallowing 22 h after surgery (Maves & Weiler 1994).

2. In patients presenting with acute abdominal pain, the diagnosis of intestinal oedema may be confirmed by a barium meal and follow-through examination.

3. If elective surgery is required, prophylaxis can be achieved with danazol, but it needs 5 days' treatment to become effective clinically. Either danazol (a progestogen) 200 mg tds, or stanozolol (an anabolic steroid) 2.5–10 mg daily, can also be given. Danazol increases the plasma levels of C1 EI and C4 (Gelfand et al 1976), probably by influencing hepatic synthesis of the inhibitor. It starts to act within 24 h, and is at a maximum at 1–2 weeks. If possible, 5 days' treatment should be given before surgery.

4. Facilities for tracheostomy should be available in life-threatening conditions.

5. In pregnancy, androgens are contraindicated unless the fetus is known to be male, therefore treatment with these drugs should be withdrawn. Any attacks should be treated with C1 EI, and its use before Caesarean section has been advised (Cox & Holdcroft 1995). Uneventful epidural analgesia has been reported for vaginal delivery (Wingtin & Hardy 1989, Cox & Holdcroft 1995, Marescal et al 1999).

6. For severe cases, purified C1 EI can be obtained from Immuno Limited (Sevenoaks, Kent, UK). It may also be useful in patients in whom danazol does not increase the C1 EI concentrations, in those who are at risk of upper airway oedema, and for children and pregnant women in whom danazol is contraindicated (Laxenaire et al 1990).

Bibliography

Bonser RS, Dave J, Morgan J et al 1991 Complement activation during bypass in acquired C1 esterase inhibitor deficiency. Annals of Thoracic Surgery 52: 541–3.

Boulos AN, Brown R, Hukin A et al 1994 Danazol prophylaxis for delivery in hereditary angioneurotic oedema. British Journal of Obstetrics and Gynaecology 101: 1094–5.

Chappatte O, de Swiet M 1988 Hereditary angioneurotic oedema and pregnancy. Case reports and review of the literature. British Journal of Obstetrics & Gynaecology 95: 938–42.

Cicardi M, Agostoni A 1996 Hereditary angioedema. New England Journal of Medicine 334: 1666–7.

Cox M, Holdcroft A 1995 Hereditary angioneurotic oedema: current management in pregnancy. Anaesthesia 50: 547–9.

Galan HL, Reedy MB, Starr J et al 1996 Fresh frozen plasma prophylaxis for hereditary angioedema during pregnancy. A case report. Journal of Reproductive Medicine 41: 541–4.

Gelfand JA, Sherins RJ, Alling DW et al 1976 Treatment of hereditary angioedema with danazol. New England Journal of Medicine 295: 1444–8.

Haering JM, Comunale ME 1993 Cardiopulmonary bypass in hereditary angioedema. Anesthesiology 79: 1429–33.

Hamilton AG, Bosley ARJ, Bowen DJ 1977 Laryngeal oedema due to hereditary angioedema. Anaesthesia 32: 265–7.

Hawthorne LA, Gooi HC 1996 Hereditary angioedema: prophylaxis in the puerperium. Anaesthesia 51: 283–4.

Jensen NF, Weiler JM 1998 C1 esterase deficiency, airway compromise, and anesthesia. Anesthesia & Analgesia 87: 480–8.

Karlis V, Glickman RS, Stern R et al 1997 Hereditary angioedema: case report and review of management. Oral Surgery, Oral Medicine, Oral Pathology, Oral Radiology & Endodontics 83: 462–4.

Krnacik MJ, Heggeness MH 1997 Severe angioedema causing airway obstruction after anterior cervical surgery. Spine 22: 2188–90.

Kunschak M, Engl W, Maritsch F et al 1998 A randomized, controlled trial to study the efficacy and safety of C1 inhibitor concentrate in treating hereditary angioedema. Transfusion 38: 540–9.

Laxenaire M-C, Audibert G, Janot C 1990 Use of purified C1 esterase inhibitor in patients with hereditary angioedema. Anesthesiology 72: 956–7.

Marescal C, Ducloy-Bouthors AS, Laurent J et al 1999 Parturition and angioneurotic oedema. International Journal of Obstetric Anesthesia 8: 135–7.

Maves KK, Weiler JM 1994 Tonsillectomy in a patient with hereditary angioedema after prophylaxis with C1 inhibitor concentrate. Annals of Allergy 73: 438–8.

Nielsen EW, Kjernlie DF, Aaseth J 1995 A fatal outcome of hereditary angio-oedema. Tidsskrift for Den Norske Laegeforening 115: 43–4.

Postnikoff IM, Pritzker KPH 1979 Hereditary angioneurotic edema: an unusual case of maternal mortality. Journal of Forensic Sciences 24: 473–8.

Sim TC, Grant JA 1990 Hereditary angioedema: its diagnostic and management perspectives. American Journal of Medicine 88: 656–64.

Visentin DE, Yang WH, Karsh J 1998 C1-esterase inhibitor transfusions in patients with hereditary angioedema. Annals of Allergy, Asthma, & Immunology 80: 457–61.

Wall RT, Frank M, Hahn M 1989 A review of 25 patients with hereditary angioedema requiring surgery. Anesthesiology 71: 309–11.

Waytes AT, Rosen FS, Frank MM 1996 Treatment of hereditary angioedema with a vapor-heated C1 inhibitor concentrate. New England Journal of Medicine 334: 1630–4.

Wingtin LN, Hardy F 1989 Epidural block during labour in hereditary angioneurotic oedema. Canadian Journal of Anaesthesia 36: 366.

Hereditary haemorrhagic telangiectasia (HHT) (Osler–Weber–Rendu disease)

An autosomal dominant disease in which there are cutaneous, mucosal and visceral vascular anomalies, accompanied by a family history of the disorder. Recent research has shown mutations in the endoglin gene on the long arm of chromosome 9 (Shovlin & Letarte 1999). Many of the problems are functional consequences of direct communications between the pulmonary and systemic sides of the circulation. Affected individuals may present with epistaxis or gastrointestinal bleeding, often after the fourth decade. Pulmonary arteriovenous fistulae are present in about 15%

of patients. These fistulae can cause hypoxia, and, if untreated, they carry a mortality which exceeds that of treatment. Anaesthesia may be required for control of epistaxis, for gastrointestinal bleeding, for balloon or coil spring embolisation, surgery to pulmonary AV fistulae, or liver transplantation.

Preoperative abnormalities

1. Telangiectasia, systemic or pulmonary arteriovenous malformations (PAVM), and aneurysms, constitute the three forms of angiodysplasia. Telangiectasia usually appear in the second or third decade, and blanch with pressure. The evolution of telangiectasia involves loss of resistance vessels in the capillary beds, dilatation, elongation, and tortuosity of the venules, and arteriolar dilatation. As a result, direct arteriovenous connections form, that have no resistance between them (Guttmacher et al 1995). There may be dilated blood vessels over the lips and fingertips, and clubbing may be present.

2. Recurrent epistaxis from nasal telangiectasia is an early sign of the disease; in 90% of patients, recurrent epistaxis started before the age of 21. A variety of treatments include Nd:YAG laser and argon plasma coagulation under local anaesthesia (Bergler et al 1999).

3. The prevalence of ocular lesions is 45%.

4. Pulmonary arteriovenous malformations occur in 15–33% of patients and tend to increase in size with time (Haitjema et al 1996). Patients may develop exertional dyspnoea, cyanosis, clubbing, palpitations, and pulmonary vascular bruits. Right to left shunting occurs, with blood flowing directly from a pulmonary artery into a pulmonary vein, since the lesions have no intervening capillary beds. There may be secondary polycythaemia. If a bruit is present it increases on inspiration. In the majority of cases in which there is an arteriovenous fistula, the CXR is abnormal. Often the abnormality shows as a peripherally placed dense area that is

attached to the hilum by vascular markings (Burke et al 1986), or there may be isolated 'coin' lesions. Pulmonary angiography will confirm the diagnosis. Haemothorax may occur and is occasionally life threatening. If the fistulae are large, the patient may develop high output cardiac failure. One-third of patients who present with a single PAVM will have HHT. If these are multiple, the chance of having the condition increases to more than 50%.

5. The incidence of cerebral vascular malformations (CVMs) is 5–11%. They may cause intracranial haemorrhage, neurological deficits, and seizures. Brain abscess formation is well documented and is probably secondary to paradoxical embolus of infected material bypassing the filtering action of the lung capillaries.

6. The incidence of digestive tract lesions is unknown, but bleeding from gastrointestinal lesions may occur, usually from diffuse angiodysplasia, and particularly in older patients. This is difficult to treat because of problems in locating the vessels responsible.

7. Haematuria may result from bladder lesions.

8. Hepatic AV malformations can lead to fibrosis or cirrhosis. Arteriovenous and portosystemic shunts may occur. Liver transplantation may be required for large shunts that are causing severe cardiopulmonary disease.

9. Cardiac valvular disease has been reported, although the cause of this is not known.

Anaesthetic problems

1. Pulmonary AV malformations were associated with hypoxia, secondary to right to left shunting of blood, in 90% of 93 patients, and polycythaemia occurred in 12. The hypoxia was only marginally improved with oxygen therapy (Swanson et al 1999). Fistulae may increase in size, or can produce paradoxical emboli of any type, including septic emboli. Hepatic

arteriovenous shunts can also occur, with cardiac failure and pulmonary hypertension.

2. Hypoxaemia has been reported after the onset of IPPV in a patient with a pulmonary arteriovenous fistula (Friedman et al 1992). This resolved when spontaneous respiration was resumed, and was thought to have resulted from a worsening of the right to left shunt by the IPPV.

3. There may be recurrent admissions for control of epistaxis (Siegel et al 1991). In a study of 73 patients, the incidence of epistaxis was 93%; the mean age of onset was 12 years; the mean frequency of bleeding was 18 episodes per month, and the mean duration of haemorrhage was 7.5 min (Aassar et al 1991).

4. Abscess formation, particularly in the brain, may occur spontaneously, or arise in association with surgery or dental treatment (Mohler et al 1991, El Houcheimi et al 1998, Brydon et al 1999). The lesions are usually solitary and sited above the tentorium. HHT may not have been diagnosed before the presentation of the abscess (El Houcheimi et al 1998, Gelfand et al 1988), therefore the condition should be considered if a solitary abscess occurs. In one patient requiring IPPV, PEEP was thought to have worsened the shunt through the PAVM and prolonged weaning time (Brydon et al 1999).

5. There is a risk of paradoxical embolism of any type, because microemboli bypass the pulmonary capillary filter.

6. There have been a number of reports of spontaneous, severe and sometimes fatal, haemothorax (Ference et al 1994). Pregnancy increases the risks of this.

7. In 23 pregnancies in which PAVMs were present at the start, ten were complicated (Shovlin et al 1995). Six women had deteriorating intrapulmonary shunts, three had cerebrovascular accidents, and two died from pulmonary haemorrhage. Pregnancy can increase the rate of growth of the PAVM (Swinburne et al 1986), probably secondary to

hormonal and cardiovascular changes (Chanatry 1992), and may be associated with the formation of new fistulae. High output cardiac failure during pregnancy has been described in association with a hepatic AVM and the diagnosis was confirmed by echocardiography and MRI (Gong et al 1988). Spontaneous haemothorax and hypoxia in the midtrimester may necessitate embolisation of the fistulae (Gammon et al 1990, Waring et al 1990).

8. Bleeding usually occurs secondary to vascular abnormalities, and in the absence of coagulation defects. However, there is an association between HHT and von Willebrand's disease. It is possible that defects in the endothelial cells may result in impaired production of Factor VIII and vWF factor (Quitt et al 1990).

Management

1. Complications of HHT should be sought, particularly the presence of PAVMs and resultant hypoxia.

2. Take care to avoid causing paradoxical emboli via sites of intravenous access. If epidural anaesthesia is required, loss of resistance to saline, rather than air, should be used to identify the epidural space.

3. Patients with PAVMs should be counselled about the hazards of pregnancy. Although an epidural infusion for labour has been described in a patient with HHT and rheumatic heart disease, epidural anaesthesia should be used with caution and the patient monitored closely for the development of an epidural haematoma. There is a possibility of abnormal epidural vessels, and a small risk of coagulation problems if there are vWF or Factor VIII abnormalities in addition.

4. Incidence of readmission for epistaxis was found to be reduced if treatment with laser therapy combined with septodermoplasty was undertaken (Siegel et al 1991).

5. In view of the risks of abscess formation,

the use of antibacterial prophylaxis, similar to that for cardiac lesions, has been suggested (Swanson & Dahl 1991).

6. Certain drugs have been reported to decrease the incidence of haemorrhage. Desmopressin has been used to treat gastrointestinal bleeding that was unresponsive to cryoprecipitate in a patient with decreased vWF, and also in those patients without deficiency (Quitt et al 1990). Aminocaproic acid 1–1.5 g bd apparently reduced the incidence of epistaxes in two patients (Saba et al 1994). However, success with medical treatment has been mixed, and caution has been advised when using prothrombotic agents (Phillips 1994). Oestrogen–progesterone therapy has also been used.

Bibliography

Aassar OS, Friedman CM, White RI Jr 1991 The natural history of epistaxis in hereditary telangiectasia. Laryngoscope 101: 977–80.

Bergler W, Reidel F, Baker-Schreyer A et al 1999 Argon plasma coagulation for the treatment of hereditary hemorrhagic telangiectasia. Laryngoscope 109: 15–20.

Brydon HL, Akinwunmi J, Selway R et al 1999 Brain abscesses associated with pulmonary arteriovenous malformations. British Journal of Neurosurgery 13: 265–9.

Burke CM, Safai C, Nelson DP et al 1986 Pulmonary arteriovenous malformations: a critical update. American Review of Respiratory Disease 134: 334–9.

Chanatry BJ 1992 Acute hemothorax owing to pulmonary arteriovenous malformation in pregnancy. Anesthesia & Analgesia 74: 613–15.

El Houcheimi I, Hardwidge C, Walter P et al 1998 Brain abscess and hereditary haemorrhagic telangiectasia: a report of three cases. British Journal of Neurosurgery 12: 15–17.

Ference BA, Shannon TM, White RI Jr et al 1994 Life-threatening pulmonary hemorrhage with pulmonary arteriovenous malformations and hereditary hemorrhagic telangiectasia. Chest 106: 1387–90.

Friedman BC, McGrath BJ, Williams JF 1992 Pulmonary arteriovenous fistula: mechanical ventilation and hypoxemia. Canadian Journal of Anaesthesia 39: 963–5.

Gammon RB, Miksa AK, Keller FS 1990 Osler–Weber–Rendu disease and pulmonary arteriovenous fistulas. Deterioration and embolotherapy during pregnancy. Chest 98: 1522–4.

Gelfand MS, Stephens DS, Howell EI et al 1988 Brain abscess: association with pulmonary arteriovenous fistula and hereditary hemorrhagic telangiectasia: report of three cases. American Journal of Medicine 85: 718–20.

Gong B, Baken L, Julian T et al 1988 High-output heart failure due to hepatic arteriovenous fistula during pregnancy: a case report. Obstetrics & Gynecology 72: 440–2.

Guttmacher AE, Marchuk DA, White RI 1995 Hereditary hemorrhagic telangiectasia. New England Journal of Medicine 333: 918–21.

Haitjema T, Westermann CJJ, Overtoom TC et al 1996 Hereditary hemorrhagic telangiectasia (Osler–Weber–Rendu disease): new insights in pathogenesis, complications, and treatment. Archives of Internal Medicine 156: 714–19.

Mohler ER, Monahan B, Canty MD et al 1991 Cerebral abscess associated with dental procedure in hereditary haemorrhagic telangiectasia. Lancet 338: 508–9.

Phillips MD 1994 Stopping bleeding in hereditary telangiectasia. New England Journal of Medicine 330: 1822–3.

Quitt M, Froom P, Veisler A et al 1990 The effect of desmopressin on massive gastrointestinal bleeding in hereditary telangiectasia unresponsive to treatment with cryoprecipitate. Archives of Internal Medicine 150: 1744–6.

Saba HI, Morelli GA, Logrono LA 1994 Brief report: treatment of bleeding in hereditary hemorrhagic telangiectasia with aminocaproic acid. New England Journal of Medicine 330: 1789–90.

Shovlin CL, Letarte M 1999 Hereditary haemorrhagic telangiectasia and pulmonary arteriovenous malformations: issues in clinical management and review of pathogenic mechanisms. Thorax 54: 714–29.

Shovlin CL, Winstock AR, Peters AM et al 1995 Medical complications of pregnancy in hereditary haemorrhagic telangiectasia. Quarterly Journal of Medicine 88: 879–87.

Siegel MB, Keane WM, Atkins JF Jr et al 1991 Control of epistaxis in patients with hereditary hemorrhagic telangiectasia. Otolaryngology—Head & Neck Surgery 105: 675–9.

Swanson DL, Dahl MV 1991 Embolic abscesses in

hereditary hemorrhagic telangiectasia. Journal of the American Academy of Dermatology 24: 580–3.

Swanson KL, Prakash UBS, Stanson AW 1999 Pulmonary arteriovenous fistulas: Mayo Clinic experience. Mayo Clinic Proceedings 74: 671–80.

Swinburne AJ, Fedullo AJ, Bangemi R et al 1986 Hereditary telangiectasia and multiple arteriovenous fistulas. Clinical deterioration during pregnancy. Chest 89: 459–60.

Waring PH, Shaw DB, Brumfield CG 1990 Anesthetic management of a parturient with Osler–Weber–Rendu syndrome and rheumatic heart disease. Anesthesia & Analgesia 71: 96–9.

Hereditary spherocytosis

A familial haemolytic anaemia of autosomal dominant inheritance in which premature destruction of intrinsically abnormal erythrocytes occurs in the spleen. Specific molecular defects have been found. The clinical severity of the disease varies considerably (Eber et al 1990). Anaesthesia may be required for splenectomy and/or cholecystectomy. However, a conservative approach to splenectomy is being adopted; avoidance of surgery in those with mild to moderate disease is now recommended. After splenectomy there are increases in haemoglobin, average platelet count, and cholesterol concentration. These are associated with a long-term increased risk of atherosclerotic events, such as stroke and myocardial infarction (Schilling 1997). The possibility of partial splenectomy is being explored (Tse & Lux 1999). If splenectomy is thought necessary, there is controversy as to whether prophylactic cholecystectomy should be undertaken at the same time, and whether or not both should be performed laparoscopically.

Preoperative abnormalities

1. Small, spherocytic red blood cells are present in the peripheral blood. The surface to volume ratio is altered and the normal discoid shape is lost. Cells have an increased osmotic fragility, their survival time is reduced, and there is marrow hyperplasia.

2. Splenomegaly, mild haemolytic anaemia, and acholuric jaundice.

3. An increased reticulocyte count of up to 20%. Haptoglobins are almost absent.

4. An increased incidence of gallstones and leg ulcers.

5. RBC survival times, which may be reduced to 60 days or less ($n = 120$ days), are improved by splenectomy.

6. Splenectomy is accompanied by an increase in average Hb, the average platelet count is above normal, and serum cholesterol concentration is increased.

7. Pregnancy is relatively rare.

Anaesthetic problems

1. In the past, the majority of patients underwent splenectomy, although this is a controversial area since the long-term effects of splenic removal have been observed. Cholecystectomy may be required.

2. Postsplenectomy complications include thrombocytosis, overwhelming sepsis, and chest infections. However, since the introduction of pneumococcal and *Haemophilus influenzae* B vaccines, the sepsis risks are much lower than previously (Schilling 1995).

3. There are long-term disadvantages of splenectomy; the average Hb level is increased, as is the platelet level and the cholesterol concentration. These are associated with an increased risk of atherosclerotic events, such as stroke and myocardial infarction (Schilling 1997).

4. Preoperative autologous blood donation is probably unwise. Although the spherocytic RBCs survive collection, they can lose membrane under optimal storage conditions (Weinstein et al 1997). However, intraoperative cell salvage is acceptable.

5. Pregnancies in women who still have their spleens may be complicated by anaemia or

haemolytic crisis (Pajor et al 1993). In 19 pregnancies, eight were complicated by anaemia, six by haemolytic crisis, and four women required blood transfusion. These complications only occurred in patients in whom splenectomy had not been undertaken.

Management

1. Surgery should be avoided in the presence of a haemolytic crisis.

2. Prophylaxis before and after splenectomy. Three vaccines should be given, preferably 2 weeks before splenectomy:

> Pneumovax 0.5 ml sc or im, and repeat once between 5 and 10 years later.

> HIB vaccine 0.5 ml sc or im once only.

> Mengivac (A+C) 0.5 ml sc or im, or Meningitec (C) 0.5 ml im. Repeat every 2 years.

Continuous antibiotic prophylaxis; benzylpenicillin 600 mg 12 hrly iv or oral penicillin V 250 mg 12 hrly. If penicillin allergic, give erythromycin 500 mg 12 hrly iv, or orally 250 mg 12 hrly.

3. Cardiac surgery has been undertaken using preoperative iron and recombinant erythropoietin, pre- and perioperative autologous transfusion, and postoperative iron therapy (Yamagishi et al 1998). Total exchange transfusion has also been used (Aykac et al 1994).

4. If pregnancy occurs, patients should be observed carefully. Folic acid should be given, infections prevented, and the haemolytic state monitored if the patient has her spleen.

Bibliography

Aykac B, Erolcay H, Dikmen Y 1994 Total exchange transfusion (TET) and open heart surgery in a patient with hereditary spherocytosis (HS). Journal of Cardiothoracic & Vascular Anesthesia 8 (3 suppl 2): 87.

Eber SW, Ambrust R, Schroter W 1990 Variable clinical severity of hereditary spherocytosis: relation to erythrocytic spectrum, concentration, osmotic fragility and autohemolysis. Journal of Pediatrics 117: 409–16.

Pajor A, Lehoczky D, Szakacs Z 1993 Pregnancy and hereditary spherocytosis. Report of 8 patients and a review. Archives of Gynecology & Obstetrics 253: 37–41.

Schilling RF 1995 Estimating the risk for sepsis after splenectomy in hereditary spherocytosis. Annals of Internal Medicine 122: 187–8.

Schilling RF 1997 Spherocytosis, splenectomy, strokes and heart attacks. Lancet 350: 1677–8.

Tse WT, Lux SE 1999 Red blood cell membrane disorders. British Journal of Haematology 104: 2–13.

Weinstein R, Martinez R, Hassoun H, Palek J 1997 Does a patient with hereditary spherocytosis qualify for preoperative autologous blood donation? Transfusion 37: 1179–83.

Yamagishi I, Sakurada T, Abe T 1998 Cardiac surgery using only autologous blood for a patient with hereditary spherocytosis. Annals of Thoracic & Cardiovascular Surgery 4: 294–7.

Hers' disease (Cori type VI glycogen storage disease)

One of the glycogen storage diseases in which there is reduced or absent liver glycogen phosphorylase activity, secondary to a gene mutation (Hers et al 1989). It is similar to types I and III, but is less severe (Burchell 1998). There are a number of different variants.

Preoperative abnormalities

1. Children may present with failure to thrive, although beyond childhood, growth is usually normal. Hepatomegaly is secondary to increased glycogen stores in the liver.

2. There is a tendency to hypoglycaemia and a variable response to glucagon and epinephrine (adrenaline) (Cox 1968).

3. Metabolic abnormalities such as hypercholesterolaemia and increased serum triglycerides occur, but metabolic acidosis is rare. Liver function tests may be mildly abnormal.

4. Tends to be less severe than type I disease.

In a series of patients having portacaval shunt surgery for metabolic diseases, the single type VI case was the only one not to require parenteral nutrition (Casson 1975).

5. High protein diets are recommended (Goldberg & Slonim 1993).

Anaesthetic problems

1. Hypoglycaemia and acidosis can occur after starvation.

Management

1. Prolonged fasting should be avoided and a dextrose infusion should be given during the period of preoperative starvation.

Bibliography

Burchell A 1998 Glycogen storage diseases and the liver. Baillieres Clinical Gastroenterology 12: 337–54.

Casson H 1975 Anaesthesia for portocaval bypass in patients with metabolic diseases. British Journal of Anaesthesia 47: 969–75.

Cox JM 1968 Anesthesia and glycogen storage disease. Anesthesiology 29: 1221–5.

Goldberg T, Slonim AE 1993 Nutrition therapy for hepatic glycogen storage disease. Journal of the American Dietetic Association 93: 1423–30.

Hers H-G, van Hoof F, de Barsy T 1989 The glycogen storage diseases. In: Scriver CR et al (eds) The metabolic basis of inherited disease. McGraw-Hill, New York. 425.

Lee PJ, Leonard JV 1995 The hepatic glycogen storage diseases—problems beyond childhood. Journal of Inherited Metabolic Disease 18: 462–72.

Wolfsdorf JI, Holm IA, Weinstein DA 1999 Glycogen storage diseases. Phenotypic, genetic, and biochemical characteristics, and therapy. Endocrine & Metabolism Clinics of North America 28: 801–23.

Homocystinuria

One of the aminoacidurias, this autosomal recessive, metabolic disease results from a deficiency of cystathionine B synthetase, which catalyses the reaction of homocystine and serine to produce cystathionine. Large amounts of homocystine and methionine are found in the blood and the urine. There is evidence that homocystine may affect the coagulation system and the resistance of endothelium to thrombosis, and that it may interfere with the vasodilator and antithrombotic functions of nitric oxide (Nygard et al 1997). The decrease in cystine, which is an important constituent of the cross linkages in collagen, produces a weakened collagen. There is fragmentation of elastic tissue of large arteries. There is evidence that vitamin E and ascorbic acid can block the effect of hyperhomocystinaemia, thus suggesting an oxidative mechanism for impairment of endothelial cell function (Nappo et al 1999).

Hyperhomocystinaemia has been found to be an independent risk factor in young individuals with vascular disease (Clarke et al 1991). After diagnostic criteria had been determined (peak serum homocystine levels following methionine loading), 123 patients with vascular disease presenting before the age of 55 were compared with 27 normal, matched individuals. Hyperhomocystinaemia was found in 42% with cerebrovascular disease, 28% with peripheral vascular disease, and 30% with coronary artery disease, but was not seen in normal subjects. In 18 of the 23 patients with hyperhomocystinaemia, deficiency of cystathionine beta-synthase deficiency was confirmed. Plasma total homocystine levels were found to be a strong predictor of mortality in patients with angiographically confirmed coronary artery disease (Nygard et al 1997).

Preoperative abnormalities

1. Abnormalities include lens dislocation, ligamentous laxity, elongated extremities similar to Marfan's syndrome, but without the hyperextensiblity of joints, kyphoscoliosis, and brittle, light-coloured hair. If the condition is not diagnosed and treated early, mental retardation occurs.

2. Homocystine, which is not normally present in the urine, occurs in large amounts, as does methionine.

3. The irritant effect on the vascular endothelium causes platelet aggregation and subsequent thromboembolism. If untreated, 50% of patients have major thromboembolic episodes, and the mortality is about 20% before the age of 30 years (Nygard et al 1997).

4. Treatment consists of a diet that is low in methionine but contains cystine supplements. Pyridoxine, dipyramidole and acetyl salicylic acid may be used to decrease platelet adhesion. Vitamin B_{12} and folic acid are also given. Anticoagulants may be required in high-risk situations.

Anaesthetic problems

1. Thomboembolism, which can be fatal, may occur in association with surgery. Problems are not confined to the homozygous individual. Cerebral infarction, which occurred 11 days after Caesarean section, was the presenting feature in a heterozygote (Minkhorst et al 1991). Three weeks after normal delivery, a 20-year-old patient thought to have Marfan's syndrome suffered near-fatal postpartum cavernous sinus thrombosis. Only after this was the diagnosis of homocystinuria made (Calvert & Rand 1995).

2. Patients may have increased insulin levels resulting in hypoglycaemia.

3. Regional anaesthesia has certain theoretical disadvantages. Penetration of a large epidural blood vessel might initiate thrombosis, as may the accompanying venous stasis of the lower limbs.

4. Anaesthesia for lensectomy is most frequently reported (Grover et al 1979, Parris & Quimby 1982, Lowe et al 1995). In a series of 45 patients having 82 operations, the majority required general anaesthesia, and more than half were mentally retarded (Harrison et al 1998).

5. A state of psychotic delirium occurred following lensectomy in a 16 year old. It was postulated that the glutamate agonist effects of methionine, homocystine and cystine interfered with cerebral glutamatergic transmission (Eschweiler et al 1997). Another patient presented with an acute psychiatric disorder that responded to pyridoxine 400 mg daily (Li & Stewart 1999).

6. There are increased risks in pregnancy and maternal deaths have been reported secondary to thromboses (Minkhorst et al 1991, Constantine & Green 1997). There is a high incidence of fetal loss and unsuccessful pregnancies (Burke et al 1992).

Management

1. Dehydration must be avoided, and a good cardiac output and peripheral perfusion maintained.

2. Blood viscosity and platelet adhesiveness can be reduced by dextran, and the prior administration of pyridoxine.

3. Dextrose infusion will prevent hypoglycaemia.

4. Early mobilisation, elastic stockings, and low-dose heparin therapy will help to decrease the chance of postoperative thromboembolism.

5. In the pregnant patient, heparin 10 000 u bd may be needed to reduce thrombotic risk. In the high-risk patient warfarin may have to be given following delivery (Calvert & Rand 1995). Pyridoxine and folic acid must be continued during pregnancy.

Bibliography

Burke G, Robinson K, Refsum H et al 1992 Intrauterine growth retardation, perinatal death, and maternal homocysteine levels. New England Journal of Medicine 326: 69–70.

Calvert SM, Rand RJ 1995 A successful pregnancy in a patient with homocystinuria and a previous near-fatal postpartum cavernous sinus thrombosis. British Journal of Obstetrics & Gynaecology 102: 751–2.

Clarke R, Daly L, Robinson K et al 1991 Hyperhomocysteinemia: an independent risk factor for vascular disease. New England Journal of Medicine 324: 1149–55.

Constantine G, Green A 1987 Untreated homocystinuria: a maternal death in a woman with four pregnancies. British Journal of Obstetrics & Gynaecology 97: 803–6.

Eschweiler GW, Rosin R, Thier P et al 1997 Postoperative psychosis in homocystinuria. European Psychiatry 12: 98–101.

Grover VK, Malhotra SK, Kaushik S 1979 Anaesthesia and homocystinuria. Anaesthesia 34: 913–14.

Harrison DA, Mullaney PB, Mesfer SA et al 1998 Management of ophthalmic complications of homocystinuria. Ophthalmology 105: 1886–90.

Li SC, Stewart PM 1999 Homocystinuria and psychiatric disorder: a case report. Pathology 31: 221–4.

Lowe S, Johnson DA, Tobias JD 1994 Anesthetic implications of the child with homocystinuria. Journal of Clinical Anesthesia 6: 142–4.

Minkhorst AG, van Dongen PW, Boers GH et al 1991 Cerebral infarction after caesarean section due to heterozygosity for homocystinuria; a case report. European Journal of Obstetrics, Gynecology & Reproductive Biology 40: 241–3.

Nappo F, De Rosa N, Marfella R et al 1999 Impairment of endothelial functions by acute hyperhomocysteinemia and reversal by antioxidant vitamins. Journal of the American Medical Association 281: 2113–18.

Nygard O, Nordrehaug JE, Refsum H et al 1997 Plasma homocysteine levels and mortality in patients with coronary artery disease. New England Journal of Medicine 337: 230–6.

Parris WCV, Quimby CW 1982 Anesthetic considerations for the patient with homocysteinuria. Anesthesia & Analgesia 61: 708–10.

Hunter's syndrome (see Hurler's syndrome and Mucopolysaccharidoses)

Huntington's disease

A degenerative neurological disorder secondary to a gene mutation, inherited as autosomal dominant. There is progressive neuronal loss in the neostriatum of the basal ganglia, and subsequently in the cerebral cortex, accompanied by a decrease in the levels of the associated neurotransmitters (Schapira 1997, Martin 1998). Onset is between 30 and 45 years, and death frequently follows within 10–15 years of the first symptoms.

Preoperative abnormalities

1. Clinical features are progressive, and include choreiform movements, ataxia, dysarthria, and dementia. Sleep and anaesthesia usually abolish the chorea, which may not return until several hours following the anaesthetic.

2. The chorea may be preceded by several years of gradually increasing personality changes and mental deterioration.

3. Patients with the clinical disease may be taking a variety of drugs to improve the chorea, including butyrophenones, phenothiazines, and tetrabenazine.

Anaesthetic problems

1. Despite the use of a variety of agents, four of the 16 cases reported in the anaesthetic literature were accompanied by prolonged apnoea or recovery (Davies 1966, Gualandi & Bonfanti 1968, Blanloeil et al 1982). Barbiturate (Davies 1966) and suxamethonium (Gualandi & Bonfanti 1968) sensitivities were suggested as the likely causes. Plasma cholinesterase measurement was not mentioned. Subsequent papers have, however, reported successful anaesthetics in which one or both of these agents were given (Farina & Raucher 1977, Browne & Cross 1981, Costarino & Gross 1985), whilst others used alternative agents (Lamont 1979, Johnson & Heggie 1985, Rodrigo 1987, Kaufman & Erb 1990). Assessment of the possible causative factors for either prolonged apnoea or delayed recovery from anaesthesia must take account of:

a) A higher than expected incidence of atypical plasma cholinesterase (the fluoride resistant gene, E_1^f) has been confirmed in patients with Huntington's disease (Whittaker 1980).

b) These patients are often receiving a variety of powerful psychotropic drugs including phenothiazines and butyrophenones, and tetrabenazine, a drug that depletes stores of cerebral biogenic amines. Any of these may interact with anaesthetic agents.

c) In advanced cases, there are gross atrophic changes in the cerebral cortex and basal ganglia.

d) Patients are frequently wasted and of poor nutritional status.

2. Dysphagia and abnormalities of pharyngeal and laryngeal function may predispose to aspiration in the perioperative period. Videofluoroscopic studies identified coughing on foods, choking on liquid, and episodes of aspiration (Kagel & Leopold 1992).

3. The problems of managing the uncooperative patient (Cangemi & Miller 1998).

Management

1. Plasma cholinesterase investigations should be carried out when patients are admitted for surgery, even if the use of suxamethonium is not intended. Their documentation may be of subsequent value. Should suxamethonium be required in the absence of the results, or if nondepolarising agents are used, neuromuscular monitoring is essential.

2. The dosages of all anaesthetic agents should be kept to a minimum, bearing in mind the pathology of the disease itself, preoperative neuroactive drugs, and the general nutrition of the patient.

3. Case reports of individul patients have promoted the use of midazolam for induction (Rodrigo 1987), and a propofol bolus for induction and an infusion for maintenance (Kaufman & Erb 1990, Soar & Matheson 1990).

4. Use of spinal anaesthesia for hernia repair has been decribed (Fernandez et al 1997).

Bibliography

Blanloeil Y, Bigot A, Dixneuf B 1982 Anaesthesia in Huntington's chorea. Anaesthesia 37: 695–6.
Browne MG, Cross R 1981 Huntington's chorea. British Journal of Anaesthesia 53: 1367.
Cangemi CF Jr, Miller RJ 1998 Huntington's disease: review and anesthetic case management. Anesthesia Progress 45: 150–3.
Costarino A, Gross JB 1985 Patients with Huntington's chorea may respond normally to succinylcholine. Anesthesiology 63: 570.
Davies DD 1966 Abnormal response to anaesthesia in a case of Huntington's chorea. British Journal of Anaesthesia 38: 490–1.
Farina J, Rauscher LA 1977 Anaesthesia and Huntington's chorea. British Journal of Anaesthesia 49: 1167–8.
Fernandez IG, Sanchez MP, Ugale AJ et al 1997 Spinal anaesthesia in a patient with Huntington's chorea. Anaesthesia 52: 391.
Gualandi W, Bonfanti G 1968 Un caso di apnea prolungata in corea di Huntington. Acta Anaesthesiologica (Padova) 19: 235–8.
Johnson MK, Heggie NM 1985 Huntington's chorea: a role for the newer anaesthetic agents. British Journal of Anaesthesia 57: 235–6.
Kagel MC, Leopold NA 1992 Dysphagia in Huntington's disease: a 16-year retrospective. Dysphagia 7: 106–14.
Kaufman MA, Erb T 1990 Propofol for patients with Huntington's chorea. Anaesthesia 45: 889–90.
Lamont ASM 1979 Brief report: anaesthesia and Huntington's chorea. Anaesthesia & Intensive Care 7: 189–90.
Martin JB 1998 Molecular basis of the neurodegenerative disorders. New England Journal of Medicine 340: 1970–80.
Rodrigo MRC 1987 Huntington's chorea: midazolam, a suitable induction agent? British Journal of Anaesthesia 59: 388–9.
Schapira AH 1997 Mitochondrial function in Huntington's disease: clues for pathogenesis and prospects for treatment. Annals of Neurology 41: 141–2.
Soar J, Matheson KH 1993 A safe anaesthetic in Huntington's disease. Anaesthesia 48: 743–4.
Whittaker M 1980 Plasma cholinesterase variants and the anaesthetist. Anaesthesia 35: 174–97.

Hurler, Hurler–Scheie, Scheie and Hunter syndromes (see also Mucopolysaccharidoses)

The mucopolysaccharidoses (MPS) are a group of inherited connective tissue syndromes that result from deficiencies of specific enzymes responsible for the degradation of mucopolysaccharides (glycoaminoglycans).

Mucopolysaccharides are constituents of normal connective tissue and are composed of repeating disaccharide units connected to protein. They are normally broken down in the cell lysosomes to monosaccharides and amino acids. In the absence of certain enzymes, intermediate products of degradation accumulate. Cell size increases and cell function is impaired. The effects depend upon the enzyme defect and the specific organs involved.

Hurler, Hurler–Scheie and Scheie syndromes are all type I MPS. Hunter's, type II, is similar to Hurler's, but less severe and with no mental retardation. All four are considered together here because they produce similar anaesthetic airway problems, and are the most difficult of the MPS types with which the anaesthetist will have to deal. Cardiac involvement is present in most patients with MPS, but the most severe changes occur in Hurler, Hunter, and Maroteaux–Lamy (Dangel 1998).

Patients often present with otolaryngological problems, including serous otitis media, sensorineural deafness and upper airway obstruction. In a study of 45 children, every patient had at least one head and neck complication (Bredenkamp et al 1992). Since airway problems increase with age, it has been suggested that, if surgery is contemplated, it should be undertaken earlier rather than later (Moores et al 1996). Anaesthesia is most likely to be required for recurrent ENT procedures, the repair of inguinal or umbilical herniae, and, since the mid 1980s, bone marrow transplantation. In selected patients, bone marrow transplantation has improved certain features of Hurler's syndrome, but the orthopaedic and corneal problems persist.

Preoperative abnormalities

Hurler's syndrome (type IH: gargoylism)

1. Craniofacial. Hypertelorism, frontal bossing, depressed nasal bridge, coarse features, irregular and broadly spaced teeth, gum hypertrophy, macroglossia, and corneal opacities.

2. Respiratory. Mouth breathing, airway obstruction, profuse secretions, pectus excavatum, frequent respiratory infections, and sleep apnoea.

3. Cardiac. Coronary artery disease resulting from intimal deposition of mucopolysaccharides, valvular lesions (Wipperman et al 1995), pulmonary hypertension, and cardiac failure.

4. Skeletal. Dwarfing, short neck, kyphoscoliosis, and claw hand. Atlantoaxial instability has been described.

5. Mental status. Subnormal.

6. Other organs. Hepatosplenomegaly, umbilical and inguinal herniae.

7. Deficient enzyme. L-iduronidase.

8. Prognosis. Death within the first decade.

Scheie (type IS)

1. Craniofacial. Corneal clouding, prognathism, and macroglossia.

2. Respiratory. Airway involvement but less severe than Hurler's syndrome.

3. Cardiac. Aortic regurgitation.

4. Skeletal. Normal stature, short neck, deformity of hands and feet.

5. Mental status. Normal.

6. Other organs. Glaucoma, herniae and carpal tunnel syndrome.

7. Deficient enzyme. L-iduronidase.

Hurler–Scheie (type IH/S)

Intermediate between Hurler and Scheie.

Hunter's (type II)

An X-linked recessive disease, similar to Hurler's but less severe. There is evidence of two distinct groups, mild and severe. This distinction is based on the presence or absence of progressive mental retardation (Young & Harper 1982).

1. Craniofacial. Coarse facies, deafness, and papilloedema.

2. Respiratory. Upper airway involvement from soft-tissue deposition, excessive secretions.

3. Cardiac. Coronary intimal thickening, valvular disease, and heart failure. Heart disease is the commonest cause of death.

4. Skeletal. Dwarfism, kyphoscoliosis, claw hands, and stiff joints.

5. Mental status. Normal in the mild form, progressive retardation in the severe.

6. Other organs. Hepatosplenomegaly. The majority of patients have either umbilical or inguinal herniae.

7. Deficient enzyme. Iduronate sulphatase.

Anaesthetic problems

1. Airway maintenance and induction difficulties. Reviews of patients with MPS have noted that more than 50% had airway-related problems (Baines & Keneally 1983, Kempthorne & Brown 1983, King et al 1984, Herrick & Rhine 1988, Walker et al 1994, Moores et al 1996). The majority of these were in Hurler, Hunter, or Maroteaux–Lamy MPS. Difficulties in airway maintenance appear to arise in part from obstruction by soft-tissue deposits in the mouth, the tongue, and the pharyngeal tissues, and in part from excess, and frequently purulent, tracheobronchial secretions. Pharyngeal tissue infiltration can assume a polypoid form and cause stridor by obstructing the laryngeal inlet (Busoni & Fognani 1999).

2. Tracheal intubation difficulties were again reported in more than 50% of cases. The above problems are compounded by the large head and hypertelorism. Complete failure to intubate occurred in three patients, another had a hypoxic cardiac arrest (Kempthorne & Brown 1983) but was resuscitated, and one died (Young & Harper 1982). It has been noted that the larynx is often smaller than anticipated. In one series, tracheostomy was required in four patients,

either for sleep apnoea or for failed intubation during induction of anaesthesia (Ruckstein et al 1990). Failure to intubate a patient before aortic and mitral valve replacement prompted the institution of cardiopulmonary bypass whilst undertaking mask ventilation of the lungs (Nicolson et al 1992). Multiple attempts to intubate the patient subsequently culminated in the use of a retrograde tracheal technique.

3. Emergency tracheostomy was required on day 6 following tonsillectomy (Yoskavitch et al 1998). The technique may be difficult or impossible to perform. Fatal postoperative respiratory obstruction occurred secondary to glottic oedema in an abnormal larynx, and emergency tracheostomy was impeded by the presence of hard, thickened cartilage (Hopkins et al 1973).

4. The airway may be obstructed by abnormal tissue and, in one patient, this was found to extend the whole length. Thus, the patient's left lower lobe collapse was found to be secondary to mucopolysaccharide thickening of the bronchial wall, rather than a mucous plug (Moores et al 1996). In an infant with Hunter's syndrome, obstruction was secondary to distal tracheobronchomalacia, and, during EUA, severe anteroposterior flattening of the trachea was seen (Morehead & Parsons 1993).

Laryngeal mask airway insertion was attempted in an 11-year-old child with stridor, but still no airway could be obtained. Rigid bronchoscopy revealed a large pedunculated polyp above the epiglottis, which had been displaced by the laryngeal mask airway (Busoni & Fognani 1999). Although use of the laryngeal mask airway has been reported to be successful in some patients, it cannot be depended upon, particularly if there are clinical signs of obstruction in the periglottic region, or in the airway distal to the vocal cords. The laryngeal mask airway failed in a 15-year-old boy having grommet insertion, in whom neither intubation nor mask ventilation was possible. The cricothyroid membrane could not be located and emergency tracheostomy was performed.

Unfortunately, cardiac arrest occurred and, although initial resuscitation was successful, the patient died 2 weeks later (Gaitini et al 1998).

5. Obstructive sleep apnoea, secondary to infiltration with myxomatous tissue around the vocal cords, was found in one patient (Orliaguet et al 1999). Removal of the tissue allowed CPAP to be used successfully.

6. Venous access may be a problem (King et al 1984).

7. Atlanto-occipital instability resulted in a spastic quadriplegia in one patient with Hurler's (Brill et al 1978).

8. Sleep apnoea secondary to upper airway obstruction, with oxygen desaturation and hypercarbia during sleep, has been reported (Ruckstein et al 1990). This may result in cardiac failure and growth retardation (Stevens 1988). In a study of 21 patients, 50% had a clinical history of sleep apnoea and 90% had evidence of it confirmed on polysonography (Semenza & Pyeritz 1988).

9. Pulmonary oedema occurred secondary to airway obstruction in a patient undergoing fibreoptic intubation (Wilder & Belani 1990).

10. Delayed recovery from anaesthesia has been reported in a 27-kg boy (Kreidstein et al 1994). This was attributed to fentanyl 25 mg, which was eventually reversed by naloxone.

Management

1. A careful assessment of the airway, and possible intubation difficulties, is essential. Examination of previous anaesthetic notes may indicate problems. Occasionally, a CT scan of the airway may be helpful. Parents should be warned of the increased risk of anaesthesia, and that tracheostomy may be required. Two experienced anaesthetists should be present.

2. Cardiological assessment is required.

3. If appropriate, the cervical spine should be screened to detect atlantoaxial instability.

4. A drying agent is essential, because of excessive secretions, and sedatives are best avoided.

5. It has been claimed that inhalation inductions are difficult, and intravenous agents are dangerous (Herrick & Rhine 1988). Awake fibreoptic intubation should be considered, but this is not free of risk (Wilder & Belani 1990), and should only be carried out by those experienced in the technique. The advantages of maintaining spontaneous respiration has been stressed (Walker & Dearlove 1997), and neuromuscular blockers should not be used until the airway is ensured.

6. A nasal airway has been suggested as being more effective than an oral one (Brown 1984), and this can be left in place until the patient is awake. Lateral X-rays in two patients have shown that an oral airway pushes the epiglottis down and backwards to occlude the laryngeal inlet, whereas a nasal airway keeps it forward. However, a nasopharyngeal airway did not help in a fatal case reported by Gaitini et al (1998). Preoperative tracheostomy has been performed in patients with known failed intubation (Baines & Keneally 1983). However, secretions may still block the tube. The domiciliary use of a nasopharyngeal tube has been described in a patient with cardiac failure and episodes of profound nocturnal hypoxia (Stevens 1988).

7. Use of the laryngeal mask airway has been reported in a 43 year old with Hunter's syndrome and a fixed flexion deformity (Henderson 1995). However, the age of the patient, and the fact that laryngoscopy at the end revealed a grade 1 view, suggests that he had a mild form of the disease. Walker and Dearlove (1997) support the use of the laryngeal mask airway, both for routine airway management and as a back-up to failed intubation. However, Moores et al (1996) suggest that the role of the laryngeal mask airway has not yet been defined in the difficult MPS cases, and have suggested that it should be used with caution because of the short neck and high larynx. Brown (1997) suggests that it may not need to be inserted as far

as usual, and that it, like the oropharyngeal airway, can push the epiglottis over the laryngeal inlet causing obstruction. As has already been pointed out, the laryngeal mask airway has limited value if the obstruction lies at glottic level or below.

8. Local anaesthetic techniques should be considered. Spinal anaesthesia has been reported in a patient with a previous failed intubation (Sjögren & Pedersen 1986). Combined continuous spinal analgesia and general anaesthesia were used for upper abdominal surgery in a patient with Hurler–Scheie syndrome (Sethna and Berde 1991).

9. Tracheostomy may be required, either for failed tracheal intubation or to treat obstructive sleep apnoea.

Bibliography

Baines D, Keneally J 1983 Anaesthetic implications of the mucopolysaccharidoses. Anaesthesia & Intensive Care 11: 198–202.

Bredenkamp JK, Smith ME, Dudley JP et al 1992 Otolaryngologic manifestations of the mucopolysaccharidoses. Annals of Otology, Rhinology & Laryngology 101: 472–8.

Brill CB, Rose JS, Godmilow L et al 1978 Spastic quadriparesis due to C1–C2 subluxation in Hurler syndrome. Journal of Pediatrics 92: 441–3.

Brown TCK 1984 The airway in mucopolysaccharidoses. Anaesthesia & Intensive Care 12: 178.

Brown TCK 1997 Anaesthesia and the mucopolysaccharidoses: reply. Anaesthesia & Intensive Care 25: 197–8.

Busoni P, Fognani G 1999 Failure of the laryngeal mask to secure the airway in a patient with Hunter's syndrome (mucopolysaccharidosis type II). Paediatric Anaesthesia 9: 153–5.

Dangel JH 1998 Cardiovascular changes in children with mucopolysaccharide storage diseases and related disorders—clinical and echocardiographic findings in 64 patients. European Journal of Pediatrics 157: 534–8.

Gaitini L, Fradis M, Vaida S et al 1998 Failure to control the airway in a patient with Hunter syndrome. Journal of Laryngology & Otology 112: 380–2.

Henderson MA 1995 Use of a laryngeal mask airway in an adult patient with the Hunter syndrome. European Journal of Anaesthesiology 12: 613–16.

Herrick IA, Rhine EJ 1988 The mucopolysaccharidoses and anaesthesia: a report of clinical experience. Canadian Journal of Anaesthesia 35: 67–73.

Hopkins R, Watson JA, Jones JH et al 1973 Two cases of Hunter's syndrome. The anaesthetic and operative difficulties in oral surgery. British Journal of Oral Surgery 10: 286–99.

Kempthorne PM, Brown TCK 1983 Anaesthesia and the mucopolysaccharidoses. Anaesthesia & Intensive Care 11: 203–7.

King DH, Jones RM, Barnett MB 1984 Anaesthetic considerations in the mucopolysaccharidoses. Anaesthesia 39: 126–31.

Kreidstein A, Boorin MR, Crespi P et al 1994 Delayed awakening from general anaesthesia in a patient with Hunter syndrome. Canadian Journal of Anaesthesia 41: 423–6.

Moores C, Rogers JG, McKenzie IM et al 1996 Anaesthesia for children with mucopolysaccharidoses. Anaesthesia & Intensive Care 24: 459–63.

Morehead JM, Parsons DS 1993 Tracheobronchomalacia in Hunter's syndrome. Journal of Pediatric Otorhinolaryngology 26: 255–61.

Nicolson SC, Black AE, Kraras CM 1992 Management of a difficult airway in a patient with Hurler–Scheie syndrome during cardiac surgery. Anesthesia & Analgesia 75: 830–2.

Orliaguet O, Pepin JL, Veale D et al 1999 Hunter's syndrome associated with sleep apnoea cured by CPAP and surgery. European Respiratory Journal 13: 1195–7.

Ruckstein MJ, Macdonald RE, Clarke JTR et al 1990 The management of otolaryngological problems in the mucopolysaccharidoses: a retrospective review. Journal of Otolaryngology 20: 177–83.

Semenza GL, Pyeritz RE 1988 Respiratory complications of mucopolysaccharide storage disorders. Medicine 67: 209–19.

Sethna NF, Berde CB 1991 Continuous subarachnoid analgesia in two adolescents with severe scoliosis and impaired pulmonary function. Regional Anesthesia 16: 333–6.

Sjögren P, Pedersen T 1986 Anaesthetic problems in Hurler–Scheie syndrome. Report of 2 cases. Acta Anaesthesiologica Scandinavica 30: 484–6.

Stevens IM 1988 Domiciliary use of nasopharyngeal intubation for obstructive sleep apnoea in a child with mucopolysaccharidosis. Anaesthesia & Intensive Care 16: 493–4.

Walker RWM, Dearlove OR 1997 Anaesthesia for children with mucopolysaccharidoses. Anaesthesia & Intensive Care 25: 197.

Walker RWM, Darowski M, Morris P et al 1994 Anaesthesia and mucopolysaccharidoses. A review of airway problems in children. Anaesthesia 49: 1078–84.

Wilder RT, Belani KG 1990 Fiberoptic intubation complicated by pulmonary edema in a 12-year-old child with Hurler syndrome. Anesthesiology 72: 205–7.

Wipperman CF, Beck M, Schranz D et al 1995 Mitral and aortic regurgitation in 84 patients with mucopolysaccharidoses. European Journal of Pediatrics 154: 98–101.

Yoskavitch A, Tewfik TL, Brouillette RT et al 1998 Acute airway obstruction in the Hunter syndrome. International Journal of Pediatric Otolaryngology 44: 273–8.

Young ID, Harper PS 1982 Mild form of Hunter's syndrome: clinical delineation based on 31 cases. Archives of Diseases in Childhood 57: 828–36.

Hydatid disease

Hydatid cysts are the larval stage of the tapeworm, *Echinococcus granulosus*. Dogs are the main hosts. Man and sheep are intermediate hosts. Hydatid disease is not uncommon amongst the mid-Wales farming communities, and up to 26% of farm dogs in this area have *E. granulosus*. The incidence is also high in some regions of the Mediterranean (Sola et al 1995), North Africa, the Middle East, and Australia. If the ova are ingested by man, embryos are released when the chitinous coat is digested. These enter the liver by the portal vein. They may be destroyed, or they may develop into a cyst. In man, the cysts are found in the liver (65%), lung (25%), muscles (5%), bone (3%), and brain (1%).

Each cyst is two layered and contains straw-coloured fluid in which there are free scolices, brood capsules containing scolices, and daughter cysts. Around the cyst is an area of compressed host tissue and fibrosis known as the pericyst. In 5–10% of cases the cyst will die, and calcification may occur (Lewis et al 1975).

Preoperative abnormalities

1. Hepatic cysts occur most frequently in the right lobe. Bacterial infection may result in a liver abscess. Rupture into a bile duct, or bile duct obstruction, can occur and produce biliary colic. There may be jaundice. The number and location of the cysts are shown on CT scan or ultrasound.

2. Pulmonary cysts can present with haemoptysis, dyspnoea, cough, or chest pain. Chest X-ray may show a variety of appearances including an oval opacity, evidence of bronchial fistula formation, or rupture of the cyst with the development of a fluid level.

3. Eosinophilia occurs in about 30% of cases. The Casoni skin test is still used for screening. Immunoelectrophoresis is the most specific test. Complement fixation test is positive in up to 80% of cases. Haemagglutination test detects a specific antibody.

Anaesthetic problems

1. Pulmonary hydatid cysts can cause bronchial obstruction, and occasionally they may rupture into the airway. If this happens, flooding of the lungs occurs, with widespread dissemination of the scolices. Boots (1998) described spontaneous rupture of a pulmonary cyst in a cattleman, who jumped into the river whilst intoxicated.

2. Hydatid fluid is highly antigenic, and rupture of a cyst has occasionally produced sudden death from an anaphylactic reaction (Jakubowski & Barnard 1971). During lung cyst puncture in another patient, a period of severe hypotension occurred, for which cardiopulmonary resuscitation measures were required (Blanco et al 1996). Anaphylaxis to hydatid was confirmed by increased serum histamine and tryptase levels, with elevated levels

of total and echinococcus-specific IgE antibodies. Aspiration of a hepatic cyst during surgery caused cardiovascular collapse and hypoxaemia in another patient (Sola et al 1995). In a study of 386 cases, 12 had allergic reactions to cyst rupture, but none were fatal (Jerray et al 1992).

3. Patients can develop anaphylaxis of unknown origin. Laglera et al (1997) described a 49-year-old woman who presented with signs of cardiogenic shock and ST elevation in leads V1–V3. Echocardiography and CT scan showed an interventricular cystic mass that was excised under cardiopulmonary bypass and found to be hydatid.

4. Cerebral cysts can cause increased intracranial pressure.

5. Scolicidal agents are potentially toxic and their use in combination with surgery may increase the complication rate.

6. Acute hyperosmolar coma from hypernatraemia (serum Na 163 mmol l^{-1}) and hyperglycaemia (42 mmol l^{-1}) occurred in a 13 year old after emergency surgery for a hepatic cyst. The area around the liver had been packed with 20% saline sponges and the remaining saline (from a 1-litre bag) had been used for irrigation of the cyst cavity (Rakic et al 1994). The hypernatraemia was probably compounded by sodium bicarbonate given to treat a metabolic acidosis.

7. Postoperative complications following surgery for hydatid cyst of the lung included prolonged air leak and aspiration pneumonia (Jerray et al 1992).

Management

1. Surgical removal is indicated, except in older patients with small cysts (Behrns & van Heerden 1991). Meticulous care must be taken to avoid rupture and spread of the fertile scolices.

2. Relatively new drugs, such as mebendazole and albendazole, are being tested as scolicidal agents. However, there is no evidence

that they are effective in the treatment of pulmonary hydatid (Aggarawal & Wali 1991).

3. Pulmonary cysts. Protective formalin-soaked packs are placed around the wound, an incision is made through the pericyst and the cyst is carefully extruded by the anaesthetist, using gentle hand ventilation (Saidi 1977).

4. Because of the risk of an anaphylactic reaction, epinephrine (adrenaline), metaraminol, isoprenaline and steroids must be immediately available (Lewis et al 1975).

Bibliography

Aggarawal P, Wali JP 1991 Albendazole in the treatment of pulmonary echinococcosis. Thorax 46: 559–60.

Behrns KE, van Heerden JA 1991 Surgical management of hepatic hydatid disease. Mayo Clinic Proceedings 66: 1193–7.

Blanco I, Cardenas E, Aguilera L et al 1996 Serum tryptase measurement in diagnosis of intraoperative anaphylaxis caused by hydatid cyst. Anaesthesia & Intensive Care 24: 489–91.

Boots RJ 1998 'Near drowning' due to hydatid disease. Anaesthesia & Intensive Care 26: 680–1.

Jakubowski MS, Barnard DE 1971 Anaphylactic shock during operation for hydatid disease. Anesthesiology 34: 197–9.

Jerray M, Benzarti M, Garrouche A et al 1992 Hydatid disease of the lungs: study of 386 cases. American Review of Respiratory Disease 146: 185–9.

Laglera S, Garcia-Enguita MA, Martinez-Gutierrez F et al 1997 A case of cardiac hydatidosis. British Journal of Anaesthesia 79: 671–3.

Lewis JW, Koss N, Kerstein MD 1975 A review of echinococcal disease. Annals of Surgery 181: 390–6.

Rakic M, Vegan B, Sprung J et al 1994 Acute hyperosmolar coma complicating anesthesia for hydatid disease surgery. Anesthesiology 80: 1175–8.

Saidi F 1977 A new approach to the surgical treatment of hydatid cyst. Annals of the Royal College of Surgeons 59: 115–18.

Sola JL, Vaquerizo A, Madariaga MJ et al 1995 Intraoperative anaphylaxis caused by a hydatid cyst. Acta Anaesthesiologica Scandinavica 39: 273–4.

Hypercalcaemia

When artefactual causes of an increased serum calcium level have been excluded, the commonest causes of hypercalcaemia are malignancy and hyperparathyroidism. Sarcoidosis, thyrotoxicosis and vitamin D toxicity are uncommon. Other causes are extremely rare. Occasionally a patient with hypercalcaemia may present for anaesthesia. Severe hypercalcaemia (>3.2 mmol l^{-1}) may be dangerous and, in consultation with a physician, urgent lowering of the level may be required.

Preoperative abnormalities

1. Any malignancy with destructive bone metastases can produce hypercalcaemia, by increased bone resorption and reduced urinary excretion of calcium. Hypercalcaemia occurs in about 10% of cancer patients and the commonest causes are breast carcinoma, myeloma, bronchial and renal carcinoma. If the serum albumin is low, the adjusted calcium = measured calcium + 0.02 × [mean normal albumin − measured albumin] where Ca is in mmol l^{-1} and albumin is in g l^{-1}.

2. The combination of hypercalcaemia and an increased parathyroid hormone (PTH) level is diagnostic of hyperparathyroidism. However, PTH levels may take several weeks to obtain and treatment may be required before the result is available.

3. Carcinoma of the lung or a renal cell carcinoma may rarely release a parathormone-like substance, leading to hypercalcaemia.

4. Symptoms of hypercalcaemia may be vague. They include general muscle weakness, apathy, gastrointestinal complaints such as nausea, vomiting and constipation, weight loss, thirst, polyuria, polydipsia, and mental disturbances, progressing to unconsciousness. Renal stones may form. Symptoms do not usually occur until the serum calcium is >3.2 mmol l^{-1}. ECG may show an abnormally short QT interval.

Anaesthetic problems

1. A hypercalcaemic patient may be severely dehydrated.

2. Hypercalcaemia may precipitate serious arrhythmias. Fatal intraoperative cardiac arrest occurred in a young man with a serum calcium level of 5.6 mmol l^{-1}, despite attempts to reduce the level (Murphy 1992).

3. Hypercalcaemia in pregnancy presented as hyperemesis gravidarum (Sharma et al 1995).

4. Digitalis toxicity is exacerbated by a high serum calcium level.

5. If rapid sequence induction is undertaken in the presence of hypercalcaemia, 1.4 times the normal dose of suxamethonium will be required (Roland et al 1991).

Management

1. Replacement of extracellular fluid by rehydration is the first and most important procedure. A diuresis causes excretion of calcium in the urine. An infusion of 1 l of sodium chloride 0.9% 3–4 hrly for 24 h should reduce the serum calcium by 0.5 mmol l^{-1}. Loop diuretics can be added, but not until adequate fluid repletion has been achieved. Thiazide diuretics should not be used because they increase tubular reabsorption of calcium. Fluid balance and serum potassium levels require careful monitoring.

2. Disodium pamidronate (60 mg if Ca <3.5 mmol l^{-1}, 90 mg if Ca >3.5 mmol l^{-1}) over 2 h, or sodium clodronate 1500 mg over 4 h, both in 500 ml 0.9% saline. Diphosphonates reduce osteoclastic bone resorption (Falk & Fallon 1997, Mundy & Guise 1997).

3. Measure serum calcium after 48 h. Treatment may take 3–5 days.

4. Corticosteroids can be used, although there is some question about their efficiency. Calcitonin (100–400 iu sc 8 hrly) reduces mobilisation of calcium from bone and will also produce an early, but transient effect (48–72 h) on calcium levels.

Bibliography
Falk S, Fallon M 1997 ABC of palliative care. Emergencies. British Medical Journal 315: 1525–8.

Mundy GR, Guise TA 1997 Hypercalcemia of malignancy. American Journal of Medicine 103: 134–45.

Murphy JP 1992 Fatal hypercalcaemic crisis. British Journal of Hospital Medicine 18: 677–8.

Roland E, Villers S, Lequeau F et al 1991 Succinylcholine dose-response in hyperparathyroidism. Anesthesiology 75: A808.

Sharma JB, Davies WAR, McConnell D 1995 Primary hyperparathyroidism in pregnancy masquerading as hyperemesis gravidarum. Journal of Obstetrics & Gynaecology 15: 185–6.

Stevenson JC 1985 Malignant hypercalcaemia. British Medical Journal 291: 421–2.

Tisell L-E, Hedback G, Jansson S et al 1991 Management of hyperparathyroid patients with grave hypercalcemia. World Journal of Surgery 15: 730–7.

Hyponatraemia

Hyponatraemia is of concern because of increasing evidence that it is a cause of significant morbidity and mortality in the hospital population (Arieff 1998, Gill & Leese 1998, Knochel 1999, Lane & Allen 1999). Even more worrying is the iatrogenic contribution to its development. There have been several studies of the distribution of low sodium levels in hospital. Flear et al (1981) showed that 15.2% of patients had levels below 134 mmol l^{-1}, 4.9% below 130 mmol l^{-1}, 1.2% below 125 mmol l^{-1} and 0.2% below 120 mmol l^{-1}. Whilst the latter figure is considered to be dangerous, chronic levels lower than this have been tolerated surprisingly well. However in the acute situation, levels between 120 and 125 mmol l^{-1} have sometimes produced convulsions.

A recent estimate from studies in the USA suggests that 20% of women who develop symptomatic hyponatraemia die or suffer serious brain damage; this may involve 10–15 000 patients (Fraser & Arieff 1997). The contribution of hypoxia to the development of irreversible brain damage is now recognised in both adults (Ayus & Arieff 1999, Knochel 1999) and children (Arieff 1998).

Hyponatraemia encountered in the perioperative period is usually secondary to water overload, and may occur preoperatively as a result of medication or underlying illness, or postoperatively secondary to enthusiastic use of non-salt-containing fluids. The contribution of thiazide diuretic therapy to chronic hyponatraemia, particularly in elderly women, has only recently been recognised (Ayus & Arieff 1999). Lane and Allen (1999) described an example in which an elderly women with borderline hyponatraemia from thiazide diuretics was given 6 l of dextrose saline over the 2 days after knee replacement. By day 2 she was in coma with a serum sodium of 115 mmol l^{-1}. Although this was then recognised and corrected over 5 days, she had residual cognitive impairment.

After operation, most patients have been shown to have increased plasma levels of ADH. In addition, a number of drugs possess antidiuretic properties. The administration of large quantities of hypotonic dextrose solution can therefore cause serious fluid retention and hyponatraemia.

Vigorous attempts should be made to determine the primary cause. Therapeutic measures, if required, differ markedly, and depend on the aetiology and degree of severity. Interpretation of states of hyponatraemia and hyposmolality are difficult, and Oster and Singer (1999) have constructed data for six different hyponatraemic states and explain their relative risks.

In many mild cases, an underlying illness may simply require treatment, whilst water intake should be restricted when appropriate. Controversy has previously existed about the necessity or otherwise to be more active and administer saline to those more severely affected. Sterns (1992) is a protagonist of the dangers of 'osmotic demyelination syndrome' and the case for conservative management of hyponatraemia with correction rates of <6–8 mmol l^{-1} day^{-1}. However, there is now persuasive evidence that failure to treat acute water intoxication adequately can be equally dangerous and has resulted in cerebral oedema, uncal herniation, and death. In particular, it has been demonstrated that the presence of concurrent hypoxia can cause severe brain damage in those untreated patients who survive (Knochel 1999).

Patients may be admitted who are receiving drugs such as thiazide diuretics and selective serotonin antagonists which are associated with hyponatraemia. Excessive beer drinking and excessive water drinking associated with Ecstasy may be a cause in young people. Hyponatraemia can occur in glucocorticoid deficiency, primary adrenal failure, or secondary pituitary ACTH deficiency.

Causes

1. *Dilutional hyponatraemia.*

a) *Excess water intake.* Water retention can occur due to the perioperative infusion of large volumes of non-salt-containing glucose solutions. Oxytocin and opiates, both of which have antidiuretic properties, given during labour or prostaglandin termination of pregnancy, can compound the problem (Feeney 1982). Use of oxytocin in dextrose 5% in labour, compared with Hartmann's solution, resulted in significantly decreased maternal and neonatal serum sodium concentrations (Higgins et al 1996). In patients treated with beta adrenoceptor stimulants to suppress premature labour, retention of water is thought to be one of the contributing factors towards the rare development of pulmonary oedema (Hawker 1984), and, in addition, recent studies have shown these drugs to have no significant benefit on preterm labour (Canadian Preterm Labour Investigation Group 1992). Surgery is normally associated with increased ADH levels. The use of certain drugs, such as vasopressin, DDAVP, and steroids, will tend to exacerbate the situation. The features of the TURP syndrome (see Section 2) are in part caused by hyponatraemia,

secondary to absorption of glycine from the prostatic venous sinuses during prostatectomy.

b) *Decreased water clearance.* May be due to appropriate, or inappropriate, secretion of ADH. The syndrome of inappropriate antidiuresis (SIAD) is said to occur with a variety of conditions. It may be associated with a tumour, most frequently bronchial carcinoma, thoracic disease, IPPV, the Guillain–Barré syndrome and a variety of cerebral problems such as injury, meningitis, or primary tumours. However, it has been suggested that the ADH secretion associated with CNS lesions is iatrogenic, occurring secondary to excessive administration of fluids (Bouzarth & Shenkin 1982).

2. *Loss of body solutes.*

a) Loss of sodium. Causes include thiazide diuretics, gastrointestinal losses, renal disease, adrenal insufficiency, withdrawal of steroid therapy, salt depletion, and severe hypothyroidism. Further causes of solute loss have been suggested (Flear et al 1981), but there is controversy about their significance.

b) Loss of intracellular anions and potassium. If solute is lost, cells become hypo-osmolar. To prevent cell shrinkage, the plasma osmolality falls and hyponatraemia is produced.

c) Membrane defects result in leakage of cellular contents. This may occur in sick cell syndrome, associated for example with heart failure.

d) In cachexia, the catabolic state results in impaired production of intracellular anions. Doubt has been cast on the concept of sick cell syndrome (Bichet & Schrier 1982), since the leakage of intracellular solute into the extracellular fluid should be capable of being demonstrated by a positive osmolal gap (measured minus calculated osmolality) and a normal serum osmolality. Some studies have failed to confirm this.

3. *Increase in solute in plasma.* Results in a redistribution of water to maintain osmotic balance. Can occur in:

a) An infusion of mannitol to reduce cerebral oedema.

b) Sudden hyperglycaemia.

c) The sick cell syndrome (see above).

It is suggested that serious illness may cause cell membrane defects which result in loss of intracellular solutes into the extracellular fluid, which in turn extracts intracellular water. Hyponatraemia occurs, but if this theory is correct, the plasma osmolality should remain normal, and an osmolal gap should be shown.

4. *Excess of large paraprotein or lipid molecules.* May decrease the fractional water content of plasma and give a falsely low sodium level (pseudohyponatraemia).

5. *Reduction of plasma proteins.* At physiological pH these contribute to the anions. A reduction may result in a compensatory decrease in serum sodium.

6. *'Drip arm' hyponatraemia.* Caused by venepuncture upstream from an infusion of hypotonic fluid.

Problems

1. Hyponatraemic encephalopathy in adults. Confusion, a decreased conscious level, and fits, may occur. The level at which this appears is variable, often depending on the rapidity with which the hyponatraemia has developed. As little as 3–4 l of dextrose-containing fluid over 2 days can be dangerous. Early symptoms, such as weakness, nausea, vomiting, and headache, are nonspecific. In acute hyponatraemia, fits can occur when plasma sodium levels are 123 mmol l^{-1} or less, but patients with chronic hyponatraemia appear to tolerate levels that are much lower than this, although brain damage

may occur (Ayus & Arieff 1999). In those who develop encephalopathy, hypoxia and respiratory failure result. Hypoxia is thought to be the cause of brain damage. Hyponatraemic fits occurred in a child treated with desmopressin for von Willebrand's disease (Allen et al 1999).

2. Encephalopathy from postoperative hyponatraemia is also recognised in children, who are more susceptible than adults. Biochemical, hormonal and anatomical differences are thought to contribute (Arieff 1998). Again, the aetiology of brain damage or death seems to be a combination of hyponatraemic iv fluids, elevated plasma ADH, and hypoxia secondary to the encephalopathy. A tendency towards hyponatraemia will occur when any intravenous fluid is given with a concentration of less than 140 mmol l^{-1}.

3. Pulmonary oedema may occur.

4. Populations at particular risk are premenopausal women and children, in whom levels of 128 mmol l^{-1} can be dangerous (Arieff 1998). Postmenopausal women are slightly less susceptible and may tolerate levels down as far as 120 mmol l^{-1}.

5. The problem lies in whether or not to treat hyponatraemia actively. At one stage it was believed that rapid correction could be dangerous and associated with an 'osmotic demyelination syndrome' (Sterns et al 1986), and the pathological changes found in the brain were described as central pontine myelinolysis. It is now thought that the risks of not treating cerebral oedema actually outweigh the small risk of osmotic demyelination (Fraser & Arieff 1997, Kumar & Berl 1998).

Diagnosis

1. *Investigations.* A number of investigations may be required for the evaluation of hyponatraemia, although in many cases not all are necessary.

a) Plasma electrolytes, urea, creatinine, and glucose.

b) Plasma osmolality (measured and calculated).

c) Urine osmolality and urinary sodium, 24 h if possible.

d) Serum proteins.

e) Plasma cortisol or short synacthen test.

f) Serum lipids.

g) Body weight changes.

2. *Dilutional hyponatraemia.* May be diagnosed on history alone. During prostaglandin termination, or in labour, the administration of more than 3.5 l of dextrose 5% with oxytocin has been associated with water intoxication and fits (Feeney 1982). Postoperative hyponatraemia may be a combination of dilution with 5% dextrose and an elevated ADH level. Hyponatraemia, low plasma osmolality, a urine osmolality of about 3–4 times that of the plasma, and a high urinary sodium is highly suggestive of SIAD. Causes of SIAD should be sought.

3. *Loss of body solutes.* When there is sodium depletion, the urinary sodium excretion may be $<20 \, mmol \, 24 \, h^{-1}$, or a single sample concentration may be $<10 \, mmol \, l^{-1}$. In renal disease or heart failure these measurements may not be reliable. Hypokalaemia and alkalosis may indicate total body potassium depletion.

4. *Increase in solute in plasma.* Iso-osmotic redistribution of water takes place when there is a sudden increase in a solute. This may occur in hyperglycaemia, mannitol administration, and possibly in the sick cell syndrome. When the integrity of the cell membrane is impaired, some leakage of organic solutes is allowed into the extracellular fluid. The movement of solute is accompanied by water. If this happens, hyponatraemia should be accompanied by a normal plasma osmolality and an osmolal gap.

5. *Pseudohyponatraemia.* Hyponatraemia in the presence of a normal plasma osmolality may also indicate a paraproteinaemia or high serum triglyceride levels. If these are removed during estimation, the sodium concentration will be found to be normal.

6. *Decrease in serum cations or increase in anions.* Hypoproteinaemia or paraproteinaemia may alter the electrochemical balance resulting in a compensatory reduction in serum sodium.

Management

1. *Dilutional hyponatraemia.* **Prevention is critically important, since iatrogenic causes predominate.**

a) Excess water intake. **Large quantities of dextrose 5% or dextrose/saline should not be administered perioperatively, at a time when antidiuretic factors are operating**. If oxytocin is required, sodium chloride 0.9% or Ringer lactate should be used as an alternative vehicle (Higgins et al 1996). Should an electrolyte solution be contraindicated, a syringe pump may be used, or the total volume of dextrose 5% limited to 2 l in 24 h. Water restriction should be used as the primary treatment. However, should symptoms of encephalopathy occur in the presence of hyponatraemia, intravenous correction is urgent. **In addition, oxygen saturation should be monitored and hypoxia treated.** A sodium correction rate to achieve an increase in serum sodium of $1–2 \, mmol \, l^{-1} h^{-1}$ has been proposed, until symptoms improve (Fraser & Arieff 1999), stopping at a level of $133 \, mmol \, l^{-1}$. It is important not to overcorrect. A loop diuretic, such as frusemide, will enhance free water secretion. For less severe cases, lower rates of $6–8 \, mmol \, l^{-1} day^{-1}$ may be sufficient (Sterns 1992).

b) Syndrome of inappropriate antidiuresis (SIAD). Water is restricted and potassium given. If unsuccessful, demeclocycline $0.9–1.2 \, g \, day^{-1}$ is given in divided doses reducing to a daily maintenance dose of $600–900 \, mg \, day^{-1}$. The renal excretion of water is enhanced by blocking the renal tubular effect of ADH.

2. *Loss of body solutes.*

a) Loss of sodium. Treatment of the underlying illness is usually sufficient. Intravenous saline 0.9% may be required. Hypertonic solutions should be avoided because of the risk of producing sudden osmotic gradients.

b) Diuretics must be discontinued if hypokalaemia is suspected.

3. *Increase in solutes in plasma.* Treatment of diabetes, if present. If a diagnosis of sick cell syndrome is confirmed, the underlying disease should be treated. Occasionally the use of glucose, insulin and potassium may assist the cell membrane to return to normal. Initially 100 ml 50% dextrose, 20 u soluble insulin, and potassium chloride should be used. Initial doses of the latter will depend on serum K^+ levels. Subsequent dosages will depend on both blood glucose and potassium.

4. *Pseudohyponatraemia.* There is an osmolar gap, which is the difference between the calculated and measured plasma osmolalities. Osmolality is a measure of the total solute content of body fluids (or the number of particles in a given weight of solvent). Since most of the measured osmolality in healthy patients comes from urea, glucose, sodium, and its anions, attempts have been made to find the best formula for the calculated osmolality, in order to detect an unmeasured osmolar component, such as alcohol, glycine, trichloroethane, hyperproteinaemia, or hyperlipidaemia. Comparing varying types of patients and five different formulae, the most appropriate was:

Calculated osmolality $= 2 \times Na + $ urea $+$ glucose.

Bibliography

Allen GC, Armfield DR, Bontempo FA et al 1999 Adenotonsillectomy in children with von Willebrand disease. Archives of Otolaryngology— Head & Neck Surgery 125: 547–51.

Arieff AI 1998 Postoperative hyponatraemic encephalopathy following elective surgery in children. Paediatric Anaesthesia 8: 1–4.

Ayus JC, Arieff AI 1999 Chronic hyponatraemic encephalopathy in postmenopausal women: association of therapies with morbidity. Journal of the American Medical Association 281: 2299–304.

Bichet D, Schrier RW 1982 Evidence against concept of hyponatraemia and 'sick cells'. Lancet i: 742.

Bouzarth WF, Shenkin HA 1982 Is 'cerebral hyponatraemia' iatrogenic? Lancet i: 1061–2.

Canadian Preterm Labour Investigation Group 1992 Treatment of preterm labor with beta-adrenergic agonist ritodrine. New England Journal of Medicine 327: 308–12.

Feeney JG 1982 Water intoxication and oxytocin. British Medical Journal 285: 243.

Flear CTG, Gill GV, Burn J 1981 Hyponatraemia: mechanisms and management. Lancet ii: 26–31.

Fraser CL, Arieff AI 1997 Epidemiology, pathophysiology, and management of hyponatremic encephalopathy. American Journal of Medicine 102: 67–77.

Gill G, Leese G 1998 Hyponatraemia: biochemical and clinical perspectives. Postgraduate Medical Journal 74: 516–23.

Hawker F 1984 Pulmonary oedema associated with beta 2 sympathomimetic treatment of premature labour. Anaesthesia & Intensive Care 12: 143–51.

Higgins J, Gleeson R, Holohan M et al 1996 Maternal and neonatal hyponatraemia: a comparison of Hartmanns solution with 5% dextrose for the delivery of oxytocin in labour. European Journal of Obstetrics, Gynecology, & Reproductive Biology 68: 47–8.

Knochel JP 1999 Hypoxia is the cause of brain damage in hyponatremia. Journal of the American Medical Association 281: 2342–3.

Kumar S, Berl T 1998 Sodium. Lancet 352: 220–8.

Lane N, Allen K 1999 Hyponatraemia after orthopaedic surgery. British Medical Journal 318: 1363–4.

Oster JR, Singer I 1999 Hyponatremia, hyposmolality, and hypotonicity. Archives of Internal Medicine 159: 333–6.

Sterns RH 1992 Severe hyponatraemia: the case for conservative management. Critical Care Medicine 20: 534–9.

Sterns RH, Riggs JE, Schochet SS Jr 1986 Osmotic demyelination syndrome following correction of hyponatraemia. New England Journal of Medicine 314: 1535–42.

Hypothyroidism

Hypothyroidism may be primary, or secondary to pituitary or hypothalamic disease.

Autoimmune thyroiditis is the commonest primary cause, whilst the sequelae of surgical or radioiodine treatment of thyroid disease are also common. Deficiency of circulating thyroid hormone results in retardation of all body functions.

The condition may be subclinical, mild or severe, and it is predominantly a disease of females (in a 10:1 ratio). It affects all systems of the body and the presentations are protean. Mild disease may be unnoticed preoperatively, but it can be responsible for delayed recovery from anaesthesia.

After successful treatment, both TSH and T_4 levels should be normal. Replacement therapy must be cautious so as not to precipitate myocardial ischaemia or heart failure. In severe, untreated hypothyroidism, elective surgery must be postponed. If emergency surgery has to be undertaken, the mortality is high.

Since thyroxine is an inotropic agent and a vasodilator, its routine use in cardiac surgery in patients without thyroid disease has been suggested. However, there is no evidence to show that it is of benefit (Bennett-Guerrero et al 1997).

Preoperative abnormalities

1. Delay in the relaxation phase of reflexes, dry skin, a husky voice, loss of the outer part of the eyebrows, and weight gain. In severe disease there is lethargy, bradycardia, hypothermia, and respiratory depression. Deposition of a mucinous substance causes thickening of the subcutaneous tissues producing a nonpitting oedema. Myxoedematous infiltration of the vocal cords and tongue can occur. Cardiovascular complications include ischaemic heart disease, bradycardia, pericardial effusion, and cardiac failure (Gomberg-Maitland & Frishman 1998). Neurological complications may involve carpal tunnel syndrome, polyneuritis, myopathy, and cerebellar syndrome. About 70% of patients have paraesthesia or sensory neuropathy. Psychiatric disturbances may predominate.

2. An increased TSH, and decreased T_4 and sometimes T_3. It should be remembered that depression of T_4 alone often occurs in ill patients who are not hypothyroid. Acute hypothyroidism has been described in a severely ill surgical patient (Mogensen & Hjortso 1988).

3. Hypothyroidism is associated with bradycardia and AV conduction blocks. Diastolic hypertension may occur and is associated with increased systemic resistance (Gammage & Franklyn 1997). Ventricular systolic and diastolic function are impaired. The ECG is of low voltage with flattened or inverted T waves, and CXR may show mild cardiac enlargement.

4. Features of myxoedema coma include anaemia, which may be microcytic or macrocytic, lactic and respiratory acidosis, inappropriate ADH secretion, with severe hyponatraemia (Hanna & Scanlon 1997), and hypoglycaemia.

5. Hyperlipidaemia, with increases in total and low-density cholesterol.

6. Associated diseases include diabetes mellitus, pernicious anaemia, and Addison's disease.

7. Patients occasionally develop hypothyroidism during pregnancy and this is associated with thyroid antibodies, preeclampsia, preterm delivery, and subsequent impairment of IQ of the child (Montoro 1997, Haddow et al 1999).

8. Most cases are iatrogenic and follow radioactive iodine or thyroidectomy, but amiodarone and lithium are other causes.

Anaesthetic problems

1. Elderly patients with undiagnosed hypothyroidism may present with acute colonic emergencies. Bergeron et al (1997) described six patients, in four of whom intestinal atony was responsible for the surgical intervention.

2. Severe hypotension, and even cardiac arrest, has been reported after induction of

anaesthesia (Abbott 1967, Levelle et al 1985). This probably results from myocardial depression, which is less responsive to catecholamines than in normal patients.

3. There is extreme sensitivity to anaesthetic agents, narcotics, and analgesics (Kim & Hackman 1977).

4. Respiratory responses are impaired and there may be obstructive sleep apnoea. Muscle weakness may predispose to respiratory failure. An obese patient with undiagnosed myxoedema had severe hypotension on induction, and postoperative respiratory failure. It was difficult to wean her off the ventilator. On the sixth day, when it was noticed that the oxygen consumption index was very low, the diagnosis of myxoedema was made and confirmed biochemically (Levelle et al 1985). Another patient presented with a perioperative respiratory rate of 3–4 breath min^{-1} and a persistent respiratory alkalosis (Lee & Levine 1999). One pregnant patient, who presented with OSA and primary hypothyroidism, had a lingual tonsillar obstruction in addition (Taibah et al 1998).

5. In the presence of a low BMR, IPPV readily results in hypocapnoea, which decreases cerebral blood flow. Since cerebral oxygen consumption is not reduced, a relative reduction in cerebral oxygenation may result.

6. Hypothermia occurs readily under anaesthesia (Abbott 1967).

7. A completely absent response to peripheral nerve stimulation has been reported (Miller et al 1989). Subsequent investigation showed a sensorimotor polyneuropathy. After treatment of the hypothyroidism, the response to nerve stimulation returned to normal.

8. Hypothyroid coma may be precipitated by anaesthesia, or intercurrent illness such as pneumonia (Sherry & Hutchinson 1984, Gilbert et al 1992, Smallridge 1992). The condition carries a mortality of 50%, even when there is optimal treatment.

9. Adrenocortical insufficiency may also be present.

10. Rapid treatment of hypothyroidism may precipitate angina, myocardial infarction, or cardiac failure.

11. Large goitres may cause tracheal compression.

12. Impaired haemostasis has been recorded secondary to Factor VII deficiency (Ford & Carter 1990).

Management

1. In severe hypothyroidism, elective surgery should be postponed whilst treatment is instituted. There is some argument about the management of patients requiring coronary artery bypass surgery. Although suggestions have been made that treatment should not be given before surgery, for fear of precipitating cardiac ischaemia or heart failure (Finlayson & Kaplan 1982, Drucker & Borrow 1985, Vanderpump et al 1996), hypothyroidism is not protective in cardiovascular disease and untreated patients have a worse recovery (Bennett-Guerrero et al 1997). With milder forms of the disease, the case for cancellation is less clear. In a study of 59 patients with mild or moderate hypothyroidism (with matched controls), the authors found no evidence to justify deferring surgery until the hypothyroidism had been corrected (Weinberg et al 1983).

2. Adequate treatment of hypothyroidism, using 50–100 μg l-thyroxine daily, takes time to achieve (Vanderpump et al 1996). Particular caution is required in the elderly, or in those with cardiac disease. In these patients, the dose should be reduced to 25 μg per day, increasing only at 3- to 4-weekly intervals. With overt hypothyroidism, it may take 6 months to restore metabolism to normal. A normal T$_4$ and TSH signals adequate treatment.

3. Perioperative therapy. It does not matter if a dose of l-thyroxine is omitted on the day of surgery because the half-life is 1–2 weeks,

whereas the half-life of triiodothyronine (T_3) is only 1.5 days.

4. Severe hypothyroidism requiring urgent surgery, and myxoedema coma, are probably the only indications for intravenous thyroid replacement.

   a) A single dose of lyothyronine sodium 50 μg slowly then 25 μg 8-hrly. ECG control should be used. Triiodothyronine should also be given.

   b) Hydrocortisone 100 mg 6-hrly and intravenous fluids, including dextrose, may also be required.

5. If urgent surgery is needed in severe disease, careful cardiovascular monitoring is essential. There is minimal reserve. Dehydration and fluid overload are poorly tolerated. Inotropic agents may produce severe arrhythmias and myocardial ischaemia.

6. Controlled ventilation with CO_2 monitoring to avoid hypocapnoea. Postoperative IPPV may be needed.

7. Core temperature should be monitored. A warming blanket, high theatre temperature, and an infusion warmer will reduce the degree of hypothermia.

8. All drugs should be administered with caution. In particular, small doses of muscle relaxants should be given, with careful neuromuscular monitoring.

9. Patients should have their thyroid status carefully monitored and treated during pregnancy (Girling et al 1994, Mestman et al 1995, Haddow et al 1999).

Bibliography

Abbott TR 1967 Anaesthesia in untreated myxoedema: report of two cases. British Journal of Anaesthesia 35: 510–14.

Bennett-Guerrero E, Kramer DC, Schwinn DA 1997 Effect of chronic and acute thyroid reduction on perioperative outcome. Anesthesia & Analgesia 85: 30–6.

Bergeron E, Mitchell A, Heyen F et al 1997 Acute colonic surgery and unrecognised hypothyroidism:

a warning. Report of six cases. Diseases of the Colon & Rectum 40: 859–61.

Drucker DJ, Burrow GN 1985 Cardiovascular surgery in the hypothyroid patient. Archives of Internal Medicine 145: 1585–7.

Finlayson DC, Kaplan JA 1982 Myxoedema and open heart surgery: anaesthesia and intensive care unit experience. Canadian Anaesthetists' Society Journal 29: 543–9.

Ford HC, Carter JM 1990 Haemostasis in hypothyroidism. Postgraduate Medical Journal 66: 280–4.

Gammage M, Franklyn J 1997 Hypothyroidism, thyroxine treatment, and the heart. Heart 77: 189–90.

Gilbert RE, Thomas GW, Hope RN 1991 Coma and thyroid dysfunction. Anaesthesia & Intensive Care 20: 86–7.

Girling JC, De Swiet M, Hall R et al 1994 The thyroid and pregnancy. British Journal of Obstetrics & Gynaecology 101: 180–1.

Gomberg-Maitland M, Frishman WH 1998 Thyroid hormones and cardiovascular disease. American Heart Journal 135: 187–96.

Haddow JE, Palomaki GE, Allan WC et al 1999 Maternal thyroid deficiency during pregnancy and subsequent neuropsychological development of the child. New England Journal of Medicine 341: 549–55.

Hanna FWF, Scanlon M 1997 Hyponatraemia, hypothyroidism, and role of arginine-vasopressin. Lancet 350: 755–6.

Kim JM, Hackman L 1977 Anaesthesia for untreated hypothyroidism: report of 3 cases. Anesthesia & Analgesia 56: 299–302.

Lee HT, Levine M 1999 Acute respiratory alkalosis associated with low minute ventilation in a patient with severe hypothyroidism. Canadian Journal of Anaesthesia 46: 185–9.

Levelle JP, Jopling MW, Sklar GS 1985 Perioperative hypothyroidism: an unusual postanesthetic diagnosis. Anesthesiology 63: 195–7.

Mestman JH, Goodwin TM, Montoro MM 1995 Thyroid disorders of pregnancy. Endocrine & Metabolism Clinics of North America 24: 41–71.

Miller LR, Benumof JL, Alexander L et al 1989 Completely absent response to peripheral nerve stimulation in an acutely hypothyroid patient. Anesthesiology 71: 779–81.

Mogensen T, Hjortso N-C 1988 Acute hypothyroidism in a severely ill surgical patient. Canadian Journal of Anaesthesia 35: 74–5.

Montoro MN 1997 Management of hypothyroidism during pregnancy. Clinical Obstetrics & Gynecology 40: 65–80.

Sherry KM, Hutchinson IL 1984 Postoperative myxoedema. A report of coma and upper airway obstruction. Anaesthesia 39: 1112–14.

Smallridge RC 1992 Metabolic and anatomic thyroid emergencies: a review. Critical Care Medicine 20: 276–91.

Taibah K, Ahmed M, Baessa E et al 1998 An unusual cause of obstructive sleep apnoea presenting during pregnancy. Journal of Laryngology & Otology 112: 1189–91.

Vanderpump MPJ, Ahlquist JAO, Franklyn JA et al 1996 Consensus statement for good practice and audit measures in the management of hypothyroidism and hyperthyroidism. British Medical Journal 313: 539–44.

Weinberg AD, Brennan MD, Gormon CA et al 1983 Outcome of anesthesia and surgery in hypothyroid patients. Archives of Internal Medicine 143: 893–7.

Infectious mononucleosis

A common viral infection caused by the Ebstein–Barr virus, in which a variety of clinical patterns and spectrum of severity can present. Three rare complications of the disease may occasionally involve the anaesthetist:

1. Acute upper airway obstruction, which can cause sudden death (Boglioli & Taff 1998).

2. Guillain–Barré syndrome and bulbar paralysis.

3. Splenic rupture requiring splenectomy.

Preoperative abnormalities

1. The three main types are:

a) Anginose: pharyngitis and adenitis.

b) Glandular: predominantly lymphadenopathy and mild fever.

c) Febrile: a prolonged generalised illness with fever.

2. Diagnosis may be confirmed by the Monospot test and specific serology, as well as the presence of a lymphocytosis, with atypical lymphocytes on blood film.

3. Rare complications include thrombocytopenia (Cyran et al 1991), acute splenic rupture, and neurological lesions.

Anaesthetic problems

1. There have been several reports of upper airway obstruction from lymphoid hyperplasia of Waldeyer's ring, and oedema of the faucial arch, epiglottis, aryepiglottic fold (Wolfe & Rowe 1980, Wohl & Isaacson 1995), and lingual tonsils (Har-El & Josephson 1990). Cardiac arrest has been reported during tracheostomy (Lee 1969), apnoea and hypoxia on inhalation induction (Konarzewski et al 1991), and fatalities have occurred (Carrington & Hall 1986). In one patient, bilateral peritonsillar abscesses necessitated awake fibreoptic intubation followed by acute tonsillectomy (Burstin & Marshall 1998).

2. In one near fatal case, a cervical and parapharyngeal abscess resulted in gross oedema of the epiglottic, subglottic and postcricoid regions (Westmore 1990).

3. Emergency tonsillectomy does not necessarily immediately improve the airway problem. Stridor and episodes of sleep apnoea persisted in one patient for 48 h after surgery (Konarzewski et al 1991).

4. Liver function may be impaired.

5. Infectious mononucleosis is occasionally complicated by the Guillain–Barré syndrome or bulbar palsies (Maddern et al 1991). Deaths have been associated with respiratory failure, aspiration, and pneumonia.

6. Acute mucosal bleeding may occur, sometimes associated with thrombocytopenia (Johnsen et al 1984).

7. Although splenic rupture is extremely rare, it is the commonest cause of death in infectious mononucleosis. Laparotomy reveals free intraperitoneal blood and multiple subcapsular haematomas (Farley et al 1992).

Management

1. Although upper airway obstruction may be a feature in patients requiring hospital admission, it is generally mild and responds to conservative treatment. In a series of 109 patients, only three required surgical intervention (Ganzel et al 1996). The use of a soft nasopharyngeal airway has been suggested, and in 25 cases of airway obstruction thus treated, only one patient required tracheostomy (Snyderman & Stool 1982). However, occasionally severe airway obstruction develops. It is therefore recommended that patients with even minimal respiratory embarrassment be observed in a place with ENT and anaesthetic facilities (Johnsen et al 1984). Acute airway obstruction has been relieved by

minitracheotomy using a Seldinger technique (Ala-Kokko et al 1996).

2. Some surgeons consider 'hot' tonsillectomy to be the treatment of choice (Stevenson et al 1992). If an anaesthetic is required for adenotonsillectomy, facilities for immediate tracheostomy must be available. A case of stridor was described in which an attempted awake visualisation of the pharynx under local anaesthetic precipitated tonsillar bleeding. Immediate tracheostomy was performed under local anaesthesia, followed by a general anaesthetic for tonsillectomy (Catling et al 1984). Cardiac arrest has also been reported during tracheostomy under local anaesthesia (Lee 1969).

3. Bulbar paralysis may be another indication for tracheostomy (Wolfe & Rowe 1980).

4. Successful treatment of thrombocytopenia using gamma globulin has been described (Cyran et al 1991).

5. Splenic rupture should be suspected if a young patient develops left upper quadrant pain in the absence of trauma. Its management is controversial. Following the nonoperative management of three cases and a review of the literature, Schuler and Filtzer (1995) questioned the assumption that surgery is the most appropriate treatment. However, since this complication can be fatal, Farley et al (1992), after reviewing nine cases out of 8116 infectious mononucleosis admissions over a 40-year period, considered emergency splenectomy to be safest.

Bibliography

Ala-Kokko TI, Kyllonen M, Nuutinen L 1996 Management of upper airway obstruction using a Seldinger minitracheotomy kit. Acta Anesthesiologica Scandinavica 40: 385–8.

Boglioli LR, Taff ML 1998 Sudden asphyxial death complicating infectious mononucleosis. American Journal of Forensic Medicine & Pathology 19: 174–7.

Burstin PP, Marshall CL 1998 Infectious mononucleosis and bilateral peritonsillar abscess resulting in airway obstruction. Journal of Laryngology & Otology 112: 1185–8.

Carrington P, Hall JI 1986 Fatal airway obstruction in infectious mononucleosis. British Medical Journal 292: 195.

Catling SJ, Asbury AJ, Latif M 1984 Airway obstruction in infectious mononucleosis. Anaesthesia 39: 699–702.

Cyran EM, Rowe JM, Bloom RE 1991 Intravenous gammaglobulin treatment for immune thrombocytopenia associated with infectious mononucleosis. American Journal of Hematology 38: 124–9.

Farley DR, Zietlow SP, Bannon MP et al 1992 Spontaneous rupture of the spleen due to infectious mononucleosis. Mayo Clinic Proceedings 67: 843–53.

Ganzel TM, Goldman JL, Padhya TA 1996 Otolaryngologic clinical patterns in pediatric infectious mononucleosis. American Journal of Otolaryngology 17: 397–400.

Har-EL G, Josephson JS 1990 Infectious mononucleosis complicated by lingual tonsillitis. Journal of Laryngology & Otology 104: 651–3.

Johnsen T, Katholm M, Stangerup S-E 1984 Otolaryngological complications in infectious mononucleosis. Journal of Laryngology & Otology 98: 999–1001.

Konarzewski W, Walker P, Donovan A 1991 Upper airway obstruction by enlarged tonsils. Anaesthesia 46: 595–6.

Lee MD 1969 Respiratory obstruction in glandular fever. Journal of Laryngology & Otolaryngology 63: 617–22.

Maddern BR, Werkhaven J, Wessel HB et al 1991 Infectious mononucleosis with airway obstruction and multiple cranial nerve paresis. Otolaryngology—Head & Neck Surgery 104: 529–32.

Schuler JG, Filtzer H 1995 Spontaneous splenic rupture: the role of nonoperative management. Archives of Surgery 130: 662–5.

Snyderman NL, Stool SE 1982 Management of airway obstruction in children with infectious mononucleosis. Otolaryngology—Head & Neck Surgery 90: 168–70.

Stevenson DS, Webster G, Stewart JA 1992 Acute tonsillectomy in the management of infectious mononucleosis. Journal of Laryngology and Otology 106: 989–91.

Westmore GA 1990 Cervical abscess: a life-threatening complication of infectious mononucleosis. Journal of Laryngology & Otology 104: 358–9.

Wohl DL, Isaacson JE 1995 Airway obstruction in children with infectious mononucleosis. Ear, Nose & Throat Journal 74: 630–8.

Wolfe JA, Rowe LD 1980 Upper airway obstruction in infectious mononucleosis. Annals of Otology, Rhinology & Laryngology 89: 430–3.

Insulinoma

A rare insulin-secreting pancreatic islet cell tumour, which may be benign or malignant. Malignancy occurs in about 10% of cases. In the majority, the tumour is solitary and resection is curative. A small number of insulinomas are associated with the MEN I syndrome, in which case they are usually multiple. Hypoglycaemia may also occur with secretion of insulin-like growth factors from tumours or other tissue situated outside the pancreas (Le Roith 1999).

Preoperative abnormalities

1. The symptoms of episodic hypoglycaemia may be suggestive of CNS disease, hysteria, epilepsy, sympathetic overactivity, behavioural problems, or intoxication. Patients may complain of sweating, hunger, palpitations, or exhibit various focal neurological deficits coinciding with cerebral hypoglycaemia. Symptoms are either spontaneous, or induced by an overnight fast, or a controlled insulin infusion. They frequently occur before breakfast, or during vigorous exercise. In a study of 25 patients, the median time of severe symptoms of cerebral hypoglycaemia was 2 years and one-third of patients had had hypoglycaemic seizures (Doherty et al 1991). Hypoglycaemia may also occur in pregnancy or postpartum. One patient was found to be comatose on the second morning after delivery (Garner & Tsang 1989). Another was found confused, hypothermic (31.3°C), and sweating at 33 weeks' gestation, with a blood sugar of 0.8 mmol l^{-1}. Difficulty was experienced maintaining her blood sugar because she had very high insulin levels. On CT scan she had low-density defects throughout the liver parenchyma, suggesting nonislet cell hypersecretion of insulin (Hyer et al 1995).

2. The diagnostic criteria for insulinomas include a fasting plasma insulin of >6 μU ml^{-1} and detectable levels of serum C-peptide, at the same times as symptoms of hypoglycaemia and a blood glucose concentration of <2.5 mmol l^{-1} (Le Roith 1999). Closely supervised fasts of up to 24 h or beyond may be required, since factitious hypoglycaemia has been produced by concealed consumption of oral hypoglycaemics (Proye et al 1998).

3. Medical control of insulin secretion may be required for those in whom tumours cannot be localised, or who are unfit for surgery (Gill et al 1997). Diazoxide probably counteracts hypoglycaemia by effects on beta-cell potassium channels, but may cause fluid retention. The somatostatin analogue octreotide, or streptozotocin, may also be used.

4. A small percentage of insulinomas form part of a multiple endocrine neoplasia syndrome (MEN I).

5. Diagnosis may be difficult. Ultrasound and CT scans are not very sensitive. MRI angiography, selective visceral angiography, or portal venous sampling, may be required (Geoghegan et al 1994).

Anaesthetic problems

1. Insulin secretion, particularly during tumour handling, may produce hypoglycaemia under anaesthesia. Permanent neurological damage may result, but the approach to management of the blood sugar during surgery remains controversial. Techniques range from administering dextrose 25% via a central venous infusion, whilst checking the plasma glucose regularly (Chari et al 1977), to the use of an artificial pancreas (Pulver et al 1980, Roizen 1994). This device performs on-line glucose estimations and automatically administers glucose/insulin iv as necessary. Others have withheld glucose except when the blood glucose decreased below 3 mmol l^{-1} (Lamont & Jones

1978). This was based on the premise that a rebound hyperglycaemia after insulinoma resection indicated complete removal of the tumour. Thus, if glucose were to be given, the sign would be masked. The reliability of this sign has, however, been questioned. Records of 38 operations for insulinomas in which glucose had not been given were studied (Muir et al 1983) They concluded that: provided the glucose was above 3.3 mmol l⁻¹, intermittent sampling at 15-min intervals was safe; the deliberate withholding of intraoperative glucose was potentially dangerous, because although rebound hyperglycaemia often occurred, it was of no predictive value during the operation.

2. Patients with high insulin secretion who have poor cardiac function may not tolerate the requisite volumes of dextrose solutions to prevent hypoglycaemia (Utas et al 1993).

3. Hyperglycaemia may occur for the first few postoperative days as a result of persistent high levels of hormones with hyperglycaemic effects.

4. A possible interaction between diazoxide and thiopental has been suggested (Burch & McLeskey 1981). Two patients receiving diazoxide infusions developed hypotension on induction of anaesthesia. Diazoxide inhibits insulin release, has systemic vasodilator effects, and is strongly protein bound. Mechanisms associated with competition for binding sites between the two drugs were postulated.

5. Intraoperative tumour localisation may be difficult. Thus surgery may have to be abandoned. Three patients out of 51 reported by Proye et al (1998), in whom tumours were not found at operation, subsequently turned out to have factitious hypoglycaemia.

Management

1. Since hyperglycaemic rebound is not predictive of complete removal of the insulinoma during operation, moderate hypoglycaemia would appear to be both

unnecessary, and potentially dangerous (Muir et al 1983). Maintenance of a plasma glucose level between 5.5 and 8.5 mmol l⁻¹, with estimations at 15-min intervals, is recommended.

2. Care must be taken to avoid either hyper- or hypoglycaemia. In patients treated with diazoxide, rapid infusion of dextrose 5% was found to produce high glucose levels (Burch & McLeskey 1981). It was suggested that the rate be limited to 2 ml kg⁻¹h⁻¹. In a patient with cardiac failure, in order to avoid large glucose infusions, octreotide 100 μg sc was given 1 h preoperatively. Blood glucose estimations, performed every 15 min, showed no hypoglycaemia (Utas et al 1993).

3. Serial intraoperative measurements of serum insulin levels have been used for retrospective (Krentz et al 1990), and intraoperative, confirmation of the success of surgery (Proye et al 1998).

4. Close cardiovascular monitoring during induction of anaesthesia is essential, especially in patients receiving diazoxide infusions, when hypotension may be a problem.

5. The use of sevoflurane anaesthesia, which is claimed to suppress insulin secretion, has been described (Matsumoto & Sakai 1992).

Bibliography
Burch PG, McLeskey CH 1981 Anesthesia for patients with insulinoma treatment with oral diazoxide. Anesthesiology 55: 472–5.
Chari P, Pandit SK, Kataria RN et al 1977 Anaesthetic management of insulinoma. Anaesthesia 32: 261–4.
Doherty GM, Doppman JL, Shawker TH et al 1991 Results of a prospective strategy to diagnose, localize, and resect insulinomas. Surgery 110: 989–96.
Garner PR, Tsang R 1989 Insulinoma complicating pregnancy presenting with hypoglycaemic coma after delivery: a case report and review of the literature. Obstetrics & Gynecology 73: 847–9.
Geoghegan JG, Jackson JE, Lewis MPN et al 1994 Localization and surgical management of insulinoma. British Journal of Surgery 81: 1025–8.
Gill GV, Rauf O, MacFarlane IA 1997 Diazoxide treatment for insulinoma. Postgraduate Medical Journal 73: 640–1.

Hyer SL, Thomas DM, Polak JM et al 1995 Malignant insulinoma in pregnancy presenting as hypothermia. Journal of Obstetrics & Gynaecology 15: 34–6.

Krentz AJ, Hale PJ, Baddeley RM et al 1990 Intra-operative blood glucose and serum insulin concentrations in the surgical management of insulinoma. Postgraduate Medical Journal 66: 24–7.

Lamont ASM, Jones D 1978 Anaesthetic management of insulinoma. Anaesthesia & Intensive Care 6: 261.

Le Roith D 1999 Tumor-induced hypoglycemia. New England Journal of Medicine 341: 757–8.

Matsumoto M, Sakai H 1992 [Sevoflurane anesthesia for a patient with insulinoma. English Abstract.] Masui 41: 446–9.

Muir JJ, Endres SM, Offord K et al 1983 Glucose management in patients undergoing operation for insulinoma removal. Anesthesiology 59: 371–5.

Proye C, Pattou F, Canraille B et al 1998 Intraoperative insulin measurement during surgical management of insulinomas. World Journal of Surgery 22: 1218–24.

Pulver JJ, Cullen BF, Miller DR et al 1980 Use of the artificial beta cell during anesthesia for surgical removal of insulinoma. Anesthesia & Analgesia 59: 950–2.

Roizen MF 1994 Preoperative evaluation. In: Miller RD (ed) Anesthesia. Churchill Livingstone, Edinburgh, p 911.

Utas C, Kelestimur F, Boyaci A et al 1993 Control of plasma glucose with somatostatin analogue (SMS 201–995) during surgical removal of insulinomas. Postgraduate Medical Journal 69: 920–1.

J

272

Jehovah's witnesses (management for surgery)

Two recent documents have been published for guidance; the Association of Anaesthetist's *Management of Anaesthesia for Jehovah's Witnesses* (1999), and the Medical Defence Union document *Consent to Treatment* (1997).

Problems

1. *Ethical, moral and practical issues* (see also Benson 1989, Layon et al 1990, Kleinman 1994). The problem of conflict between *autonomy*, the individual's right to accept or reject recommendations, and *benificence*, the obligation to promote the well-being of others.

   a) The limitations placed on the physician and their effects. Jehovah's Witnesses will not accept the transfusion of blood or blood products on religious grounds. If an adult is accepted for elective surgery, the surgeon and anaesthetist must also accept the limitations placed on their practice of medicine by the patient's wishes. In the case of an emergency, or in the situation of essential treatment, if the practitioner is the only suitably qualified person available, there may be no choice but to undertake treatment. In general, however, it is the anaesthetist who has to administer blood, and, as the likely resuscitator in the event of life-threatening haemorrhage, has to face the impact of these restrictions to his/her normal practice. The devastating effect of watching a patient exsanguinate, and to be unable to administer blood, cannot be underestimated. Another problem is that the original agreement to surgery was usually made between the surgeon and the patient. The anaesthetist, who may only be involved at a later stage, is external to this agreement and may not be party to its exact terms. Not only must he/she know whether or not the patient understands the full implications of his/her decision but, almost more importantly, whether the surgeon does as well.

   b) The type of surgery. These days, blood transfusion is undertaken in fewer operations. In addition, substantial blood loss is unlikely for many types of surgery. As a result, the fact that a Jehovah's Witness has signed a form to say that he/her refuses blood transfusion often has little impact on the anaesthetist's relationship with his/her patient. If, on the other hand, substantial blood loss is anticipated, there is likely to have been extensive discussion. Thus, all parties in the agreement will have accepted the remote possibility of the patient's death. Practical preparation of the patient, for example by haemodilution techniques, is also likely to have taken place. The worst scenario is when completely unexpected bleeding occurs in a situation in which transfusion would be most unusual.

2. In the UK, legal issues have been decided by case, not statute, law (Cox & Lumley 1995).

   a) *The child for blood transfusion.* Apply via Trust's legal department for a Specific Issue Order from the High Court, provided that two doctors of consultant status decide that transfusion is essential.

   b) *The child in an emergency situation.* Courts have been consistent in their support of children against parental objection. When a child's life is in danger, transfusion is allowed despite religious objections by the parents. Technically, application can be made to the Official Solicitor, via the Trust's legal department, although this may not be possible in the time.

   c) *The adult for elective surgery.* If a fully informed adult has refused blood transfusion and subsequently dies, the physician is legally protected. Unless the physician believes that the patient did not understand the implications, the undertaking to give blood should not be reversed.

d) *Adults and third party problems.* Certain situations may modify the legal judgements in the case of adults. These involve innocent third parties; for example, the protection of a mature fetus, or the prevention of abandonment of a child, and these may take precedence over an individual's expression of religious freedom. However, this is not always so, and opinions differ, particularly if there is family support for the child (Sacks & Koppes 1994). Adults have rights to refuse (for details, see Benson 1989).

e) *Unconscious or incompetent adult.* The situation may be different in the case of an emergency, or with an unconscious patient, when the physician becomes an 'involuntary host'. However, the courts have been inconsistent in their judgments. In Ontario, a Canadian doctor was found guilty of battery when he transfused an unconscious patient who was in possession of an undated card indicating that she would not accept blood transfusion (Brahams 1989). By contrast, in Pennsylvania, the courts upheld the appointment of a guardian who authorised a transfusion, because there was reasonable doubt about the validity of the patient's treatment refusal (Kleinman 1994).

3. *Problems with administration of treatment which may result in increased bleeding.* A patient with a myocardial infarction, randomised in a clinical trial to receive streptokinase, subsequently died from haemorrhagic complications (Sugarman et al 1991).

4. *Acceptance of products or techniques.* On certain issues, in the past, there was some lack of clarity. However, many Jehovah's Witness Hospital Liaison Committees now produce Health-Care Advance Directives that identify individual products or techniques. These are signed by the patient, and witnessed by two individuals. In them, he/she can sign separate clauses to indicate whether or not they will accept:

a) 'Minor blood fractions', such as clotting factors, immunoglobulins, or products that may contain a small amount of albumin (eg streptokinase, some forms of erythopoietin).

b) 'Non-stored autologous blood' that *'does not involve storage'* but is *'constantly linked to my circulatory system'* (eg haemodialysis, heart–lung machines, haemodilution). In general, autologous intra- or postoperative blood salvage of blood lost during or after surgery is acceptable, as long as it *'does not involve storage or more than brief interruption of blood flow, provided any equipment used is not primed with stored blood'*. In fact, some Hospital Liaison Committees have assisted hospitals to fund cell salvage machines.

c) It also suggests *'non-blood medical or surgical management to stop, avoid or minimise blood loss'* or *'to build up or conserve my own blood'* that would be acceptable (eg dextran, saline, Ringer's lactate, modified fluid gelatin, hetastarch, perflurochemicals, oral and parenteral iron).

5. *Mortality.* This was found to be dependent on the blood loss at surgery, not on the preoperative Hb (Spence et al 1990). Mortality is increased only in cardiac and vascular surgery (Kitchens 1993). However, in trauma cases, a patient may die who would otherwise have lived had blood been given (Finfer et al 1994).

6. *Haematological problems.*

a) Circulating volume.

b) Oxygen carriage.

c) Platelets and coagulation.

d) Oncotic pressure.

e) Immune status.

7. *Reactions to plasma expanders.* Transfusion of hydroxyethyl starch 2.66 g kg^{-1} in a child (which represented 60% of the patient's blood volume) undergoing scoliosis correction resulted in a severe coagulopathy that did not revert to normal until 72 h later (Lockwood et al 1988).

Defects included prolonged PT and APTT, and decreased levels of Factor X, VII, Factor VIII:C, and vWF:Ag. In clinical studies, up to $1.4\,g\,kg^{-1}$ had been used with only minor laboratory abnormalities.

8. The problems of managing postspinal headache.

Management

1. *Preliminary discussions.* For an elective procedure, a physician may decide not to accept the limitations placed on his/her treatment, but to refer the patient to a colleague, or to a hospital specialising in the treatment of Jehovah's Witnesses.

a) For a child who needs transfusion, support in writing from a colleague should be obtained first. If time allows, and in the presence of the colleague, the reason for transfusion and the risks if blood is not given are discussed with the parents. In the event of refusal by the parents, a record is made in the case notes. Both physicians should sign this record. In an emergency, an application to a magistrate for custody of the child is not usually necessary (Medical Defence Union 1997) bu if there is particular concern, the practitioner may consult a defence union for advice.

b) If in adults a decision is made to proceed, there should be a proper assessment of risk factors. Both the patient and the surgeon must understand the consequences of refusal (Editorial 1992). Even if blood loss is thought to be unlikely, detailed information about acceptable products must be documented, since this may subsequently be lifesaving (Dasen et al 2000). It has been suggested that an adult should also be interviewed alone at some point, without the presence of relatives or a minister.

c) The anaesthetist must be involved at an early stage, so that the options for

treatment can be discussed with the patient or family. It is important to establish exactly what the individual is willing to accept. In particular, the patient's views on albumin, haemophiliac factors, and autologous intraoperative transfusion must be clarified absolutely.

d) Proper informed consent in the presence of a witness and, if wished, a relative or adviser. A full explanation of the benefits of surgery, and the hazards if blood transfusion is refused, must be undertaken. Consent or refusal should be witnessed and signed by a relative.

e) If a patient is accepted for elective surgery, the physician must accede to the individual's decision.

2. *Preoperative preparation.* For elective surgery, the patient's Hb and Hct may be improved by restoration of iron stores, nutritional support and, if acceptable, treatment with erythropoietin. There have been several reports of its use in patients requiring major, elective surgery (Atabek et al 1992, Connor & Olsson 1992, Tsuji et al 1995). In a patient accepted for liver transplantation, after 35 days' treatment, the Hb had increased from $11\,g\,dl^{-1}$ to $14\,g\,dl^{-1}$ (Snook et al 1996). It is particularly useful to overcome the low reticulocyte count associated with bone marrow suppression by inflammation (Wolff et al 1997). Seven weeks treatment with erythropoietin (r-HuEPO), $100\,u\,kg^{-1}$ 2–3 times a week given to an adolescent for scoliosis surgery improved the Hct from 39.5% to 47% and increased the Hb by $2\,g\,dl^{-1}$ (Rothstein et al 1990). Erythropoietin shortens the response time from 7 days to 4 days (Busuttil & Copplestone 1995).

a) Treatment of patients on the ITU. Erythropoietin (r-HuEPO) was given to a Jehovah's Witness with an Hb of $3.2\,g\,dl^{-1}$ following multiple trauma, to expedite weaning from mechanical ventilation

(Kraus & Lipman 1992), and to a patient with an Hb of 2.8 g dl⁻¹ after repair of a leaking aortic aneurysm (Baker et al 1998). In this patient, total parenteral nutrition, folinic acid and intravenous iron (Venofer, an iron saccharate preparation, which is only available on a named patient basis), were also given. Hypertension and thrombocythaemia may occur as a side effect of treatment.

b) Limit blood withdrawal after admission, by only performing essential investigations, by the use of paediatric sample tubes, and, in the case of ITU patients, by returning the flush from arterial lines.

3. *Methods of minimising blood loss.* Techniques that minimise surgical blood loss should be employed. These include a meticulous surgical technique with extensive use of diathermy, ligation of vessels before cutting them, the use of sharp dissection, and dissection along anatomical tissue planes (Spence et al 1990).

a) If blood losses of greater than 500 ml are anticipated, monitor the CVP and replace losses with colloid as they occur.

b) Induced hypotension to 50–55 mmHg may be considered if a blood loss of greater than 20% of the blood volume is anticipated. Careful technique in 100 Jehovah's Witnesses undergoing total hip arthoplasty, 89 of whom had hypotensive anaesthesia, showed a reduction in blood loss when compared with a control group of patients who were not Jehovah's Witnesses and who had had surgery under normotensive anaesthesia (Nelson & Bowen 1986).

c) Haemodilution techniques with a glucose crystalloid prime were used for cardiopulmonary bypass in surgery for congenital heart disease in 110 children of Jehovah's Witnesses. Only one death was attributed to blood loss (Henling et al 1985).

d) Acute hypervolaemic haemodilution at the start of surgery has been used to achieve a moderate (20–25%) or low (<20%) Hct, so that any blood lost involves a decreased loss of blood cells. Haemodilution to a Hct of 0.20 was induced in an anaemic patient who required emergency surgery, after full invasive monitoring was established (Trouwborst et al 1990). Dextran 40 500 ml and Ringer's lactate 500 ml were infused on two occasions over a period of 40 min and measurements repeated each 15 min. During surgery, blood loss was replaced by equal volumes of gelatin and Ringer's lactate, given as urine volume plus 500 ml h⁻¹.

4. *Methods of treating blood loss:*

a) Use of plasma expanders to replace blood loss as it occurs. Blood substitutes (Fluosol, a perfluorocarbon emulsion) may increase dissolved oxygen in the first 12 h (Atabek et al 1992), but are probably of little use otherwise.

b) Use of the patient's own blood in a continuous system. Autotransfusion of blood collected just before surgery (Schaller et al 1983). Blood was removed and replaced with three times the volume of a balanced electrolyte solution. The blood remained in continuity, and after most of the surgical blood loss had stopped, it was returned and furosemide (frusemide) was given.

c) Return of blood by intraoperative use of a cell saver and autotransfusion. In this case, a continuous circuit is made from the patient to the cell saver device, and back to the patient. A dedicated line is 'piggybacked' from the autotransfusion device to the patient and kept open with a saline infusion via a three-way tap until enough blood is collected to transfuse. The three-way tap is then turned to re-establish flow. Again, this technique is acceptable to most Jehovah's Witnesses because blood never leaves a continuous circuit with the body. In all haemodilution techniques there is the question of whether crystalloid or colloid should be used for dilution. A mixture may be appropriate.

5. *Reducing oxygen requirement or maximising oxygenation:*

a) Oxygenation and IPPV.

b) Hypothermia to reduce oxygen consumption, with simultaneous haemodilution. A patient with a haematocrit of 4% was treated with hypothermia, isovolaemic haemodilution, muscular paralysis, IPPV, and sedation for 4 h, whilst awaiting a court decision concerning transfusion (Lichenstein et al 1988).

6. *Use of DDAVP and antifibrinolytics for oozing.* The prophylactic use of DDAVP $0.3 \mu g kg^{-1}$ iv over 20 min has been suggested (Stone & DiFazio 1988). DDAVP may also correct vWF and platelet abnormalities after large infusions of colloids. Other antifibrinolytics, such as tranexamic acid and aprotinin, have also been used.

7. *Spinal headache.* A blood patch was performed in a patient with a postspinal headache, using manometer tubing, a three-way tap and a syringe, so that no continuity of blood was lost (Tyers 1988).

8. *Management of postpartum/postoperative anaemia.* Postpartum anaemia which resulted from multiple vaginal tears has been treated with r-HuEPO $100 iu kg^{-1}$ (Rasanayagam & Cooper 1996).

Bibliography
Association of Anaesthetists of Great Britain and Ireland 1999 Management of anaesthesia for Jehovah's Witnesses. Association of Anaesthetists of Great Britain and Ireland, London.

Atabek U, Spence RK, Pello M et al 1992 Pancreatico-duodenectomy without homologous blood transfusion in an anemic Jehovah's Witness. Archives of Surgery 127: 349–51.

Baker CE, Kelly GD, Perkins GD 1998 Perioperative care of a Jehovah's Witness with a leaking abdominal aortic aneurysm. British Journal of Anaesthesia 81: 256–9.

Benson KT 1989 The Jehovah's Witness patient: considerations for the anesthesiologist. Anesthesia & Analgesia 69: 647–56.

Brahams D 1989 Jehovah's witness transfused without consent: a Canadian case. Lancet ii: 1407–8.

Busuttil D, Copplestone A 1995 Management of blood loss in Jehovah's Witnesses. British Medical Journal 311: 1115–16.

Connor JP, Olsson CA 1992 The use of recombinant human erythropoietin in a Jehovah's Witness requiring major reconstructive surgery. Journal of Urology 147: 131–2.

Cox M, Lumley J 1995 No blood or blood products. Anaesthesia 50: 583–5.

Dasen KR, Niswander DG, Schlenker RE 2000 Autologous and allogenic blood products for unanticipated massive blood loss in a Jehovah's Witness. Anesthesia & Analgesia 90: 553–5.

Editorial 1992 When a patient says no. Lancet 340: 345.

Finfer S, Howell S, Miller J et al 1994 Managing patients who refuse blood transfusions: an ethical dilemma. British Medical Journal 308: 1423–4.

Henling CE, Carmichael MJ, Keats AS et al 1985 Cardiac operation for congenital heart disease in children of Jehovah's Witnesses. Journal of Thoracic & Cardiovascular Surgery 89: 914–20.

Kitchens CS 1993 Are transfusions overrated? Surgical outcome of Jehovah's Witnesses. American Journal of Medicine 94: 117–19.

Kleinman I 1994 Written advance directives refusing blood transfusion: ethical and legal consideration. American Journal of Medicine 96: 563–7.

Kraus P, Lipman J 1992 Erythropoietin in a patient following multiple trauma. Anaesthesia 47: 962–4.

Layon AJ, D'Amico R, Caton D et al 1990 And the patient chose: medical ethics and the case of the Jehovah's Witness. Anesthesiology 73: 1258–62.

Lichtenstein A, Eckhart WF, Swanson KJ et al 1988 Unplanned intraoperative and postoperative hemodilution: oxygen transport and consumption during severe anemia. Anesthesiology 69: 119–22.

Lockwood DN, Bullen C, Machin SJ 1988 A severe coagulopathy following volume replacement with hydroxyethyl starch. Anaesthesia 43: 391–3.

Medical Defence Union 1997 Consent to Treatment. MDU Ltd, London.

Nelson CL, Bowen WS 1986 Total hip arthroplasty in

Jehovah's Witnesses without blood transfusion. Journal of Bone & Joint Surgery 68: 350–3.

Rasanayagam SR, Cooper GM 1996 Two cases of severe postpartum anemia in Jehovah's witnesses. International Journal of Obstetric Anesthesia 5: 302–5.

Rothstein P, Roye D, Verdisco L et al 1990 Preoperative use of erythropoietin in an adolescent Jehovah's witness. Anesthesiology 73: 568–70.

Sacks DA, Koppes RH 1994 Caring for the female Jehovah's Witness: balancing medicine, ethics, and the First Amendment. American Journal of Obstetrics & Gynecology 170: 452–5.

Schaller RT, Schaller J, Morgan A et al 1983 Hemodilution anesthesia: a valuable aid to major cancer surgery in children. American Journal of Surgery 146: 79–84.

Snook NJ, O'Beiren HA, Enright S et al 1996 Use of recombinant erythropoietin to facilitate liver transplantation in a Jehovah's Witness. British Journal of Anaesthesia 76: 740–3.

Spence RK, Carson JA, Poses R et al 1990 Elective surgery without transfusion: influence of preoperative hemoglobin level and blood loss on mortality. American Journal of Surgery 159: 320–4.

Stone DJ, DiFazio CA 1988 DDAVP to reduce blood loss in Jehovah's Witnesses. Anesthesiology 69: 1028.

Sugarman J, Churchill LR, Moore JK et al 1991 Medical, ethical and legal issues regarding thrombolytic therapy in the Jehovah's witness. American Journal of Cardiology 68: 1525–9.

Trouwborst A, Hagenouw RRPM, Jeekel J et al 1990 Hypervolaemic haemodilution in an anaemic Jehovah's witness. British Journal of Anaesthesia 64: 646–8.

Tsuji Y, Kambayashi J, Shiba E et al 1995 Effect of recombinant erythropoietin on anaemia after gastrectomy: a pilot study. European Journal of Surgery 161: 29–33.

Tyers M 1988 Blood patch in a Jehovah's witness. Anaesthesia & Intensive Care 16: 127–8.

Wolff M, Fandrey J, Hirner A et al 1997 Perioperative use of recombinant human erythropoietin in patients refusing blood transfusions. Pathophysiological considerations based on 5 cases. European Journal of Haematology 58: 154–9.

Juvenile hyaline fibromatosis

A rare autosomal recessive condition in which there are defects in the synthesis and metabolism of type I and III collagen (Brier et al 1997). Abnormal material accumulates in soft tissues. Features include the appearance of tumorous lesions of the skin from infancy, gingival hypertrophy, flexion contractures of joints, and destruction of bone. Anaesthesia may be required for Nissen's fundoplication, tumour resection, orthopaedic, or skin surgery.

Preoperative abnormalities

1. Painful flexion contractures of all large joints and the radiological appearance of osteopenia and cortical defects, particularly in the humerus and femur (O'Neill & Kasser 1989). Patients become wheelchair bound.

2. Oral lesions, in particular gingival hyperplasia, and sometimes anal mucosal hypertrophy (Aldred & Crawford 1987).

3. Multiple tumorous, mucocutaneous lesions presenting as firm brown nodules of the face, nose, palate, ears, and neck.

4. Growth retardation secondary to vomiting and feeding difficulties. Recurrent infections which may be fatal (Bedford et al 1991).

5. Kidney, lung and gastrointestinal tract may be involved.

Anaesthetic problems

1. Difficulties in intubation can result from gingival hypertrophy, infiltration of tissues, circumoral polypoidal masses, and contracture involving the cervical spine and temporomandibular joints (Sugahara et al 1993, Norman et al 1996). These may progress with age. Growths on the head may cause problems in positioning, and facial abnormalities can prevent the mask from fitting. Tissue hyperplasia may involve the larynx.

2. In one adult, resistance to suxamethonium had been noted on several previous anaesthetics. A mechanomyograph was used before laparoscopic cholecystectomy. There was

difficulty in mouth opening after succinylcholine 1.5 mg kg^{-1}, no fasciculations occurred, and only a 50% block was achieved. EMG, nerve conduction and plasma cholinesterase levels were all normal (Baraka 1997). The significance of this finding is not known.

3. Flexion contractures of joints, which are not lessened under anaesthesia, and may interfere with positioning and patient monitoring.

4. Gastric reflux may occur.

Management

1. Assessment of organ involvement.

2. Estimation of intubation difficulties.

3. Techniques for airway management have included the use of the laryngeal mask airway, and nasal fibreoptic bronchoscopy whilst spontaneous respiration was maintained via an airway in the other nostril (Norman et al 1996). Awake fibreoptic intubation has also been performed in a 13-month-old child using a bronchoscopically placed stylet as a guide (Vaughn et al 1990).

Bibliography

Aldred MJ, Crawford PJ 1987 Juvenile hyaline fibromatosis. Oral Surgery, Oral Medicine & Oral Pathology 63: 71–7.

Baraka AS 1997 Succinylcholine resistance in a patient with juvenile hyaline fibromatosis. Anesthesiology 87: 1250–2.

Bedford CD, Sills JA, Sommelet-Olive D et al 1991 Juvenile hyaline fibromatosis: a report of two severe cases. Journal of Pediatrics 119: 404–10.

Brier F, Fang-Kircher S, Wolff K et al 1997 Juvenile hyaline fibromatosis: impaired collagen metabolism in human skin. Archives of Disease in Childhood 77: 436–40.

Norman B, Soni N, Madden N 1996 Anaesthesia and juvenile hyaline fibromatosis. British Journal of Anaesthesia 76: 163–6.

O'Neill DB, Kasser JR 1989 Juvenile hyaline fibromatosis. A case report and review of musculoskeletal manifestations. Journal of Bone & Joint Surgery 71A: 941–4.

Sugahara S, Ikezaki H, Abe K et al 1993 [Anesthetic management of a patient with juvenile hyaline fibromatosis: a case report. Japanese] Masui— Japanese Journal of Anaesthesiology 42: 1853–5.

Vaughn GC, Kaplan RF, Tieche S, Downs JB 1990 Juvenile hyaline fibromatosis: anesthetic management. Anesthesiology 72: 201–3.

Kawasaki disease (mucocutaneous lymph node syndrome)

An acute inflammatory illness of young children manifesting as a systemic febrile vasculitis. In the UK it is relatively rare, but it is three times more common in the USA and 30 times more common in Japan. The aetiology is not known, but bacterial superantigen toxin may be involved, similar to the mechanism in staphylococcal toxic shock syndrome. A rapidly reversible process secondary to toxins or cytokines is suggested by the fact that myocardial contractility was seen to improve over a period of 4 days' treatment with gamma globulin (Moran et al 2000).

If the patient is treated within 10 days with immunoglobulin and aspirin, the complication rate is reduced. Untreated, coronary arteritis progresses to the development of aneurysms, thrombosis, or myocardial infarction. The diagnosis is easily missed, because the clinical picture is similar to that of many other infectious/inflammatory diseases. However, the fever extends beyond 5 days and the child is extremely miserable.

Preoperative abnormalities

1. Diagnostic criteria; at least five of six of the following:

   a) A fever for 5 days or more.

   b) Bilateral nonpurulent conjunctivitis.

   c) A polymorphous rash.

   d) Mucous membrane changes; reddened, dry, cracked lips, strawberry tongue, and redness of oral or pharyngeal mucosa.

   e) Extremity changes: reddening of palms or soles; oedema of hands or feet; skin desquamation during convalescence.

   f) Cervical lymphadenopathy >1.5 cm diameter, painful *plus exclusion of diseases with similar presentation* (Curtis 1997).

2. Thombocytosis.

3. Cardiovascular complications. At presentation, more than 50% of patients have abnormal myocardial function (Moran et al 2000). About 10% progress to coronary giant aneurysms, arrhythmias, myocarditis, and 4% eventually develop ischaemic heart disease, often with calcified stenosis (Sugimura et al 1997). Recurrent episodes of disease are more likely to result in cardiac complications (Nakamura et al 1998). Late-stage vasculitis may occur (Takahashi 1998), and one child died suddenly, in association with the use of the beta-2 agonist albuterol for asthma, 17 weeks after the disease had apparently resolved

4. Treatment. Intravenous gamma globulin $2\,g\,kg^{-1}$, within 10 days of onset, and aspirin $3-5\,mg\,kg^{-1}\,day^{-1}$.

5. Significant long-term morbidity, in terms of coronary artery scarring and accelerated atherosclerosis, may occur in untreated patients.

6. Pregnancy has been reported in a patient following Kawasaki disease (Shear & Leduc 1999).

Anaesthetic problems

1. Cardiovascular complications. Myocardial dysfunction occurs early in the disease (Moran et al 2000). Patients may require anaesthesia for complications of the disease. Kowaleski et al (1996) described anaesthesia for CABG surgery in a 10 year old with coronary artery aneurysms and stenoses following Kawasaki disease at the age of 1 year.

2. Anaesthesia was required for bleeding after injury to the tongue in a 13 month old, who was anticoagulated to prevent extension of a coronary artery thrombus (Thomas & McEwan 1998).

3. Those with tonsillar enlargement may need tonsillectomy (Ravi & Brooks 1997). Massive lymphadenopathy has caused respiratory obstruction. A 4 year old required tracheal

intubation and IPPV after swelling in the right side of the neck progressed to dysphagia and respiratory embarrassment (Burgner et al 1996). Another 4 year old had prevertebral and retropharyngeal swelling that regressed dramatically after pulsed steroid therapy (Shetty et al 1998).

4. Patients with coronary artery aneurysms after childhood Kawasaki disease have become pregnant (Alam et al 1995, Shear & Leduc 1999).

Management

1. Assessment of cardiac disease, if present.

2. Management of airway obstruction from tonsillar swelling.

3. Coronary artery bypass surgery has been reported in a 10 year old using sufentanil and isoflurane supplemented by subarachnoid bupivacaine and morphine (Kowalewski et al 1996).

4. Caesarean section under epidural anaesthesia has been reported in a patient with a giant aneurysm of the left coronary artery and complete occlusion of the right coronary artery (Alam et al 1995). Epidural anaesthesia has also been used for assisted vaginal delivery in a patient with two coronary artery aneurysms and stenosis of the right coronary artery (Shear & Leduc 1999).

Bibliography

Alam S, Sakura S, Kosaka Y 1995 Anaesthetic management for Caesarean section in a patient with Kawasaki disease. Canadian Journal of Anaesthesia 42: 1024–6.

Burgner D, Festa M, Isaacs D 1996 Delayed diagnosis of Kawasaki disease presenting with massive lymphadenopathy and airway obstruction. British Medical Journal 312: 1471–2.

Curtis N 1997 Kawasaki disease. Early recognition is vital to prevent cardiac complications. British Medical Journal 315: 322–3.

Kowalewski R, MacAdams C, Froelich J et al 1996 Anesthesia supplemented with subarachnoid bupivacaine and morphine for coronary artery bypass surgery in a child with Kawasaki disease. Journal of Cardiothoracic & Vascular Anesthesia 10: 243–6.

Moran AM, Newburger JW, Sanders SP et al 2000 Abnormal myocardial mechanics in Kawasaki disease: rapid response to gamma-globulin. American Heart Journal 139: 217–23.

Nakamura Y, Yanagawa H, Ojima T et al 1998 Cardiac sequelae of Kawasaki disease among recurrent cases. Archives of Disease in Childhood 78: 163–5.

Ravi KV, Brooks JR 1997 Peritonsillar abscess—an unusual presentation of Kawasaki disease. Journal of Laryngology & Otology 111: 73–4.

Shear R, Leduc L 1999 Successful pregnancy following Kawasaki disease. Obstetrics & Gynecology 94: 841.

Shetty AK, Homsi O, Ward K et al 1998 Massive lymphadenopathy and airway obstruction in a child with Kawasaki disease: success with pulse steroid therapy. Journal of Rheumatology 25: 1215–17.

Sugimura T, Yokoi H, Sato N et al 1997 Interventional treatment for children with severe coronary artery stenosis with calcification after long-term Kawasaki disease. Circulation 96: 3928–33.

Takahashi M 1998 The endothelium in Kawasaki disease: the next frontier. Journal of Pediatrics 133: 177–9.

Thomas ML, McEwan A 1998 The anaesthetic management of a case of Kawasaki's disease (mucocutaneous lymph node syndrome) and Beckwith–Weidemann syndrome presenting with a bleeding tongue. Paediatric Anaesthesia 8: 500–2.

Waldron RJ 1993 Kawasaki disease and anaesthesia. Anaesthesia & Intensive Care 21: 213–17.

Kearns–Sayre syndrome (see also Mitochondrial encephalomyopathies)

One of the oxidative phosphorylation (OXPHOS) diseases, a group of rare multisystem disorders, in which there are mutations of mitochondrial DNA (mitochondrial cytopathies). They are increasingly being recognised as causes of multisystem disorders in children (Sokol 1996). In Kearns–Sayre, external ophthalmoplegia is associated with neural, retinal and cardiac abnormalities (Tulinius et al 1991). It is the most severe of the mitochondrial DNA rearrangements (Shoffner 1996).

Preoperative abnormalities

1. Progressive ophthalmoplegia develops in infancy, childhood, or early adulthood, but usually before the age of 20 years (Johns 1995).

2. Retinal pigmentation occurs.

3. There may be proximal limb muscle weakness, and sometimes bulbar involvement and cerebellar ataxia. Patients may develop respiratory failure, chest infections, and require ventilatory support (Lauwers et al 1994).

4. Heart block. The incidence of cardiac conduction defects increases with age, and syncope or sudden death may occur in the fourth decade. A study of 17 patients with confirmed mitochondrial diseases showed a variation in the type of cardiac involvement. The three patients with Kearns–Sayre disease had AV conduction defects, but normal cardiothoracic ratios. One patient had RBBB which progressed to complete AV block over a period of 2 years (Anan et al 1995).

5. Cerebral infarction is a known complication and may arise from a thrombus in the left atrium (Kosinski et al 1995).

6. Endocrinopathies may occur. Renal tubular acidosis and tetany have been reported (Eviatar et al 1990).

7. Diagnosis is made on muscle biopsy.

Anaesthetic problems

1. Conduction defects, including bundle branch block and complete heart block, have been described (Kenny & Wetherbee 1990, Williams 1995). The patient may already have had a pacemaker implanted.

2. In the presence of muscle weakness, an abnormal response to muscle relaxants might be anticipated. However, D'Ambra et al (1979) performed neuromuscular studies in one patient using both suxamethonium and pancuronium. There was a normal response to both relaxants, and no hyperkalaemia after suxamethonium.

However, postoperative respiratory depression and metabolic acidosis occurred in a 51 year old, despite documented recovery of neuromuscular function to 80% of control (Kitoh et al 1995).

3. Abnormalities of swallowing may occur secondary to impairment of pharyngeal and oesophageal peristalsis (Shaker et al 1992).

Management

1. Conduction defects may necessitate preoperative transvenous pacemaker insertion.

2. The problems of anaesthesia in patients with permanent pacemakers (see Heart block).

3. Neuromuscular monitoring is advisable, although delays in recovery may occur even when neuromuscular function has apparently returned to normal.

4. Postoperative respiratory support may be required (Kitoh et al 1995).

5. Epidural anaesthesia and assisted ventouse delivery was reported in a 31-year-old woman with a history of ophthalmoplegia, ptosis, and progressive muscle weakness (Blake & Shaw 1999). Her resting serum lactate was 1.6 mmol l^{-1} (N 0.8–1.2 mmol l^{-1}).

Bibliography

Anan R, Nakagawa M, Miyata M et al 1995 Cardiac involvement in mitochondrial diseases. A study on 17 patients with documented mitochondrial defects. Circulation 91: 955–61.

Blake LL, Shaw RW 1999 Mitochondrial myopathy in a primigravid pregnancy. British Journal of Obstetrics & Gynaecology 106: 871–3.

Chinnery PF, Turnbull DM 1997 Mitochondrial medicine. Quarterly Journal of Medicine 90: 657–67.

D'Ambra MN, Dedrick D, Savarese JJ 1979. Kearns–Sayre syndrome and pancuronium-succinylcholine-induced neuromuscular blockade. Anesthesiology 51: 343–5.

Eviatar L, Shanske S, Gauthier B et al 1990 Kearns–Sayre syndrome presenting as renal tubular acidosis. Neurology 40: 1761–3.

Johns DR 1995 Mitochondrial DNA and disease. New England Journal of Medicine 333: 638–44.

Kenny D, Wetherbee J 1990 Kearns–Sayre syndrome in the elderly: mitochondrial myopathy with advanced heart block. American Heart Journal 120: 440–3.

Kitoh T, Mizuno K, Otagiri T et al 1995 Anesthetic management for a patient with Kearns–Sayre syndrome. Anesthesia & Analgesia 80: 1240–2.

Kosinski C, Mull M, Lethen H et al 1995 Evidence for cardioembolic stroke in a case of Kearns–Sayre syndrome. Stroke 26: 1950–2.

Lauwers MH, Van Lersberghe C, Camu F 1994 Inhalation anaesthesia and the Kearns–Sayre syndrome. Anaesthesia 49: 876–8.

Shaker R, Kupla JI, Kidder TM et al 1992 Manometric characteristics of cervical dysphagia in a patient with the Kearns–Sayre syndrome. Gastroenterology 103: 1328–31.

Shoffner JM 1996 Maternal inheritance and the evaluation of oxidative phosphorylation diseases. Lancet 384: 1283–8.

Sokol RJ 1996 Expanding spectrum of mitochondrial disorders. Journal of Pediatrics 128: 597–9.

Tulinius MH, Holme E, Kristiansson B et al 1991 Mitochondrial encephalomyopathies in childhood II Clinical manifestations and syndromes. Journal of Pediatrics 119: 251–9.

Williams RS 1995 Cardiac involvement in mitochondrial diseases, and vice versa. Circulation 91: 1266–8.

Klippel–Feil syndrome

An inherited symptom complex in which skeletal abnormalities, particularly in the cervical spine, may be associated with genitourinary and cardiac anomalies. An increasing variety of other anomalies are being described (Pizzutillo et al 1994). About one-third of patients are at increased risk of progressive neurological damage, mostly those in whom upper cervical fusion and occipitocervical instability are present, and surgery may be required (Baba et al 1995).

Preoperative abnormalities

1. A short, webbed neck with restricted movement, and undescended, winged scapulae. The hairline is usually low. Several cervical vertebrae may be fused or reduced in number. The base of the skull may be flattened (platybasia), and the thoracic vertebrae are occasionally involved. Spinal cord anomalies may occur. The syndrome has been classified according to the pattern of vertebral fusion:

Type I   Block fusion of all cervical and some upper thoracic vertebrae.

Type II   Fusion of one or two parts. Often C2–3 and C5–6.

Type III   Types I and II combined with lower thoracic or lumbar involvement.

Type II is the commonest, and is most likely to be associated with neurological changes (Pizzutillo et al 1994, Baba et al 1995).

2. In a small number of patients there may be associated hindbrain malformations and syringobulbomyelia. The more numerous the abnormalities, the more likely it is that neurological problems will arise that require surgery.

3. Scoliosis is common. In a study of 57 patients, 70% had scoliosis (Thomsen et al 1997).

4. Significant genitourinary abnormalities were found in 64% of patients in one series (Moore et al 1975). Problems included renal agenesis, ectopia and malrotation, and penile hypospadias.

5. An incidence of congenital heart disease of 4–14% has been reported. Lesions include patent ductus arteriosus, coarctation of the aorta, and mitral valve prolapse.

6. Maxillofacial abnormalities may occur.

7. Deafness occurs in about one-third of patients, although audiological testing shows abnormalities in more than 75%.

Anaesthetic problems

1. A short neck and fused cervical vertebrae may contribute to difficulties in tracheal intubation.

2. In some patients with upper cervical spine abnormalities, hypermobility may be associated with neurological complications (Pizzutillo et al 1994, Baba et al 1995). By contrast, decreased motion of the lower cervical spine predisposed to degenerative disease. If cervical instability is present, there is a risk of spinal cord injury. Quadriplegia has been reported after minor trauma (Elster 1984). In one patient, paraesthesia and weakness occurred on neck extension (Hall et al 1990). Magnetic resonance imaging of the spinal canal undertaken in 20 children showed stenoses of 9 mm or less in 25% of patients (Ritterbusch et al 1991), and subluxation of 5 mm or greater in 25%. Several children had spinal cord abnormalities in addition.

3. Sleep apnoea from craniocervical compression may be misdiagnosed as being secondary to tonsillar enlargement (Rosen et al 1993). A child underwent adenotonsillectomy for severe sleep apnoea. Polysomnography 6 days later showed no improvement and, in view of the presence of neurological signs, tracheostomy was planned. However, before this could be undertaken, the child had a respiratory arrest during sleep, and autopsy showed syringobulbomyelia and displacement of the odontoid process against the medulla and upper cervical cord. In a second child with similar symptoms, Arnold–Chiari malformation was detected, by chance before tonsillectomy, and subsequent suboccipital craniectomy resulted in improvement in sleep apnoea.

4. The trachea may be short (15 or fewer rings compared with the normal 17). This increases the risk of accidental bronchial intubation (Wells et al 1989).

5. Kyphoscoliosis may reduce respiratory reserve.

6. A single case of muscle rigidity and rhabdomyolysis after halothane induction followed by suxamethonium has been reported, in which the CK increased to 20 470 iu l^{-1} (Khalil et al 1999). The significance of this is unknown.

Management

1. Plain X-rays of the cervical spine to show the types of cervical anomaly, and flexion and extension views to demonstrate the presence of any instability. If, on questioning, any symptoms suggestive of spinal cord compression are elicited, the use of MRI should be considered to evaluate the abnormalities more accurately (Ritterbusch et al 1991).

2. Potential intubation difficulties must be assessed. Awake intubation may be appropriate and was used for cholecystectomy (Daum & Jones 1988), and for Caesarean section in patients with Klippel–Feil syndrome, congenital hydrocephalus, and preeclampsia (Burns et al 1988). An inhalation induction was described in a neonate with coincidental Klippel–Feil and a craniocervical encephalocoele (Naguib et al 1986).

3. One pregnant patient requested regional anaesthesia for her Caesarean section. After gentle laryngoscopy under local anaesthesia had shown that intubation would be possible in the event of a problem, a microspinal technique, with incremental doses of heavy bupivacaine, was used (Dresner & Maclean 1995). Two patients underwent epidural anaesthesia for vaginal delivery (Singh et al 1996).

4. If cardiac defects are diagnosed, prophylactic antibiotic therapy will be necessary.

Bibliography

Baba H, Maezawa Y, Furusawa N et al 1995 The cervical spine in Klippel–Feil syndrome. International Orthopaedics 19: 204–8.

Burns AM, Dorje P, Lawes EG et al 1988 Anaesthetic management of Caesarean section for a mother with pre-eclampsia, the Klippel–Feil syndrome and congenital hydrocephalus. British Journal of Anaesthesia 61: 350–4.

Daum REO, Jones DJ 1988 Fibreoptic intubation in Klippel-Feil syndrome. Anaesthesia 43: 18–21.

Dresner MR, Maclean AR 1995 Anaesthesia for Caesarean section in a patient with Klippel–Feil syndrome. Anaesthesia 50: 807–9.

Elster AD 1984 Quadriplegia after minor trauma in the Klippel–Feil syndrome. Journal of Bone & Joint Surgery 66A: 1473–4.

Hall JE, Simmons ED, Danylchuk K et al 1990 Instability of the cervical spine and neurological involvement in Klippel–Feil syndrome. A case report. Journal of Bone & Joint Surgery 72A: 460–2.

Khalil SN, Youngblood B, Campos C et al 1999 Signs of an MH reaction. Paediatric Anaesthesia 9: 277–8.

Moore WB, Matthews TJ, Rabinowitz R 1975 Genitourinary anomalies associated with Klippel–Feil syndrome. Journal of Bone & Joint Surgery 57A: 355–7.

Naguib M, Farag H, Ibrahim AEW 1986 Anaesthetic considerations in Klippel–Feil syndrome. Canadian Anaesthetists' Society Journal 33: 66–70.

Norman B, Stambach T, Vreede E et al 1997 Anaesthetic management of labour associated with Klippel–Feil syndrome. International Journal of Obstetric Anesthesia 6: 68.

Pizzutillo PD, Woods M, Nicholson L et al 1994 Risk factors in Klippel–Feil syndrome. Spine 19: 2110–16.

Ritterbusch JF, McGinty LD, Spar J, et al 1991 Magnetic resonance imaging for stenosis and subluxation in Klippel–Feil syndrome. Spine 16: S539–41.

Rosen CL, Novotny EJ, D'Andrea LA et al 1993 Klippel–Feil sequence and sleep disordered breathing in two children. American Review of Respiratory Disease 147: 202–4.

Singh D, Mills GH, Caunt JA et al JD 1996 Anaesthetic management of labour in two patients with Klippel–Feil syndrome. International Journal of Obstetric Anesthesia 5: 198–201.

Thomsen MN, Schneider U, Weber M et al 1997 Scoliosis and congenital anomalies associated with Klippel–Feil syndrome types I–III. Spine 22: 396–401.

Wells AL, Wells TR, Landing BH et al 1989 Short trachea, a hazard in tracheal intubation of neonates: syndromal associations. Anesthesiology 71: 367–73.

Klippel–Trenaunay–Weber syndrome

Related to Sturge–Weber syndrome, with which it may coexist. A congenital, generalised mesodermal abnormality. The classical triad consists of superficial haemangiomas of the lower extremity, ipsilateral varicose veins, and asymmetrical hypertrophy of soft and bony tissues of the lower limb, but other anomalies may occur. Mixed vascular malformations involve the capillary, venous, arterial and lymphatic systems.

Preoperative abnormalities

1. In a series of 252 patients, capillary malformations occurred in 98%, varicosities or venous malformations in 72%, and limb hypertrophy in 67% (Jacob et al 1998). All three anomalies featured in 63% of patients. Lymphatic and arteriovenous malformations may also occur.

2. Rarely, spinal arteriovenous malformations are present.

3. Almost half of the patients required surgery, which included epiphysiodesis for leg length discrepancies, stripping of varicose veins, excision of venous malformations, and amputations or debulking procedures.

4. More than 80% of angiomas bleed spontaneously at some time during the patient's life. In the presence of visceral or pelvic haemangiomas, bleeding may occur from the bladder, rectum, colon, vagina, vulva, and penis (Markos 1987, Samuel & Spitz 1995).

5. There is an increased incidence of deep venous thrombosis and recurrent pulmonary embolism, which can be fatal (Christie et al 1998, Gianlupi et al 1999).

6. Children may present with high output cardiac failure secondary to arteriovenous shunts.

7. There are risks of invasion of abdominal angiomas with enteric organisms. Several cases of gram-negative bacteraemia have been reported in children with haemangiomas involving the skin of the abdominal wall (Bird et al 1996).

Anaesthetic problems

1. Two children with features of both the Klippel–Trenaunay–Weber and the

Sturge–Weber syndromes presented with severe upper airway obstruction (Reich & Wiatrak 1995). The 10 year old required tracheostomy under local anaesthesia for an enlarging mass that had expanded to replace the hard palate and maxilla. The 9 year old, who had recurrent pneumonia and difficulty in breathing, was found to have a high arched palate, narrowed choanae, and a hypoplastic and hypotonic pharynx. A tracheostomy under general anaesthesia relieved his obstruction.

2. If by any small chance spinal AV malformations are present, regional anaesthesia is hazardous. Sometimes they can occur in the same dermatome as the cutaneous lesions, and can bleed spontaneously after straining or coughing (Eastwood 1991).

3. Thrombophlebitis and thromboembolic phenomenon that are associated with the venous varicosities may occur. A 45-year-old woman developed right heart failure and multiple perfusion defects on lung scan. Having declined treatment, she eventually agreed to insertion of an IVC filter, but died on the eighth day (Gianlupi et al 1999).

4. The Kasabach–Merritt syndrome is an acute bleeding diathesis characterised by thrombocytopenia and a consumptive coagulopathy. It may be precipitated by hypovolaemia and is thought to result from a combination of venous stasis and the presence of abnormal cells within a haemangioma. Platelets pool within the lesion and are destroyed; this activates the coagulation cascade. Severe bleeding from coagulopathy occurred on the fourth day after Caesarean section (Neubert et al 1995), and recurrently after gynaecological surgery (Aronoff & Roshon 1998). A state of chronic thrombocytopenia has been reported (Poon et al 1989).

5. High output cardiac failure.

6. Venous malformations of the vulva and abdominal wall may present problems in pregnancy and delivery (Neubert et al 1995). Haemangiomas of the uterus can also occur (Andreasen et al 1999).

Management

1. Although regional anaesthesia was originally thought to be contraindicated, because of the rare possibility of spinal AV malformations (de Leon Casasola & Lema 1991), there are now techniques that can identify these, or at least can exclude their presence, in the spinal cord. These include MRI, CT scan, and colour flow mapping. Regional anaesthesia has been reported for Caesarean section (Gaiser et al 1995, Neubert et al 1995), vaginal delivery (Dobbs et al 1999), and reconstructive surgery to the leg (Christie et al 1998).

2. In pregnancy, the presence of venous abnormalities in the lower half of the body may determine the mode of delivery (Verheijen et al 1989). In view of localised angiomatous changes in the lower half of the uterus, the cervix, and the labia, Caesarean section by a classical incision was carried out under spinal anaesthesia. Sequential ultrasound scans mapped the increased size of a uterine haemangioma as pregnancy advanced (Andreasen et al 1999). In the absence of lower genitourinary AV malformations, vaginal delivery should be aimed for (Pollack et al 1995).

3. Hypovolaemia and extremes of blood pressure should be avoided.

4. Prevention of thromboembolic disease may require antithrombotic therapy and compression stockings.

5. Treatment for Kasabach–Merritt syndrome will need expert haematological advice. A patient with chronic profound thrombocytopenia (platelet count $6 \times 10^9 l^{-1}$) and documented pooling of platelets within a vascular malformation of the lower limb, responded dramatically to gradually increasing doses of epsilon-aminocaprioc acid, given to inhibit fibrinolysis. After 7 weeks the platelet count had returned to normal and organised clot was demonstrated within the lesion. Surgery was then undertaken (Poon et al 1989). The use of tranexamic acid for bleeding from inoperable lesions has also been reported. Another patient who bled repeatedly following surgery to the

cervix, eventually stopped following administration of low-dose heparin and antithrombin III given as a desperate measure (Aronoff & Roshon 1998).

Bibliography

Andreasen KR, Tabor A, Weber T 1999 Klippel–Trenaunay–Weber syndrome in pregnancy and at delivery. Journal of Obstetrics & Gynaecology 19: 78–9.

Aronoff DM, Roshon M 1998 Severe hemorrhage complicating the Klippel–Trenaunay–Weber syndrome. Southern Medical Journal 91: 1073–5.

Bird LM, Jones MC, Kupperman N et al 1996 Gram-negative bacteremia in four patients with Klippel–Trenaunay–Weber syndrome. Pediatrics 97: 739–41.

Christie IW, Ahkine PA, Holland RL 1998 Central regional anaesthesia in a patient with Klippel–Trenaunay syndrome. Anaesthesia & Intensive Care 26: 319–21.

de Leon-Casasola OA, Lema MJ 1991 Anesthesia for patients with Sturge–Weber disease and Klippel–Trenaunay syndrome. Journal of Clinical Anesthesia 3: 409–13.

de Leon Casasola OA, Lema MJ 1992 Epidural anesthesia in patients with Klippel–Trenaunay syndrome. Anesthesia & Analgesia 74: 353–62.

Dobbs P, Caunt A, Alderson TJ 1999 Epidural analgesia in an obstetric patient with Klippel–Trenaunay syndrome. British Journal of Anaesthesia 82: 144–6.

Eastwood DW 1991 Hematoma after epidural anesthesia: relationship of skin and spinal angiomas. Anesthesia & Analgesia 73: 352–4.

Gaiser RR, Cheek TG, Gutsche BB 1995 Major conduction anesthesia in a patient with Klippel–Trenaunay syndrome. Journal of Clinical Anesthesia 7: 316–19.

Gianlupi A, Harper RW, Dwyre DM et al 1999 Recurrent pulmonary embolism associated with Klippel–Trenaunay–Weber syndrome. Chest 115: 1199–201.

Jacob AG, Driscoll DJ, Shaughnessy WJ et al 1998 Klippel–Trenaunay syndrome: spectrum and management. Mayo Clinic Proceedings 73: 28–36.

Markos AR 1987 Klippel–Trenaunay syndrome—a rare cause of severe menorrhagia. British Journal of Obstetrics & Gynaecology 94: 1105–6.

Neubert GA, Golden MA, Rose NC 1995 Kasabach–Merritt coagulopathy complicating Klippel–Trenaunay–Weber syndrome in pregnancy. Obstetrics & Gynecology 85: 831–3.

Pollack RN, Quance DR, Shatz RM 1995 Pregnancy complicated by the Klippel–Trenaunay syndrome. A case report. Journal of Reproductive Medicine 40: 240–7.

Poon M-C, Kloiber R, Birdsell DC 1989 Epsilon-aminocaproic acid in the reversal of consumptive coagulopathy with platelet sequestration in vascular malformation in Klippel–Trenaunay syndrome. American Journal of Medicine 87: 211–13.

Reich DS, Wiatrak BJ 1995 Upper airway obstruction in Sturge–Weber and Klippel–Trenaunay–Weber syndromes. Annals of Otology, Rhinology & Laryngology 104: 364–8.

Samuel M, Spitz L 1995 Klippel–Trenaunay syndrome: clinical features, complications and management in children. British Journal of Surgery 82: 757–61.

Verheijen RHM, Van Rijen-De Rooij HJM, Van Zundert AAJ et al 1989 Pregnancy in a patient with the Klippel–Trenaunay–Weber syndrome: a case report. European Journal of Obstetrics, Gynecology & Reproductive Biology 33: 89–94.

Lambert–Eaton syndrome (see

Eaton–Lambert syndrome)

Laryngeal papillomatosis

Benign, warty tumours of the larynx that occur mainly in children, but sometimes in adults, and are caused by one or more of the human papillomaviruses, the majority type 11, but sometimes type 6. They arise most commonly on the true vocal cords with extension onto the ventricles. Frequently recurrent, they may be present in other parts of the respiratory tract. Extension into the subglottis is common, but involvement of the trachea, proximal bronchus and lung parenchyma is rare. In children, transmission is thought to occur from the mother. In adults it may be sexually transmitted. It has been suggested that the old terms 'juvenile' and 'adult' be replaced by aggressive and nonaggressive, since the aggressive form can occur in adults and vice versa (Doyle et al 1994). Analysis of 399 children from a national registry concluded that those diagnosed before the age of 3 years had more severe disease than those who were 3 years or older (Armstrong et al 1999). A staging system has been suggested (Derkay et al 1998).

Preoperative abnormalities

1. Usually presents in early childhood with hoarseness, cough, respiratory distress, stridor or sleep disturbances, secondary to upper airway obstruction. Patients are often labelled as having 'croup' or 'asthma' before the true nature of the condition is recognised. Of 90 patients whose symptoms presented between birth and age 11, nearly half occurred before the age of 2 years, 90% had a voice change, 44% airway obstruction, and 39% stridor (Cohen et al 1980). The most aggressive form occurs in the young, at an average age of 2 years.

2. Obstructive sleep apnoea with snoring may be a presenting symptom. A 10 year old with OSA since birth, an apnoea index of 50,

and oxygen saturations as low as 47%, was found on sleep nasendoscopy to have a granular mass of viral papillomas in the nasopharynx (Wheatley et al 1997).

3. Chronic airway obstruction may lead to pulmonary hypertension, right ventricular hypertrophy, cor pulmonale, and polycythaemia.

4. The theory that regression occurs at puberty has been challenged (Doyle et al 1994).

5. Tracheal involvement is more frequent than was previously thought, although current techniques in management are reducing the incidence of tracheal spread (Crockett et al 1987b).

6. Laryngeal malignancy may occur subsequently.

Anaesthetic problems

1. Upper respiratory tract obstruction in young infants. Total airway obstruction on induction of anaesthesia has been described in a 18 month old, as a result of multiple papillomas completely occluding the larynx. Emergency tracheostomy was required (Dalmeida et al 1996). Several cases have been described in which children could maintain their airways during spontaneous respiration, but total obstruction occurred when manual ventilation was attempted on a mask (Theroux et al 1998). In one case, even though the infant could be ventilated on a mask initially, this was not possible following attempts (and subsequent failure) to intubate.

2. During difficult intubation or rigid bronchoscopy, papillomas may obstruct the tube or be forced distal to the larynx.

3. Multiple anaesthetics may be required. In one series, 66% of the patients had multiple diffuse disease and each had required an average of 15.9 anaesthetics (Cohen et al 1980).

4. Tracheobronchial papillomatosis has been reported in 2–26% of cases of laryngeal papillomatosis. Subglottic involvement usually

occurs in very young children. A case was reported in which an absence of ventilation of the right lung was noticed during resection of laryngeal papillomata in a 10 year old child. At bronchoscopy, a large papilloma was found to be occluding the right main bronchus. Tracheostomy had been performed in this child at an earlier stage (Callander 1986).

5. It has been suggested that tracheostomy seeds papillomas and causes distal spread of the disease. However, a recent study found that those with tracheostomy were younger children with more aggressive disease, and that spread had often predated the tracheostomy (Shapiro et al 1996). The combination of laser treatment with Venturi and jet ventilation techniques may minimise viral spread (Crockett et al 1987b). However, Venturi techniques carry the risk of barotrauma. In one patient, a Carden's tube was displaced into the oesophagus during jet ventilation and, at laparotomy, tears in the gastroduodenal junction and posterior wall of the stomach were found (Braverman et al 1994).

6. Laser treatment is not complication free. In a study of 890 resections in 66 patients, although the immediate complication rate was low, delayed tissue damage occurred in 36% of children and 17% of adults (Crockett et al 1987b). The more severe the disease, the more the likelihood of late complications.

7. Airway fires have been described with laser treatment. Ignition of the surgeon's glove resulted in entrainment of burning vapours into the airway by the Venturi (Wegryznowicz et al 1992), and burns were sustained by both patient and surgeon.

8. There is a small risk of virus being spread to the staff. A laser surgeon who had previously treated anogenital condylomas developed laryngeal papillomatosis. Both of these tumours harbour papillomaviruses of the same viral types, therefore it was speculated that the laser plume had carried virus particles (Hallmo & Naess 1991). However, analysis of the smoke plume from laser-treated laryngeal papillomas did not reveal the presence of human papillomavirus,

unless direct suction contact had been made with the lesion (Abramson et al 1991). It has also been suggested from experiments on papilloma specimens that viral particles do not survive continuous mode carbon dioxide laser irradiation (Kunachak et al 1996).

9. A fatal case of laryngeal papillomatosis in pregnancy has been described (Helmrich et al 1992).

10. Iatrogenic airway stenosis may occur following recurrent treatment (Perkins et al 1998).

Management

1. There should be an index of suspicion if children present with recurrent problems associated with the upper airway.

2. Anticipation of airway difficulties under anaesthesia. Nasendoscopy, or indirect laryngoscopy, performed before admission, can give diagnostic information about aetiology. However, visualisation of the vocal cords with the patient awake and positioned upright does not guarantee that intubation will be easy. In case of failure of mask ventilation or tracheal intubation, facilities for rigid bronchoscopy and tracheostomy should be available. If severe obstructive symptoms are present, the airway must be secured before general anaesthesia is given. In one obese patient, in whom laryngeal polyps were found by chance during incidental surgery, intubation and ventilation were impossible. However, passage of a laryngeal mask airway saved the deteriorating situation and allowed gentle positive pressure ventilation, whilst the surgeon performed emergency tracheostomy (Pennant et al 1994).

3. The use of tracheostomy is controversial, but it may be needed in children with aggressive disease. Cohen et al (1980) found the incidence of tracheobronchial papillomas to be related to the incidence of tracheostomy and suggested that tracheostomy seeded the virus and was contraindicated. However, subsequent papers

have demonstrated the presence of distal spread before the tracheostomy was undertaken.

4. A variety of techniques have been suggested. Inhalation anaesthesia, local anaesthetic spray, or insufflation of halothane and oxygen (or air in the case of laser surgery), have been reported. Apnoeic techniques with intermittent ventilation (Weisberger & Emhardt 1996), and tubeless techniques via a jet ventilation laryngoscope in infants and children (Grasl et al 1997), have also been described. However, care should be taken to avoid airway fires and barotrauma. If safe airway maintenance is a problem, a range of laser-proof tubes are now available.

5. Precautions to prevent spread of the virus to staff include the use of eye protection and gloves. Since the aspirate is potentially infective, disposable suction canisters and tubing should be used.

6. Postoperative humidification of oxygen is recommended.

7. Perioperative corticosteroids have been claimed to reduce postoperative oedema, but their use is arguable. Laser techniques are increasingly being used for laryngeal lesions and seem to be associated with fewer immediate postoperative complications, although delayed pain may be a problem.

8. Interferon has been reported to eliminate papilloma in 40% of children and reduce their growth rate in 30% (Crockett et al 1987a). However, in the case of lesions that are unresponsive to interferon, endoscopy and resection or laser excision may be required regularly.

Bibliography

Abramson AL, DiLorenzo TP, Steinberg BM 1991 Is papillomavirus detectable in the plume of laser-treated laryngeal papilloma? Archives of Otolaryngology & Head & Neck Surgery 116: 604–7.

Armstrong LR, Derkay CS, Reeves WC 1999 Initial results from the national registry for juvenile-onset recurrent respiratory papillomatosis. RRP Task Force. Archives of Otolaryngology & Head & Neck Surgery 125: 743–8.

Braverman I, Sichel J-Y, Halimi P et al 1994 Complications of jet ventilation during microlaryngeal surgery. Annals of Otology, Rhinology & Laryngology 103: 624–7.

Callander CC 1986 Tracheobronchial papillomatosis: anaesthetic implications. Anaesthesia & Intensive Care 14: 201–2.

Cohen SR, Geller KA, Seltzer S et al 1980 Papilloma of the larynx and tracheobronchial tree in children. Annals of Otolaryngology 89: 497–503.

Crockett DM, Scamman FL, McCabe BF et al 1987a Venturi jet ventilator for microlaryngoscopy: technique, complications, pitfalls. Laryngoscopy 97: 1326–30.

Crockett DM, McCabe BF, Shive CJ 1987b Complications of laser surgery for recurrent respiratory papillomatosis. Annals of Otology, Rhinology and Laryngology 96: 639–44.

Dalmeida RE, Mayhew JF, Driscoll B et al 1996 Total airway obstruction by papillomas during induction of general anesthesia. Anesthesia & Analgesia 83: 1332–4.

Derkay CS, Mails DJ, Zalzal G et al 1998 A staging system for assessing severity of disease and response to therapy in recurrent papillomatosis. Laryngoscope 108: 935–7.

Doyle DJ, Gianoli GJ, Espinola T et al 1994 Recurrent respiratory papillomatosis: juvenile versus adult form. Laryngoscope 104: 523–7.

Grasl MC, Donner A, Schragl E et al 1997 Tubeless laryngotracheal surgery in infants and children via jet ventilation laryngoscope. Laryngoscope 107: 277–81.

Hallmo P, Naess O 1991 Laryngeal papillomatosis with human papillomavirus DNA contracted by a laser surgeon. European Archives of Otolaryngology 248: 425–7.

Helmrich G, Stubbs TM, Stoeker J 1992 Fatal maternal laryngeal papillomatosis in pregnancy: a case report. American Journal of Obstetrics & Gynecology 166: 524–5.

Kunachak S, Sithisarn P, Kulapaditharom B 1996 Are laryngeal papilloma virus-infected cells viable in the plume derived from a continuous mode carbon dioxide laser, and are they infectious? A preliminary report in one laser mode. Journal of Laryngology & Otology 110: 1031–3.

Pennant JH, Gajraj NM, Yamanouchi KJ 1994 The laryngeal mask airway and laryngeal polyposis. Anesthesia & Analgesia 74: 1206–7.

Perkins JA, Inglis AF Jr, Richardson MA 1998
Iatrogenic airway stenosis with recurrent respiratory
papillomatosis. Archives of Otolaryngology & Head
& Neck Surgery 124: 281–7.

Shapiro AM, Rimell FL, Shoemaker D et al 1996
Tracheotomy in children with juvenile-onset
recurrent respiratory papillomatosis: the Children's
Hospital of Pittsburgh experience. Annals of
Otology, Rhinology & Laryngology 105: 1–5.

Theroux MC, Grodecki V, Reilly JS et al 1998
Juvenile laryngeal papillomatosis: scary anaesthetic.
Paediatric Anaesthesia 8: 357–61.

Wegrzynowicz ES, Jensen NF, Pearson KS et al 1992
Airway fire during jet ventilation for laser excision
of vocal cord papillomata. Anesthesiology 76:
468–9.

Weisberger EC, Emhardt JD 1996 Apneic anesthesia
with intermittent ventilation for microsurgery of
the upper airway. Laryngoscope 106: 1099–102.

Wheatley AH, Temple RH, Camilleri AE 1997
Childhood obstructive sleep apnoea syndrome due
to nasopharyngeal viral papillomatosis. Journal of
Laryngology & Otology 111: 976–7.

Latex allergy (see Section 2 for emergency presentation)

This is an increasing problem amongst both
patients and health workers. Reports of latex
allergy began in the mid 1980s, predominantly
from the USA. Gloves, particularly those that
were starch containing, were the most common
cause (Hirshman 1992). At that time there was a
substantial demand for latex gloves because of
universal precautions for hepatitis and HIV, new
chemicals were being used in the manufacturing
processes, and production standards in the USA
may have been less stringent. Hospitals are now
required to develop a strategy, for prevention of
the problem and protection of both staff and
patients (Dakin & Yentis 1998). This may be led
by a dermatologist, and involve the occupational
therapy department, the risk management group,
and the operating theatre directorate. Education
of all groups is important, and there must be a
high index of suspicion when untoward events
occur some time after the start of surgery.
Reactions can be immediate type I or delayed
type IV (contact dermatitis).

In addition to surgery, reactions have developed
during barium enema, urethral catheterisation
(Stewart & Bogod 1995), and dental procedures.
Routes of exposure can involve the skin, mucous
membranes, by inhalation, intravascular or
internally. Latex-free gloves are expensive and
difficult to use.

Analysis of 162 children with latex allergy
undergoing 267 procedures showed that they
could be safely anaesthetised without the use of
prophylactic medications (Holzman 1997). The
patients had undergone an average of 10.2 (4.7)
surgical procedures. Only one problem was
encountered; that of an epidural syringe which
had been prepared in pharmacy 10 days earlier. It
has been suggested that there is a difference in
immune expression between adults and children,
and that adults may require preoperative
prophylaxis.

The use of testing in high-risk patients has been
recommended, but this is controversial
(Moneret-Vautrain & Laxenaire 1991).

Preoperative identification

1. *Known history of anaphylaxis to latex*. It does
not always occur to patients that their rubber
allergy might be of relevance to the anaesthetist.
Two patients who denied allergies developed
delayed responses of intraoperative hypotension
and flushing. Both had increases in tryptase levels
($10.4\,\mathrm{mg\,l^{-1}}$ and $8.5\,\mathrm{mg\,l^{-1}}$; normal $2\,\mu\mathrm{g\,l^{-1}}$), and
positive skin prick tests to latex. Only at this
stage did each patient declare their cutaneous
reactions to latex (Fisher 1997). Another had
hives after the use of gloves and sneezing during
vaginal examinations (Ballantine & Brown
1995). She had undergone IVF for infertility,
which involved regular use of a latex-covered
vaginal probe.

2. *High-risk groups*. Repeat bladder
catheterisation.

   a) Spina bifida and congenital urogenital
      abnormalities such as bladder and cloacal
      exstrophy.

b) Multiple surgical procedures.

c) Occupational exposure.

d) Healthcare workers.

e) History of atopy, drugs allergies, food allergies such as bananas, kiwi fruit, and avocados.

3. *Routine questioning.* Specific questions about skin reactions to rubber gloves, or lip swelling after dental examinations, or blowing up balloons, would have identified reactors in several case reports (Ballantine & Brown 1995, Fisher 1997, Rae et al 1997).

Preoperative preparation

1. All ward and operating staff should be alerted to the existence of a latex allergy in a patient.

2. Premedication with antihistamines and steroids has been suggested. However, this is controversial and may not be required in children (Holzman 1997). One adult, pretreated with ranitidine for gastro-oesophageal reflux, developed 3 : 1 heart block during an unexpected reaction, found to be secondary to latex anaphylaxis (Patterson & Milne 1999). Since H_1 receptors are involved in AV conduction delay, it was suggested that the use of H_2 antagonists alone may increase the risk of AV conduction defects occurring in the presence of high levels of circulating histamine.

3. The patient should be first on the theatre list, preferably in a latex-free environment (Kam et al 1997).

4. Drugs for the treatment of anaphylaxis should be drawn up in advance.

Intraoperative precautions

1. Use of latex-free anaesthetic masks, ECG electrodes and wires, blood pressure cuffs, self-inflating bag, elastic bandages, catheters, ileostomy bags, instrument mats, adhesive tapes, dental instruments and material, rectal balloons, airborne latex proteins from glove powder. Powderless gloves should be used and drugs should not be drawn from ampoules with rubber stoppers.

2. Each department should have a database of latex-free equipment (Dakin & Yentis 1998).

Bibliography

Ballantine JC, Brown E 1995 Latex anaphylaxis: another case, another cause. Anesthesia & Analgesia 81: 1303–4.

Dakin MJ, Yentis SM 1998 Latex allergy: a strategy for management. Anaesthesia 53: 774–81.

Fisher MMCD 1997 Latex allergy during anaesthesia: cautionary tales. Anaesthesia & Intensive Care 25: 302–3.

Hirshman CA 1992 Latex anaphylaxis. Anesthesiology 77: 223–5.

Holzman RS 1997 Clinical management of latex-allergic children. Anesthesia & Analgesia 85: 529–33.

Kam PCA, Lee MSM, Thompson JF 1997 Latex allergy: an emerging clinical and occupational problem. Anaesthesia 52: 570–5.

Moneret-Vautrin DA, Laxenaire MC 1991 Routine testing for latex allergy in patients with spina bifida is not recommended. Anesthesiology 74: 391–2.

Patterson LJ, Milne B 1999 Latex anaphylaxis causing heart block: role of ranitidine. Canadian Journal of Anaesthesia 46: 776–8.

Rae SM, Milne MK, Wildsmith JAW 1997 Anaphylaxis associated with, but not caused by, extradural bupivacaine. British Journal of Anaesthesia 78: 224–6.

Stewart PD, Bogod D 1995 Latex anaphylaxis during late pregnancy. International Journal of Obstetric Anesthesia 4: 48–50.

Lesch–Nyhan disease

An X-linked recessive disorder of purine metabolism in which there is an absence of hypoxanthine guanine phosphoribosyl transferase (HGPRT) activity. There is primary purine overproduction, with hyperuricaemia, gout, and choreoathetoid spasticity. Neurological features may be associated with abnormalities of dopaminergic function in the basal ganglia (Nyhan & Wong 1996). MRI studies have shown consistently reduced basal ganglia volumes, and positron-emission tomography has demonstrated abnormally few dopaminergic nerve terminals and cell bodies, deficits that are not restricted to the basal ganglia alone (Ernst et al 1996). Anaesthesia may be required for orthopaedic surgery, diagnostic imaging, and dental extraction.

Preoperative abnormalities

1. Mental retardation, choreoathetoid and dystonic movements, spasticity, and bizarre episodes of self mutilation and aggression.

2. Hyperuricaemia can cause a nephropathy and urinary tract calcification. Death frequently results from renal failure in the third decade.

3. Arthritis and gouty tophi occur.

4. A B-lymphocyte immune deficiency may result in an increased susceptibility to infection.

5. Urinary uric acid is always increased and serum urate usually so.

Anaesthetic problems

1. Self mutilation may result in scarring of the mouth region.

2. Patients are susceptible to aspiration pneumonitis.

3. Abnormal adrenergic responses and decreased monoamine oxidase activity have been reported (Larson & Wilkins 1985).

4. Atlantoaxial instability has been described in two brothers. The 5 year old had neck pain and progressive quadriplegia, and CT scan showed fracture of the odontoid tip and forward subluxation of the atlas. The 16-year-old brother was screened and had similar findings, but without quadriplegia (Shewell et al 1996).

Management

1. Teeth extraction may be required to reduce the trauma from self mutilation.

2. Suxamethonium should probably not be used (Larson & Wilkins 1985).

3. Williams et al (1997) have described outpatient anaesthesia for diagnostic imaging using a propofol infusion and spontaneous respiration.

Bibliography
Ernst M, Zametkin AJ, Matochik JA 1996 Presynaptic dopaminergic deficits in Lesch–Nyhan disease. New England Journal of Medicine 334: 1568–72.
Larson LO, Wilkins RG 1985 Anesthesia and the Lesch–Nyhan Syndrome. Anesthesiology 63: 197–9.
Nyhan WL, Wong DF 1996 New approaches to understanding Lesch–Nyhan disease. New England Journal of Medicine 334: 1602–4.
Shewell PC, Thompson AG, Hensinger RN 1996 Atlantoaxial instability in Lesch–Nyhan syndrome. Spine 21: 757–62.
Williams KS, Hankerson JG, Ernst M et al 1997 Use of propofol anesthesia during outpatient radiographic imaging studies in patients with Lesch–Nyhan syndrome. Journal of Clinical Anesthesia 9: 61–5.

Ludwig's angina

A rapidly spreading cellulitis of the floor of the mouth that can be produced by any infection. It involves the submandibular, sublingual and submental spaces. Gram-positive cocci (usually streptococci), *Staphylococcus aureus* and *Staphylococcus epidermidis* are now the most common organisms (Har-El et al 1994), but sometimes gram-negative rods or anaerobes are responsible. In 50% of cases more than one organism is isolated (Moreland et al 1988). It is frequently precipitated by dental infection involving the second and third lower molars, but trauma may be contributory.

The frequency is generally decreasing, but there is now a higher incidence in patients with associated systemic diseases. Before the advent of antibiotics, or in the untreated patient, fatalities have occurred, and occasionally still do occur. Antibiotics and aggressive surgical treatment have dramatically improved the mortality rate. In the postantibiotic era, the mean age of patients is 29 years; they are usually previously fit, but most have dental disease (Iwu 1990). Airway management is controversial, as is shown by recent debate (Marple 1999, Quinn 1999, Shockley 1999). However, as Quinn comments, airway compromise develops insidiously, but actual obstruction is abrupt.

Preoperative abnormalities

1. The condition usually arises from the teeth, but tongue piercing with metal barbels has provided a novel source of infection (Perkins et al 1997). Bilateral submandibular swelling proceeds to brawny induration of the neck. Although the submandibular space is primarily involved in Ludwig's angina, spread into adjacent fascial spaces may occur. A detailed account of the anatomy of spread of infection can be consulted (Lindner 1986).

2. Elevation of the tongue caused by cellulitis of the floor of the mouth.

3. Dysphagia secondary to swelling, and trismus.

4. Gradual onset, or sudden, upper airway obstruction.

5. There is frequently an underlying systemic condition, such as diabetes, AIDS, or substance abuse.

6. Other complications include bacteraemia, aspiration, retropharyngeal abscess, empyema, mediastinitis, internal jugular vein thrombosis, and pericarditis.

7. Fever, leucocytosis, and increased ESR.

Anaesthetic problems

1. Trismus, not necessarily relieved by muscle relaxants, may make oral intubation difficult or impossible.

2. Sudden total upper airway obstruction producing hypoxia.

3. Intravenous induction of anaesthesia may be hazardous because it can result in apnoea and an inability to maintain ventilation on a mask (Loughnan & Allen 1985).

4. After fibreoptic intubation with a polyvinylchloride nasotracheal tube, difficulties were experienced in withdrawing the bronchoscope (Chung & Liban 1991). When the bronchoscope was successfully removed, obstruction again occurred, and was found to be the result of compression of the tube caused by severe supraglottic swelling.

5. Sepsis may track down through the retropharyngeal space into the posterior mediastinum. A young man with a 2-week history of dental sepsis required awake oral intubation, ventilatory support, and an eventual thoracotomy for a thoracic empyema (Dugan et al 1998).

Management

1. Aggressive early treatment with antibiotics reduces airway problems and the need for surgical intervention.

2. Less severely affected patients may be managed by close observation, but only provided that staff are available who can manage acute obstruction. Some argue the case for early tracheostomy (Har-El et al 1994).

3. Surgical drainage with or without tooth extraction.

4. Anaesthesia for surgery in which there is trismus, but **without** compromise of the upper airway:

   a) Awake fibreoptic nasal intubation but with facilities for emergency tracheostomy available. Reusche and Egan (1999) used a low-dose remifentanil infusion as part of a 'sedation–analgesia' regimen, in a man with trismus and diffuse oedema, but without airway compromise.

b) Inhalation induction and laryngoscopy (Gupta & Wilson 1998). If the trismus relaxes and the vocal cords can be seen, a neuromuscular blocker can be given.

c) Tracheostomy may be required in the presence of spreading oedema.

5. **Airway maintenance in the compromised airway.** Signs of airway obstruction, including stridor, dyspnoea, dysphagia, difficulty with secretions, and deteriorating oxygen saturations, may indicate the need for rapid, active intervention. In these patients, sedative premedication should be avoided and a drying agent given. If there is significant stridor, a tracheostomy under local anaesthesia may be considered. Emergency cricothyroidotomy under local anaesthesia has also been reported (Busch & Shah 1997).

Bibliography

Busch RF, Shah D 1997 Ludwig's angina: improved treatment. Otolaryngology—Head & Neck Surgery 117: S172–5.

Chung RA, Liban JB 1991 Ludwig's angina and tracheal tube obstruction. Anaesthesia 46: 228–9.

Dugan MJ, Lazow SK, Berger JR 1998 Thoracic empyema resulting from direct extension of Ludwig's angina. A case report. Journal of Oral & Maxillofacial Surgery 56: 968–71.

Gupta S, Wilson JU 1998 Sevoflurane for inhalational induction in patients with anticipated difficult intubation. Acta Anaesthesiologica Scandinavica 42: 1232.

Har-El, G, Aroesty JH, Shaha A et al 1994 Changing trends in neck abscesses. A retrospective study of 110 patients. Oral Surgery, Oral Medicine, Oral Pathology 1994 77: 446–50.

Iwu CO 1990 Ludwig's angina: report of seven cases and review of current concepts of management. British Journal of Oral & Maxillofacial Surgery 28: 189–93.

Lindner HH 1986 The anatomy of the fasciae of the face and neck with particular reference to the spread and treatment of intraoral infections (Ludwig's) that have progressed into adjacent fascial spaces. Annals of Surgery 204: 705–14.

Loughman TE, Allen DE 1985 Ludwig's angina. The anaesthetic management of nine cases. Anaesthesia 40: 295–7.

Marple BF 1999 Ludwig angina: a review of current airway management. Archives of Otolaryngology—Head & Neck Surgery 125: 596–9.

Moreland LW, Corey J, McKenzie R 1988 Ludwig's angina. Report of a case and review of the literature. Archives of Internal Medicine 148: 461–6.

Perkins CS, Meisner J, Harrison JM 1997 A complication of tongue piercing. British Dental Journal 182: 147–8.

Quinn FB 1999 Ludwig angina [comment]. Archives of Otolaryngology—Head & Neck Surgery 125: 599.

Reusche MD, Egan TD 1999 Remifentanil for conscious sedation and analgesia during awake fiberoptic tracheal intubation. A case report with pharmacokinetic simulations. Journal of Clinical Anesthesia 11: 64–8.

Sethi DS, Stanley RE 1994 Deep neck abscesses—changing trends. Journal of Laryngology & Otology 108: 138–43.

Shockley WW 1999 Ludwig angina: a review of current airway management. Archives of Otolaryngology—Head & Neck Surgery 125: 600.

Lysergic acid diethylamide (LSD) abuse

LSD is a psychedelic drug, which can either be synthesised, or obtained naturally from the seeds of *Rivea corymbosa* (morning glory), or ergot fungus on rye. Its effect is almost entirely on the CNS, where it modifies serotonin metabolism by acting on $5HT_2$ receptors, and it rapidly produces tolerance. Intoxicated patients are liable to injure themselves and be unaware of it. Respiratory depression has been reported.

Preoperative abnormalities

1. The onset of CNS effects occurs 40 min after an oral dose. Hallucinations may last for 2 h and the biological half-life is 3 h (Caldwell 1990).

Effects (Caldwell 1990):

0.5–$1\,\mu g\,kg^{-1}$—euphoria and a degree of visual, auditory or tactile disturbances.

$1 \mu g\,kg^{-1}$—increases sensory distortion.

$2 \mu g\,kg^{-1}$—alarming hallucinations.

$0.2\,mg\,kg^{-1}$—possible lethal threshold.

2. Central autonomic stimulation occurs, probably mediated via the hypothalamus. Parasympathetic and sympathetic effects include tremors, tachycardia, hypertension, fever, piloerection, mydriasis, lacrimation, and hyperreflexia.

3. LSD has analgesic properties.

4. Tolerance to both autonomic and psychic effects is produced rapidly, but dependence does not occur.

5. LSD produces EEG changes.

Anaesthetic problems

1. Injury may be sustained without the patient being aware of it.

2. Hypertension, tachycardia and fever occur with toxic doses.

3. Interaction with belladonna alkaloids may occur.

4. Some inhibition of cholinesterase activity has been reported and theoretically it may prolong the action of suxamethonium.

5. Exaggerated responses to other sympathomimetic amines may occur.

6. Increased toxicity of ester-type local anaesthetics has been suggested (McGoldrick 1980).

Management

1. Heart rate, blood pressure and temperature should be monitored continuously.

2. Persistent sympathetic effects during general anaesthesia can be treated with alpha and beta blockers:

Phentolamine 1–2 mg and repeat, or infusion of $0.1–2\,mg\,min^{-1}$.

Propranolol 0.5 mg at 10-min intervals to a maximum of 5 mg.

Metoprolol $1–2\,mg\,min^{-1}$ up to 5 mg. Repeat at 5-min intervals to a total of 10–15 mg.

3. If sedatives are required, a benzodiazepine or chlorpromazine have been suggested as being suitable.

4. Anticholinergics should be avoided if the patient shows signs of toxicity, because the effects of LSD may be enhanced.

5. Recent work on animals has shown that the calcium channel blocker nifedipine may prevent some of the behavioural consequences of chronic LSD abuse (Antkiewicz-Michaluk et al 1997). If the effects of LSD are still present, less analgesia will be needed. Opiates should be used cautiously in case of respiratory depression (McCammon 1986).

6. The concomitant use of other sympathomimetics should be avoided.

Bibliography

Antkiewicz-Michaluk L, Romanska I, Vetulani J 1997 Ca^{2+} channel blockade prevents lysergic acid diethylamide-induced changes in dopamine and serotonin metabolism. European Journal of Pharmacology 332: 9–14.

Caldwell T 1990 Anesthesia for patients with behavioral and environmental disorders. In: Katz J, Benumol JL, Kadis LB, eds. Anesthesia and uncommon diseases. WB Saunders, Philadelphia, pp 841–50.

McCammon RL 1986 Anesthesia for the chemically dependent patient. International Anesthesia Research Society Review Course Lectures 47–55.

McGoldrick KE 1980 Anesthetic implications of drug abuse. Anesthesiology Review 7: 12–17.

Malignant hyperthermia

A rare pharmacogenetic condition, or possibly a spectrum of conditions, of complex inheritance. Malignant hyperthermia (MH) usually presents during general anaesthesia with a syndrome indicative of greatly accelerated muscle metabolism. Occasionally, it has been induced by severe exercise (Britt 1988, Hackl et al 1991). The exact defect is unknown. Dysfunction of the sarcoplasmic reticulum and abnormalities of intracellular ionic calcium are thought to play an important role, with the secondary, and possibly synergistic effects of the sympathetic nervous system (Gronert et al 1988). The primary release of calcium is normal, but there is thought to be an enhanced calcium-induced release of calcium from the sarcoplasmic reticulum, by agents known to induce MH. Studies on erythrocytic membranes suggest that there may be a generalised membrane permeability defect. Genetic studies indicate that one of the MH genes is on chromosome 19, in a position close to the ryanodine receptor gene (Levitt et al 1991).

Ryanodine (Ry_1) receptors form a major component of the calcium release pathway, although other associated proteins are also involved in the processes. The receptors are named after a plant alkaloid, ryanodine, which binds to the sarcoplasmic reticulum calcium release channel. Since this alkaloid was important in identification of the protein, which forms a 'foot' structure at the T tubule/SR junction, it was termed the ryanodine receptor. The Ry_1 receptor is encoded by at least three distinct genes and has become important in current research into the genetics of MH. Opening and closing of the receptors can be modified by many physiological ligands and a wide variety of drugs. Volatile agents increase Ry_1 activity and disturb calcium regulation, particularly in MH susceptible individuals. The effect is probably dose dependent and is possibly the basis of initiation of metabolic disturbances when drug and genetic susceptibility meet. In fact, it may be the common cellular basis for stimulation of rhabdomyolysis by a number of different disease/drug processes.

However, other genetic linkages have been found apart from the one on chromosome 19, which makes the picture more complex than was previously thought, and DNA testing not, as yet, achievable (Hopkins et al 1994, Robinson et al 1998). It is probable that the mutation in the ryanodine receptor only accounts for about 20% of susceptible families (Denborough 1998). There also appears to be variations between laboratories in their results from ryanodine contracture tests (Hopkins et al 1998).

Diagnosis, therefore, is still by *in vitro* contracture tests, performed according to either the European Malignant Hyperthermia Group protocol or the North American Malignant Hyperthermia Group protocol.

Dantrolene sodium is a direct acting muscle relaxant which is used in the treatment and prophylaxis of MH. It blocks calcium release from intracellular storage sites and recent studies have suggested action on at least two binding sites on the Ry_1 receptor, which respond to different concentrations (Nelson et al 1996). Whilst one reduces channel gating, an action in accord with its effect as a muscle relaxant, the other appears to activate the channel. The clinical significance of this finding is not known, but the authors raise the possibility that under certain conditions dantrolene could have adverse effects on susceptible muscle.

The cardinal signs of MH include hyperthermia, and respiratory and metabolic acidosis, with or without muscle rigidity. It can be precipitated by a number of drugs, known as 'trigger' agents. In the past, the mortality was high, but it has now been reduced dramatically from about 70% to 5% today (Denborough 1998). The reduction has been achieved by:

1. An increased awareness of the condition.

2. More intensive patient monitoring for sensitive indicators, such as $ETCO_2$, which assist early diagnosis.

3. Availability of an iv form of dantrolene sodium, a drug that has played an important role in the treatment of MH. In the past, the

diagnosis was made too readily on clinical grounds alone. In retrospect, a number of cases previously identified as 'MH' in the literature may well not have been so. In 1984, the European MH Group (Ellis et al 1984) agreed a protocol for the diagnosis of the condition. This was subsequently modified (European MH Group 1985). In 1990, A North American MH Group also reported (Allen et al 1990). It is hoped that the standardisation of *in vitro* tests and diagnostic classification will allow further elucidation of the precise defect. Case reports should now be given credence only when the diagnosis has been confirmed according to these criteria.

Is MH associated with other conditions?

During anaesthesia, patients with a number of other disorders have developed clinical syndromes which have certain features in common with MH, and as a result have been labelled as being 'associated with an increased risk of MH'.

These assertions have in general proved not to be true (Brownell 1988, Ellis et al 1990), except in the case of central core disease (see Central core disease). However, there are certain other neuromuscular conditions which are associated with acute rhabdomyolysis, hyperkalaemia, a high serum CK, mild pyrexia and acidosis, and yet *in vitro* testing usually shows the patient not to be MH susceptible. These include the muscular dystrophies, spinal muscular atrophy, the myotonias and periodic paralyses, and the neuroleptic malignant syndrome.

Muscular dystrophies

The muscular dystrophies are most prone to present with features similar to those of MH under anaesthesia, sometimes with a fatal outcome. Contracture testing for MH was negative in two children, one with Becker's muscular dystrophy and the other with Duchenne's muscular dystrophy (Gronert et al

1992). It was considered that the MH-like features seen during anaesthesia were a result of alterations in the muscle membrane secondary to the dystrophy itself. Exposure to volatile agents and suxamethonium might increase membrane permeability, and it is suggested that compensatory hypermetabolism results from attempts to re-establish membrane stability and prevent calcium flux.

Spinal muscular atrophy

A 13-year-old child developed acute rhabdomyolysis in association with dental anaesthesia and halothane (personal observation). On the day following surgery, the serum CK was in excess of $252\,000$ u l^{-1}. Investigation 4 years later was negative for MH, but electron microscopy suggested a subclinical spinal muscular atrophy. Rhabdomyolysis had presumably been precipitated by suxamethonium.

Myotonia syndromes and the periodic paralyses

Lehmann-Horn and Iaizzo (1990) subjected muscle from patients with myotonia or periodic paralysis to *in vitro* contracture tests for MH. Four out of 44 tests gave positive tests and ten were equivocal. All the positive tests were in patients with myotonic dystrophy, and eight patients with hyperkalaemic periodic paralysis had equivocal results. The significance of this is not known. However, neither the patients nor their families had experienced problems with general anaesthesia.

Neuroleptic malignant syndrome

Investigation of six survivors of the neuroleptic malignant syndrome (NMS) revealed that five were negative for MH, and one result was equivocal (Krivosic-Horber et al 1987). This would suggest that NMS is a distinct entity, but sharing with MH common clinical features, and a response to dantrolene.

Heat stroke

Heat stroke may produce a picture similar to that of MH. Muscle biopsy and *in vitro* contracture tests were performed in two patients who had developed severe exercise-induced rhabdomyolysis. In one, this proved to be positive (Britt 1988, Hackl et al 1991), although the clinical patterns were indistinguishable. The frequency of exercise-induced symptoms (muscle pains, cramps, and stiffness) is reported to be greater in those patients undergoing muscle biopsy who are MHS than those who are MHN (Hackl et al 1991).

Presentation

1. A family history of MH may be elicited. Confirmatory tests may or may not have been performed. According to standard criteria agreed by members of the European MH Group (1985), the current diagnoses are:

    a) MHS: definite susceptibility to MH.

    b) MHN: nonsusceptible subject from a proven MH pedigree.

    c) MHE: equivocal result; consider as MHS.

2. The clinical signs and symptoms of MH can be broadly divided into two:

    a) signs of metabolic stimulation, and

    b) signs of abnormal muscle activity.

    However, it must be remembered that other conditions may cause one, or other, or both. Signs of both may occur with Duchenne and Becker muscular dystrophy, spinal muscle atrophy, myotonia congenita, and McArdle's disease.

3. Signs of metabolic stimulation:

    a) Hypercarbia. Tachypnoea occurs in a spontaneously breathing patient, whilst in the paralysed patient there is an apparently increased requirement for muscle relaxants. Both states are initially due to stimulation of respiration by a rising alveolar CO_2. An increase in $ETCO_2$ may be the earliest sign of MH.

    b) Metabolic acidosis. In early reports of fulminating cases, an arterial pH of less than 7.0 was not uncommon. Severe acidosis may have been responsible for the cases in which sudden death occurred unexpectedly in the operating theatre.

    c) Arrhythmias.

    d) Hyperthermia.

    e) Hypoxaemia. In the later stages, cyanosis may result from the combination of a massive increase in oxygen consumption, and ventilation perfusion defects.

4. Signs of abnormal muscle activity:

    a) Failure of the jaw to relax after suxamethonium. An increase in tone in the masseter muscle is a normal response to suxamethonium, and in some patients the tension developed may be significant (Leary & Ellis 1990, Saddler et al 1990). However, jaw rigidity may also be an early sign of MH. Susceptibility to MH was found in about half of a series of 77 patients who developed masseter muscle rigidity (MMR) (Rosenberg & Fletcher 1986). In view of this it was suggested that any patient who developed MMR after suxamethonium should be assumed to be MH susceptible and anaesthesia terminated. However, a 1% incidence of MMR was found in children receiving halothane and suxamethonium (Carroll 1987) and soon it became apparent that MMR was not exclusive to MH. (See also Section 2, Masseter muscle rigidity.)

A 25 year old involved in major trauma developed masseter muscle spasm after suxamethonium, when tracheal intubation was performed for resuscitation. He was later transferred to the operating theatre, and isoflurane was given 2.5 h after suxamethonium, following which an episode of MH was triggered (Ramirez-R et al 1998).

b) Rigidity of certain, but not necessarily all, groups of muscles. Although a non-rigid group has been described, it is not yet known whether this is a different biochemical process, or an earlier stage of the same process. A contracture of the muscle actually takes place and if the process is not aborted, oedema, and subsequently ischaemia, of the muscle can develop.

c) Hyperkalaemia: potassium may be released in large quantities, particularly after the use of suxamethonium.

d) Myoglobinuria and renal failure may result.

e) A greatly elevated serum CK; this may be in excess of $100\,000\,\text{iu}\,\text{l}^{-1}$.

5. A consumption coagulopathy may occur in advanced cases.

6. Cerebral and pulmonary oedema can occur.

Management

1. Criteria for preoperative diagnosis. Following a strict protocol (Ellis et al 1984, European MH Group 1985, North American Malignant Hyperthermia Group 1989, Allen et al 1990), a quadriceps muscle biospy, which includes the motor point, is subjected to:

a) A static caffeine test.

b) A static halothane test.

c) A dynamic halothane test.

2. The results should allow classification of patients into the three groups: MHS, MHN, and MHE.

3. Comparison between these two major protocols shows reasonable accordance, except near the cutoff limits (Fletcher et al 1999, Islander & Twetman 1999).

4. A patient who is known to be MHS, MHE, or possibly has a family history of MH, should be given a nontriggering anaesthetic.

a) Known triggering agents include:

   i) All the inhalational agents including desflurane (Wedel et al 1991) and sevoflurane (Otsuka et al 1991).

   ii) Suxamethonium.

b) Agents not definitely implicated but avoidance suggested (Gronert 1980):

   i) Ketamine (Derschwitz et al 1989).

   ii) Phenothiazines.

5. Discussion continues over the safety of giving calcium, which may be needed to treat severe hyperkalaemia. Its avoidance has been suggested, but there is clinical and experimental evidence against it acting as a trigger agent (Gronert et al 1986, Murakawa et al 1988).

a) Agents thought to be safe, or for use if necessary, include:

   i) Thiopentone/propofol.

   ii) Nitrous oxide.

   iii) Any analgesics.

   iv) Droperidol/metoclopramide.

   v) Atracurium/vecuronium (any nondepolarising).

   vi) Benzodiazepines.

   vii) Any local anaesthetic (plain).

   viii) Atropine/glycopyrrolate/ neostigmine.

6. The routine use of dantrolene preoperatively in MHS and MHE patients remains controversial. There is now no indication for the use of oral dantrolene, in view of its side effects and the uncertainty of achieving therapeutic levels (Harrison 1988). Most believe that it is sufficient to give a nontriggering anaesthetic, provided that an entirely volatile agent free anaesthetic machine is used, the monitoring of $ETCO_2$ is available, and iv dantrolene is to hand. Decontamination of a machine may be achieved by flushing it with oxygen $12\,\text{l}\,\text{min}^{-1}$ for 6 min (McGraw & Keon

3. Plasma histamine levels did not increase during a portacaval shunt in a patient who was treated with histamine antagonists and cromoglycate (Smith et al 1987). However, plasma histamine has a short half-life and is difficult to measure. Plasma tryptase may be a better indicator of mast cell activation in systemic mastocytosis, since it is released together with histamine from mast cells and is present in blood for several hours (Schwartz et al 1987, 1995).

4. Preoperative intradermal skin testing, with drugs likely to be used during anaesthesia, has been suggested (Parris et al 1986). Positive skin tests occurred in 15 out of a series of 42 patients. Drugs likely to produce reactions should be avoided. It has been suggested that, since most patients are receiving histamine antagonists at the time of surgery, greater concentrations of drugs should be used than those employed for testing after anaphylactoid reactions (Lerno et al 1990). The standard procedure of 0.01–0.02 ml of a dilute solution (10^{-4}–10^{-6}) to raise a 1–2-mm wheal is recommended for drug-related anaphylactoid reactions (Fisher 1984). Lerno et al (1990) recommend that concentrations of 10^{-2} or 10^{-3} should be used in systemic mastocytosis. A positive reaction is a wheal appearing within 10 min, lasting at least 30 min, and of at least 10 mm diameter. Alternatively, skin prick testing may be used using clinical dilutions (Pepys et al 1994).

5. Sedation with a benzodiazepine helps to reduce anxiety.

6. It is recommended that epinephrine (adrenaline), both as a 1 in 10000 dilution and as an infusion of 1 mg in 25 ml saline, should be available for immediate use to treat severe hypotension (Parris et al 1986). An initial dose of 5–8 μg kg^{-1} followed by an infusion of 5–10 μg kg^{-1} min^{-1} is recommended (Lerno et al 1990). Volume replacement with warmed fluids will also be required.

7. There have been no reports of inhalational agents causing degranulation of mast cells. In fact it has been suggested that ether-linked anaesthetics, such as isoflurane, may actually inhibit degranulation. Total intravenous anaesthesia with propofol, fentanyl and vecuronium has been used for a patient undergoing splenectomy, during which plasma tryptase levels remained normal (Borgeat & Ruetsch 1998). However, histamine levels from the spleen were ten times normal and the increased basal turnover of histamine demonstrated the magnitude of the reserve, had mast cell degranulation occurred.

8. Care should be taken to avoid precipitating factors such as trauma, hypothermia, and hyperthermia (Parris et al 1981).

9. Dextrans and blood transfusion are probably best avoided (Scott et al 1983).

10. Uneventful epidural anaesthesia with bupivacaine and fentanyl, for vaginal delivery in a patient with urticaria pigmentosa, has been described (Gupta et al 1998).

Bibliography

Austen KF 1992 Systemic mastocytosis. New England Journal of Medicine 326: 639–40.

Borgeat A, Ruetsch YA 1998 Anesthesia in a patient with malignant systemic mastocytosis using a total intravenous anesthetic technique. Anesthesia & Analgesia 86: 442–4.

Cherner JA, Jensen RT, Dubois A et al 1985 Gastrointestinal dysfunction in systemic mastocytosis: a prospective study. Gastroenterology 95: 657–67.

Coleman MA, Liberthson RR, Crone RK et al 1980 General anesthesia in a child with urticaria pigmentosa. Anesthesia & Analgesia 59: 704–6.

Desborough JP, Taylor I, Hattersley A et al 1990 Massive histamine release in a patient with systemic mastocytosis. British Journal of Anaesthesia 65: 833–6.

Editorial 1992 Systemic mastocytosis. New England Journal of Medicine 326: 639–40.

Fisher MM 1984 Intradermal testing after anaphylactoid reaction to anaesthetic drugs: practical aspects of performance and interpretation. Anaesthesia & Intensive Care 12: 115–20.

Golkar L, Bernhard JD 1997 Mastocytosis. Lancet 349: 1379–85.

f) Give dantrolene sodium iv 1 mg kg^{-1}. Repeat at 10-min intervals, if necessary up to a maximum of 10 mg kg^{-1}.

g) If the syndrome is severe, treat the symptoms. Cool the patient and treat hyperkalaemia if necessary.

h) Keep the first urine sample for myoglobin estimation. Measure urine output. If obvious myoglobinuria occurs, give intravenous fluids, and mannitol or furosemide (frusemide) to promote urine flow. Remember, each 20 g dantrolene contains 3 g mannitol. Haemodialysis may be required.

i) The use of steroids is controversial, but may be indicated for cerebral oedema in the severe case.

(j) Repeat the serum CK estimation at 24 h.

(k) Treat a coagulopathy if it occurs.

(l) Dantrolene may need to be repeated for up to 24 h, since retriggering may occasionally occur. Its half-life is only 5 h.

(m) If problems persist, exclude other causes (eg thyrotoxicosis, phaeochromocytoma, infection). Do not forget the possibility of other myopathies or myotonic syndromes.

12. With general awareness of MH and increased use of monitoring, the occurrence of postoperative pyrexia sometimes results in a patient being informed that 'there might be a small chance that you are susceptible to malignant hyperthermia'. Whilst such caution is commendable, in the absence of other positive features of MH this statement has enormous implications for the patient, the family, and for their subsequent anaesthetists. With such a history, the odds of the patient being MHS are negligible, yet once this spectre has been raised, subsequent anaesthetists may feel obliged to treat the patient as MHS. Since, on the basis of such a vague history, *in vitro* testing would never be undertaken, the ghost cannot be laid to rest.

Under such circumstances, my preference is to administer an anaesthetic in which ventilation is controlled, but an inhalational agent is given. Blood is taken for serum CK levels before and after operation, and ETCO$_2$ and temperature are monitored continuously during surgery. If these prove to be normal, the patient is told that he/she is not susceptible, and is given a letter outlining the strategy that was undertaken.

13. The social implications for a family, particularly in certain cultures, may be devastating (Fletcher 1987, Ellis 1988). In addition, despite warning their surgeons in advance, they frequently face surgical delays or cancellations by anaesthetists who are unfamiliar with administration of nontriggering agents.

14. At present, the *in vitro* contracture tests using halothane and caffeine on muscle samples are the gold standard. The complexity of the genetics of the disease means that, at present, DNA linkage tests are not sufficiently reliable (Hopkins et al 1994, Robinson et al 1998).

Bibliography

Allen GC, Fletcher JE, Huggins FJ et al 1990 Caffeine and halothane contracture testing in swine using the recommendations of the North American Malignant Hyperthermia Group. Anesthesiology 72: 71–6.

Britt BA 1988 Combined anesthetic- and stress-induced malignant hyperthermia in two offspring of malignant hyperthermia-susceptible parents. Anesthesia & Analgesia 67: 393–9.

Brownell AKW 1988 Malignant hyperthermia: relationship to other diseases. British Journal of Anaesthesia 60: 303–8.

Carroll JB 1987 Increased incidence of masseter spasm in children with strabismus anaesthetised with halothane and succinyl choline. Anesthesiology 67: 559–61.

Cunliffe M, Lerman J, Britt BA 1987 Is prophylactic dantrolene indicated for MHS patients undergoing elective surgery? Anesthesia & Analgesia 66: S35.

Denborough M 1998 Malignant hyperthermia. Lancet 352: 1131–6.

Dershwitz M, Sreter FA, Ryan JF 1989 Ketamine does not trigger malignant hyperthermia in susceptible swine. Anesthesia & Analgesia 69: 501–3.

Ellis FR 1988 The diagnosis of MH: its social implications. British Journal of Anaesthesia 60: 251–2.

Ellis FR, Halsall PJ 1984 Suxamethonium spasm. British Journal of Anaesthesia 56: 381–4.

Ellis FR, Fletcher R, Halsall P 1984 A protocol for the investigation of malignant hyperpyrexia by the European Malignant Hyperpyrexia Group. British Journal of Anaesthesia 56: 1267–9.

Ellis FR, Halsall PJ, Harriman DGF 1986 The work of the Leeds Malignant Hyperpyrexia Unit, 1971–1984. Anaesthesia 41: 809–15.

Ellis FR, Halsall PJ, Christian AS 1990 Clinical presentation of suspected malignant hyperthermia during anaesthesia in 402 probands. Anaesthesia 45: 838–41.

European MH Group 1985 Laboratory diagnosis of malignant hyperpyrexia susceptibility (MHS). British Journal of Anaesthesia 57: 1038.

Fletcher JE, Rosenberg H, Aggarwal M 1999 Comparison of European and North American malignant hyperthermia protocol outcomes for use in genetic studies. Anesthesiology 90: 654–61.

Fletcher R 1987 4th International Hyperpyrexia Workshop. Report of a meeting. Anaesthesia 42: 206.

Gronert GA 1980 Malignant hyperthermia. Anesthesiology 53: 395–423.

Gronert GA, Ahern CP, Milde J et al 1986 Effect of CO_2, calcium, digoxin and potassium on cardiac and skeletal muscle in malignant hyperthermia susceptible swine. Anesthesiology 64: 24–8.

Gronert GA, Mott J, Lee J 1988 Aetiology of malignant hyperthermia. British Journal of Anaesthesia 60: 253–67.

Gronert GA, Fowler W, Cardinet GH et al 1992 Absence of malignant hyperthermia contractures in Becker–Duchenne dystrophy at age 2. Muscle & Nerve 15: 52–6.

Hackl W, Winkler M, Mauritz W et al 1991 Muscle biopsy for diagnosis of malignant hyperthermia susceptibility in two patients with severe exercise-induced myolysis. British Journal of Anaesthesia 66: 138–40.

Harrison GG 1988 Dantrolene—dynamics and kinetics. British Journal of Anaesthesia 60: 279–86.

Hopkins PM, Halsall PJ, Ellis FR 1994 Diagnosing malignant hyperthermia susceptibility. Anaesthesia 49: 373–5.

Hopkins PM, Hartung E, Wappler F 1998 Multicentre evaluation of ryanodine contracture testing in malignant hyperthermia. The European Malignant Hyperthermia Group. British Journal of Anaesthesia 80: 389–94.

Islander G, Twetman ER 1999 Comparison between the European and North American protocols for diagnosis of malignant hyperthermia. Anesthesia & Analgesia 88: 1155–60.

Krivosic-Horber R, Adnet P, Guevart E et al 1987 Neuroleptic malignant syndrome and malignant hyperthermia. British Journal of Anaesthesia 59: 1554–6.

Leary NP, Ellis FR 1990 Masseteric muscle spasm as a normal response to suxamethonium. British Journal of Anaesthesia 64: 488–92.

Lehmann-Horn F, Iaizzo PA 1990 Are myotonias and periodic paralyses associated with susceptibility to malignant hyperthermia. British Journal of Anaesthesia 65: 692–7.

Levitt RC, Meyers D, Fletcher JE et al 1991 Molecular genetics and malignant hyperthermia. Anesthesiology 75: 1–3.

McGraw TT, Keon TP 1989 Malignant hyperthermia and the clean machine. Canadian Journal of Anaesthesia 36: 530–2.

Murakawa M, Hatano Y, Magaribuchi T et al 1988 Should calcium administration be avoided in treatment of hyperkalaemia in malignant hyperthermia? Anesthesiology 67: 604–5.

Nelson TE, Lin M, Zapata-Sudo G et al 1996 Dantrolene sodium can increase or attenuate activity of skeletal muscle ryanodine receptor calcium release channel. Clinical implications. Anesthesiology 84: 1368–79.

North American Malignant Hyperthermia Group 1989 Standardization of the caffeine halothane muscle contracture test. Anesthesia & Analgesia 69: 511–19.

Otsuka H, Komura Y, Mayumi T et al 1991 Malignant hyperthermia during sevoflurane anesthesia in a child with central core disease. Anesthesiology 75: 699–700.

Ramirez-R JA, Cheetham ED, Laurence AS et al 1998 Suxamethonium, masseter spasm and later malignant hyperthermia. Anaesthesia 53: 1111–16.

Robinson R, Curran JL, Hall WJ et al 1998 Genetic heterogeneity and HOMOG analysis in British malignant hyperthermia families. Journal of Medical Genetics 35: 196–201.

Rosenberg H, Fletcher JE 1986 Masseter muscle rigidity and malignant hyperthermia susceptibility. Anesthesia & Analgesia 65: 161–4.

Saddler JM, Bevan JC, Plumley MH et al 1990 Jaw muscle tension after succinylcholine in children undergoing strabismus surgery. Canadian Journal of Anaesthesia 37: 21–5.

Wedel DJ, Iaizzo PA, Milde JH 1991 Desflurane is a trigger of malignant hyperthermia in susceptible swine. Anesthesiology 74: 508–12.

Marcus Gunn jaw winking phenomenon

A rare congenital abnormality in which there appears to be abnormal connections between the external pterygoid and ocular muscles. This results in ptosis, which can be partly corrected by the patient either opening the jaw, or moving it to the contralateral side. A number of other abnormal reflexes may be present. The Marcus Gunn phenomenon can be associated with other defects, in particular in the congenital fibrosis syndrome, a form of myopathy associated with external ophthalmoplegia (Brodsky 1998). In this condition, there may be abnormalities in the extraocular muscle lower motor neurone system (Engle et al 1997).

Preoperative abnormalities

1. Ptosis is present, but lid retraction is associated with jaw opening.

2. Abnormal pupillary reflexes may occur.

Anaesthetic problems

1. Unusual oculocardiac reflexes were reported during three separate operations on the eyelid in a young man with Marcus Gunn syndrome (Kwik 1980). Arrhythmias, which appeared on manipulation of the eyelid and also occurred in the recovery room, included premature atrial contractions, wandering pacemaker, and bradycardia.

2. A myopathy may be present (Brodsky 1998).

Management

1. It has been suggested that the use of IPPV and a retrobulbar block may decrease the incidence of arrhythmias (Kwik 1980).

2. ECG monitoring should begin in the anaesthetic room and be continued in the recovery room.

Bibliography

Brodsky MC 1998 Hereditary external ophthalmoplegia, synergistic divergence, jaw winking, and oculocutaneous hypopigmentation: a congenital fibrosis syndrome caused by deficient innervation to extraocular muscles. Ophthalmology 105: 717–25.

Engle EC, Goumnerov BC, McKeown CA et al 1997 Oculomotor nerve and muscle abnormalities in congenital fibrosis of the extraocular muscles. Annals of Neurology 41: 314–25.

Kwik RSH 1980 Marcus Gunn syndrome associated with an unusual oculo-cardiac reflex. Anaesthesia; 35: 46–9.

Marfan syndrome

An autosomal dominant, inherited condition involving a connective tissue deficit, secondary to mutations within the fibrillin gene on chromosome 15. It affects the microfibrillar component of elastic fibres. The abnormal fibrillin alters the functional relationship between blood flow and vascular endothelial cell response (Westaby 1999). The tensile strength of collagen is reduced, while its elasticity is increased and the wall becomes weakened. Skeletal, cardiovascular and ocular features occur. The diagnosis is made on clinical grounds and phenotypic heterogeneity means that there are widely variable manifestations of the condition. At least two of the following four criteria should be present: a family history of the condition, the ocular, cardiovascular or skeletal features (Pyeritz & McKusick 1979).

In the past, premature death in the third to fifth decade was common; the biochemical defect makes the aorta susceptible to dilatation and dissection, such that aortic dissection and valvular regurgitation were responsible for about 90% of these deaths. However, with the use of regular noninvasive cardiovascular assessment, more aggressive surgical treatment, and prophylactic beta blockade (Adams & Trent 1998), the prognosis has improved. It has been suggested that elective resection of an aneurysm should occur when the diameter approaches 5.5 cm (Baumgartner et al 1999). In a study of

675 patients who underwent replacement of the aortic root, the 30-day mortality was 1.5% for elective surgery, 2.6% for urgent repair, and 11.7% for emergency repair (Gott et al 1999). Late deaths occurring after 30 days were mostly from rupture of other parts of the aorta, or cardiac arrhythmias. Data have shown that mean [SD] age at death has increased from 32 [16] years in 1972 to 41 [18] years in 1993 (Silverman et al 1995).

Surgery may be required for the correction of the ophthalmic, cardiovascular and orthopaedic features of the disease. This may include elective or emergency aortic surgery, or cardiac valve replacement. Aortic valve-sparing procedures, which avoid the need for long-term anticoagulation, are at present being assessed (Devereux & Roman 1999).

Pregnant patients with Marfan's syndrome should be monitored closely for aortic dilatation. A longitudinal study of 45 pregnancies in 21 patients showed that, provided the aortic root diameter remains <40 mm, pregnancy was tolerated well (Rossiter et al 1995).

Preoperative abnormalities

1. Skeletal abnormalities include arachnodactyly, a high arched palate, increased length of tubular bones, scoliosis (40–70%), pectus excavatus, and ligamentous laxity.

2. Ectopia lentis occurs in up to 80% of cases and lensectomy may be required. Patients are prone to myopia and retinal detachment.

3. Cardiovascular complications are the most common cause of death. Structural changes in the heart and great vessels may be present and can result in mitral or aortic incompetence, dissecting aortic aneurysm, aortic root or pulmonary artery dilatation, and coronary artery disease. Mitral valve prolapse and acute aortic valve prolapse can also occur. Pathological changes in arteries include cystic degeneration of the media and replacement of elastic fibres by mucoid material. Assessment of aortic size and valvular dysfunction may require

echocardiography, cardiac catheterisation, or MRI. In young people <20 years old, the prevalence of serious cardiovascular complications is low, but aortic root diameter does increase with age and serious complications are similar to those in adults (El Habbal 1992). Mitral valve prolapse and aortic root dilatation are the commonest (Hirata et al 1992). Mitral valve prolapse tends to be symptomatic, but aortic root dilatation is silent, unless there is dissection or aortic regurgitation.

4. In the pregnant patient there is a risk of aortic arch dissection during labour or in the postpartum period. This risk is greatest in those who have significant cardiovascular disease at the start of pregnancy. However, in a recent random sample of 36 patients from one clinic, none of whom had symptoms related to a cardiovascular abnormality before conception, significant aortic events occurred in only six (four dissections and two progressive aortic root dilatations) (Lipscomb et al 1997). Two of the dissections occurred at 14 and 16 days after delivery. Obstetric problems include cervical incompetence, an abnormal placental site, and postpartum haemorrhage.

5. There is a high incidence of sleep apnoea, in part as a result of maxillary abnormalities causing high nasal airway resistance (Cistulli et al 1996), and in part secondary to increased upper airway collapsibility (Cistulli & Sullivan 1995).

6. The use of long-term beta adrenoceptor blockers slows the rate of aortic dilatation and reduces the development of complications in some patients (Shores et al 1994).

Anaesthetic problems

1. Young patients may present to the emergency department in a collapsed state secondary to aortic dissection. If this affects the coronary ostia, signs of myocardial infarction may be evident on ECG (Ward 1996).

2. A number of deaths have been reported in association with nonvascular surgery, but there was no consistent cause of death. In a study of 13

patients, two of four who died had been assessed as having no cardiovascular involvement (Verghese 1984). Neither had, however, undergone echocardiography.

3. Hypotonia and ligamentous laxity may predispose the patient to accidental injury during anaesthesia. Joints, including the temporomandibular, are prone to dislocation.

4. Scoliosis, sleep apnoea, hypotonia, a high incidence of emphysema, lung cysts, spontaneous pneumothoraces, and honeycomb lungs, all increase the risk of intra- and postoperative pulmonary complications. Midtracheal obstruction and respiratory distress occurred after Harrington rod placement in a patient with scoliosis (Mesrobian & Epps 1986). This was attributed to a combination of structural weakness of cartilage, and skeletal abnormalities. Obstructive sleep apnoea is thought to be caused by increased upper airway collapsibility secondary to the connective tissue defect (Cistulli & Sullivan 1995).

5. If ascending aortic dilatation already exists, especially if it is greater than 6 cm in an adult, the risk of rupture is high and hypertensive peaks may predispose to aortic dissection (Pyeritz & McKusick 1979).

6. Management of pregnancy and delivery presents a challenge. A patient with an aortic root measurement of 4.8 cm and mitral valve regurgitation undergoing epidural anaesthesia, became unstable during delivery, despite receiving beta blockers (Gordon & Johnson 1993). However, in another patient, the aortic root diameter increased from 8.1 cm to 8.9 cm at 38 weeks, by which stage she had developed severe aortic regurgitation. She had refused surgery, but accepted beta blockers and epidural analgesia, and survived (Mayet et al 1998).

7. There is an increased risk of postpartum haemorrhage. In one patient, recurrent bleeding followed elective Caesarean section. Three weeks later, at total abdominal hysterectomy, hugely dilated vessels were found, with some thrombosis and fragmentation of the elastic lamina (Irons & Pollard 1993).

Management

1. Detailed examination of the cardiovascular system is essential and should include assessment of aortic size, and a search for evidence of aortic or mitral regurgitation, coronary artery disease, and heart failure. A recent echocardiograph is mandatory in all patients requiring surgery.

2. High pulsatile pressures must be avoided to reduce the risks of aortic dissection. Beta adrenoceptor blockers have been shown to decrease aortic stiffness and mean blood pressure. However, haemodynamic studies suggest that acute beta blockade is not necessarily beneficial (Yin et al 1989). Dynamic aortic studies in patients given iv beta blockers (propranolol 0.15 mg kg^{-1}) showed that short-term beta blockers exacerbated the primary abnormality of Marfan's, which is an increase in the magnitude of the wave reflections, causing additional stress to the aortic wall. The abnormality was ameliorated by sodium nitroprusside, a vasodilator.

3. Direct arterial monitoring may assist in the process of controlling sudden increases in blood pressure, but may carry a higher than normal risk of damage to the artery.

4. Those with known cardiovascular involvement should be advised to delay pregnancy until after aortic root replacement (Oakley 1997); if already pregnant, therapeutic abortion may be prudent. In the absence of cardiovascular disease, the risks of aortic dissection are less, but monthly transthoracic echocardiography is recommended from the 6th week of gestation onwards (Lipscomb et al 1997). Vaginal delivery with epidural anaesthesia is advised for those with stable aortic measurements of <40 mm during pregnancy. However, those patients with changes in aortic root diameter during pregnancy, and for those with an aortic root >40 mm, an elective LSCS with epidural anaesthesia will minimise the aortic wall stress (Elkayam et al 1995, Oakley 1997). Hypertension must be treated aggressively and

beta blockade should be considered from midtrimester onwards. Each pregnancy is potentially high risk, and therefore needs combined obstetric, cardiology and anaesthetic care. There is a 50% risk of transmission to offspring (Lipscomb et al 1997). One patient with aortic dissection was treated medically using glyceryl trinitrate, hydralazine, nifedipine, and labetalol (Jayaram et al 1995). It was repaired 6 months after delivery under partial bypass. The use of total intravenous anaesthesia with propofol has been described for elective Caesarean section, to stabilise maternal haemodynamics (Llopis et al 1997).

5.   Prophylactic antibiotics are probably warranted.

Bibliography

Adams JN, Trent RJ 1998 Aortic complications of Marfan's syndrome. Lancet 352: 1722–3.

Baumgartner WA, Cameron DE, Redmond JM et al 1999 Operative management of Marfan syndrome: the Johns Hopkins experience. Annals of Thoracic Surgery 67: 1859–60.

Cistulli PA, Sullivan CE 1995 Sleep apnea in Marfan's syndrome. Increased upper airway collapsibility during sleep. Chest 108: 631–5.

Cistulli PA, Richards GN, Palmisano RG et al 1996 Influence of maxillary construction on nasal resistance and sleep apnea severity in patients with Marfan's syndrome. Chest 110: 1184–8.

Deveraux RB, Roman MJ 1999 Aortic disease in Marfan's syndrome. New England Journal of Medicine 340: 1358–9.

El Habbal MH 1992 Cardiovascular manifestations of Marfan's syndrome in the young. American Heart Journal 123: 752–7.

Elkayam U, Ostrzega E, Shotan A et al 1995 Cardiovascular problems in pregnant women with the Marfan syndrome. Annals of Internal Medicine 123: 117–22.

Gordon CF, Johnson MD 1993 Anesthetic management of the patient with Marfan syndrome. Journal of Clinical Anesthesia 5: 248–51.

Gott VL, Greene PS, Alejo DE et al 1999 Replacement of the aortic root in patients with Marfan's syndrome. New England Journal of Medicine 340: 1307–13.

Hirata K, Triposkiadis F, Sparks E et al 1992 The Marfan syndrome: cardiovascular physical findings and diagnostic correlates. American Heart Journal 123: 743–52.

Irons DW, Pollard KP 1993 Postpartum haemorrhage secondary to Marfan's disease and uterine vasculitis. British Journal of Obstetrics & Gynaecology 100: 279–301.

Jayaram A, Carp HM, Davis L et al 1995 Pregnancy complicated by aortic dissection: caesarean delivery during extradural anaesthesia. British Journal of Anaesthesia 75: 358–60.

Lipscomb KJ, Clayton Smith J, Clarke B et al 1997 Outcome of pregnancy in women with Marfan's syndrome. British Journal of Obstetrics & Gynaecology 104: 201–6.

Llopis JE, Garcia-Aguado R, Sifre C et al 1997 Total intravenous anaesthesia for Caesarean section in a patient with Marfan's syndrome. International Journal of Obstetric Anesthesia 6: 59–62.

Mayet J, Steer P, Somerville J 1998 Marfan syndrome, aortic dilatation and pregnancy. Obstetrics & Gynecology 92: 713.

Mesrobian RB, Epps JL 1986 Midtracheal obstruction after Harrington rod placement in a patient with Marfan's syndrome. Anesthesia & Analgesia 65: 411–13.

Oakley CM 1997 Pregnancy and congenital heart disease. Heart 78: 12–14.

Pyeritz RE, McKusick VA 1979 The Marfan syndrome: diagnosis and management. New England Journal of Medicine 300: 772–7.

Rossiter JP, Repke JT, Morales AJ et al 1995 A prospective longitudinal evaluation of pregnancy in the Marfan syndrome. American Journal of Obstetrics & Gynecology 173: 1599–606.

Shores J, Berger KR, Murphy EA et al 1994 Progression of aortic dilatation and the benefit of long-term beta-adrenergic blockade in Marfan's syndrome. New England Journal of Medicine 330: 1335–41.

Silverman DI, Burton KJ, Gray J et al 1995 Life expectancy in the Marfan syndrome. American Journal of Cardiology 75: 157–60.

Verghese C 1984 Anaesthesia in Marfan's syndrome. Anaesthesia 39: 917–22.

Ward SJ 1996 Marfan's syndrome: a case report. Hospital Update April: 134–6.

Westaby S 1999 Aortic dissection in Marfan's syndrome. Annals of Thoracic Surgery 67: 1861–3.

Yin FCP, Brin KP, Ting C-T et al 1989 Arterial hemodynamic indexes in Marfan's syndrome. Circulation 79: 854–62.

Maroteaux–Lamy syndrome (see also Hurler's syndrome, Hunter's syndrome)

One of the mucopolysaccharidoses (Type VI), this connective tissue disorder results from the abnormal metabolism of certain polysaccharides. It is associated with a deficiency of arylsulphatase B. Although patients are of normal IQ, the facial features resemble those of Hurler/Hunter syndromes, with which it also shares tracheal intubation and mask ventilation difficulties. Anaesthesia may be required for ENT, ophthalmological, and cardiac valvular surgery. Some improvement has occurred after bone marrow transplantation.

Preoperative abnormalities

1. Coarse features and macroglossia, but with normal intelligence.

2. Kyphoscoliosis, flat vertebrae, genu valgum.

3. Cardiac involvement, including valvular heart disease and cardiomyopathy, may be severe (Dangel 1998). Surgery for aortic and mitral valve stenoses has been reported (Marwick et al 1992, Tan et al 1992).

4. Corneal opacities.

Anaesthetic problems

1. In three series, five out of eight patients had either a difficult airway or difficult intubation (Baines & Keneally 1983, Kempthorne & Brown 1983, Walker et al 1994). The degree of difficulty depends upon severity. Four patients with valvular heart disease had problems. In the first, multiple attempts at intubation resulted in hypoxaemia and pulmonary oedema. In the second, fibreoptic intubation was performed before hip replacement, but on the fourth postoperative day, when respiratory distress occurred, emergency tracheostomy was needed after failed intubation. In the third, failed intubation necessitated tracheostomy, and in the fourth,

difficulties were experienced during fibreoptic intubation under sedation (Tan et al 1992).

2. Cervical problems. In an asymptomatic patient, MRI showed a hypoplastic odontoid and critical narrowing of the spinal canal. Three hours into surgery, sensory-evoked potentials (SEP) disappeared. Repositioning of the head caused immediate SEP reappearance, suggesting that spinal cord compression had occurred (Linstedt et al 1994).

Management

1. Airway and difficult intubation assessment.

2. Cervical spine assessment.

3. Appropriate management of difficult airway/intubation (see Hurler's/Hunter's syndrome).

4. Antibiotics as prophylaxis for valvular heart disease.

Bibliography

Baines D, Keneally J 1983 Anaesthetic implications of the mucopolysaccharidoses. Anaesthesia & Intensive Care 11: 198–202.

Dangel JH 1998 Cardiovascular changes in children with mucopolysaccharide storage diseases and related disorders—clinical and echocardiographic findings in 64 patients. European Journal of Pediatrics 157: 534–8.

Kempthorne PM, Brown TCK 1983 Anaesthesia and the mucopolysaccharidoses. Anaesthesia & Intensive Care 11: 203–7.

Linstedt U, Maier C, Joehnk H et al 1994 Threatening spinal cord compression during anesthesia in a child with mucopolysaccharidosis VI. Anesthesiology 80: 227–9.

Marwick TH, Bastian B, Hughes CF et al 1992 Mitral stenosis in the Maroteaux–Lamy syndrome: a treatable cause of dyspnoea. Postgraduate Medical Journal 68: 287–8.

Tan CTT, Schaff HV, Miller Jr FA et al 1992 Valvular heart disease in four patients with Maroteaux–Lamy syndrome. Circulation 85: 188–95.

Walker RWM, Darowski M, Morris P et al 1994 Anaesthesia and mucopolysaccharidoses. A review of airway problems in children. Anaesthesia 49: 1078–84.

Mastocytoses

A rare group of diseases in which there is overproliferation and abnormal aggregations of mast cells within the skin, and in other organs (Austen 1992). The disorders range from cutaneous mastocytosis, through systemic mastocytosis to mast-cell leukaemia (Golkar & Bernhard 1997). When the skin alone is involved, the condition is known as urticaria pigmentosa. This mostly occurs in infants and children, may be associated with mastocytomas, and is relatively benign (Coleman et al 1980). In the systemic diseases, bone, liver, spleen and lymph nodes are most commonly affected.

Systemic mastocytosis occurs in about 10% of cases. The various forms that occur in adult life may be associated with intermittent symptoms, varying from a mild disturbance to the occasional fatal attack. These episodes are associated with mast cell disruption and the resultant release of one or more of a number of biochemical substances from granules within the cells. Histamine and heparin were thought to be the most important of these, although other enzymes, such as chymases, tryptases, and hydrolases, may be released. Prostaglandin D2 has also been implicated as a cause of symptoms in certain patients who failed to respond to histamine antagonists (Roberts et al 1980). Mast cells also produce cytokines (such as the interleukins) involved in adaptive immunity and tissue inflammatory response (Austen 1992). Other substances that may be released in small amounts include the leukotrienes, serotonin, antiplatelet factor, and hyaluronic acid. Amongst the precipitating factors are trauma, surgery, extremes of temperature, toxins, alcohol, and a variety of drugs.

Preoperative abnormalities

1. Symptoms are variable, and can include episodic attacks of itching, urticaria, dermographia, headache, flushing, syncope, palpitations, abdominal pain, diarrhoea, nausea, and vomiting. The flush is bright red and lasts for about 20 min, in contrast with that associated with carcinoid, which is more cyanotic and lasts for less than 10 min. Delay in diagnosis is frequent. In a series of 26 patients, the mean duration of symptoms before diagnosis was found to be 2 years (Webb et al 1982).

2. Attacks can be precipitated by alcohol, aspirin, NSAIDS, exposure to friction, pressure, temperature extremes, and insect stings.

3. Skin lesions vary in type and colour, but small, reddish brown maculopapular lesions are common. A positive Darier's sign may be demonstrated. Light stroking of the affected skin with a blunt, but pointed, object produces dermographia (secondary to localised urticaria), and a flare.

4. When bones are affected, the patient may present with unexpected bone loss, or compression fractures secondary to osteoporosis.

5. In a study of 41 patients, two-thirds had evidence of liver disease (Mican et al 1995). Hepatomegaly was detected in 24% and splenomegaly in 41%.

6. Increased gastric acid secretion is associated with duodenal ulceration. In one study, all patients with gastrointestinal symptoms were found to have increased plasma histamine levels, and these correlated with basal gastric acid output (Cherner et al 1985).

7. Skin biopsy shows an increased number of mast cells (>5 per high power field). Diagnosis may also be made on bone or liver biopsy.

8. Tryptase, a protease produced by all mast cells, is a clinical marker of systemic mastocytosis. Two types have been identified, a B12-measured and a G5-measured. Most patients with the systemic disease have B12 tryptase levels that are $>20\,ng\,ml^{-1}$, and are at least 10-fold greater than the corresponding G5-measured tryptase level, whereas most of those subjects with B12 tryptase $<20\,ng\,ml^{-1}$ had only cutaneous manifestations (Schwartz et al 1995). By contrast, in patients with systemic anaphylaxis without mastocytosis, the ratio of B12- to G5-

measured tryptase was always <5 and approached unity (Schwartz et al 1994). Increased blood and urinary levels of histamine, and urinary prostaglandin D2 metabolite levels, may be demonstrated in systemic mastocytosis.

9. Certain groups of patients may develop haematological abnormalities, including malignancies. Anaemia, leucocytosis and thrombocytopenia were the commonest problems (Horny et al 1990), although thrombocythaemia has been reported (Le Tourneau et al 1991). Coagulation studies are occasionally abnormal.

10. Treatment is symptomatic only, and is aimed at blocking mast cell degranulation, or the effects of mast cell mediators on organs (Golkar & Bernhard 1997).

Anaesthetic problems

1. Mast cell degranulation during anaesthesia may release huge reserves of histamine to produce severe cardiovascular effects. Drugs reported to have precipitated symptoms in individual patients include salicylates, NSAIDs, opiates, polymyxin, thiopental, lidocaine (lignocaine), dextrans, gallamine, d-tubocurarine, and X-ray contrast media. Large fluid shifts can occur from the intravascular compartment.

2. Surgery, endoscopy (Schwab et al 1999), regional and general anaesthesia can also produce life-threatening complications. In one series, complications occurred in six out of 42 patients (Parris et al 1986). Hypotension and bronchospasm were the most frequently encountered. Intraoperative cardiovascular collapse occurred during pancreatic biopsy. A massive increase in plasma histamine levels was associated with hypotension, flushing, and a profound decrease in systemic vascular resistance. This patient had experienced a similar, but less severe episode during upper gastrointestinal endoscopy (Desborough et al 1990).

Gradually decreasing oxygen saturation followed by cardiac arrest occurred in a 43 year old during emergency orthopaedic surgery (Vaughan & Jones 1998). Cutaneous mastocytosis had been diagnosed 2 years before and an intraoperative plasma tryptase level of $18\,ng\,l^{-1}$ with normal plasma IgE levels was said to imply an anaphylactoid reaction and mast cell degranulation. This is a relatively low plasma tryptase level for the diagnosis of systemic disease (Schwartz et al 1995), but signs of systemic mastocytosis were found at postmortem.

3. Although heparin may also be released, it has rarely produced clinically significant problems. However, in the patient described by Desborough et al (1990), the APTT became prolonged (to 150 s) during pancreatectomy, subsequent to his episode of cardiovascular collapse.

4. If systemic mastocytosis is present and an anaphylactoid reaction occurs, it is likely to be more severe than in a normal patient. It has been suggested that this applies particularly to blood transfusion reactions (Scott et al 1983).

5. The presence of cutaneous lesions alone does not guarantee freedom from anaesthetic problems. Profound hypotension and flushing were reported during surgery in a patient with asymptomatic urticaria pigmentosa (Hosking & Warner 1987).

Management

1. A full history and examination. Evidence of organ involvement should be sought and liver function tests, platelet count and coagulation checked.

2. Symptoms should be controlled preoperatively by the use of H_1 receptor antagonists (chlorphenamine (chlorpheniramine), terfenadine), and H_2 receptor antagonists (cimetidine, ranitidine, or famotidine), and prostaglandin inhibitors (indometacin or salicylates). If salicylates are used, they should be introduced gradually, in case they precipitate an attack. Sodium cromoglycate, a mast cell stabiliser, improves preoperative symptoms.

3. Plasma histamine levels did not increase during a portacaval shunt in a patient who was treated with histamine antagonists and cromoglycate (Smith et al 1987). However, plasma histamine has a short half-life and is difficult to measure. Plasma tryptase may be a better indicator of mast cell activation in systemic mastocytosis, since it is released together with histamine from mast cells and is present in blood for several hours (Schwartz et al 1987, 1995).

4. Preoperative intradermal skin testing, with drugs likely to be used during anaesthesia, has been suggested (Parris et al 1986). Positive skin tests occurred in 15 out of a series of 42 patients. Drugs likely to produce reactions should be avoided. It has been suggested that, since most patients are receiving histamine antagonists at the time of surgery, greater concentrations of drugs should be used than those employed for testing after anaphylactoid reactions (Lerno et al 1990). The standard procedure of 0.01–0.02 ml of a dilute solution (10^{-4}–10^{-6}) to raise a 1–2-mm wheal is recommended for drug-related anaphylactoid reactions (Fisher 1984). Lerno et al (1990) recommend that concentrations of 10^{-2} or 10^{-3} should be used in systemic mastocytosis. A positive reaction is a wheal appearing within 10 min, lasting at least 30 min, and of at least 10 mm diameter. Alternatively, skin prick testing may be used using clinical dilutions (Pepys et al 1994).

5. Sedation with a benzodiazepine helps to reduce anxiety.

6. It is recommended that epinephrine (adrenaline), both as a 1 in 10 000 dilution and as an infusion of 1 mg in 25 ml saline, should be available for immediate use to treat severe hypotension (Parris et al 1986). An initial dose of 5–8 μg kg^{-1} followed by an infusion of 5–10 μg kg^{-1} min^{-1} is recommended (Lerno et al 1990). Volume replacement with warmed fluids will also be required.

7. There have been no reports of inhalational agents causing degranulation of mast cells. In fact it has been suggested that ether-linked anaesthetics, such as isoflurane, may actually inhibit degranulation. Total intravenous anaesthesia with propofol, fentanyl and vecuronium has been used for a patient undergoing splenectomy, during which plasma tryptase levels remained normal (Borgeat & Ruetsch 1998). However, histamine levels from the spleen were ten times normal and the increased basal turnover of histamine demonstrated the magnitude of the reserve, had mast cell degranulation occurred.

8. Care should be taken to avoid precipitating factors such as trauma, hypothermia, and hyperthermia (Parris et al 1981).

9. Dextrans and blood transfusion are probably best avoided (Scott et al 1983).

10. Uneventful epidural anaesthesia with bupivacaine and fentanyl, for vaginal delivery in a patient with urticaria pigmentosa, has been described (Gupta et al 1998).

Bibliography

Austen KF 1992 Systemic mastocytosis. New England Journal of Medicine 326: 639–40.

Borgeat A, Ruetsch YA 1998 Anesthesia in a patient with malignant systemic mastocytosis using a total intravenous anesthetic technique. Anesthesia & Analgesia 86: 442–4.

Cherner JA, Jensen RT, Dubois A et al 1985 Gastrointestinal dysfunction in systemic mastocytosis: a prospective study. Gastroenterology 95: 657–67.

Coleman MA, Liberthson RR, Crone RK et al 1980 General anesthesia in a child with urticaria pigmentosa. Anesthesia & Analgesia 59: 704–6.

Desborough JP, Taylor I, Hattersley A et al 1990 Massive histamine release in a patient with systemic mastocytosis. British Journal of Anaesthesia 65: 833–6.

Editorial 1992 Systemic mastocytosis. New England Journal of Medicine 326: 639–40.

Fisher MM 1984 Intradermal testing after anaphylactoid reaction to anaesthetic drugs: practical aspects of performance and interpretation. Anaesthesia & Intensive Care 12: 115–20.

Golkar L, Bernhard JD 1997 Mastocytosis. Lancet 349: 1379–85.

Gupta S, Gilder F, Glazebrook C 1998 Intrapartum management of a patient with urticaria pigmentosa. International Journal of Obstetric Anesthesia 7: 261–2.

Horny HP, Ruck M, Wehrmann M et al 1990 Blood findings in generalized mastocytosis: evidence of frequent occurrence of myeloproliferative disorders. British Journal of Haematology 76: 186–93.

Hosking MP, Warner MA 1987 Sudden intraoperative hypotension in a patient with asymptomatic urticaria pigmentosa. Anesthesia & Analgesia 66: 344–6.

James PD, Krafchik BR, Johnston AE 1987 Cutaneous mastocytosis in children: anaesthetic considerations. Canadian Journal of Anaesthesia 34: 522–4.

Lerno G, Slaats G, Coenen E et al 1990 Anaesthetic management of systemic mastocytosis. British Journal of Anaesthesia 65: 254–7.

Le Tourneau A, Gaulard P, D'Agay MF et al 1991 Primary thrombocythaemia associated with systemic mastocytosis: a report of five cases. British Journal of Haematology 79: 84–9.

Mican JM, Di Bisceglie AM, Fong T-L et al 1995 Hepatic involvement in mastocytosis: clinicopathologic correlations in 41 cases. Hepatology 22: 1163–70.

Parris WCV, Sandidge PC Petrinely G 1981 Anesthetic management of mastocytosis. Anesthesiology Review 8: 32–5.

Parris WCV, Scott HW, Smith BE 1986 Anesthetic management of systemic mastocytosis: experience with 42 cases. Anesthesia & Analgesia 65: S117.

Pepys J, Pepys EO, Baldo BA et al 1994 Anaphylactic/anaphylactoid reactions to anaesthetic and associated agents. Skin prick tests. Anaesthesia 49: 470–5.

Roberts LJ, Sweetman BJ, Lewis RA et al 1980 Increased production of prostaglandin D2 in patients with systemic mastocytosis. New England Journal of Medicine 303: 1400–4.

Rosenbaum KJ, Strobel GE 1973 Anesthetic considerations in mastocytosis. Anesthesiology 38: 398–401.

Schwab D, Raithel M, Ell C et al 1999 Severe shock during upper GI endoscopy in a patient with systemic mastocytosis. Gastrointestinal Endoscopy 50: 264–7.

Schwartz LB, Metcalfe DD, Miller JS et al 1987 Tryptase levels as an indicator of mast cell activation in systemic anaphylaxis and mastocytosis. New England Journal of Medicine 316: 1622–6.

Schwartz LB, Bradford TR, Rouse C et al 1994 Development of a new, more sensitive immunoassay for human tryptase: use in systemic anaphylaxis. Journal of Clinical Immunology 14: 190–204.

Schwartz LB, Sakai K, Bradford TR et al 1995 The alpha form of human tryptase is the predominant type present in blood at baseline in normal subjects and is elevated in those with systemic mastocytosis. Journal of Clinical Investigation 96: 2702–10.

Scott HW, Parris WCV, Sandidge PC et al 1983 Hazards in operative management of patients with systemic mastocytosis. Annals of Surgery 197: 507–14.

Smith GB, Gusberg RJ, Jordan RH et al 1987 Histamine levels and cardiovascular responses during splenectomy and splenorenal shunt formation in a patient with systemic mastocytosis. Anaesthesia 42: 861–7.

Vaughan STA, Jones GN 1998 Systemic mastocytosis presenting as profound cardiovascular collapse during anaesthesia. Anaesthesia 53: 804–9.

Webb TA, Li C-Y, Yam LT 1982 Systemic mast cell disease: a clinical and hematopathologic study of 26 cases. Cancer 49: 927–38.

McArdle's syndrome (myophosphorylase deficiency)

A type V glycogen storage disease that appears as an autosomal recessive myopathy. Skeletal muscle is mainly involved, although reports of cardiac muscle and ECG abnormalities have appeared. It results from the single enzyme defect of muscle phosphorylase. Failure of conversion of glycogen into lactate results in increased muscle glycogen. Patients with myophosphorylase deficiency do not become acidotic during exercise and it has been suggested that hyperkalaemia may contribute significantly to the drive to breathe, especially during heavy exercise (Paterson et al 1990). It is possible that impairment of mitochondrial function contributes to the exercise-related symptoms (De Stefano et al 1996). Males are more commonly affected than females. There was one report of dual pathology in a patient with excess muscle fatiguability— McArdle's disease coexisted with MH (Isaacs et al 1989). Attempts to improve exertional myalgia in McArdle's using dantrolene have been unsuccessful.

Preoperative abnormalities

1. Symptoms of cramp, stiffness, muscle pains and fatiguability on exercise may appear in childhood. Muscle contractions are relieved by rest. A family history may be elicited.

2. Occasional episodes of myoglobinuria can occur after strenuous exercise. Rhabdomyolysis was associated with the development of renal failure in a patient who had previously been asymptomatic (McMillan et al 1989).

3. Progressive atrophy of muscle may occur in the fifth decade.

4. The diagnosis can be made with neurohistochemical techniques, or by demonstrating decreased venous lactate and pyruvate concentrations with ischaemic exercise. NMR can be used to demonstrate muscle phosphorylase deficiency and EMG shows a decrease in evoked muscle response, after supramaximal stimuli.

Anaesthetic problems

1. Suxamethonium may cause myoglobinuria, with the risk of renal failure.

2. The use of a limb tourniquet may result in muscle atrophy.

3. Shivering can produce muscle damage.

4. Pyrexia, pulmonary oedema and renal failure occurred in association with repair of tetralogy of Fallot in a 2 year old. Autopsy showed McArdle's disease, but the pulmonary oedema and rhabdomyolysis were thought to be adverse reactions to protamine (Lobato et al 1999).

Management

1. Suxamethonium should not be given. Atracurium has been used in a child (Rajah & Bell 1986), and vecuronium in an adult (Tzabar & Ross 1990), without producing myoglobinuria or serum CK elevation. The use

of alcuronium during a Caesarean section has also been reported (Coleman 1984). A peripheral nerve stimulator must be used.

2. A tourniquet should only be applied if absolutely essential.

3. Core temperature should be monitored. The operating theatre must be warm. A heated mattress and blood warmer are required for long operations, to avoid shivering and heat loss. Patients are intolerant of a hypermetabolic state.

4. A usable, exogenous energy source such as dextrose, fructose or lactate should be given during the procedure and continued until oral intake is resumed.

5. Adequate systemic blood flow should be maintained.

6. If myoglobinuria occurs, iv fluids and mannitol should be given to reduce the possibility of renal failure.

Bibliography

Coleman P 1984 McArdle's disease. Problems of anaesthetic management for Caesarean section. Anaesthesia 39: 784–7.

De Stefano N, Argov Z, Matthews PM et al 1996 Impairment of muscle glycogenolysis in McArdle's disease (myophosphorylase deficiency). Muscle & Nerve 19: 764–9.

Isaacs H, Badenhorst ME, Du Sautoy C 1989 Myophosphorylase B deficiency and malignant hyperthermia. Muscle & Nerve 12: 203–5.

Lobato EB, Janelle GM, Urdaneta F et al 1999 Noncardiogenic pulmonary edema and rhabdomyolysis after protamine administration in a patient with unrecognized McArdle's disease. Anesthesiology 91: 303–5.

McMillan MA, Hallworth MJ, Doyle D et al 1989 Acute renal failure due to McArdle's disease. Renal Failure 11: 23–5.

Paterson DJ, Friedland JS, Bascom DA et al 1990 Changes in arterial K^+ and ventilation during exercise in normal subjects and subjects with McArdle's syndrome. Journal of Physiology 429: 339–48.

Rajah A, Bell CF 1986 Atracurium and McArdle's disease. Anaesthesia 41: 93.

Tzabar Y, Ross DG 1990 Vecuronium and McArdle's disease. Anaesthesia 45: 697.

Wolfsdorf JI, Holm IA, Weinstein DA 1999 Glycogen storage diseases. Phenotypic, genetic, and biochemical characteristics, and therapy. Endocrine & Metabolism Clinics of North America 28: 801–23.

Mediastinal masses

The mediastinum lies between the right and left pleural cavities and is divided at the level of the sternal angle into the superior and inferior mediastinum. The latter is further divided into posterior, middle or anterior mediastinum. When a patient presents with a mediastinal mass, two features provide clues to the nature of the mass—the site of the mass and the age of the patient. In babies they are likely to be bronchial cysts, teratomas, or secondary to oesophageal duplication. In infants and children, the commonest masses are neurogenic in origin, and are in the posterior mediastinum. In adults, middle mediastinal masses are usually carcinoma or lymphoma, although achalasia of the oesophagus has been reported (King and Strickland 1979). Anterior masses are frequently related to the thymus or thyroid. Posterior masses are often neurogenic in origin.

Patients with mediastinal masses may present for diagnostic procedures or thoracotomy. Bronchoscopy, lymph node biopsy, mediastinoscopy, and staging laparotomy are the commonest operations. Anaesthesia may also be required for laser surgery for near obstructing carcinomas of the bronchus (Conacher et al 1999). Patients may also present in late pregnancy (Boyne et al 1999).

Anaesthesia in a patient with a large mediastinal mass may be extremely hazardous because several important structures can be compressed. The superior vena cava, the trachea and tracheal bifurcation, the pulmonary artery, and the aortic arch are all adjacent. Fatalities and major morbidity in association with anaesthesia in patients with superior vena caval (SVC) obstruction, or compression of the trachea or a main bronchus, continue to be reported (Mackie 1987, Viswanathan et al 1995).

Preoperative abnormalities

1. *SVC obstruction.* This is diagnosed on clinical examination. It is four times more likely to occur with right-sided lesions than with those on the left, and it will be more severe when the obstruction is below the azygos vein. At postmortem examination, actual venous thrombosis has been found to be present in more than one-third of cases of SVC obstruction (Lokich & Goodman 1975). The majority of masses that cause SVC obstruction are malignant.

Initially, there is dilatation of the veins in the neck and upper thorax. Distension is most prominent when the patient is supine, and the veins do not collapse on sitting or standing. Subsequently there is progression to oedema of the face (with periorbital and conjunctival oedema, and proptosis), and the arms and the breasts, to give a peau d'orange appearance. In these latter cases, signs and symptoms of cerebral oedema may develop, and increasing respiratory difficulty secondary to laryngeal oedema may indicate the need for urgent radiotherapy or chemotherapy.

2. *Signs of airway obstruction or invasion.* A careful history, and, in particular, direct questioning about positional respiratory difficulty, stridor, dyspnoea, and nonproductive cough. Obstruction is often intermittent, worse on lying supine, during sleep, or on first waking, all of which suggest positional compression (Power et al 1997). Patients often prefer to sit up. Possibly, the supine position is associated with a decrease in thoracic volume (Pullerits & Holzman 1989). One child with intermittent upper airway obstruction was mistakenly diagnosed as having inhaled a foreign body (Ahktar et al 1991). Children with mediastinal masses are particularly at risk. Lesions may progress rapidly, therefore a recent CXR is essential. A normal PA view does not exclude obstruction. Anteroposterior compression of the trachea may only be seen on a penetrated lateral view, but nowadays a CT scan of the airway is mandatory, since the diameter of the trachea and

the site of obstruction can be measured accurately (Azizkhan et al 1985, Barker et al 1991). A reduction of tracheal diameter by 50% or more is usually associated with symptoms. Sometimes it may be helpful to examine dynamic airway function in addition. This can be seen directly, during fibreoptic bronchoscopy under local anaesthesia, or by constructing flow–volume loops. Reductions in maximum expiratory flows may warn of the possibility of obstruction after tracheal extubation.

3. *Myocardial or pericardial involvement.* Arrhythmias can occur, or the patient may have signs of a pericardial effusion. If cardiac tamponade is present, there is respiratory distress and pulsus paradoxicus. There may be cyanosis and syncope on straining (Keon 1981). Echocardiography should confirm the diagnosis.

4. *Obstruction of the pulmonary artery.* As a result of direct compression.

5. *Spinal cord involvement.* Can occur in posterior mediastinal tumours.

6. *Recurrent laryngeal nerve problems.* Predominantly occur with left-sided lesions.

7. *Systemic nonmetastatic effects of tumours.* These include hormone secretion, neuropathies, and myasthenia gravis.

Anaesthetic problems

1. In the presence of SVC obstruction, if a venous wall is breached anywhere in the area that drains into the SVC, severe haemorrhage can occur. Drugs given via venous access in the arm will have a significantly delayed action. Cyanosis of the face and upper trunk and increased central venous pressure occurred following general anaesthesia in a patient subsequently found to have a tumour encasing and obstructing the superior vena cava (Riley et al 1992).

2. In severe obstruction, cerebral and glottic oedema may occur. Acute superior vena caval syndrome, and difficulty in breathing followed by pulmonary oedema, occurred in a patient with a paratracheal mass encroaching on the superior vena cava (Power et al 1997).

3. There can be tracheal compression or invasion. Sudden respiratory obstruction can happen at any stage of the anaesthetic. It most commonly occurs after administration of a muscle relaxant and tracheal intubation (Bray & Fernandes 1982, O'Leary & Tracey 1983, Azizkhan et al 1985), but problems have also been encountered during reversal of neuromuscular blockade and tracheal tube removal (Prakash et al 1988), during inhalation induction (Mackie & Watson 1985), after extubation (Power et al 1997), and in the recovery room (Bittar 1975). Deaths continue to be reported (Neuman et al 1984, Levin et al 1985, Northrip et al 1986).

4. Difficulty in inflation of the lungs after tracheal intubation might be a result of external pressure, producing distortion or obstruction of the tube. However, it most probably results from the changes in lung mechanics that occur during anaesthesia, particularly after administration of a muscle relaxant. During spontaneous respiration there is a subatmospheric intrapleural pressure and widening of the airways on inspiration. Administration of a muscle relaxant alters the support of the bronchial tree, such that, in the presence of external pressure, collapse of the airway can occur and cause complete obstruction. Softening of the tracheal wall may contribute to this. In most of the cases described, partial relief of the obstruction coincided with the return of spontaneous respiration or recovery of consciousness.

5. Pulmonary oedema occurred after tracheal extubation in patients following biopsy of an anterior mediastinal tumour (Price & Hecker 1987) and mediastinoscopy (Power et al 1997).

6. Pulmonary artery involvement will decrease pulmonary perfusion and cardiac output.

7. Myocardial or pericardial involvement may result in arrhythmias, and occasionally

cardiac tamponade. Fatal collapse on induction of anaesthesia has been described in two children (Keon 1981, Halpern et al 1983), both of whom were found to have lymphomas involving the heart and infiltrating the pericardium and pulmonary artery at autopsy. Cardiovascular collapse has also occurred on induction of anaesthesia without evidence of tracheal obstruction or tamponade. Animal models have shown that the decrease in cardiac index associated with a mediastinal mass results from right ventricular afterload, causing right ventricular enlargement. This affects left ventricular volume because of the interventricular interdependence (Johnson et al 1991).

8. Spinal cord involvement occurs most commonly in children with neurogenic tumours.

Management

1. Detailed history taking is essential. Many authors admit that disaster might have been avoided had careful questioning been undertaken (Power et al 1997). Full assessment, as outlined above, and in particular CT or MRI scan, is important before embarking on general anaesthesia. In patients with major airway compression involving the lower trachea or bronchi, discussion between all the relevant specialties is essential (Mason & Fielder 1999). Children are particularly at risk (Azizkhan et al 1985). Masses may grow rapidly and the importance of recent X-rays has been emphasised. Death from tracheal obstruction occurred after day case lymph node biopsy in an asymptomatic 10-year-old boy, whose CXR had been reported as normal 3 weeks before (Viswanathan et al 1995). The use of CT scan to ascertain the optimal patient position for surgery has been suggested. The lateral position was shown to produce least compression of the bronchus in a 13 year old (Frawley et al 1995).

2. If there are obvious signs of SVC obstruction, urgent radiotherapy (Sold et al 1989), or chemotherapy is probably indicated before surgical intervention, although this has been disputed (Yellin et al 1990). Radiotherapy reduces the size of the tumour, as well as the degree of venous obstruction, provided that actual venous thrombosis has not occurred. If thrombosis is suspected, fibrinolytic agents or anticoagulants may be given. Temporary extracorporeal bypass can reduce the high venous pressure before induction of anaesthesia (Shimokawa et al 1996). Use of a stent has been described (Jackson & Brooks 1995).

3. Should there be any suggestion of tracheal obstruction, surgery ought to be performed under local anaesthetic, if possible. After the passage of a double lumen tube under local anaesthesia, a patient breathed spontaneously until the chest was opened (Younker et al 1989). If general anaesthesia is essential, endoscopy and awake fibreoptic intubation will provide information about the degree and nature of compression (Lewer & Torrance 1996, Boyne et al 1999, Goh et al 1999). Spontaneous ventilation should be maintained and no muscle relaxants given. A variety of techniques have been described including inhalational agents, and midazolam and ketamine infusions (Frawley et al 1995). In a 13 year old with bronchial compression, anaesthesia was induced with ketamine $2\,mg\,kg^{-1}$ and midazolam $0.1\,mg\,kg^{-1}$ with atropine $0.01\,mg\,kg^{-1}$. This was followed by infusions of ketamine and midazolam of $2\,mg\,kg^{-1}h^{-1}$ and $0.1\,mg\,kg^{-1}h^{-1}$ respectively. When the patient is symptomatic, radiotherapy may need to be undertaken before surgery. Five life-threatening complications were associated with intubation anaesthesia in 74 cases of untreated mediastinal or hilar Hodgkin's disease (Piro et al 1976). By contrast, no complications were seen in 24 cases with mediastinal involvement when anaesthesia took place after initial radiotherapy, or in the 78 anaesthetics in patients in whom there was no mediastinal disease. Planned extracorporeal oxygenation may be indicated under certain circumstances (Hall & Friedman 1975, Shimokawa et al 1996). It has been suggested that those with greater than 50%

obstruction of the airway at the level of the lower trachea and main bronchi should have their femoral vessels cannulated in readiness for cardiopulmonary bypass (Goh et al 1999).

4. If severe airway obstruction occurs unexpectedly, an improvement may be obtained by moving the patient from the supine to the lateral or prone position (Prakash et al 1988, Ahktar et al 1991), or in children, lifting the sternum manually (Cheung & Lerman 1998). Direct laryngoscopy, which straightens the trachea, may relieve the obstruction, and rigid bronchoscopy has been lifesaving (McMahon et al 1997).

5. Laser surgery for central airway obstruction (Conacher et al 1998).

Bibliography

Akhtar TM, Ridley S, Best CJ 1991 Unusual presentation of acute upper airway obstruction caused by an anterior mediastinal mass. British Journal of Anaesthesia 67: 632–4.

Azizkhan RG, Dudgeon DL, Buck JR et al 1985 Life-threatening airway obstruction as a complication to the management of mediastinal masses in children. Journal of Pediatric Surgery 20: 816–22.

Barker P, Mason RA, Thorpe MH 1991 Computerised axial tomography of the trachea. A useful investigation when a retrosternal goitre causes symptoms. Anaesthesia 46: 195–8.

Bittar D 1975 Respiratory obstruction associated with induction of general anesthesia in a patient with mediastinal Hodgkin's disease. Anesthesia & Analgesia 54: 399–403.

Boyne IC, O'Connor R, Marsh D 1999 Awake fibreoptic intubation, airway compression and lung collapse in a parturient: anaesthetic and intensive care management. International Journal of Obstetric Anaesthesia 8: 138–41.

Bray RJ, Fernandes FJ 1982 Mediastinal tumour causing airway obstruction in anaesthetised children. Anaesthesia 37: 571–5.

Cheung SLW, Lerman J 1998 Mediastinal masses and anesthesia in children. Anesthesiology Clinics of North America 16: 893–910.

Conacher ID, Paes LL, McMahon CC et al 1998 Anesthetic management of laser surgery for central airway obstruction: a 12-year case series. Journal of Cardiothoracic & Vascular Anesthesia 12: 153–6.

Frawley G, Low J, Brown TCK 1995 Anaesthesia for an anterior mediastinal mass with ketamine and midazolam infusion. Anaesthesia & Intensive Care 23: 610–12.

Goh MH, Liu XY, Goh YS 1999 Anterior mediastinal masses: an anaesthetic challenge. Anaesthesia 54: 670–3.

Hall DK, Friedman M 1975 Extracorporeal oxygenation for induction of anesthesia in a patient with an intrathoracic tumor. Anesthesiology 42: 493–5.

Halpern S, Chatten J, Meadows AT et al 1983 Anterior mediastinal masses: anesthesia hazards and other problems. Journal of Pediatrics 102: 407–10.

Jackson JE, Brooks DM 1995 Stenting of superior vena caval obstruction. Thorax 50 (Suppl 1): S31–6.

John RE, Narang VPS 1988 A boy with an anterior mediastinal mass. Anaesthesia 43: 864–6.

Johnson D, Hurst T, Cujec B et al 1991 Cardiopulmonary effects of an anterior mediastinal mass in dogs anesthetized with halothane. Anesthesiology 74: 725–36.

Keon TP 1981 Death on induction of anesthesia for cervical node biopsy. Anesthesiology 55: 471–2.

King DM, Strickland B 1979 An unusual case of thoracic inlet obstruction. British Journal of Radiology 52: 910–13.

Levin H, Bursztein S, Heifetz M 1985 Cardiac arrest in a child with an anterior mediastinal mass. Anesthesia & Analgesia 64: 1129–30.

Lewer BM, Torrance JM 1996 Anaesthesia for a patient with a mediastinal mass presenting with acute stridor. Anaesthesia & Intensive Care 24: 605–8.

Lokich JJ, Goodman R 1975 Superior vena cava syndrome. Journal of the American Medical Association 231: 58–61.

Mackie A 1987 Anesthetic management of mediastinal masses—again. Anesthesia & Analgesia 66: 696.

Mackie AM, Watson CB 1984 Anaesthesia and mediastinal masses. Anaesthesia 39: 899–903.

McMahon CC, Rainey L, Fulton B et al 1997 Central airway compression. Anaesthetic and intensive care consequences. Anaesthesia 52: 158–62.

Mason RA, Fielder CP 1999 The obstructed airway in head and neck surgery. Anaesthesia 54: 625–8.

Neuman GG, Weingarten AE, Abramowitz RM et al 1984 The anesthetic management of the patient with an anterior mediastinal mass. Anesthesiology 60: 144–7.

Northrip DR, Bowman KB, Tsueda K 1986 Total airway occlusion and superior vena cava syndrome in a child with an anterior mediastinal mass. Anesthesia & Analgesia 65: 1079–82.

O'Leary HT, Tracey JA 1983 Mediastinal tumours causing airway obstruction. Anaesthesia 38: 66–7.

Piro AJ, Weiss DR, Hellman S 1976 Mediastinal Hodgkin's disease: a possible danger for intubation anaesthesia. International Journal of Radiation, Oncology, Biology, Physics 1: 415–19.

Power CK, Buggy D, Keogh J 1997 Acute superior vena caval syndrome with airway obstruction following elective mediastinoscopy. Anaesthesia 52: 989–92.

Prakash VBS, Abel MD, Hubmayr RD 1988 Mediastinal mass and tracheal obstruction during general anesthesia. Mayo Clinic Proceedings 63: 1004–11.

Price SL, Hecker BR 1987 Pulmonary oedema following obstruction in a patient with Hodgkin's disease. British Journal of Anaesthesia 59: 518–21.

Pullerits J, Holzman R 1989 Anaesthesia for patients with mediastinal masses. Canadian Journal of Anaesthesia 36: 681–8.

Riley RH, Harris LA, Davis WJ et al 1992 Superior vena cava syndrome following general anaesthesia. Anaesthesia & Intensive Care 20: 229–32.

Shimokawa S, Yamashita T, Kinjyo T et al 1996 Extracorporeal venous bypass: a beneficial device in operation for superior vena caval syndrome. Annals of Thoracic Surgery 62: 1863–4.

Sold MJ, Feyerabend T, Lazarus G 1989 Emergency radiotherapy in a patient with mediastinal lymphoblastoma. Anaesthesia 44: 450–1.

Vas L, Naregal F, Naik V 1999 Anaesthetic management of an infant with anterior mediastinal mass. Paediatric Anaesthesia 9: 439–43.

Viswanathan S, Campbell CE, Cork RC 1995 Asymptomatic undetected mediastinal mass: a death during ambulatory anesthesia. Journal of Clinical Anesthesia 7: 151–5.

Yellin A, Rosen A, Reichert N et al 1990 Superior vena cava syndrome—the myth—the facts. American Review of Respiratory Diseases 141: 1114–18.

Younker D, Clark R, Coveler L 1989 Fiberoptic endobronchial intubation for resection of a mediastinal mass. Anesthesiology 70: 144–6.

Miller's syndrome

A recently described syndrome of postaxial acrofacial dysostosis (Barbuti et al 1989).

Preoperative abnormalities

1. Craniofacial abnormalities similar to those found in Treacher Collin's syndrome, and include micrognathia, malar hypoplasia, cleft lip and palate, low set ears, and eyelid coloboma. Partial upper airway obstruction may be a problem during infancy.

2. Limb hypoplasia and cardiac defects, including ASD, VSD and PDA, also occur.

3. The patient is usually of normal intelligence.

4. Multiple anaesthetics may be required for plastic surgery.

Anaesthetic problems

1. Intubation difficulties secondary to micrognathia. Gaseous induction resulted in complete airway obstruction in one infant. Intubation was performed blindly after suxamethonium (Richards 1987). Difficult awake intubation was performed using a straight blade (Stevenson et al 1991).

2. Upper airway obstruction may lead to difficulties in the postoperative period (Richards 1987).

3. Limb shortening causing venous access problems.

4. Difficulties with positioning of the patient.

Management

1. Identification of cardiac problems, if present.

2. Anticipation of intubation difficulties. Awake intubation with a straight blade modified for oxygen administration has been described (Stevenson et al 1991). On the second occasion, difficulties were overcome by using a right lateral approach to the larynx. If there is upper airway obstruction and multiple anaesthetics are anticipated, a tracheostomy may be considered (Stevenson et al 1991).

3. Support for the limbs is required to prevent stress on joints, nerves, and blood vessels.

Bibliography

Barbuti D, Orazi C, Reale A et al 1989 Postaxial acrofacial dysostosis or Miller syndrome: a case report. European Journal of Pediatrics 148: 445–6.

Richards M 1987 Miller's syndrome. Anaesthetic management of postaxial acrofacial dysostosis. Anaesthesia 42: 871–4.

Stevenson GW, Hall SC, Bauer BS et al 1991 Anaesthetic management of Miller's syndrome. Canadian Journal of Anaesthesia 38: 1046–9.

Mitochondrial encephalomyopathies (see also

Kearns–Sayre syndrome)

A heterogeneous group of multisystem diseases, the basis of which involves abnormalities of the mitochondrial metabolic pathways. They form part of a group now known as the OXPHOS (oxidative phosphorylation) diseases (Shoffner 1996). The OXPHOS diseases are associated with deletions and mutations of mitochondrial DNA, which is maternally inherited, or less commonly, nuclear DNA, which is not. Such mutations may also be part of the ageing process and Parkinson's disease. In aerobic metabolism, adenosine triphosphate is produced by the mitochondrial respiratory chain and oxidative phosphorylation systems. A variety of enzyme–protein complexes are involved, complexes I–V, that are located in the mitochondrial inner membrane. Mutations may result in dysfunctional aerobic metabolism and a large number of organs can be affected. There may be characteristic pathological muscle changes seen in mitochondrial myopathies. When some muscle fibres are stained with a special Gomori stain, 'ragged red fibres' are seen. However, classification of mitochondrial diseases is a complex subject since genotypes are not necessarily related to phenotypes. For further details see Shoffner (1996). In many diseases, there is progressive deterioration in cardiac, muscle, and nervous system function and reserve (Ciccotelli et al 1997). Anaesthesia may be required for biopsies of muscle, skin and liver, and eye surgery.

The following are some of the better known phenotypes:

1. Kearns–Sayre; ophthalmoplegia, cardiac conduction defects, retinopathy, and ataxia (see also Kearns–Sayre syndrome).

2. Mitochondrial encephalopathy with lactic acidosis and stroke-like episodes (MELAS). Presents as strokes in the young. Cerebellar ataxia may precede the disease by some years. Migraine headache, seizures, deafness, and dementia. Increased risk of cardiomyopathy, diabetes mellitus, retinitis pigmentosa, renal tubular defects, lactic acidaemia, and hyperalaninaemia. Thompson and Wahr (1997) have reported anaesthesia for cochlear implant.

3. Myoclonic epilepsy with red-ragged fibres (MERRF). The onset is late childhood to adulthood and involves a myopathy in association with red ragged fibres. Multifocal neurological diseases, including deafness, optic atrophy, and cerebellar ataxia. Other features include cardiomyopathy, renal tubular dysfunction, lactic acidaemia, and hyperalaninaemia.

4. NARP (neuropathy, ataxia, and retinitis pigmentosa), and Leigh's disease involve maternally inherited DNA mutations, probably involving complex V of the chain.

5. Pearson's syndrome (neonatal pancreatic and hepatic insufficiency, pancytopenia, and lactic acidosis) again involves mitochondrial DNA mutations. Infants require frequent blood transfusions.

6. Leber's hereditary optic neuropathy. Features are painless visual loss and abnormal colour vision. Although it was the first disease to be linked to maternally inherited DNA mutations, it is clinically unlike the other mitochondrial diseases.

Preoperative abnormalities

1. For features of individual diseases, see above.

2. In children, the diagnosis should be considered in any child with a multisystem or complex neurological disorder (Nissenkorn et al 1999), or who is being investigated for hypotonia (Keyes et al 1996).

3. The following systems may be involved (Johns 1995):

a) Skeletal muscle. Patients may have muscle cramps and are intolerant of exercise. Acute exacerbations with lactic acidosis may be particularly related to fasting and exercise. Myopathy and neuropathy can occur.

b) Brain. Seizures, ataxia, myoclonus, strokes, migraine, and dementia. Calcification of basal ganglia. Elevated levels of CSF protein.

c) Heart. Involvement varies between the subgroups, but particular mutations can have characteristic disorders (Anan et al 1995). These include Wolff-Parkinson-White syndrome, conduction disorders, and cardiomyopathy.

d) Eyes. External ophthalmoplegia, optic neuropathy, retinopathy, ptosis, visual field defects, and cataracts.

e) Pancreas. Diabetes mellitus.

f) Kidney. Glomerulitis, Fanconi's syndrome, lactic acidosis, and acid–base disturbances.

g) Liver. Dysfunction and failure.

h) GI tract. Dysphagia and colonic pseudo-obstruction.

i) Ear. Sensorineural deafness.

4. Diagnosis is made by blood and CSF lactate, muscle biopsy, molecular genetic analysis, and respiratory chain studies (Chinnery & Turnbull 1997).

5. Treatment is symptomatic and supportive.

Anaesthetic problems

1. Neuromuscular blockade. Reports of responses to muscle relaxants have been variable.

Wiesel et al (1991), using a cumulative dose–response technique, found no sensitivity to vecuronium in a 13-month-old boy. However, Finsterer et al (1998) found sensitivity to both rocuronium and atracurium in a 29-year-old woman, and this observation led to her diagnosis of mitochondrial myopathy first being made. Naguib et al (1996) found extreme sensitivity to mivacurium. Before mivacurium was given, the initial TOF (train-of-four) response demonstrated fade that was not improved by edrophonium 10 mg. A dose of $15\,\mu g\,kg^{-1}$ produced 98% inhibition of T1, and recovery of T1 to 100% took 38 min. It took another 10 min for the TOF ratio to reach 60%, close to the initial value before mivacurium was given.

2. Cardiac muscle. Conduction defects and cardiomyopathy. Patients may have pacemakers.

3. Metabolic problems. Exercise intolerance may occur. Light exercise testing was performed in a young woman with a defect in complex III of the electron transport chain. Impaired oxygen utilisation was shown, and the patient developed a profound metabolic acidosis as a result of lactate accumulation (Rosaeg et al 1996). Later, when pregnant, after 2 h in labour she developed a compensated metabolic acidosis. An epidural was sited, sodium bicarbonate was given, and Caesarean section performed.

4. Cerebral problems. White matter degeneration was found on a brain scan in a sick 13 month old, who underwent surgery for a gangrenous gall bladder, and developed neurological signs postoperatively. A scan 3 months before had not shown any gross abnormality, and the child had had four previous anaesthetics without problem. He died 5 weeks later (Casta et al 1997). Patients may present to ITU with respiratory failure, partly due to diaphragmatic weakness, partly as a result of decreased central respiratory drive, and often precipitated by a chest infection (Howard et al 1995). In a study of 11 patients, the mean age at admission was 28 years (range 22 months to 54 years), and mortality was high.

5. Laryngeal involvement was found in a 36

year old. She presented with proximal myopathy and bulbar symptoms, and laryngoscopy showed incomplete adduction of the vocal cords, a weak voice, and a poor cough (Hartley & Ascott 1994).

6. Reduced ventilatory drive, secondary to altered neural control, that may cause episodes of life-threatening hypoventilation. It was suggested that this is likely to be exacerbated in relation to surgery, sedation, and infections (Barohn et al 1990). Patients are more sensitive than normal to sedatives (Wallace et al 1998). Admission to the ITU may be required for respiratory failure, metabolic support, or control of status epilepticus (Howard et al 1995, Naguib et al 1996).

7. Hyperthermia has been reported (Thompson & Wahr 1997), although there is no evidence of any relationship with MH.

Management

1. History, examination and investigation for individual organ involvement, in particular cardiac, neurological, and musculoskeletal. In some phenotypes echocardiography may be needed.

2. Optimise oxygenation and avoid metabolic stresses that may provoke or worsen any lactic acidosis.

3. Cautious use of small doses of nondepolarising agents with neuromuscular monitoring.

4. In pregnancy, in patients with lactic acidosis, it has been suggested that labour be avoided by performing elective Caesarean section under epidural anaesthesia. This prevents the increase in oxygen consumption associated with painful uterine contractions (Rosaeg et al 1996). However, vaginal delivery may be preferable, provided adequate pain relief is given. Epidural anaesthesia and assisted ventouse delivery was reported in a 31 year old with a history of ophthalmoplegia, ptosis, and progressive muscle weakness (Blake & Shaw

1999). Resting serum lactate was 1.6 mmol l^{-1} (N 0.8–1.2 mmol l^{-1}).

5. Spinal anaesthesia was performed for orthopaedic surgery in a patient with multisystem disease and a family history of MELAS (Maslow & Lisbon 1993). A propofol infusion, a laryngeal mask airway and caudal analgesia were used for a 6-year-old child with a fractured hip (Cheam & Critchley 1998).

6. Close monitoring in the postoperative period for respiratory depression.

Bibliography

Anan R, Nakagawa M, Miyata M et al 1995 Cardiac involvement in mitochondrial diseases: a study on 17 patients with documented mitochondrial DNA defects. Circulation 91: 955–61.

Barohn RJ, Clanton T, Sahenk Z et al 1990 Recurrent respiratory insufficiency and depressed ventilatory drive complicating mitochondrial myopathies. Neurology 40: 103–6.

Blake LL, Shaw RW 1999 Mitochondrial myopathy in a primigravid pregnancy. British Journal of Obstetrics & Gynaecology 106: 871–3.

Burns AM, Shelly MP 1989 Anaesthesia for patients with mitochondrial myopathy. Anaesthesia 44: 975–7.

Casta A, Quackenbush EJ, Houck CS et al 1997 Perioperative white matter degeneration and death in a patient with a defect in mitochondrial oxidative phosphorylation. Anesthesiology 87: 420–5.

Cheam EWS, Critchley LAH 1998 Anesthesia for a child with complex I respiratory chain enzyme deficiency. Journal of Clinical Anesthesia 10: 524–7.

Chinnery PF, Turnbull DM 1997 Mitochondrial medicine. Quarterly Journal of Medicine 90: 657–67.

Ciccotelli KK, Prak EL, Muravchick S 1997 An adult with inherited mitochondrial encephalomyopathy: report of a case. Anesthesiology 87: 1240–2.

Finsterer J, Stratil U, Bittner R et al 1998 Increased sensitivity to rocuronium and atracurium in mitochondrial myopathy. Canadian Journal of Anaesthesia 45: 781–4.

Hartley C, Ascott F 1994 Laryngeal involvement in mitochondrial myopathy. Journal of Laryngology & Otology 108: 685–7.

Howard RS, Russell S, Losseff N et al 1995

Management of mitochondrial disease on an intensive care unit. Quarterly Journal of Medicine 88: 197–207.

Johns DR 1995 Mitochondrial DNA and disease. New England Journal of Medicine 333: 638–43.

Keyes MA, Van de Wiele BV, Stead SW 1996 Mitochondrial myopathies: an unusual cause of hypotonia in infants and children. Paediatric Anaesthesia 6: 329–35.

Maslow A, Lisbon A 1993 Anesthetic considerations in patients with mitochondrial dysfunction. Anesthesia & Analgesia 76: 884–6.

Naguib M, el Dawlatly AA, Ashour M et al 1996 Sensitivity to mivacurium in a patient with mitochondrial myopathy. Anesthesiology 84: 1506–9.

Nissenkorn A, Zeharia A, Lev D et al 1999 Multiple presentations of mitochondrial disorders. Archives of Disease in Childhood 81: 209–14.

Rosaeg OP, Morrison S, MacLeod JP 1996 Anaesthetic management of labour and delivery in the parturient with mitochondrial myopathy. Canadian Journal of Anaesthesia 43: 403–7.

Shoffner JM 1996 Maternal inheritance and the evaluation of oxidative phosphorylation diseases. Lancet 348: 1283–8.

Thompson VA, Wahr JA 1997 Anesthetic considerations in patients presenting with mitochondrial myopathy, encephalopathy, lactic acidosis, and stroke-like episodes (MELAS) syndrome. Anesthesia & Analgesia 85: 1404–6.

Wallace JJ, Perndt H, Skinner M 1998 Anaesthesia and mitochondrial disease. Paediatric Anaesthesia 8: 249–54.

Wiesel S, Bevan JC, Samuel J et al 1991 Vecuronium neuromuscular blockade in a child with mitochondrial myopathy. Anesthesia & Analgesia 72: 696–9.

Mitral valve disease

Two main problems confront the anaesthetist when dealing with a patient with cardiac valvular disease. The first is that of the preoperative assessment of the severity of the lesion, and the degree of myocardial dysfunction resulting from it. The second, and crucial to the conduct of anaesthesia, is an understanding of the compensatory mechanisms which may have taken place. These will depend on whether the valvular disease is acute or longstanding.

The pathophysiology and compensatory mechanisms when an acute valve lesion follows endocarditis or myocardial infarction, are very different from those of chronic valve disease, in which gradual compensatory cardiac hypertrophy or dilatation has taken place. In either case, the aim is to give an anaesthetic that will cause as little disturbance as possible to these compensatory mechanisms.

The serious effects of decompensation range from pulmonary oedema and hypoxia, to a severe decrease in left ventricular output resulting in myocardial ischaemia, infarction, or arrhythmias. Whilst in mild disease there may be few problems, severe valvular disease requires close cardiovascular monitoring, a careful choice of anaesthetic technique, and anticipation and cautious correction of the factors causing decompensation.

Mitral regurgitation

Causes include rheumatic endocarditis (in which the lesion is frequently mixed), mitral valve prolapse, papillary muscle dysfunction, or rupture of the chordae tendinae. The latter conditions usually follow myocardial ischaemia or infarction. There is a difference in pathophysiology between chronic mitral regurgitation and that of acute onset. In the acute event, the regurgitated volume depends upon the duration of systole, the size of the orifice, and the systolic pressure gradient across the valve. Volume loading will increase the size of the orifice, but if the volume is too low the contractility will be suboptimal. An improved systematic examination of the mitral valve before surgery has been described, using transoesophageal echocardiography (Lambert et al 1999).

Preoperative abnormalities

1. An apical pansystolic murmur radiating to the axilla.

2. During systole, part of the stroke volume

enters the aorta, whilst the rest is regurgitated into the left atrium. The ratio between the two depends upon the degree of incompetence and the impedance of each pathway.

3. There is left ventricular hypertrophy secondary to increased work, but it progresses insidiously, so that damage occurs before the onset of symptoms. In severe, chronic cases, left ventricular failure may eventually occur. However, in acute mitral regurgitation, pulmonary oedema appears early (McLintic et al 1992).

4. During diastole the left atrium has to eject the normal pulmonary venous flow in addition to the regurgitated fraction. Left atrial dilatation therefore takes place. Once the left ventricular ejection fraction decreases below 60%, the prognosis worsens (Carabello & Crawford 1997).

5. AF usually only occurs in mixed lesions or in advanced cases.

6. Chest X-ray shows left atrial dilatation and left ventricular hypertrophy. Echocardiography provides precise information about chamber dimensions, wall thickness and movement, and will demonstrate a rheumatic or prolapsing valve.

7. In general, in a patient with rheumatic mitral regurgitation, the progression of exercise intolerance is slow, unless complications such as heart failure or bacterial endocarditis occur. If, however, the incompetence follows myocardial infarction, there may be sudden onset of acute pulmonary oedema and death.

Anaesthetic problems

1. Even when the disease is mild, there is a greater risk of bacterial endocarditis than with any other valve lesion.

2. There is a risk of systemic embolism and the patient may be anticoagulated.

3. An increase in systemic vascular resistance will augment the regurgitated volume and decrease the cardiac output.

4. Hypovolaemia will decrease the LAP and the stroke work.

5. A bradycardia can worsen the regurgitation, since distortion of the valve may be enhanced by an increased diameter of the ventricle during diastole.

6. In pregnancy, deterioration may take place in the last trimester (Scott et al 1998). Difficulties may occur when lying flat. Decompensation occurred with the onset of atrial fibrillation at 37 weeks in a parturient with known mixed mitral valve disease, predominantly regurgitation, but with a valve area of $2\,cm^2$. Increments of digoxin 0.25 mg iv were given, followed by quinidine $400\,mg\,day^{-1}$, with a view to cardioversion, but the patient spontaneously reverted to sinus rhythm. An epidural infusion was started 10 days later for induction of labour, with invasive haemodynamic monitoring in place (Sharma et al 1994).

Management

1. Prophylactic antibiotics are required when appropriate.

2. Situations of heat loss, untreated pain and hypovolaemia, all of which produce systemic vasoconstriction, should be avoided.

3. Left atrial filling pressure should be maintained to increase the forward output of the left ventricle. Hypovolaemia must therefore be avoided.

4. Acute isovolaemic haemodilution to a haemoglobin value of $10.3\,g\,dl^{-1}$ was studied in 20 patients with mitral regurgitation about to undergo mitral valve surgery, ten in sinus rhythm and ten in AF. It was well tolerated in both groups, with compensatory increases in cardiac index and oxygen extraction and no signs of ischaemia (Spahn et al 1998).

5. A mild tachycardia is advantageous, to avoid excess diastolic filling of the ventricle and valve distortion.

6. Remifentanil infusion was used for Caesarean section in a patient with mixed mitral valve disease (predominantly regurgitation), asthma, and preeclampsia (Scott et al 1998). The remifentanil infusion was continued with IPPV until analgesia was re-established with an epidural infusion.

Mitral stenosis

Normal left ventricular filling is restricted by the decreased area across the stenosed valve. The normal area of the valve is $4\,cm^2$. Symptoms appear when this is reduced to about $2.5\,cm^2$; below $1\,cm^2$ the symptoms are severe.

Compensation is normally achieved by increasing the pressure gradient across the mitral valve, and is dependent upon atrial contraction and the duration of diastole. Decompensation often begins with the onset of atrial fibrillation, associated with a fast ventricular rate. Deterioration may also occur during pregnancy.

Echocardiography allows assessment of the severity of the stenosis and of any other valvular disease.

Preoperative abnormalities

1. The pulse may be irregular as a result of atrial fibrillation. Palpation of the precordium may reveal a palpable first sound ('tapping' apex beat). On auscultation there may be an opening snap (the closer to the second sound, the more severe the stenosis), followed by a mid-diastolic murmur, with presystolic accentuation if the patient remains in sinus rhythm. The loudness of the murmur is no guide to severity, and may be inaudible if the cardiac output is low, in neglected disease. Atrial fibrillation causes decompensation by decreasing the left ventricular filling time and by reducing cardiac output. This is manifest clinically by cool, possibly cyanosed peripheries, and a low volume pulse. A malar flush is common.

2. LAP is increased, while dilatation and hypertrophy of the left atrium occurs. When LAP increases, so does pulmonary capillary pressure, and when this exceeds the colloid osmotic pressure (25–30 mmHg), pulmonary oedema develops. A sudden increase in LAP may be precipitated by tachycardia secondary to exercise, emotion, fever, pregnancy, or by an arrhythmia. A proportion of the patients will develop irreversible pulmonary hypertension, right ventricular hypertrophy, pulmonary and tricuspid incompetence, and occasionally right heart failure.

3. Chest X-ray shows left atrial enlargement, with a prominent left atrial appendage and double contour of the right heart border. Kerley B lines may be present. ECG may show P mitrale. Definitive diagnosis is by echocardiography, which allows precise measurement of left atrial dimensions and demonstration of the abnormal movement of the thickened or calcified valve cusps. If combined with Doppler techniques, valve area can be estimated.

4. In the presence of AF, systemic thromboembolism may occur.

5. The patient is usually taking digoxin, and sometimes beta blockers, calcium channel blockers, and anticoagulants.

6. Symptomatic history is a good guide to severity. Dyspnoea on mild exertion, with episodes of paroxysmal nocturnal dyspnoea, indicate a LAP of 15–20 mmHg. Occasionally angina occurs.

7. Worsening stenosis and signs of pulmonary hypertension are indications for mechanical relief of the stenosis. Balloon valvotomy, open commissurotomy or mitral valve replacement may be indicated (Carabello & Crawford 1997).

Anaesthetic problems

1. Tachycardia or fast atrial fibrillation reduces diastolic filling time and may precipitate pulmonary oedema.

2. Large decreases in systemic vascular resistance may result in severe hypotension, since there is limited capacity to increase cardiac output in compensation.

3. Volume overload may produce pulmonary oedema; conversely, hypovolaemia, accentuated by diuretics, may reduce cardiac output. Mitral stenosis may be a cause of intractable pulmonary oedema in patients undergoing IPPV (Davis et al 1996).

4. Myocardial depressant drugs can cause severe hypotension.

5. The Trendelenburg position may result in hypoxia and pulmonary oedema.

6. Hypoxia and acidosis can cause pulmonary vasoconstriction.

7. Nitrous oxide may be unsafe if pulmonary vascular resistance is high (Schulte-Sasse et al 1982).

8. Bacteraemia during surgery or instrumentation carries the risk of endocarditis.

9. Mitral stenosis may first present, or the condition may decompensate, during pregnancy. A 34-year-old woman presented with abdominal pain and hypoglycaemia at 35 weeks' gestation. She rapidly developed cardiac failure, which was found to be secondary to severe mitral stenosis (area 0.75 cm^2), deteriorated and died, despite maximum inotropic support (Sia et al 1998).

In the immediate postpartum period, autotransfusion secondary to uterine contraction can cause circulatory overload. Pulmonary oedema and collapse occurred after therapeutic abortion of twins at 15 weeks' gestation, probably secondary to the autotransfusion following oxytocin administration. Emergency mitral valve replacement was performed (Tio et al 1998). Problems may also occur when the vasodilator effects of epidural anaesthesia are wearing off.

Problems may not stop with delivery of the child. One patient with severe disease and preeclampsia developed pulmonary oedema 1

day after Caesarean section, and pulmonary thromboembolism 4 weeks later (Afrangui & Malinow 1998).

Management

1. Prophylactic antibiotics are required for any surgery which carries a risk of producing a bacteraemia. This includes dental, genitourinary, and bowel operations, and childbirth.

2. AF must be controlled before surgery.

3. Whilst digoxin is the mainstay of treatment, care should be taken to prevent tachycardia. Atropine should be avoided. A sedative premedication reduces anxiety. An adequate depth of anaesthesia and good analgesia are essential.

4. Inotropic agents, particularly a dilating inotrope such as dobutamine, may be required to treat hypotension, although they can worsen pulmonary vasoconstriction.

5. Myocardial depressants should be avoided if possible.

6. Prevention of systemic vasoconstriction, secondary to cold, pain, and hypovolaemia, is essential. A CVP will assist the assessment of volume requirement for optimal right ventricular function. In severe mitral stenosis, and before corrective surgery, it may be necessary to use dilating agents such as sodium nitroprusside or nitrates. IPPV may be life saving.

7. The complexity of monitoring used depends upon the severity of the lesion and the magnitude of the surgery. In the absence of pulmonary hypertension the changes in CVP will mirror those in the left atrium. However, if PH is present, the PAWP correlates poorly with the LAP.

8. If there is right ventricular dysfunction, nitrous oxide should be avoided.

9. Oakley (1996) stresses the important role of beta blockers in the treatment of pulmonary

oedema secondary to mitral stenosis. If intractable pulmonary oedema occurs in elderly patients with severe mitral stenosis, balloon mitral valve dilatation may provide temporary relief before valve replacement (Davis et al 1996). Failure to respond to medical treatment during pregnancy may be another indication (Kalra et al 1994, Deshpande 1998).

10. Pregnant patients with mitral stenosis should be assessed by a cardiologist early in pregnancy and their management planned. Surgical intervention may occasionally be required for severe cases (Yaryura et al 1996). In the less severe, epidural anaesthesia may be appropriate for delivery or Caesarean section. The beneficial effects of epidural anaesthesia in a patient during delivery has been demonstrated using PAP monitoring (Hemmings et al 1987). Ngan Kee et al (1999) described three patients who had vaginal delivery under combined spinal-epidural anaesthesia. Fentanyl $25\,\mu g$ was followed by an epidural infusion of bupivacaine and fentanyl, and preloading was deliberately avoided. High-dose alfentanil was used for emergency Caesarean section in a patient with severe mitral stenosis, and the baby responded to a single dose of naloxone (Batson et al 1990). Epidural opiates were used for postoperative pain.

Mitral valve prolapse (MVP)

The recognition of this condition has increased with the advent of echocardiography, although there is argument about its diagnosis, significance, and prognosis (Freed et al 1999, Nishimura & McGoon 1999). It has been reported to occur in up to 5% of healthy patients. However, the diagnosis is a nonspecific one, and would appear to cover a wide spectrum, with considerable variations in significance. A chance finding on echocardiography in thin, young patients who are asymptomatic, and in whom there is no regurgitation, is probably not of importance. In older patients who are symptomatic, and who have elongated or ruptured chordae tendinae, or

pathological valve changes in association with mitral regurgitation, the prognosis may be less good. Each patient should be assessed in relation to the clinical symptoms and findings. However, in some patients, regurgitation may be provoked by exercise, and in this group there appears to be a higher risk (Stoddard et al 1995). In children, arrhythmias may also be precipitated by exercise. Patients with previously undiagnosed MVP may occasionally present with arrhythmias during anaesthesia.

Preoperative abnormalities

1. Abnormalities vary from slight prolapse of the posterior mitral valve leaflet with no regurgitation, to gross prolapse associated with large volume regurgitation when the ventricles contract. The first is probably an anatomical variation; the second can arise from pathological changes in the chordae tendinae or valve leaflets.

2. MVP has also been found in a number of genetic conditions in which there are connective tissue defects. These include Marfan's, Ehlers–Danlos syndrome, osteogenesis imperfecta, pseudoxanthoma elasticum, and scleroderma.

3. The patient is frequently asymptomatic, but symptoms such as syncope, chest pain and palpitations may feature. Complications include progressive mitral regurgitation, bacterial endocarditis, orthostatic syncope, cerebral ischaemia and arrhythmic sudden death (Zuppiroli et al 1995). Complications were found to be higher in men, those >45 years, those with a family history, and those with left atrial or left ventricular diameter ≥4 mm, or ≥6 mm, respectively.

4. Clinical signs may include a midsystolic click and a late systolic murmur. As valve function deteriorates, the click may disappear and the murmur become pansystolic. If gross regurgitation occurs during systole, left atrial dilatation and left ventricular hypertrophy may be present. Atrial and ventricular arrhythmias can occur and there are occasional reports of sudden death.

5. Echocardiographic criteria require at least a 2-mm posterior movement in late systole.

6. Patients with arrhythmias may be receiving beta blockers, and those with severe regurgitation, diuretics, digoxin, and ACE inhibitors.

Anaesthetic problems

1. The degree of valve prolapse is increased by anything that reduces ventricular volume, thus resulting in redundancy of the mitral leaflet. Some patients with mitral valve prolapse and no regurgitation at rest were found to have exercise-induced regurgitation (Stoddard et al 1995). Conversely prolapse is reduced by increases in ventricular volume. The following situations may accentuate mitral valve prolapse:

a) Increased myocardial contractility.

b) Decreased preload secondary to hypovolaemia.

c) Vasoconstriction, decreasing LV emptying, and increasing LV volume.

d) Tachycardia, which reduces the time for ventricular filling.

e) High airways pressure produced by straining.

2. Most case reports are of unexpected atrial or ventricular arrhythmias arising in the perioperative period, and in more than half of the cases the diagnosis was made postoperatively on echocardiography (Krantz et al 1980, Thiagarajah & Frost 1983, Berry et al 1985). There have been occasional reports of ventricular fibrillation, profound bradycardia, and actual cardiac arrest (Cheng 1990). In one patient, two episodes of asystole occurred during attempted diagnostic extradural block (Abrahams & Lees 1989), although its association with mitral valve prolapse was unclear. In a child undergoing tonsillectomy, ventricular fibrillation occurred after halothane induction followed by atropine 0.2 mg iv (Moritz et al 1997).

Management

1. Evaluation of functional MVP versus symptomatic and haemodynamically significant disease (Hanson et al 1996). If regurgitation exists, distinction must also be made between chronic regurgitation, and the acute state secondary to sudden chordal rupture.

2. The anaesthetic technique in known cases of MVP should aim to minimise the effects of factors known to worsen the prolapse.

a) Avoid sympathetic stimulation and increases in myocardial contractility. A good premedication relieves anxiety. Atropine, and agents producing arrhythmias, are avoided. Hypoxia, hypercarbia and acidosis are prevented. Avoid light anaesthesia. If tachycardia occurs in spite of these manoeuvres, propranolol can be used.

b) Prevent hypovolaemia. Circulating blood volume is maintained by expansion of the intravascular volume. A fluid challenge will reverse echocardiographic evidence of prolapse (Lax et al 1993).

c) A combination of opioids with judicious, low-dose volatile agents.

d) Minimise decreases in systemic vascular resistance. Sympathetic blockade produced by regional anaesthesia may worsen the prolapse. However, sometimes there may be no choice. Epidural anaesthesia was required for Caesarean section in a patient with MVP, asthma, and pneumonia (Alcantara & Marx 1987). The importance of adequately preloading the patient, and fractionating the doses of local anaesthetic, were stressed. Hypotension secondary to sympathetic blockade should be treated with a dilute phenylephrine solution, or metaraminol, rather than ephedrine (adrenaline). Induced hypotension may also worsen the prolapse and should preferably not be used.

3. High airway pressures should be avoided.

4. Prophylactic antibiotics for bacterial endocarditis are required with MVP in the presence of a systolic murmur.

Bibliography

Abrahams ZA, Lees DC 1989 Two cardiac arrests after needle puncture in a patient with mitral valve prolapse: psychogenic? Anesthesia & Analgesia 69: 126–8.

Afrangui B, Malinow AM 1998 Severe preeclampsia complicating mitral valve stenosis. Regional Anesthesia & Pain Medicine 23: 204–9.

Alcantara LG, Marx GF 1987 Cesarean section under epidural analgesia in a parturient with mitral valve prolapse. Anesthesia & Analgesia 66: 902–3.

Batson MA, Longmire S, Csontos E 1990 Alfentanil for urgent caesarean section in a patient with severe mitral stenosis and pulmonary hypertension. Canadian Journal of Anaesthesia 37: 685–8.

Berry FA, Lake CL, Johns RA et al 1985 Mitral valve prolapse—another cause of intraoperative arrhythmias in the pediatric patient. Anesthesiology 62: 662–4.

Carabello BA, Crawford FA 1997 Valvular heart disease. New England Journal of Medicine 337: 32–41.

Cheng TO 1990 Cardiac arrest and mitral valve prolapse. Anesthesia & Analgesia 70: 229.

Davis G, Khan RM, Randall N et al 1996 Balloon mitral valve dilatation as an aid to weaning from ventilatory support in patients with intractable pulmonary oedema caused by severe mitral stenosis. British Journal of Anaesthesia 76: 879–80.

Deshpande S 1998 Epidural analgesia for term vaginal delivery after balloon valvotomy for mitral stenosis at 24 weeks gestation. International Journal of Obstetric Anesthesia 7: 177–80.

Freed LA, Levy D, Levine RA et al 1999 Prevalence and clinical outcome of mitral-valve prolapse. New England Journal of Medicine 341: 1–7.

Hanson EW, Neerhut RK, Lynch III C 1996 Mitral valve prolapse. Anesthesiology 85: 178–95.

Hemmings GT, Whalley DG, O'Connor PJ et al 1987 Invasive monitoring and anaesthetic management of a parturient with mitral stenosis. Canadian Journal of Anaesthesia 34: 182–5.

Kalra GS, Arora R, Khan JA et al 1994 Percutaneous mitral commissurotomy for severe mitral stenosis during pregnancy. Catheterization & Cardiovascular Diagnosis 33: 28–30.

Krantz JM, Viljoen JF, Schermer R et al 1980 Mitral valve prolapse. Anesthesia & Analgesia 59: 379–83.

Lambert AS, Miller JP, Merrick SH et al 1999 Improved evaluation of the location and mechanism of mitral valve regurgitation with a systematic transoesophageal echocardiography examination. Anesthesia & Analgesia 88: 1205–12.

Lax D, Eicher M, Goldberg SJ 1993 Effects of hydration on mitral valve prolapse. American Heart Journal 126: 415–18.

McLintic AJ, Metcalfe MJ, Ingram KS et al 1992 Acute mitral regurgitation: physiological and pharmacological considerations in the management of a critically ill patient. Anaesthesia & Intensive Care 20: 373–6.

Moritz HA, Parnass SM, Mitchell JS 1997 Ventricular fibrillation during anesthetic induction in a child with undiagnosed mitral valve prolapse. Anesthesia & Analgesia 85: 59–61.

Ngan Kee WD, Shen J, Chui ATO et al 1999 Combined spinal-epidural analgesia in the management of labouring parturients with mitral stenosis. Anaesthesia & Intensive Care 27: 523–6.

Nishimura RA, McGoon MD 1999 Perspectives on mitral valve prolapse. New England Journal of Medicine 341: 48–50.

Oakley CM 1996 Beta blockers have important role in pulmonary oedema due to mitral stenosis. British Medical Journal 312: 376.

Savage RM, Cosgrove DM 1999 Systematic transesophageal echocardiographic examination in mitral valve repair: the evolution of a discipline into the twenty-first century. Anesthesia & Analgesia 88: 1197–9.

Schulte-Sasse U, Hess W, Tarnow J 1982 Pulmonary vascular responses to nitrous oxide in patients with normal and high pulmonary vascular resistance. Anesthesiology 57: 9–13.

Scott H, Bateman C, Price M 1998 The use of remifentanil in general anaesthesia for Caesarean section in a patient with mitral valve disease. Anaesthesia 53: 695–7.

Sharma SK, Gambling DR, Gajraj NM et al 1994 Anesthetic management of a parturient with mixed mitral valve disease and uncontrolled atrial fibrillation. International Journal of Obstetric Anesthesia 3: 157–62.

Sia ATH, Chong JL, Tan CGM 1998 Severe mitral stenosis in a parturient with congestive cardiac failure and hypoglycaemia. International Journal of Obstetric Anesthesia 7: 173–6.

Spahn DR, Seifert B, Pasch T et al 1998 Haemodilution tolerance in patients with mitral regurgitation. Anaesthesia 53: 20–4.

Stoddard MF, Prince CR, Dillon S et al 1995
Exercise-induced mitral regurgitation is a predictor
of morbid events in subjects with mitral valve
prolapse. Journal of the American College of
Cardiology 25: 693–9.

Thiagarajah S, Frost EAM 1983 Anaesthetic
considerations in patients with mitral valve
prolapse. Anaesthesia 38: 560–6.

Tio I, Tewari K, Balderston KD et al 1998 Emergency
mitral valve replacement in the setting of severe
pulmonary hypertension and acute cardiovascular
decompensation after evacuation of twins at 15
weeks. American Journal of Obstetrics &
Gynecology 179: 270–2.

Yaryura RA, Carpenter RJ Jr, Duncan JM et al 1996
Management of mitral valve stenosis in pregnancy:
case presentation and review of the literature.
Journal of Heart Valve Disease 5: 16–19.

Zuppiroli A, Rinaldi M, Kramer-Fox R et al 1995
Natural history of mitral valve prolapse. American
Journal of Cardiology 75: 1028–32.

Morquio's syndrome (see also

Mucopolysaccharidoses)

One of the mucopolysaccharidoses (type IV),
this autosomal recessive connective tissue
disorder results from the abnormal metabolism
of certain polysaccharides (Baines & Keneally
1983, Kempthorne & Browne 1983). Morquio A
involves deficiency of n-acetyl-galactosamine-6-
sulphate sulphatase. Morquio B, in which there is
a deficiency of β galactosidase, is less severe.
Excessive amounts of some metabolites of these
substances are laid down in the body tissues and
result in a variety of defects. Skeletal, cardiac, eye
and hearing problems develop, but the individual
is of normal intelligence. Death frequently
occurs before the age of 30. Bone marrow
transplantation has had variable effects on the
course of the disease.

Preoperative abnormalities

1. Skeletal abnormalities include dwarfism,
kyphosis, genu valgum, hand deformity, joint
mobility, pigeon chest, vertebral flattening with
wide disc spaces, and neck instability secondary
to hypoplasia of the odontoid peg. Spinal cord
compression may develop in late childhood with
slow-onset paraplegia. The face is flattened, and
the teeth may be widely spaced and have
defective enamel.

2. Restrictive lung disease secondary to
kyphoscoliosis.

3. Cardiac infiltration can affect both
the mitral and aortic valves, and late-onset
aortic regurgitation may occur. In an
echocardiographic study of ten patients, 60% had
abnormalities mainly involving the aortic or
mitral valves (John et al 1990). However, these
lesions were haemodynamically relatively mild
and, in a study of Doppler flow mapping, only
33% were affected (Wipperman et al 1995).
Heart disease may also develop secondary to the
progressive chest deformity.

4. Hepatosplenomegaly.

5. Corneal opacities commonly develop.

6. Nerve deafness may occur.

7. Inguinal herniae are common and may
require surgery.

8. Excess keratin sulphate is found in the
urine.

Anaesthetic problems

1. Atlantoaxial subluxation may occur and
result in spinal cord transection (Lipson 1977),
although this may not always be the cause of
neurological problems. In a myelographic study
of 13 patients, odontoid dysplasia and a
hypoplastic dens were found in every case
(Stevens et al 1991). However, the atlantoaxial
stability was said to be mild and, if severe spinal
cord compression was present, it was secondary
to anterior extradural soft tissue thickening,
rather than the subluxation. An MRI study of 11
patients showed that all had normal brains, but
abnormalities of the odontoid were present, with
varying degrees of cord compression, that were
worse than neurological signs had suggested
(Hughes et al 1997). Instability and cord
compression were described in a child who

developed a hemiparesis after a fall (Ashraf et al 1991). Acute tetraplegia, and subsequent death from pneumonia, was reported in an 8-year-old girl having a myelogram under general anaesthesia (Beighton & Craig 1973). Forward displacement of the atlas on the axis was found to have occurred. This was attributed to excess movement of the head during the anaesthetic.

2. Respiratory function may be impaired (Hope et al 1973), and upper airway obstruction and chest deformities can contribute to postoperative respiratory problems. Respiratory failure and subsequent death from pneumonia occurred in a patient following radical cervical lymph node resection for melanoma of the scalp (Jones & Croley 1979). Intrathoracic obstruction may occur. Infiltration of upper airway structures with glycosaminoglycans may cause upper airway obstruction in the perioperative period (Berkowitz et al 1990).

3. Intubation difficulty may result from a potential, or actual, unstable neck (Walker et al 1994, Moores et al 1996), or a previous cervical fusion (Bartz et al 1999). Occasionally it may result from facial deformity and redundant pharyngeal mucosa, but this occurs much less commonly than in the other mucopolysaccharidoses (Jones & Croley 1979).

4. Upper airway obstruction may be provoked by head flexion (Pritzker et al 1980).

5. Obstructive sleep apnoea.

Management

1. A careful assessment of respiratory function is required, so as to detect those patients with seriously impaired reserve. In view of the increased risk of major postoperative problems, and the reduced life expectancy, a decision to embark on nonessential major surgery should not be made lightly.

2. Cervical spine X-rays should be examined for signs of C1–2 instability, and pre-existing neurological defects documented. If hypoplasia of the dens or instability is suspected, some

means of immobilising the neck, such as manual inline stabilisation or a halo frame, is required to prevent flexion damage to the spinal cord. The management of appendicectomy in a young boy, who already had paraplegia secondary to cord compression, was described (Birkinshaw 1975). The child lay prone with his head propped on his hands and a plaster cast was applied to his head, back, and sides. When the plaster was dry the patient was carefully rolled into a supine position. After an inhalation induction with halothane, intubation was achieved with deep ether anaesthesia. Nasal fibreoptic intubation under ketamine/midazolam sedation has been reported in a 23-month-old girl for cervical decompression (Tzanova et al 1993). Awake fibreoptic intubation was performed in a 9-year-old boy undergoing posterior spinal fusion for spinal cord compression (Bartz et al 1999). Prophylactic or early cervical fusion has been suggested, because late surgery carries a poor prognosis (Ransford et al 1996).

3. If intubation difficulties are suspected, either an inhalation induction or an awake intubation should be considered.

4. Continuous spinal anaesthesia has been reported for orthopaedic surgery in an 8-year-old girl (Tobias 1999). The spinal catheter was inserted under ketamine sedation and anaesthesia was maintained with a propofol infusion.

5. If there are cardiac lesions prophylaxis for endocarditis is required.

Bibliography

Ashraf J, Crockard HA, Ransford AO et al 1991 Transoral decompression and posterior stabilisation in Morquio's disease. Archives of Diseases in Childhood 66: 1318–21.

Baines D, Keneally J 1983 Anaesthetic implications of the mucopolysaccharidoses: a fifteen year experience in a Children's Hospital. Anaesthesia & Intensive Care 11: 198–202.

Bartz H-J, Wiesner L, Wappler F 1999 Anaesthetic management of patients with mucopolysaccharidosis IV presenting for major orthopaedic surgery. Acta Anaesthesiologica Scandinavica 43: 679–83.

Beighton P, Craig J 1973 Atlanto-axial subluxation in the Morquio syndrome. Journal of Bone & Joint Surgery 55B: 478–81.

Berkowitz ID, Raja SN, Bender KS et al 1990 Dwarfs: pathology and anesthetic implications. Anesthesiology 73: 739–59.

Birkinshaw KJ 1975 Anaesthesia in a patient with an unstable neck: Morquio's syndrome. Anaesthesia 30: 46–9.

Hope EOS, Farebrother MJB, Bainbridge D 1973 Some aspects of respiratory function in three siblings with Morquio–Brailsford disease. Thorax 28: 335–43.

Hughes DG, Chadderton RD, Cowie RA et al 1997 MRI of the brain and craniocervical junction in Morquio's disease. Neuroradiology 39: 381–5.

John RM, Hunter D, Swanton RH 1990 Echocardiographic abnormalities in type IV mucopolysaccharidoses. Archives of Diseases in Childhood 65: 746–9.

Jones AEP, Croley TF 1979 Morquio syndrome and anesthesia. Anesthesiology 51: 261–2.

Kempthorne PM, Brown TCK 1983 Anaesthesia and the mucopolysaccharidoses: a survey of techniques and problems. Anaesthesia & Intensive Care 11: 203–7.

Lipson SJ 1977 Dysplasia of the odontoid process in Morquio's syndrome causing quadriparesis. Journal of Bone & Joint Surgery 59A: 340–4.

Moores C, Rogers JG, McKenzie et al 1996 Anaesthesia for children with mucopolysaccharidoses. Anaesthesia & Intensive Care 24: 459–63.

Pritzker MR, King RA, Kronenberg RS 1980 Upper airway obstruction during head flexion in Morquio's disease. American Journal of Medicine 69: 467–70.

Ransford AO, Crockard HA, Stevens JM et al 1999 Occipito-atlanto-axial fusion in Morquio–Brailsford syndrome. A ten-year experience. Journal of Bone & Joint Surgery 78: 307–13.

Stevens JM, Kendall BE, Crockard HA et al 1991 The odontoid process in Morquio–Brailsford's disease. The effects of spinal fusion. Journal of Bone & Joint Surgery 73: 851–8.

Tobias JD 1999 Anesthesia care for the child with Morquio syndrome: general versus regional. Journal of Clinical Anesthesia 11: 242.

Tzanova I, Schwartz M, Jantzen JP 1993 [Securing the airway in children with the Morquio–Brailsford syndrome. German.] Anaesthesist 42: 477–81.

Walker RWM, Darowski M, Morris P et al 1994 Anaesthesia and mucopolysaccharidoses. A review of airway problems in children. Anaesthesia 49: 1078–84.

Wipperman CF, Beck M, Schranz D et al 1995 Mitral and aortic regurgitation in 84 patients with mucopolysaccharidoses. European Journal of Pediatrics 154: 98–101.

Motor neurone disease (amyotrophic lateral sclerosis)

A progressive degenerative disease of the motor system of unknown aetiology. It involves both upper and lower motor neurones and presents in late middle age with muscle weakness and fasciculations. Bulbar palsies are a common and distressing feature and involvement of nonmotor pathways is increasingly being recognised (Tandan & Bradley 1985). A defect in the high-affinity glutamate transport system has been found (Kaplan & Hollander 1994). The prognosis is poor, and in about 50% of cases death occurs within 3 years of onset. In the early stages there is an increased risk of bony injury from falls and subsequently anaesthetists may be involved in ventilatory assistance. The importance of supportive treatment in terminal care has been emphasised (O'Brien et al 1992).

Preoperative abnormalities

1. A combination of signs and symptoms of upper and lower motor neurone disease. Muscle cramps, weakness, wasting, fasciculations, spasticity, hyperreflexia and extensor plantar reflexes may coexist with bulbar signs. These include impairment of speech, swallowing and laryngeal reflexes, which cause distressing symptoms such as dysphagia, drooling, choking, and dysarthria. The extraocular muscles and sphincters are spared. The disease is progressive.

2. Inspiratory muscle weakness determines respiratory failure and its symptoms, whilst abdominal muscle weakness affects the ability to generate an effective cough. Weakness in both

may coexist. In the sniff test, fluoroscopy may demonstrate a lack of descent of the diaphragm during inspiration. In some patients there may be vocal cord dysfunction (Polkey et al 1998).

3. The autonomic system may be involved and sometimes cardiac sympathetic denervation may develop early.

4. EMG indicates muscle denervation and shows fibrillation potentials.

5. Riluzole and gabapentin may slow the progression of the disease.

6. A form of the disease may occur in conjunction with a carcinoma, usually bronchial.

Anaesthetic problems

1. Administration of suxamethonium has produced hyperkalaemic cardiovascular collapse (Beach et al 1971).

2. Patients may be sensitive to the effects of nondepolarising muscle relaxants (Rosenbaum et al 1971).

3. There is a risk of perioperative aspiration and airway obstruction when bulbar signs are present. Obstructive sleep apnoea has been reported.

4. Postoperative respiratory insufficiency may occur (Jacka & Sanderson 1998).

5. The ethical problems involved in the conflict between preserving life and minimising suffering in the later stages of the disease (Newrick & Langton Hewer 1984).

6. Chronic respiratory insufficiency may not be recognised as being secondary to motor neurone disease. Difficulty in weaning from IPPV occurred in two patients aged 60 and 65 years respectively. Only after neurological examination and electromyography was the diagnosis of MND made (Kuisma et al 1993).

7. Pregnancy may be associated with neurological deterioration. A patient was first diagnosed at 8 weeks' gestation, when she developed progressive leg weakness. By 32 weeks

she was dyspnoeic at rest, with an FVC 26% of predicted and an arterial $P\text{co}_2$ of 7.3 kPa. Caesarean section was performed under epidural anaesthesia, after which she had noninvasive respiratory support. One week later she required full ventilatory support and was discharged home with a tracheostomy for long-term ventilation (Jacka & Sanderson 1998).

Management

1. In view of the report of cardiovascular collapse secondary to hyperkalaemia, suxamethonium should not be used.

2. If nondepolarising drugs are essential, small doses are given initially and neuromuscular function monitored.

3. If bulbar muscle function is impaired, precautions should be taken to prevent perioperative pulmonary aspiration.

4. The use of epidural anaesthesia for lower abdominal surgery has been reported in four patients (Kochi et al 1989, Hara et al 1996). No worsening of pulmonary function was documented.

5. Silverstein et al (1991) stress the importance of regularly giving patients the opportunity to discuss ventilatory support and express their views about cardiopulmonary resuscitation.

6. In advanced disease, careful consideration should be given to the appropriateness of surgery, particularly when there is bulbar involvement. Difficult problems may arise once a patient is committed to IPPV. However, in some patients, respiratory muscle weakness may present as shortness of breath early in the disease. In these patients, noninvasive respiratory support at night may produce symptomatic benefit (Howard et al 1989). The use of phrenic nerve pacing is being tried for ventilatory support (Editorial 1990).

7. Muscle pains may be a prominent and distressing feature. The response to opiates has been shown to be good and there is no evidence

that the course or duration of the disease is affected (O'Brien et al 1992). Oral morphine, either as an elixir or a slow-release preparation, is the opioid of choice, accompanied by a laxative. An antiemetic may be needed in the early stages.

Bibliography

Beach TP, Stone WA, Hamelberg W 1971 Circulatory collapse following succinylcholine: report of a patient with diffuse lower motor neurone disease. Anesthesia & Analgesia 50: 431–7.

Editorial 1990 Phrenic nerve pacing in quadriplegia. Lancet 336: 88–90.

Hara K, Sakura S, Saito Y et al 1996 Epidural anesthesia and pulmonary function in a patient with amyotrophic lateral sclerosis. Anesthesia & Analgesia 83: 878–9.

Howard RS, Wiles CM, Loh L 1989 Respiratory complications and their management in motor neuron disease. Brain 112: 1155–70.

Jacka MJ, Sanderson F 1998 Amyotrophic lateral sclerosis presenting during pregnancy. Anesthesia & Analgesia 86: 542–3.

Kaplan LM, Hollander D 1994 Respiratory dysfunction in amyotrophic lateral sclerosis. Clinics in Chest Medicine 15: 675–81.

Kimura K, Tachibana N, Kimura J et al 1999 Sleep-disordered breathing at an early stage of amyotrophic lateral sclerosis. Journal of the Neurological Sciences 164: 37–43.

Kochi T, Oka T, Mizuguchi T 1989 Epidural anesthesia for patients with amyotrophic lateral sclerosis. Anesthesia & Analgesia 68: 410–12.

Kuisma MJ, Saarinen KV, Teirmaa HT 1993 Undiagnosed amyotrophic lateral sclerosis and respiratory failure. Acta Anaesthesiologica Scandinavica 37: 628–30.

Newrick PG, Langton-Hewer R 1984 Motor neurone disease: can we do better? British Medical Journal 289: 539–42.

O'Brien T, Kelly M, Saunders C 1992 Motor neurone disease: a hospice perspective. British Medical Journal 304: 471–3.

Polkey MI, Lyall RA, Green M et al 1998 Expiratory muscle function in amyotrophic lateral sclerosis. American Journal of Respiratory & Critical Care Medicine 158: 734–41.

Rosenbaum KJ, Neigh JL, Strobel GE 1971 Sensitivity to non depolarising muscle relaxants in amyotrophic lateral sclerosis. Anesthesiology 35: 638–41.

Silverstein MD, Stocking CB, Antel JP 1991 Amyotrophic lateral sclerosis and life-sustaining therapy: patients' desires for information, participation in decision making, and life-sustaining therapy. Mayo Clinic Proceedings 66: 906–13.

Tandan R, Bradley WG 1985 Amyotrophic lateral sclerosis. Part I. Clinical features, pathology and ethical issues in management. Annals of Neurology 18: 271–80.

Moyamoya disease

A rare abnormality of the cerebral circulation, first described, and predominantly seen, in Japan. There is gradual occlusion or severe stenosis of the internal carotid arteries and cerebral angiography shows a fine hazy network of vessels (the moyamoya collaterals) around the base of the brain. Patients usually present with signs of cerebrovascular insufficiency, either in childhood, or as adults. Surgery, which can be divided into direct anastomotic and indirect nonanastomotic techniques, carries the risk of postoperative stroke. Many papers have discussed the role of anaesthesia (in particular hypocapnoea) in the development of strokes. However, in one retrospective analysis of 368 cases, the severity of the disease and the type of surgical procedure were found to be the major determinants of postoperative cerebral ischaemia. The frequency of preoperative TIAs and the use of indirect, nonanastomotic revascularisation techniques were the main risk factors, rather than the anaesthetic management (Sakamoto et al 1997). In another study of 124 cases, the incidence of preoperative TIAs was again cited as an important risk factor, but in combination with perioperative hypercapnoea of >45 mmHg (Iwama et al 1996). The disease in children is said to differ from that in adults. Soriano et al (1993) reported a series of 22 encephalodural arteriosynangiosis procedures in 13 children, seven of whom had concurrent disease. Whilst this is mainly a Japanese disease, Caucasians have been affected (Farrugia et al 1997).

Preoperative abnormalities

1. The patient may present with a variety of features suggestive of inadequate cerebral blood

flow. These may range from TIAs to fixed neurological deficits. Adults have headaches and may develop intracranial haemorrhages (Henderson & Irwin 1995). Children develop TIAs and strokes, usually between infancy and 5 years, after which they deteriorate rapidly. The occurrence of TIAs may, in particular, be associated with hypercapnoea, crying, or exercising.

2. Cerebral angiography demonstrates the occluded arteries and the abnormal 'net-like' collateral circulation. The autoregulatory response to hypotension is decreased in children, but not in adults (Soriano et al 1993). In children, hyperventilation is accompanied by slow wave patterns on EEG, similar to those produced by cerebral hypoperfusion, and these persist even after the episode of hyperventilation stops.

3. Normal cerebral blood flow may be reduced by as much as a half.

4. In adults there is an increased incidence of intracranial aneurysms.

Anaesthetic problems

1. Hyperventilation can cause a reduction in arterial $P\text{CO}_2$ that may compromise the already poor cerebral circulation. Patients have been described in whom hypocapnoea during anaesthesia was associated with a deterioration in neurological status. No deterioration occurred in those patients in whom normocapnoea was maintained (Sumikawa & Nagai 1983, Bingham & Wilkinson 1985). Anaesthesia using pancuronium, fentanyl, and 0.5–1% isoflurane, while maintaining normocapnoea, was used in eight procedures on seven patients (Brown & Lam 1987). An increased CO_2 may also be deleterious. The effects of hypercapnoea on cortical blood flow were examined by Kurehara et al (1993). Continuous measurement using laser Doppler techniques showed a significant decrease in cortical blood flow between a $Pa\text{CO}_2$ of 5.2 kPa and one of 6.3 kPa.

2. In one series, four out of seven patients were found to have abnormal ECGs. One 27 year old developed a ventricular tachycardia during surgery (Brown & Lam 1987).

3. Postoperatively, subjects are prone to develop fits.

4. The diagnosis may not always be known before surgery. A 5-year-old child was given spinal anaesthesia for circumcision. Two hours after surgery he developed recurrent seizures and a left hemiparesis lasting for 10 days (Yasukawa et al 1988). The development of subsequent TIAs was suggestive of a compromised cerebral circulation and carotid angiography showed the picture of moyamoya disease.

5. The diagnosis was also unknown in a pregnant patient, who presented with a grand mal fit that was assumed to be eclamptic (Amin-Hanjani et al 1993). Magnesium sulphate was given and Caesarean section performed. However, in the absence of other signs of eclampsia, and the presence of left lower extremity weakness and xanthochromic CSF, carotid angiography was undertaken. This showed not only a subarachnoid haemorrhage, but an overall picture consistent with moyamoya disease.

Management

1. Surgical treatment is directed towards increasing the cerebral blood flow. Various surgical manoeuvres have been tried, including anastomosis of the superficial temporal to the middle cerebral artery, encephalo-duroarteriosynangiosis, and encephalo-omental synangiosis (Havlik et al 1992). Direct anastomotic procedures seem to produce the best results.

2. Both hypo- and hypercapnoea should be avoided in the perioperative period. Normocapnoea and normothermia should be maintained.

3. There is a suggestion that inhalational anaesthetics are more likely to decrease regional

cortical blood flow than total intravenous anaesthesia with propofol (Sato et al 1999). Soriano et al (1993) used a technique of fentanyl and isoflurane. However, there is little evidence that any one particular anaesthetic influences the outcome.

4. In children, avoidance of pain, crying and dehydration in the postoperative period, has been suggested to reduce later neurological deficits (Sakamoto et al 1998).

5. Relatively little has been reported about the course of pregnancy and the effect of normal delivery on the cerebral blood flow. However, use of a technetium brain scan to assess cerebral blood flow during hyperventilation in a girl who had undergone surgical treatment during childhood, suggested that her cerebrovascular reserve was adequate to allow natural delivery (Kume et al 1999). Furuya et al (1998) used nimodipine 1 mg iv prior to induction for Caesarean section under general anaesthesia using a propofol infusion and normocapnoea. Caesarean section under epidural anaesthesia has also been reported. Continuous monitoring of cerebral oxygenation by near infrared spectroscopy took place during surgery (Ngan Kee & Gomersall 1996).

6. Similar preoperative studies of the effects of hyperventilation, but this time using EEG monitoring, were described in a child who required cardiopulmonary bypass for ASD repair (Wang et al 1997). Nimodipine was again used before surgery, for its cerebral vasodilator and protectant properties. Thiopentone was given before going on bypass and the blood pressure was maintained with a phenylephrine infusion.

Bibliography

Amin-Hanjani S, Kuhn M, Sloane N et al 1993 Moyamoya disease in pregnancy: a case report. American Journal of Obstetrics & Gynecology 169: 395–6.

Bingham RM, Wilkinson DJ 1985 Anaesthetic management in Moya-moya disease. Anaesthesia 40: 1198–202.

Brown SC, Lam A 1987 Moya-moya disease. A review of clinical experience and anaesthetic management. Canadian Journal of Anaesthesia 34: 71–5.

Farrugia M, Howlett DC, Saks AM 1997 Moyamoya disease. Postgraduate Medical Journal 73: 549–52.

Furuya A, Matsukawa T, Ozaki M et al 1998 Propofol anesthesia for cesarean section successfully managed in a patient with moyamoya disease. Journal of Clinical Anesthesia 10: 242–5.

Havlik RJ, Fried I, Chyatte D et al 1992 Encephalo-omental synagiosis in the management of moyamoya disease. Surgery 111: 156–62.

Henderson MA, Irwin MG 1995 Anaesthesia and moyamoya disease. Anaesthesia & Intensive Care 23: 503–6.

Iwama T, Hashimoto N, Yonekawa Y 1996 The relevance of hemodynamic factors to perioperative ischemic complications in childhood moyamoya disease. Neurosurgery 38: 1120–5.

Kume N, Hayashida K, Shimotsu Y et al 1999 Hyperventilation technetium-99m-HMPAO brain SPECT in moyamoya disease to assess risk of natural childbirth. Journal of Nuclear Medicine 38: 1894–7.

Kurehara K, Ohnishi H, Touho H et al 1993 Cortical blood flow response to hypercapnia during anaesthesia in Moyamoya disease. Canadian Journal of Anaesthesia 40: 709–13.

Ngan Kee WD, Gomersall CD 1996 Extradural anaesthesia for Caesarean section in a patient with moyamoya disease. British Journal of Anaesthesia 77: 550–2.

Sakamoto T, Kawaguchi M, Kurehara K et al 1997 Risk factors for neurologic deterioration after revascularization surgery in patients with moyamoya disease. Anesthesia & Analgesia 85: 1060–5.

Sakamoto T, Kawaguchi M, Kurehara K et al 1998 Postoperative neurological deterioration following the revascularization surgery in children with moyamoya disease. Journal of Neurosurgical Anesthesiology 10: 37–41.

Sato K, Shirane R, Kato M et al 1999 Effect of inhalational anesthesia on cerebral circulation in Moyamoya disease. Journal of Neurosurgical Anesthesiology 11: 25–30.

Soriano SG, Sethna NF, Scott RM 1993 Anesthetic management of children with moyamoya disease. Anesthesia & Analgesia 77: 1066–70.

Sumikawa K, Nagai H 1983 Moya-moya disease and anesthesia. Anesthesiology 58: 204–5.

Wang N, Kuluz J, Barron M et al 1997 Cardiopulmonary bypass in a patient with moyamoya disease. Anesthesia & Analgesia 84: 1160–3.

Yasukawa K, Akagawa S, Nakagawa Y et al 1988
Convulsions and temporary hemiparesis following
spinal anesthesia in a child with moya moya disease.
Anesthesiology 69: 1023.

Mucopolysaccharidoses (MPS)

(see also individual syndromes)

A group of inherited connective tissue
syndromes that result from enzyme deficiencies.
The mucopolysaccharides (or
glycoaminoglycans) are constituents of
connective tissue, and are made up of repeating
disaccharide units connected to protein. They are
normally broken down in the cell lysosomes to
monosaccharides and amino acids. In the
absence of certain enzymes, accumulation of
intermediate products of degradation process
takes place. These substances increase cell size
and cause impairment of function. The effects
depend upon the enzyme defect, and the specific
organs involved. The disease progresses with age,
and life expectancy is greatly reduced.

Surgery is required most frequently for inguinal
and umbilical herniae, ENT, orthopaedic or
neurosurgical operations. In a review of 43
children, every patient was found to have at least
one complication involving the head and neck,
and in more than a half, ENT surgery was
required (Bredenkamp et al 1992). There have
been attempts to replace missing enzymes by
regular implantation of tissue such as human
amnion, but with little evidence of success.
Bone marrow transplantation has had more
success in modifying the course of the disease in
some patients. Although these syndromes are
rare, the more commonly encountered ones
provide a considerable anaesthetic challenge,
primarily because of airway problems. The
classification of syndromes is shown below.
Some are dealt with under their individual
names. Abnormalities in the least common types
are included here.

Type I

Type I H: Hurler's syndrome (gargoylism)
(see Hurler).

Type I S: Scheie's syndrome (see Hurler).

Type I H/S: Hurler–Scheie (see Hurler).

Type II: Hunter's syndrome (see Hurler).

Type III: Sanfilippo's syndrome.

Craniofacial: mild coarsening of facial
features.

Skeletal: none.

Cardiac: mitral and aortic regurgitation
may occur.

Mental: severe progressive retardation,
aggression, sleep problems.

Other organs: none.

Anaesthetic: although difficult intubation
has been reported in one case
(Kempthorne & Brown 1983), it is not
usually a problem.

Type IV: Morquio's syndrome (see
Morquio's).

Type VI: Maroteaux–Lamy syndrome (see
Maroteaux–Lamy).

Type VII: β-glucuronidase.

Type VIII: ? like Morquio's and Sanfilippo.

Bibliography

Baines D, Keneally J 1983 Anaesthetic implications of
the mucopolysaccharidoses. Anaesthesia & Intensive
Care 11: 198–202.
Bredenkamp JK, Smith ME, Dudley JP et al 1992
Otolaryngologic manifestations of the
mucopolysaccharidoses. Annals of Otology,
Rhinology & Laryngology 101: 472–8.
Herrick IA, Rhine EJ 1988 The
mucopolysaccharidoses and anaesthesia. Canadian
Journal of Anaesthesia 35: 67–73.
Kempthorne PM, Brown TCK 1983 Anaesthesia and
the mucopolysaccharidoses. Anaesthesia & Intensive
Care 11: 203–7.
Moores C, Rogers JG, McKenzie et al 1996
Anaesthesia for children with
mucopolysaccharidoses. Anaesthesia & Intensive
Care 24: 459–63.
Ruckenstein MJ, MacDonald RE, Clarke JT et al
1991 The management of otolaryngological

problems in the mucopolysaccharidoses: a retrospective review. Journal of Otolaryngology 20: 177–83.

Walker RWM, Darowski M, Morris P et al 1994 Anaesthesia and mucopolysaccharidoses. A review of airway problems in children. Anaesthesia 49: 1078–84.

Wipperman CF, Beck M, Schranz D et al 1995 Mitral and aortic regurgitation in 84 patients with mucopolysaccharidoses. European Journal of Pediatrics 154: 98–101.

Multiple endocrine neoplasia (see also Sipple's syndrome)

A group of dominantly inherited cancer syndromes associated with mutations of tumour suppressor genes. Multiple endocrine neoplasia (MEN) is defined as the occurrence of tumours in two or more endocrine glands (Thakker 1998).

MEN 1: An autosomal dominant condition in which the tumour suppressor locus is on chromosome 11 and the gene 'menin' has been identified (Heath 1998).

MEN 2A: Caused by mutations of the receptor tyrosine kinase (RET) proto-oncogene on chromosome 10.

MEN 2B: Also caused by mutations of the RET proto-oncogene on chromosome 10, it differs from MEN 2A by its extra-endocrine features. Also characterised by early onset of tumours and more aggressive thyroid carcinomas.

Preoperative abnormalities

1. MEN 1. Parathyroid adenomas may be associated with one or more of a variety of enterohepatic endocrine tumours (gastrinoma, vipoma, glucagonoma, pancreatic polypeptidoma), and pituitary tumours (prolactinoma, GH-releasing factor tumour). Symptoms, which present in early adulthood, are usually related to primary hyperparathyroidism (95%). Islet cell tumours occur in about 50%,

and pituitary tumours in a third. There is often a family history.

2. MEN 2A. Tumours of the thyroid C cells (medullary thyroid carcinoma), with tumours of the adrenal medulla (phaeochromocytoma), and sometimes parathyroid hyperplasia or adenoma. May present at any time during adulthood, and medullary thyroid carcinoma is the commonest initial presentation (see Sipple's syndrome).

3. MEN 2B features early and aggressive medullary thyroid carcinomas, multiple mucosal ganglioneuromas (of tongue, eyelids, conjunctivae, buccal mucosa, and gastrointestinal tract), phaeochromocytomas, a Marfanoid habitus with a high arched palate, severe colonic dysfunction associated with megacolon, more aggressive thyroid carcinomas that are of earlier onset, and bilateral phaeochromocytomas.

Anaesthetic problems

1. Those of phaeochromocytomas, if present.

2. Patients who have total bilateral adrenalectomies are susceptible to Addisonian crises (de Graaf et al 1999). In a long-term follow-up of 22 patients, nine had a total of 19 Addisonian crises, one of which was fatal because it was unrecognised.

3. Problems of hypercalcaemia, if untreated.

Management

1. In general, since these are rare conditions, surgical treatment is best undertaken in specialist units (Heath 1998). Management requires screening and investigation of the patients' families because the disease will occur in about 50% of first degree relatives.

2. A somatostatin analogue, Octreotide, can be used in MEN-1 patients. It produces a symptomatic and biochemical response, with reduction in size of hepatic metastases (Burgess et al 1999).

3. It is suggested that some adrenal tissue be

left following surgery for phaeochromocytomas, to reduce the morbidity from Addisonian crises (de Graaf et al 1998).

Bibliography

Burgess JR, Greenaway TM, Parameswaran V et al 1999 Octreotide improves biochemical, radiologic, and symptomatic indices of gastroenteropancreatic neoplasia in patients with multiple endocrine neoplasia type 1 (MEN-1). Implications for an integrated model of MEN-1 tumorigenesis. Cancer 86: 2154–9.

de Graaf JS, Dullaart RP, Zwierstra RP 1999 Complications after bilateral adrenalectomy for phaeochromocytoma in multiple endocrine neoplasia type 2—a plea to conserve adrenal function. European Journal of Surgery 165: 843–6.

Heath D 1998 Multiple endocrine neoplasia. Journal of the Royal College of Physicians of London 32: 98–101.

Thakker RV 1998 Multiple endocrine neoplasia—syndromes of the twentieth century. Journal of Clinical Endocrinology & Metabolism 83: 2617–20.

Multiple system atrophy (MSA)

(formerly Shy–Drager syndrome) (see also Autonomic failure)

A progressive condition presenting in later life, in which autonomic failure or dysfunction is associated with, or precedes, the onset of widespread central neuronal degeneration. The old term 'Shy–Drager syndrome' has been replaced by the broader term multiple system atrophy (MSA). This has been divided into three categories (Schatz 1996):

1. Striatonigral degeneration, which produces a Parkinsonian form with some cerebellar dysfunction.

2. Olivopontocerebellar atrophy with primarily cerebellar signs and minor Parkinsonian features.

3. The old Shy–Drager syndrome, with predominantly autonomic failure.

There may be considerable overlap between these categories and in the early stages it can be difficult to distinguish between them. Manifestations of autonomic failure include: orthostatic hypotension, anhidrosis, constipation, bladder disturbances and retention, erectile and ejaculatory failure, Horner's syndrome, stridor, and apnoeic episodes (Mathias 1997).

Preoperative abnormalities

1. Neurological symptoms and signs of widespread neuronal involvement, the clinical features of which depend upon the category of MSA. These include autonomic failure, cerebellar ataxia, and Parkinsonism.

2. Postural hypotension and an inability, in response to stress, to produce the normal pressor response which depends on reflex vasoconstriction and tachycardia. There is reversal of the usual diurnal pattern of blood pressure, and that normally produced by postural changes.

3. Anhidrosis, incontinence and impotence can occur.

4. Fluid and electrolyte homeostasis is disturbed, resulting in a failure to concentrate urine at night, and producing a nocturnal diuresis and sodium loss.

5. Vocal cord paralysis, secondary to abductor palsy, may result in stridor and respiratory failure. In some cases isolated palsy has preceded the disease by as much as two years (Kew et al 1990). Sudden deaths have been reported.

6. There may be a disordered nocturnal respiratory pattern, sleep apnoea, and glottic snoring.

7. Denervation hypersensitivity has been reported.

8. Osteoporosis and aseptic necrosis of bone are thought to result from impaired periosteal vascular control. Orthopaedic surgery may therefore be required.

9. Patients may be receiving a wide range of drugs including fludrocortisone, levodopa, and bromocriptine.

Anaesthetic problems

1. The failure of the cardiovascular system to respond to stress by vasoconstriction and tachycardia results in significant cardiovascular instability. The heart rate may be relatively fixed. An inability to release catecholamines has been suggested. A lack of pressor response to painful stimuli under light anaesthesia has been noted (Sweeney et al 1985). Systolic hypertension occurs in the supine position, but standing produces systolic hypotension and an absence of tachycardia.

2. Decreased sensitivity of the respiratory system to increased carbon dioxide levels under anaesthesia may make techniques using spontaneous respiration difficult to achieve (Sweeney et al 1985). Pulmonary respiratory reflexes are impaired.

3. Defective lacrimation, decreased sweating and sluggish pupillary reflexes may be present. The unreliability of these reflexes may cause difficulties in assessing the depth of anaesthesia.

4. A denervation hypersensitivity type of response to the infusion of catecholamines (Malan & Crago 1979), and a lack of response to indirectly acting amines such as ephedrine, methylamphetamine and tyramine have been reported. However, it has been suggested that these features should only be seen in conditions in which there is peripheral, not central, autonomic dysfunction (Stirt et al 1982).

5. Sensitivity to the effects of intravenous and volatile anaesthetics (Sweeney et al 1985).

6. Bilateral abductor vocal cord paralysis contributed to the occurrence of postoperative respiratory failure, with subsequent difficulties in weaning from IPPV and removing the tracheostomy tube (Drury & Williams 1991). A neurologist was consulted and MSA was diagnosed. Emergency tracheostomy may be required for stridor (Bawa et al 1993).

7. Sleep-related breathing disorders are common and may result in death during sleep (Sadaoka et al 1996).

Management

1. The blood pressure abnormalities can be detected by Shellong's test, in which the blood pressure is taken, first supine, then standing. In the case of severe symptoms, a tilting table should be used.

2. If there is stridor, snoring, or other signs suggestive of laryngeal abductor palsy, endoscopy should be undertaken. Bilateral vocal cord paralysis raises the possibility of multiple system atrophy. Tracheostomy may be the only effective long-term treatment (Bawa et al 1993).

3. Anaesthestic agents with minimal cardiovascular depression should be chosen.

4. Regional anaesthesia has been used, despite the problems with cardiovascular instability. Hip surgery was performed under continuous spinal anaesthesia followed by a 3-in-1 femoral nerve block for postoperative pain relief (Niquille et al 1998). A single shot spinal anaesthetic was used for prostatectomy (Konarzewski & Knorr 1997), and caudal anaesthesia for cystoscopy (Gomesz & Montell 1992). Problems are presumably minimised by the relative systolic hypertension in the supine position. However, precautions should be taken during mobilisation; one patient was unable to stand for 24 h following surgery because of postural hypotension.

5. Hypovolaemia should be corrected promptly.

6. Techniques using spontaneous respiration should probably be avoided.

7. Careful monitoring of blood pressure is essential for the correction of hypotension. Use of elastic bandages applied to the legs reduces vasodilatation.

8. Postoperative observation to detect respiratory insufficiency.

9. Treatment with fludrocortisone may increase extracellular fluid volume (Watson 1987). One patient, bedridden from severe orthostatic hypotension, was given an ambulatory norepinephrine (noradrenaline)

solution at a rate of $30 \, ng \, kg^{-1} \, min^{-1}$ (Kribben et al 1998).

Bibliography

Bawa R, Ramadan HH, Wetmore SJ 1993 Bilateral vocal cord paralysis with Shy–Drager syndrome. Otolaryngology—Head & Neck Surgery 109: 911–14.

Drury PME, Williams EGN 1991 Vocal cord paralysis in the Shy–Drager syndrome. A cause of postoperative respiratory obstruction. Anaesthesia 46: 466–8.

Gomesz FAR, Montell M 1992 Caudal anaesthesia in Shy–Drager syndrome. Anaesthesia 47: 1100.

Kew J, Gross M, Chapman P 1990 Shy–Drager syndrome presenting as isolated paralysis of vocal cord abductors. British Medical Journal 300: 1441.

Konarzewski WH, Knorr C 1997 Spinal anaesthesia and Shy–Drager syndrome. Anaesthesia 52: 1020–1.

Kribben A, Bremer C, Fritschka E et al 1998 Ambulatory infusion of noradrenaline for long-term treatment of Shy–Drager syndrome. Kidney & Blood Pressure Research 21: 70–3.

Malan MD, Crago RR 1979 Anaesthetic considerations in idiopathic orthostatic hypotension and the Shy–Drager syndrome. Canadian Anaesthetists' Society Journal 26: 322–7.

Mathias CJ 1997 Autonomic disorders and their recognition. New England Journal of Medicine 336: 721–4.

Niquille M, Van Gessel E, Gamulin Z 1998 Continuous spinal anesthesia for hip surgery in a patient with Shy–Drager syndrome. Anesthesia & Analgesia 87: 366–9.

Sadaoka T, Kakitsuba N, Fujiwara Y et al 1996 Sleep-related disorders in patients with multiple system atrophy and vocal fold palsy. Sleep 19: 479–84.

Schatz IJ 1996 Farewell to the 'Shy–Drager syndrome'. Annals of Internal Medicine 125: 74–5.

Stirt JA, Frantz RA, Gunz EF et al 1982 Anesthesia, catecholamines and haemodynamics in autonomic dysfunction. Anesthesia & Analgesia 61: 701–4.

Sweeney BP, Jones S, Langford RM 1985 Anaesthesia in dysautonomia: further complications. Anaesthesia 40: 783–6.

Watson RDS 1987 Treating postural hypotension. British Medical Journal 294: 390–1.

Muscular dystrophy (see also under Duchenne, Becker and Emery–Dreifuss muscular dystrophies)

A group of inherited muscle disorders, now known as the dystrophinopathies. The severe Duchenne type, which is the most common, and the less severe Becker type, produce the most serious anaesthetic problems. Precise diagnosis is not always possible, but the other types are not as severe. In general, these other dystrophies do not affect the muscles of respiration or swallowing, and cardiac involvement is less common, except with Emery–Dreifuss. However, sensitivity to curare was reported with ocular muscular dystrophy (Robertson 1984), therefore neuromuscular monitoring is mandatory in these patients.

X-linked

1. Duchenne (severe). In this condition, anaesthesia has been associated with a number of serious and sometimes fatal complications (see Duchenne muscular dystrophy).

2. Becker (mild). Although this dystrophy is less severe than the Duchenne type, anaesthetic deaths associated with acute rhabdomyolysis, hyperkalaemia and hypocalcaemia have been reported (see also Becker muscular dystrophy).

3. Emery–Dreifuss. Flexion of the elbow and shortening of tendo Achilles, limitation of neck flexion, progressive muscle weakness and wasting (humero-peroneal), cardiomyopathy with heart block, and atrial arrhythmias. Although the muscle dystrophy itself is relatively benign, sudden death may occur (see also Emery–Dreifuss muscular dystrophy).

Autosomal recessive

1. Severe type.

2. Mild limb girdle; with facial involvement and without facial involvement. Cardiac abnormalities are present in 10% of patients with limb girdle muscular dystrophy. These include dilated cardiomyopathy and AV conduction defects (van der Kooi et al 1998).

Autosomal dominant

1. Facioscapulohumeral (Landouzy–Dejerine, FSHD) has onset in adolescence, first affecting the shoulders, facial weakness, winging of scapulae, proximal arm wasting. It is slowly progressive. There is an increased incidence of cardiac arrhythmias suggesting that conduction tissue may be involved. Uneventful anaesthesia using atracurium (Dressner et al 1989), and vecuronium (Nitahara et al 1999), showed no increased sensitivity, but more rapid recovery times than normal.

2. Distal.

3. Ocular.

4. Oculopharyngeal (Landrum & Eggers 1992).

Bibliography

Dressner DL, Ali HH 1989 Anaesthetic management of a patient with facioscapulohumeral muscular dystrophy. British Journal of Anaesthesia 62: 331–4.

Emery AE 1998 The muscular dystrophies. British Medical Journal 317: 991–5.

Landrum AL, Eggers GWN 1992 Oculopharyngeal dystrophy: an approach to anesthetic management. Anesthesia & Analgesia 75: 1043–5.

Nitahara K, Sakuragi T, Matsuyama M et al 1999 Response to vecuronium in a patient with facioscapulohumeral muscular dystrophy. British Journal of Anaesthesia 83: 499–500.

Robertson JA 1984 Ocular muscular dystrophy. A cause of curare sensitivity. Anaesthesia 39: 251–3.

van der Kooi AJ, de Voogt WG, Barth PG et al 1998 The heart in limb girdle muscular dystrophy. Heart 79: 73–7.

Myasthenia gravis (MG)

An autoimmune disease of the neuromuscular junction involving the postjunctional acetylcholine receptors. Specific autoantibodies have been identified and microscopic changes in the membrane demonstrated. Not only is there a reduction in the number of acetylcholine receptors at the postjunctional membrane, so that the safety margin is decreased, but also there appears to be a variation in the functional ability of the antibodies to block the receptors. In addition there seem to be two populations of receptors, with half-lives of 12 days and 12 h. Both may be decreased in MG. The condition is characterised by muscle weakness and fatiguability on repeated use of that muscle. Females are more commonly affected than males, in a two to one ratio. There is an association with thymic enlargement and thymomas, both benign and malignant.

Anaesthesia may be required for thymectomy. There is dispute about the approach, which can be transsternal or transcervical.

Preoperative abnormalities

1. Symptoms are primarily those of increasing muscle weakness and neuromuscular fatigue, which improve after resting. Muscles of the eye and face are affected early in the disease, producing ptosis and diplopia. Bulbar palsy may result in swallowing and speech difficulties, and neck muscles may be affected. Sometimes respiratory muscle involvement occurs early. Variable progression or remission may occur. The involvement of particular muscle groups is inconstant, but proximal muscles of the upper limbs are affected more frequently than the lower limbs.

2. Extrathoracic upper airway obstruction has recently been reported in some patients (Putman & Wise 1996). This is thought to be secondary to bulbar and upper airway muscle weakness and can be demonstrated on flow–volume loops.

3. Antibodies against acetylcholine receptors are found in 80–90% of patients with myasthenia gravis.

4. Diagnosis may be confirmed by demonstrating an improvement in weakness within 10–30 s of giving edrophonium iv 2–10 mg. This lasts for about 5 min.

5. Current treatment includes:

a) Immunological suppression to eliminate the antibody. Azathioprine or steroids are used and benefit 90% of cases. This has become the first line of treatment.

b) Thymectomy, increasingly via the transcervical approach.

c) Symptomatic relief with anticholinesterase preparations that potentiate the effects of acetylcholine. Pyridostigmine and neostigmine are most commonly used. Concurrent use of atropine or propantheline may be required to block muscarinic effects, such as intestinal colic.

d) Plasma exchange, for short-term treatment, particularly in a crisis.

Anaesthetic problems

1. *Anaesthesia in the presence of undiagnosed myasthenia.* The myasthenic state is usually unmasked by anaesthesia in which nondepolarising blockers are used. Failure to reverse neuromuscular blockade, or hypoventilation or apnoea in the recovery room, are the commonest modes of presentation (Prior & Swanston 1994, Fraser & Chalkiadis 1995, Haider-Ali et al 1998).

2. *Type of surgery.* Anaesthesia may be required for thymectomy, or for other incidental surgery. Thymectomy is performed either via a median sternotomy or a transcervical approach. The former produces the greater anaesthetic difficulties.

3. *The variables during surgery.* The main problem revolves around the anaesthetist's ability to anticipate and manage three variables:

a) The muscle weakness produced by the patient's disease.

b) The preoperative anticholinesterase medication.

c) The surgeon's requirement for muscle relaxation. Adequate respiratory function must be maintained in the pre- and postoperative period, yet reasonable intraoperative muscle relaxation may be needed for surgical access.

4. *The use of neuromuscular blockers.* Myasthenics may or may not have an increased sensitivity to nondepolarising blockers. Unexpected sensitivity or apnoea may represent the first signs of myasthenia. In one patient with an undiagnosed thymoma, total paralysis after pancuronium 1 mg was associated with a high titre of antiacetylcholine receptor antibodies, but without clinical manifestations of the disease (Enoki et al 1989). A patient with seronegative ocular myasthenia was profoundly sensitivity to only 2 mg of vecuronium (Kim & Mangold 1989). Sensitivity may also occur when the patient is in remission (Lumb & Calder 1989).

The blockade of the acetylcholine receptors by antibody resembles partial curarisation, therefore the amount of a drug required to produce effective paralysis is often reduced. There is, however, wide patient variation in response. The actual amount of drug needed will depend upon factors such as the stage of the disease, the presence or absence of a remission, the actual muscles being tested, and whether or not anticholinesterase medication has been given preoperatively. In addition, the responses of the peripheral and bulbar muscles may be very different, particularly when there is bulbar involvement (Baraka 1992a). Using a cumulative dose plus infusion technique, Eisenkraft et al (1989) found that the ED_{50} and ED_{95} of vecuronium in ten myasthenics was 53% and 56% respectively. Responses to suxamethonium vary widely. Resistance to suxamethonium has been reported (Wainwright & Broderick 1987). However, the use of 1.5 mg kg^{-1} has been reported to give good intubating conditions with recovery in 10–15 min (Baraka & Tabboush 1991). Resistance may not occur if the patient is in remission (Abel et al 1991). Baraka (1992b) studied the plasma cholinesterase in three myasthenic patients about to undergo thymectomy, two of whom were receiving pyridostigmine therapy. He found that the levels correlated with the recovery time from suxamethonium. Both patients treated with pyridostigmine had decreased plasma cholinesterase activity and in these patients there was prolongation of neuromuscular block with suxamethonium.

5. *The use of volatile agents.* These will increase muscle weakness, and isoflurane has twice as potent a depressant effect on neuromuscular transmission in myasthenics as halothane (Nilsson & Muller 1990).

6. *Excess anticholinesterase.* An excessive amount of an anticholinesterase may itself cause increased muscle weakness. This can be confused with weakness from the myasthenia. Experimentally, an excess of anticholinesterase has been shown to reduce the number of functioning receptors. Patients in a cholinergic crisis may require a period of IPPV.

7. *Respiratory dysfunction or prolonged apnoea.* Respiratory muscle or bulbar weakness may occur pre- or postoperatively and can predispose the patient to pulmonary aspiration, chest infection, or respiratory failure. In 125 consecutive patients undergoing transsternal thymectomy, the incidence of postoperative pneumonia was related to the severity of the disease, varying from 0% in class 1 to 44% in class 2 (Machens et al 1998). The development of tracheal stenosis at the site of a previous tracheostomy provided an additional problem in one patient (Froelich & Eagle 1996).

8. *Immunosuppression.* This may lead to neutropenia and serious infection.

Management

1. *Management of neuromuscular blockade.* The method of management depends on the severity of the myasthenia, the type of operation, and the anaesthetist's personal preference. Whilst some surgery can be undertaken using analgesics and inhalational agents, abdominal surgery requires a greater degree of muscle relaxation than can be produced by inhalation agents alone. Reliable neuromuscular monitors and relaxant infusions allow good control to be achieved with minimal doses of a nondepolarising relaxant. Atracurium, in five patients with moderate to severe myasthenia, was found to be 1.7–1.9 times more potent than in normal individuals (Smith et al 1989). The satisfactory use of atracurium in incremental doses has been reported (MacDonald et al 1984, Ward & Wright 1984). While the final doses required to produce 90–95% blockade varied from 0.05 mg kg^{-1} to 0.33 mg kg^{-1}, it was agreed that with atracurium, a relatively rapid rate of spontaneous recovery took place when compared with other relaxants. Sensitivity to vecuronium has been shown, and its degree was related to the titre of acetylcholine receptor antibodies (Nilsson & Meretoja 1990). Vecuronium 0.02–0.04 mg kg^{-1} has been used in six patients for thymectomy, without problems in reversal (Hunter et al 1985). The cumulative dose of mivacurium required to establish full neuromuscular block in four myasthenics varied from 60 to 90 μg kg^{-1} (Paterson et al 1994). Alternatively, if a rapid sequence induction is required, suxamethonium 1.5 mg kg^{-1} will give good intubating conditions.

2. *Techniques without muscle relaxants.* Several techniques have been reported for surgery that required opening the chest. Thoracic epidural anaesthesia was given in combination with light general anaesthesia, and epidural fentanyl allowed early extubation (Burgess & Wilcosky 1989). A thoracic epidural using bupivacaine 0.5% combined with 0.4% isoflurane produced adequate relaxation (Akpolat et al 1997). Intrathecal morphine (10 μg kg^{-1}), given at induction, produced effective analgesia and better postoperative respiratory function when compared with iv morphine (30 μg kg^{-1}) at induction (Nilsson et al 1997). The use of remifentanil and propofol infusions was reported to provide stable anaesthesia and early awakening (Lorimer & Hall 1998). Cardiopulmonary bypass was performed under propofol and fentanyl anaesthesia (Ishimura et al 1998).

3. *Muscle relaxant reversal and anticholinesterases.* Either reversal of muscle relaxants, or restoration of respiration in the myasthenic, may be achieved by the routine use of neostigmine and atropine. However, care must be taken not to give a dose in excess of the patient's normal requirements, otherwise a cholinergic crisis may occur. Equivalent doses are:

Neostigmine iv	1 mg.
Neostigmine oral	30 mg.
Pyridostigmine iv	4 mg.
Pyridostigmine oral	120 mg.

The patient's usual anticholinesterases may have to be given iv until oral medication can be taken.

4. *Postoperative care.* All patients require postoperative high-dependency facilities. Some patients will need postoperative IPPV. The surgical approach to the thymus is still controversial. A transcervical technique is being increasingly used, rather than the more traumatic transsternal route. The cervical approach is associated with a reduced requirement for prolonged postoperative IPPV. Thoracic epidural bupivacaine 0.5% has been used for postoperative analgesia (Akpolat et al 1997). Intrathecal morphine was found to improve ventilatory function compared with PCA morphine and provided adequate analgesia for sternotomy pain (Nilsson et al 1997).

5. *Tracheostomy.* Occasionally tracheostomy may be required, but only if IPPV is prolonged and excess secretions are a problem.

6. *Respiratory failure in myasthenia.* Respiratory failure in myasthenic patients may be secondary to either a myasthenic or a cholinergic crisis. IPPV should be instituted, anticholinesterase therapy stopped, then only cautiously reintroduced after testing with iv edrophonium. An improvement suggests a myasthenic cause; a deterioration indicates a cholinergic crisis. Facilities should be available for the rapid institution of IPPV. Isoflurane sedation has been used for prolonged ventilation in a 3 year old with congenital myasthenia gravis and pneumonia (McBeth & Watkins 1996).

Bibliography

Abel M, Eisenkraft, Patel N 1991 Response to suxamethonium in a myasthenic patient during remission. Anaesthesia 46: 30–2.

Akpolat N, Tilgen H, Gursoy F et al 1997 Thoracic epidural anaesthesia and analgesia with bupivacaine for transsternal thymectomy for myasthenia gravis. European Journal of Anaesthesiology 14: 220–3.

Baraka A 1992a Anaesthesia and myasthenia gravis. Canadian Journal of Anaesthesia 39: 476–86.

Baraka A 1992b Suxamethonium block in the myasthenic patient. Correlation with plasma cholinesterase. Anaesthesia 47: 217–19.

Baraka A, Tabboush Z 1991 Neuromuscular response to succinylcholine-vecuronium sequence in three myasthenic patients undergoing thymectomy. Anesthesia & Analgesia 72: 827–30.

Burgess FW, Wilcosky B 1989 Thoracic epidural anesthesia for transsternal thymectomy in myasthenia gravis. Anesthesia & Analgesia 69: 529–31.

Eisenkraft JB, Book WJ, Papatestas AE et al 1989 Sensitivity to vecuronium in myasthenia gravis: a dose–response study. Anesthesia & Analgesia 68: S80.

Enoki T, Naito Y, Hirokawa Y et al 1989 Marked sensitivity to pancuronium in a patient without clinical manifestations of myasthenia gravis. Anesthesia & Analgesia 69: 840–2.

Fraser RS, Chalkiadis GA 1995 Anaesthesia and undiagnosed myasthenia gravis. Anaesthesia & Intensive Care 23: 114–16.

Froelich J, Eagle CJ 1996 Anaesthetic management of a patient with myasthenia gravis and tracheal stenosis. Canadian Journal of Anaesthesia 43: 84–9.

Haider-Ali AM, MacGregor FB, Stewart M 1998 Myasthenia gravis presenting with dysphagia and postoperative ventilatory failure. Journal of Laryngology & Otology 112: 1194–5.

Hunter JM, Bell CF, Florence AM et al 1985 Vecuronium in the myasthenic patient. Anaesthesia 40: 848–53.

Ishimura H, Sata T, Matsumoto T et al 1998 Anesthetic management of a patient with myasthenia gravis during hypothermic cardiopulmonary bypass. Journal of Clinical Anesthesia 10: 228–31.

Kim J-M, Mangold J 1989 Sensitivity to both vecuronium in a sero-negative myasthenic patient. British Journal of Anaesthesia 63: 497–500.

Lorimer M, Hall R 1998 Remifentanil and total intravenous anaesthesia for thymectomy in myasthenia gravis. Anaesthesia & Intensive Care 26: 210–12.

Lumb AB, Calder I 1989 'Cured' myasthenia gravis and neuromuscular blockade. Anaesthesia 44: 828–30.

McBeth C, Watkins TG 1996 Isoflurane for sedation in a case of congenital myasthenia gravis. British Journal of Anaesthesia 77: 672–4.

MacDonald AM, Keen RI, Pugh ND 1984 Myasthenia gravis and atracurium. British Journal of Anaesthesia 56: 651–4.

Machens A, Emskotter T, Busch C et al 1998 Postoperative infection after transsternal thymectomy for myasthenia gravis: a retrospective analysis of 125 cases. Surgery Today 28: 808–10.

Nilsson E, Meretoja OA 1990 Vecuronium dose–response and maintenance requirements in patients with myasthenia gravis. Anesthesiology 73: 28–32.

Nilsson E, Muller K 1990 Neuromuscular effects of isoflurane in patients with myasthenia gravis. Acta Anaesthesiologica Scandinavica 34: 126–31.

Nilsson E, Perttunen K, Kalso E 1997 Intrathecal morphine for post-sternotomy pain in patients with myasthenia gravis: effects on respiratory function. Acta Anaesthesiologica Scandinavica 41: 549–56.

Paterson IG, Hood JR, Russell SH et al 1994 Mivacurium in the myasthenic patient. British Journal of Anaesthesia 73: 494–8.

Prior AJ, Swanston AR 1994 Myasthenia gravis presenting during general anaesthesia for oesophagoscopy—a cautionary tale. Journal of Laryngology & Otology 108: 599–600.

Putman MT, Wise RA 1996 Myasthenia gravis and upper airway obstruction. Chest 109: 400–4.

Smith CE, Donati F, Bevan DR 1989 Cumulative dose–response curves for atracurium in patients with myasthenia gravis. Canadian Journal of Anaesthesia 36: 402–6.

Wainwright AP, Broderick PM 1987 Suxamethonium in myasthenia gravis. Anaesthesia 42: 950–7.

Ward S, Wright DJ 1984 Neuromuscular blockade in myasthenia gravis with atracurium besylate. Anaesthesia 39: 51–3.

Myasthenic syndrome (see

Eaton–Lambert syndrome)

Myeloma, multiple

This plasma cell neoplasm is one of the paraproteinaemias, the peak incidence of which is in the seventh decade. It erodes bone and infiltrates bone marrow. The diagnosis requires two of the three following criteria: plasma cells in the bone marrow to be >20% of marrow nucleated cells, a paraprotein to be present in the serum and/or urine, and lytic bone lesions.

Preoperative abnormalities

1. Myeloma may present with bone pain, pathological fractures, anaemia, renal disease, or hypercalcaemia. Hypercalcaemia causes drowsiness, vomiting, constipation, dehydration, confusion, and coma. Punched-out lytic lesions may occur anywhere in the skeleton, but are most frequent in the skull, vertebrae, ribs, and long bones. Peripheral neuropathy may occur, or paraplegia may arise from an extradural plasmacytoma or vertebral collapse. A variety of patients have presented with head and neck manifestations (Nofsinger et al 1997).

2. The hyperviscosity syndrome can produce neurological (confusion, vertigo, headaches, fits), ocular (visual disturbances and blindness), haematological (bleeding problems), and cardic failure.

3. There is usually anaemia, a high ESR, excretion of Bence Jones protein in the urine, and abnormal protein electrophoresis. Bone marrow is infiltrated with plasma cells. The diagnosis requires >20% of total marrow nucleated cells.

4. Patients may be taking steroids or a variety of cytotoxic agents. Other treatment includes allogeneic or autologous transplantation, biphosphonates, antioestrogen therapy, and interferon (Gahrton 1999).

5. Renal impairment occurs in 50% of patients during the course of the disease (Alexanian et al 1990), secondary to difficulties in salt and water conservation, to hypercalcaemia or to renal amyloid. In a study of 56 patients

with myeloma and severe renal failure, renal failure was the initial presentation of myeloma in 50% (Irish et al 1997).

Anaesthetic problems

1. Bone involvement may result in rib fracture or vertebral collapse, either spontaneously or with relatively minor trauma.

2. Urgent treatment may be required for spinal cord compression, hyperviscosity, or hypercalcaemia, all of which may be life-threatening. Hypercalcaemia, which results from widespread bone disease, is present in about 30% of cases and may be associated with severe dehydration (see Hypercalcaemia).

3. Renal impairment occurs in almost half of the cases, and actual renal failure in 25%.

4. There is an increased susceptibility to infection as a result of impairment of the normal production of IgG.

5. Thrombocytopenia or coagulopathies occasionally occur.

6. Hyperviscosity may produce vascular and CNS problems, which include headaches, visual disturbances, and retinopathy.

7. A high-output cardiac state may occur and result in cardiac failure. Its occurrence was shown in eight out of 36 patients, and was thought to be related to extensive bone disease.

Management

1. Hb, WCC and platelets should be checked. A coagulation screen should be performed if there is any suggestion of abnormal bleeding.

2. Dehydration should be prevented and early renal impairment should be treated with a high fluid intake.

3. Hypercalcaemia $>3.2\,mmol\,l^{-1}$ is dangerous and requires urgent treatment (see Hypercalcaemia). An infusion of 1 litre of

sodium chloride 0.9% 3–4 hrly for 24 h should reduce the serum calcium by $0.5\,mmol\,l^{-1}$. In patients susceptible to fluid load, CVP monitoring may be required. Biphosphonates, given iv, reduce serum calcium by inhibiting bone resorption. Disodium pamidronate (as a single treatment), disodium etidronate (daily for 5 days) and sodium clodronate (daily for 5 days) are all licenced in the UK.

4. Patients should be moved and positioned with care during anaesthesia, to prevent pathological fractures.

5. Regional anaesthesia should be avoided if a neuropathy or a coagulation abnormality is suspected.

6. Steroid supplements may be required.

Bibliography

Alexanian R, Barlogie B, Dixon D 1990 Renal failure in multiple myeloma. Archives of Internal Medicine 150: 1693–5.
Gahrton G 1999 Treatment of multiple myeloma. Lancet 353: 85–6.
Irish AB, Winearls CG, Littlewood T 1997 Presentation and survival of patients with severe renal failure and myeloma. Quarterly Journal of Medicine 90: 773–80.
McBride W, Jackman JD, Grayburn PA 1990 Prevalence and clinical characteristics of a high output cardiac state in patients with multiple myeloma. American Journal of Medicine 89: 21–4.
Nofsinger YC, Mirza N, Rowan PT et al 1997 Head and neck manifestations of plasma cell neoplasms. Laryngoscope 107: 741–6.

Myoglobinuria (see Rhabdomyolysis)

Myotubular (centronuclear) myopathy

An X-linked, severe myopathy in which survival beyond infancy had initially been thought not to occur. However, three forms are now recognised, one of which results in long-term survival. The form with autosomal dominant inheritance has a later onset and milder course. The condition is so called because on electron microscopy the muscle appearance is that of fetal myotubules (Thompson & Wallgren-Pettersson 1996).

Preoperative abnormalities

1. There are three different forms with different clinical features and prognoses.

2. Those surviving infancy may present in childhood with slowly progressive weakness which can affect extraocular, facial, neck and limb muscles.

3. Those with the X-linked form that survive often develop other medical problems, which suggests that the protein abnormality may not affect muscle alone. In a study of 55 males who survived beyond 1 year, 80% were partially or completely ventilator dependent, four had pyloric stenosis, six had evidence of liver dysfunction, four gallstones, two spherocytosis, and two renal calculi (Herman et al 1999).

4. Presence of central nuclei in biopsy specimens.

Anaesthetic problems

1. The patient may be, or may become, ventilator dependent. Restrictive lung defects or recurrent chest infections can develop.

2. Patients may be extremely sensitive to nondepolarising muscle relaxants. Breslin et al (2000), using a force transducer and myograph in a 53-year-old male, showed a profound decrease in single twitch height and TOF (train-of-four), without any muscle relaxants having been given. Subsequent nerve conduction studies demonstrated normal amplitude and conduction velocity, but electromyography showed small motor units suggesting a mild to moderately severe abnormality, and with a distribution that indicated 'myopathic type' changes.

3. Apnoea following droperidol and fentanyl occurred in one wheelchair-bound patient with sleep apnoea (Gottschalk et al 1998). In a subsequent anaesthetic for arthroplasty for

bilateral ankylosis of the temporomandibular joint, awake fibreoptic intubation was followed by a propofol infusion.

Management

1. Assessment of respiratory function.

2. It may be unnecessary to use muscle relaxants, since Breslin et al (2000) showed the electromyographic responses to be poor.

Bibliography
Breslin D, Reid J, Hayes A et al 2000 Anaesthesia in myotubular (centronuclear) myopathy. Anaesthesia 55: 471–4.

Gottschalk A, Heiman-Patterson T, deQuevedo R et al 1998 General anesthesia for a patient with centronuclear (myotubular) myopathy. Anesthesiology 89: 1018–20.

Herman GE, Finegold M, Zhao W et al 1999 Medical complications in long-term survivors with X-linked myotubular myopathy. Journal of Pediatrics 134: 206–14.

Thomas N, Wallgren-Pettersson C 1996 X-linked myotubular myopathy. Neuromuscular Disorders 6: 129–32.

Myxoedema (see Hypothyroidism)

Myxoma (cardiac)

A benign cardiac tumour, often rapidly growing, that accounts for about one-third of primary intracardiac tumours. It occurs more frequently in females than in males, in a ratio of about 2:1, and in the age range 20–50 years. Myxomas most commonly arise in the left atrium (more than 75%), from the rim of the fossa ovalis, and are usually pedunculated; 20–25% originate in the right atrium; the ventricle is rarely involved. Symptoms are protean and myxomas mimic other, much more common, diseases, including infective, immunological and malignant processes (Reynen 1996). The tumour may cause intracardiac obstruction, valvular dysfunction, or emboli of thrombotic or myxomatous tissue.

Syncope may occur as a result of sudden obstruction to intracardiac blood flow and its effects may be life threatening. Diagnosis by clinical means alone is difficult, but the advent of echocardiography (including transoesophageal used during surgery) has increased the rate of diagnosis (Hodgins et al 1995).

Preoperative abnormalities

1. Dyspnoea is the commonest symptom, followed by constitutional disturbances, embolisation, palpitations, syncope, oedema of the legs, and chest pain. Intracardiac obstruction may produce pulmonary oedema or right heart failure. Cardiac failure was the commonest presenting feature in one series and occurred in 24 out of 33 cases (Hanson et al 1985). Obstruction may be positional in nature and can also cause syncope or sudden death.

2. Almost all are attached to the interatrial septum. The pedunculated tumour may move through the mitral valve during diastole; there may be intermittent signs of mitral valve disease, of sudden onset, again sometimes positionally related.

3. Tachyarrhythmias, such as atrial fibrillation, may be the presenting sign.

4. Hypoxaemia, which may also be positional, can occur secondary to low cardiac output, a right to left shunt, or tumour embolisation.

5. Systemic embolisation of myxomatous material, or thrombi from the tumour surface, occurs in about one-third of patients, most commonly to the cerebral or coronary vessels, but also to the legs. Pulmonary emboli can originate from right-sided lesions (Bitner et al 1998).

6. Pulmonary hypertension may occur with left-sided lesions.

7. A proportion of patients have systemic, constitutional symptoms, such as fever, anaemia, raised ESR, and hyperglobulinaemia. Infected

cardiac myxomas may occur rarely (Revankar & Clark 1998).

8. The possibility that myxomas can produce hormones or vasoactive substances has been suggested (Johns et al 1988). High levels of VIP, a potent vasodilator, were found in one atrial myxoma.

9. An augmented first heart sound is common and apical pansystolic and early diastolic sounds are often present. However, both auscultatory and CXR findings are, in general, unhelpful in making the diagnosis.

10. Investigations include echocardiography (which is now the method of choice), cardiac catheterisation, or MRI.

Anaesthetic problems

1. Sudden cardiovascular collapse. Ventricular filling may be compromised by outflow obstruction. Cardiovascular collapse occurred on induction of anaesthesia in one patient who had a right atrial myxoma (Moritz & Azad 1989), and in another with a right ventricular myxoma (Lebovic et al 1991). Hypotension occurred in one patient undergoing surgery for popliteal artery occlusion, and transoesophageal echocardiography, performed to examine the patient's left ventricular function, showed a mobile mass in the left atrium (Brooker et al 1995). Chest pain and cardiorespiratory arrest, immediately after emergency orthopaedic surgery, was caused by a large atrial myxoma attached to the septum (Asai et al 1999). Fragmentation and embolisation of part of a right atrial myxoma resulted in circulatory arrest during laparotomy for pain in a 17 year old (Bitner et al 1998). Fatal pulmonary embolism was precipitated during manipulation of a transoesophageal echocardiography probe (Cavero et al 1998). However, even patients with large tumours may be asymptomatic. Three uneventful anaesthetics occurred in a woman subsequently found to have a large atrial myxoma (Carr et al 1988). The absence of problems was attributed to the fact that the

patient was in the Trendeleburg position. However, rapid growth of a myxoma over 8 months has been shown (Rodaut et al 1987), so it might not necessarily have been present at previous surgery.

2. Surgery may cause conduction defects, particularly complete heart block.

3. Valvular dysfunction.

4. A tachycardia in the presence of a large atrial myxoma may increase both the pressure gradient across the mitral valve and the pulmonary artery pressure.

5. If a right atrial myxoma is present, pulmonary artery catheterisation may be contraindicated. Tumour embolisation, or passage of the catheter through a right-to-left shunt may occur.

6. Supraventricular arrhythmias may occur during anaesthesia (Carr et al 1988), and have been reported in the postoperative period in up to 70% of cases.

Management

1. Diagnosis may be made with 2-D echocardiography, cardiac catheterisation, or MRI. Two cases were diagnosed intraoperatively by transoesophageal echocardiography (Brooker et al 1995, Swenson & Bailey 1995). This procedure, however, is not entirely without complication, since fragmentation of the myxoma mass, producing a fatal pulmonary embolism, has been reported during attempts at oesophageal intubation (Cavero et al 1998).

2. If atrial fibrillation is present, the ventricular response should be controlled.

3. If there is positional dyspnoea, give oxygen.

4. The haemodynamic management depends upon the location of the tumour. In the presence of a left atrial myxoma, a tachycardia must be avoided, the rate of AF controlled, preload should be maintained, and vasodilators used

cautiously (Moritz & Azad 1989). Anaesthesia for lung biopsy in the presence of a large right atrial myxoma, which extended into the right ventricle, has been described (Kay & Koch 1989). The trachea was intubated whilst the patient was awake, and the effect of IPPV tested before anaesthesia was induced. Maintenance was with ketamine, pancuronium, and nitrous oxide.

Bibliography

Asai Y, Ichimura K, Kaneko M et al 1999 Treatment of life-threatening huge atrial myxoma: report of two cases. Surgery Today 29: 813–16.

Bitner M, Jaszewsaki R, Wojtasik L et al 1998 Unusual course of right atrial myxoma, masked by acute abdominal pain, and complicated by pulmonary embolus. Scandinavian Cardiovascular Journal 32: 371–3.

Brooker RF, Butterworth JF, Klopfenstein HS 1995 Intraoperative diagnosis of left atrial myxoma. Anesthesia & Analgesia 80: 183–4.

Carr CME, Waller DA, Ettles DF 1988 Repeated general anaesthetics in the presence of a large undiagnosed left atrial myxoma. Anaesthesia 43: 1058.

Cavero MA, Cristobal C, Gonzalez M et al 1998 Fatal pulmonary embolization of a right atrial mass during transesophageal echocardiography. Journal of the American Society of Echocardiography 11: 397–8.

Hanson EC, Gill CC, Razavi M et al 1985 The surgical treatment of atrial myxomas. Journal of Thoracic and Cardiovascular Surgery 89: 298–303.

Hodgins L, Kisslo JA, Mark JB 1995 Perioperative transesophageal echocardiography: the anesthesiologist as cardiac diagnostician. Anesthesia & Analgesia 80: 4–6.

Johns RA, Kron OL, Carey RM et al 1988 Atrial myxoma: case report, brief review, and recommendations for anesthestic management. Journal of Cardiothoracic Anesthesia 2: 207–12.

Kay J, Koch J-P 1989 Anesthesia for open lung biopsy in a patient with intracardiac tumour. Anesthesiology 71: 607–10.

Lebovic S, Koorn R, Reich DL 1991 Role of two-dimensional transoesophageal echocardiography in the management of a right ventricular tumour. Canadian Journal of Anaesthesia 38: 1050–4.

Moritz HA, Azad SS 1989 Right atrial myxoma: case report and anaesthetic considerations. Canadian Journal of Anaesthesia 36: 212–14.

Revankar SG, Clark RA 1998 Infected cardiac myxoma. Case report and literature review. Medicine 77: 337–44.

Reynen K 1996 Cardiac myxomas. New England Journal of Medicine 333: 1610–17.

Roudaut R, Gosse P, Dallocchio M 1987 Rapid growth of a left atrial myxoma shown by echocardiography. British Heart Journal 58: 413–16.

Swenson JD, Bailey PL 1995 The intraoperative diagnosis of atrial myxoma by transesophageal echocardiography. Anesthesia & Analgesia 80: 180–2.

Myxoma (cardiac)

Nemaline myopathy

An autosomal dominant, congenital myopathy associated with the presence in skeletal muscle of rod-like structures, composed, in part, of alpha-actinin. Recent linkage studies have assigned the gene for nemaline rod myopathy to chromosome 1 (Laing et al 1992). The condition affects all skeletal muscle, including the diaphragm.

Preoperative abnormalities

1. Weakness, hypotonia, and abnormal gait presenting in early childhood.

2. Swallowing difficulty, aspiration of food, and weakness of respiratory muscles.

3. Skeletal abnormalities, including scoliosis, dislocation of the hips, pes cavus, and pectus excavatum.

4. Micrognathia, hypertelorism, and high arched palate.

5. Cardiac abnormalities, including septal defects, aortic regurgitation, and patent ductus arteriosus.

6. Increased serum CK, serum aldolase and LDH levels.

Anaesthetic problems

1. Possible difficulties in tracheal intubation. A pregnant patient undergoing general anaesthesia had a failed intubation, copious secretions, and atelectasis (Stackhouse et al 1994).

2. Patients are prone to pulmonary aspiration.

3. Recurrent respiratory infections and poor pulmonary reserve. Lung complications are the most frequent cause of death. In some patients, the onset of respiratory insufficiency is the first sign of the disease (Falga-Tirado et al 1995, Sasaki et al 1997).

4. Bradycardias on tracheal intubation were described in three patients undergoing cardiac surgery (Asai et al 1992). Mild temperature increases were also reported.

5. Abnormal resistance to suxamethonium has been demonstrated on a chart recorder, although there was no difficulty with tracheal intubation (Heard & Kaplan 1983).

6. In the presence of scoliosis secondary to muscle weakness, technical difficulties may be experienced during regional anaesthesia (Wallgren-Pettersson et al 1995).

Management

1. It has been suggested that neuromuscular blocking agents should be avoided, if possible (Cunliffe & Burrows 1985). However, their uneventful use has also been reported (Heard & Kaplan 1983, Asai et al 1992).

2. Atropine should be available to treat bradycardia.

3. After major surgery, particularly for cardiac lesions, IPPV may be required. Chest infections should be treated vigorously.

4. Elective Caesarean section under epidural anaesthesia has been described in a 28 year old with contractures, severe muscle weakness, scoliosis, and micrognathia. Insertion of the needle at an angle of 20 degrees towards the concave side of the scoliosis resulted in a successful block (Wallgren-Pettersson et al 1995).

Bibliography

Asai T, Fujise K, Uchida M 1992 Anaesthesia for cardiac surgery in children with nemaline myopathy. Anaesthesia 47: 405–8.

Cunliffe M, Burrows FA 1985 Anaesthetic implications of nemaline rod myopathy. Canadian Anaesthetists' Society Journal 32: 543–7.

Falga-Tirado C, Perez-Peman P, Ordi-Ros J et al 1995 Adult onset nemaline myopathy as respiratory insufficiency. Respiration 62: 353–4.

Heard SO, Kaplan RF 1986 Neuromuscular blockade in a patient with nemaline myopathy. Anesthesiology 59: 588.

Laing NG, Majda BT, Akkari PA et al 1992
Assignment of a gene (NEMI) for autosomal
dominant nemaline myopathy to chromosome 1.
American Journal of Human Genetics 50: 576–83.

Sasaki M, Takeda M, Kobayashi K et al 1997
Respiratory failure in nemaline myopathy. Pediatric
Neurology 16: 344–6.

Stackhouse R, Chelmow D, Dattel BJ 1994 Anesthetic
complications in a pregnant patient with nemaline
myopathy. Anesthesia & Analgesia 79: 1195–7.

Wallgren-Pettersson C, Hiilesmaa VK, Paatero H 1995
Pregnancy and delivery in congenital nemaline
myopathy. Acta Obstetrica et Gynecologica
Scandinavica 74: 659–61.

Neurofibromatosis (NF type 1 and NF type 2)

A term for at least two separate autosomal dominant inherited conditions, associated with the occurrence of neurofibromas, but involving genes on different chromosomes. Neurofibromatosis 1 (NF-1, formerly known as von Recklinghausen's disease), which accounts for 90% of cases, is localised on chromosome 17, and neurofibromatosis 2 (NF-2) to chromosome 22 (Gutmann et al 1997). There are now strict criteria for the diagnosis of each, and this is important because of the differences in prognosis. Neurofibromas may occur anywhere in the body and can cause a variety of symptoms. A wide spectrum of associated abnormalities has been described. The condition is progressive and the effects vary from mild to severe. There is an increased incidence of malignancies. The exact aetiology of the condition is unknown, but the abnormalities may originate from neural crest defects.

Preoperative abnormalities

1. The major features are the cafe au lait spots, the peripheral neurofibromas, and the Lisch nodules. Short stature and macrocephaly may also occur. There is now consensus on the diagnostic criteria for each condition.

2. For *neurofibromatosis-1* (NF-1) there should be two or more of the following:

a) Cafe au lait spots, at least six, having one diameter of more than 1.5 cm in adults, or 5 mm before puberty, should be present.

b) Freckling in the inguinal or axillary regions.

c) Two or more neurofibromas or one plexiform neurofibroma.

d) Optic glioma.

e) Two or more iris hamartomas (Lisch nodules).

f) A distinctive osseous lesion, such as sphenoid dysplasia or thinning of long bone cortex with or without pseudoarthrosis.

g) A first degree relative who fulfils the same criteria for NF-1.

3. The complications of NF-1 can affect any system in the body:

a) Nervous system. In a recent series, 55% of 158 cases of NF-1 had some neurological involvement (Creange et al 1999). Neurofibromas may appear in the vertebral foramina and cause dumbell tumours. Cerebral tumours such as optic path gliomas and meningiomas occur in 5–15% of patients with NF-1. There is some intellectual impairment in 40% of cases, 2–5% of patients have frank mental retardation, and epilepsy is common. MRI is now used for localising nervous system lesions. Pain is the leading symptom in adults and was related to neurofibromas and malignant nerve sheath tumours.

b) Pulmonary: an associated fibrosing alveolitis may occur in up to 20% of cases.

c) Skeletal: kyphoscoliosis develops in 2% of patients and bone sarcoma can occur. Pseudoarthrosis of the tibia and fibula.

d) Endocrine: phaeochromocytomas are present in up to 1% of patients and medullary thyroid carcinomas have been described.

e) Renal: there may be renal artery stenosis and hypertension.

f) Airway: oral and upper airway tumours have been reported.

4. For *neurofibromatosis-2* (NF-2) there are:

a) Bilateral VIII nerve masses on imaging, or

b) A first degree relative with the condition, and either a unilateral VIII nerve mass, or

c) Two of the following: neurofibroma, meningioma, glioma, schwannoma or acoustic neuromas, a juvenile posterior subcapsular lens opacity.

5. In a study of 150 patients with NF-2, the mean age of onset was 21 years. Patients presented with symptoms of vestibular schwannomas, cranial meningiomas, and spinal tumours (Evans et al 1993). The mean age of death was 36 years and all but one died from a complication of the disease.

6. The complications of NF-2 depend on the progression of the acoustic neuroma. In a rapidly progressive lesion, deafness may proceed to cerebellar ataxia, visual disturbances, and eventually death from brainstem compression.

Anaesthetic problems

1. Airway difficulties can occur with neurofibromas in the neck or upper respiratory tract. Seven children between 2 months and 13 years old presented with stridor secondary to neural tumours of the larynx and required partial laryngectomy (Garabedian et al 1999). Failed awake fibreoptic intubation occurred in a patient with a giant malignant schwannoma of the neck that was obstructing the pharynx and compromising respiration. A tracheostomy under local anaesthesia was performed (Wulf et al 1997). A laryngeal tumour caused difficulty during laryngoscopy in a 13-year-old boy (Fisher 1975). Tracheostomy was required for a benign tumour that deformed the right half of the larynx and extended into the neck (Czinger & Fekete-Szabo 1994). Such tumours are very

rare. Emergency cricothyroidotomy had to be performed in one patient, whose lungs could not be ventilated after induction of anaesthesia for stabilisation of a mandibular fracture (Crozier 1987). Subsequently a large neurofibroma of the tongue was removed. Oral lesions are said to be present in 5% of cases (Baden et al 1955, Gutteridge 1991).

2. Regional anaesthesia is contraindicated in the presence of spinal tumours. Difficulty in performing a spinal block, thought to be secondary to the presence of a neurofibroma in the needle path, has been reported (Fisher 1975).

3. If kyphoscoliosis and pulmonary disease coexist, they may contribute to postoperative respiratory complications.

4. There is a 10-fold higher incidence of phaeochromocytoma than in the normal population, so signs of this should be sought, particularly if hypertension is also present. In a study of 18 patients with both conditions, phaeochromocytomas were all associated with the adrenal glands, and each secreted both epinephrine (adrenaline) and norepinephrine (noradrenaline). Convulsions, cardiovascular collapse and death occurred in late pregnancy in a patient with neurofibromatosis who, at autopsy, was found to have a phaeochromocytoma (Harper et al 1989).

5. Vasculopathy is a less well recognised complication and is probably related to structural abnormalities of the vessel wall. Spontaneous haemothorax has resulted in sudden deaths (Miura et al 1997, Griffiths et al 1998), and subclavian and intercostal vessels rupture most commonly.

6. Pregnancy is likely to be complicated by hypertensive disorders and fetal outcome is poor (Sharma et al 1991). There is a higher than normal Caesarean section and stillbirth rate (Segal et al 1999). Maternal arterial rupture can occur. Rupture of a pancreaticoduodenal artery (Serleth et al 1998), and a brachial artery (Tidwell & Copas 1998), have been reported.

7. Cervical spine involvement may result in

instability. An asymptomatic, grossly unstable dislocation at C4–5 was found 2 days after hand surgery using a laryngeal mask airway in a 16 year old. Previous laminectomy and fusion of C5–T1 had been performed for multiple cervical neurofibromatosis (Lovell et al 1994). The patient remembered hearing a loud crack in his neck followed by clicking, a couple of weeks before his hand surgery. The absence of pain was attributed to damage to the nerve supply by the neuromas.

8. A small number of patients have had prolonged neuromuscular blockade from neuromuscular blocking agents (Nagao et al 1983, Baraka 1974). However, normal responses have also been shown (McCarthy et al 1990, Richardson et al 1996).

9. Obstructive hydrocephalus occasionally occurs, as a result of aqueduct stenosis. A 21 year old had a seizure 12 h after removal of a large neurofibroma of the neck, following which his pupils became fixed and dilated. A CT scan showed severe obstructive hydrocephalus and transtentorial herniation. Despite ventriculostomy he died. A diagnosis of aqueduct stenosis was made and the acute increase in intracranial pressure was attributed to his convulsion (Pivalizza et al 2000). Decompression surgery for hydrocephalus resulted in airway obstruction from inability of the patient to control his airway when asleep. This was attributed to changes in brainstem position caused by the surgery, and eventually a tracheostomy had to be performed (Davidson et al 1997).

Management

1. Careful preoperative assessment is essential, with particular attention being paid to mouth and airway lesions, chest, and neurological complications.

2. If phaeochromocytoma is suspected, urinary catecholamine estimation should be performed.

3. Neuromuscular monitoring is essential.

4. In patients with NF-2 undergoing schwannoma surgery, it has been suggested that a spinal scan be done to exclude an asymptomatic spinal tumour (Evans et al 1993). Surgery for NF-2 is very specialised and should be limited to a few centres (Evans et al 1993).

5. There is no contraindication to pregnancy and no evidence that it worsens the disease, but Caesarean section may be required. However, antenatal assessment should be undertaken in a tertiary centre (Segal et al 1999).

Bibliography

Baden E, Pierce HE, Jackson WF 1955 Multiple neurofibromatosis with oral lesions; review of the literature. Oral Surgery 8: 263–80.

Baraka A 1974 Myasthenic response to muscle relaxants in von Recklinghausen's disease. British Journal of Anaesthesia 46: 701–3.

Creange A, Zeller J, Rostaing-Rigattieri S et al 1999 Neurological complications of neurofibromatosis type 1 in adulthood. Brain 122: 473–81.

Crozier WC 1987 Upper airway obstruction in neurofibromatosis. Anaesthesia 42: 1209–11.

Czinger J, Fekete-Szabo G 1994 Neurofibroma of the supraglottic larynx in childhood. Journal of Laryngology & Otology 108: 156–8.

Davidson E, Minkowitz HS, Abramson DC 1997 Airway obstruction after ventriculoperitoneal shunt insertion in a patient with neurofibromatosis. Anesthesia & Analgesia 84: 223–4.

Evans DG, Ramsden R, Huson SM et al 1993 Type 2 neurofibromatosis: the need for supraregional care? Journal of Laryngology & Otology 107: 401–6.

Fisher M McD 1975 Anaesthetic difficulties in neurofibromatosis. Anaesthesia 30: 648–50.

Garabedian EN, Ducroz V, Ayache D et al 1999 Results of partial laryngectomy for benign neural tumors of the larynx in children. Archives of Otolaryngology– Head & Neck Surgery 108: 666–71.

Griffiths AP, White J, Dawson A 1998 Spontaneous haemothorax: a cause of sudden death in von Recklinghausen's disease. Postgraduate Medical Journal 74: 679–81.

Gutmann DH, Aylsworth A, Carey JC et al 1997 The diagnostic evaluation and multidisciplinary management of neurofibromatosis 1 and neurofibromatosis 2. Journal of the American Medical Association 278: 51–7.

Gutteridge DL 1991 Neurofibromatosis: an unusual oral manifestation. British Dental Journal 170: 303–4.

Harper MA, Murnaghan GA, Kennedy L et al 1989 Phaeochromocytoma in pregnancy. Five cases and a review of the literature. British Journal of Obstetrics & Gynaecology 96: 594–606.

Lovell AT, Alexander R, Grundy EM 1994 Silent, unstable cervical spine injury in multiple neurofibromatosis. Anaesthesia 49: 453–4.

McCarthy GJ, McLoughlin C, Mirakhur RK 1990 Neuromuscular blockade in von Recklinghausen's disease. Anaesthesia 45: 340–1.

Miura H, Taira O, Uchida O et al 1997 Spontaneous haemothorax associated with von Recklinhausen's disease: review of occurrence in Japan. Thorax 52: 577–8.

Miyamoto RT, Campbell RL, Roos KL et al 1991 Contemporary management of neurofibromatosis. Annals of Otology, Rhinology & Laryngology 100: 38–43.

Nagao H, Yamashita M, Shinozaki Y et al 1983 Hypersensitivity to pancuronium in a patient with von Recklinghausen's disease. British Journal of Anaesthesia 55: 253.

Pivalizza EG, Rabb MF, Johnson S 2000 Fatal hydrocephalus in a patient with neurofibromatosis. Anesthesiology 92: 630.

Richardson MG, Setty GK, Rawoof SA 1996 Responses to nondepolarizing neuromuscular blockers and succinylcholine in von Recklinghausen neurofibromatosis. Anesthesia & Analgesia 82: 382–5.

Segal D, Holcberg G, Sapir O et al 1999 Neurofibromatosis in pregnancy. Maternal and perinatal outcome. European Journal of Obstetrics, Gynecology, & Reproductive Biology 84: 59–61.

Serleth HJ, Cogbill TH, Gundersen SB 3rd 1998 Ruptured pancreaticoduodenal artery aneurysms and pheochromocytoma in a pregnant patient with neurofibromatosis. Surgery 124: 100–2.

Sharma JB, Gulati N, Malik S 1991 Maternal and perinatal complications in neurofibromatosis during pregnancy. International Journal of Gynecology & Obstetrics 34: 221–7.

Tidwell C, Copas P 1998 Brachial artery rupture complicating a pregnancy with neurofibromatosis. American Journal of Obstetrics & Gynecology 179: 832–4.

Wulf H, Brinkmann G, Rautenberg M 1997 Management of the difficult airway. A case of failed fibreoptic intubation. Acta Anaesthesiologica Scandinavica 41: 1080–2.

Neurogenic pulmonary oedema

(see Pulmonary oedema)

Neuroleptic malignant syndrome (NMS)

A rare, but serious, idiosyncratic complication of treatment with neuroleptic drugs, characterised by the development of catatonic, extrapyramidal and autonomic effects. Its aetiology is unknown, but appears to be related to the antidopaminergic activity of the precipitating drug on dopamine receptors in the striatum and hypothalamus. Its occurrence in a patient after treatment with a tricyclic antidepressant has led to a suggestion that the syndrome involves a central imbalance between norepinephrine (noradrenaline) and dopamine, rather than dopamine depletion alone (Baca & Martinelli 1990). Brain-damaged individuals are thought to be more susceptible to NMS (Turk & Lask 1991). Its occurrence in Parkinsonian patients after L-Dopa withdrawal (Gibb 1988), and its spontaneous appearance in a patient with Hallervorden–Spatz disease (Hayashi et al 1993), both of which disorders involve the striatonigral systems of the basal ganglia, is of interest. Permanent cerebellar damage was evident in one patient following a severe episode of NMS (Lal et al 1997).

Clinical features include hyperthermia, muscle rigidity, sympathetic overactivity, and a variable conscious level. A mortality of 20% has been reported (Caroff et al 1983). The concept that NMS is related to anaesthetic-induced malignant hyperthermia was supported in some quarters (Caroff et al 1983, Denborough et al 1985), but most now agree that, despite the superficial clinical similarities, MH and NMS are two distinct and unrelated entities. When the criteria of the European MH Group for muscle testing were applied to six NMS survivors, five were found to be normal and one was equivocal (Krivosic-Horber et al 1987). In addition, a retrospective study of 20 patients with NMS suggested no cross vulnerability (Hermesh et al

1989). A patient with severe asthma, unresponsive to conventional treatment and IPPV, developed hyperthermia and rhabdomyolysis following treatment with halothane. The problem resolved on stopping the halothane. Eight days later he developed severe NMS following droperidol, which responded to dantrolene. Unfortunately, no MH contracture test was performed, so the diagnosis remained unresolved (Portel et al 1999).

Presentation

1. Haloperidol and fluphenazine are the drugs most frequently reported as being associated with NMS. Others include chlorpromazine, trifluoperazine, droperidol, thioridazine, thiapride, and metoclopramide. In most cases these drugs have been given for a variety of psychiatric disorders. Some of them have long elimination times and are tightly protein bound (Gaitini et al 1997). NMS has also occurred with tetrabenazine, desipramine, a tricyclic antidepressant, and after stopping treatment with levodopa in a patient with striatonigral degeneration (Gibb 1988). The condition may occur within hours of starting the drug, or after some months of treatment. Concurrent lithium therapy may facilitate its development. The episode may occur after normal doses, but sometimes after an overdose of the drug.

2. NMS may present in association with drugs given during the perioperative period. A probable case has been described in which a young man was given normal doses of droperidol and metoclopramide (Patel & Bristow 1987). A 6 year old given droperidol 2.5 mg as premedication and metoclopramide 2.5 mg for nausea developed signs of NMS. Her CK was 28 000 iu l^{-1} and she had myoglobinuria and hyponatraemia. Hyponatraemia could have been associated with infusions of dextrose 5% which were given for 48 h (Shaw & Matthews 1995). Another patient developed NMS while receiving chlorpromazine suppositories when he was undergoing IPPV on the ITU (Montgomery and Ironside 1990). A schizophrenic who took an overdose of cyclizine and perphenazine was admitted with hyperthermia, thrombocytopenia, coagulopathy, and rhabdomyolysis, which rapidly progressed to renal failure and death (Lenler-Petersen et al 1990).

3. Hyponatraemia may precipitate NMS (Shaw & Matthews 1995, Sechi et al 1996).

4. Clinical features include catatonia, hyperthermia, sweating, stupor, tremor, muscle rigidity, akinesia, autonomic dysfunction, incontinence, and renal failure.

5. Rhabdomyolysis may occur. The CK is usually increased and levels in excess of 10 000 iu l^{-1} have been reported. LFTs may be abnormal and leucocytosis often occurs.

6. In cases in which muscle biopsy has been performed, areas of necrosis and hypercontraction have been seen, but with muscle fibres of normal size and normal fibre type distribution (Montgomery & Ironside 1990).

7. It has been suggested that patients with Parkinson's disease are more susceptible to neuroleptic malignant syndrome, and that the susceptibility is in direct relationship to the severity of the disease (Ueda et al 1999).

Management

1. The relevant medication is discontinued.

2. The patient is cooled, rehydrated, and acidosis or electrolyte imbalance corrected (Bristow & Kohen 1993). In one patient, correction of hyponatraemia was associated with complete recovery of an NMS episode within 6 h.

3. The role of specific drugs in the management is controversial. There have been a large number of individual case reports recommending the use of dantrolene sodium and bromocriptine to accelerate recovery. Dantrolene sodium, 50 mg qds for 5 days and

bromocriptine mesylate, 5 mg tds increasing to 10 mg tds, are typical regimens recommended to treat NMS (Mueller et al 1983). In one patient who had failed to respond to small doses, larger doses were given for a further 10 days (Tsujimoto et al 1998). However, there have been dissenting voices. Rosebush et al (1991) claimed that there was no evidence that dantrolene or bromocriptine were useful, and even suggested that they might prolong the course of the illness and increase the likelihood of sequelae. They prospectively studied 20 patients with their first episode of NMS, some of whom were treated with dantrolene, bromocriptine, or both. However, the treatments were not randomised and depended on the individual physician's familiarity with the literature. Resolution of the issue must await a properly controlled trial.

4.   In severe cases, IPPV, fluid replacement and intensive care facilities will be required. Neuromuscular blocking agents abolish the rigidity associated with NMS (Prager et al 1994). Plasmapheresis was claimed to have arrested the syndrome in a patient unresponsive to other treatment. However, a week later he bled from a duodenal ulcer and ultimately died from surgery (Gaitini et al 1997).

5.   Whether or not a survivor of NMS who requires an anaesthetic should be treated as MH susceptible is arguable. Two papers have reported positive MH testing in NMS survivors (Denborough et al 1985, Caroff et al 1987), whereas two others could not confirm any association between the two conditions (Krivosic-Horber et al 1987, Hermesh et al 1989).

Bibliography

Baca L, Martinelli L 1990 Neuroleptic malignant syndrome: a unique association with a tricyclic antidepressant. Neurology 40: 1797–8.

Bristow MF, Kohen D 1993 How 'malignant' is the neuroleptic malignant syndrome? British Medical Journal 307: 1223–4.

Caroff S, Rosenberg H, Gerber JC 1983 Neuroleptic malignant syndrome and malignant hyperpyrexia. Lancet i: 244.

Caroff SN, Rosenberg H, Fletcher JE et al 1987 Malignant hyperthermia susceptibility in neuroleptic malignant syndrome. Anesthesiology 67: 20–5.

Denborough MA, Collins SP, Hopkinson KC 1985 Rhabdomyolysis and malignant hyperpyrexia. British Medical Journal 288: 1878–9.

Gaitini L, Fradis M, Vaida S et al 1997 Plasmapheresis in neuroleptic malignant syndrome. Anaesthesia 52: 165–8.

Gibb WRG 1988 Neuroleptic malignant syndrome in striatonigral degeneration. British Journal of Psychiatry 153: 254–5.

Hayashi K, Chihara E, Sawa T et al 1993 Clinical features of neuroleptic syndrome in basal ganglia disease. Spontaneous presentation in a patient with Hallervorden–Spatz syndrome in the absence of neuroleptic drugs. Anaesthesia 48: 499–502.

Hermesh H, Aizenberg D, Lapidot M et al 1989 The relationship between malignant hyperthermia and neuroleptic malignant syndrome. Anesthesiology 70: 171.

Krivosic-Horber R, Adnet P, Guevart E et al 1987 Neuroleptic malignant syndrome and malignant hyperthermia. British Journal of Anaesthesia 59: 1554–6.

Lal V, Sardana V, Thussu A et al 1997 Cerebellar degeneration following neuroleptic malignant syndrome. Postgraduate Medical Journal 73: 735–6.

Lenler-Petersen P, Hansen BD, Hasselstrom L 1990 A rapidly progressing case of neuroleptic malignant syndrome. Intensive Care Medicine 16: 267–8.

Montgomery JN, Ironside JW 1990 Neuroleptic malignant syndrome in the intensive care unit. Anaesthesia 45: 311–13.

Mueller PS, Vester JW, Fermaglich J 1983 Neuroleptic malignant syndrome: successful treatment with bromocriptine. Journal of the American Medical Association 249: 386–8.

Patel P, Bristow G 1988 Postoperative neuroleptic malignant syndrome. A case report. Canadian Journal of Anaesthesia 34: 515–18.

Portel L, Hilbert G, Gruson D et al 1999 Malignant hyperthermia and neuroleptic malignant syndrome in a patient during treatment for acute asthma. Acta Anaesthesiologica Scandinavica 43: 107–10.

Prager LM, Millham FH, Stern TA 1994 Neuroleptic malignant syndrome: a review for intensivists. Journal of Intensive Care Medicine.

Rosebush PI, Stewart T, Mazurek MF 1991 The treatment of neuroleptic malignant syndrome. Are dantrolene and bromocriptine useful adjuncts to supportive care? British Journal of Psychiatry 159: 709–12.

Sechi G, Manca S, Deiana GA et al 1996 Acute hyponatremia and neuroleptic malignant syndrome in Parkinson's disease. Progress in Neuro-Psychopharmacology & Biological Psychiatry 20: 533–42.

Shaw A, Matthews EE 1995 Postoperative neuroleptic malignant syndrome. Anaesthesia 50: 246–7.

Tsujimoto S, Maeda K, Sugiyama T et al 1998 Efficacy of prolonged large-dose dantrolene for severe neuroleptic malignant syndrome. Anesthesia & Analgesia 86: 1143–4.

Turk J, Lask B 1991 Neuroleptic malignant syndrome. Archives of Disease in Childhood 66: 91–2.

Ueda M, Hamamoto M, Nagayama H et al 1999 Susceptibility to neuroleptic malignant syndrome. Neurology 52: 777–81.

Noonan's syndrome

A hereditary condition, inherited as autosomal dominant, that is similar to Turner's syndrome. However, it affects both males and females, and chromosomes are normal. It is associated with characteristic facial features. The child is usually mentally retarded and under height and weight for age. Right-sided cardiac lesions predominate, most commonly pulmonary stenosis, with or without septal defects, and some patients have either a hypertrophic or restrictive cardiomyopathy. Musculoskeletal abnormalities are common. Undescended testis occurs in 77% of males. Anaesthesia may be required for orchidopexy, orthopaedic abnormalities, cardiac investigation, or corrective cardiac surgery. There is increasing evidence that Noonan's syndrome and cardio-facio-cutaneous syndrome are variable manifestations of the same entity.

Preoperative abnormalities

1. Abnormal facies are present in 100% of patients. Features include hypertelorism, high arched eyebrows, downward slanting palpebral fissures, low set ears, and short stature. Severe ptosis is present in 42%, webbing of the neck in 23%, and dental malocclusion is common.

2. Failure to thrive, a high incidence of gastro-oesophageal reflux, and poor gut motility, which improves with age (Shah et al 1999).

3. Cardiac abnormalities. In a recent study of 151 cases, only 12.5% had normal echocardiographic findings. Sixty-two percent had pulmonary valvular stenosis, which was sometimes associated with septal defects (Sharland et al 1992a). A hypertrophic cardiomyopathy was present in 20% in this particular series, but others quote higher percentages of cardiac muscle abnormalities. Although the cardiomyopathy is not always obstructive or symptomatic, it is the main risk factor for sudden death. Restrictive cardiomyopathy has also been recognised (Kushwaha et al 1997).

4. Hepatosplenomegaly is present in 50%, and undescended testis occurs in 77% of males.

5. Musculoskeletal abnormalities are common. Sternal defects occur, with pectus excavatus inferiorly, and pectus carinatus superiorly. There may be a narrow spinal canal, a lumbar lordosis, and kyphoscoliosis. General hypotonia is present, with abnormal joint hyperextensibility.

6. Although fertility in females is normal, males frequently do not reproduce. This may be because of the high incidence of cryptorchism and the greater severity of the cardiac lesions, which may determine survival (Collins & Turner 1973).

7. Lymphangiomatosis can occur, with abnormal lymph vessels of the chest wall, pleura, and lungs.

Anaesthetic problems

1. Webbed neck, micrognathia, high arched palate and dental malocclusion may contribute to intubation difficulties (Schwartz & Eisenkraft 1992).

2. Problems of anaesthesia in the presence of cardiac disease, particularly cardiomyopathies

(Campbell & Bousfield 1992, Schwartz & Eisenkraft 1992, McLure & Yentis 1996).

3. A history of easy bruising and bleeding has been elicited from 65% of 72 patients with Noonan's syndrome, and 50% had specific abnormalities of the intrinsic coagulation pathway (partial factor XI:C, XII:C, and VIII:C). However, there was a lack of correlation between the history of bleeding and the coagulation abnormalities, which makes prediction of bleeding in any individual patient difficult (Editorial 1992, Sharland et al 1992b). This also limits the use of regional anaesthesia during labour. Grange et al (1998) reported the management of labour in a 19 year old with Factor XI deficiency and thrombocytopenia. Severe intra- and postoperative bleeding occurred in a 22 year old with low fibrinogen and Factors XI and XII deficiency having orthognathic surgery, despite preoperative administration of fresh frozen plasma. Further severe bleeding occurred 10 days later and carotid artery ligation was required (Sugar et al 1994).

4. If spinal canal stenosis is a feature, care should be taken when performing regional anaesthetic techniques. Coagulation defects should be excluded beforehand.

5. Severe problems following airway surgery have been described (Yellon 1997). In two infants with subglottic obstruction, incision into lymphangiomatous tissue in the neck resulted in chylothorax and massive loss of proteins. One child became septic and died 28 days postoperatively. Ligation of the thoracic duct does not necessarily resolve the problem in these patients because chylous leakage continues from abnormal lymphatics.

6. Parturients must be identified in early pregnancy, so that management can be decided by a multidisciplinary team.

Management

1. Full cardiovascular assessment to determine the extent of any cardiac lesions.

2. Evaluation of airway and anticipation of difficult intubation. Cervical spine X-rays may be required if neck movements are a problem (Schwartz & Eisenkraft 1992). Fibreoptic intubation has been described for Caesarean section for intrauterine death (McLure & Yentis 1996), and direct laryngoscopy under local anaesthesia and sedation for postpartum evacuation of the uterus (Grange et al 1998).

3. Management of hypertrophic or restrictive cardiomyopathy if present (see appropriate sections in Cardiomyopathies). In patients with the hypertrophic form, outlet obstruction is worsened by tachycardia, increased contractility, arterial vasodilatation, and decreased pre-load, therefore management should be directed towards minimising these (Campbell & Bousfield 1992). A child with hypertrophic cardiomyopathy was treated with an esmolol infusion, a pre-induction fluid load, inhalational induction with halothane, and intubation under deep anaesthesia (Schwartz & Eisenkraft 1992).

4. Assessment and treatment of potential bleeding disorders. One child with Noonan's syndrome and cherubism was given desmopressin for abnormal Ristocetin cofactor activity (Addante & Breen 1996).

5. Epidural anaesthesia has been described for both labour (McLure & Yentis 1996) and Caesarean section (Dadabhoy & Winnie 1988), in patients whose coagulation tests were normal. In a patient with Factor XI deficiency and thrombocytopenia, labour was managed using PCA with $25\,\mu g$ fentanyl bolus and a lockout time of 5 min (Grange et al 1998).

Bibliography

Addante RR, Breen GH 1996 Cherubism in a patient with Noonan's syndrome. Journal of Oral & Maxillofacial Surgery 54: 210–13.

Campbell AM, Bousfield JD 1992 Anaesthesia in a patient with Noonan's syndrome and cardiomyopathy. Anaesthesia 47: 131–3.

Collins E, Turner G 1973 The Noonan syndrome—a review of the clinical and genetic features of 27 cases. Journal of Pediatrics 83: 941–50.

Dadabhoy ZP, Winnie AP 1988 Regional anesthesia

for cesarean section in a parturient with Noonan's syndrome. Anesthesiology 68: 636–8.

Editorial 1992 Noonan's syndrome. Lancet 340: 22–3.

Grange CS, Heid R, Lucas SB et al 1998 Anaesthesia in a parturient with Noonan's syndrome. Canadian Journal of Anaesthesia 45: 332–6.

Kushwaha SS, Fallon JT, Fuster V 1997 Restrictive cardiomyopathy 336: 267–76.

McLure HA, Yentis SM 1996 General anaesthesia for Caesarean section in a parturient with Noonan's syndrome. British Journal of Anaesthesia 77: 665–8.

Schwartz N, Eisenkraft JB 1992 Anesthetic management of a child with Noonan's syndrome and idiopathic hypertrophic subaortic stenosis. Anesthesia & Analgesia 74: 464–6.

Shah N, Rodriguez M, Louis DS et al 1999 Feeding difficulties and foregut dysmotility in Noonan's syndrome. Archives of Disease in Childhood 81: 28–31.

Sharland M, Burch M, McKenna WM et al 1992a A clinical study of Noonan's syndrome. Archives of Disease in Childhood 67: 178–83.

Sharland M, Patton MA, Talbot S et al 1992b Coagulation-factor deficiencies and abnormal bleeding in Noonan's syndrome. Lancet 339: 19–21.

Sugar AW, Ezsias A, Bloom AL et al 1994 Orthognathic surgery in a patient with Noonan's syndrome. Journal of Oral & Maxillofacial Surgery 52: 421–5.

Yellon RF 1997 Complications following airway surgery in Noonan syndrome. Archives of Otolaryngology—Head & Neck Surgery 123: 1341–3.

O

Obesity

Morbid obesity can be defined as occurring when a subject's weight is more than 70% greater than the ideal weight for his or her age and height. Body mass index (BMI) is an alternative useful measure (weight/height^2), and obesity is defined as a BMI $>30\,kg\,m^{-2}$, and morbid obesity as a BMI $>39\,kg\,m^{-2}$. Insurance statistics show a greatly increased mortality rate for such patients, and surgery and anaesthesia carry a number of risks. In addition to incidental procedures, the obese patient may be subjected to weight-reducing intestinal bypass operations, particularly in North America. A number of studies have been undertaken to identify the problems and determine the best methods of anaesthesia. Recently, laparoscopic techniques have been used for gastroplasty.

Preoperative abnormalities

1. *Respiratory*. FRC is reduced, mainly because of a decrease in expiratory reserve volume. Tidal ventilation occurs below the closing volume, particularly in the supine position. The Pa_{O_2} may be reduced, and the work and oxygen cost of respiration are increased. The Pickwickian syndrome, characterised by hypoventilation, somnolence, cor pulmonale, and hypoxia, is very rare.

2. *Cardiovascular*. An increased incidence of hypertension and coronary artery disease. Significant hypertrophy of the left ventricle is found in pregnant obese patients compared with nonobese patients (Veille & Hanson 1994).

3. *Metabolic*. Increased glucose intolerance and diabetes.

Anaesthetic problems

1. Difficulties with venous access.

2. Mechanical problems resulting from the size and weight of the patient.

3. Difficulties in locating the epidural or subarachnoid space. Standard length needles may be too short.

4. There is a more extensive spread of local anaesthetic solutions in the subarachnoid space when compared with patients of normal weight (Taivainen et al 1990).

5. Tracheal intubation problems. Obesity is a significant risk factor, particularly in obstetric anaesthesia (Rocke et al 1992).

6. Cyanosis develops rapidly, especially in the supine position, as a result of a reduced FRC. The tidal volume may approach, or fall within, the closing volume. There is a 50% reduction in FRC at the onset of anaesthesia (Damia et al 1988). Apnoea is associated with an increased risk of hypoxia (Jense et al 1991), the effectiveness of preoxygenation is considerably reduced, and desaturation may occur before tracheal intubation has been achieved (Berthoud et al 1991).

7. Rapid dehydration and a poor response to hypovolaemia results from a reduced blood volume per unit weight.

8. Reliable indirect blood pressure monitoring is difficult to achieve.

9. Difficulties in maintaining an airway during mask anaesthesia.

10. Problems with intraoperative oxygenation during abdominal surgery, particularly when in the head-down position, or when intra-abdominal packs are in place.

11. For the first 48 h postoperatively, the supine position is associated with a significant decrease in Pa_{O_2} (Vaughan et al 1976).

12. Obstructive sleep apnoea is very common (Kyzer & Charuzi 1998). Hypertension, heart block, left and right ventricular hypertrophy, and brain infarction may result.

13. Sensitivity to postoperative analgesia may occur. Respiratory failure was reported in an obese patient receiving PCA together with a background infusion of morphine (VanDercar et al 1991). Following episodes of obstructive

apnoea, periods of hyperpnoea associated with arousal were interpreted by the nursing staff as pain, and supplementary analgesia was given.

14. Increased incidence of postoperative respiratory problems.

15. Venous thrombosis and pulmonary embolism (PE). Despite thromboprophylaxis with heparin, DVT and PE may still occur. In a series of 200 patients, there were three cases of PE (one fatal), and four DVTs confirmed by venogram (Goulding & Hovell 1995).

16. An increased risk of wound infection (8–28%).

17. Pregnancy may be complicated by all of the above problems. It may not be recognised. In 117 morbidly obese women, 62% underwent Caesarean section compared with only 24% of controls (Hood & Dewan 1993). Pregnancy in those treated with bariatric surgery may be complicated by severe anaemia resulting from malabsorption (Gurewitsch et al 1996). Another patient had haematemesis at 26 weeks' gestation due to erosion of the synthetic graft from a vertical banded gastroplasty performed 4 years previously (Ramirez & Turrentine 1995).

Management

1. Detailed cardiovascular and respiratory assessment is required. If there is pre-existing hypoxia or hypercarbia, then some weight loss is advisable before elective surgery. Mandibular wiring has been suggested to aid this, before abdominal weight-reducing surgery.

2. If intubation difficulties are anticipated, awake intubation may be advisable. The incidence of difficult intubation under general anaesthesia lies between 6% and 13%. Even if difficulties are not anticipated, the ineffectiveness of preoxygenation may be another indication for awake intubation (Berthoud et al 1991). Little difference was found between preoxygenation with 3 min of 100% oxygen or four vital capacity breaths of 100% oxygen (Goldberg et al 1989). With the former technique, slight carbon

dioxide retention was found. Awake fibreoptic intubation was performed in a 300-kg woman with a 78-kg ovarian cyst. Surgery lasted 13 h, there was a blood loss of 7.5 l, and weaning from IPPV took place over several days (Trempy & Rock 1993).

3. Thoracic epidural anaesthesia has been recommended as an adjunct to general anaesthesia. The rationale is that, as a consequence, only light general anaesthesia is required, good postoperative pain relief is provided, and early extubation and mobilisation are permitted. Epidural analgesia was given to 70 patients in a series of 110 undergoing weight-reducing surgery (Fox et al 1981). There was an incidence of postoperative lung collapse of 18.5% in these patients, compared with 27.5% for those just receiving pethidine im. However, there was a suggestion that pulmonary emboli might be slightly more common in the epidural group.

Others do not consider that epidural analgesia offers significant advantages. Thoracic epidurals are technically difficult to perform in the very obese and there was a 20% failure rate in one series (Buckley et al 1983). Some improvement in cardiovascular function, as evidenced by a decrease in left ventricular stroke volume and myocardial oxygen requirement, was reported in patients with a thoracic epidural block and general anaesthesia, when compared with opiates and general anaesthesia (Gelman et al 1980). However it was found to be no better than iv morphine in terms of postoperative pain relief, vital capacity, and gas exchange. Fewer pulmonary complications were experienced with epidural analgesia, but a greater incidence of intraoperative hypotension and bradycardia (Buckley et al 1983).

Care must be taken to avoid giving an excessive volume of local anaesthetic to the morbidly obese. The reduced dose of bupivacaine required for epidural anaesthesia in obese pregnant patients (Hodgkinson & Husain 1980) has been confirmed by others (Buckley et al 1983). This is probably a result of venous engorgement in the epidural space.

4. The use of antacids and H_2 receptor antagonists as a precaution against acid aspiration syndrome is recommended.

5. A comparison of adjuvants with IPPV were made in 67 patients for gastric stapling (Cork et al 1981). There was no difference between halothane, enflurane or fentanyl in terms of early postoperative recovery. However, the use of isoflurane or sevoflurane, which are the least metabolised, would seem rational.

6. During abdominal surgery, frequent blood gas sampling is advisable and an increased inspired oxygen concentration is required when the head-down position is employed. The use of subdiaphragmatic intra-abdominal packs may produce severe hypoxia and should be avoided if possible. Oxygenation in otherwise healthy obese subjects having abdominal surgery was studied (Vaughan & Wise 1976). Fourteen per cent of patients in the supine position, and 77% with a 15 degrees head-down tilt, had a Pao_2 of <10.6 kPa on 40% oxygen. In 23% of those in the latter group, the Pao_2 decreased to <8.0 kPa. In all four patients in whom subdiaphragmatic packs were used, the Pao_2 was <8.6 kPa.

7. Whilst PCA may be valuable in the obese, the avoidance of a background infusion, the use of smaller bolus doses, and the setting of a 4-hrly dose limit, would seem advisable (Levin et al 1992).

8. The increasing use of laparoscopic techniques has improved the immediate postoperative course (Juvin et al 1999).

9. Nasal CPAP may benefit patients with OSA in the postoperative period. Bilevel positive airway pressure, which combines pressure support ventilation and PEEP via a nasal mask, given for the first 24 h after gastroplasty, reduced pulmonary dysfunction (Joris et al 1997).

10. Thromboprophylaxis should be started preoperatively. Since both DVT and PE can occur despite this, the signs and symptoms should be looked for closely. Systemic urokinase therapy was used to treat a PE on the fourth day after an umbilical hernia repair (Hartmannsgruber et al 1996).

11. Caesarean section has been reported under local anaesthetic infiltration (Gautam et al 1999), and under epidural anaesthesia (Patel 1999). Three patients were reported in whom continuous spinal anaesthesia was used for Caesarean section; in two of the patients, conversion from an epidural was necessary because of accidental dural puncture (Milligan & Carp 1992).

Bibliography

Bardoczky GI, Yernault JC, Houben JJ et al 1995 Large tidal volume ventilation does not improve oxygenation in morbidly obese patients during anesthesia. Anesthesia & Analgesia 81: 385–8.

Berthoud MC, Peacock JE, Reilly CS 1991 Effectiveness of preoxygenation in morbidly obese patients. British Journal of Anaesthesia 67: 464–6.

Buckley FP, Robinson NB, Simonowitz DA et al 1983 Anaesthesia in the morbidly obese. Anaesthesia 38: 840–51.

Cork RC, Vaughan RW, Bentley JB 1981 General anesthesia for morbidly obese patients: an examination of postoperative outcomes. Anesthesiology 54: 310–13.

Damia G, Mascheroni D, Croci M et al 1988 Perioperative changes in functional residual capacity in morbidly obese patients. British Journal of Anaesthesia 60: 574–8.

Fox GS, Whalley DG, Bevan DR 1981 Anaesthesia for the morbidly obese, experience with 110 patients. British Journal of Anaesthesia 53: 811–16.

Gautam PL, Kathuria S, Kaul TK 1999 Infiltration block for caesarean section in a morbidly obese parturient. Acta Anaesthesiologica Scandinavica 43: 580–1.

Gelman S, Laws HL, Potzick J et al 1980 Thoracic epidural versus balanced anesthesia in morbid obesity. An intraoperative and postoperative hemodynamic study. Anesthesia & Analgesia 59: 902–8.

Goldberg ME, Norris MC, Larijani GE et al 1989 Preoxygenation in the morbidly obese: a comparison of two techniques. Anesthesia & Analgesia 68: 520–2.

Goulding ST, Hovell B 1995 Anaesthetic experience of vertical banded gastroplasty. British Journal of Anaesthesia 75: 301–6.

Gurewitsch ED, Smith-Levitin M, Mack J 1996 Pregnancy following gastric bypass surgery for morbid obesity. Obstetrics & Gynecology 88: 658–61.

Hartmannsgruber MW, Trent FL, Stolzfus DP 1996 Thrombolytic therapy for treatment of pulmonary embolism in the postoperative period: case report and review of the literature. Journal of Clinical Anesthesia 8: 669–74.

Hodgkinson R, Husain FJ 1980 Obesity and the cephalad spread of analgesia following epidural administration of bupivacaine for Cesarean section. Anesthesia & Analgesia 59: 89–92.

Hood DD, Dewan DM 1993 Anesthetic and obstetric outcome in morbidly obese parturients. Anesthesiology 79: 1210–18.

Jense HG, Dubin SA, Silverstein PI et al 1991 Effect of obesity on safe duration of apnea in anesthetized humans. Anesthesia & Analgesia 72: 89–93.

Joris JL, Sottiaux TM, Chiche JD et al 1997 Effect of bi-level positive airway pressure (BiPAP) nasal ventilation on the postoperative pulmonary restrictive syndrome in obese patients undergoing gastroplasty. Chest 111: 665–70.

Juvin P, Marmuse JP, Delerme S et al 1999 Post-operative course after conventional or laparoscopic gastroplasty in morbidly obese patients. European Journal of Anaesthesiology 16: 400–3.

Kyzer S, Charuzi I 1998 Obstructive sleep apnea in the obese. World Journal of Surgery 22: 998–1001.

Levin A, Klein SL, Brolin RE et al 1992 Patient-controlled analgesia for morbidly obese patients: an effective modality if used correctly. Anesthesiology 76: 857–8.

Milligan KH, Carp H 1992 Continuous spinal anaesthesia for caesarean section in the morbidly obese. International Journal of Obstetric Anesthesia 1: 111–13.

Patel J 1999 Anaesthesia for LSCS in a morbidly obese patient. Anaesthesia & Intensive Care 27: 216–19.

Ramirez MM, Turrentine MA 1995 Gastrointestinal hemorrhage during pregnancy in a patient with a history of vertical banded gastroplasty. American Journal of Obstetrics & Gynecology 173: 1630–1.

Rocke DA, Murray WB, Rout CC et al 1992 Relative risk analysis of factors associated with difficult intubation in obstetric anesthesia. Anesthesiology 77: 67–73.

Taivainen T, Tuominen M, Rosenberg PH 1990 Influence of obesity on the spread of spinal analgesia after injection of plain 0.5% bupivacaine at the L3–4 or L4–5 interspace. British Journal of Anaesthesia 64: 542–6.

Trempy GA, Rock P 1993 Anesthetic management of a morbidly obese woman with a massive ovarian cyst. Journal of Clinical Anesthesia 5: 62–8.

VanDercar DH, Martinez AP, DeLisser EA 1992 Sleep apnea syndromes: a potential contraindication for patient-controlled analgesia. Anesthesiology 74: 623–4.

Vaughan RW, Wise L 1976 Intraoperative arterial oxygenation in obese patients. Annals of Surgery 184: 35–42.

Vaughan RW, Bauer S, Wise L 1976 Effect of position (semirecumbent versus supine) on postoperative oxygenation in markedly obese subjects. Anesthesia & Analgesia 55: 37–41.

Veille JC, Hanson R 1994 Obesity, pregnancy, and left ventricular functioning during the third trimester. American Journal of Obstetrics & Gynecology 171: 980–3.

Obstructive sleep apnoea

A term used for recurrent hypoxaemic respiratory disturbances during sleep, which result from varying combinations of anatomical airway obstruction, functional control of airway musculature, and central apnoea. A variety of definitions have been used. 'Apnoea' is a 10-s or more pause in nasal/oral airflow during sleep, whereas 'hypopnoea' is one in which a 50% or greater reduction in tidal volume occurs for 10 s or more. The apnoea–hypopnoea index (AHI) is the number of abnormal respiratory events that occur each hour of sleep (Boushra 1996). The sleep apnoea syndrome is said to occur when more than 30 of these episodes occur during 7 h sleep (Hanning 1989, Davies & Stradling 1993). It is a common condition, although frequently undiagnosed, and up to 2% of the adult population may be affected. The multiplicity of contributing factors presumably accounts for the fact that OSA has been associated with such a wide variety of conditions. OSA in children is increasingly being recognised, and is commonly secondary to adenotonsillar hypertrophy. It has been suggested that the syndrome in children is a separate entity, and for a detailed review of OSA in children see Warwick and Mason (1998).

Contributing factors

1. *Reduction in pharyngeal area.* The area of the pharynx is reduced compared with that of

normal individuals. Increased adipose tissue, thickened pharyngeal mucosa, large tonsils and adenoids, and mandibular hypoplasia may all contribute. The small pharyngeal space in the awake patient is reduced even further during sleep, or in the supine posture. Thus, in the anaesthetised patient total obstruction often occurs. Obstruction in the supine position is also related to FRC. The actual site of obstruction may vary (see Pierre Robin syndrome), and can be single or multiple. The pharynx is the commonest site, and the larynx is the least common. MRI studies in volunteers showed that during administration of propofol, the commonest cause of obstruction was approximation of the soft palate to the posterior pharyngeal wall (Mathru et al 1996).

2. *Impairment of muscle function.* Muscular function depends on neurological control and coordination, particularly of the genioglossus, geniohyoid, and tensor palati muscles. The pharynx is prone to collapse and this is associated with a decrease in activity of the pharyngeal muscles. During inspiration, the subatmospheric pressure may abolish muscle splinting, so that the pharynx is obliterated. There is also lack of coordination between the pharyngeal and thoracic muscles, and an associated reduction in FRC.

3. *Central control.* Obstructive sleep apnoea is made worse by diseases in which there is CNS involvement.

4. *Sleep cycles.* Cycles during sleep include nonrapid eye movement (NREM) sleep and rapid eye movement (REM) sleep. REM sleep is associated with generalised loss of muscle tone, which tends to increase upper airway obstruction. In the early postoperative period, sleep disturbance with suppression of REM sleep occurs. The return of REM on day 4–5 results in excessively deep sleep (Knill et al 1990).

Preoperative abnormalities

1. In adults, men are affected predominantly, whereas in children the gender incidence is equal. In adults, features include snoring, often vividly described by the patient's partner, obesity, nocturnal sleep disturbance, and excessive daytime sleepiness. In children, nocturnal snoring and noisy breathing, restlessness during sleep, and apnoeas, alternate with frequent awakening. Obesity is unusual in children, and low weight, small stature and facial changes secondary to obstruction, are more common. Primary craniofacial abnormalities, hypotonia and neuromuscular disorders may also be associated with OSA. In severe, long-term upper airway obstruction in both adults and children, hypoxia, hypercarbia and right ventricular failure may ensue.

2. Decreased nocturnal, and sometimes diurnal, oxygen saturation and secondary polycythaemia (Messinezy et al 1991).

3. Diagnosis is by polysomnography and continuous oxygen saturation measurements.

4. An increased neck circumference has been found in adult patients with OSA compared with nonapnoeic, snoring controls (Katz et al 1990). Increased mass loading in the upper airway was thought to contribute to the pathogenesis of the condition.

5. Systemic and pulmonary hypertension (Dark 1996). There is an increased incidence of OSA in the hypertensive adult population. In children there may be evidence of right ventricular strain; cor pulmonale with large P waves in II and V1, a large R wave in V1, and a deep S wave in V6.

6. Cardiac arrhythmias may be a feature. In 458 patients with OSA, a 58% prevalence of arrhythmias was found (Hoffstein & Mateika 1994). In addition, heart block occurs in 20% of patients with severe sleep apnoea and 7.5% of total patients (Becker et al 1998). Nasal CPAP prevented these episodes in 80–90% of individuals.

Anaesthetic problems

1. Periods of apnoea and desaturation during normal sleep that are worse and more frequent

in the postoperative period. Such episodes are increased in incidence and severity in REM sleep. REM sleep is almost completely abolished for the first 2–3 days after surgery, but a rebound occurs on night 5 (Knill et al 1990). Physiological accompaniments of REM sleep are episodic breathing disturbances, with fluctuations in heart rate and blood pressure. These factors may account for delayed cardiovascular and cerebrovascular complications after surgery. During such episodes, saturations may decrease to below 50%. In one patient, even before surgery, 33 min of the night were spent with saturations of less than 85% (Reeder et al 1991). Subsequent computer studies of his postoperative nights showed three types of respiratory events, each ranging from 10 to 30 s in duration: 'obstructive'; 'mixed' (cycles beginning with central apnoea, then obstruction with increasing respiratory effort, and finally sudden awakening); and 'apnoeic'. The last event was the least common. Patients having nasal surgery followed by nasal packing are particularly at risk from these problems (Tierney et al 1989).

2. Periodic fluctuations in heart rate and blood pressure, associated with episodes of obstruction and the resultant major swings in intrathoracic pressure (Reeder et al 1991). The obstructive phase was associated with a decrease in systemic pressure, whereas hypertension tended to be associated with arousal and relief of obstruction. Nasal CPAP corrects these sleeping blood pressure disturbances (Davies 1998).

3. Episodes of heart block have been reported in 20% of patients with severe sleep apnoea, and 7.5% of an unselected group (Becker et al 1998). Again, this may be prevented in 80–90% of individuals using nasal CPAP.

4. There is an increased incidence of intubation problems in those undergoing OSA surgery. In a study of 182 patients, 18.6% had difficult intubation (Riley et al 1997). Awake fibreoptic intubation may also prove to be impossible, especially if the patient has been sedated (Biro et al 1995).

5. In children following tonsillectomy with or without adenoidectomy for OSA, the risk factors for postoperative complications were: age <2 years, craniofacial abnormalities, failure to thrive, hypotonia, and morbid obesity (Rosen et al 1994).

6. Sensitivity to postoperative analgesia. Respiratory failure occurred after nephrectomy in an obese patient who was receiving a PCA and a background infusion of morphine (VanDercar et al 1991). Nursing staff may interpret periods of hyperpnoea, associated with arousal and relief of obstruction, as pain, and consequently give supplementary analgesia. Surgery for OSA may be very painful and a difficult balance exists between providing satisfactory analgesia and avoiding hypoxia.

7. Postoperative epidural analgesia, although recommended in OSA, may also produce respiratory depression. Ostermeier et al (1997) reported three postoperative deaths from delayed respiratory depression (up to 48 h), whilst the patients were receiving epidural bupivacaine and fentanyl $10 \mu g \, ml^{-1}$. The onset of depression was sudden, the patients had pain scores of zero, and none was being nursed in a high-dependency area at the time.

8. Wound healing is reduced and infection more likely when wound oxygen tension is low.

9. Patients with severe OSA may die during sleep, possibly secondary to hypoxaemia or arrhythmias. There appears to be a high incidence of obstructive sleep apnoea in patients with coronary artery disease who require intensive/coronary care, compared with controls (Peker et al 1999).

10. The problems of the airway do not end following surgery. Recurrent episodes of airway obstruction, each requiring reintubation, was reported in a 38-year-old man. He was ultimately admitted to the ITU for CPAP. Subsequent questioning revealed severe snoring and OSA (Vidhani & Langham 1997). Acute obstruction occurred during emergence from anaesthesia after uvulopalatopharyngoplasty

(Gabrielczyk 1988). The patient pulled out his own tracheal tube while still on the operating table and divested himself of cannulae and monitoring. This episode underlines the importance of retaining key personnel and equipment close to the patient until successful extubation has been accomplished.

Management

1. Preoperative identification of patients with OSA. If the diagnosis is suspected from the patient's habitus, neck size and weight, the question 'do you snore' may confirm the suspicion. It should also prompt a thorough examination for potential intubation difficulties.

2. Monitoring with apnoea alarms or pulse oximetry.

3. Supplementary oxygen at night, particularly in the perioperative period.

4. Treatment of the underlying cause, for example obesity, by weight loss.

5. Total intravenous anaesthesia with propofol provided a more rapid recovery and better oxygen saturations in the first postoperative hour compared with a technique using isoflurane (Hendolin et al 1994).

6. Avoidance, or at least the cautious use, of sedatives and narcotics in the perioperative period. If PCA is used, a background continuous infusion is unwise, unless there is continuous observation of the patient at the same time.

7. OSA surgery. Riley et al (1997) have suggested a protocol for patients undergoing significant surgery for OSA. This includes:

a) CPAP for 2 weeks before surgery in patients with severe disease shown on polysomnography.

b) The presence of the surgeon for induction and intubation.

c) Awake fibreoptic intubation if there are airway concerns.

d) HDU/ITU care for patients with significant concurrent disease, or having multiple procedures.

e) Continued nasal CPAP for those needing it preoperatively, humidified oxygen for all others.

f) Strictly controlled use of iv morphine by a nurse on an HDU.

g) No PCA use.

h) Only im or oral analgesics on the ward.

8. Local anaesthetic blocks may help reduce the need for opioid analgesics, but are more difficult to perform and have a higher complication rate in the obese.

9. Nasal continuous positive airway pressure (CPAP) given by nasal mask abolishes obstructions, by acting as a splint to maintain airway patency (Polo 1999). It also decreased blood pressure postoperatively in a surgical patient in whom preoperative obstructive sleep apnoea and desaturation had been demonstrated (Reeder et al 1991). Thomas et al (1992) describe one such system. These systems can generate pressures of 2.5–20 cmH$_2$O and reduce sleep disturbances, hypoxia, and cardiovascular changes. The probable effect of CPAP is to open up the airway and prevent collapse, but the positive pressure may also cause reflex activation of pharyngeal muscles. In a study of 182 patients undergoing OSA surgery, it was found that nasal CPAP abolished hypoxaemia and allowed adequate oral or parenteral analgesics to be given (Riley et al 1997).

10. Nasopharyngeal airways or other mechanical devices are of limited value.

11. Surgery for OSA. Detailed discussion is beyond the scope of this book. However, if palatal surgery is considered, direct measurements of intra-airway pressure at different sites to locate the sites of obstruction beforehand are essential.

a) Tracheostomy; effective, but limited by side effects, particularly in the obese.

b) Minitracheotomy was used for 4 months as a temporary measure in a patient with OSA awaiting tonsillectomy (Hassan et al 1989). This allowed resolution of cor pulmonale and papilloedema, and weight loss.

c) Uvulopalatoplasty, the commonest definitive procedure, involves removal of the uvula, tonsils, part of the soft palate, and excess pharyngeal tissue. Complications are not insignificant and at the present time the benefits are questionable.

12. Associated conditions, such as respiratory disease, obesity, heart failure and pulmonary hypertension, must be treated before surgery.

13. Drugs are of limited value, but protryptiline may reduce REM sleep in which most of the apnoeic episodes occur.

14. These patients can sometimes be difficult, demanding, and occasionally litiginous. Potential medicolegal problems should be anticipated. The use of a fact sheet may be advisable.

Bibliography

Becker HF, Keohler U, Stammnitz A et al 1998 Heart block in patients with sleep apnoea. Thorax 53(suppl 3): S29–32.

Biro P, Kaplan V, Bloch KE 1995 Anesthetic management of a patient with obstructive sleep apnea syndrome and difficult airway access. Journal of Clinical Anesthesia 7: 417–21.

Boushra NN 1996 Anaesthetic management of patients with sleep apnoea syndrome. Canadian Journal of Anaesthesia 43: 599–616.

Dark DS 1996 Sleep apnoea and pulmonary hypertension. Chest 109: 300–1.

Davies RJ 1998 Cardiovascular aspects of obstructive sleep apnoea and their relevance to the assessment of efficacy of nasal continuous positive pressure therapy. Thorax 53: 416–18.

Davies RJ, Stradling JR 1993 Acute effects of obstructive sleep apnoea. British Journal of Anaesthesia 71: 725–9.

Gabrielczyk MR 1988 Acute airway obstruction after uvulopharyngoplasty for obstructive sleep apnea syndrome. Anesthesiology 69: 941–3.

Hanning CD 1989 Obstructive sleep apnoea. British Journal of Anaesthesia 63: 477–88.

Hassan A, Mcguigan J, Morgan MDL et al 1989 Minitracheotomy: a simple alternative to tracheostomy in obstructive sleep apnoea. Thorax 44: 224–5.

Hendolin H, Kansanen M, Koski E et al 1994 Propofol-nitrous oxide versus thiopentone-isoflurane-nitrous oxide anaesthesia for uvulopalatopharyngoplasty in patients with obstructive sleep apnea. Acta Anaesthesiologica Scandinavica 38: 694–8.

Hoffstein V, Mateika S 1994 Cardiac arrhythmias, snoring, and sleep apnoea. Chest 106: 466–71.

Katz I, Stradling JR, Slutsky AS et al 1990 Do patients with obstructive sleep apnea have fat necks? American Review of Respiratory Disease 141: 1228–31.

Knill RL, Moote CA, Skinner MI et al 1990 Anesthesia with abdominal surgery leads to intense REM sleep during the first postoperative week. Anesthesiology 73: 52–61.

Mathru M, Esch O, Lang J et al 1996 Magnetic resonance imaging of the upper airway. Effects of propofol anesthesia and nasal continuous positive airway pressure in humans. Anesthesiology 84: 252–5.

Messinezy M, Aubry S, O'Connell G et al 1991 Oxygen desaturation in apparent and relative polycythaemia. British Medical Journal 302: 216–17.

Ostermeier AM, Roizen MF, Hautkappe M et al 1997 Three sudden postoperative respiratory arrests associated with epidural opioids in patients with sleep apnea. Anesthesia & Analgesia 85: 452–60.

Peker Y, Kraiczi H, Hedner J et al 1999 An independent association between obstructive sleep apnoea and coronary artery disease. European Respiratory Journal 14: 179–84.

Polo O 1999 Continuous positive airway pressure for treatment of sleep apnoea. Lancet 353: 2086–7.

Reeder MK, Goldman MD, Loh L et al 1991 Postoperative obstructive sleep apnoea. Haemodynamic effects of treatment with nasal CPAP. Anaesthesia 46: 849–53.

Riley RW, Powell NB, Guilleminaut C et al 1997 Obstructive sleep apnea surgery: risk management and complications. Otolaryngology—Head & Neck Surgery 117: 648–52.

Rosen GM, Muckle RP, Mahowald MW et al 1994 Postoperative respiratory compromise in children with obstructive sleep apnea syndrome: can it be anticipated? Pediatrics 93: 784–8.

Thomas AN, Ryan JP, Doran B et al 1992 A nasal CPAP system. Description and comparison with facemask CPAP. Anaesthesia 47: 311–15.

Tierney NM, Pollard BJ, Duran BRH 1989 Obstructive sleep apnoea. Anaesthesia 44: 235–7.

VanDercar DH, Martinez AP, De Lisser EA 1991 Sleep apnea syndrome: a potential contraindication for patient-controlled analgesia. Anesthesiology 74: 623–4.

Vidhani K, Langham BT 1997 Obstructive sleep apnoea syndrome: is this an overlooked cause of desaturation in the immediate postoperative period? British Journal of Anaesthesia 78: 442–3.

Warwick JP, Mason DG 1998 Obstructive sleep apnoea in children. British Journal of Anaesthesia 53: 571–9.

Opiate addiction

Dependence on opiates is present when a physical withdrawal state occurs on abrupt cessation of the drug, and when tolerance to the drug develops. Psychological dependence can also occur. The anaesthetist may be involved, either because a dependent patient requires surgery, or for resuscitation when accidental or deliberate overdosage occurs. The problem may be admitted by the patient, or concealed. He/she may or may not be registered as an addict. Occasionally, a cured addict may come for surgery. Opiates should be scrupulously avoided in these patients. Alternatives such as continuous epidural analgesia should be considered for postoperative pain.

The absence of a history of drug abuse, bizarre behaviour, malnutrition or social deterioration in a patient under 40 should prompt the search for injection marks.

Preoperative abnormalities

1. Malnutrition, skin infection, superficial venous thrombosis, anaemia, or jaundice may be present.

2. There is a high incidence of liver disease to which malnutrition may contribute. A 10% incidence of hepatitis has been reported. There is a significant risk of transmission of hepatitis and possibly AIDS.

3. An increased risk of bacterial or fungal endocarditis, most frequently due to *Staphylococcus aureus*, but sometimes to pseudomonas. Arterial emboli, sometimes septic, can result.

4. Pulmonary infection, infarction and atelectasis are common. Pulmonary hypertension or oedema can occur.

5. Tetanus may be seen, in part due to additives such as quinine which allow the growth of anaerobes (McGoldrick 1980).

6. Adrenocortical function is suppressed.

Anaesthetic problems

1. Venous access may be difficult.

2. Problems of management of HBV- or HIV-positive patients.

3. Physical dependence and withdrawal signs and symptoms. Symptoms include yawning, sweating, lacrimation, and rhinorrhoea. Signs include tachycardia, tremors, acute anxiety, sweating, piloerection, mydriasis, nausea, and vomiting. There is evidence to suggest that brain catecholamines play some part in the aetiology of this syndrome (McGoldrick 1980). Signs begin about 12 h after the last dose of opioid and peak at about 48–72 h.

4. Tolerance to all the effects of opiates occurs. Anaesthetic techniques relying on opioids may be unsuitable, because very high doses will be required to suppress sympathetic responses to surgical stimulation.

5. The administration of partial or pure narcotic antagonists may precipitate a withdrawal state.

6. Hypotension may occur.

7. Problems of the pregnant opioid user who appears in late pregnancy (Gerada et al 1990).

8. Morphine tolerance can occur in patients

undergoing long-term use of opiates on the ITU. Two children undergoing IPPV for severe thermal injury and treated with morphine had dramatically increased requirements for sedation (Williams et al 1998). The mechanism for this is unknown. However, substitution of methadone for morphine produced rapid control of sedation.

9. The time course of the individual abstinence syndromes has been described (McCammon 1980):

Drug	Onset	Peak	Duration
Pethidine	3 h	8–12 h	4–5 days
Morphine	8–12 h	36–48 h	7–10 days
Heroin	8–12 h	36–48 h	7–10 days
Methadone	1–2 days	3–6 days	2–3 weeks

Management

1. A careful history should be taken, and a thorough examination made. If the patient is registered, then the drug centre, the GP or the psychiatrist should be contacted to verify details. Expert advice on management may be necessary. If doubt exists, urine may be tested for the presence of drugs. Belongings should be checked for concealed drugs.

2. Patients should be presumed to be HBV and HIV positive unless proved otherwise.

3. Most authorities are agreed that the perioperative period is not the correct time to institute detoxification. Opiates will therefore need to be given. This may be the preparation already being used, or the equivalent dose of methadone might be substituted. Approximately equivalent dosages (DHSS 1984) are reported as:

a) Methadone: 10 mg (some authorities quote 5 mg).

b) Morphine: 10 mg.

c) Pethidine: 100 mg.

d) Dextromoramide: 5 mg.

e) Heroin: 10 mg.

f) Dipipanone: 20 mg.

g) Buprenorphine: 0.8 mg.

h) Pentazocine: 125 mg.

If genuine organic pain does exist then, as a result of tolerance, higher than normal doses of opiates will be required. There is also a variability in cross tolerance to opioids, such that when patients still have uncontrolled pain in spite of intolerable side effects, an alternative drug may be substituted with success (Collett 1998).

4. If there is venous thrombosis, internal jugular or subclavian venous cannulation, or a venous cutdown, may be required.

5. Partial opiate antagonists such as pentazocine, or pure antagonists such as naloxone, should not be used since they may produce severe acute withdrawal symptoms.

6. The use of other drugs with addictive potential, such as the benzodiazepines, should be avoided.

7. Hypotension has been described preoperatively in opiate addicts. When it occurs during surgery, responses to various forms of treatment including opiates, fluids, vasoconstrictors or hydrocortisone have been reported.

8. Opioids should continue to be given in labour, calculated as a minimum daily requirement (Birnbach 1998). There is little evidence that opiates are harmful to a fetus already exposed to opiates during pregnancy and respiratory depression is thought not to be a feature. There is no contraindication to epidural analgesia.

Bibliography

Birnbach DJ 1998 Anesthesia and the drug abusing parturient. Anesthesiology Clinics of North America 16: 385–95.

Caldwell T 1990 Anesthesia for patients with behavioral and environmental disorders. In: Katz J, Benumof J, Kadis L, (eds). Anesthesia and uncommon diseases. WB Saunders, Philadelphia, pp 794–812.

Collett B-J 1998 Opioid tolerance: the clinical perspective. British Journal of Anaesthesia 81: 58–68.

DHSS 1984 Guidelines of good clinical practice in the treatment of drug misuse. Report of the Medical Working Group on Drug Dependence. HMSO, London.

DHSS 1991 Drug misuse and dependence. Guidelines on clinical management. HMSO, London.

Gerada C, Dawe S, Farrell M 1990 Management of the pregnant opiate user. British Journal of Hospital Medicine 43: 138–41.

McCammon RL 1986 Anesthesia for the chemically dependent patient. Anesthesia & Analgesia Review Course Lectures 47–55.

McGoldrick KE 1980 Anesthetic implications of drug abuse. Anesthesiology Review 7: 12–17.

Williams PI, Sarginson RE, Ratcliffe JM 1998 Use of methadone in the morphine-tolerant burned paediatric patient. British Journal of Anaesthesia 80: 92–5.

Opitz–Frias syndrome

A rare congenital disorder involving a number of midline abnormalities (Wilson & Oliver 1988). Features include craniofacial and genital defects, and functional swallowing and laryngeal problems. Males are more severely affected than females.

Preoperative abnormalities

1. Hypertelorism, prominent parietal and occipital areas, micrognathia, a high arched or cleft palate, bifid uvula.

2. Hypospadias and bifid scrotum, imperforate anus.

3. Dysphagia, probably of neuromuscular origin, oesophageal achalasia, hiatus hernia, gastric aspiration, and pulmonary problems.

4. Posterior laryngeal cleft, wheezing and inspiratory stridor, with a hoarse cry.

5. Cardiac defects.

Anaesthetic problems

1. Recurrent gastric aspiration may cause cyanotic episodes, apnoea, and asystole.

2. Craniofacial abnormalities can lead to intubation problems.

Management

1. Assessment of abnormalities described above.

2. Anaesthetic management of a 9-month-old child for fundoplication and feeding jejunostomy has been reported (Bolsin & Gilbe 1985). Several episodes of cyanosis and CXR changes had occurred after birth. A scan of an isotopic milk feed demonstrated reflux, and the child was fed through a nasogastric tube. Before surgery, two admissions for respiratory distress and inhalation had been required. Some intubation difficulty was reported secondary to an immature larynx.

Bibliography

Bolsin SN, Gillbe C 1985 Opitz–Frias syndrome. A case with potentially hazardous anaesthetic implications. Anaesthesia 40: 1189–93.

Wilson GN, Oliver WJ 1988 Further delineation of the G syndrome: a manageable genetic cause of infantile dysphagia. Journal of Medical Genetics 25: 157–63.

Osler–Weber–Rendu syndrome

(see Hereditary haemorrhagic telangiectasia)

Osteogenesis imperfecta

The general term given to a heterogeneous group of inherited disorders of collagen, caused by mutations of one of the two genes encoding collagen type 1, *COL1A1* and *COL1A2*. Predominant features are osteopenia, multiple fractures, severe bony deformities, and short stature. Four broad types have been identified, but increased knowledge of the large number of genetic mutations suggests that further expansion of groupings will be needed (Cole & Cohen 1991, Marini 1998). In less severe cases, diagnosis may be delayed, but the resultant bony fragility, and propensity to fractures, may result in

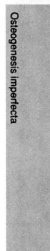
the mistaken diagnosis of child abuse (Gahagan & Rimsza 1991). In severe cases, cardio-respiratory failure and basilar invagination of the skull are the most frequent causes of death. Anaesthesia may be required for reduction of fractures, scoliosis surgery, neurosurgery, and other corrections of skeletal deformities.

Type I is of autosomal dominant inheritance and present in 80% of cases. Extraskeletal tissues are mainly involved and the bone disease is mild. Fractures mainly occur in childhood but become less common after puberty. The joints are hypermobile, and the tendons susceptible to rupture. Patients are almost normal in stature. The sclera are blue, 50% have early-onset deafness and only some children have dental problems. The aortic valve is thin, and sometimes incompetent.

Type II have severe skeletal abnormalities and usually die in the perinatal period.

Type III have severe skeletal deformities that are progressive. Chest deformity, with kyphoscoliosis and prominent sternum, often results in respiratory problems. Long bones are narrow and bent. The skull is large and asymmetrical and there may be cortical atrophy. Sclera are usually white, but can be blue in childhood. Dentinogenesis imperfecta is frequent. Hearing defects are common.

Type IV is similar to type I, but with more bone abnormalities and some dwarfing. Teeth are frequently involved. Sclera are white.

Preoperative abnormalities

1. Individual features have been described above. A number of other defects occur in addition. Dentinogenesis imperfecta is present in about 50% of patients.

2. Severe skeletal injuries may occur with minor trauma, often in the absence of physical signs of bruising, swelling, or contusion. A UK survey showed that out of 804 patients, in 113 the diagnosis of nonaccidental injury had been made at some stage (Patterson 1990).

3. Hearing loss is common. Thirty-one out of 57 patients with osteogenesis imperfecta had conductive or mixed loss, therefore anaesthesia may be required for middle ear surgery (Bergstrom 1977).

4. There is some evidence of hypermetabolism, with excessive sweating and metabolic acidosis. Half of the patients have increased serum thyroxine levels.

5. Platelet dysfunction may occur and produce a mild bleeding tendency, although the platelet count may be normal.

6. Aortic and mitral valve insufficiency results from the defective connective tissue formation, but may be clinically inapparent. Sometimes cardiac surgery may be required (Wong et al 1995). Aortic root dilatation was found in 12% of patients in one survey, but unlike that seen in Marfan's syndrome, it is mild and nonprogressive (Hortop et al 1986). However, congenital cardiac lesions have been reported.

7. Kidney stones and renal papillary calcification may occur and dietary supplementation with calcium and vitamin D may predispose to this.

8. Cranial developmental defects may cause brainstem compression, hydrocephalus, or vascular disruption. Softening of the basal portion of the occipital bone and upward movement of the cervical spine can combine to cause secondary basilar impression which mainly occurs in type III disease (Engelbert et al 1998). Warning signs include cough, headache, vertigo, and trigeminal neuralgia (Hayes et al 1999). Patients with severe type III osteogenesis imperfecta with macrocephaly and cortical atrophy have been reported.

9. Those patients with kyphoscoliosis may have restrictive pulmonary defects. Sixty per cent have significant chest wall deformities. A thoracic scoliosis of more than 60 degrees will have severe effects on lung function, with a reduction in vital capacity to below 50% (Widmann et al 1999).

10. There is some evidence that in children with type III and IV disease, iv pamidronate improves signs and symptoms and decreases the fracture rate (Marini 1998).

Anaesthetic problems

1. Bones and teeth are easy to break. The mandible is prone to fracture, but the facial bones are less so. Inadvertent rib fractures were followed by fatal haemorrhage in a young girl during spinal fusion surgery (Sperry 1989).

2. In the severest form, forced extension of the head during intubation carries a risk of vertebral fracture.

3. Airway problems may occur if the head is large, if there is macroglossia, or if the skeletal deformities are severe. Difficult intubation was reported secondary to limited mouth opening (Edge et al 1997). Awake fibreoptic intubation failed, a laryngeal mask airway was passed, and eventually tracheal intubation was achieved after 2 h.

4. Thoracic scoliosis of greater than 60 degrees may result in pulmonary morbidity (Widmann et al 1999).

5. Hypermetabolic states, with hyperthermia, acidosis, sweating and cardiovascular instability, have been reported, but these are unrelated to MH (Masuda et al 1990). An MH-like syndrome that was terminated with dantrolene was described in a young man who subsequently refused further investigation. His sister had died aged 14 after a prolonged mask anaesthetic for reduction of a fracture (Rampton et al 1984). Postoperative hyperthermia, hypoxia and acidosis without hypercarbia, which responded to active cooling, occurred in a child. There was biochemical evidence of mild rhabdomyolysis (Ryan et al 1989). A 9-year-old child, who had developed a high fever during a previous anaesthetic, was given an anaesthetic that was nontriggering for MH, for osteosynthesis surgery. After nearly 3 h of anaesthesia, tachycardia, hypercarbia and metabolic acidosis developed suddenly and, although the CO_2 was

starting to decrease spontaneously, dantrolene sodium was given. On the ITU the temperature increased to a maximum of 40.0°C, although the CK was only 595 U l^{-1}. Two years later, MH testing proved to be negative (Porsborg et al 1996). Only one patient with osteogenesis imperfecta has been shown to be MH susceptible on muscle testing (Rosenberg 1988), and in this case it is assumed that the hyperthermia associated with osteogenesis imperfecta was a separate entity.

6. A coagulopathy has occurred during scoliosis correction and was associated with the sudden development of widespread petechiae (Edge et al 1997). Fatal haemorrhage occurred in a young girl during spinal fusion surgery, secondary to accidental rib fractures (Sperry 1989).

7. Multiple general anaesthetics may be required for orthopaedic or ENT procedures.

8. Violent suxamethonium fasciculations can cause fractures.

Management

1. Patients should be positioned on the operating table and handled with extreme care. Padding should be used. If the head is large, a pillow placed under the chest may assist tracheal intubation.

2. Surgery should be avoided in the pyrexial patient. Core temperature, oxygen saturation and $ETCO_2$ should be monitored throughout surgery. Hyperthermia is reported to have responded to cooling alone (Cho et al 1992).

3. In the severe types of the disease, concern has been expressed that a blood pressure cuff may damage the humerus. Direct arterial monitoring has been suggested as an alternative (Libman 1981).

4. Suxamethonium should be avoided when the risk of fractures is high.

5. The use of ketamine has been reported (Oliverio 1973, Robison & Wright 1986). This

offers a convenient method of avoiding mask and intubation anaesthesia. A woman with type 1 disease and previous problems with weaning after umbilical hernia surgery, was anaesthetised using a laryngeal mask airway, IPPV, and a propofol infusion. The laryngeal mask airway was removed on the ITU 40 min after surgery (Kostopanagiotou et al 2000).

6. Although skeletal deformity may make regional anaesthesia technically difficult, epidural anaesthesia has been used for the management of a Caesarean section (Cunningham et al 1984). In this patient, platelet studies were normal. One patient with type I disease had five Caesarean sections, three under epidural anaesthesia and two under spinal (Yeo & Paech 1999). However, such techniques must be managed with extreme care if serious intubation difficulties are anticipated. In one patient for Caesarean section who refused regional anaesthesia, neuromuscular block was achieved with vecuronium (Cho et al 1992). One 5-month-old child with type II disease was given caudal anaesthesia for herniorrhaphy (Barros 1995), and in another child, TIVA (total intravenous anaesthesia) was described (Baines 1995).

Bibliography

Baines D 1995 Total intravenous anaesthesia for patients with osteogenesis imperfecta. Paediatric Anaesthesia 5: 144.

Barros F 1995 Caudal block in a child with osteogenesis imperfecta, type 2. Paediatric Anaesthesia 5: 202–3.

Bergstrom L 1977 Osteogenesis imperfecta. Otological and maxillofacial aspects. Laryngoscope 87 (suppl 6): 1–42.

Cho E, Dayan SS, Marx GF 1992 Anaesthesia in a parturient with osteogenesis imperfecta. British Journal of Anaesthesia 68: 422–3.

Cole DEC, Cohen MM 1991 Osteogenesis imperfecta: an update. Journal of Pediatrics 119: 73–4.

Cunningham AJ, Donnelly M, Comerford J 1984 Osteogenesis imperfecta: anesthetic management of a patient for Cesarean section. Anesthesiology 61: 91–3.

Edge G, Okafor B, Fennelly ME et al 1997 An unusual manifestation of bleeding diathesis in a patient with osteogenesis imperfecta. European Journal of Anaesthesiology 14: 215–19.

Engelbert RH, Gerver WJ, Breslau-Siderius LJ et al 1998 Spinal complications in osteogenesis imperfecta: 47 patients 1–16 years of age. Acta Orthopaedica Scandinavica 69: 283–6.

Gahagan S, Rimsza ME 1991 Child abuse or osteogenesis imperfecta: how can we tell? Pediatrics 88: 987–92.

Hayes M, Parker G, Ell J et al 1999 Basilar impression complicating osteogenesis imperfecta type IV: the clinical and radiological findings in four cases. Journal of Neurology, Neurosurgery & Psychiatry 66: 357–64.

Hortop J, Tsipouras P, Hanley JA et al 1986 Cardiovascular involvement in osteogenesis imperfecta. Circulation 73: 54–61.

Kostopanagiotou G, Coussi T, Tsaroucha N et al 2000 Anaesthesia using a laryngeal mask airway in a patient with osteogenesis imperfecta. Anaesthesia 55: 506.

Libman RH 1981 Anaesthetic considerations for the patient with osteogenesis imperfecta. Clinical Orthopaedics & Related Research 159: 123–5.

Marini JC 1998 Osteogenesis imperfecta—managing brittle bones. New England Journal of Medicine 339: 986–7.

Masuda Y, Harada Y, Honma E et al 1990 Anesthetic management of a patient with osteogenesis imperfecta congenita [English abstract]. Masui 39: 383–7.

Oliverio RO 1973 Anesthetic management of intramedullary nailing in osteogenesis imperfecta. Anesthesia & Analgesia 52: 232–6.

Patterson CR 1990 Osteogenesis imperfecta and other bone disorders in the differential diagnosis of unexplained fractures. Journal of the Royal Society of Medicine 83: 72–4.

Porsborg P, Astrup G, Bendixen D et al 1996 Osteogenesis imperfecta and malignant hyperthermia. Is there a relationship? Anaesthesia 51: 863–5.

Rampton AJ, Kelly DA, Shanahan EC et al 1984 Occurrence of malignant hyperpyrexia in a patient with osteogenesis imperfecta. British Journal of Anaesthesia 56: 1443–6.

Robison C, Wright DJ 1986 Anaesthesia for osteogenesis imperfecta. Today's Anaesthetist 1(2): 22–3.

Rodrigo C 1995 Anesthesia for maxillary and mandibular osteotomies in osteogenesis imperfecta. Anesthesia Progress 42: 17–20.

Rosenberg H 1988 Clinical presentation of malignant hyperthermia. British Journal of Anaesthesia 60: 268–73.

Ryan CA, Al-Ghamdi AS, Gayle M et al 1989 Osteogenesis imperfecta and hyperthermia. Anesthesia & Analgesia 68: 811–14.

Sperry K 1989 Fatal intraoperative haemorrhage during spinal fusion surgery for osteogenesis imperfecta. American Journal of Forensic Medicine & Pathology 10: 54–9.

Widmann RF, Bitan FD, Laplaza FJ et al 1999 Spinal deformity, pulmonary compromise, and quality of life in osteogenesis imperfecta. Spine 24: 1673–8.

Wong RS, Follis FM, Shively BK et al 1995 Osteogenesis perfecta and cardiovascular disease. Annals of Thoracic Surgery 60: 1439–43.

Yeo ST, Paech MJ 1999 Regional anaesthesia for multiple caesarean sections in a parturient with osteogenesis imperfecta. International Journal of Obstetric Anesthesia 8: 284–7.

Pacemakers (see Heart block)

Paget's disease

A metabolic bone disease which may be either focal or diffuse. The aetiology is unknown, but epidemiological studies and the presence of inclusion bodies in osteoclasts suggest a viral origin. The primary process appears to be unusually active resorption of bone by abnormal osteoclasts, and although osteoblasts replace it, the architecture is disorganised and mineralisation is defective. There is fibrosis of the marrow, and both marrow and bone are extremely vascular. In the later, sclerotic stage, vascularity decreases and the bone becomes dense and hard. Suppression of the disease is now possible using specific inhibitors of osteoclast-mediated bone resorption (Delmas & Meunier 1997).

Preoperative abnormalities

1. The patient can be asymptomatic, or have bone pain. There may be localised bone enlargement; affected bones can become deformed and the overlying skin warm. The pelvis, femur, tibia, skull, and spine, are the most commonly involved.

2. The bone is more vulnerable to fractures than normal bone. About 1% of patients develop bone sarcoma.

3. Bone enlargement and deformity may encroach on either the central or peripheral nervous system, and produce a variety of neurological symptoms. Basilar invagination can cause compression of the brainstem, cerebellum or cranial nerves, to produce deafness, headache, or hydrocephalus. Hypertrophy of the spine can cause nerve entrapment, spinal compression, and cauda equina syndrome. Ossification of extradural structures can produce spinal stenosis or result in ischaemic neuropathy.

4. If the disease is widespread, the vascular stage may be associated with a high cardiac output. In severe Paget's disease, there is a high prevalence of calcific aortic stenosis (22%), heart block, and bundle branch block (Hultgren 1998). These abnormalities are absent in less severe cases.

5. Most patients require no treatment or mild analgesics only. Specific treatment is indicated in those with bone pain, complications of deformity, neurological symptoms, or heart failure. Mithramycin has been used for the rapid relief of pain and in spinal cord compression. Calcitonin (im or iv) reduces the vascularity of bone before orthopaedic procedures, and is used for bone pain and in osteolytic disease. Etidronate is increasingly used. It reduces bone turnover and may interfere with mineralisation. Treatment is usually limited to 6 months, but the effects may be prolonged. Newer drugs such as pamidronate and alendronate are even more effective (Delmas & Meunier 1997).

375

Anaesthetic problems

1. Bone fracture is a common complication of Paget's disease (Guyer 1980). It can occur with minimal trauma. In view of the increased vascularity of the bone, there may be considerable blood loss during orthopaedic procedures. A spontaneous epidural haematoma was thought to be secondary to increased vascularity of bone, resulting in greater blood flow through the epidural veins (Hanna et al 1989).

2. Venous air embolism occurred when a pulsed saline lavage was used during hip replacement (Sides 1996). It was thought that a combination of air in the system when the saline bag was changed, and a tight fit between the cannula and the femoral canal, resulted in high pressures in the shaft. The fact that air could be entrained in the tubing was later demonstrated. The increased vascularity in Paget's disease may have exacerbated the problem.

3. Paget's disease may affect the atlas and axis (Brown et al 1971). Cervical spine disease can be associated with serious neurological

complications. Bone hypertrophy and narrowing of the spinal canal may cause cord compression, or interference with the blood supply. Vertebral displacement can occur secondary to fracture or subluxation. Invagination of the foramen magnum into the posterior fossa is present in one-third of patients with Paget's disease of the skull (Guyer 1980).

4. The lumbar spine is often involved, particularly at the L3–4 level, therefore regional anaesthesia may be technically difficult. Midline puncture failed in three patients undergoing spinal anaesthesia for hip arthroplasty and paramedian placement was required in all three (Murphy & Shorten 1999).

Management

1. To avoid fractures, patients should be moved and positioned very gently under anaesthesia. Limbs should be supported and padded.

2. Treatment with calcitonin has been reported to decrease the bone vascularity. However, its effect is maximal in the early stages of treatment but may progressively diminish after the first 3 months.

3. Patients with cervical spine and skull disease should be treated with extreme care. Neurological symptoms and signs should be sought and documented in advance. Atlantoaxial subluxation must be excluded.

4. Spinal anaesthesia may be more easily achieved using the paramedian approach (Murphy & Shorten 1999).

5. Cardiac failure, if present, should be treated.

Bibliography

Brown HP, LaRocca H, Wickstrom JK 1971 Paget's disease of the atlas and axis. Journal of Bone & Joint Surgery 53B: 1441–4.

Delmas PD, Meunier PJ 1997 The management of Paget's disease of bone. New England Journal of Medicine 336: 558–66.

Guyer PB 1980 Radiology in Paget's disease. Hospital Update 6: 1079–91.

Hanna JW, Ball MR, Lee KS et al 1989 Spontaneous hematoma complicating Paget's disease of the spine. Spine 14: 900–2.

Hultgren HN 1998 Osteitis deformans (Paget's disease) and calcific disease of the heart valves. American Journal of Cardiology 81: 1461–4.

Murphy CM, Shorten G 1999 Spinal anaesthesia in three patients with Paget's disease of bone. Anaesthesia 54: 1227.

Sides CA 1996 Pulsed saline lavage causing venous air embolism in a patient with Paget's disease. British Journal of Anaesthesia 76: 330–1.

Papillomatosis (see Laryngeal papillomatosis)

Parkinson's disease

A disorder of the extrapyramidal motor system of unknown aetiology. Onset is gradual, and usually occurs after the age of 50. Pathological changes include degeneration of cells and loss of pigmented neurones in the substantia nigra, in excess of the rate normally associated with ageing. These cells synapse with dopamine receptors in the striatum (Mason et al 1996). Biochemical abnormalities in brain neurotransmitters, and in particular a deficiency of dopamine in the striatum and substantia nigra, have been demonstrated. Balance and movement are particularly affected by these changes. Parkinson's disease has also occurred following insults to the brain such as encephalitis lethargica, trauma, certain chemicals, major psychotropic drugs, cerebrovascular disease, or hypoxia. Parkinsonian features may occur in other degenerative CNS diseases that may exhibit additional signs such as autonomic failure (eg multiple system atrophy).

Dopamine/acetylcholine imbalance occurs and the aim of drug treatment is to increase dopamine concentrations in the basal ganglia, or to decrease the effects of acetylcholine; that is to redress the balance between central dopaminergic and cholinergic activity. The introduction of levodopa, which increases the dopamine levels in the striatum, has produced a considerable improvement in the quality of life for many patients, although long-term therapy may cause a reduction in response, resulting in fluctuations in mobility. Dopamine agonists such as bromocriptine, lisuride and pergolide are also used. Monoamine oxidase B inhibitors, such as selegiline hydrochloride, improve the duration of action of brain dopamine. This latter drug has been shown to have a protective effect in early Parkinson's disease. Symptomatic relief and side effects have to be balanced to find the optimum dosage. Improvements in drug therapy had decreased the requirement for stereotactic surgery, although there is a resurgence of interest in surgical treatment (Quinn & Bhatia 1998).

Autologous adrenal medulla transplant has been attempted, although improvements were not long term and the risks of surgery were thought to outweigh the benefits produced (Marsden 1990). The future of embryonic brain tissue transplants is at present unknown. Pallidotomy, through a frontal burr hole, is primarily for bradykinesia and rigidity, and thalamotomy for tremor.

For any surgery, the major perioperative problems for patients with Parkinson's disease are: (1) stopping drugs that allow them to function and (2) drug interactions.

Preoperative abnormalities

1. This is a clinical diagnosis and the main features are progressive akinesia, increased muscle tone with 'cogwheel' rigidity, and tremor that is increased with stress, decreased during action, and absent during sleep. Postural changes involve flexion of the head and body. Symptoms may be asymmetrical. The facies becomes expressionless, giving a false impression of disinterest or poor cerebral function. However, the subject is usually intellectually unimpaired, although dementia or depression may occur in the later stages of the disease.

2. Drug therapy depends on the symptoms and stage of the disease. In the early stages, anticholinergics may ameliorate tremor and rigidity. Levodopa is appropriate when postural changes and akinesia develop, but large doses have to be given because only 5% of the drug crosses the blood–brain barrier, and the rest is broken down by dopa decarboxylase. However, the dose, and hence the side effects secondary to high peripheral levels of levodopa metabolites, can be reduced by as much as 75% when it is combined with an inhibitor of extracerebral dopa decarboxylase, such as carbidopa or benserazide.

3. Gastrointestinal function is abnormal, and disturbances of deglutition, oesophageal motility, and colonic movement occur (Edwards et al 1992).

Anaesthetic problems

1. Abnormalities of swallowing have been demonstrated in 92% of Parkinsonian patients studied using videofluoroscopy, and tracheal aspiration was seen in 46% (Stroudley & Walsh 1991). This has implications for the perioperative period.

2. Arrhythmias may occur in patients receiving high doses of levodopa alone without a decarboxylase inhibitor, because of its metabolism to dopamine. However, the half-life is only 4 h. The concomitant use of carbidopa reduces dopaminergic side effects.

3. Orthostatic hypotension may occur in patients taking chronic levodopa therapy. This may result from a combination of decreased intravascular volume, decreased norepinephrine (noradrenaline) production, and reduction of norepinephrine stores.

4. Intraoperative exacerbation of the disease in a patient whose levodopa had been given 5 h beforehand has been described (Reed & Han 1992). The artefact produced on the ECG resembled coarse ventricular fibrillation.

5. Upper airway muscles may also be involved in extrapyramidal disorders producing

dysfunctional airway obstruction with abnormal flow/volume loops.

6. If levodopa is stopped completely in the perioperative period, the patient will become rigid and immobile. Maintenance of adequate ventilation may be difficult and venous thrombosis is a risk. Respiratory dyskinesia has also been reported. Several episodes of severe upper respiratory obstruction occurred in a patient whose levodopa/carbidopa combination had been omitted for five doses (Fitzpatrick 1995). Nasotracheal intubation immediately relieved the problem, but it recurred again the next day after extubation. Postextubation laryngeal spasm occurred in another patient (Backus et al 1991).

7. Phenothiazines and butyrophenones antagonise levodopa and may cause a deterioration in the Parkinson's disease.

8. Levodopa can interact with direct-acting sympathomimetic amines and monoamine oxidase inhibitors, to cause severe hypertension. The monoamine oxidase B inhibitor selegiline has been reported to have interacted with pethidine to give muscle rigidity, hyperthermia, and death (Zornberg et al 1991).

9. Autonomic dysfunction has been described in advanced disease (see Autonomic failure).

10. Suxamethonium-induced hyperkalaemia ($4.2–7.6\,mmol\,l^{-1}$) occurred in a patient with poorly controlled Parkinsonism (Gravlee 1980). This took place during induction of anaesthesia for CABG, when a number of drugs had been given. Levodopa had been stopped for 5 days. However, there is little evidence that this is generally a problem (Ho 1989, Muzzi et al 1989).

11. The theoretical possibility that high-dose opioid/nitrous oxide anaesthesia may be dangerous, on the grounds that opioid-induced rigidity resembles Parkinson's disease, has been suggested (Severn 1988). An acute dystonia occurred after the use of alfentanil 1 mg in a patient with untreated Parkinson's disease (Mets

1991). This was thought to result from decreased central dopaminergic transmission.

12. The use of local anaesthetic techniques may be limited by the extrapyramidal movements. Certain sedatives, such as the phenothiazines and butyrophenones, should be avoided because they block central dopaminergic receptors.

13. Venous air embolism occurred in two patients who were in a semisitting position undergoing stereotactic pallidotomy with light sedation and spontaneous respiration (Suarez et al 1999). Symptoms that suggested the diagnosis included coughing, chest pain, tachypnoea, decrease in SpO_2, and $ETCO_2$. Another patient who had similar symptoms during pallidotomy developed respiratory distress. Air bubbles in the right side of the heart were seen on echocardiography and a brain scan showed a significant volume of air in the subdural space where the twist drill had entered (Swartz et al 1997). In stereotactic surgery, the use of Doppler is not possible because of interference with neural recording.

14. After surgery, patients are more likely to develop confusional states and hallucinations (Golden et al 1989). Postoperative unmasking of Parkinson's disease has also been reported. A 54-year-old, otherwise healthy man, was admitted for cholecystectomy. His only complaint was a previous dystonic reaction to prochlorperazine. Despite having received no drugs known to induce extrapyramidal side effects, for 2 h postoperatively he exhibited a severe, dystonic, Parkinsonian-like syndrome. Eighteen months later he developed overt Parkinson's disease (Muravchick & Smith 1995).

15. Patients with Parkinson's disease are more susceptible to NMS than normal (Ueda et al 1999), and NMS may occur after withdrawal of anti-Parkinsonian drugs (Sechi et al 1996).

Management

1. The patient's current drug therapy must be known. If levodopa is being given in

combination with a dopa decarboxylase inhibitor, as occurs in most cases, the drugs can be given up to the time of surgery. If it is being given alone, it should be stopped 12–24 h before surgery. In order to prevent exacerbation of the disease, it has been suggested that the oral preparation should be given 20 min before surgery (Reed & Han 1992). Medication should be continued after surgery, by nasogastric tube if necessary. Furuya et al (2000) suggested 1 tablet of carbidopa/levodopa crushed in 10 ml saline every 2 h.

2. Avoid the use of drugs that can exacerbate extrapyramidal symptoms such as metoclopramide, phenothiazines, or butyrophenones. If extrapyramidal symptoms develop, diphenhydramine or levodopa can be given.

3. Evidence of autonomic neuropathy should be sought.

4. Careful cardiovascular monitoring for arrhythmias, hypotension, and hypertension. If intravascular volume is decreased, colloids may be required.

5. The use of regional anaesthesia has been suggested. However, it may be inadvisable in certain patients, if they are receiving complex drug regimens, or if there is a suggestion of autonomic neuropathy.

6. The use of ketamine in one patient with severe disease taking levodopa was reported to have greatly improved tremor and rigidity for several hours (Hetherington & Rosenblatt 1980).

7. Diphenhydramine, which possesses central anticholinergic effects, has been used during ophthalmic surgery under local anaesthesia. It was found to produce sedation with minimal tremor (Stone & DiFazio 1988).

8. For stereotactic pallidotomy or thalamotomy, anti-Parkinsonian medications are withheld for 12–24 h. Local anaesthesia and minimal sedation is usually given to allow communication. However, the use of the laryngeal mask airway for stereotactic surgery

and MRI has been reported (Silva & Brimacombe 1996). The anaesthetist should be prepared to deal with airway access should a CNS bleed occur, or with hypertension and excess tremor (Mason et al 1996). Abolition of tremor has been reported in two patients following anaesthesia. It was suggested that should general anaesthesia be required for stereotactic procedures, propofol be avoided (Anderson et al 1994).

Bibliography

Anderson BJ, Marks PV, Futter ME 1994 Propofol—contrasting effects in movement disorders. British Journal of Neurosurgery 8: 387–8.

Backus WW, Ward RR, Vitkun SA et al 1991 Postextubation laryngeal spasm in an unanesthetized patient with Parkinson's disease. Journal of Clinical Anesthesia 3: 314–16.

Edwards LL, Quigley EM, Pfeiffer RF 1992 Gastrointestinal function in Parkinson's disease: frequency and pathophysiology. Neurology 42: 726–32.

Fitzpatrick AJ 1995 Upper airway obstruction in Parkinson's disease. Anaesthesia & Intensive Care 23: 367–9.

Furuya R, Hirai A, Andoh T et al 1998 Successful perioperative management of a patient with Parkinson's disease by enteral levodopa administration under propofol anesthesia. Anesthesiology 89: 261–3.

Golden WE, Lavender RC, Metzen WS 1989 Acute postoperative confusion and hallucinations in Parkinson's disease. Annals of Internal Medicine 111: 218.

Gravlee GP 1980 Succinylcholine-induced hyperkalemia in a patient with Parkinson's disease. Anesthesia & Analgesia 59: 444–6.

Hetherington A, Rosenblatt RM 1980 Ketamine and paralysis agitans. Anesthesiology 52: 527.

Ho AM-H 1989 Parkinsonism and the anaesthetist. British Journal of Anaesthesia 62: 580.

Marsden CD 1990 Parkinson's disease. Lancet i: 948–52.

Mason LJ, Cojocaru TT, Cole DJ 1996 Surgical intervention and anesthetic management of the patient with Parkinson's disease. International Anesthesiology Clinics 34: 133–50.

Mets B 1991 Acute dystonia after alfentanil in untreated Parkinson's disease. Anesthesia & Analgesia 72: 557–8.

Muravchick S, Smith DS 1995 Parkinsonian symptoms during emergence from general anesthesia. Anesthesiology 82: 305–7.

Muzzi DA, Black S, Cucchiara RF 1989 The lack of effect of succinylcholine on serum potassium in patients with Parkinson's disease. Anesthesiology 71: 322.

Quinn N, Bhatia K 1998 Functional neurosurgery for Parkinson's disease. Has come a long way, though much remains experimental. British Medical Journal 316: 1259–60.

Reed AP, Han DG 1992 Intraoperative exacerbation of Parkinson's disease. Anesthesia & Analgesia 75: 850–3.

Sechi G, Manca S, Deiana GA et al 1996 Acute hyponatremia and neuroleptic malignant syndrome in Parkinson's disease. Progress in Neuro-Psychopharmacology & Biological Psychiatry 20: 533–42.

Severn A 1988 Parkinsonism and the anaesthetist. British Journal of Anaesthesia 61: 761–70.

Silva LCE, Brimacombe JR 1996 The laryngeal mask airway for stereotactic implantation of fetal hypophysis. Anesthesia & Analgesia 82: 430–1.

Stone DJ, DiFazio CA 1988 Sedation for patients with Parkinson's disease undergoing ophthalmic surgery. Anesthesiology 68: 821.

Stroudley J, Walsh M 1991 Radiological assessment of dysphagia in Parkinson's disease. British Journal of Radiology 64: 890–3.

Suarez S, Ornaque I, Fabregas N et al 1999 Venous air embolism during Parkinson surgery in patients with spontaneous ventilation. Anesthesia & Analgesia 88: 793–4.

Swartz MA, Munz M, Stern MB 1997 Respiratory failure following stereotactic neurosurgery in a 53-year-old woman. Chest 111: 1112–14.

Ueda M, Hamamoto M, Nagayama H et al 1999 Susceptibility to neuroleptic malignant syndrome in Parkinson's disease. Neurology 52: 777–81.

Zornberg GI, Bodkin JA, Colon BM 1991 Severe adverse reaction between pethidine and selegiline. Lancet 337: 246. Neurology 52: 777–81.

Paroxysmal nocturnal haemoglobinuria (PNH)

An acquired, clonal haematological disorder of stem cells, involving erythrocytes, leucocytes and platelets, which results in abnormal haematopoiesis, a reduction in life span of cells, and haemolytic anaemia. Various biochemical abnormalities have been reported, including deficiencies in a number of membrane proteins that interact with complement (Editorial 1992). The gene has now been identified. Cells of the paroxysmal nocturnal haemoglobinuria (PNH) clone are vulnerable to the haemolytic action of complement, acting either by the classic or alternative pathways. Cyclical lysis of PNH cells occurs, resulting in a reduction in the life span of the cell, although there is usually a population of normal cells present as well. Sometimes bone marrow aplasia develops, producing aplastic anaemia, although the precise relationship between the two diseases is not known. The presentations of PNH are very variable, attacks ranging from mild and intermittent to severe. It is mainly a disease of adults, but sometimes it occurs in children, in whom the disease tends to be more severe (Ware et al 1991). Those with venous thrombosis have the worst prognosis. Gallstones are common and patients may present for open or laparoscopic cholecystectomy, surgery for Budd–Chiari syndrome, or sometimes bone marrow transplantation.

Preoperative abnormalities

1. The median age of presentation is 42 years, with a range of 16–75 (Hillmen et al 1995).

2. Irregular episodes in which reddish-brown urine is passed. This may occur at night, or may be precipitated by exercise, surgery or infections, pregnancy and drugs. There may be recurrent attacks of abdominal pain, symptoms of anaemia, recurrent infection, and headaches.

3. Haematological abnormalities include haemolytic anaemia, nocturnal haemoglobinuria, variable but mild jaundice, haemosiderin in the urine leading to iron deficiency, leucopenia, thrombocytopenia, and reticulocytosis. Occasionally, acute renal failure occurs secondary to massive haemolysis. Aplastic anaemia sometimes develops.

4. Isolated venous thrombosis may occur, possibly triggered by platelet activation. In a study of 80 patients, venous thrombosis occurred in 39% and was sometimes recurrent (Hillmen et al 1995). Hepatic venous thrombosis (Budd–Chiari syndrome) is found in about 20%; intestinal thromboses and renal infarcts may also occur (see Budd–Chiari syndrome).

5. Patients are prone to recurrent infections because of leucopenia and defective leucocyte function.

6. Even in the presence of a normal glomerular filtration rate, there are defects in urinary concentrating ability.

7. Diagnosis may be suspected if haemosiderin is present in the urine. The Ham acid haemolysis test is used for the definitive diagnosis.

8. Supportive treatment includes blood and platelet transfusion, iron and folic acid therapy, antibiotics, long-term anticoagulants, and occasionally steroids (Rosse 1997). In some patients there may be an indication for bone marrow transplantation, although restoration of normal bone marrow function occurs in only about 50%, and the risks of the procedure may outweigh the benefits.

9. A poor survival is associated with thrombosis, pancytopenia, myelodysplastic or leukaemic syndromes, thrombocytopenia, or age above 50 years at diagnosis (Socie et al 1996).

Anaesthetic problems

1. There is an increased incidence of postoperative venous thrombosis, which is particularly high in the older age groups.

2. Pregnancy may be complicated by Budd–Chiari syndrome, fetal loss, and prematurity (Bais et al 1994). In a study of 38 pregnancies, both during pregnancy and postpartum, acute haemolysis and haemorrhage were the commonest complications. In another analysis of 65 pregnancies, 24.6% had acute haemolysis, 18.8% had obstetric haemorrhage, 7.7% septicaemia, and 4.6% pulmonary embolism (Svigos & Norman 1994). Three patients had hepatic venous thrombosis, two had intracerebral haemorrhage, and one had cerebral thrombosis. Nearly one-third of pregnancies end in miscarriage (De Gramont et al 1987).

3. Reactions that involve complement are more serious than usual, because of the vulnerability of the red cells to lysis (Taylor et al 1987).

4. Severe haemolysis and renal failure has been precipitated by ABO-incompatible plasma in pooled platelets (Jackson et al 1992).

Management

1. The importance of cooperation between the surgeon, haematologist, and anaesthetist has been emphasised.

2. Treatment of infection.

3. Prevention of dehydration by intravenous infusion the night before surgery with saline, glucose, with or without potassium, but not with Ringer lactate solution. A urine output of greater than $100\,\mathrm{ml\,h^{-1}}$ should be maintained. Acidosis must be prevented because it may enhance haemolysis. For major surgery, a catheter should be inserted to monitor the urine for haemoglobinuria (Ogin et al 1990).

4. If blood transfusion is required, the use of washed red cells reduces the chance of reactions (Jackson et al 1992). In anaemic patients, blood transfusion will decrease the proportion of abnormal cells.

5. All iv drugs should be given cautiously. It has been suggested that those known to have a low incidence of anaphylactoid reactions should be used (Taylor et al 1987).

6. Should hepatic venous thrombosis develop, anticoagulants or thrombolytic therapy may be required. However, heparin protamine complexes activate the classical complement pathway, therefore protamine should be avoided.

7. Corticosteroids may abort haemolytic episodes in some patients, but should only be given for short intervals. Prednisone given at 6 pm can prevent the noctural haemolytic episode in responders. Hydration should be maintained and transfusion may suppress the production of complement-sensitive cells. Tissue plasminogen activator is under evaluation (Wyatt et al 1995).

8. In pregnancy, regular haematological monitoring is essential, because transfusions of washed red cells or platelets, anticoagulants, treatment of infections, and screening for Budd–Chiari syndrome may be needed (Bais et al 1994).

Bibliography

Bais J, Pel M, von dem Borne A et al 1994 Pregnancy and paroxysmal nocturnal hemoglobinuria. European Journal of Obstetrics, Gynecology, & Reproductive Biology 53: 211–14.

De Gramont A, Krulik M, Debray J 1987 Paroxysmal nocturnal haemoglobinuria and pregnancy. Lancet i: 868.

Editorial 1992 Paroxysmal nocturnal haemoglobinuria. Lancet 339: 395–6.

Hillmen P, Lewis SM, Bessler M et al 1995 Natural history of paroxysmal noctural hemoglobinuria. New England Journal of Medicine 333: 1253–8.

Jackson GH, Noble RS, Maung ZT et al 1992 Severe haemolysis and renal failure in a patient with paroxysmal nocturnal haemoglobinuria. Journal of Clinical Pathology 45: 176–7.

Ogin GA 1990 Cholecystectomy in a patient with paroxysmal nocturnal hemoglobinuria. Anesthetic implications and management in the perioperative period. Anesthesiology 72: 761–4.

Rosse WF 1997 Paroxysmal nocturnal hemoglobinuria as a molecular disease. Medicine 76: 63–93.

Socie G, Mary JY, de Gramont A et al 1996 Paroxysmal nocturnal haemoglobinuria: long term follow-up and prognostic factors. French Society of Haematology. Lancet 348: 573–7.

Svigos JM, Norman J 1994 Paroxysmal nocturnal haemoglobinuria and pregnancy. Australian & New Zealand Journal of Obstetrics & Gynaecology 34: 104–6.

Taylor MB, Whitwam JG, Worsley A 1987 Paroxysmal nocturnal haemoglobinuria. Perioperative management of a patient with Budd–Chiari syndrome. Anaesthesia 42: 639–42.

Ware RE, Hall SE, Rosse WF 1991 Paroxysmal nocturnal hemoglobinuria with onset in childhood and adolescence. New England Journal of Medicine 325: 991–6.

Wyatt HA, Mowat AP, Layton M 1995 Paroxysmal nocturnal haemoglobinuria and the Budd–Chiari syndrome. Archives of Disease in Childhood 72: 241–2.

Pemphigus vulgaris (and foliaceous)

An autoimmune, bullous disease, caused by autoantibodies against adhesion molecules of the skin and mucous membranes. In pemphigus vulgarus, the blister is intra-epidermal and can affect skin and any mucous membrane covered by squamous epithelium (Nousari & Anhalt 1999). This contrasts with pemphigus foliaceous, which affects skin only and tends to be superficial. Vulgaris involves the protein desmoglein 3, whereas foliaceous affects desmoglein 1. A high incidence occurs in Ashkenazi Jews. The mortality has improved since the use of steroids, but steroids themselves can produce serious complications. However, in severe cases death often occurs within 5 years and is commonly associated with infection.

Preoperative abnormalities

1. Onset is usually in the fifth or sixth decade. It is a blistering disease involving skin and mucous membranes. Vesicles, erosions and ulceration are characteristic, although lesions tend to heal without scarring. Presentation is usually with painful mouth lesions, and in many patients, mucous membranes alone are affected. If it spreads, the skin of the head and neck are involved first, followed by the trunk and flexor surfaces (Nousari & Anhalt 1999). Lateral pressure on the skin causes separation of the epidermis (Nickolsky sign).

2. Oesophageal involvement may produce blisters and strictures (Mignogna et al 1997). Unlike pemphigoid, which can produce upper

airway obstruction from scarring (Drenger et al 1986), the larynx is usually spared.

3. Treatment with high-dose corticosteroids, azathioprine, intravenous gamma globulin, or plasmapheresis. Topical therapy plays no part in the treatment.

4. There is a correlation between antibody titre and severity of disease.

5. Infection is the most frequent cause of death, and in a study of 48 patients, 25% of deaths were related to the disease (Mourellou et al 1995).

Anaesthetic problems

1. Difficulty with venous access.

2. Friction and pressure may cause trauma.

3. Problems with mask application on induction.

4. Bleeding may occur at intubation from lesions within the oropharynx (Mahalingam et al 2000).

5. Side effects from treatment with high-dose steroids may necessitate surgery. Peritonitis from a perforated chronic duodenal ulcer occurred in a 45 year old receiving steroids for pemphigus vulgaris that had only erupted 20 days before (Mahalingam et al 2000).

6. Infection.

7. Although less common in the child-bearing age group, pemphigus may first appear, or worsen, during pregnancy (Daniel et al 1995). Severe disease is associated with a poor fetal outcome (Ruach et al 1995). Infants may have transient pemphigus.

8. In one patient, pemphigus was precipitated by emergency resection of colonic carcinoma. The onset of blistering around the stoma was followed by relentless spread over the next 6 days. High-dose steroids controlled the blisters, but death occurred on day 14 (Harries et al 1997).

Management

1. Assessment of general condition and nutrition.

2. Prevention of friction and trauma; suture cannulae, cover facial lesions with hydrocortisone cream and cotton sponges (see also Epidermolysis bullosa).

3. A variety of managements have been described, including diazepam and ketamine (Vatashsky & Aronsen 1982), epidural anaesthesia and ketamine for cholecystectomy (Jeyaram & Torda 1974), continuous spinal anaesthesia for hysterectomy (Gilsanz et al 1992), general anaesthesia and tracheal intubation for emergency laparotomy (Mahalingam et al 2000).

4. In pregnancy, regular antibody tests will show if the disease is progressing. It is recommended that patients should be delivered vaginally, because Caesarean section incisions may develop secondary infection (Daniel et al 1995). However, spinal anaesthesia for Caesarean section has been reported in pemphigus foliaceous (Abouleish et al 1997). No local anaesthesia was used and an area was chosen for incision that was free of lesions.

Bibliography

Abouleish EI, Elias MA, Lopez M et al 1997 Spinal anesthesia for cesarian section in a case of pemphigus foliaceous. Anesthesia & Analgesia 84: 449–50.

Daniel Y, Shenhav M, Botchan A et al 1995 Pregnancy associated with pemphigus. British Journal of Obstetrics & Gynaecology 102: 667–9.

Drenger B, Zidenbaum M, Reifen E et al 1986 Severe upper airway obstruction and difficult intubation in cicatricial pemphigoid. Anaesthesia 41: 1029–31.

Gilsanz F, Meilan ML, Roses R et al 1992 Regional anaesthesia in pemphigus vulgaris. Anaesthesia 47: 74.

Harries K, Owen C, Mills C et al 1997 Acute stomal "contact dermatitis or pemphigus. British Journal of Surgery 84: 685.

Jeyaram C, Torda TA 1974 Anesthetic management of cholecystectomy in a patient with buccal pemphigus. Anesthesiology 40: 600–1.

Mahalingam TG, Kathirvel S, Sidhi P 2000 Anaesthetic management of a patient with pemphigus vulgaris for emergency laparotomy. Anaesthesia 55: 160–2.

Mignogna MD, Lo Muzio L, Galloro G et al 1997 Oral pemphigus: clinical significance of esophageal involvement: report of eight cases. Oral Surgery, Oral Medicine, Oral Pathology, Oral Radiology, & Endodontics 84: 179–84.

Mourellou O, Chaidemenos GC, Koussidou T et al 1995 The treatment of pemphigus vulgaris. Experience with 48 patients seen over a 11-year period. British Journal of Dermatology 133: 83–7.

Nousari HC, Anhalt GJ 1999 Pemphigus and bullous pemphigoid. Lancet 354: 667–72.

Ruach M, Ohel G, Rahav D, Samueloff A 1995 Pemphigus vulgaris and pregnancy. Obstetrical & Gynecological Survey 50: 755–80.

Vatashsky E, Aronson HB 1982 Pemphigus vulgaris: anaesthesia in the traumatised patient. Anaesthesia 37: 1195–7.

384

Pericardial disease (see Cardiac tamponade)

Phaeochromocytoma (see also Section 2 for emergency presentation)

A rare catecholamine-secreting tumour, which usually originates in the adrenal gland, but may arise from anywhere in the sympathetic chain. Secretion of norepinephrine (noradrenaline) is more common than epinephrine (adrenaline). Extra-adrenal phaeochromocytomas are usually below the diaphragm, most commonly in the superior para-aortic region (Goldfarb et al 1989). Diagnosis may be made preoperatively, in which case adrenoceptor blockade must be instituted before surgery, or as soon as the diagnosis is made. Rarely, it may present unexpectedly during operation, or in labour as a life-threatening crisis (see Section 2, Phaeochromocytoma). In these cases, presenting features include tachycardia, hypertension, pulmonary oedema, and sudden death. In a retrospective survey of 62 autopsies, the diagnosis was only made before death in 17 (27%) patients (Platts et al 1995). Phaeochromocytomas may feature in a number of rare syndromes that include neurofibromatosis, von Hippel–Lindau disease, carotid body tumours, and the multiple endocrine neoplasias.

The existence of a catecholamine-induced myocarditis is increasingly being recognised (Editorial 1990). Initially, the myocardium is infiltrated with acute inflammatory cells, but this may be succeeded by a frank cardiomyopathy. The precise aetiology is unknown, but changes in cardiac adrenoceptors, the chronic effects of catecholamines on lipids, and direct damage from free radicals, are possible contributing factors.

Adequate preparation of the patient before surgery is essential. In a significant number of reports it is apparent that this has not always been achieved. The importance of anaesthetic involvement in the process has been emphasised (Shupak 1999).

Preoperative abnormalities

1. Episodes of headache, sweating and palpitations are the commonest presenting symptoms. The majority of patients have two or more of these complaints. If none of the three is present, or if flushing is a feature, then phaeochromocytoma is almost certainly not the cause (Bravo & Gifford 1984). Other useful markers are flank pain, visual symptoms, and pallor (Stein & Black 1991).

2. Persistent hypertension occurs in 50% of cases. In most of the remaining patients it is episodic.

3. Patients are frequently thin, appear anxious, and are peripherally vasoconstricted. Preoperative adrenoceptor blockade, with the accompanying expansion of the vascular volume, often causes the patient's face to fill out.

4. A number of cases have been reported in which cardiac failure has presented in conjunction with a phaeochromocytoma. Sometimes this may occur in normotensive patients (Sardesai et al 1990). Six patients were reported, five of whom died of pulmonary

oedema. It has been suggested that a cardiomyopathy, secondary to the chronic high levels of catecholamines, occurs more frequently than has been recognised. The reversibility of the cardiomyopathy, first by treatment with alpha-methyl-para-tyrosine, and subsequently by surgery, has been demonstrated (Imperato-McGinley et al 1987).

5. Biochemical diagnosis involves the initial screening of at least three 24-h urine collections for catecholamine metabolites. Measurement of urinary HMMA (3-hydroxy 4-methoxymandelic acid; sometimes called VMA or vanillylmandelic acid), or urinary metanephrines can be performed. The latter is more accurate. Levels may be mildly increased in a proportion of individuals without a phaelochromocytoma, but if the values are 1.5–2 times the upper limit of normal, this suggests that a phaeochromocytoma is present (Stein & Black 1991).

Should the screening tests prove positive, then direct plasma epinephrine (adrenaline) and norepinephrine (noradrenaline) estimations can be performed, but special laboratory facilities may be required. If the levels are only slightly elevated in the presence of hypertension, the diagnosis is unlikely. Patients with phaeochromocytomas become less sensitive than normal patients to catecholamines. Thus, in a patient with a phaeochromocytoma who has hypertension, plasma catecholamines are likely to be at least twice normal levels (Brown 1987).

A number of drugs, including levodopa, methyl dopa and MAOIs, may interfere with the biochemical tests.

Several provocation and suppression tests have been described for cases in which the diagnosis is in doubt. However, the provocation tests are dangerous and should not be used. Suppression of plasma catecholamine levels with pentolinium and clonidine will occur with physiologically raised levels, but not when the catecholamines are tumour generated.

6. Ninety per cent of tumours are adrenal in origin; they are bilateral in 10% of cases. If epinephrine (adrenaline) constitutes at least 20% of the total plasma catecholamines, the tumour is likely to be in the adrenal (Brown 1987). This is so because the synthesis of epinephrine (adrenaline) from norepinephrine (noradrenaline) is dependent on the presence of high levels of glucocorticoids, which are carried to the medulla in blood from the cortex.

For accurate localisation, a CT scan is now the first line of investigation. Provided that the tumours are greater than 1 cm in diameter, more than 90% of tumours will be identified.

Radioisotope *meta*-iodobenzylguanidine (mIBG) scanning has been reported to assist in both diagnosis and treatment of malignant tumours. mIBG is similar to norepinephrine (noradrenaline) in structure and is taken up and concentrated in the storage granules of chromaffin tissue. Imaging takes place at 24, 48 and 72 h. Adrenergic tissue is thus located. In cases in which the site is still in doubt, selective venous sampling from the inferior vena cava, or arteriography, may be necessary. Adrenoceptors must be blocked before any invasive investigation.

Anaesthetic problems

1. *Problems during anaesthesia in the untreated patient.* The undiagnosed, or the diagnosed but unblocked patient, is greatly at risk from hypertensive crises, particularly during arteriography (Platts et al 1995, Brueckel & Boehm 1998), anaesthesia, surgery, or delivery (Botchan et al 1995). Whilst the previous high mortality has been greatly reduced by preoperative adrenoceptor blocking, patients are still reported in whom surgery is embarked on before adequate control of blood pressure has been achieved. This is most likely to occur when agents other than phenoxybenzamine have been used (Mann et al 1996). The risks in the undiagnosed case having incidental surgery (Sutton et al 1981), or when it occurs in association with pregnancy (Mitchell et al 1987), remain high. Major problems are:

a) Severe hypertension, with the risk of cerebral haemorrhage, encephalopathy, pulmonary oedema, myocardial infarction, ventricular fibrillation, and renal failure. Hypertension may occur at induction and intubation, during handling of the tumour, or in labour during uterine contractions. It can also be precipitated if a beta blocker is administered alone, before alpha blockade has been established (Ambesh 1993, Sheaves et al 1995). This is because removal of the beta vasodilator effects leaves the alpha vasoconstrictor effects totally unopposed.

b) Severe hypotension following removal of the tumour, from a combination of hypovolaemia and the sudden decrease in circulating catecholamines. An inadequately prepared patient had asystole following ligation of the venous drainage and subsequently died from brain damage (Shupak 1999). Before adrenoceptor blockade, hypotension was usually treated with norepinephrine (noradrenaline) or epinephrine (adrenaline) infusions, and the patient frequently died in a state of profound vasoconstriction and hypotension.

c) Severe and protracted hypoglycaemia following removal of the tumour has been reported (Levin & Heifetz 1990).

2. Formerly, a request for only partial preoperative blockade was often made by the surgeon, in order to assess, after initial tumour removal, whether or not a second was present. Improved methods of tumour location have now made this much less necessary. In practice, however, some hypertensive response to tumour handling usually occurs.

3. At laparoscopic adrenalectomy, peritoneal insufflation can produce large increases in catecholamine output with intense vasoconstriction (Mann et al 1996). This was confirmed in eight consecutive patients treated preoperatively with a variety of antihypertensive medications. Significant catecholamine release occurred during the creation of the pneumoperitoneum and adrenal gland manipulation. Cardiac output increased twofold, but the blood pressure was controlled with a nicardipine infusion in all eight patients, and tachycardia controlled with boluses of atenolol in the six patients who had not received preoperative beta blockade (Joris et al 1999).

4. Incidentally detected, asymptomatic, apparently nonfunctioning adrenal tumours have occasionally turned out during surgery to be functioning phaeochromocytomas (Linos et al 1996, Harioka et al 1999).

Management

1. *Diagnosis and location.* See above.

2. *Preoperative preparation.* Pharmacological treatment with adrenoceptor blocking agents. This is the most crucial part of the patient's management. Preparation with oral drugs should be undertaken for at least 10–14 days to allow gradual re-expansion of vascular volume. Postural hypotension often indicates that the patient is volume-depleted. Thus, during the period of vasodilatation, iv repletion may be necessary. Criteria for the adequacy of blockade have been specified (Roizen et al 1982). These require that there must be control of blood pressure without undue postural hypotension, control of major symptoms, and 2 weeks' freedom from ST- and T- wave changes on ECG. A number of regimens have been described. However, in this author's opinion, no new agent has yet proved superior to phenoxybenzamine, a well-tested agent, given according to Roizen's specifications. Single daily blood pressure measurements are inadequate and unreliable. Although mean ambulatory blood pressure was said to be satisfactory in a patient with an epinephrine(adrenaline)-secreting tumour, two episodes of severe hypertension occurred during the day that were coincident with symptoms (Gallen et al 1994).

a) Phenoxybenzamine oral 10 mg bd initially, increasing gradually until hypertension is controlled. Between 80 and 200 mg may be required. At least 10 days' treatment will be needed. Despite the fashion for newer agents, the use of phenoxybenzamine as the basis of treatment appears to result in the best intraoperative stability (Russell et al 1998).

b) If a tachycardia develops, a beta blocker, such as propranolol 40–80 mg daily, increasing gradually if necessary, should be given.

If ischaemic heart disease is present, blocking should be instituted cautiously, to prevent sudden hypotension or tachycardia.

Occasionally, intravenous blocking may be required. This should take a minimum of 3 days. There should be close monitoring by medical staff throughout the procedure, particularly in patients with a degree of myocardial ischaemia.

Day 1:

Phenoxybenzamine $1 \, mg \, kg^{-1}$ in 500 ml saline over 2 h.

Propranolol orally if pulse rate above 120 beat min^{-1}.

Day 2:

Phenoxybenzamine $1–1.5 \, mg \, kg^{-1}$ over 2 h.

Propranolol to keep pulse rate below 100 beat min^{-1}.

Day 3:

Phenoxybenzamine $1–2 \, mg \, kg^{-1}$ over 2 h.

Propranolol as necessary.

Day of operation:

Phenoxybenzamine 50 mg.

Propranolol as necessary.

At this stage the BP should be 110/70 and pulse rate <90 beat min^{-1}.

c) Other suggested methods of preoperative adrenoceptor blocking:

i) Prazosin, an alpha$_1$ receptor antagonist. There is more than one alpha adrenoceptor site. Alpha$_1$

receptors are postsynaptic whereas alpha$_2$ are presynaptic. It appears that stimulation of the alpha$_2$ receptors has an inhibiting effect on the release of norepinephrine (noradrenaline) from the nerve terminal. Blocking of these receptors therefore will enhance the release of norepinephrine (noradrenaline) (Hoffman & Lefkowitz 1980). Phentolamine and phenoxybenzamine block both types of receptor, and the resultant tachycardia from the use of these drugs is said to result from cardiac beta receptor stimulation. Since prazosin is a selective alpha$_1$ blocker, it does not usually produce a tachycardia. Its use for preoperative preparation has been reported in four patients (Nicholson et al 1983). An initial test dose of prazosin 1 mg only was given, because sudden hypotension has been described in some subjects (Wallace & Gill 1978). On the basis of the response to this, further doses were prescribed. Apparently satisfactory preoperative stabilisation was produced with between 6 and 16 mg prazosin. However, all four patients had severe hypertensive responses during surgery that required phentolamine infusion, and in one case, surgery was abandoned to allow treatment with phenoxybenzamine for 2 weeks. Prazosin alone therefore may not provide the best protection from the effects of high catecholamine levels produced during surgery.

ii) Labetalol, a combined alpha and beta blocker. Its beta effects are three to seven times those of its alpha effects and it is therefore potentially dangerous in patients with phaeochromocytomas. Paradoxical severe hypertension has been reported following its use (Navaratnarajah & White 1984, Sheaves et al 1995).

iii) Management of phaeochromocytoma with magnesium sulphate (James 1989, Pivalizza 1995).

iv) Calcium channel blockers have been used for their systemic vasodilator effects, either alone or in combination with other drugs. Colson et al (1998) used nicardipine intraoperatively in 19 consecutive patients, but hypertension was sustained in seven out of 11. There is other evidence that, as sole therapy, calcium channel blockers may be inadequate to control swings in pressure (Munro et al 1995). Joris et al (1999) used it in conjunction with sufentanil and boluses of atenolol in eight patients undergoing laparoscopic adrenalectomy.

v) Alpha methylparatyrosine can achieve blockade by generation of a false transmitter.

3. *Anaesthetic techniques.* A wide variety of techniques and drugs have been recommended. After a randomised trial of four anaesthetic methods, it was concluded that the choice of technique was not the crucial factor in patient outcome (Roizen et al 1982). Adequacy of preoperative adrenoceptor blockade was probably of more importance.

The aim is to provide conditions under which catecholamine release by the tumour, or the effect of any catecholamines released, is kept to a mimimum. Tracheal intubation, creation of pneumoperitoneum, handling of the tumour, and certain drugs, are known stimuli. A sedative premedication and a quiet, unhurried induction of anaesthesia are essential.

Both morphine and pethidine release histamine, and atropine gives a tachycardia. Droperidol has been reported to produce pressor responses, possibly from inhibition of catecholamine uptake (Sumikawa & Amakata 1977). Suxamethonium is traditionally avoided, since fasciculations increase intra-abdominal pressure.

Epidural anaesthesia is often combined with general anaesthesia (Hopkins et al 1989). However, it should be remembered that patients with epidural blockade are sensitive to circulating catecholamines (Hull 1986), and that an epidural does not suppress the release of catecholamines (Liem et al 1991). Tonnesen et al (1989) measured killer cell activity during surgery in a patient who had not received preoperative adrenoceptor blocking drugs and showed a strong relationship between plasma catecholamines and natural killer cell activity. In this patient, despite the use of epidural anaesthesia, glyceryl trinitrate and phentolamine to control blood pressure during surgery, mean arterial pressures of up to 155 mmHg occurred during tumour handling.

Although pancuronium has been used on many occasions, hypertension has been reported (Jones & Hill 1981). Vecuronium is a more logical substitute since it avoids the hypertension and tachycardia produced by pancuronium.

Halothane sensitises the heart to the effect of catecholamines. Sufentanil infusions have been reported (Joris et al 1999). Desflurane has been used to control swings of blood pressure in a patient with high norepinephrine (noradrenaline) levels, who had been well prepared with phenoxybenzamine and metyrosine. In view of the ability of desflurane to cause sympathetic activation, the authors emphasised the importance of proper preoperative preparation, if is to be used (Lippmann et al 1994).

4. *Monitoring.* Direct arterial monitoring should begin in the anaesthetic room. Measurement of central venous pressure, $ETCO_2$, urine output and neuromuscular monitoring are required in addition. A recent report described the use of laser Doppler flowmetry, by which the authors demonstrated a correlation between skin blood flow and plasma norepinephrine (noradrenaline) levels (Sakuragi et al 1996). Transoesophageal echocardiography has also been used to monitor fluid administration and left ventricular function (Ryan et al 1993).

5. *Treatment of intraoperative complications*

a) *Hypertension.* Phentolamine, sodium nitroprusside and glyceryl trinitrate have all been given. The choice depends on individual preference. Phentolamine causes a tachycardia, whereas sodium nitroprusside may produce swings in blood pressure, with hypotension occurring when tumour stimulation stops. Magnesium sulphate has been used to control the blood pressure in a pregnant patient (James et al 1988). Magnesium inhibits the release of catecholamines from the adrenal medulla, decreases the sensitivity of alpha adrenoceptors, and causes direct vasodilatation. Nicardipine was used as a vasodilator to maintain SVR at less than $1600 \, \text{dyn s cm}^{-5}$ in 19 consecutive patients (Colson et al 1998). However, in seven out of 11 patients, sustained increases in blood pressure persisted. Esmolol and nicardipine infusions were used during laparoscopic adrenalectomy in a child (Pretorius et al 1998).

b) *Tachycardia.* This usually responds to beta blockers, propranolol iv 1–2 mg being the most frequently used. Bronchospasm has been noticed in one nonasthmatic patient, occurring 2 h after operation (personal observation). In asthmatic patients, a cardioselective blocker, such as atenolol or metoprolol, may be more appropriate. Esmolol, a short-acting beta adrenoreceptor blocker given by infusion, has attractions because it can be stopped easily (Zakowski et al 1989, Ryan et al 1993).

If heart failure is a problem, beta blockers may not be suitable. Amiodarone has been given to treat a tachycardia in a patient with phaeochromocytoma and a cardiomyopathy (Solares et al 1986).

c) *Hypotension.* May occur after ligation of the main veins from the tumour. Sudden reduction in catecholamine output by the tumour is in part responsible, but hypovolaemia may contribute. Patients with adrenoceptor blockade are very sensitive to changes in blood volume. Rapid infusion and CVP monitoring will usually correct the hypotension. If this fails, the use of phenylephrine or dopamine has been suggested (Roizen et al 1982). An infusion of angiotensin II (2.5 mg in 100–1000 ml saline at a rate of $1–20 \, \mu \text{g min}^{-1}$) has been used (Sommerville & McKellar 1989). It is an octapeptide produced by the breakdown of angiotensin I, with a half life of 1–2 min. Its vasoconstrictor action is powerful.

d) *Phaeochromocytoma during pregnancy.* If a phaeochromocytoma is diagnosed before delivery, its removal is frequently combined with Caesarean section (Hopkins et al 1989, Takahashi et al 1998). However, there may be the necessity to remove it earlier (Hamilton et al 1997). Medical therapy alone was given in one patient who had recurrence during pregnancy (Sweeney & Katz 1994). Antepartum diagnosis reduces the mortality, but unfortunately is only made in about half of the patients (Harper et al 1989).

Bibliography

Ambesh SP 1993 Occult pheochromocytoma in association with hyperthyroidism presenting under general anesthesia. Anesthesia & Analgesia 77: 1074–6.

Botchan A, Hauser R, Kupfermine M et al 1995 Pheochromocytoma in pregnancy: case report and review of the literature. Obstetrical & Gynecological Survey 50: 321–7.

Bravo EL, Gifford RW 1984 Pheochromocytoma: diagnosis, localisation and management. New England Journal of Medicine 311: 1298–303.

Brown M J 1987 The measurement of autonomic function in clinical practice. Journal of the Royal College of Physicians 21: 206–9.

Brueckel J, Boehm BO 1998 Crisis after angiography. Lancet 352: 1278.

Colson P, Ryckwaert F, Ribstein J et al 1998 Haemodynamic heterogeneity and treatment with the calcium channel blocker nicardipine during phaeochromocytoma surgery. Acta Anaesthesiologica Scandinavica 42: 1114–19.

Editorial 1990 Phaeochromocytoma still surprises. Lancet 335: 1189–90.

Gallen IW, Taylor RS, Salzmann MB et al 1994 Twenty-four hour ambulatory blood pressure and heart rate in a patient with predominantly adrenaline secreting phaeochromocytoma. Postgraduate Medical Journal 70: 589–91.

Goldfarb DA, Novick AC, Bravo EL et al 1989 Experience with extra-adrenal pheochromocytoma. Journal of Urology 142: 931–6.

Hamilton A, Sirrs S, Schmidt N et al 1997 Anaesthesia for phaeochromocytoma in pregnancy. Canadian Journal of Anaesthesia 44: 654–7.

Harioka T, Nomura K, Hosoi S et al 1999 Laparoscopic resection of unsuspected pheochromocytoma. Anesthesia & Analgesia 89: 1068.

Harper MA, Murnaghan GA, Kennedy L et al 1989 Phaeochromocytoma in pregnancy. Five cases and a review of the literature. British Journal of Obstetrics & Gynaecology 96: 594–606.

Hoffman BB, Lefkowitz RJ 1980 Alpha-adrenergic receptor subtypes. New England Journal of Medicine 302: 1390–6.

Hopkins PM, Macdonald R, Lyons G 1989 Caesarean section at 27 weeks gestation with removal of phaeochromocytoma. British Journal of Anaesthesia 63: 121–4.

Hull CJ 1986 Phaeochromocytoma. Diagnosis, preoperative preparation and management. British Journal of Anaesthesia 58: 1453–68.

Imperato-McGinley J, Gautier T, Ehlers K et al 1987 Reversibility of catecholamine-induced dilated cardiomyopathy in a child with pheochromocytoma. New England Journal of Medicine 316: 793–7.

James MFM 1989 Use of magnesium sulphate in the management of phaeochromocytoma: a review of 17 anaesthetics. British Journal of Anaesthesia 62: 616–23.

James MFM, Huddle KRL, Owen AD et al 1988 Use of magnesium sulphate in the anaesthetic management of phaeochromocytoma. Canadian Journal of Anaesthesia 35: 178–82.

Jones RM, Hill AB 1981 Severe hypertension associated with pancuronium in a patient with phaeochromocytoma. Canadian Anaesthetists' Society Journal 28: 394–6.

Joris JL, Hamoir EE, Hartstein GM et al 1999 Hemodynamic changes and catecholamine release during laparoscopic adrenalectomy for pheochromocytoma. Anesthesia & Analgesia 88: 16–21.

Levin H, Heifetz M 1990 Phaeochromocytoma and severe protracted hypoglycaemia. Canadian Journal of Anaesthesia 37: 477–8.

Liem TH, Moll JE, Booij LHDJ 1991 Thoracic epidural analgesia in a patient with bilateral phaeochromocytoma undergoing coronary artery bypass grafting. Anaesthesia 46: 654–8.

Linos DA, Stylopoulos N, Raptis SA 1996 Adrenaloma: a call for more aggressive management. World Journal of Surgery 20: 788–93.

Lippmann M, Ford M, Lee C et al 1994 Use of desflurane during resection of phaeochromocytoma. British Journal of Anaesthesia 72: 707–9.

Mann C, Millat B, Boccara G et al 1996 Tolerance of laparoscopy for resection of phaeochromocytoma. British Journal of Anaesthesia 77: 795–7.

Mitchell SZ, Freilich JD, Brant D et al 1987 Anesthetic management of pheochromocytoma resection during pregnancy. Anesthesia & Analgesia 66: 478–80.

Munro J, Hurlbert BJ, Hill GE 1995 Calcium channel blockade and uncontrolled blood pressure during phaeochromocytoma surgery. Canadian Journal of Anaesthesia 42: 228–30.

Navaratnarajah M, White DC 1984 Labetalol and phaeochromocytoma. British Journal of Anaesthesia 56: 1179.

Nicholson JP, Vaughn ED, Pickering TG et al 1983 Pheochromocytoma and prazosin. Annals of Internal Medicine 99: 477–9.

Pivalizza EG 1995 Magnesium sulfate and epidural anesthesia in pheochromocytoma and severe coronary artery disease. Anesthesia & Analgesia 81: 414–16.

Platts JK, Drew PJ, Harvey JN 1995 Death from phaeochromocytoma: lessons from a post-mortem survey. Journal of the Royal College of Physicians of London 29: 299–306.

Pretorius M, Rasmussen GE, Holcomb GW 1998 Hemodynamic and catecholamine responses to laparoscopic adrenalectomy for pheochromocytoma in a pediatric patient. Anesthesia & Analgesia 87: 1268–70.

Roizen MF, Horrigan RW, Koike M et al 1982 A prospective randomised trial of four anesthetic techniques for resection of pheochromocytoma. Anesthesiology 57: A43.

Russell WJ, Metcalfe IR, Tonkin AL et al 1998 The preoperative management of phaeochromocytoma. Anaesthesia & Intensive Care 26: 196–200.

Ryan T, Timoney A, Cunningham AJ 1993 Use of transoesophageal echocardiography to manage beta-adrenoceptor block and assess left ventricular function in a patient with a phaeochromocytoma. British Journal of Anaesthesia 70: 101–3.

Sakuragi T, Okamoto I, Fujiki T et al 1996 Skin blood flow and plasma catecholamines during removal of pheochromocytoma. Anesthesiology 85: 1485–8.

Sardesai SH, Mourant AJ, Sivathandon Y et al 1990 Phaeochromocytoma and catecholamine-induced cardiomyopathy presenting as heart failure. British Heart Journal 63: 234–7.

Sheaves R, Chew SL, Grossman AB 1995 The dangers of unopposed beta-adrenergic blockade in phaeochromocytoma. Postgraduate Medical Journal 71: 58–9.

Shupak RC 1999 Difficult anesthetic management during pheochromocytoma surgery. Journal of Clinical Anesthesia 11: 247–50.

Solares G, Ramos F, Martin-Duran R et al 1986 Amiodarone, phaeochromocytoma and cardiomyopathy. Anaesthesia 41: 186–90.

Sommerville KJ, McKellar JBM 1989 Angiotensin II in the management of excision of phaeochromocytoma. Anaesthesia 44: 841–2.

Stein PP, Black HR 1991 A simplified diagnostic approach to pheochromocytoma. Medicine 70: 46–66.

Sumikawa K, Amakata Y 1977 The pressor effect of droperidol on a patient with pheochromocytoma. Anesthesiology 46: 359–61.

Sutton MStJ, Sheps SG, Lie JT 1981 Prevalence of clinically unsuspected pheochromocytoma. Mayo Clinic Proceedings 56: 354–60.

Sweeney WJ, Katz VL 1994 Recurrent pheochromocytoma during pregnancy. Obstetrics & Gynecology 83: 820–2.

Takahashi K, Sai Y, Nosaka S 1998 Anaesthetic management for caesarean section combined with removal of phaeochromocytoma. European Journal of Anaesthesiology 15: 364–6.

Tonnesen E, Knudsen F, Nielsen HK et al 1989 Natural killer cell activity in a patient undergoing resection of phaeochromocytoma. British Journal of Anaesthesia 62: 327–30.

Wallace JM, Gill DP 1978 Prazosin in diagnosis and treatment of pheochromocytoma. Journal of the American Medical Association 240: 2752–3.

Zakowski M, Kaufman B, Berguson P et al 1989 Esmolol use during resection of pheochromocytoma: report of three cases. Anesthesiology 70: 875–7.

Phenylketonuria

One of a group of inborn errors of amino acid metabolism of autosomal recessive inheritance, that involves the essential amino acid, phenylalanine. There is absence of phenylalanine hydroxylase, which catalyses the conversion of phenylalanine to tyrosine, a reaction that only takes place in the liver, kidney, and pancreas. There is impairment of protein synthesis, and the accumulation of phenylalanine in the blood and urine inhibits a number of enzyme systems. There are decreased catecholamine levels, alterations in the metabolism of 5-hydroxytryptamine, and interference with melanin synthesis. Early diagnosis and treatment of phenylketonuria (PKU) is essential, otherwise irreversible brain damage occurs. Mental retardation is not present at birth, but the metabolic defect becomes evident soon afterwards and, if untreated, brain damage ensues. Nowadays, mass screening means that the majority of cases will have been diagnosed and treated before the onset of brain damage. It had been thought that the diet could be relaxed, but not stopped, after the age of 8 years, except during pregnancy (Phenylketonuria: diagnosis and management 1989). However, on the basis of white matter abnormalities shown on MRI scan in adults, a recent MRC working party has suggested that phenylalanine restriction should continue throughout life, and that blood concentrations of phenylalanine should be maintained at $700\,\mu\,\mathrm{mol\,l^{-1}}$ or less (Walter 1995). There is also a suggestion that some noncompliant patients may be severely B_{12} deficient, so that there should be caution in the use of nitrous oxide.

Preoperative abnormalities

1. In the undiagnosed or untreated patient there is diffuse and focal demyelination. Clinical

features include hyperreflexia, hypertonia, seizures, behavioural problems, microcephaly, decreased pigmentation secondary to inhibition of melanin synthesis, eczematous skin, progressive loss of hair, and a musty smell. The maxilla is prominent, with gaps between the teeth, and enamel abnormalities.

2. The diagnosed patient will have a dietary regimen that includes protein restriction, the administration of supplementary amino acids with extra tyrosine, together with all essential amino acids apart from phenylalanine (Editorial 1991a,b). A blood phenylalanine level of $100–400 \mu \, mol \, l^{-1}$ is aimed at and this requires close monitoring. However, excessive restriction of phenylalanine will result in protein catabolism causing delayed growth, hypoglycaemia, and neurological damage. Adults should have levels not exceeding $700 \mu \, mol \, l^{-1}$. Vitamin B_{12} should also be taken.

3. There is evidence that performance on neuropsychological tests and blood phenylalanine levels are inversely correlated (Scriver et al 1989).

Anaesthetic problems

1. If the patient was not diagnosed early, seizures and mental retardation may be a problem.

2. Prolonged perioperative fasting may stimulate catabolism.

3. High blood levels of phenylalanine predispose to fits and behavioural abnormalities.

4. A 14-year-old, noncompliant phenylketonuric developed acute neurological problems that started 1 week following nitrous oxide anaesthesia for myringoplasty. A spastic paraparesis, an Hb of $8.4 \, g \, dl^{-1}$, a low serum B_{12} and folate, and a serum phenylalanine that was double the recommended level, were found. It was suggested that nitrous oxide had precipitated a myeloneuropathy that was associated with lack of B_{12} (Lee et al 1999). Nitrous oxide irreversibly inactivates the active form of B_{12}, therefore

patients who are cobalamin deficient may be at risk from demyelination, subacute combined degeneration of the cord, and encephalopathy (Guttormsen et al 1994, Rosener & Dichgans 1996, Takacs 1996). Guttormsen et al described five patients (without PKU) with unexpected cobalamin deficiencies who developed myelopathy after nitrous oxide anaesthesia of less than 4 h duration.

5. The fragile skin is vulnerable to pressure and friction stresses.

6. Hyperphenylalaninaemia can cause severe fetal damage, including microcephaly and congenital heart disease, even if the fetus does not have PKU itself (Walter 1995).

Management

1. It is suggested that blood phenylalanine and serum B_{12} levels be checked within 72 h of elective surgery to assess adequacy of dietary therapy. Preoperative review by a metabolic team may be appropriate, so that any nutritional abnormalities can be identified and corrected (Anders & Dearlove 1999).

2. The patient should be first on the operating theatre list. A glucose infusion should be started in advance, to prevent a catabolic state and the resultant increased phenylalanine levels.

3. If delayed diagnosis has resulted in cerebral impairment, the management is that of a retarded child with a seizure disorder.

Bibliography

Anders NRF, Dearlove O 1999 Need for preoperative visit before general anaesthesia. Lancet 353: 1446.

Editorial 1991a Phenylketonuria grows up. Lancet 337: 1256–7.

Editorial 1991b Phenylketonuria—genotypes and phenotypes. New England Journal of Medicine 324: 1280–1.

Guttormsen AB, Refsum H, Ueland PM 1994 The interaction between nitrous oxide and cobalamin. Biochemical effects and clinical consequences. Acta Anaesthesiologica Scandinavica 38: 753–6.

Lee P, Smith I, Piesowicz A et al 1999 Spastic paraparesis after anaesthesia. Lancet 353: 554.

Phenylketonuria: diagnosis and management 1989 Proceedings of a symposium. Postgraduate Medical Journal 65 (suppl 2): S1–26.

Rosener M, Dichgans J 1996 Severe combined degeneration of the spinal cord after nitrous oxide anaesthesia in a vegetarian. Journal of Neurology, Neurosurgery & Psychiatry 60: 354.

Scriver CR, Kaufman S, Woo SLC 1989 The hyperphenyl-alaninemias. In: Scriver CR et al (eds) The metabolic basis of inherited disease. McGraw Hill, New York, pp 495–546.

Takacs J 1996 [N₂O-induced funicular myelosis in latent B₁₂ deficiency.] Anasthesiologie, Intensivmedizin, Notfallmedizin, Schmerztherapie 31: 525–8.

Walter JH 1995 Late effects of phenylketonuria. Archives of Disease in Childhood 73: 485–6.

Pierre Robin syndrome and the

Robin sequence

A rare syndrome in which the combination of severe micrognathia and posterior prolapse of the tongue results in respiratory obstruction in infancy, failure to thrive, and, occasionally, cor pulmonale. Other congenital abnormalities, such as cleft palate and oesophageal atresia, may occur. The 'Robin sequence', a term that is increasingly being used in the specialist surgical literature, describes a spectrum of anomalies, the common features of which include mandibular hypoplasia, glossoptosis and incomplete cleft palate, although all three are not necessarily present. The Robin sequence may be an isolated abnormality, or it may be part of a syndrome. Since there may be airway and intubation problems in any of these patients, several authors have considered them together.

These patients frequently require anaesthesia at a young age. In a retrospective analysis of airway endoscopy in those less than 1 month old, the Pierre Robin sequence was the most common associated anomaly (Ungkanont et al 1998). Management of long-term airway obstruction is a matter for debate, but at present tracheostomy seems to be back in favour. The mortality from paediatric tracheostomy has declined and it increases the safety of subsequent anaesthetics (Bath & Bull 1997, Myer et al 1998).

Preoperative abnormalities

1. Many present as difficult or failed intubation during resuscitation at delivery. Hypoxic brain damage may be sustained at this stage. The remainder usually present within a few hours of birth when the micrognathia and glossoptosis cause breathing and feeding difficulties, with episodes of cyanosis when the child is in the supine position. Feeding difficulties correlate with the severity of airway obstruction. Subsequently there is failure to thrive.

2. In a retrospective review of 62 neonates undergoing airway endoscopy, the Robin sequence was found to be the most common indication. There was a high incidence of concomitant problems, which included gastro-oesophageal reflux, congenital heart disease, and pulmonary disease (Ungkanont et al 1998).

3. A new index for defining micrognathia has been described (van der Haven et al 1997). Measurement of three facial dimensions produces a jaw index; children with Pierre Robin have an average index more than 3.6 times the normal value.

4. Cleft palate occurs in 60%, and eye problems in 40% of patients with the Pierre Robin syndrome.

5. Chronic upper airway obstruction can result in cor pulmonale. An increased pulmonary artery pressure may produce right to left shunting through a patent foramen ovale or a persistent ductus arteriosus.

6. Obstructive sleep apnoea may occur (Brouillette et al 1982). The use of nasal CPAP has been reported in a 12-year-old child (Deegan et al 1995).

7. A sequence of strategies is recommended in an attempt to minimise respiratory obstruction and allow safe feeding. The treatment required depends upon severity. Initially, the infant is nursed in the prone position. If this fails, prolonged nasopharyngeal intubation may help to protect the airway (Sher

1992). If respiratory distress and failure to thrive persists, and lateral X-ray of the neck in the supine position shows upper airway obstruction, suturing of the tongue to the lower gum or lip (tongue to lip adhesion) may be needed (Augarten et al 1990). Modified nasopharyngeal tubes or splints have been described (Smyth 1998, Masters et al 1999). Feeding may be undertaken via a nasogastric tube or a gastrostomy. Respiration and oxygen saturation are monitored, and appropriate oxygen supplementation given.

Sometimes tracheostomy may be required, although previously there has been reluctance to resort to this. Benjamin and Walker (1991), in a 10-year retrospective study of 26 patients, classified them into three groups according to the treatment required: mild (needing posture alone), moderate (needing nasopharyngeal tube), and severe (needing tracheal intubation or tracheostomy). All of the deaths occurred in this latter group (seven out of 11); one from hypoxic brain damage at birth, two while still intubated, and two who had tracheostomies.

As the child grows, the obstruction tends to improve, partly from growth of the mandible and the size of the airway, and partly as a result of better neurological control of the tongue muscles. Problems mainly seem to resolve by the time the child is 6 months old. In one series (Benjamin & Walker 1991), mild cases could be nursed supine from 3 to 6 months (mean 5.6 months). In the moderate group, nasopharyngeal intubation was required for between 14 days and 14 weeks, after which they were nursed prone. All could sleep supine by 6 months.

Anaesthetic problems

1. Even in the unanaesthetised infant, during the first few months of life, respiratory obstruction occurs in the supine position. The main mechanism for this was thought to be glossoptosis, prolapse of the tongue backwards, but it is now realised that there are multiple factors. Sher (1992) believes obstruction to be related to a combination of the anatomical abnormalities of the mandible, with functional impairment of the genioglossus and other pharyngeal muscles that are concerned with maintenance of the airway. Varying degrees of obstruction exist, ranging from none at all, to obstruction when the infant is asleep and, in the worst cases, obstruction in the awake state. In any infant, obstruction worsens during an upper respiratory tract infection, feeding, and crying. In addition, studies suggest that the site of obstruction varies from patient to patient. From endoscopic observations, these have been classified (Sher 1992).

> Type 1: A true glossoptosis in which the dorsum of the tongue is opposed to the posterior pharyngeal wall.
>
> Type 2: The tongue compresses the soft palate against the posterior pharyngeal wall, so that all three structures meet in the upper oropharynx.
>
> Type 3: Medial apposition of the lateral pharyngeal walls.
>
> Type 4: A sphincteric constriction of the pharynx.

2. Oxygen desaturation and obstructive sleep apnoea, detected by pulse oximetry and polysonography, occurs in the majority of infants and contributes to the mortality from obstruction (Bull et al 1990).

3. Gastro-oesophageal reflux may be present (Bull et al 1990).

4. The unusual facial configuration, in particular the receding lower jaw, makes it difficult to maintain an airtight fit with an anaesthetic mask.

5. Many cases of difficult or failed intubation have been reported (Hansen et al 1995). Difficulties in tracheal intubation result from a combination of micrognathia, and prolapse or inward sucking of the posteriorly attached, and often enlarged, tongue. This may be compounded by the presence of tongue-tie which, paradoxically, may prevent airway

obstruction. In one infant, intubation problems were underestimated because of the lack of preoperative airway obstruction (Jones & Derrick 1998). However, once the tongue-tie had been corrected, subsequent intubation became easy.

6. Pulmonary oedema has occurred after relief of airway obstruction following palatal repair in an 8-month-old baby (Lynch & Underwood 1991).

Management

1. Monitoring by pulse oximetry, to detect airway obstruction, is crucial.

2. The importance of an individualised approach to airway management for assessment or surgery has been stressed (Benjamin & Walker 1991). Several methods have been proposed to overcome the problem of difficult intubation, some under general anaesthesia, and some in the awake patient. The consensus of opinion now seems to favour awake techniques.

a) *Asleep technique with a special laryngoscope.* Handler and Keon (1983) described a technique for intubation for the anaesthetised spontaneously breathing patient, in which a Jackson anterior commissure laryngoscope is used. The head is elevated above the shoulders, with flexion of the lower cervical vertebrae and extension at the atlanto-occipital joint. The laryngoscope is introduced into the right side of the mouth. Only the tip is directed towards the midline, the proximal end remaining laterally, so that a further 30 degrees of anterior angulation can be obtained. The narrow, closed blade prevents the tongue from falling in and obscuring the view of the larynx. When visualised, the epiglottis is elevated, and the larynx entered. Intubation is then achieved by passing a lubricated tube, without its adaptor, down the laryngoscope. It is held in place with alligator forceps whilst the laryngoscope is withdrawn.

b) *Asleep technique in the prone position.* The appreciation of the problems in the supine position led to the description of a successful blind nasal intubation with the patient prone (Populaire et al 1985). This position allows the tongue and mandible to fall forward under the effect of gravity and leave the larynx exposed.

c) *Fibreoptic bronchoscopic techniques.* A variety of fibreoptic techniques have been described (Howardy-Hansen & Berthelsen 1988, Scheller & Schulman 1991, Sher 1992). In small infants, the 'tube over bronchoscope' technique is not always possible because of the small size of the tube, therefore a Seldinger type approach may be necessary (paediatric bronchoscopes of 2.5 mm diameter are now available, but their very fineness makes them less easy to handle than the 4-mm bronchoscopes). After the administration of atropine, ketamine im, and topical lidocaine (lignocaine), a fibreoptic bronchoscope (OD 3.6 mm, L 60 cm, and suction channel 1.2 mm) was passed through one nostril. The tongue was held forward with Magill forceps, until the vocal cords were seen, but not entered, because of the risk of total obstruction. Under direct vision, a Teflon-coated guidewire with a flexible tip was passed via the suction channel into the trachea. The bronchoscope was carefully removed leaving the wire in place, and a 3-mm nasotracheal tube then passed over it into the trachea.

d) *Awake techniques using a special laryngoscope.* The use of a special purpose, slotted laryngoscope (Holiger paediatric anterior commissure laryngoscope Karl Storz, Tuttlingen, FRG) has been described (Benjamin & Walker 1991).

e) *Laryngeal mask techniques.* The use of a laryngeal mask airway to guide an introducer for subsequent intubation was used as an emergency (Chadd et al 1992,

Baraka 1995), and electively (Hansen et al 1995, Osses et al 1999, Selim et al 1999). Elective placement of the laryngeal mask airway following topical anaesthesia in three awake infants has been described (Markakis et al 1992).

f) *The use of a lighted stylet* (Cook–Sather & Schreiner 1997).

Bibliography

Augarten A, Sagy M, Yahav J et al 1990 Management of upper airway obstruction in the Pierre Robin syndrome. British Journal of Oral & Maxillofacial Surgery 28: 105–8.

Baraka A 1995 Laryngeal mask airway for resuscitation of a newborn with Pierre Robin syndrome. Anesthesiology 83: 645–6.

Bath AP, Bull PD 1997 Management of upper airway obstruction in Pierre Robin sequence. Journal of Laryngology & Otology 111: 1155–7.

Benjamin B, Walker P 1991 Management of airway obstruction in the Pierre Robin sequence. Internal Journal of Pediatric Otorhinolaryngology 22: 29–37.

Brouillette RT, Fernbach SK, Hunt CE 1982 Obstructive sleep apnea in infants and children. Journal of Pediatrics 100: 31–40.

Bull MJ, Givan DC, Sadove AM et al 1990 Improved outcome in Pierre Robin sequence: effect of multidisciplinary evaluation and management. Pediatrics 86: 294–301.

Chadd GD, Crane DL, Phillips PM et al 1992 Extubation and reintubation guided by the laryngeal mask airway in a child with Pierre Robin syndrome. Anesthesiology 76: 640–1.

Cook-Sather SD, Schreiner MS 1997 A simple homemade lighted stylet for neonates and infants: a description and case report of its use in an infant with the Pierre Robin anomalad. Paediatric Anaesthesia 7: 233–5.

Deegan PC, McGlone B, McNicholas WT 1995 Treatment of Robin sequence with nasal CPAP. Journal of Laryngology and Otology 109: 328–30.

Handler SD, Keon TP 1983 Difficult laryngoscopy/ intubation: the child with mandibular hypoplasia. Annals of Otology, Rhinology & Laryngology 92: 401–4.

Hansen TG, Joensen H, Henneberg SW et al 1995 Laryngeal mask airway guided tracheal intubation in a neonate with the Pierre Robin syndrome. Acta Anaesthesiologica Scandinavica 39: 129–31.

Howardy-Hansen P, Berthelsen P 1988 Fibreoptic bronchoscopic nasotracheal intubation of a neonate with Pierre Robin syndrome. Anaesthesia 43: 121–2.

Jones SE, Derrick GM 1998 Difficult intubation in an infant with Pierre Robin syndrome and concomitant tongue tie. Paediatric Anaesthesia 8: 510–11.

Lynch M, Underwood S 1991 Pulmonary oedema following the relief of upper airway obstruction in the Pierre Robin syndrome. British Journal of Anaesthesia 66: 391–3.

Markakis DA, Sayson SC, Schreiner MS 1992 Insertion of the laryngeal mask airway in awake infants with the Robin sequence. Anesthesia & Analgesia 75: 822–4.

Masters IB, Chang AB, Harris M et al 1999 Modified nasopharyngeal tube for upper airway obstruction. Archives of Disease in Childhood 80: 186–7.

Myer CM 3rd, Reed JM, Cotton RT et al 1998 Airway management in Pierre Robin sequence. Otolaryngology—Head & Neck Surgery 118: 630–5.

Osses H, Poblete M, Asenjo F 1999 Laryngeal mask for difficult intubation in children. Paediatric Anaesthesia 9: 399–401.

Populaire C, Lundi JN, Pinaud M et al 1985 Elective tracheal intubation in the prone position for a neonate with Pierre Robin syndrome. Anesthesiology 62: 214–15.

Selim M, Mowafi H, Al-Ghamdi A et al 1999 Intubation via LMA in pediatric patients with difficult airways. Canadian Journal of Anaesthesia 46: 891–3.

Scheller JG, Schulman SR 1991 Fiber-optic bronchoscopic guidance for intubating a neonate with Pierre Robin syndrome. Journal of Clinical Anesthesia 3: 45–7.

Sher AE 1992 Mechanisms of airway obstruction in Robin sequence: implications for treatment. Cleft Palate—Craniofacial Journal 29: 224–31.

Smyth AG 1998 A simple nasal splint to assist the stability of nasopharyngeal tubes in the Pierre Robin sequence associated with airway obstruction: technical innovation. Journal of Cranio-Maxillo-Facial Surgery 26: 411–14.

Ungkanont K, Friedman EM, Sulek M 1998 A retrospective analysis of airway endoscopy in patients less than 1 month old. Laryngoscope 108: 1724–8.

van der Haven I, Mulder JW, van der Wal KG et al 1997 The jaw index: new guide defining micrognathia in newborns. Cleft Palate—Craniofacial Journal 34: 240–1.

Pituitary apoplexy

A term used to describe a complication of a pituitary adenoma. Sudden enlargement secondary to haemorrhage, infarction, or both, in a previously undiagnosed (or known) tumour, results in symptoms and signs of compression of adjacent intracranial structures (Gaillard 1992). The optic chiasma and cranial nerves, in particular the third, fourth, fifth and sixth cranial nerves, may be involved. Pituitary apoplexy can be of sudden onset and life threatening in nature, or symptoms and signs may gradually evolve over a couple of weeks. A number of predisposing factors have been suggested. Pituitary apoplexy has been described after surgery, mostly cardiopulmonary bypass, but pituitary stimulation tests, renal dialysis, head injury and myocardial infarction have also precipitated it. Anatomical factors, particularly the nature of the blood supply, make the abnormal pituitary more susceptible to infarction under hypotensive conditions.

Presentation

1. The symptoms may result from pressure effects, leakage of blood into the subarachnoid space, or endocrinopathy. Rolih and Ober (1993) found the commonest presentations to be headache (75.8%), visual disturbances (62.1%), and ophthalmoplegias (40.4%). These may be associated with meningism, vomiting, and impaired conscious level, all of which are suggestive of subarachnoid haemorrhage.

2. There may be a varying pattern of associated endocrine disorders. However, these are usually mild and previously unnoticed.

3. There may be radiological signs of an expanded pituitary fossa or an empty sella turcica.

4. The differential diagnosis includes intracranial or subarachnoid haemorrhage, emboli, brain abscess, cavernous sinus thrombosis, or encephalitis.

5. Diagnosis may be made by CT scan, which is most helpful in the early days after haemorrhage, or MRI, which is more sensitive in the subacute or chronic stages (Ostrov et al 1989).

6. A number of predisposing factors have been described, including trauma, anticoagulation, radiotherapy, IPPV, surgery, dialysis, and CSF leak following lumbar puncture.

Presentation and problems

1. Pituitary apoplexy has presented with a variety of neurological signs and symptoms after surgery, sometimes up to several days later. The majority of cases have been associated with cardiac surgery (Cooper et al 1986, Shapiro 1990), although not exclusively. In one patient the pituitary tumour had already been diagnosed, but pituitary surgery had been postponed in favour of coronary artery grafting (Absalom et al 1993). Signs of pituitary apoplexy occurred 40 h after bypass and craniotomy revealed bleeding into the tumour, but the patient died from myocardial infarction. In one patient a pituitary crisis occurred after cholecystectomy performed under combined general and epidural anaesthesia (Yahagi et al 1992). In another, severe headache started 6 h after total hip replacement under spinal anaesthesia. A blood patch at 18 h failed to relieve the headache and progressive vision loss and partial third nerve palsy developed (Lennon et al 1998). Two patients died after partial resection of giant pituitary tumours and, at re-exploration, massive swelling of the remaining tumour and haemorrhagic infarction were found (Goel et al 1995). The exact sequence of events leading to pituitary apoplexy is unknown. However, since the anterior pituitary has no direct arterial supply, it depends upon adequate portal venous perfusion (Slaughter et al 1993). Because of this, an adenoma may have a relatively compromised blood supply, possibly secondary to tumour compression, or pathological abnormalities of the vessels. It is thus susceptible to ischaemia, secondary to

reduced perfusion pressure during surgery, portal venous thrombosis, microemboli or haemorrhage, as a result of incomplete reversal of anticoagulants. The nonpulsatile flow and decreased perfusion pressure that occurs when a patient is on cardiopulmonary bypass may account for the high incidence of association with cardiac surgery.

2. Signs include ophthalmoplegia, visual loss, endocrine failure, severe headache, and sudden loss of consciousness.

3. Timing in relation to surgery. Symptoms and signs have appeared immediately (Meek et al 1998), after several hours, or several days. One patient presented with deep coma and dilated pupils 3 weeks after cardiac surgery (Wiesmann et al 1999). The tumour was removed 5 days later.

4. The problems of making a differential diagnosis of the sudden onset of cerebral symptoms and signs, including deterioration in conscious level, following surgery. They may be confused with emboli, air, cerebral ischaemia, or hypotension.

5. Hormone abnormalities may be present. These include panhypopituitarism with amenorrhoea, galactorrhoea, elevated prolactin levels, and hypothyroidism. Acute adrenal insufficiency is the most serious problem and occurs in about two-thirds of patients; in one patient, acute hyponatraemia of 122 mmol l^{-1}, and hypotension was thought to be secondary to this (Lennon et al 1998).

Management

1. If neurological symptoms and signs follow surgery, a neurosurgeon or neurologist should be consulted. Urgent CT or MRI scans may be necessary to establish the diagnosis.

2. Treatment may be conservative or operative. Initial treatment to reduce the oedema using dexamethasone 2–16 mg day^{-1} has been suggested, after which decisions should be made on clinical and tomographic findings

(Maccagnan et al 1995). In a proportion of cases, signs will resolve and immediate surgery will be avoided. Resolution of nerve palsies has been also reported after treatment with bromocriptine (Brisman et al 1996). In the event of impairment of vision or consciousness, or evidence of an expanding adenoma, pituitary decompression surgery may be required (Shapiro 1990, Yahagi et al 1992).

3. Replacement therapy for adrenal insufficiency will be needed in a substantial number of patients.

4. Pituitary hormone function should be investigated, since other hormonal replacement may be required.

Bibliography

Absalom M, Rogers KH, Moulton RJ 1993 Pituitary apoplexy after coronary artery surgery. Anesthesia & Analgesia 76: 470–1.

Brisman MH, Katz G, Post KD 1996 Symptoms of pituitary apoplexy rapidly reversed with bromocriptine. Case report. Journal of Neurosurgery 85: 1153–5.

Cooper DM, Bazarae MG, Furlan AJ et al 1986 Pituitary apoplexy: complication of cardiac surgery. Annals of Thoracic Surgery 41: 547–50.

Gaillard RC 1992 Pituitary gland emergencies. Baillières Clinical Endocrinology & Metabolism 6: 57–75.

Goel A, Deogaonkar M, Desai K 1995 Fatal postoperative "pituitary apoplexy": its cause and management. British Journal of Neurosurgery 9: 37–40.

Lennon M, Seigne P, Cunningham AJ 1998 Pituitary apoplexy after spinal anaesthesia. British Journal of Anaesthesia 81: 616–18.

Maccagnan P, Macedo CL, Kayath MJ 1995 Conservative management of pituitary apoplexy: a prospective study. Journal of Clinical Endocrinology & Metabolism 80: 2190–7.

Meek EN, Butterworth J, Kon ND et al 1998 Pituitary apoplexy following mitral valve repair. Anesthesiology 89: 1580–2.

Ostrov SG, Quencer RM, Hoffman JC et al 1989 Hemorrhage within pituitary adenomas: how often associated with pituitary apoplexy syndrome? American Journal of Roentgenology 153: 153–60.

Rolih CA, Ober KP 1993 Pituitary apoplexy. Endocrinology & Metabolism Clinics of North America 22: 291–302.

Shapiro LM 1990 Pituitary apoplexy following coronary artery bypass surgery. Journal of Surgical Oncology 44: 66–8.

Slaughter TF, Mark JB, Reves JG 1993 Pituitary apoplexy and the conflicting perioperative goals of anticoagulation and hemostasis. Anesthesia & Analgesia 76: 648–9.

Wiesmann M, Gliemroth J, Kehler U et al 1999 Pituitary apoplexy after cardiac surgery presenting as deep coma with dilated pupils. Acta Anaesthesiologica Scandinavica 43: 236–8.

Yahagi N, Nishikawa A, Matsui S et al 1992 Pituitary apoplexy following cholecystectomy. Anaesthesia 47: 234–6.

Plasma cholinesterase abnormalities (see also Section 2, Suxamethonium apnoea)

Plasma cholinesterase (ChE) is present in plasma and most other tissues, apart from erythrocytes, and is an enzyme capable of hydrolysing many esters. It must be distinguished from acetylcholinesterase (AChE), which is found in erythrocytes and at the neuromuscular junction. ChE is a protein manufactured in the liver and its half-life is thought to be approximately 8–12 days. No physiological role for the enzyme has as yet been unequivocally demonstrated.

Its anaesthetic significance lies in the fact that it hydrolyses the depolarising neuromuscular blocker suxamethonium (thus terminating its action after 1–5 min), and the short-acting nondepolarising blocker mivacurium (Bevan 1993). In the presence of normal ChE activity, a two-stage hydrolysis of suxamethonium occurs.

$$succinyl\ dicholine + water \rightarrow succinyl\ monocholine +$$
$$\downarrow\ \ \ \ \ \ \ \ \ \ \ \ \ \ \ choline$$
$$succinic\ acid + choline$$

If there is a low level of normal plasma cholinesterase (normal level 3700–11 500 iu l^{-1}), or if the cholinesterase is abnormal, prolonged apnoea may occur. In either case, following suxamethonium administration, the duration of muscle paralysis can vary from about 10 min to 2 h. Decreased ChE activity may be due to genetic variants of the enzyme, pre-existing disease, or iatrogenic causes.

For further details of the relevance of plasma cholinesterase to anaesthetic practice, see the review by Davis et al (1997).

Genetic variants

Plasma cholinesterase synthesis is controlled by two allelic genes, the normal genotype being designated $E_1^u E_1^u$. There are several genetic defects which result in an individual having a diminished ability to metabolise suxamethonium (Whittaker 1980, Davis et al 1997).

Differentiation between the normal and an atypical cholinesterase was first demonstrated by comparing the rates at which each hydrolysed benzoylcholine, in the presence of varying concentrations of an inhibitor, dibucaine. The percentage inhibition by a 10^{-5} molar concentration of dibucaine is known as the dibucaine number. Homozygous individuals for the atypical (or dibucaine-resistant) genotype ($E_1^a E_1^a$) have a dibucaine number about 20, heterozygotes ($E_1^u E_1^a$) about 60, and those with normal enzyme, about 80. Further genetic variants have subsequently been found. These include a 'silent' gene, E_1^s, which has little or no enzymic activity, and a fluoride-resistant gene, E_1^f. The fluoride number is determined in a similar way to the dibucaine number, but sodium fluoride is used as the inhibitor.

The distribution of the genotypes in suxamethonium-sensitive individuals has been studied by Whittaker and Britten (1987) and Davis et al (1997). So far, more than 12 genotypes have been recognised. Since ChE is a large molecule of four polypeptide chains, it is likely that further variants will be described.

The main categories of subjects sensitive to suxamethonium have the genotypes $E_1^a E_1^a$ and $E_1^a E_1^s$, and their frequency is about 1 in 1800.

Disease states

Low levels of normal enzyme have been reported in association with a number of pathological conditions. These include severe liver disease, malnutrition, renal failure, malignant disease, tetanus, Huntington's chorea, and collagen disorders. It has also been described in Churg–Strauss syndrome (Taylor et al 1990), although in the cases reported, it may have been associated with the immunosuppressive therapy.

Pregnancy

In pregnancy, from about 10 weeks' gestation, there is a reduction in ChE activity of about 20%. From 2 to 4 days postpartum, this is further reduced, and normal levels are only achieved at about 6 weeks. Normally this does not produce clinical problems. However, there are three circumstances in which problems have arisen.

1. The use of plasmapheresis in the treatment of rhesus isoimmunisation is associated with profound reduction in maternal ChE activity (Whittaker et al 1988). A patient with a normal phenotype was reported to have been apnoeic for 50 min following suxamethonium 75 mg. This was given during a Caesarean section undertaken 2 days after the seventh plasmapheresis, and was associated with very low ChE activity (Evans et al 1980).

2. The heterozygous patient. Pregnancy can also cause clinically detectable apnoea in a heterozygous patient that would not normally be manifested in the nonpregnant patient, and especially if a suxamethonium infusion is used (Whittaker et al 1988).

3. A pregnant patient with retained placenta received both suxamethonium 75 mg and mivacurium 30 mg, after which she required IPPV overnight for prolonged neuromuscular blockade. Her plasma cholinesterase was $1.6 \, \text{iu} \, \text{l}^{-1}$ (normal range 4.1–$8.8 \, \text{iu} \, \text{l}^{-1}$). Fluoride and dibucaine numbers were normal and a month later, a repeat ChE level was just within the normal range (Davies & Landy 1998). Presumably, the blockade was potentiated by the two drugs being given in combination.

Iatrogenic causes

Reported iatrogenic associations include radiotherapy, renal dialysis, plasmapheresis, cardiac bypass, cytotoxic drugs, ecothiopate eye drops, oral contraceptives, propanidid, neostigmine, pyridostigmine, chlorpromazine, pancuronium, metoclopramide, and exposure to organophosphorus compounds.

Anaesthetic problems

1. In individuals with suxamethonium sensitivity, varying lengths of apnoea can follow the administration of suxamethonium. With a peripheral nerve stimulator, apnoea from this cause may be distinguished from that due to other causes. A cumulative dose–response curve in a patient with low plasma cholinesterase activity showed the increased potency of the drug of four to seven times that of a normal individual (Smith et al 1989). One 3.5-kg infant of 2 days old has been reported (Pasquariello & Schwartz 1993).

2. There are changes in plasma cholinesterase levels during pregnancy, so that heterozygous individuals may become sensitive to suxamethonium. There is evidence that metoclopramide is a powerful inhibitor of plasma cholinesterase, therefore patients receiving both this and suxamethonium should be carefully monitored (Kao et al 1990).

3. If suxamethonium sensitivity is confirmed, subsequent investigation of the patient, and if possible the close relatives, is required.

4. Mivacurium, a synthetic, nondepolarising blocker, is also metabolised by plasma cholinesterase and the rate of hydrolysis is about 70–88% that of suxamethonium. The duration of action is therefore increased in patients with reduced plasma cholinesterase activity (Maddineni & Mirakhur 1993, Petersen et al 1993, Fox & Hunt 1995, Goudsouzian 1997, Lejus et al 1998). Doses as low as $0.03 \, \text{mg} \, \text{kg}^{-1}$ have caused prolonged response in patients homozygous for the atypical gene (Ostergaard et al 1995). Lengths of apnoea recorded with doses

of $0.12–0.2\,mg\,kg^{-1}$ vary from 3 h in a heterozygous patient to 8 h in a homozygous patient. One teenager had homozygous atypical plasma cholinesterase deficiency (2.5-h block) following liver transplantation, although both parents had a normal phenotype. The girl had received suxamethonium previously without unduly prolonged block. It is suggested that she had 'acquired' the abnormal gene from the donor liver (Sockalingham & Green 1995).

Antagonising the block with anticholinesterases may hasten recovery; two cases had blocks of 4–6 h, whereas in another in whom block was not reversed, the recovery time was 8 h (Goudsouzian et al 1993). A group of patients with known cholinesterase abnormalities were also used in a phase 3 study of mivacurium (Ostergaard et al 1995). The effects of administration of human plasma cholinesterase were studied, with and without anticholinesterases. In the first (heterozygous) patient, mivacurium $0.1\,mg\,kg^{-1}$ was given. A PTC (post-tetanic count) of 1 was seen at 123 min and human cholinesterase given at 144 min, but without anticholinesterases. Recovery to TOF ratio 0.75 only finally occurred at 200 min from the original dose of mivacurium. In the second (homozygous) patient, mivacurium $0.03\,mg\,kg^{-1}$ caused complete disappearance of the TOF, and a PTC of 4 was not seen until 145 min later. Human plasma cholinesterase was given and T1 appeared in 10 min. After a further 5 min T1 had reached 20%, and on this occasion reversal with anticholinesterase was used, and head lift achieved at 170 min.

5. Local anaesthetics, in particular cocaine, are partially metabolised by plasma cholinesterase. There is now definite evidence that those with cocaine-induced complications have a significantly lower level of plasma cholinesterase than those without complications (Hoffman et al 1992, Om et al 1993).

Management

1. When spontaneous respiration fails to return after the administration of

suxamethonium, IPPV should be continued. Light anaesthesia or sedation must be maintained to prevent the patient becoming distressed. The presence of a neuromuscular blockade should be confirmed with a peripheral nerve stimulator. This is most important, since about 30% of patients referred to the Cholinesterase Research Unit have a normal phenotype. The routine use of a nerve stimulator might influence this figure. IPPV should be continued until there is evidence of a reversible block (at least two twitches of the TOF) using a nerve stimulator, and adequate head lift and respiration can be maintained. It is important that anticholinesterases should not be given until there is some return of neuromuscular activity.

2. Fresh frozen plasma (Gill et al 1991) and a purified form of human cholinesterase (Ostergaard et al 1995) have both been given, to expedite recovery, but the use of these products is extremely controversial (Davis et al 1997).

3. When the patient has recovered, detailed anaesthetic, family and drug histories should be taken. A simple explanation of the need for further investigation should be given.

4. Plasma cholinesterase activity, dibucaine and fluoride numbers should be investigated. While this may be done in a local laboratory, there are advantages of using the service provided by the Cholinesterase Research Unit.

5. A rapid service can be obtained, by sending 10 ml heparinised or whole blood, or separated plasma or serum, by first class post, to the Cholinesterase Research Unit, Royal Postgraduate Medical School, Hammersmith Hospital, London (Whittaker & Britten 1987).

6. If the results are abnormal, the patient's notes should be clearly marked and the general practitioner informed.

Bibliography

Bevan DR 1993 Prolonged mivacurium-induced neuromuscular block. Anesthesia & Analgesia 77: 4–6.
Davies P, Landy M 1998 Suxamethonium and mivacurium sensitivity from pregnancy-induced

plasma cholinesterase deficiency. Anaesthesia 53: 1109–11.

Davis L, Britten JJ, Morgan M 1997 Cholinesterase: its significance in anaesthetic practice. Anaesthesia 52: 244–60.

Evans RT, MacDonald R, Robinson A 1980 Suxamethonium apnoea associated with plasmaphoresis. Anaesthesia 35: 198–201.

Fox MH, Hunt PCW 1995 Prolonged neuromuscular block associated with mivacurium. British Journal of Anaesthesia 74: 237–8.

Gill RS, O'Connell N, Scott RPF 1991 Reversal of prolonged suxamethonium apnoea with fresh frozen plasma in a six-week-old infant. Anaesthesia 46: 1036–8.

Goudsouzian NG 1997 Mivacurium in infants and children. Paediatric Anaesthesia 7: 183–90.

Goudsouzian NG, d'Hollander A, Viby-Mogensen J 1993 Prolonged neuromuscular block from mivacurium in two patients with cholinesterase deficiency. Anesthesia & Analgesia 77: 183–5.

Hoffman RS, Henry GC, Howland MA et al 1992 Association between life-threatening cocaine toxicity and plasma cholinesterase activity. Annals of Emergency Medicine 21: 247–53.

Kao YJ, Tellez J, Turner DR 1990 Dose-dependent effect of metoclopramide on cholinesterases and suxamethonium metabolism. British Journal of Anaesthesia 65: 220–4.

Lejus C, Blanloeil Y, Le Roux N 1998 Prolonged mivacurium neuromuscular block in children. Paediatric Anaesthesia 8: 433–5.

Maddineni VR, Mirakhur RK 1993 Prolonged neuromuscular block following mivacurium. Anesthesiology 78: 1181–4.

Om A, Ellahham S, Ornato JP et al 1993 Medical complications of cocaine: possible relationship to low plasma cholinesterase enzyme. American Journal of Cardiology 125: 1114–17.

Ostergaard D, Jensen FS, Viby-Mogensen J 1995 Reversal of intense mivacurium block with human plasma cholinesterase in patients with atypical plasma cholinesterase. Anesthesiology 82: 1295–8.

Pasquariello CA, Schwartz RE 1993 Plasma cholinesterase deficiency in an infant. Canadian Journal of Anaesthesia 40: 529–31.

Petersen RS, Bailey PL, Kalameghan R et al 1993 Prolonged neuromuscular block after mivacurium. Anesthesia & Analgesia 194–6.

Smith CE, Lewis G, Donati F et al 1989 Dose–response relationship for succinylcholine in a patient with genetically determined low plasma

cholinesterase activity. Anesthesiology 70: 156–8.

Sockalingham I, Green DW 1995 Mivacurium-induced prolonged neuromuscular block. British Journal of Anaesthesia 74: 234–6.

Taylor BL, Whittaker M, Van Heerden V et al 1990 Cholinesterase deficiency and the Churg–Strauss syndrome. Anaesthesia 45: 649–52.

Whittaker M 1980 Plasma cholinesterase variants and the anaesthetist. Anaesthesia 35: 174–97.

Whittaker M, Britten JJ 1987 Phenotyping of individuals sensitive to suxamethonium. British Journal of Anaesthesia 59: 1052–5.

Whittaker M, Crawford JS, Lewis M 1988 Some observations of levels of plasma cholinesterase activity within an obstetric population. Anaesthesia 43: 42–5.

Polycythaemia vera

Polycythaemia is a general term for an increased haemoglobin (Hb >17 g dl^{-1} in men and >16 g dl^{-1} in women), an increased red cell count, or haematocrit (>0.51 in men and >0.47 in women). It can be *relative* (in which there is an increased Hb and PCV, a normal red cell mass but a reduction in plasma volume), *apparent* (an increased Hb and PCV, a normal red cell mass and normal plasma volume), or *absolute* (in which the increased Hb and PCV is associated with an increased red cell mass). Apparent polycythaemia, also known as stress polycythaemia, may be associated with smoking, alcohol, obesity, hypoxia, fluid loss, hypertension, renal disease, and phaeochromocytoma (Pearson & Messinezy 1996). Absolute polycythaemia can be primary or secondary. Causes of secondary polycythaemia include pulmonary disease, cyanotic heart disease, and inappropriate production of erythropoietin.

According to Thorne (1998), there are misconceptions about the polycythaemia (more correctly termed erythrocytosis) that is associated with cyanotic congenital heart disease. Unlike the situation in polycythaemia vera (PV), there is no evidence that routine venesection prevents stroke in these patients. In fact, since recurrent venesection causes iron deficiency anaemia, venesection in adults should only take place if there are symptoms of hyperviscosity with a haematocrit >65, and only provided volume replacement takes place at the same time.

The primary disease, PV, is a neoplastic condition and is one of the chronic myeloproliferative disorders. This condition is associated with impaired haemostasis, abnormal platelet function, hyperviscosity, and reduced organ blood flow. As a result of these abnormalities, surgery in untreated PV carries a high risk of either thrombotic or bleeding complications.

A study was conducted into the differences between patients with PV and polycythaemia secondary to smoking (Schwarcz et al 1993). Forty-three patients with PV were compared with 27 patients with polycythaemia secondary to smoking, groups having been matched for age and haematocrit. The platelet counts were significantly different (mean $605 \times 10^9 l^{-1}$ vs. $233 \times 10^9 l^{-1}$). Although the incidence of cardiac and cerebrovascular events were similar, there were significantly more thromboembolic events, and more peripheral arterial thomboemboli, in the patients with PV.

Treatment of PV reduces the risk of complications. Of 1213 patients, 41% had arterial and venous thromboses, about one-third of these occurred after treatment and two-thirds before (Gruppo Italiano Studio Policitemia 1995). However, aggressive treatment is associated with an increased risk of neoplasia.

Preoperative abnormalities

1. Occurs most commonly in men, usually over 50 years of age. Patients can present with a range of symptoms secondary to hyperviscosity, a thrombotic, or a bleeding episode, or a high haemoglobin level found on routine testing.

2. Splenomegaly, hepatomegaly, and hypertension are common.

3. Haematological abnormalities include an elevated haemoglobin level, an increased red cell mass and packed cell volume (50–70%), and often a leucocytosis and thrombocythaemia. A venous haematocrit of >0.50 in males and >0.47 in females is suggested as being sufficient to warrant further investigation. A higher incidence of vascular occlusion is found when the platelet count is $>400 \times 10^9 l^{-1}$. The diagnosis should also be considered in patients with a normal haemoglobin, but a microcytosis. This may be secondary to slow blood loss from the gastrointestinal tract, resulting in severe iron deficiency.

4. Spontaneous haematomas can occur in a variety of sites, and platelet function may be abnormal.

5. Hyperuricaemia and secondary gout is common.

6. The method of treatment is controversial. It may involve venesection to keep the PCV below 50%, radioactive phosphorus, busulfan (busulphan), or hydroxyurea.

Anaesthetic problems

1. Polycythaemia vera carries an increased surgical and anaesthetic risk. The level at which this risk begins is debatable, but it has been suggested that levels above $17 \, g \, dl^{-1}$ for men and above $16 \, g \, dl^{-1}$ for women require an explanation (Irving 1991). An early study showed that 79% of untreated patients whose haemoglobin was greater than $17 \, g \, dl^{-1}$ had postoperative thrombotic or haemorrhagic problems, with a 43% morbidity and a 36% mortality (Wasserman & Gilbert 1964). These figures contrasted with a group whose polycythaemia had been controlled for more than 4 months, in whom there was a morbidity of only 5%, and no deaths.

2. Polycythaemia vera is associated with thrombotic complications, and the patient's first presentation may be for emergency surgery. In a study involving 200 patients, nearly 50% presented with vascular problems (Barabas 1980). Seventy-eight arterial complications occurred in 68 patients, 66 venous complications

in 57 patients, and there were 27 patients who had both. Distal arterial disease is more common than that involving major vessels. A patient with ulcerative colitis presented with Budd–Chiari syndrome following colorectal surgery. Iron deficiency had masked the polycythaemia (Whiteford et al 1999).

3. Despite the fact that PV is primarily a thrombotic condition, bleeding can also occur as a result of abnormal platelet function. A history of recurrent epistaxis is common and gastrointestinal haemorrhage may occur. Two patients presented with a spontaneous retropharyngeal haematoma (Mackenzie & Jellicoe 1986, DiFrancesco et al 1999), and in one of them, emergency tracheal intubation for airway obstruction was required. Another developed a paraplegia from a large spinal haematoma (Kalina et al 1995). Patients with polycythaemia may occasionally be anaemic, secondary to bleeding, in which case the diagnosis may not be immediately obvious.

4. Increases in total blood volume and the presence of a high blood viscosity increase both the cardiac output, and the work of the heart. Cerebral blood flow is low, and this contributes to the high incidence of cerebrovascular occlusion.

5. Cyanosis occurs readily.

6. In the emergency case, the main problem is to decide whether or not a patient with a high haemoglobin and an increased haematocrit has the primary condition, or a polycythaemia secondary to respiratory disease or smoking. In the first instance, cerebral blood flow will be low, and venesection is appropriate, whilst in the second, cerebral blood flow may actually be increased. One hundred patients with Hb $>16\,\mathrm{g\,dl^{-1}}$ resulting from chronic obstructive pulmonary disease, and 100 matched controls, were compared for thrombotic and haemorrhagic complications in the first postoperative month (Lubarsky et al 1991). No differences were found between the groups and it was concluded that secondary polycythaemia did not increase postoperative risk, although the

authors acknowledged that the study was retrospective, the groups were small, and few patients with extreme Hb values were included. However, these results might have been expected simply on consideration of the basic pathological processes; secondary polycythaemia is not accompanied by abnormal haemostasis or reduced cerebral blood flow, both of which are characteristics of PV, and are most probably responsible for the complications.

7. However, secondary polycythaemia may be associated with other problems, since it may result from daytime and nocturnal hypoxaemia. More recently, it has been shown that nocturnal oxygen desaturation can also occur in some patients with apparent and relative polycythaemia (Messinezy et al 1991). Sixteen patients were studied, and in the four who had nocturnal desaturation, supine daytime oximetry showed an oxygen saturation of less than 92% on air.

Management

1. Differential diagnosis. If a high haemoglobin level and an increased haematocrit is found, arterial blood gases may assist in the diagnosis. The presence of hypoxia or hypercarbia suggests a respiratory cause. Other causes of secondary polycythaemia should be sought; the commonest cause of polycythaemia is probably smoking; nocturnal oximetry may indicate obstructive sleep apnoea, and correction of hypoxia may abolish polycythaemia. If PV is likely, elective surgery should be postponed until there is medical control of the condition. It has been suggested that the peripheral blood picture and the blood volume should be normal for at least 4 months preoperatively (Barabas 1980).

2. If emergency surgery is required, venesection should be performed, and the blood replaced with the same volume of PPF or colloid. It has been suggested that patients with PV and peripheral vascular complications should have a haematocrit of 30–40%. Cerebral blood flow is increased as the venous haematocrit is reduced.

3. Treatment with hydroxyurea, radioactive phosphorus, or alkylating agents (Terasako & Sasai 1998).

4. Prevention of venous stasis.

5. Extremes of hypotension and hypertension should be avoided.

6. Anticoagulants are inadvisable, since bleeding may occur.

7. In the presence of bleeding, platelet transfusion may be required (Terasako & Sasai 1998). Although the platelet count is high, platelet function appears to be abnormal.

8. For management of adults with erythrocytosis and cyanotic congenital heart disease, see Thorne (1998). Venesection is not usually needed unless the patient is symptomatic.

Bibliography

Barabas AP 1980 Surgical problems associated with polycythaemia. British Journal of Hospital Medicine 23: 289–94.

DiFrancesco RC, Escamilla JS, Sennes LU et al 1999 Spontaneous cervical hematoma: report of two cases. Ear, Nose, & Throat Journal 78: 168–5.

Gruppo Italiano Studio Policitemia 1995 Polycythemia vera: the natural history of 1213 patients followed for 20 years. Annals of Internal Medicine 123: 656–64.

Irving G 1991 Polycythaemia and the anaesthetist. South African Medical Journal 80: 418–19.

Kalina P, Drehobl KE, Black K et al 1995 Spinal cord compression by spontaneous spinal subdural haematoma in polycythemia vera. Postgraduate Medical Journal 71: 378–9.

Lubarsky DA, Gallagher CJ, Berend JL 1991 Secondary polycythemia does not increase the risk of perioperative hemorrhagic or thrombotic complications. Journal of Clinical Anesthesia 3: 99–103.

Mackenzie JW, Jellicoe JA 1986 Acute upper airway obstruction. Spontaneous retropharyngeal haemorrhage in a patient with polycythaemia rubra vera. Anaesthesia 41: 57–9.

Messinezy M, Aubry S, O'Connell G et al 1991 Oxygen desaturation in apparent and relative polycythaemia. British Medical Journal 302: 216–17.

Pearson TC, Messinezy M 1996 Investigation of patients with polycythaemia. Postgraduate Medical Journal 72: 519–24.

Schwarcz TH, Hogan LA, Endean ED et al 1993 Thromboembolic complications of polycythemia vera versus smokers' polycythemia. Journal of Vascular Surgery 17: 518–23.

Terasako K, Sasai S 1998 Platelet transfusion for surgery in the presence of polycythemia vera. Acta Anaesthesiologica Scandinavica 42: 270–1.

Thorne SA 1998 Management of polycythaemia in adults with cyanotic congenital heart disease. Heart 79: 315–16.

Wasserman LR, Gilbert HS 1964 Surgical bleeding in polycythemia vera. New England Journal of Medicine 269: 216–17.

Whiteford MH, Moritz MJ, Ferber A et al 1999 Budd–Chiari syndrome complicating restorative proctocolectomy for ulcerative colitis: report of a case. Diseases of the Colon & Rectum 42: 1220–4.

405

Pompe's disease (and adult-onset acid maltase deficiency)

A glycogen storage disease, type IIa, in which there is a deficiency of lysosomal alpha-1,4-glucosidase (acid maltase) (Reuser et al 1995). This enzyme is involved in glycogen breakdown, therefore glycogen accumulates with the lysosomes. Three different modes of presentation are now recognised. The most severely affected patients present with cardiac failure in the first 3 months of life, and usually die in the first year. This was the type described by Pompe. There is a less severe form appearing in infancy, with death before adulthood. In these forms, glycogen deposits are found in cardiac, skeletal and smooth muscle, kidney, liver, spleen, brain, spinal cord, and tongue. A third form, adult-onset acid maltase deficiency, presents as a myopathy in the 20–40-year age group. Anaesthesia may be required for diagnostic muscle biopsy, cardiac catheterisation, or bronchoscopy.

Preoperative abnormalities

1. Infantile form:

a) There is generalised hypotonia and muscle weakness, although muscle mass is normal.

b) The heart is greatly enlarged as a result of a hypertrophic cardiomyopathy. Outflow obstruction secondary to enlargement of the interventricular septum occurs in 50% of patients. Murmurs are usually absent. Cardiac failure rapidly supervenes.

c) CXR shows massive biventricular hypertrophy. Lobar collapse is common secondary to bronchial obstruction.

d) ECG shows a short PR interval (<0.09 s) and massive, wide QRS complexes.

e) Glucose, lactate and lipid levels are normal. Muscle enzymes are moderately increased.

f) In the most severe form of the disease, cardiorespiratory failure, pulmonary aspiration and pneumonia all contribute towards death.

2. Adult-onset acid maltase deficiency (Felice et al 1995):

a) Progressive weakness, mainly involving proximal muscles of both upper and lower extremities.

b) Exercise intolerance.

c) Involvement of respiratory muscles and diaphragm, with a reduction in FVC.

d) An abnormal EMG.

e) Increased CK of two- to ten-fold (Ausems et al 1999).

f) Other features may include a family history, mild macroglossia, tongue weakness, and muscle atrophy.

Anaesthetic problems

1. Pompe's disease:

a) Problems associated with cardiomyopathies and cardiac failure. Inhalational induction with halothane resulted in bradycardia and ventricular fibrillation in a 5-month-old baby (McFarlane & Soni 1986), and cardiac arrest occurred in a child having a muscle biopsy (Ellis 1980). In the latter case, the diagnosis of Pompe's disease was only made at postmortem examination. Outflow tract obstruction often occurs, and the diseased muscle of the ventricles cannot compensate by hypertrophy and increased contractility. Massive cardiomegaly may produce lobar collapse by bronchial compression.

b) Macroglossia may occur and can cause upper airway obstruction and difficult intubation. It has also been suggested that protrusion of the tongue secondary to respiratory distress gives a false impression of macroglossia (McFarlane & Soni 1986).

c) Impaired neurological function depresses cough and swallowing reflexes and predisposes to aspiration, atelectasis, and pneumonia. All these factors may contribute to hypoxia.

d) Patients are sensitive to respiratory depressants.

2. Later-onset forms:

a) Patients with progressive muscle weakness may require postoperative IPPV. An 11-year-old boy with primary hyperparathyroidism required ventilation for 15 days after surgery, despite having not been given muscle relaxants (Kotani et al 1996).

b) Muscle weakness can predispose to respiratory failure in the absence of surgery. A 51-year-old woman, diagnosed only 5 years before, was admitted with respiratory insufficiency and received a short period of IPPV. She was discharged with a tracheostomy after 6 weeks, but died at home 3 days later (Felice et al 1995).

Management

1. Pompe's disease:

a) The importance of monitoring and the avoidance of hypoxia has been stressed

(McFarlane & Soni 1986). Two anaesthetics were given to the same patient a week apart. The first, a halothane induction, began without monitoring and ended with ventricular fibrillation and the abandonment of the procedure. In the second, uneventful anaesthetic, there was direct arterial monitoring and subsequent induction was established with ketamine and vecuronium and the patient's lungs were ventilated.

b) Ketamine, halothane and suxamethonium were used successfully on different occasions in two patients (Kaplan 1980). However, on the evidence of a limited number of case reports, induction with halothane in these patients may be hazardous. Whether this is an effect of halothane on the myocardium, or to hypoxia secondary to airway obstruction, is impossible to judge. Undoubtedly, if tracheal intubation and control of respiration are achieved rapidly, this will reduce the potential for hypoxia and the need for high concentrations of inhalation agents.

c) In view of the risk of hyperkalaemia or rhabdomyolysis, the use of suxamethonium in a patient with any myopathy is inadvisable.

d) It has been suggested that neuromuscular blockers may not be required, since muscle hypotonia facilitates IPPV.

e) A local anaesthetic technique should be considered. Diagnostic muscle biopsy has been described using a modified femoral nerve block and a peripheral nerve stimulator. Ketamine was used for sedation (Rosen & Broadman 1986). Caudal anaesthesia has also been suggested as a suitable technique (Kaplan 1980).

f) If macroglossia is present, and the possibility of difficult intubation exists, awake intubation may be indicated.

2. Adult form:

a) Assessment of respiratory function and reserve.

b) Avoidance of suxamethonium.

Bibliography

Ausems MG, Lochman P, van Diggelen OP et al 1999 A diagnostic protocol for adult-onset glycogen storage type II. Neurology 52: 851–3.

Ellis FR 1980 Inherited muscle disease. British Journal of Anaesthesia 52: 153–64.

Felice KJ, Alessi AG, Grunnet ML 1995 Clinical variability in adult-onset acid maltase deficiency: report of affected sibs and review of the literature. Medicine 74: 131–5.

Kaplan R 1980 Pompe's disease presenting for anesthesia. Anesthesiology Review 7: 21–8.

Kotani N, Hashimoto H, Hirota K et al 1996 Prolonged respiratory depression after anesthesia for parathyroidectomy in a patient with juvenile type of acid maltase deficiency. Journal of Clinical Anesthesia 8: 620.

McFarlane HJ, Soni N 1986 Pompe's disease and anaesthesia. Anaesthesia 41: 1219–24.

Reuser AJ, Kroos MA, Hermans MM et al 1995 Glycogenosis type II (acid maltase deficiency). Muscle & Nerve 3S: 61–9.

Rosen KR, Broadman LM 1986 Anaesthesia for diagnostic muscle biopsy in an infant with Pompe's disease. Canadian Anaesthetists' Society Journal 33: 790–4.

Porphyria

A group of disorders of porphyrin metabolism resulting from defects in certain enzymes involved in the synthesis of haem. They may be inherited or acquired. Although porphyria is very rare in the UK, one type, variegate porphyria (VP), is common in certain regions of South Africa, whilst in Sweden and Finland both acute intermittent porphyria (AIP) and VP are relatively common. As a result, much of the clinical and experimental work on the subject originates from these countries.

Haem, which is synthesised in the liver, bone marrow and erythrocytes, is required for the manufacture of haemoglobin, myoglobin and a number of other respiratory pigments, such as the cytochrome enzymes.

In the hepatic porphyrias, only the liver is involved in the abnormality of haem synthesis. It is this group of porphyrias that is of particular concern to the anaesthetist, and only they are discussed. In each of these, there is a different relative deficiency of one of the enzymes involved in the hepatic synthesis of haem. The majority of haem manufactured by the liver is used in the biosynthesis of the cytochrome P-450 enzyme system. This system is important for drug metabolism.

The administration of certain drugs to patients with porphyria can, on occasions, result in serious neurological defects. Most of the drugs which are potentially dangerous in porphyria can increase delta-aminolaevulinic acid (ALA) synthase activity. This is the first enzyme required to initiate the sequence that results in the manufacture of haem. These drugs are usually lipid soluble, and to assist their excretion by the kidneys, they require transformation into water-soluble compounds by the cytochrome P-450 enzyme system. The presence of any of these drugs can therefore increase the activity of this system. In other words, they share the common property of being enzyme inducers of the cytochrome P-450 system. A demand for haem secondary to this induction of cytochrome P-450 results in a feedback mechanism stimulating further production of ALA synthase. The hepatic haem metabolic pathway is thus stimulated, but because the underlying enzyme deficiencies cannot fully cope with this additional activity, there is accumulation of certain porphyrins or precursors at specific levels in the metabolic chain. These levels will vary according to the particular relative enzyme deficiency.

The exact relationship between the biochemistry, and the clinical features of the porphyric crises and neurological deficits, is still not known. However, there are characteristic pathological lesions in the CNS, the spinal cord, and the autonomic ganglia. Axon degeneration and demyelination are particular features. It has been suggested that the signs and symptoms of porphyria can be entirely attributed to neurological damage (Laiwah et al 1987).

However, porphyrin precursors do not seem to be the main cause of the neurotoxicity, as has been previously postulated. Existing evidence suggests that the nervous system lesions primarily result from a deficiency of haem, while neurotoxicity secondary to increased levels of ALA may be an additional factor in their evolution.

Although some patients still die within acute attacks, recent long-term studies show that the frequency of attacks is less than before 1967, and the mortality lower (Kauppinen & Mustajoki 1992). Morbidity and mortality is most often associated with delay in diagnosis or failure of treatment. Porphyria has been associated with an increased incidence of hepatocellular carcinoma, hypertension, and acute renal failure.

Preoperative abnormalities

1. The clinical and biochemical features of the hepatic porphyrias rarely appear before puberty, and some patients remain permanently asymptomatic. Symptoms, which depend on the particular type of porphyria, may involve the gastrointestinal tract, the nervous system, and the skin. Intermittent acute crises, which may result in severe neurological deficits and occasionally death, can be precipitated by a variety of drugs, including alcohol. Crises may also be associated with menstruation, acute infection, fasting, and pregnancy (Harrison & McAuley 1992).

2. Clinical features of the individual types of porphyria:

a) *Acute intermittent porphyria (AIP)* is an autosomal dominant condition in which there is a reduction in porphobilinogen deaminase. It is the most common cause of acute attacks. During an attack there are increased amounts of ALA and porphobilinogen (PBG) produced and excreted. AIP often presents in adult life with episodes of acute abdominal pain, vomiting, and pyrexia. Peripheral sensory and motor deficits, cranial nerve palsies and autonomic disturbances may occur.

There may be severe neuropsychiatric manifestations, including hallucinations, mental changes, and epilepsy. In adults with AIP, the risk of attacks has been found to correlate with the excretion of PBG in the urine. A low excretion of porphyrins predicted low risk (Kauppinen & Mustajoki 1992).

b) *Hereditary coproporphyria (HC)* is a rare condition which is similar to AIP. There is a deficiency of coproporphyrinogen oxidase, so that coproporphyrin III levels may be elevated, in addition to those of ALA and PBG.

c) *Variegate porphyria (VP)* results from a deficiency of protoporphyrinogen oxidase; the enzymatic block is therefore one step further on from that in HC. It usually presents with blistering skin lesions, commonly on the hands and face. Photosensitivity causing blisters is due to the presence of certain porphyrins in the skin. Urinary PGB, ALA (acute phase) and coproporphyrin III (acute phase) are increased. In the plasma porphyrin–protein conjugate is present with a fluorescence emission peak at 624–6 nm.

3. In the screening test for PBG, the patient's urine turns dark red on the addition of Ehrlich's aldehyde. Specific tests exist for different precursors and/or porphyrins, to elicit the exact type of porphyria.

4. Acute crises can vary in length from hours to days. The commonest symptoms are abdominal pain, vomiting, hypertension, tachycardia, and hyponatraemia (Elder et al 1997).

5. Haematin, which suppresses ALA synthase activity, has been used to relieve the symptoms of porphyria.

Anaesthetic problems

1. *Drug porphyrinogenicity.* A wide range of drugs possess a potential for increasing the production of porphyrins or their precursors, thus precipitating an acute attack. The use of any of these drugs may result in severe neurological deficits, including paraplegia or quadriplegia. In a survey of Finnish patients with AIP, 2% of surgical operations and 4% of pregnancies were associated with acute attacks (Kauppinen & Mustajoki 1992). Since the overall number of patients with porphyria presenting for anaesthesia is small, experience with any individual anaesthetic drug is limited. In addition, a patient's response to a particular drug will vary according to the state of their porphyria. A retrospective analysis of 78 anaesthetics given to 47 patients suggested that if the patient was in a latent period, the risks of using thiopentone were small. By contrast, seven out of ten patients given thiopentone during an acute episode had a worsening of porphyric symptoms (Mustajoki & Heinonen 1980). However, with such potentially devastating complications, the scope for prospective human 'studies' is limited. For this reason, experimental models are used to assess the porphyrinogenicity of certain anaesthetic drugs. Rats primed with 3,5-dicarbethoxy-1,4-dihydrocolidine (DDC) provide a model for latent variegate porphyria. With this system, various drugs have been tested for their ability to increase hepatic ALA synthase activity and produce intermediate porphyrins (Blekkenhorst et al 1980, Harrison et al 1985). Although animal studies cannot necessarily be extrapolated to man, additional testing with known safe and unsafe drugs has provided some measure of control (Blekkenhorst et al 1980).

A simple method of drug classification has been suggested as a clinical guide to therapy in porphyria (Disler et al 1982).

Category A:
Drugs reported in terms of clinical experience as dangerous or safe by three or more authorities.

Category B:
As Category A, but reported by only two or fewer authorities.

These two categories are usually associated with corroborated experimental animal data.

Category C:

Drugs evaluated only in the experimental rat model.

Category D:

Drugs evaluated in chick embryo liver cell culture or 'in ovo'.

Neither Categories C nor D have corroborative reports of human cases.

In some drugs the data are conflicting.

For detailed information on general prescribing, Disler's article is recommended.

Probably dangerous drugs include: barbiturates, carbamazepine, carbromal, chloramphenicol, chlordiazepoxide, cimetidine, ergot alkaloids, erythromycin, flunitrazepam, furosemide (frusemide), glutethimide, griseofulvin, hydantoins, imipramine, meprobamate, methyl dopa, metoclopramide, nalidixic acid, nikethimide, nitrazepam, pargyline, pentazocine, phenoxybenzamine, steroids, sulphonamides, sulphonylurea antidiabetic agents, theophylline, and tranylcypromine.

Possibly dangerous drugs: A number of drugs have often been used without complication, but a single case report, or experimental data exist, implicating it as being porphyrinogenic. This group includes corticosteroids, diazepam, enflurane★, etomidate★, fentanyl★, halothane★, hydralazine, ketamine★, lidocaine (lignocaine)★, pancuronium★, paraldehyde, pethidine★, and the sex hormones.(★ Specific reference to these drugs is made below.)

Barbiturates, as is well known, are contraindicated. Between 1950 and 1971, 31 out of 145 admissions for acute attacks to the Groote Schuur Hospital in Cape Town were precipitated by anaesthesia with thiopentone, and two of the patients died (Harrison et al 1993). Although a

single dose of etomidate produced equivocal results using the DDC-primed rat model, a continuous infusion of etomidate caused an increase in ALA synthase, coproporphyrin, and protoporphyrin levels. The authors of this study believed it should be considered as category C, and thus potentially porphyrinogenic (Harrison et al 1985). In this same study, ketamine did not produce any change. A single case report has implicated ketamine as porphyrinogenic, but there is clinical and experimental evidence suggesting that it is safe (Rizk et al 1977, Blekkenhorst et al 1980, Capouet et al 1987).

Propofol following epidural blockade with lidocaine (lignocaine) and fentanyl produced urinary porphobilinogen levels above the upper limit of normal, but with no porphyric symptoms (Kantor & Rolbin 1992).

Halothane, lidocaine (lignocaine), fentanyl, pethidine and pancuronium have been implicated in single case reports only, and have been used on other occasions without complications (Disler et al 1982). Pancuronium has been suggested as being unsafe on animal data, but as yet there is nothing to incriminate vecuronium, which has been used clinically. Enflurane is porphyrogenic in the rat model, but there have been no clinical reports of problems. Isoflurane has been used in humans without problems, but no experimental data exist.

2. Acute abdominal crises can cause undiagnosed porphyrics to be subjected to surgery. There may be an accompanying tachycardia and hypertension.

3. A porphyric crisis may last for several days and result in dehydration, hyponatraemia, and hypokalaemia.

4. Fasting before surgery induces cytochrome P-450 enzyme activity.

Management

1. *Nonanaesthetic drugs.* These should only be prescribed after reference to a drug list (such as found in the British National Formulary), and

detailed information about anaesthetic drugs (Harrison et al 1993, Jensen et al 1995). All drugs known to precipitate acute crises should be avoided. However, recommendations are not absolute and individual clinical judgements must be made about the controversial ones, taking into account the presence or absence of an acute attack (see above). Nevertheless, new drugs that have not yet been tested for porphyrogenicity should be avoided, unless no satisfactory alternative exists (Harrison et al 1993).

Nonanaesthetic drugs that are reported to be safe in porphyrics (Disler et al 1982, Harrison et al 1993) include: epinephrine (adrenaline), aminoglycosides, aspirin, atropine, beta blockers, biguanides, bupivacaine, buprenorphine, cephalosporins, chlorphenamine (chlorpheniramine), chlorpromazine, codeine, coumarins, diazoxide, digitalis, droperidol, erythromycin, heparin, hyoscine, insulin, labetalol, lorazepam, morphine, neostigmine, nitroglycerin, paracetamol, penicillins, procaine, prochlorperazine, promazine, promethazine, propranolol, sodium nitroprusside, thyroxine, and trifluoperazine.

2. *Anaesthetic drugs.*

a) *Premedication.* If this is essential, temazepam and midazolam appear to be safe (Harrison et al 1993).

b) *Intravenous agents.* Clinical and experimental reports have suggested that propofol may be safe for anaesthesia (Mitterschiffthaler et al 1988, Meissner et al 1991, Pazvanska et al 1999), for sedation on the ITU (Harrison & McAuley 1992), and for repeated use for ECT (Shaw & McKeith 1998), although patients should be observed carefully postoperatively. In the rat model, Bohrer et al (1995) concluded that propofol was safe as a single bolus dose, but suggested caution with large cumulative doses. Midazolam appeared to be safe in the experimental model and in clinical reports. Ketamine also appears to be safe, although it possesses disadvantages as an agent for routine use.

c) *Volatile agents.* Halothane, although contentious, has been used clinically and experimentally. Harrison et al (1993) recommend it as the inhalational agent of choice. Enflurane has experimental data to implicate it as porphyrogenic, but no acute attacks in humans have been attributed to it. Nitrous oxide is safe.

d) *Muscle relaxants.* Suxamethonium and tubocurarine are known to be safe. The clinical use of atracurium has been reported but no porphyrin metabolites were measured (Lin & Chen 1990). Although vecuronium is related to pancuronium, which is unsafe, the use of vecuronium has been supported clinically, although there are no experimental data.

e) *Analgesics.* Fentanyl, morphine, pethidine and codeine are generally considered safe.

f) *Local anaesthetics.* The use of bupivacaine and lignocaine (lidocaine) is contentious, but they are thought to be safe, because there are no clinical reports of any local anaesthetic ever having induced an acute crisis (Harrison et al 1993).

g) *Reversal agents.* Neostigmine and atropine are considered to be safe.

3. *Drugs for symptomatic use in an acute crisis.* Opiate analgesics can be given and may be needed in high doses. Chlorpromazine is useful as a sedative and prochlorperazine for vomiting. Intravenous dextrose or nasogastric feeding should be given. Tachycardia and hypertension may be treated with beta adrenergic blockers. A patient admitted in a porphyric crisis may require correction of fluid and electrolyte balance.

4. *Specific treatment for an acute crisis.* Haematin has been reported to be effective in aborting clinical episodes of porphyria, by decreasing ALA synthase activity. A haematin infusion has been used to treat increased urinary porphobilinogen levels in a patient following cardiopulmonary bypass (Roby and Harrison 1982). Haem arginate has been used with

success, but it needs to be given early in the attack (Elder et al 1997).

5. *Preoperative management.* If neurological deficits exist, a careful history and examination must be made. Carbohydrate loading suppresses the synthesis of porphyrins. Glucose administration inhibits enzyme induction and fasting increases it. Administration of dextrose 10% should therefore begin before a period of starvation.

6. *Regional anaesthesia.* This may be appropriate on occasions. Caesarean section under both spinal and epidural anaesthesia using bupivacaine has been described (Brennan et al 1990, McNeill & Bennet 1990). However, the importance of early antenatal assessment is emphasised so that a plan for the emergency situation can be documented in the patient's notes.

7. *The postoperative period.* The patient should be observed for an acute attack and, if symptoms occur, urine, faeces or plasma should be collected for evidence of porphyrinogenesis.

8. *Urgent expert advice.* Additional advice can be obtained from the Porphyria Research Unit, Western Infirmary, Glasgow G11 6NT.

Bibliography

Asokumar B, Kierney C, James TW et al 1999 Anaesthetic management of a patient with erythropoietic porphyria for ventricular septal defect closure. Paediatric Anaesthesia 9: 356–8.

Blekkenhorst GH, Harrison GG, Cook ES, Eales L 1980 Screening of certain anaesthetic agents for their ability to elicit acute porphyric phases in susceptible patients. British Journal of Anaesthesia 52: 759–62.

Bohrer H, Schmidt H, Martin E et al 1995 Testing the porphyrinogenicity of propofol in a primed rat model. British Journal of Anaesthesia 75: 334–8.

Brennan L, Halfacre JA, Woods SD 1990 Regional anaesthesia in porphyria. British Journal of Anaesthesia 65: 594.

Capouet V, Dernovoi B, Azagra JS 1987 Induction of anaesthesia with ketamine during an acute crisis of hereditary coproporphyria. Canadian Journal of Anaesthesia 34: 388–90.

Disler PB, Blekkenhorst GH, Eales L et al 1982 Guidelines for drug prescription in patients with the acute porphyrias. South African Medical Journal 61: 656–60.

Dover SB, Plenderleith L, Moore MR et al 1994 Safety of general anaesthesia and surgery in acute hepatic porphyria. Gut 35: 1112–15.

Elder GH, Hift RJ, Meissner PN 1997 The acute porphyrias. Lancet 349: 1613–17.

Harrison GG, Moore MR, Meissner PN 1985 Porphyrinogenicity of etomidate and ketamine as continuous infusions. British Journal of Anaesthesia 57: 420–3.

Harrison GG, Meissner PN, Hift RJ 1993 Anaesthesia for the porphyric patient. Anaesthesia 48: 417–21.

Harrison JC, McAuley FT 1992 Propofol sedation in intensive care in a patient with an acute porphyric attack. Anaesthesia 47: 355–6.

Jensen NF, Fiddler DS, Striepe V 1995 Anesthetic considerations in porphyrias. Anesthesia & Analgesia 80: 591–9.

Kantor G, Rolbin SH 1992 Acute intermittent porphyria and Caesarean delivery. Canadian Journal of Anaesthesia 39: 282–5.

Kauppinen R, Mustajoki P 1992 Prognosis of acute porphyria: occurrence of acute attacks, precipitating factors, and associated diseases. Medicine 74: 1–13.

Laiwah ACY, Moore MR, Goldberg A 1987 Pathogenesis of acute porphyria. Quarterly Journal of Medicine 241: 377–92.

Lin Y, Chen L 1990 Atracurium in a patient with acute intermittent porphyria. Anesthesia & Analgesia 71: 440–5.

McNeill MJ, Bennet A 1990 Use of regional anaesthesia in a patient with acute porphyria. British Journal of Anaesthesia 64: 371–3.

Meissner PN, Harrison GG, Hift RJ 1991 Propofol as an iv induction agent in variegate porphyria. British Journal of Anaesthesia 66: 60–5.

Mitterschiffthaler G, Theiner A, Hetzel H et al 1988 Safe use of propofol in a patient with acute intermittent porphyria. British Journal of Anaesthesia 60: 109–11.

Mustajoki P, Heinonen J 1980 General anesthesia in "inducible" porphyrias. Anesthesiology 53: 15–20.

Pazvanska EE, Hinkov OD, Stojnovska LV 1999 Uneventful propofol anaesthesia in a patient with acute intermittent porphyria. European Journal of Anaesthesiology 16: 485–92.

Rizk SK, Jacobsen JH, Silva G 1977 Ketamine as an induction agent for acute intermittent porphyria. Anesthesiology 46: 305–6

Roby HP, Harrison GA 1982 Anaesthesia for coronary artery bypass in a patient with porphyria variegata. Anaesthesia & Intensive Care 10: 276–8.

Shaw IH, McKeith IG 1998 Propofol and electroconvulsive therapy in a patient at risk from acute intermittent porphyria. British Journal of Anaesthesia 80: 260–2.

Sneyd JR, Kreimer-Birnbaum M, Lust MR et al 1995 Use of sufentanil and atracurium anesthesia in a patient with acute porphyria undergoing coronary artery bypass surgery. Journal of Cardiothoracic & Vascular Anesthesia 9: 75–8.

Prader–Willi syndrome

A multisystem genetic disorder of unknown aetiology, in which obesity is associated with disturbances of carbohydrate and fat metabolism. In some cases, abnormalities of chromosome 15 are thought to be involved. It is a two-stage disorder and the clinical features change with age: 0–36 months, and 3 years to adulthood. Consensus criteria have been agreed and diagnosis is based on a scoring system (Holm et al 1993).

In infancy the disorder presents with hypotonia, feeding and respiratory difficulties, and growth retardation. Beyond 3 years, there is excessive weight gain, hyperphagia, hypogonadism, and developmental delay. Despite the hypotonia, no histological, biochemical or neurophysiological abnormalities of the muscle have been demonstrated. A CNS, possibly hypothalamic, lesion has been postulated. Abnormal ventilatory responses to hypoxia and hypercarbia have been shown to improve after treatment with growth hormone (Lindgren et al 1999). Orchidopexy is commonly required for undescended testes. Dental and orthopaedic surgery may also be needed.

Preoperative abnormalities

1. Initially, the infant is hypotonic, feeds poorly, coughs, and has episodes of asphyxia. Children are of small stature with hypermobile joints. Mental retardation is usual. Amongst other features that assist diagnosis at an early stage are an abnormal cry, characteristic facies, genital hypoplasia, and alveolar ridge abnormalities (Aughton & Cassidy 1990). Obesity and hyperphagia develop from about the age of three.

2. Abnormal glucose tolerance curves are recorded and episodes of hypoglycaemia may occur. About 20% develop noninsulin-dependent diabetes that may be secondary to obesity.

3. There is thick, viscous saliva; enamel defects and dental caries are common.

4. Skeletal abnormalities include kyphosis, scoliosis, narrow bifrontal diameter, small hands and feet, a straight ulnar border, and hand and finger anomalies. In one child, kyphosis and spinal canal stenosis resulted in cervical myelopathy (Tsuji et al 1991).

5. A restrictive ventilatory impairment occurs that is probably secondary to respiratory muscle weakness (Hakonarson et al 1995). This predisposes to infection, airway obstruction, hypoventilation, and cor pulmonale.

Anaesthetic problems

There have been at least 28 reports of anaesthetics given to these patients (Milliken & Weintraub 1975, Palmer & Atlee 1976, Mayhew & Taylor 1983, Yamashita et al 1983, Mackenzie 1991, Dearlove et al 1998). Some have been uneventful, in others a variety of complications have been described.

1. The general problems of obesity, including difficult venepuncture.

2. Disturbances of thermoregulation may occur. Two cases had fever and acidosis during anaesthesia, and in six, fever occurred in the postoperative period (Yamashita et al 1983). In one child, intubation difficulty was experienced after suxamethonium (Mayhew & Taylor 1983). The anaesthetic was continued with halothane and curare, but was terminated because the

413

patient's temperature increased. However, the postoperative CK was only 240 u l⁻¹. A subsequent anaesthetic, in which pancuronium, nitrous oxide and fentanyl were used, was uneventful. Although comparisons with MH patients have been made, there is nothing to suggest that the episodes of fever originate from abnormal muscle metabolism. A hypothalamic mechanism seems to be more likely.

3. Cardiac arrhythmias were reported in five cases. A sixth, an 8-year-old child, was having a pacemaker implanted for sick sinus syndrome.

4. Difficulties in intubation were reported in two patients, but the causes were not stated. Mild micrognathia and a large head circumference are features in infants that may contribute (Aughton et al 1990).

5. Regurgitation of gastric secretions and rumination have been observed (Sloan & Kaye 1991), and it has been suggested that these may contribute to the development of dental caries and aspiration pneumonitis.

6. Abnormal ventilatory responses to hypoxia and hypercarbia have been shown, and thought to be central in origin (DiMario et al 1996, Menendez 1999). One 16-month-old, 8-kg infant developed alarming periods of apnoea associated with hypoxia and bradycardia for several days following surgery (Dearlove et al 1998). Snoring, sleep apnoea, hypersomnolence, and daytime hypoventilation have been described, although polysomnography in five patients showed the disorder to be mild (Kaplan et al 1991). In another study of 14 subjects, the lowest oxygen saturation ranged from 41% to 95%; the lowest results were often related to BMI and collar size. However, ENT examination was often unremarkable, and central disturbances are thought to contribute (Richards et al 1994). This was supported by a study of children before they had reached the obesity stage (Schluter et al 1997), which again suggested the primary disturbance to be one of central respiratory control, which may be worsened by obesity.

7. Episodes of hypoglycaemia have been reported.

8. Micrognathia, high arched palate and scoliosis are sometimes associated.

9. Convulsions have been recorded.

10. Examination of the autonomic nervous system suggested that diminished parasympathetic nervous system activity may be the basis of some of the features of the condition (DiMario et al 1994).

Management

1. Blood glucose should be observed carefully, and a glucose infusion given pre- and intraoperatively.

2. ECG, core temperature and $ETCO_2$ should be monitored from the beginning of the anaesthetic.

3. In view of the obesity and restrictive lung problems, a technique using IPPV is advisable. No prolongation of response to muscle relaxants has been reported, despite depolarising and nondepolarising drugs having been used.

4. Patients should be assumed to be at high risk from aspiration of gastric contents and appropriate precautions should be taken to reduce and neutralise acid secretions, and to secure the airway rapidly.

5. Analgesics should be administered with care in those with evidence of hypoventilation. Careful postoperative observation is required. CPAP may improve obstructive sleep apnoea, especially in patients in whom daytime ventilatory failure is associated with sleep-disordered breathing (Smith et al 1998).

Bibliography

Aughton DJ, Cassidy SB 1990 Physical features of Prader–Willi syndrome in neonates. American Journal of Disease in Childhood 144: 1251–4.

Dearlove OR, Dobson A, Super M 1998 Anaesthesia and Prader–Willi syndrome. Paediatric Anaesthesia 8: 267–71.

DiMario FJ Jr, Dunham B, Burleson JA et al 1994 An evaluation of autonomic nervous system function in patients with the Prader–Willi syndrome. Pediatrics 93: 76–81.

DiMario FJ Jr, Bauer L, Volpe J et al 1996 Respiratory sinus arrhythmias in patients with Prader–Willi syndrome. Journal of Child Neurology 11: 121–5.

Hakonarson H, Moskovitz J, Daigle KL et al 1995 Pulmonary function abnormalities in Prader–Willi syndrome. Journal of Pediatrics 126: 565–70.

Holm VA, Cassidy SB, Butler MG et al 1993 Prader–Willi syndrome: consensus diagnostic criteria. Pediatrics 91: 398–402.

Kaplan J, Frederickson PA, Richardson JW 1991 Sleep and breathing in patients with the Prader–Willi syndrome. Mayo Clinic Proceedings 66: 1124–6.

Lindgren AC, Hellstrom LG, Ritzen EM et al 1999 Growth hormone treatment increases CO_2 response, ventilation and central inspiratory drive in children with Prader–Willi syndrome. European Journal of Pediatrics 158: 936–40.

Mackenzie JW 1991 Anaesthesia and the Prader–Willi syndrome. Journal of the Royal Society of Medicine 84: 239.

Mayhew JF, Taylor B 1983 Anaesthetic considerations in the Prader–Willi syndrome. Canadian Anaesthetists' Society Journal 30: 565–6.

Menendez AA 1999 Abnormal ventilatory responses in patients with Prader–Willi syndrome. European Journal of Pediatrics 158: 941–2.

Milliken RA, Weintraub DM 1975 Cardiac abnormalities during anesthesia in a child with Prader–Willi syndrome. Anesthesiology 43: 590–2.

Palmer SK, Atlee JL 1976 Anesthetic management of the Prader–Willi syndrome. Anesthesiology 44: 161–3.

Richards A, Quaghebeur G, Clift S et al 1994 The upper airway and sleep apnoea in the Prader–Willi syndrome. Clinical Otolaryngology & Allied Sciences 19: 193–7.

Schluter B, Buschatz D, Trowitzsch E et al 1997 Respiratory control in children with Prader–Willi syndrome. European Journal of Pediatrics 156: 65–8.

Sloan TB, Kaye CI 1991 Rumination risk of aspiration of gastric contents in the Prader–Willi syndrome. Anesthesia & Analgesia 73: 492–5.

Smith IE, King MA, Siklos PW et al 1998 Treatment of ventilatory failure in the Prader–Willi syndrome. European Respiratory Journal 11: 1150–2.

Tsuji M, Kurihara A, Uratsuji M et al 1991 Cervical myelopathy with Prader–Willi syndrome in a 13-year-old boy. A case report. Spine 16: 1342–4.

Yamashita M, Koishi K, Yamaya R et al 1983 Anaesthetic considerations in the Prader–Willi syndrome. Canadian Anaesthetists' Society Journal 30: 179–84.

Protein C deficiency

In the normal subject, protein C is an essential anticoagulant. It acts by selective inhibition of activated Factors V and VIII, and by stimulation of fibrinolysis. Synthesis occurs in the liver and is vitamin K dependent.

Inherited and acquired deficiencies may occur. Since the first report in 1981 by Griffin et al, a number of families have been described in which relatively young members have had recurrent spontaneous venous thromboses in association with reduced levels (between 35% and 65% of normal) of protein C. In affected families, thromboembolic disease usually develops from the age of 20 years onwards (Cavenagh & Colvin 1996).

However, the situation has proved to be more complex than was initially thought. When attempting to define the normal range of values of protein C, it was found that one in 60 of healthy adults had levels of 55–65%, and conversely, one in 200–300 patients with heterozygous protein C deficiency had no history of venous thrombosis (Miletich et al 1986). It is therefore possible that heterozygous subjects with venous thromboses have some additional predisposing abnormality, or conversely, heterozygous subjects without venous thrombosis have some compensating mechanism. A recently developed technique for functional assay has helped to detect patients who have reduced protein C activity, but normal levels of protein C as measured by immunological assay.

Severe congenital homozygous protein C deficiency (often with no detectable levels) has been described in infants of parents who both had heterozygous deficiency. These presented with widespread skin lesions and necrosis secondary to thrombosis of small veins.

Levels of protein C may also be reduced in liver disease, ARDS, and following surgery. They may be very low, or even undetectable, in coagulopathies.

Preoperative abnormalities

1. When the condition presents in infancy, it is usually homozygous, and often fatal, because it is associated with purpura fulminans, cutaneous necrosis, and extensive venous thrombosis.

2. In heterozygous disease, there is an increased risk of deep venous thrombosis and pulmonary embolism. In adults or children with the familial deficiency, the first event may be in association with another predisposing factor (Freed 1991). Thus, pulmonary embolism may occur in the perioperative period (Sternberg et al 1991), during pregnancy (Morrison et al 1989), or in association with oral contraceptives, or infection. Superficial thrombophlebitis also features.

3. Patients may present with conditions that are secondary to thromboses at unusual sites. Mesenteric (peritonitis), cerebral, axillary, hepatic venous (Budd–Chiari) and penile thromboses (priapism) have been recorded.

4. Protein C deficiency appears to be a risk factor for myocardial infarction (Bux-Gewehr et al 1999).

5. Patients known to have the condition, and who have already had venous thromboses, will usually be taking long-term coumarin therapy. Warfarin, despite one of its actions being to lower protein C levels, has been found to be beneficial in preventing recurrent venous thromboembolism in protein C deficiency (Broekmans et al 1983). Occasionally, warfarin-induced skin necrosis, particularly in the skin overlying fatty areas, has been reported, and is secondary to capillary thrombosis.

6. Serious obstetric complications are associated with an increased frequency of genetic thrombophilia, of which protein C deficiency is one example (Kupferminc et al 1999). In a young patient who has had a previous spontaneous venous thrombosis, or who has a family history of thromboses, the possible presence of this condition should be considered (Melissari & Kakkar 1989). It is thought to account for 5–8% of such cases. Other inherited thrombophilias include protein S deficiency, Factor V Leiden, antithrombin deficiency, high concentration of Factor VIII, hyperhomocystinaemia, and prothrombin 20210A (Rosendaal 1999).

7. Fetal loss is increased.

Anaesthetic problems

1. *Homozygous infant*:

a) Skin necrosis over pressure points.

b) There is a theoretical risk of tracheal damage during the period of tracheal intubation.

2. *Heterozygous adult or child*:

a) The problems of the management of a patient for anaesthesia and surgery who is receiving anticoagulants.

b) The increased risk of venous thrombosis and pulmonary embolism in the perioperative period. Fatal pulmonary embolism occurred in an 8-year-old child following laparotomy (Sternberg et al 1991), and in a 19-year-old man after knee surgery (Rick 1990).

3. *Pregnancy*. The problems of management during pregnancy, a state that constitutes a risk factor for venous thrombosis in these patients (Morrison et al 1989). In addition, pregnancy appears to be associated with a poor fetal outcome (Bertault et al 1991), with intrauterine growth retardation probably secondary to insufficiency of the uteroplacental circulation.

Management

1. *Homozygous infant*:

a) The anaesthetic literature is limited. Three consecutive anaesthetics were reported for partial omentectomy and insertion of a Tenkhoff catheter, in a homozygous infant with renal failure (Wetzel et al 1986). Despite the theoretical risks, tracheal

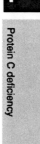
intubation was employed, using a small tube to reduce tracheal pressure. The trachea was examined with a flexible laryngoscope at subsequent anaesthetics and no damage was found.

b) The advice of a haematologist should be sought for the correction of the protein C deficiency. Protein C concentrate is now available and has been given both intravenously and subcutaneously (Dreyfus et al 1991, Minford et al 1996).

2. *Heterozygous adult or child*:

a) If the patient is taking warfarin, a heparin infusion should be substituted to obtain more flexible control. Anticoagulants should be restarted as soon as the surgery allows.

b) If the patient is not anticoagulated, low-dose heparin should be given preoperatively.

3. *Pregnancy*:

a) In pregnancy, management will have to be decided in each individual case. A patient presenting for the first time with venous thrombosis will initially require full anticoagulation with heparin.

b) Those without venous thrombosis are increasingly being managed with subcutaneous heparin (Bertault et al 1991). Low molecular weight heparin 7500 u daily was given to one patient from 4 months' gestation until postpartum. Another patient with recurrent fetal loss received protein C concentrate during the first and third trimesters of her pregnancy (Richards et al 1997).

Bibliography

Bertault D, Mandelbrot L, Tchobroutsky C et al 1991 Unfavourable pregnancy outcome associated with congenital protein C deficiency. Case reports. British Journal of Obstetrics & Gynaecology 98: 934–6.

Broekmans AW, Veltkamp JJ, Bertina RM 1983 Congenital protein C deficiency and venous thromboembolism. New England Journal of Medicine 309: 340–4.

Bux-Gewehr I, Nacke A, Feurle GE 1999 Recurring myocardial infarction in a 35 year old woman. Heart 81: 316–17.

Cavenagh JD, Colvin BT 1996 Guidelines for the management of thrombophilia. Postgraduate Medical Journal 72: 87–94.

Dreyfus M, Magny JF, Bridey F et al 1991 Treatment of homozygous protein C deficiency and neonatal purpura fulminans with a purified protein C concentrate. New England Journal of Medicine 325: 1565–8.

Freed JA 1991 Hypercoagulability. Should every patient with venous thrombosis be tested? Postgraduate Medicine 90: 157–60.

Griffin JH, Evatt B, Zimmerman TS et al 1981 Deficiency of protein C in congenital thrombotic disease. Journal of Clinical Investigation 68: 1370–3.

Kupferminc MJ, Eldor A, Steinman N et al 1999 Increased frequency of genetic thrombophilia in women with complications of pregnancy. New England Journal of Medicine 340: 9–13.

Melissari E, Kakkar VV 1989 Congenital severe protein C deficiency in adults. British Journal of Haematology 72: 222–8.

Miletich J, Sherman L, Broze G 1986 Absence of thrombosis in subjects with heterozygous protein C deficiency. New England Journal of Medicine 317: 991–6.

Minford AM, Parapia LA, Stainforth C et al 1996 Treatment of homozygous protein C deficiency with subcutaneous protein C concentrate. British Journal of Haematology 93: 215–16.

Morrison AE, Walker ID, Black WP 1989 Protein C deficiency presenting as deep venous thrombosis in pregnancy. British Journal of Obstetrics & Gynaecology 95: 1077–80.

Richards EM, Makris M, Preston FE 1997 The successful use of protein C concentrate during pregnancy in a patient with type 1 protein C deficiency, previous thrombosis and recurrent fetal loss. British Journal of Haematology 98: 660–1.

Rick ME 1990 Protein C and protein S. Vitamin K-dependent inhibitors of blood coagulation. Journal of the American Medical Association 263: 701–3.

Rosendaal FR 1999 Venous thrombosis: a multicausal disease. Lancet 353: 1167–73.

Sternberg TL, Bailey MK, Lazarchick J et al 1991 Protein C deficiency as a cause of pulmonary embolism in the perioperative period. Anesthesiology 74: 364–6.

Wetzel RC, Marsh BR, Yaster M et al 1986 Anesthetic implications of protein C deficiency. Anesthesia & Analgesia 65: 982–4.

Protein S deficiency

An inherited thrombophilia. Protein S is a nonenzymatic, vitamin K-dependent plasma protein that inhibits coagulation by functioning as a cofactor for activated protein C. Protein S can be in a free form, the only form in which it can act as a cofactor, or a protein-bound, inactive form. Inflammatory processes reduce protein S activity (Cavenagh & Colvin 1996).

In the absence of protein S, protein C is almost depleted of its functional ability as an anticoagulant. Protein S deficiency is an autosomal dominant condition associated with an increased incidence of thrombotic events, and an increase in spontaneous abortions. A comparison of the thrombotic risk associated with different inherited thrombophilias has been studied (Martinelli et al 1998).

Preoperative abnormalities

1. Homozygous disease is rare and, as with protein C deficiency, associated with neonatal purpura fulminans.

2. Heterozygous disease is associated with a high incidence of venous thrombosis and thromboembolic disease. In a review of children, 57% had venous thrombosis, 20% had arterial thrombosis, and 14% had both (Blanco et al 1994).

3. It has been suggested that in pregnancy, thrombophiliac disorders may increase the risk of early-onset preeclampsia. In a series of 101 women with this history, 24.7% had protein S deficiency (Dekker et al 1995). A primigravida with early-onset preeclampsia and postpartum thrombosis of the left femoral vein was found to have both Factor V Leiden mutation and protein S deficiency. Heparin prophylaxis was used in the two subsequent pregnancies, in which neither thromboembolism nor preeclampsia recurred (Kahn 1998).

4. Warfarin-induced skin necrosis may occur.

5. The diagnosis is made by measurement of protein S antigen; most patients have normal coagulation tests.

6. Acquired protein S deficiency can occur in liver disease, SLE, coagulopathies, and pregnancy.

Anaesthetic problems

1. Although thromboses usually occur spontaneously, there is an even greater risk during pregnancy and surgery. A 4-year-old boy having craniofacial reconstruction developed an ischaemic upper arm following intraoperative radial artery and peripheral venous cannulation (Zimmerman et al 1998).

2. Death occurred in an unfortunate parturient with protein S deficiency, after elective Caesarean section during which severe hypertension and tachycardia occurred. Postmortem showed a phaeochromocytoma of the right adrenal and myocardial infarction from undiagnosed phaeochromocytoma (Zangrillo et al 1999).

3. In pregnancy, protein S levels are reduced, and continue to be functionally less efficient until about 2 weeks' postpartum. Decisions will have to be made about the method of anaesthesia for operative delivery. In one patient, subcutaneous heparin was stopped 12 h beforehand and a combined spinal/epidural performed (Abramowitz & Beilin 1999). In another patient, whose protein S level had decreased during pregnancy, the risks of stopping heparin were considered to be too high, therefore Caesarean section was performed under general anaesthesia (Fan et al 1995). One patient had a combination of protein S deficiency and hypofibrinogenaemia (Funai et al 1997).

Management

1. Prophylaxis with low molecular weight heparin (Andrew et al 1998).

2. Hypovolaemia, hypotension and hypothermia should be avoided.

3. It has been suggested that intravascular catheters should be heparin bonded, to reduce the incidence of catheter-associated thrombosis, and that the duration of their use should be limited (Zimmerman et al 1999).

4. There must be multidisciplinary involvement during pregnancy. Decisions will have to be made about thromboprophylaxis, and whether or not it should be stopped to enable regional anaesthesia to be used for vaginal or operative delivery.

Bibliography

Abramovitz SE, Beilin Y 1999 Anesthetic management of the parturient with protein S deficiency and ischemic heart disease. Anesthesia & Analgesia 89: 709–10.

Andrew M, Michelson AD, Bovill E et al 1998 Guidelines for antithrombotic therapy in pediatric patients. Journal of Pediatrics 132: 575–88.

Blanco A, Bonduel M, Penalva L et al 1994 Deep venous thrombosis in a 13-year-old boy with hereditary protein S deficiency and a review of the pediatric literature. American Journal of Hematology 45: 330–4.

Cavenagh JD, Colvin BT 1996 Guidelines for the management of thrombophilia. Postgraduate Medical Journal 72: 87–94.

Dekker GA, de Vries JL, Doelitzsch PM et al 1995 Underlying disorders associated with severe early-onset preeclampsia. American Journal of Obstetrics & Gynecology 173: 1042–8.

Fan SZ, Yeh M, Tsay W 1995 Caesarean section in a patient with protein S deficiency. Anaesthesia 50: 251–3.

Funai EF, Klein SA, Lockwood CJ 1997 Successful pregnancy outcome in a patient with both congenital hypofibrinogenemia and protein S deficiency. Obstetrics & Gynecology 89: 858.

Grocott HP, Clements F, Landolfo K 1996 Coronary artery bypass graft surgery in a patient with hereditary protein S deficiency. Journal of Cardiothoracic & Vascular Anesthesia 10: 915–17.

Kahn SR 1998 Severe preeclampsia associated with coinheritance of Factor V Leiden mutation and protein S deficiency. Obstetrics & Gynecology 91: 812–14.

Martinelli I, Mannuccio PM, De Stefano V et al 1998 Different risk factors of thrombosis in four vaginal deliveries associated with inherited thrombophilias. A study of 150 families. Blood 92: 2353–8.

Zangrillo A, Valentini G, Casati A et al 1999 Myocardial infarction and death after Caesarean section in a woman with protein S deficiency and undiagnosed phaeochromocytoma. European Journal of Anaesthesiology 16: 268–71.

Zimmerman AA, Watson RS, Williams JK 1999 Protein S deficiency presenting as an acute postoperative arterial thrombosis in a four-year-old child. Anesthesia & Analgesia 88: 535–7.

Pulmonary hypertension (PH)

Can be applied to any condition in which the pulmonary artery pressure is increased above 35/15 mmHg, or a mean of 15–18 mmHg ($n = 15$–$30/5$–12 mmHg). Can be primary or secondary. Secondary pulmonary hypertension may result from pulmonary emboli, chronic hypoxic lung disease, left to right shunts, sickle cell anaemia, increased left ventricular filling pressures, left atrial outflow obstruction and vasculitis associated with connective tissue diseases, particularly scleroderma and SLE.

Primary pulmonary hypertension (PPH) is a rare disease of the pulmonary vasculature and is of unknown aetiology. After elimination of other causes, the diagnosis is one of exclusion. It is more common in women than in men and there may be a family history. There is an increased pulmonary artery pressure and pulmonary vascular resistance. The mortality in PPH is high and the average survival time is 2 years (Rich & Brundage 1984). Heart–lung transplantation has been successful. The effects of pulmonary vasodilators are being investigated. These include nitric oxide (Pepke-Zaba et al 1991), nifedipine, and diltiazem. The prognosis is poor. Sudden death, and deaths secondary to right ventricular failure, are common.

Preoperative abnormalities

1. Increasing dyspnoea and intense fatigue occurs, initially on exertion, but later at rest. Chest pain and haemoptysis may feature. In advanced disease, hypoxaemia occurs at rest.

2. Signs of a low cardiac output, signs of the original disease, an elevated JVP, and a right ventricular heave. A loud pulmonary second sound, right ventricular gallop (loud third sound at the left sternal edge), and possibly an early diastolic murmur from pulmonary regurgitation. Right heart failure will develop, with hepatomegaly, and peripheral oedema. Tricuspid incompetence may occur.

3. ECG shows right axis deviation, right ventricular hypertrophy, and right atrial hypertrophy (p pulmonale). Right bundle branch block is common.

4. Chest X-ray shows a prominent pulmonary artery and, at a later stage, an increased cardiothoracic ratio. There are oligaemic lung fields, except when the secondary disease results from increased blood flow, in which case the lung fields are plethoric.

5. Certain conditions are more commonly associated with PH. These include the collagen vascular diseases (mostly scleroderma and SLE), Raynaud's disease, hepatic cirrhosis, and sickle cell disease.

6. Treatment varies with the cause:

a) Primary PH includes chronic anticoagulation with warfarin and vasodilator treatment. Calcium antagonists in high doses are currently being used (Rich et al 1992). More recently, chronic iv prostacyclin has been added for those unresponsive to oral vasodilators (Barst 1997). Patients receive them permanently, or until lung transplantation.

b) PH secondary to connective tissue diseases (Sanchez et al 1999). Warfarin to maintain the INR around 2.0 (or 3.0 if there are lupus antibodies). Immunosuppressive therapy with steroids, cyclophosphamide, cyclosporin, or methotrexate. Nifedipine or diltiazem may be used in those patients shown to respond to vasodilators.

c) PH secondary to chronic hypoxic lung disease. Treatment as for airway obstruction, with anticholinergic agents, oxygen, and steroids.

7. The following features are associated with a poor prognosis: right ventricular failure; a cardiac index of less than $2-2.5 \, l \, min^{-1}$, right atrial pressure >10 mmHg; a pulmonary vascular resistance of $>1-1500 \, dyn \, s \, cm^{-5}$ (D'Alonzo et al 1991).

Anaesthetic problems

1. The pre-existing high pulmonary vascular resistance (PVR) may be further increased by hypoxaemia, acidosis, hypercarbia, cold, alpha adrenoceptor stimulation, nitrous oxide, anxiety, and PEEP.

2. A further elevation of PVR during anaesthesia can worsen right ventricular failure, or decrease venous return to the left heart, thus causing systemic hypotension. Sudden hypotension and hypoxaemia occurred on induction of anaesthesia in a child undergoing ventriculoatrial shunt. Subsequent investigation showed pulmonary hypertension secondary to recurrent pulmonary thromboembolism (Butler et al 1990).

3. There is a poor correlation between RAP and LAP, therefore measurement of PAP and PCWP has been suggested for severe cases. However, the risk of pulmonary vessel perforation is increased during PAWP measurement in patients with acute pulmonary hypertension (Kranz & Viljoen 1979).

4. The patient is often anticoagulated, and cardiologists may press to resume treatment soon after surgery. However, death from haemorrhage occurred in a patient in whom heparin was restarted within hours of a Caesarean section performed using the classical approach (Roessler & Lambert 1986).

5. Childbirth is associated with a high mortality. In a review of reports of 27 parturients with PPH and 25 with secondary PH, the respective maternal mortalities were 30% and 56%. All deaths occurred within 35 days of delivery, and often early in the postpartum period (Weiss et al 1998). Severe preeclampsia and pulmonary hypertension culminated in death within 24 h of Caesarean section (Rubin et al 1995). Acute deterioration, necessitating emergency CPB and mitral valve replacement, took place in another parturient with PH secondary to mitral valve disease, who underwent termination of twin pregnancy at 15 weeks. The patient became critically ill immediately following evacuation of the uterus under epidural anaesthesia. Autotransfusion was thought to have precipitated a sequence of pulmonary oedema, tachycardia, inadequate diastolic filling, decreased cardiac output, and profound hypotension (Tio et al 1998).

Management

1. The cause should be established, since this influences the therapy. For example, PH secondary to chronic hypoxic lung disease responds to reversal of airway obstruction, anticholinergics, oxygen and steroids, rather than to vasodilators (Peacock 1990). Secondary PH is not necessarily a contraindication to liver transplantation (Liu et al 1996, Taura et al 1996).

2. The severity of the PH must also be assessed. Hypoxaemia on air suggests advanced disease. Cardiac catheterisation and pulmonary angiography produce the best information on the degree of pulmonary hypertension and the effect of vasodilators.

3. The risks of surgery must be weighed against the benefits. There are relatively few case reports of anaesthesia in patients with PPH. In those reported, the perioperative mortality was high, especially in the pregnant patient, for whom the prognosis is poor (Nelson et al 1983, Roberts & Keast 1990).

4. For the pregnant patient, a multidisciplinary team of obstetrician, cardiologist, anaesthetist, intensivist and paediatrician is required. Roberts and Keast (1990) suggest that assessment of disease severity, plans for method and timing of delivery, management of circulatory stability, and provision of analgesia or anaesthesia, all need to be discussed and agreed early in pregnancy. Such a policy would require frequent reviews. Vaginal delivery is associated with a better chance of maternal survival. Epidural analgesia with an infusion of low-dose fentanyl and bupivacaine has been reported (Power & Avery 1989).

5. An adequate preoperative assessment of the degree of cardiorespiratory impairment is required. Treatment is difficult. Diuretics improve peripheral oedema, but decrease right ventricular, and hence cardiac, output. Pulmonary vasodilators are not always effective.

6. For major surgery, in severe disease, pulmonary artery, pulmonary capillary wedge and systemic artery pressures need to be monitored, with extreme care to avoid pulmonary vessel perforation. Monitoring of pulmonary pressures, particularly pulmonary vascular resistance, allows rational treatment of perioperative pressure changes with appropriate vasodilators, or fluid replacement.

7. Factors known to increase pulmonary vascular resistance are avoided. A sedative premedication relieves anxiety. Oxygenation should be maintained and hypercarbia and acidosis avoided. The theatre should be warm, and a heated water blanket and blood warmer used. Nitrous oxide has been shown to produce a significant elevation of PAP in patients with pre-existing high levels, but not in those with normal PAP (Schulte-Sasse et al 1982).

8. Pulmonary vasodilators may be required during anaesthesia. It has been suggested that patients should be admitted to the ITU before surgery or delivery, to assess the effect of various forms of therapy on the above parameters.

9. Regional anaesthesia. A patient for Caesarean section under epidural anaesthesia was

tested for the haemodynamic effects of a fluid load, changes in inspired oxygen percentage, tolazoline, sodium nitroprusside, and glyceryl trinitrate (Roessler & Lambert 1986). In this patient, sodium nitroprusside was the most effective drug in terms of reducing pulmonary artery pressure, but it was achieved at the expense of systemic hypotension. Similar management in another parturient demonstrated a reduction in PAP and PVR with an isoprenaline infusion of $2\,mg\,h^{-1}$ (Slomka et al 1988). In this patient, a double catheter extradural analgesia technique was used for vaginal delivery. Another patient with PPH had two Caesarean sections under epidural anaesthesia, 3 years apart. On the second occasion, onset of block was associated with a reduction in pulmonary artery pressure and an increase in cardiac index (Khan et al 1996). A parturient became severely dyspnoeic at 31 weeks' gestation and at 34 weeks needed Caesarean section. An epidural block was established gradually over 70 min and aerosolised iloprost $20\,\mu g$, given in saline 2 ml, reduced the PAP. This was given six times a day for 48 h (Weiss et al 2000).

10. General anaesthesia. In a patient scheduled for aortic aneurysm repair and hysterectomy, the pulmonary responses to oxygen, nitric oxide, iv glyceryl trinitrate and oral nifedipine were assessed. Significant decreases in PAP and PVR occurred with oxygen and glyceryl trinitrate (Rodriguez & Pearl 1998). Epidural anaesthesia was also reported in a patient undergoing vascular surgery (Davies & Beavis 1984). Although hypotension responded to colloid and metaraminol, a simultaneous moderate increase in PAP occurred. Isoflurane has been reported to have a beneficial effect on pulmonary pressures. (Cheng & Edelist 1988). A young man with PPH, whose pre-induction PAP was equal to his systemic pressure, showed a significant decrease in PVR and PAP during oxygen/isoflurane anaesthesia.

11. If an inotropic agent is required, norepinephrine (noradrenaline) has been suggested as being the most suitable. It increases

SVR without causing a tachycardia, and in animal studies has been shown to decrease PVR.

12. Adequate pain relief is important and a thoracic epidural block for intraoperative and postoperative analgesia has been used (Armstrong 1992).

13. Since deaths with PH often occur during the first few postoperative days, monitoring and IPPV have been suggested to be continued for 5 days (Rodriguez & Pearl 1998).

Bibliography

Armstrong P 1992 Thoracic epidural anaesthesia and primary pulmonary hypertension. Anaesthesia 47: 496–9.

Barst RJ 1997 Treatment of primary pulmonary hypertension with continuous intravenous prostacyclin. Thorax 77: 299–301.

Butler PJ, Wheeler RA, Spargo PM 1990 Life-threatening complications during anaesthesia in a patient with ventriculo-atrial shunt and pulmonary hypertension. Anaesthesia 45: 946–8.

Cheng DCH, Edelist G 1988 Isoflurane and primary pulmonary hypertension. Anaesthesia 43: 22–4.

D'Alonzo GE, Barst RA, Spargo PM et al 1991 Survival in patients with primary pulmonary hypertension: results from a National Prospective Registry. Annals of Internal Medicine 115: 343–9.

Davies MJ, Beavis RE 1984 Epidural anaesthesia for vascular surgery in a patient with primary pulmonary hypertension. Anaesthesia & Intensive Care 12: 165–7.

Khan MJ, Bhatt SB, Krye JJ 1996 Anesthetic considerations for parturients with primary pulmonary hypertension: review of the literature and clinical presentation. International Journal of Obstetric Anesthesia 5: 36–43.

Kranz EM, Viljoen JF 1979 Haemoptysis following insertion of a Swan–Ganz catheter. British Journal of Anaesthesia 51: 457–9.

Liu G, Knudsen KE, Secher NH 1996 Orthotopic liver transplantation in a patient with primary pulmonary hypertension. Anaesthesia & Intensive Care 24: 714–16.

Nelson DM, Main E, Crafford W et al 1983 Peripartum heart failure due to primary pulmonary hypertension. Obstetrics & Gynecology 62: 58S–62S.

Peacock A 1990 Pulmonary hypertension due to chronic hypoxia. Treat the lung not the pressure. British Medical Journal 300: 763.

Pepke-Zaba J, Higenbottam TW, Dinh-Xuan AT et al 1991 Inhaled nitric oxide as a cause of selective pulmonary vasodilation in pulmonary hypertension. Lancet 338: 1173–4.

Power K, Avery AF 1989 Extradural analgesia in the intrapartum management of a patient with pulmonary hypertension. British Journal of Anaesthesia 63: 116–20.

Rich S, Brundage BH 1984 Primary pulmonary hypertension. Journal of the American Medical Association 251: 2252–4.

Rich S, Kaufmann E, Levy PS 1992 The effect of high doses of calcium channel blockers on survival in primary pulmonary hypertension. New England Journal of Medicine 327: 76–81.

Roberts NV, Keast PJ 1990 Pulmonary hypertension and pregnancy—a lethal combination. Anaesthesia & Intensive Care 18: 366–74.

Rodriguez RM, Pearl RG 1998 Pulmonary hypertension and major surgery. Anesthesia & Analgesia 87: 812–15.

Roessler P, Lambert TF 1986 Anaesthesia for Caesarean section in the presence of primary pulmonary hypertension. Anaesthesia & Intensive Care 14: 317–20.

Rubin LA, Geran A, Rose TH et al 1995 A fatal pulmonary complication of lupus in pregnancy. Arthritis & Rheumatism 38: 710–14.

Sanchez O, Humbert M, Sitbon O et al 1999 Treatment of pulmonary hypertension secondary to connective tissue diseases. Thorax 54: 273–7.

Schulte-Sasse U, Hess W, Tarnow J 1982 Pulmonary vascular responses to nitrous oxide in patients with normal and high pulmonary vascular resistance. Anesthesiology 57: 9–13.

Slomka F, Salmeron S, Zetlaoui P et al 1988 Primary pulmonary hypertension and pregnancy: anesthetic management for delivery. Anesthesiology 69: 959–61.

Taura P, Garcia-Valdecasas JC, Beltran J et al 1996 Moderate pulmonary hypertension in patients undergoing liver transplantation. Anesthesia & Analgesia 83: 675–80.

Tio I, Tewari K, Balderston KD et al 1998 Emergency mitral valve replacement in the setting of severe pulmonary hypertension and acute cardiovascular decompensation after evacuation of twins at fifteen weeks' gestation. American Journal of Obstetrics & Gynecology 179: 270–2.

Weiss BM, Atanassoff PG 1993 Cyanotic congenital heart disease and pregnancy: natural selection, pulmonary hypertension, and anesthesia. Journal of Clinical Anesthesia 5: 332–41.

Weiss BM, Zemp L, Seifert B et al 1998 Outcome of pulmonary vascular disease in pregnancy: a systematic overview from 1978 through to 1996. Journal of the American College of Cardiology 31: 1650–7.

Weiss BM, Maggiorini M, Jenni R et al 2000 Pregnant patient with primary pulmonary hypertension: inhaled pulmonary vasodilator and epidural anesthesia for Cesarean section. Anesthesiology 92: 1191–4.

Pulmonary oedema

The causes of acute pulmonary oedema occurring in the perioperative period can be divided broadly into two groups; those of cardiogenic, and those of noncardiogenic, origin. There are some cases in which the aetiology cannot be defined clearly, and in which a number of factors may contribute. In general, one of two basic abnormalities may develop to produce pulmonary oedema. The first is an increase in the gradient between hydrostatic and colloid osmotic pressures across the pulmonary capillary wall, and the second is an increase in capillary permeability.

1. Increased pulmonary hydrostatic pressure may arise from:

a) Increase in right atrial pressure or preload as a result of fluid retention or fluid overload.

b) Decreased myocardial contractility secondary to myocardial infarction or cardiomyopathy.

c) Increase in left atrial pressure, for example in mitral stenosis.

d) Increased afterload secondary to severe hypertension, systemic vasoconstriction, anatomical or pathological obstruction.

2. Increased capillary permeability may result from:

a) Pulmonary aspiration of acid gastric contents.

b) Air, gas or amniotic fluid embolism.

c) Allergic reactions to drugs or blood products.

d) Poisoning with higher oxides of nitrogen.

e) Pneumonias and septicaemias.

f) Shock lung or ARDS.

There are a number of specific types of noncardiogenic pulmonary oedema whose mechanisms have not been completely elucidated, but which may present in the perioperative period. These include neurogenic pulmonary oedema, oedema associated with the relief of severe, acute or chronic upper airway obstruction, the therapeutic use of beta-2 sympathomimetics for premature labour, or naloxone for opiate antagonism, and gas or amniotic fluid embolism. Since the treatment required may differ, these conditions will be considered separately.

Differentiation between cardiogenic and permeability pulmonary oedema

1. *History.* In many cases the diagnosis will be obvious. There may be history of previous myocardial infarction, hypertension, valvular heart disease, or episodes of cardiac failure. The sudden onset of an arrhythmia, such as atrial fibrillation, may cause sudden cardiac decompensation. If none of these is found, the presence of a known precipitating factor for noncardiogenic oedema should be sought.

2. *Clinical examination.* Physical signs tend to be similar. Tachycardia, cool peripheries, respiratory distress, frothy sputum, cyanosis, and basal and parasternal crepitations, feature in both. In primary cardiac disease there may be obvious cardiac enlargement, murmurs or an arrhythmia. An added third sound points to a cardiac cause.

3. Chest X-ray may show cardiac enlargement in addition to the pulmonary oedema.

4. ECG may show evidence of infarction, an arrhythmia, or chamber hypertrophy.

5. In difficult cases, measurement of PAP and PCWP may be required.

6. Measurement of protein levels in pulmonary oedema fluid. This can only be done if there is copious, uncontaminated fluid for sampling. A number of studies have shown that, depending on the cause, the protein content in oedema fluid varies. When it is secondary to an increased hydrostatic pressure, i.e. cardiogenic, there is a low protein content, whereas when it results from permeability problems, the protein content tends to be high.

A study of 21 patients showed that all patients with a PCWP of <20 mmHg had an oedema fluid to plasma protein ratio >0.6, whereas the mean ratio in four patients with cardiogenic oedema was 0.46 (Fein et al 1979). When permeability problems exist, large protein molecules such as globulins will be present in oedema fluid and the protein content will approach that of blood. It has been suggested that the use of globulin ratios in conjunction with total protein ratios gives better differentiation between cardiac and noncardiac causes (Sprung et al 1981).

If oedema protein levels are high, and pulmonary artery catheterisation is unavailable, it is reasonable to assume that the cause is likely to be a permeability problem.

Bibliography

Fein A, Grossman RF, Jones JG et al 1979 The value of edema fluid protein measurement in patients with pulmonary edema. American Journal of Medicine 67: 32–8.

Sprung CL, Rackow EC, Fein A et al 1981 The spectrum of pulmonary oedema. American Review of Respiratory Diseases 124: 718–22.

Cardiogenic pulmonary oedema

This is secondary to an increase in pulmonary capillary pressure as a result of a high left atrial pressure. As a consequence, the lung water increases. This may be due to left atrial outflow obstruction (mitral valve disease, myxoma); left ventricular dysfunction (ischaemic or myopathic); left ventricular outflow obstruction; or an increased afterload. Cardiogenic pulmonary oedema may be associated with a fluid overload, or with normovolaemia.

Presentation

In a patient with cardiac disease, pulmonary oedema may occur at any time during the perioperative period.

1. In the preoperative period it presents as a sudden onset of dyspnoea, tachycardia, a third heart sound (gallop rhythm), sweating and hypertension, with bilateral basal or parasternal crepitations on auscultation. It is most likely to occur in a patient with known ischaemic, hypertensive or rheumatic heart disease, and may be associated with overenthusiastic fluid therapy before emergency surgery. A young man with known ischaemic heart disease developed acute pulmonary oedema following emergency orthopaedic surgery (Duane et al 1996). Considerable difficulties were experienced in achieving extubation.

2. Pulmonary oedema is relatively rare intraoperatively, since IPPV and the decreased systemic vascular resistance during anaesthesia tend to oppose the hydrostatic forces and reduce the afterload. Early signs are tachycardia, decreased compliance and reduced oxygen saturation. The patient may try to breathe against the ventilator. In severe cases, pulmonary oedema fluid may emerge from the tracheal tube.

3. In the postoperative period, a combination of factors may precipitate a patient from borderline into florid pulmonary oedema, usually within the first half hour of the recovery period. The redistribution of fluid from the systemic into the pulmonary circulation is the main factor. Systemic vasoconstriction may result from pain or cold, coinciding with the vasodilator effects of the inhalation anaesthetics, or regional anaesthesia, receding. In addition, iv fluids administered during the operation may compound the problem. In obstetrics, in the

past, the use of ergometrine was associated with pulmonary oedema in patients with cardiac lesions.

Differential diagnosis

1. Inhalation of gastric contents.

2. Following relief of acute or chronic upper airway obstruction.

3. Neurogenic pulmonary oedema.

4. Pulmonary oedema associated with naloxone administration.

Management

1. A conscious patient should be placed in an upright position and oxygen administered. If not, IPPV should be continued or started.

2. Morphine iv, should be given in 2-mg increments at 2-min intervals to a total of 10 mg. This reduces preload by venodilatation and relieves agitation.

3. Furosemide (frusemide) iv or im 20–50 mg, especially if there is fluid overload. Acute venodilatation and subsequent diuresis results.

4. A vasodilator, such as isosorbide dinitrate, glyceryl trinitrate or sodium nitroprusside, may be used. An isosorbide infusion (diluted) can be given at a rate of 2–10 mg h^{-1} .

5. If the patient is in rapid AF, control of the heart rate with verapamil or digoxin is required. With ECG control, verapamil 5–10 mg iv is given slowly. Note: verapamil iv is contraindicated if the patient is taking beta adrenoceptor blockers.

6. Oakley (1996) has stressed the important role of beta blockers in treatment of pulmonary oedema secondary to mitral stenosis.

7. If myocardial dysfunction is severe, a dilating inotrope such as dobutamine may be required.

8. An esmolol infusion was used in a patient in whom difficulties in weaning and extubation were experienced secondary to tachycardia (Duane et al 1996).

Bibliography

Duane DT, Redwood SR, Grounds RM 1996 Esmolol aids extubation in intensive care patient with ischaemic pulmonary oedema. Anaesthesia 51: 474–7.

Oakley CM 1996 Beta blockers have important role in pulmonary oedema due to mitral stenosis. British Medical Journal 312: 376.

Neurogenic pulmonary oedema (NPO)

A rare complication associated with intracranial damage, which may be from a head injury, tumour or cerebrovascular accident. It is postulated that the primary brain insult increases intracranial pressure and causes a secondary disturbance in hypothalamic function. A massive sympathetic discharge results in profound systemic vasoconstriction, which diverts blood from the systemic into the pulmonary circulation (Theodore & Robin 1975). Pulmonary oedema results from the sequential increase in left heart pressures, as a result of the left ventricle attempting to eject against a greatly increased systemic vascular resistance (i.e. increased LVEDP, LAP, and pulmonary venous pressures), together with an increased pulmonary blood volume. Both will result in increased pulmonary capillary pressure. There is some evidence that altered pulmonary capillary permeability resulting from capillary damage may subsequently contribute to the oedema. However, hydrostatic mechanisms seem to predominate. Retrospective analysis of 12 patients who had NPO suggested that pulmonary venoconstriction or transient elevation of left-sided pressures contributed to the syndrome. Cases of NPO have been reported in which pulmonary oedema persisted after pulmonary pressures returned to normal, and in which the oedema protein content was similar to that of plasma (Harari et al 1976). It is possible that the onset of NPO may be precipitated by noxious stimuli such as tracheal intubation or

suction, if they are performed in the lightly unconscious patient. In the past NPO has been associated with a high mortality (Casey 1983). However, with the better understanding of the pathophysiology of the condition, and the general improvement in intensive care facilities, this may change.

Presentation

1. The patient (often a young adult or child who is unconscious after a head injury) develops sudden dyspnoea, cyanosis, tachycardia or bradycardia, and hypertension, intraoperatively or postoperatively. This occurred at induction of anaesthesia in a patient with a malfunctioning ventriculoperitoneal shunt in whom the intraventricular pressure was subsequently found to be >300 mmH$_2$O (22.8 mmHg) (Braude & Ludgrove 1989).

2. Clinical signs of intense systemic vasoconstriction occur, with pallor, sweating, and cold extremities.

3. If the patient's trachea is intubated, profuse, frothy pink pulmonary secretions will pour out of the tracheal tube. If the patient is receiving IPPV, there will be a sudden decrease in lung compliance, and, unless fully paralysed, the patient will attempt to breathe against the ventilator. Oxygen saturation decreases rapidly.

Differential diagnosis

1. Inhalation of gastric contents.

2. Fluid overload during resuscitation.

Management

1. Maintenance of oxygenation.

2. If not already instituted, IPPV with a high inspired oxygen is required. PEEP may be needed.

3. Manoeuvres to reduce intracranial pressure (if raised).

a) Pa_{CO_2} should be kept around 3–4 kPa. A Pa_{CO_2} of 3.4 kPa reduces cerebral blood flow by 33%.

b) An infusion of thiopentone.

c) Surgical decompression, if necessary.

d) High-dose steroids. Dexamethasone is often used, but its value is doubtful.

4. Reduction of systemic vasoconstriction.

a) Diuretics will assist in reducing the overall blood volume, especially if large amounts of crystalloid solution have been used in resuscitation. Furosemide (frusemide) $2\,mg\,kg^{-1}$ may be used. Mannitol is usually only indicated immediately before surgical decompression, since it causes a subsequent rebound increase in intracranial pressure.

b) Alpha adrenoceptor blockers such as phenoxybenzamine $0.5–2\,mg\,kg^{-1}$ in 300 ml 5% dextrose have been recommended on the basis of the syndrome being secondary to massive sympathetic discharge. Experimentally, neurogenic pulmonary oedema can be produced in certain animals by the inflation of a balloon in the epidural space to produce a sudden increase in intracranial pressure. Pretreatment with alpha adrenoceptor blockers can prevent this occurrence of pulmonary oedema. Large doses of chlorpromazine were used successfully in a 17-month-old child with NPO following a head injury (Wauchob et al 1984). Other drugs which have been used are droperidol iv $200–300\,\mu g\,kg^{-1}$, or an infusion of phentolamine $30\,\mu g\,kg^{-1}min^{-1}$.

c) Vasodilators, such as sodium nitroprusside, $1–8\,\mu g\,kg^{-1}$ as a short-term infusion, have also been recommended to reduce systemic vascular resistance. Direct arterial monitoring is essential. The haemodynamic responses of a patient with intractable neurogenic pulmonary oedema were assessed, using sodium nitroprusside and isoprenaline in turn (Loughnan et al 1980). Both drugs transiently reduced PCWP and LVEDP, although the Pa_{O_2} did not improve. However, when phenoxybenzamine was given (see b), the Pa_{O_2} improved and the pulmonary oedema resolved rapidly.

5. Inotropic support may occasionally be required. Isoprenaline and dobutamine are both suitable, since neither has alpha adrenoceptor stimulating properties.

6. Control of fits with benzodiazepines or thiopentone.

Bibliography

Braude N, Ludgrove T 1989 Neurogenic pulmonary oedema precipitated by induction of anaesthesia. British Journal of Anaesthesia 62: 101–3.

Casey WF 1983 Neurogenic pulmonary oedema. Anaesthesia 38: 985–8.

Harari A, Rapin M, Regnier B et al 1976 Normal pulmonary capillary pressures in the late stage of neurogenic pulmonary oedema. Lancet i: 494.

Loughnan PM, Brown TCK, Edis B et al 1980 Neurogenic pulmonary oedema in man: aetiology and management with vasodilators based upon haemodynamic studies. Anaesthesia & Intensive Care 8: 65–71.

Smith WS, Matthay MA 1997 Evidence for a hydrostatic mechanism in human neurogenic pulmonary edema. Chest 111: 1326–33.

Theodore J, Robin ED 1975 Pathogenesis of neurogenic pulmonary oedema. Lancet ii: 749–51.

Wauchob TD, Brooks RD, Harrison KM 1984 Neurogenic pulmonary oedema. Anaesthesia 39: 529–34.

Pulmonary oedema associated with severe upper airway obstruction

A well-recognised complication of acute or chronic upper airway obstruction. In more than half of the reported cases, the onset of clinical pulmonary oedema followed relief of the obstruction (Barin et al 1986). The exact mechanism is not known, but it has been suggested that the intense negative pressure produced by attempted inspiration against a closed glottis may permit either transudation of fluid into the alveoli, or increased capillary permeability (Weissman et al 1984). It has been proposed that there are two types: one following acute airway obstruction, the other following relief of chronic airway obstruction (Guffin et al 1995). Other factors such as gastric inhalation and hypoxic pulmonary vasoconstriction may contribute. Although potentially dangerous because of the hypoxia produced, this type of pulmonary oedema is usually relatively shortlived. In a retrospective study of 30 surgical patients, the most common causes were postoperative laryngospasm, and a preoperative upper airway pathology. Healthy, middle-aged men were thought to be most likely to be affected (Deepika et al 1997), although a preceding cardiac problem has now been postulated (Goldenberg 1997).

Presentation

1. The onset of pulmonary oedema is preceded by an episode of severe upper respiratory tract obstruction. There may have been chronic obstruction before the event. Recognised causes include laryngeal spasm or oedema (Barin et al 1986, Wilson & Bircher 1995), epiglottitis (Galvis et al 1980, Wiesel et al 1993), malignancy, bilateral vocal cord paralysis (Dohi et al 1991), a pseudomembraneous cast (DeSio & Bacon 1993), and attempted strangulation. In one patient, brief application of wall suction (100 mmHg) down the tracheal tube to improve the surgeon's view at thoracoscopy resulted in negative pressure pulmonary oedema (Pang et al 1998). One young man, during emergence, occluded his tracheal tube by biting it (Dicpinigaitis & Mehta 1995). Unilateral pulmonary oedema may occur after sudden re-expansion of a lung which has been compressed by a pneumothorax, a pulmonary effusion, or a tumour (Khoo & Chen 1988, Matsumiya et al 1991). Re-expansion pulmonary oedema is thought to be associated with increased pulmonary capillary permeability, and may be related both to the duration of the collapse, and to the rate and force with which the lung is re-expanded. Unilateral pulmonary

oedema, possibly secondary to amiodarone pulmonary toxicity, may occur (Herndon et al 1992).

2. Relief of the obstruction is usually accompanied by the outpouring of large amounts of pink, frothy oedema fluid. There is cyanosis, tachycardia, and respiratory distress.

Diagnosis

1. Bilateral basal crepitations are heard on auscultation.

2. Chest X-ray shows diffuse pulmonary oedema. The heart size is usually normal.

3. Blood gases show a large arterial/alveolar Po_2 difference.

Management

1. Oxygenation, either via a mask or tracheal intubation. A review of cases showed that more than 50% of patients had a Pao_2 of <8 kPa at the time of intubation or soon after (Barin et al 1986).

2. CPAP, or IPPV with PEEP, may be required to improve oxygenation. A pneumo-thorax may occur as a complication of this.

3. The use of diuretics has been suggested. However, in cases in which intracardiac pressures have been measured, these have not usually been found to be elevated (Weissman et al 1984).

4. It is possible that some of these individuals may have an underlying cardiac defect that makes them more susceptible to negative pressure pulmonary oedema than others. In a study of six patients, echocardiography showed an underlying cardiac anomaly in three, hypertrophic cardiomyopathy in one, and pulmonary and tricuspid valvular incompetence in two (Goldenberg et al 1997).

Bibliography

Barin ES, Stevenson IF, Donnelly GL 1986 Pulmonary oedema following acute airway obstruction. Anaesthesia & Intensive Care 14: 54–7.

Deepika K, Kenaan CA, Barrocas AM et al 1997 Negative pressure pulmonary edema after acute upper airway obstruction. Journal of Clinical Anesthesia 9: 403–8.

DeSio JM, Bacon DR 1993 Complete airway obstruction caused by a pseudomembranous cast with subsequent negative pressure pulmonary edema. Anesthesia & Analgesia 76: 1142–3.

Dicpinigaitis PV, Mehta DC 1995 Postobstructive pulmonary edema induced by endotracheal tube occlusion. Intensive Care Medicine 21: 1048–50.

Dohi S, Okubo N, Kondo Y 1991 Pulmonary oedema after airway obstruction due to bilateral vocal cord paralysis. Canadian Journal of Anaesthesia 38: 826–7.

Galvis AG, Stool SE, Bluestone CD 1980 Pulmonary edema following relief of acute upper airway obstruction. Annals of Otology, Rhinology & Laryngology 89: 124–8.

Goldenberg JD, Portugal LG, Wenig BL et al 1997 Negative-pressure pulmonary edema in the otolaryngology patient. Otolaryngology—Head & Neck Surgery 117: 62–6.

Guffin TN, Har-el G, Sanders A et al 1995 Acute postobstructive pulmonary edema. Otolaryngology—Head & Neck Surgery 112: 235–7.

Herndon JC, Cook AO, Ramsay MAE et al 1992 Postoperative unilateral pulmonary edema: possible amiodarone toxicity. Anesthesiology 76: 308–11.

Khoo SY, Cheng FG 1988 Acute localized pulmonary oedema. Re-expansion pulmonary oedema following the surgical repair of a ruptured hemidiaphragm. Anaesthesia 43: 486–9.

Matsumiya N, Dohi S, Kimura T, Naito H 1991 Reexpansion pulmonary edema after mediastinal tumor removal. Anesthesia & Analgesia 73: 646–8.

Pang WW, Chang DP, Lin CH et al 1998 Negative pressure pulmonary oedema induced by direct suctioning on endotracheal tube adapter. Canadian Journal of Anaesthesia 45: 785–8.

Weissman C, Damask MC, Yang J 1984 Non-cardiogenic pulmonary edema following laryngeal obstruction. Anesthesiology 60: 163–5.

Wiesel S, Gutman JB, Kleiman SJ 1993 Adult epiglottitis and postobstructive pulmonary edema in a patient with severe coronary artery disease. Journal of Clinical Anesthesia 5: 158–62.

Wilson GW, Bircher NG 1995 Acute pulmonary edema developing after laryngospasm: report of a case. Journal of Oral & Maxillofacial Surgery 53: 211–14.

Pulmonary oedema associated with beta-2 sympathomimetics for premature labour

Seventy-three case reports of pulmonary oedema associated with the use of beta-2 sympathomimetic agents (tocolytics) to suppress premature labour were reviewed (Hawker 1984a). There were seven deaths. After this paper, the fetal and maternal benefits of its use were questioned.

The aetiology is unknown, although a number of mechanisms have been considered as possibly contributing. The few haemodynamic studies in patients with pulmonary oedema following tocolytics are consistent with the oedema being primarily of a noncardiogenic, permeability type (Hawker 1984a,b, Brown & Mullis 1985). However, there is evidence to suggest that fluid overload and persistent adrenoceptor stimulation are potent contributing factors (Hawker 1984a). In a study of 8709 women prescribed terbutaline infusions, pulmonary oedema developed in 28 patients. Seventeen of these were also receiving large amounts of intravenous fluids, and were being given from one to three other tocolytics (Perry et al 1995).

There is now evidence that the use of ritodrine in preterm labour has no significant effects on premature labour (Canadian Preterm Labour Investigation Group 1992).

Predisposing factors and problems

1. Drugs thought to be linked with this type of pulmonary oedema include terbutaline, ritodrine, isoxuprine, salbutamol, and fenoterol. Tachycardia is a prominent feature.

2. It is known that the beta-2 agonists do have inotropic effects on the heart via beta-1 receptors, particularly as the dose is increased. Indeed, tachycardia can be a very common and troublesome side effect of the tocolytics. A further contributing feature may be a 'downgrading' of the beta receptors during continued stimulation. After chronic exposure to catecholamines, cardiac beta receptors may

become 'downregulated', resulting in a decreased adrenoceptor support for the heart. This may occur in severe heart failure, and is supported by the discovery of a decreased beta adrenoceptor population in failing hearts (Bristow et al 1982). Myocardial changes have been found to be associated with chronic administration of catecholamines, both experimentally and clinically. Patients with phaeochromocytoma can develop a cardiomyopathy, which is usually reversible after removal of the tumour.

3. Beta-2 stimulation also causes vasodilatation and a compensatory tachycardia. There is decreased excretion of sodium, glycogenolysis which stimulates insulin secretion, and hypokalaemia secondary to the effects on the sodium/potassium pump which increases intracellular potassium (Rodgers & Morgan 1994).

4. Pulmonary oedema has been reported with oral, sc and iv routes of administration. The duration of treatment before its onset varied from 6 to 96 h (Hawker 1984a). The rates of infusion were similarly variable. Of those cases in which information was adequate, pulmonary oedema occurred in 29 before delivery, and in 17 within a further 11 h. In one patient, it developed at 5 days and she died at home on day 60. Late development may suggest a cardiomyopathy. Thirty-three percent of cases involved twin pregnancy, and in 63% of patients, steroids were given in addition. In the four cases which had haemodynamic monitoring, three had a normal or low PAWP.

5. In 21 cases in which fluid balance was recorded, 15 had a positive balance of at least 1 litre. Fluid overload can easily occur. In normal pregnancy, blood volume is already increased by 45%. Tocolytics, which are often given in large volumes of hypotonic diluent, can increase ADH secretion. Fluid retention is a feature of treatment with steroids and indometacin, both of which may be given in premature labour.

6. Acute redistribution of vascular volumes can sometimes be the precipitating factor in the development of pulmonary oedema, when volume overload is present. The administration of ergometrine has been known to cause pulmonary oedema secondary to vasoconstrictor effects. During recovery from anaesthesia, vasoconstriction from cold or pain can also cause movement of fluid from the systemic into the central circulation.

7. There are problems in giving anaesthesia in patients receiving tocolytics (Rodgers & Morgan 1994). Fenoterol and terbutaline have relatively long half-lives (6–7 h and 14–18 h respectively), therefore even when stopped, the effects continue.

Presentation

1. A history of a sudden onset of dyspnoea, cyanosis and expectoration of pink frothy sputum, during or after suppression of premature labour with beta-2 tocolytics. There is usually a pre-existing tachycardia and the patient is usually in positive fluid balance.

2. On auscultation, bilateral basal crepitations are heard. CXR shows signs of pulmonary oedema, and blood gases will indicate hypoxia.

Management

1. There is now little justification for the use of tocolytics for preterm labour. If they are given, intravenous fluid therapy should be restricted and the patient will require careful observation for the detection of a positive fluid balance. A persistent tachycardia during therapy may be a warning sign of impending pulmonary oedema.

2. If evidence of early pulmonary oedema occurs, the infusion should be stopped immediately.

3. Oxygen should be administered and, if necessary, IPPV established. It usually resolves rapidly, except in the presence of infection, or when glyceryl trinitrate has been given after open fetal surgery (DiFederico et al 1998).

4. Diuretics are required.

5. Should anaesthesia be required and tachycardia be a problem, the use of esmolol should be considered.

Bibliography

Bristow MR, Ginsberg R, Minobe W et al 1982 Decreased catecholamine sensitivity and beta adrenergic receptor density in failing human hearts. New England Journal of Medicine 307: 205–11.

Brown M, Mullis S 1985 Pulmonary oedema associated with tocolytic therapy. Anaesthesia & Intensive Care 13: 102–3.

Canadian Preterm Labour Investigation Group 1992 Treatment of preterm labor with beta-adrenergic agonist ritodrine. New England Journal of Medicine 327: 308–12.

DiFederico EM, Burlingame JM, Kilpatrick SJ et al 1998 Pulmonary edema in obstetric patients is rapidly resolved except in the presence of infection or of nitroglycerin tocolysis after open fetal surgery. American Journal of Obstetrics & Gynecology 179: 925–33.

Hawker F 1984a Pulmonary oedema associated with beta 2 sympathomimetic treatment of premature labour. Anaesthesia & Intensive Care 12: 143–51.

Hawker F 1984b Five cases of pulmonary oedema associated with beta 2 sympathomimetic treatment of premature labour. Anaesthesia & Intensive Care 12: 159–71.

Perry KG Jr, Morrison JC, Rust OA et al 1995 Incidence of adverse cardiopulmonary effects with low-dose continuous terbutaline infusion. American Journal of Obstetrics & Gynecology 173: 1273–7.

Rodgers SJ, Morgan M 1994 Tocolysis, beta$_2$ agonists and anaesthesia. Anaesthesia 49: 185–7.

Pulmonary oedema associated with naloxone reversal of opiates

Naloxone was originally thought to be a pure opiate antagonist, with no agonist action, and no side effects. This does not appear to be correct. A number of cases have occurred, in which opiate reversal with naloxone has been associated with a state of acute central adrenoceptor stimulation, resulting in cardiovascular complications. Pulmonary oedema is one of these, and appears to most closely resemble neurogenic pulmonary oedema.

In view of suggestions that opiates may in some way modulate the release of catecholamines, the report that a large dose (10 mg) of naloxone caused catecholamine release in a patient with a proven phaeochromocytoma is of interest (Mannelli et al 1983). In a recent prospective study of 463 patients given naloxone for heroin intoxication, six developed severe side effects within 10 min of administration; one asystole, three generalised convulsions, one pulmonary oedema, and one violent behaviour (Osterwalder 1996).

Presentation

The onset of pulmonary oedema has been reported in close association with the administration of naloxone to reverse the effect of opiates in the recovery period. It was first described in a 70-year-old man after cardiac surgery in which high-dose morphine was used (Flacke et al 1977). In view of the patient's pre-existing cardiac disease, this might not be considered to be remarkable. However, pulmonary oedema has also been reported after small doses of naloxone in eight healthy patients having elective surgery (Andree 1980, Taff 1983, Prough et al 1984, Partridge & Ward 1986, Brimacombe et al 1991, Johnson et al 1996). One patient died.

Management

1. Before naloxone is administered, consider the justification, in view of its extremely short action.

2. Oxygenation, and IPPV if necessary.

Bibliography

Andree RA 1980 Sudden death following naloxone administration. Anesthesia & Analgesia 59: 782–8.

Brimacombe J, Archdeacon J, Newell S et al 1991 Two cases of naloxone-induced pulmonary oedema— the possible use of phentolamine in management. Anaesthesia & Intensive Care 19: 578–80.

Flacke JW, Flacke WE, Williams SGD 1977 Acute pulmonary edema following naloxone reversal of high dose morphine anesthesia. Anesthesiology 47: 376–8.

Johnson C, Mayer P, Grosz D 1995 Pulmonary edema following naloxone in a healthy orthopedic patient. Journal of Clinical Anesthesia 7: 356–7.

Mannelli M, Maggi M, DeFeo ML et al 1983 Naloxone administration releases catecholamines in a patient with pheochromocytoma. New England Journal of Medicine 308: 654–5.

Osterwalder JJ 1996 Naloxone—for intoxications with intravenous heroin and heroin mixtures—harmless or hazardous? A prospective clinical study. Journal of Toxicology—Clinical Toxicology 34: 409–16.

Partridge BL, Ward CF 1986 Pulmonary edema following low-dose naloxone administration. Anesthesiology 65: 485–6.

Prough DS, Roy R, Bumgarner J et al 1984 Acute pulmonary edema in healthy teenagers following conservative doses of i.v. naloxone. Anesthesiology 60: 485–6.

Taff RH 1983 Pulmonary edema following naloxone administration in a patient without heart disease. Anesthesiology 59: 576–7.

Wride SRN, Smith RER, Courtney PG 1989 A fatal case of pulmonary oedema in a healthy young male following naloxone administration. Anaesthesia & Intensive Care 17: 374–7.

QT interval syndrome, prolonged

(previously known as Romano–Ward, Jervell and Lange–Nielsen syndromes, familial ventricular tachycardia)

The QT interval represents depolarisation and repolarisation of the ventricle; that is, one complete ventricular contraction. The long QT syndrome (LQTS) describes a group of inherited disorders in which there are repolarisation abnormalities that result in a long QT interval on ECG, together with other unusual features. Affected individuals may have episodes of syncope associated with serious ventricular arrhythmias, and those who are untreated have a high incidence of sudden death.

Three clinical syndromes were described originally. The first, recognised by Jervell and Lange–Nielsen, is double dominant and associated with nerve deafness, but the second, the Romano–Ward syndrome, a dominant condition, is not. The third, familial ventricular tachycardia, is also autosomal dominant. However, genetic studies have recently shown a larger number of clinical variants.

The precise aetiology is uncertain, but abnormalities of cardiac ionic channel function, and imbalance in the sympathetic nervous system between the right and left sides of the heart, are both thought to be involved. The prolonged duration of repolarisation is associated with abnormal T wave morphology. Genetic studies have shown at least five different loci for the disorders, which involve mutations of different genes influencing cardiac ionic channel function (some of which are potassium channels), and each mutation appears to be associated with different T wave patterns on ECG (Moss 1997, Ackerman et al 1999).

In some affected patients, ventricular tachyarrhythmias can be precipitated by sudden increases in sympathetic activity, mostly mediated by the left stellate ganglion (Schwartz et al 1991). Emotion or exercise can thus provoke syncopal attacks that are associated with either VT or VF, and can result in death if spontaneous termination of the arrhythmia does not occur. There is often a family history of sudden deaths, but the degree of QT_c prolongation is not an independent predictor of risk.

More recently, a high incidence of echocardiographic abnormalities has been demonstrated in patients with LQTS compared with matched healthy controls (Nador et al 1991). These consisted of unusual ventricular wall motion abnormalities, which were more likely to be seen in patients who were symptomatic. In addition, right stellate ganglionectomy in dogs produced the same abnormality.

International studies of LQTS originally helped to increase the understanding of the pathophysiology, and the prognosis has improved with active management. The effects of long-term therapy on mortality in LQTS were examined in 203 patients (Schwartz et al 1975). Untreated patients had a mortality of 73%, while in those treated with beta blockers it was only 6%. A third group, who were treated, but not with beta blockers, had a mortality of 64%. In some patients, left cervical sympathectomy shortened the QT interval and reduced the incidence of syncopal attacks (Yanagida et al 1976). Other drugs which have been used for treatment include phenytoin, verapamil, bretylium, and primidone. However, beta blockers prevent syncope in about 75–80% of patients. Those patients refractory to therapy with beta blockers have received other treatment, such as left cervicothoracic ganglionectomy (Schwartz et al 1991), or permanent pacing (Moss et al 1991). In patients who cannot tolerate beta blockers, or if this treatment is ineffective in controlling episodes of syncope, automatic implantable cardioverter defibrillators (AICDs) have been shown to reduce the incidence of syncope and tachyarrhythmias (Groh et al 1996, Lloyd Jones & Mason 2000). Children are particularly likely to be refractory to treatment (Weintraub et al 1990), therefore it has been suggested that those children who survive into adulthood are the least severely affected.

The condition, and its treatment, has considerable anaesthetic significance. There have been a number of case reports in which VT, torsade de pointes, VF, or cardiac arrest have occurred during anaesthesia in otherwise fit young patients. Most patients have been of the age at which preoperative ECGs are unlikely to have been performed, or even if they have, the condition may not have been recognised. A history of recurrent syncope (which may be diagnosed as epilepsy), congenital deafness, or a family history of sudden deaths, should alert the anaesthetist to the possibility of this condition (Adu-Gyamfi et al 1991, Holland 1993). Although the condition is rare, its mere existence illustrates the importance of initiating ECG monitoring from the start of the anaesthetic, whatever the age of the patient.

Preoperative abnormalities

1. There may be a known family history of the condition, or a history of sudden and unexpected deaths in young members of a family. Congenital sensorineural deafness may be associated.

2. The patient may give a history of syncopal or panic attacks, or, as sometimes happens, has been diagnosed as being epileptic (Ponte & Lund 1981) or hysterical. In a study of 23 children, the mean time to diagnosis was 10 years (range 4 days to 19 years), and initial symptoms included syncope, aborted sudden death, and near drowning (Weintraub et al 1990).

3. ECG abnormalities. The QT interval is measured from the beginning of the QRS complex to the end of the T wave. It varies with heart rate, shortening as heart rate increases, and therefore must be corrected for rate (see below). In general, the normal QT interval should be less than 0.42 s, while in the prolonged QT interval syndrome it may be as long as 0.6 s. T waves are also usually abnormal, being broad and diphasic or altering in polarity. There is often a bradycardia, a feature that is unusual in children.

Whilst the diagnosis is usually made when syncope is associated with a $QT_c > 0.44$ s, it is not always possible to rely on ECG criteria alone. In a recent genetic study of families affected by the LQTS, there was an overlap of QT_c intervals between carriers and noncarriers. Not all patients affected by LQTS will necessarily have discernable repolarisation abnormalities on the ECG (Moss 1997, Ackerman et al 1999).

Approximate relationship between heart rate and QT interval in a normal subject:

50 beat min^{-1}	0.38–0.42 s
60 beat min^{-1}	0.35–0.41 s
70 beat min^{-1}	0.33–0.39 s
80 beat min^{-1}	0.29–0.37 s
90 beat min^{-1}	0.28–0.36 s
100 beat min^{-1}	0.26–0.34 s

4. Treadmill testing in children has shown that the QT_c interval is significantly prolonged during exercise (Weintraub et al 1990).

5. An abnormal ventricular contraction pattern was seen on echocardiography in 55% of LQTS patients, and consisted of a rapid early contraction and a prolonged phase of slow ventricular thickening before rapid relaxation (Nador et al 1991). This feature may provide a noninvasive marker for screening patients with stress-induced syncope.

6. Some patients with long QT syndrome have a prolapsed mitral valve (Forbes & Morton 1979).

7. Beta blockers are the mainstay of drug therapy for congenital LQTS, particularly for those in whom ventricular arrhythmias are precipitated by sympathetic stimulation. Left cervicosympathetic ganglionectomy may be added in the high-risk patients who continue to have syncope or cardiac arrest, despite the use of beta blockers, or for those in whom beta blockers are contraindicated. Recently, high-risk patients have received AICD devices.

8. Molecular genetic studies enable the diagnosis to be confirmed and affected members of a family to be identified. Postmortem examination of frozen myocardial tissue in a case of unexpected drowning showed the genetic mutation responsible (Ackerman et al 1999).

Anaesthetic problems

1. The risks of anaesthesia in the undiagnosed and untreated patient are well known, and a number of individuals have presented for the first time because VT, torsade de pointes, VF or cardiac arrest has occurred unexpectedly during anaesthesia. In ten anaesthetics in which the diagnosis of LQTS had not been made, there were four episodes of VF, four of VT, one of asystole, and one of heart block (Forbes & Morton 1979, Wig et al 1979, Brown et al 1981, Ponte & Lund 1981, Medak & Benumof 1983, Adu-Gyamfi et al 1991, Richardson et al 1992, Holland 1993, Joseph-Reynolds et al 1997, Pleym et al 1999). One patient died, the others were resuscitated. In patients who received beta blockers, or who had had a left cervical sympathetic block, no such episodes occurred (Owitz et al 1979, O'Callaghan et al 1982, Medak & Benumof 1983, Carlock et al 1984, Galloway & Glass 1985).

However beta blockers may not always be protective against arrhythmias in the LQTS. Recently, a subgroup of patients has been described in whom LQTS, syndactyly and congenital heart disease is associated with a particularly high risk of sudden death (Marks et al 1995). An infant with syndactyly and a patent ductus arteriosus was only diagnosed as having LQTS after two anaesthetics had been complicated by serious arrhythmias and conduction defects (Joseph-Reynolds et al 1997). Treatment with propranolol was instituted, but in spite of this, torsade de pointes and VF occurred during the third anaesthetic for change of dressing.

2. Not all arrhythmias in association with surgery have actually presented during general anaesthesia. In one patient, unexpected cardiac arrest occurred in the postoperative period. A 29-year-old woman developed VF one day after uneventful partial thyroidectomy, but extensive cardiological examination at that time revealed no cause. No other symptoms appeared until 5 years later, when she suddenly developed recurrent syncope. During monitoring in hospital she had documented asystole, VF, and several episodes of torsade de pointes ventricular tachycardia. These arrhythmias only finally resolved after administration of a beta blocker. At this stage a QT_c of 0.545 s was noted and subsequently an AICD was implanted (Cieslinski et al 1995).

3. The risk of transient attacks of VT or VF is increased by sympathetic stimulation, emotion, exercise, or alcohol.

4. There are conflicting reports about the effects of anaesthetic agents on the QT interval and the production of arrhythmias. Two studies have shown that sevoflurane prolongs the QT interval (Gallagher et al 1998, Kleinsasser et al 2000). In the first, sevoflurane was found to lengthen the QT interval in a 17-year-old girl with a presumptive diagnosis of LQTS, but no ventricular arrhythmias occurred during its administration. In the second study of normal patients, sevoflurane increased the QT interval, but propofol did not. Reported effects of inhalation agents vary, but may depend on whether normal or affected individuals are studied. Michaloudis et al (1998) found that isoflurane prolonged the QT interval in children with LQTS, whereas halothane shortened it. However, in normal individuals, Schmeling et al (1991) found that halothane, isoflurane and enflurane, when used for slow inhalation induction, caused significant increases in QT interval, suggesting that they directly affected ventricular repolarisation. Thiopentone (Martineau & Nadeau 1987), and large doses of opiates, may also prolong the QT interval. Propofol was found to produce less prolongation than thiopentone (McConachie et al 1989, Giraud et al 1991). In one child, the use of epinephrine (adrenaline) (for caudal anaesthesia

and infiltration by the surgeon) resulted in torsade de pointes tachycardia. Treatment with lidocaine (lignocaine) produced VF (Richardson et al 1992).

5. The problems of anaesthesia for patients with automatic implantable defibrillators (Lloyd Jones & Mason 2000).

6. Pregnancy in patients with LQTS has occasionally been described. There is an increased risk of cardiac events in probands with LQTS, but not in first degree relatives (Rashba et al 1998). In probands, therefore, beta blockers should be continued. In one patient, beta adrenoceptor blockade produced problems in interpretation of cardiotocography, and the ability to detect a fetal conduction defect. In fact both twins were found to have congenital LQTS (Wilkinson et al 1991).

In Jervell and Lange–Nielsen syndrome, profound deafness proved to be a problem in two women requiring Caesarean section, one under general anaesthesia (Freshwater 1984), the other under epidural anaesthesia (Ryan 1988).

7. Communication problems, other than deafness, may prevent a significant family history being established before anaesthesia. Ventricular fibrillation occurred at the end of anaesthesia in a deaf Sikh child, whose parents spoke little English (Holland 1993). Later, a family history of unexplained deaths was discovered. Consanguinity of parents may predispose to the syndrome and another Sikh patient has been described (Freshwater 1984).

8. Side effects of treatment. Hypoglycaemia occurred in the preoperative starvation period in an infant who was receiving beta blockers for Jervell and Lange–Nielsen syndrome (Baines & Murrell 1999).

Management

1. Preoperative family history-taking is important. A child with sensorineural deafness, a history of syncope, a family history of sudden deaths, or unexpected drowning, should alert the anaesthetist to the possibility of familial LQTS.

2. If the patient has congenital LQTS, he/she should have full beta adrenoceptor blockade, usually with propranolol, before anaesthesia. Propranolol can be given orally 20–80 mg 6-hrly, or iv 1–5 mg 6-hrly. (Sotalol is not advisable because it has occasionally been associated with torsade de pointes VT.)

3. For the emergency situation an infusion of esmolol can be used. Dilute two ampoules of esmolol 2.5 g concentrate in 500 ml saline to give a solution 10 mg ml^{-1}. Give a loading dose of 500 μg kg^{-1} followed by 50–200 μg kg^{-1} min^{-1}.

4. ECG monitoring should be continued through the perioperative period, or during labour, and a defibrillator should be available.

5. A good premedication and reassurance helps to relieve anxiety.

6. Left stellate ganglion block may shorten the QT interval and increase the threshold for ventricular fibrillation.

7. Tracheal intubation and extubation cause sympathetic stimulation, and should not be performed during very light anaesthesia.

8. Although it has been suggested that any drug known to produce a tachycardia, or to prolong the QT interval, should be avoided, if the diagnosis is known, the patient should not be given anaesthesia without beta blockade having been established first.

9. For anaesthesia in a patient with an AICD, see under Automatic implantable cardioverter defibrillator.

10. Although atrial pacing has been used for treatment, electrophysiological studies have suggested that propranolol is more effective than pacing in suppressing repolarisation abnormalities during sympathetic stimulation (Shimizu et al 1997).

Bibliography

Ackerman MJ, Tester DJ, Porter CJ et al 1999 Molecular diagnosis of the inherited long-QT syndrome in a woman who died after near drowning. New England Journal of Medicine 341: 1121–5.

Adu-Gyamfi Y, Said A, Chawdhury UM et al 1991 Anaesthetic-induced ventricular tachyarrhythmias in Jervell and Lange–Nielsen syndrome. Canadian Journal of Anaesthesia 38: 345–6.

Baines DB, Murrell D 1999 Preoperative hypoglycaemia, propranolol and the Jervell and Lange–Neilsen syndrome. Paediatric Anaesthesia 9: 156–8.

Brown M, Liberthson RR, Ali HA et al 1981 Perioperative management of a patient with long Q–T interval syndrome. Anesthesiology 55: 586–9.

Callaghan ML, Nichols AB, Sweet RB 1977 Anesthetic management of prolonged Q–T interval syndrome. Anesthesiology 47: 67–9.

Carlock FJ, Brown M, Brown EM 1984 Isoflurane anaesthesia for a patient with long Q–T syndrome. Canadian Anaesthetists' Society Journal 31: 83–5.

Cieslinski G, Kadel C, Schrader R et al 1995 Implantable defibrillator in the long QT syndrome. Deutsche Medizinische Wochenschrift 120: 283–8.

Forbes RB, Morton GH 1979 Ventricular fibrillation in a patient with unsuspected mitral valve prolapse and prolonged Q–T interval. Canadian Anaesthetists' Society Journal 26: 424–7.

Freshwater JV 1984 Anaesthesia for Caesarean section and the Jervell, Lange–Nielsen syndrome (prolonged Q–T interval syndrome). British Journal of Anaesthesia 56: 655–7.

Gallagher JD, Weindling SN, Anderson G et al 1998 Effects of sevoflurane on QT interval in a patient with congenital long QT syndrome. Anesthesiology 89: 1569–73.

Galloway PA, Glass PSA 1985 Anesthetic implications of prolonged Q–T interval syndrome. Anesthesia & Analgesia 64: 612–20.

Giraud M, Chassard D, Gelas P et al 1991 QT interval during intubation with propofol or thiopental. Anesthesiology 75: A83.

Groh WJ, Silka MJ, Oliver RP et al 1996 Use of implantable cardioverter-defibrillators in the congenital long QT syndrome. American Journal of Cardiology 78: 703–6.

Holland RR 1993 Cardiac arrest under anaesthesia in a child with previously undiagnosed Jervell and Lange–Nielsen syndrome. Anaesthesia 48: 149–51.

Joseph-Reynolds AM, Auden SM, Sobczyzk WL 1997 Perioperative considerations in a newly described type of congenital long QT syndrome. Paediatric Anaesthesia 7: 237–41.

Kleinsasser A, Kuenszberg E, Loeckinger A et al 2000 Sevoflurane, but not propofol, significantly prolongs the Q–T interval. Anesthesia & Analgesia 90: 25–7.

Lloyd Jones S, Mason RA 2000 Laser surgery in a patient with Romano–Ward (long QT) syndrome and an automatic implantable defibrillator. Anaesthesia 55: 362–6.

McConachie I, Keaveny JP, Healy TEJ et al 1989 Effect of anaesthesia on the QT interval. British Journal of Anaesthesia 63: 558–60.

Marks ML, Whisler SL, Clericuzio C et al 1995 A new form of long QT syndrome associated with syndactyly. Journal of the American College of Cardiology 25: 59–64.

Martineau RJ, Nadeau SG 1987 Q–Tc interval changes during induction of anaesthesia. Canadian Journal of Anaesthesia 34: S61–2.

Medak R, Benumof JL 1983 Perioperative management of the prolonged Q–T interval syndrome. British Journal of Anaesthesia 55: 361–4.

Michaloudis D, Fraidakis O, Lefaki T et al 1998 Anaesthesia and the QT interval in humans: effects of halothane and isoflurane in premedicated children. European Journal of Anaesthesiology 15: 623–8.

Moss AJ 1997 The long QT syndrome revisited. Pacing and Clinical Electrophysiology 20: 2879–80.

Moss AJ, Liu JE, Gottlieb S et al 1991 Efficacy of permanent pacing in the management of high risk patients with long QT syndrome. Circulation 84: 1524–9.

Nador F, Beria G, De Ferrari GM et al 1991 Unsuspected echocardiographic abnormality in the long QT syndrome. Circulation 84: 1530–42.

Nagakura S, Shirai Y, Yamai K et al 1997 Sudden perioperative death in an adult with undiagnosed Jervell and Lange–Nielsen syndrome. Surgery 122: 645–6.

O'Callaghan AC, Normandale JP, Lowenstein E 1982 The prolonged Q–T syndrome. A review with anaesthetic implications and the report of two cases. Anaesthesia & Intensive Care 10: 50–5.

Owitz S, Pratilas V, Pratila MG et al 1979 Anaesthetic considerations in the prolonged Q–T interval (LQTS). Canadian Anaesthetists' Society Journal 26: 50–4.

Pleym H, Bathen J, Spigset O et al 1999 Ventricular fibrillation related to reversal of the neuromuscular blockade in a patient with long QT syndrome. Acta Anaesthesiologica Scandinavica 43: 352–5.

Ponte J, Lund J 1981 Prolongation of the Q–T interval (Romano Ward syndrome): anaesthetic management. British Journal of Anaesthesia 53: 1347–50.

Rashba EJ, Zareba W, Moss AJ et al 1998 Influence of

pregnancy on the risk for cardiac events in patients with hereditary long QT syndrome. LQTS investigators. Circulation 97: 451–6.

Richardson MG, Roark GL, Helfaer MA 1992 Introperative epinephrine-induced torsades de pointes in a child with long QT syndrome. Anesthesiology 76: 647–9.

Ryan H 1988 Anaesthesia for Caesarean section in a patient with Jervell, Lange–Nielsen syndrome. Canadian Journal of Anaesthesia 35: 422–4.

Schmeling WT, Warltier DC, McDonald DJ et al 1991 Prolongation of the QT interval by enflurane, isoflurane and halothane in humans. Anesthesia & Analgesia 72: 137–42.

Schwartz PJ, Locati E, Moss AJ et al 1991 Left cardiac sympathetic denervation in the therapy of congenital long QT syndrome. Circulation 84: 503–11.

Schwartz J, Periti M, Malliani A 1975 The long Q–T syndrome. American Heart Journal 89: 378–90.

Shimizu W, Kamakura S, Kurita T et al 1997 Influence of epinephrine, propranolol, and atrial pacing on spatial distribution of recovery time measured by body surface mapping in congenital long QT syndrome. Journal of Cardiovascular Electrophysiology 8: 1102–14.

Weintraub RG, Gow RM, Wilkinson JL 1990 The congenital long QT syndromes in childhood. Journal of the American College of Cardiology 16: 674–80.

Wig J, Bali IM, Singh RG et al 1979 Prolonged Q–T interval syndrome. Sudden cardiac arrest during anaesthesia. Anaesthesia 34: 37–40.

Wilkinson C, Gyaneshwar R, McCusker C 1991 Twin pregnancy in a patient with idiopathic long QT syndrome. Case report. British Journal of Obstetrics & Gynaecology 98: 1300–2.

Yanagida H, Kemi C, Suwa K 1976 The effects of stellate ganglion block on the idiopathic prolongation of the Q–T interval with cardiac arrhythmia (the Romano–Ward syndrome). Anesthesia & Analgesia 55: 782–7.

Relapsing polychondritis

A rare, autoimmune, systemic inflammatory disease in which there is gradual destruction of the cartilage of the nose, ears, joints, larynx, and trachea. Inflammation, oedema, and scarring of the tracheal rings results in tracheal narrowing and dynamic airway obstruction. The condition usually presents between the ages of 40 and 60 years. Anaemia, early-onset, laryngotracheal stricture, saddle nose and systemic vasculitis are associated with a poor prognosis (Trentham & Le 1998). Anaesthesia may be required for surgical reconstruction of the nose or ear, or occasionally for treatment of upper airway obstruction, or lower airway collapse. In severe cases endobronchial stenting may be required (Faul et al 1999). Occasionally, patients with relapsing polychondritis become pregnant. In a series of 25 pregnancies in 11 patients, although about 30% of patients had a flare up of the disease that required treatment, none had significant involvement of the respiratory tract (Papo et al 1997).

Preoperative abnormalities

1. The most common features are nasal and auricular chondritis, with saddle nose and cauliflower ears, and polyarthritis. Ocular inflammation and audiovestibular damage may also occur.

2. Cutaneous vasculitis and systemic symptoms, such as fever and anaemia.

3. In a study of airway complications of relapsing polychondritis, symptoms included breathlessness, cough, stridor, wheezing, hoarseness and tenderness over the laryngo-tracheal cartilages (Eng & Sabanathan 1991). Although respiratory involvement is uncommon early in the disease, up to 50% of patients are eventually affected. Respiratory complications are responsible for significant morbidity and mortality. A detailed clinical, endoscopic and CT study of nine patients showed that CT scan was a more reliable method than endoscopy for identifying tracheal and bronchial involvement, particularly early in the disease (Tillie-Leblond et al 1998). Pathological and mechanical processes causing airway obstruction include cartilage collapse, thickened tracheal walls, and fibrous masses (Faul et al 1999).

4. The incidence of cardiovascular involvement is 15–46% (VanDecker & Panidis 1988), and includes aortic and mitral regurgitation and myocarditis. Regurgitation is probably secondary to dilatation of the aortic root and annulus, as a result of degenerative changes, therefore the improvement after valve replacement may be shortlived. Valve thickening and myxomatous degeneration may also contribute to the problem.

5. Chest X-ray and CT scan may show subglottic or tracheal narrowing, although if the obstruction is dynamic these may be normal. Inspiratory and expiratory flow–volume loops will show dynamic obstruction and indicate whether it is primarily intrathoracic or extrathoracic. Intrathoracic obstruction is worse during expiration, and extrathoracic obstruction worse on inspiration (Eng & Sabanathan 1991). MRI examination may assist in the diagnosis.

6. Increased ESR and the presence of fetal cartilage antibodies.

7. Biopsy of cartilage involved will confirm the diagnosis.

8. Treatment is with steroids and immuno-suppressives. Although the management of airway problems is mainly medical, surgical intervention may be required.

Anaesthetic problems

1. Tracheomalacia results in tracheal collapse on forced inspiration and expiration. Since the obstruction is dynamic, it may be difficult to demonstrate on conventional static investigations. A CT scan does not reliably predict the degree of airway obstruction and the airway may be reported to be normal. Thus,

inspiratory and expiratory flow–volume curves may be needed.

2. The diagnosis may sometimes be missed. A pregnant patient whose dyspnoea had been attributed to chronic asthma was found to have tracheal narrowing and stenosis of the left main bronchus (Gimovsky & Nishiyama 1989). Biopsy of the auricular cartilage confirmed relapsing polychondritis.

3. Anaesthesia may precipitate airway obstruction. During bronchoscopy, the tracheal lumen was observed to collapse almost completely on each inspiration (Burgess et al 1990).

4. There is a high incidence of subglottic stenosis, on which inflammation and oedema can be superimposed. In one patient during general anaesthesia for tracheostomy, a size 3 mm tube was passed with the aid of a metal introducer. Later, the tracheostomy tube became dislodged, and on this occasion, when anaesthesia was required, the larynx would only admit a 14-G Harris catheter (Hayward & Al-Shaikh 1988). Acute stridor followed microlaryngoscopy and biopsy in one patient and emergency tracheostomy was performed. In another, it was impossible to pass a fibreoptic bronchoscope, therefore, after a difficult intubation, tracheostomy was again undertaken (Spraggs et al 1997).

5. The tracheal and laryngeal disease may result in difficulty in clearing secretions; one patient had a respiratory arrest immediately after reconstruction of his nose, and subsequent bronchoscopy showed thick secretions and inflammation of the tracheal mucosa (Eng & Sabanathan 1991).

6. Sudden death may occur following tracheal cartilage collapse, in association with endoscopy or intubation.

7. One patient developed respiratory insufficiency in the recovery room after cataract surgery under local anaesthesia alone. Tracheostomy was performed and endoscopy showed a collapsing tracheal lumen and extensive destruction of cartilage (Biro et al 1994).

8. The use of intratracheal stents is not always satisfactory and may be associated with displacement and respiratory obstruction. Death has occurred secondary to blockage of the stent by a mucous plug (Goddard et al 1991).

Management

1. If airway problems exist, assessment of the severity with CXR, CT scan, bronchoscopy, and flow–volume loops.

2. Corticosteroids are the mainstay of treatment, particularly when the disease is active. Other treatment includes immunosuppressives and NSAIDs. Plasmapheresis may have a role.

3. Surgery may occasionally be required for respiratory complications, but experience is limited and results uncertain. Posterior membrane fixation of the bronchial tree, internal stenting with a tracheal prosthesis, such as a Montgomery tube, and self-expanding stents, have been used (Neville et al 1990, Shah et al 1995, Sarodia et al 1999). Stenting may be lifesaving (Faul et al 1999). However, intracheal stents may be associated with asphyxia secondary to their displacement and obstruction.

4. In severe cases, difficult tracheal intubation and problems with tracheal or bronchial collapse might be anticipated. If the patient already has a stent in place, care must be taken not to dislodge it. A rigid bronchoscope should always be available. Awake fibreoptic intubation and introduction of a 6-mm tube was undertaken in a patient with a previous difficult intubation and severe respiratory distress. Anaesthesia was continued with propofol and sevoflurane, whilst a further stent was introduced (Fitzmaurice et al 1999).

5. Tracheostomy may be required, but is only of use when the disease is confined to the larynx or subglottis (Spraggs et al 1997).

6. Intensive physiotherapy, humidification and suction are necessary in the perioperative

period. In one patient, acute exacerbations of stridor were improved by the use of nebulised racemic ephedrine, 0.5 mg in 0.5 ml saline (Gaffney et al 1992).

7. In one patient with tracheobronchitis, who had extensive airway collapse during extubation, nasal CPAP was used until stenting could be performed (Adliff et al 1997).

Bibliography

Adliff M, Ngato D, Keshavjee S et al 1997 Treatment of diffuse tracheomalacia secondary to relapsing polychondritis with continuous airway pressure. Chest 112: 1701–4.

Biro P, Rohling R, Schmid S et al 1994 Anesthesia in a patient with acute respiratory insufficiency due to relapsing polychondritis. Journal of Clinical Anesthesia 6: 59–62.

Burgess FW, Whitlock W, Davis MJ et al 1990 Anesthetic implications of relapsing polychondritis: a case report. Anesthesiology 73: 570–2.

Eng J, Sabanathan S 1991 Airway complications in relapsing polychondritis. Annals of Thoracic Surgery 51: 686–92.

Faul JL, Kee ST, Rizk NW 1999 Endobronchial stenting for severe airway obstruction in relapsing polychondritis. Chest 116: 825–7.

Fitzmaurice BG, Brodsky JB, Kee ST et al 1999 Anesthetic management of a patient with relapsing polychondritis. Journal of Cardiothoracic & Vascular Anesthesia 13: 309–11.

Gaffney RJ, Harrison M, Blayney AW 1992 Nebulised racemic ephedrine in the treatment of acute exacerbations of laryngeal relapsing polychondritis. Journal of Laryngology & Otology 106: 63–4.

Gimovsky ML, Nishiyama M 1989 Relapsing polychondritis in pregnancy: a case report and review. American Journal of Obstetrics & Gynecology 161: 332–4.

Goddard P, Cook P, Laszlo G et al 1991 Relapsing polychondritis: report of an unusual case and a review of the literature. British Journal of Radiology 64: 1064–7.

Hayward AW, Al-Shaikh B 1988 Relapsing poly-chrondritis and the anaesthetist. Anaesthesia 43: 573–7.

Isenberg SF 1997 Relapsing polychondritis. Otolaryngology—Head & Neck Surgery 116: 138.

Neville WE, Bolanowski PJP, Kotia GG 1990 Clinical experience with the silicone tracheal prosthesis. Journal of Thoracic and Cardiovascular Surgery 99: 604–13.

Papo T, Wechsler B, Bletry O et al 1997 Pregnancy in relapsing polychondritis: twenty-five pregnancies in eleven patients. Arthritis & Rheumatism 40: 1245–9.

Sarodia BD, Dasgupta A, Mehta AC 1999 Management of airway manifestations of relapsing polychondritis. Chest 116: 1669–75.

Shah R, Sabanathan S, Mearns AJ et al 1995 Self-expanding tracheobronchial stents in the management of major airway problems. Journal of Cardiovascular Surgery 36: 343–8.

Spraggs PD, Tostevin PM, Howard DJ 1997 Management of laryngotracheobronchial sequelae and complications of relapsing polychondritis. Laryngoscope 107: 936–41.

Tillie-Leblond I, Wallaert B, Leblond D et al 1998 Respiratory involvement in relapsing polychondritis: clinical, functional, endoscopic, and radiographic evaluations. Medicine 77: 168–76.

Trentham DE, Le CH 1998 Relapsing polychondritis. Annals of Internal Medicine 129: 114–22.

VanDecker W, Panidis IP 1988 Relapsing polychondritis and cardiovascular involvement. Annals of Internal Medicine 109: 340–1.

Rett syndrome

A progressive neurodevelopmental disorder, predominant in females. Generalised brain atrophy occurs, with an increased density of serotoninergic receptors in the brainstem. Possibly secondary to a primary deficit in cholinergic function.

Preoperative abnormalities

1. Normal development occurs until 6–18 months of age, after which there is deterioration in cerebral function. Features include stereotyped hand movements, severe mental deficiency, cortical and extrapyramidal dysfunction, microcephaly, seizures, and poor teeth.

2. A characteristic abnormal breathing pattern that is observed only when awake, and is associated with movement disorders and agitation. During hyperventilation there is generalised activation of the ventrolateral

medulla, and blood pressure and heart rate lability occurs (Kerr & Julu 1999). Awake hyperventilation and breath-holding are associated with decreased cerebral oxygenation.

3. Neurogenic scoliosis, for which surgery may be required.

4. There is an increased incidence of sudden, unexplained death. Girls with Rett syndrome have significantly longer QT_c intervals and T wave abnormalities than were found in age-matched healthy girls and, as the syndrome advanced, the proportion of these abnormalities increased (Sekul et al 1994). This was confirmed by Ellaway et al (1999), although 24-h Holter monitor in 34 girls showed no significant arrhythmias.

5. Inappropriate autonomic reactions occur, particularly during hyperventilation episodes.

6. Increase beta-endorphins in the CSF (Myer et al 1992).

Anaesthetic problems

1. An increased incidence of pulmonary infections (Dearlove & Walker 1996), and the need for IPPV.

2. Respiratory impairment, possibly secondary to increase in beta-endorphin concentrations. Prolonged respiratory depression occurred 12 h after epidural analgesia was stopped. This was reversed by a naloxone infusion without increasing the intensity of pain (Konen et al 1999).

3. Prolonged recovery from a brief halothane anaesthetic following oral premedication with alimemazine (trimeprazine) $2\,mg\,kg^{-1}$ and ketamine $5\,mg\,kg^{-1}$ was reported (Konarzewski & Misso 1994).

4. Anaesthesia may be required for scoliosis surgery (Maguire & Bachman 1989). Sudden death occurred 1 month after scoliosis surgery in one of three girls, although no evidence of LQTS was seen on ECG (Dearlove & Walker 1996).

Management

1. Examination of the ECG for evidence of LQTS.

2. Individuals seem to be sensitive to the depressant effects of hypnotics, sedatives, and opiates. Small doses and close perioperative observation is recommended.

3. Epidural analgesia was used in a 14 year old for pain relief after spine stabilisation (Konen et al 1999). However, since prolonged respiratory depression subsequently occurred, the use of local anaesthesia only has been suggested.

Bibliography

Dearlove OR, Walker RW 1996 Anaesthesia for Rett syndrome. Paediatric Anaesthesia 6: 155–8.

Ellaway CJ, Sholler G, Leonard H et al 1999 Prolonged QT interval in Rett syndrome. Archives of Disease in Childhood 80: 470–2.

Kerr AM, Julu PO 1999 Recent insights into hyperventilation from the study of Rett syndrome. Archives of Disease in Childhood 80: 384–7.

Konarzewski WH, Misso S 1994 Rett syndrome and delayed recovery from anaesthesia. Anaesthesia 49: 357.

Konen AA, Joshi GP, Kelly CK 1999 Epidural analgesia for pain relief after scoliosis in a patient with Rett's syndrome. Anesthesia & Analgesia 89: 451–2.

Maguire D, Bachman C 1989 Anaesthesia and Rett syndrome: a case report. Canadian Journal of Anaesthesia 36: 478–81.

Myer EC, Tripathi HL, Brase DA et al 1992 Elevated CSF beta-endorphin immunoreactivity in Rett syndrome: report of 158 cases and comparison with leukaemic children. Neurology 42: 357–60.

Sekul EA, Moak JP, Schultz RJ 1994 Electrocardiographic findings in Rett syndrome: an explanation for sudden death? Journal of Pediatrics 125: 80–2.

Rhabdomyolysis

Injury to skeletal muscle producing myoglobinaemia and myoglobinuria, associated with an increase, sometimes massive, of the CK levels. Free myoglobin appears in the blood soon after exposure to the cause. It may be detected in blood and urine almost immediately, but its transient appearance means that it is frequently missed, whereas the CK takes several hours to increase. A degree of rhabdomyolysis occurs after any muscle-cutting operation. After 30 operations in which suxamethonium was not used, serum myoglobin reached a maximum of $1390\,\mu\,g\,l^{-1}$ (median $345\,\mu\,g\,l^{-1}$), and serum CK a maximum of $1339\,iu\,l^{-1}$ (median $422\,iu\,l^{-1}$ for major surgery) (Laurence 2000). However, renal failure does not usually occur until levels in excess of $50\,000\,\mu\,g\,l^{-1}$ are reached. The exact mechanism of the renal damage is unclear.

Rhabdomyolysis of varying degrees of severity can be precipitated by a wide range of conditions, including drug overdoses, and the administration of certain anaesthetic agents. It is more likely to occur when there is muscle disease, but drug overdoses may precipitate rhabdomyolysis in apparently normal muscle. However, during surgery and anaesthesia the commonest causes are compartment syndrome, secondary to pressure/stretch injury during prolonged surgery in one position, tourniquet use for a long time, or at a high pressure, and reperfusion injury after acute ischaemic damage.

Factors not associated with anaesthesia and surgery

1. Predisposing factors that are not associated with anaesthesia include crush and burns injury, ischaemia, viral infections, polymyositis, heat stroke, marathon running, McArdle's syndrome (McMillan et al 1989), Taurius' syndrome, neuroleptic malignant syndrome, and carnitine palmityl transferase deficiency (Kelly et al 1989). Occasionally it has been reported following status epilepticus accompanied by lactic acidosis (Winocour et al 1989).

2. Drug overdose may be accompanied by rhabdomyolysis, and reports have included theophylline (Parr & Willatts 1991), ecstasy and other related amphetamines (Singarajah & Lavies 1992, Tehan et al 1993), cocaine and beta-2 adrenoreceptor agonists. In a study of cocaine

users presenting to an emergency department, 24% had rhabdomyolysis, defined as a CK $>1000\,u\,l^{-1}$, although symptoms were often absent (Welch et al 1991). Massive rhabdomyolysis and acute renal failure has been reported. Rhabdomyolysis, acute renal failure and compartment syndrome have been described in young alcoholics undergoing treatment with benzodiazepines (Rutgers et al 1991). Rhabdomyolysis and acute renal failure occurred from a beta-2 adrenoreceptor agonist terbutaline (Blake & Ryan 1989), secondary to intense beta receptor stimulation.

3. Pre-existing conditions in which rhabdomyolysis may be precipitated during anaesthesia include malignant hyperthermia myopathy, Duchenne and Becker muscular dystrophies, myotonia congenita, spinal muscle atrophy, Guillain–Barré syndrome (Scott et al 1991), burns, and polyneuropathy.

4. The CK levels are greatly increased and the passage of dark brown urine, positive for blood on reagent strip, but with no RBCs on microscopy, is suggestive of the diagnosis. Myoglobin levels are increased, but only in the early stages.

Intraoperative factors

1. *Positional, pressure/stretch damage.* The mechanism of muscle damage that occurs when patients with normal muscle have surgery for long periods in certain positions is not known precisely. However, pressure/stretch damage, followed by ischaemia and reperfusion may all contribute. Large numbers of reports of rhabdomyolysis have occurred, in association with prolonged surgery in the following positions. The majority of the operations lasted in excess of 6 h and evidence of compartment syndrome could be found in the relevant muscles.

a) The Lloyd-Davies/extended/exaggerated lithotomy position for rectal or prostate surgery (Lydon & Spielman 1984, Ali et al 1993). A patient in the lithotomy position for 10 h 10 min, with compression stockings intermittently being inflated to 40 mmHg, developed severe lateral and anterior compartment syndromes in both legs and required fasciotomy (Verdolin et al 2000).

b) In the lateral decubitus position for revision hip surgery (Lachiewicz & Latimer 1991, Targa et al 1991), or renal surgery (Mathes et al 1996).

c) Knee–elbow position for spinal surgery (Keim & Weinstein 1970).

2. *Tourniquet-induced.* Compartment syndrome, rhabdomyolysis and occasionally renal failure have been reported following use of a tourniquet (Shenton et al 1990, Hirvensalo et al 1992). There may be persistent neurological defects and occasionally amputation is required (Falk et al 1973). Factors affecting damage are tourniquet time, tourniquet pressure, accidental tourniquet slippage and reinflation without allowing a period of recirculation, and the size and shape of the tourniquet in relation to the limb.

3. *Reperfusion of ischaemic muscle.* Rhabdomyolysis and renal failure may occur in association with revascularisation of an acutely ischaemic limb. Patients with ischaemia for >6 h had a median CK following surgery of 29 370 iu l⁻¹, compared with insignificant increases in those who had not (Adiseshiah et al 1992).

4. *Anaesthetic drug-induced rhabdomyolysis.* This is most frequently precipitated by suxamethonium. It may occasionally occur after suxamethonium in an otherwise normal patient. Children are more susceptible to muscle injury after suxamethonium than adults, particularly if a volatile agent has been used first (McKishnie et al 1983). However, those individuals who have a significant degree of muscle destruction are usually found subsequently to have some underlying muscle disorder.

5. *Muscle diseases associated with rhabdomyolysis.* Although rhabdomyolysis is one feature of the

malignant hyperthermia (MH) syndrome, other features usually predominate initially. However, it has also occurred in association with anaesthesia in patients with DMD, Becker muscular dystrophy, Guillain–Barré syndrome, spinal muscular atrophy, myotonia congenita, McArdle's syndrome, and carnitine palmitoyl transferase deficiency (see individual diseases).

6. *Masseter muscle rigidity (MMR).* This is a term applied to severe spasm of the muscles of mastication lasting for 2–3 min following suxamethonium. This may be accompanied by varying degrees of rhabdomyolysis. About 50% of patients with severe MMR were reported to be susceptible to MH (Rosenberg & Fletcher 1986). However, increased tone in the masseter muscle is known to be a normal effect of suxamethonium, and MMR has been reported to occur in 1% of normal children, particularly when an inhalational agent has been given first. (See also Section 2, Masseter muscle rigidity.)

Intraoperative problems

1. Sometimes the first sign of muscle breakdown is the occurrence of a serious cardiac arrhythmia, or cardiac arrest, secondary to acute hyperkalaemia. Early cardiac arrest has been reported in Guillain–Barré syndrome (Hawker et al 1985), Duchenne muscular dystrophy (Seay et al 1978, Linter et al 1982, Chalkiadis & Branch 1990), or nonspecific myopathy (Schaer et al 1977).

2. During rhabdomyolysis, muscle cell integrity is lost and there is release of contents. Biochemical markers are myoglobin, creatine kinase, lactic acid dehydrogenase, aldolase, phosphate, potassium, aspartate aminotransferase, alanine aminotransferase, and neutral proteases. These move from muscle into the ECF. At the same time, sodium chloride and calcium move from the ECF into the cells, resulting in hypovolaemia, shock, metastatic calcification, prerenal and renal failure. Features include hyperkalaemia, hyperphosphataemia, hypocalcaemia, hyperuricaemia, a high

creatinine, and hypoalbuminaemia. There will be a metabolic acidosis and a coagulopathy may develop. Myoglobinuria occurs early and may be missed unless it is looked for. The CK increase begins later and is sustained for a longer period; it reaches its maximum at 24–36 h. A level of 500 iu l^{-1} indicates significant muscle damage, but in trained, muscular athletes, or in myopathic individuals, levels in excess of 250 000 iu l^{-1} may occur. When levels are high, myoglobinuria may present unexpectedly in the postoperative period (Hool et al 1984, Rubiano et al 1987), and if severe, or untreated, may progress to renal failure. Postoperative myoglobinuria and renal failure after suxamethonium and halothane was reported in a 3 year old with a strong family history of DMD (McKishnie et al 1983). This author has seen severe rhabdomyolysis in a 13-year-old boy after dental anaesthesia accompanied by a maximum CK of 252 000 iu l^{-1}. A presumptive diagnosis of MH was made, but investigations 4 years later were negative for MH and electron microscopy suggested an asymptomatic spinal muscular atrophy.

3. Compartment syndrome. This is a term used to describe the muscle tamponade and ischaemic myoneural damage secondary to increases in interstitial pressure within a limited area, such as a fascial compartment or osteofascial space. Compromise of blood flow occurs and a vicious circle of rhabdomyolysis, swelling, ischaemia and secondary reperfusion damage takes place. The limb is painful and swollen, but arterial pulses may be present, and the skin warm. Irreversible muscle damage occurs if the pressure is not relieved and amputation may subsequently be required.

4. In less severe, or treated rhabdomyolysis, postoperative muscle weakness or stiffness may occur in the affected muscles.

Management

1. *Anticipation of a potential problem.* In patients with myopathic or neuropathic types of disease, suxamethonium should be avoided, particularly in those who are immobile. It should certainly not be given in DMD, Becker's dystrophy, Guillain–Barré syndrome, McArdle's syndrome, MH myopathy, or after thermal injury. Should sudden cardiac arrest occur after suxamethonium, and T waves become peaked with a wide QRS, hyperkalaemia must be assumed and glucose 50% 50 ml with soluble insulin 10–20 u, and calcium chloride 10% 10 ml given urgently. Sodium bicarbonate 50 mmol (8.4% 50 ml) may be added. Blood samples should be taken for serum potassium and, if levels remain high, emergency treatment continued to lower it. In myopathic muscle, it may take a long time to restore the serum potassium to normal (Chalkiadis & Branch 1990). In these cases, myoglobinaemia and myoglobinuria should be anticipated.

2. *Positioning in prolonged surgery.* Awareness of the problem and preventive measures are paramount. When prolonged surgery is anticipated, care must be taken with the initial positioning, so that direct pressure or stretching of muscle is reduced. Extreme lithotomy positions, in which the thighs approach or touch the chest, should be avoided. When the patient is in the lithotomy position, it is not appropriate to use compression stockings or wrap the legs tightly (Verdolin et al 2000). In lateral positions, the posterior pelvic clamp should be positioned over the sacrum rather than the gluteal muscles, and posterior rotation of the operating table avoided.

Intraoperative diagnosis cannot usually be made, since much of the damage occurs only once reperfusion of the muscle has taken place, and compartment pressures only increase later. Distal pulses and capillary refill are usually normal. Although pulse oximetry of the peripheries has been suggested, this too is normal. However, in the postoperative period, signs and symptoms which suggest compartment syndrome should be taken seriously and orthopaedic advice about possible intramuscular pressure monitoring or fasciotomy should be sought early. Urine output should be observed and the urine examined early if myoglobinuria is suspected. Should this stage be missed, serum CK levels, which achieve a maximum at 24–36 h, will provide a diagnosis, and indicate the severity of muscle breakdown. Compartment syndrome cannot be divorced from rhabdomyolysis, therefore if significant compartment syndrome develops, aggressive early treatment with iv fluids and mannitol may prevent renal failure. Once renal failure is established, dialysis will be needed until recovery occurs. Even with established leg compartment syndrome, venography is normal and peripheral pulses remain intact. In the case of the gluteal or spinal muscles, clinical diagnosis is more difficult but major muscle damage can be confirmed by scanning procedures (Uratsuji et al 1999). Once compartment syndrome has been diagnosed, raising the legs to promote venous drainage will not help, since it lowers the driving pressure to the limb.

3. *Limitation of tourniquet times and pressures.* There are a large number of clinical and experimental papers on this subject. The exact safe tourniquet times and pressures are arguable. However, there is evidence that systolic arterial pressure plus 50–75 mmHg is sufficient to provide a bloodless field, and that the time should be limited to 1.5–2 h. In fat patients, conical cuffs may provide better occlusion.

4. *Anticipation of muscle breakdown, and prophylaxis.* If myoglobinuria occurs or is suspected, intravenous fluid therapy and an osmotic diuretic such as mannitol should be given to maintain an adequate urine flow. Urine output, serum CK, urea, creatinine and electrolytes should be checked regularly in the acute phase.

5. *Treat renal failure early.* If renal failure is already established, haemodialysis should be instituted until renal function recovers.

6. *Other measures.* Dantrolene sodium has been used in the treatment of hyperthermia and rhabdomyolysis caused by theophylline overdose (Parr & Willatts 1991), that secondary to the consumption of synthetic amphetamines

'Ecstasy' (Singarajah & Lavies 1992), and 'Eve' (Tehan et al 1993), and in the neuroleptic malignant syndrome. However, its effectiveness is dubious in these situations; its only proven use is in the treatment of malignant hyperthermia.

Bibliography

Adiseshiah M, Round JM, Jones DA 1992 Reperfusion injury in skeletal muscle: a prospective study in patients with acute limb ischaemia and claudicants treated by revascularization. British Journal of Surgery 79: 1026–9.

Ali H, Nieto JG, Rhamy RK et al 1993 Acute renal failure due to rhabdomyolysis associated with the extreme lithotomy position. American Journal of Kidney Diseases 22: 865–9.

Blake PG, Ryan F 1989 Rhabdomyolysis and acute renal failure after terbutaline overdose. Nephron 53: 76–7.

Chalkiadis GA, Branch KG 1990 Cardiac arrest after isoflurane anaesthesia in a patient with Duchenne's muscular dystrophy. Anaesthesia 45: 22–5.

Falk K, Rayyes AN, David SD et al 1973 Myoglobinuria with reversible acute renal failure. New York State Journal of Medicine 73: 537–43.

Hawker F, Pearson IY, Soni N et al 1985 Rhabdomyolytic renal failure and suxamethonium. Anaesthesia & Intensive Care 13: 208–9.

Hirvensalo E, Tuominen H, Lapinsuo M et al 1992 Compartment syndrome of the lower limb caused by tourniquet: a report of two cases. Journal of Orthopaedic Trauma 6: 469–72.

Hool GJ, Lawrence PJ, Sivaneswaran N 1984 Acute rhabdomyolytic renal failure due to suxamethonium. Anaesthesia & Intensive Care 12: 360–4.

Keim HA, Weinstein JD 1970 Acute renal failure—a complication of spinal fusion in the tuck position. Journal of Bone & Joint Surgery 52: 1248–9.

Kelly KJ, Garland JS, Tang TT et al 1989 Fatal rhabdomyolysis following influenza infection in a girl with familial carnitine palmityl transferase deficiency. Pediatrics 84: 312–16.

Lachiewicz PF, Latimer HA 1991 Rhabdomyolysis following total hip arthroplasty. Journal of Bone & Joint Surgery 73B: 576–9.

Laurence AS 2000 Serum myoglobin and creatine kinase following surgery. British Journal of Anaesthesia 84: 763–9.

Linter SPK, Thomas PR, Withington PS et al 1982 Suxamethonium hypertonicity and cardiac arrest in unsuspected pseudohypertrophic muscular dystrophy. British Journal of Anaesthesia 54: 1331–3.

Lydon JC, Spielman FJ 1984 Bilateral compartment syndrome following prolonged surgery in the lithotomy position. Anesthesiology 60: 236–8.

McKishnie JD, Muir JM, Girvan DP 1983 Anaesthesia induced rhabdomyolysis. Canadian Anaesthetists' Society Journal 30: 295–8.

McMillan MA, Hallworth MJ, Doyle D et al 1989 Acute renal failure due to McArdle's disease. Renal Failure 11: 23–5.

Mathes DD, Assimos DG, Donofrio PD 1996 Rhabdomyolysis and myonecrosis in a patient in the lateral decubitus position. Anesthesiology 84: 727–9.

Parr MJA, Willatts SM 1991 Fatal theophylline poisoning with rhabdomyolysis. A potential role for dantrolene treatment. Anaesthesia 46: 557–9.

Rosenberg H, Fletcher JE 1986 Masseter muscle rigidity and malignant hyperthermia susceptibility. Anesthesia & Analgesia 65: 161–4.

Rubiano R, Chang J-L, Carroll J et al 1987 Acute rhabdomyolysis following halothane anesthesia without succinylcholine. Anesthesiology 67: 856–7.

Rutgers PH, van der Harst E, Koumans RK 1991 Surgical implications of drug-induced rhabdomyolysis. British Journal of Surgery 78: 490–2.

Schaer H, Steinmann B, Jerusalem S et al 1977 Rhabdomyolysis induced by anaesthesia with intraoperative cardiac arrest. British Journal of Anaesthesia 49: 495–9.

Scott AJ, Duncan R, Henderson L et al 1991 Acute rhabdomyolysis associated with atypical Guillain–Barré syndrome. Postgraduate Medical Journal 67: 73–4.

Seay AR, Ziter FA, Thompson JA 1978 Cardiac arrest during induction of anaesthesia in Duchenne muscular dystrophy. Journal of Pediatrics 93: 88–90.

Shenton DW, Spitzer SA, Mulrennan BM 1990 Tourniquet-induced rhabdomyolysis. Journal of Bone & Joint Surgery 72A: 1405–6.

Singarajah C, Lavies NG 1992 An overdose of ecstasy. A role for dantrolene. Anaesthesia 46: 686–7.

Targa L, Droghetti I, Caggese G et al 1991 Rhabdomyolysis and operating position. Anaesthesia 46: 141–3.

Tehan B, Hardem R, Bodenham A 1993 Hyperthermia associated with 3,4-methylene dioxymethamphetamine ('Eve'). Anaesthesia 48: 507–10.

Uratsuji Y, Ijichi K, Irie J et al 1999 Rhabdomyolysis after abdominal surgery in the hyperlordotic position enforced by pneumatic support. Anesthesiology 91: 310.

Verdolin MH, Toth AS, Schroeder R 2000 Bilateral lower extremity compartment syndromes following prolonged surgery in the low lithotomy position with serial compression stockings. Anesthesiology 92: 1189–91.

Welch RD, Todd K, Krause GS 1991 Incidence of cocaine-associated rhabdomyolysis. Annals of Emergency Medicine 20: 154–7.

Winocour PH, Waise A, Young G et al 1989 Severe, self-limiting lactic acidosis and rhabdomyolysis accompanying convulsions. Postgraduate Medical Journal 65: 321–2.

Rheumatoid arthritis

A common, autoimmune connective tissue disease, primarily involving joints, but with widespread systemic effects. There is hypergammaglobulinaemia, and rheumatoid factors, which are autoantibodies of IgE, IgA and IgM classes, are present.

Preoperative abnormalities

1. The joint disease involves inflammation, formation of granulation tissue, fibrosis, joint destruction, and deformity. Any joint may be affected. Those of particular concern to the anaesthetist are the cervical, the temporo-mandibular, and the cricoarytenoid joints. Airway obstruction can occur from closely adducted, immobile vocal cords, or from laryngeal amyloidosis. Rheumatoid nodules can affect the larynx.

2. Extra-articular problems occur in more than 50% of patients.

a) *Lungs.* May be affected by effusions, nodular lesions, diffuse interstitial fibrosis, or Caplan's syndrome. This is a form of massive pulmonary fibrosis seen in coal miners with rheumatoid arthritis or positive rheumatoid factor, and probably represents an abnormal tissue response to inorganic dust. There may be a restrictive lung defect, with a contribution from reduced chest wall compliance.

b) *Kidney.* Twenty-five per cent of patients eventually die from renal failure. Renal damage may be related to the disease process itself, from secondary amyloid disease, or from drug treatment.

c) *Heart.* Is involved in up to 44% of cases. Small pericardial effusions are common, but are not usually of clinical significance. Rarely, pericarditis and tamponade may occur, usually in seropositive patients and those with skin nodules. Other problems include endocarditis or left ventricular failure. Occasionally heart valve lesions occur and are of two types; rheumatoid granulomas involving the leaflets and ring, and nongranulomatous valvular inflammation with thickening and fibrosis of the leaflets.

d) *Blood vessels.* A widespread vasculitis can occur. Small arteries and arterioles are often involved, frequently in the presence of relatively disease-free main trunk vessels. Significant ischaemia may result, the actual effects depending on the tissue or organ supplied.

e) *Autonomic involvement* (Louthrenoo et al 1999).

f) *Gastrointestinal.* Swallowing problems and dysphagia were found in eight of 29 patients with classical rheumatoid arthritis compared with only one in a control group (Geterud et al 1991b). Oesophageal manometry showed upper oesophageal dysfunction in the rheumatoid group, but there was no correlation between the results of manometry and the symptoms of dysphagia.

g) *Peripheral neuropathy.*

3. Chronic anaemia, which has been shown to respond to erythropoietin therapy, is common (Salvarani et al 1991).

Anaesthetic problems

1. *Disease of the cervical vertebrae.* Cervical involvement, and damage to the cervical spinal cord, has been associated with neck manipulation during anaesthesia and sedation. Instability is said to occur in 25% of patients with rheumatoid arthritis. Of these, one-quarter will have no neurological symptoms to alert the physician (Norton & Ghanma 1982). The presenting symptoms of 31 patients with cervical myelopathy were analysed (Marks & Sharp 1981). Sensory disturbances occurred in 74%, but these were often dismissed and attributed to peripheral neuropathy. Weakness occurred in 19%, flexor spasms in 16%, and incontinence in 6%. By the time the diagnosis was made, 77% had spastic paraparesis or quadriparesis. The problem of instability is not necessarily confined to those with longstanding disease.

The commonest lesion is that of atlantoaxial subluxation, although subaxial subluxations may occur in addition. Destruction of bone, and weakening of the ligaments, allow the odontoid peg to migrate backwards and upwards, compressing the spinal cord against the posterior arch of the atlas. Thus, the main danger lies in cervical flexion. In an MRI study of 34 patients with atlantoaxial instability, the relationships between spinal cord diameter in the neutral and flexed positions, the clinical signs, and latency of motor evoked potentials, were all examined. Thickening of inflammatory tissue of greater than 3 mm behind the odontoid peg was observed in 22 patients and this contributed to a decreased spinal cord diameter when the neck was in the flexed position. A spinal cord diameter in flexion of less than 6 mm, severe pain and cranial migration of the axis, were suggested to indicate the need for surgical intervention (Dvorak et al 1989).

The potential dangers of anaesthesia and endoscopy have been emphasised. Flexion of the head and reduction in muscle tone may result in cervical cord damage (McConkey 1982, Norton & Ghanma 1982). Dislocation of the odontoid process and spinal cord damage was discovered in a patient undergoing postoperative IPPV on the ITU (Bollensen et al 1991). It was not known exactly when this had occurred. In an analysis of 113 rheumatoid patients having total hip or knee arthroplasty, cervical spine X-rays were examined for signs of atlantoaxial subluxation, atlantoaxial impaction, and subaxial subluxation (Collins et al 1991). One or more of these findings were present in 61% of patients.

2. *Cervical instability below the level of a fusion.* Those who have previously undergone occipital cervical fusion may develop cervical instability below the level of the original arthrodesis (Kraus et al 1991). Two groups of patients were compared: one group had undergone occipitocervical fusion for atlantoaxial subluxation and superior migration of the odontoid; the other group had undergone atlantoaxial fusion for isolated axial subluxation. In the first group, 36% of patients developed subaxial subluxation requiring surgery at an average of 2.6 years, whereas in the second group 5.5% of patients developed subaxial subluxation requiring surgery after an average of 9 years. Occipitocervical fusion is thought to generate a greater force at lower cervical level, that in turn stresses the unfused facet joints.

3. *Laryngeal problems.* A constant pattern of laryngeal and tracheal deviation is reported to occur in some patients, particularly those with proximal migration of the odontoid peg (Keenan et al 1983). The larynx is tilted forwards, displaced anteriorly and laterally to the left, and the vocal cords rotated clockwise. Involvement of the larynx in the rheumatoid process is more common than was previously thought. In a study of 29 females, one or more signs of laryngeal involvement were found in 69% of patients; physical signs were seen on fibreoptic examination in 59%, there was evidence of extrathoracic airway obstruction in 14%, and 10% had abnormal X-rays (Geterud et al 1991a). Although symptoms of breathing difficulty occurred in 75% of the group studied, cricoarytenoid joint involvement only rarely produces actual upper airway obstruction.

However, fatal airway obstruction occurred following cervical spine fusion, secondary to massive oedema in the meso- and hypopharynx (Lehmann et al 1997). Acute obstruction in a 4 year old with juvenile RA also resulted from gross swelling of the arytenoids; unlike those with epiglottitis, the obstruction was improved in the supine position (Vetter 1994).

4. *The laryngeal mask airway should not be relied upon to overcome failed tracheal intubation.* It was impossible to insert a laryngeal mask airway into a patient with a grade 4 laryngoscopic view. Subsequent cervical X-rays with the head maximally extended showed that the angle between the oral and pharyngeal axes at the back of the tongue was only 70 degrees, compared with 105 degrees in five normal patients. A simulation of different angles using an aluminium plate showed that at an angle less than 90 degrees, the laryngeal mask airway could not be advanced without kinking at the corner (Ishimura et al 1995).

5. *Sleep apnoeas.* Medullary compression associated with major atlantoaxial subluxation may result in nocturnal oxygen desaturation (Howard et al 1994).

6. *Limitation of mouth opening* may occur secondary to arthritis of the temporomandibular joints. This is a particular problem in juvenile rheumatoid arthritis (Hodgkinson 1981).

7. A pericardial effusion and tamponade presented as an acute abdominal emergency in a young patient with seropositive rheumatoid arthritis (Bellamy et al 1990). Hypoxia and hypotension occurred at induction of anaesthesia. Laparotomy showed gross hepatic congestion and ascites, CXR revealed cardiomegaly, and 1 litre of turbid fluid was drained at pericardial fenestration.

8. Rheumatoid aortic valve involvement may be more rapidly progressive than aortic valve disease from other causes, so that there is little time for compensatory hypertrophy of the ventricle to occur. Acute aortic regurgitation caused sudden cardiac failure in a young woman

and required urgent valve replacement (Camilleri et al 1991).

9. Lung disease can result in reduced pulmonary reserve and hypoxia.

10. An increased sensitivity to anaesthetic agents may occur.

Management

1. Clinical assessment of neck and jaw mobility. The Sharp and Purser test gives some indication of cervical spine instability (Norton & Ghanma 1982). The patient should be upright, relaxed and with the neck flexed. With a finger on the spinous process of the axis, the forehead should be pressed backwards with the other hand. Normally there is minimal movement. If subluxation is present, the head moves backwards as reduction occurs.

2. A lateral view of the cervical spine in flexion and extension will show the distance between the odontoid peg and the posterior border of the anterior arch of the atlas. If subluxation is present, this distance is greater than 3 mm. Neutral lateral cervical views alone are insufficient, since they failed to confirm the diagnosis of subluxation in 48% of 65 rheumatoid patients with unstable atlantoaxial subluxations (Kauppi & Neva 1998). Frontal views of the odontoid and entire cervical spine have also been suggested (Kwek et al 1998).

3. Cervical X-rays of patients who have previously undergone occipital spinal fusions should be carefully examined for evidence of cervical instability at a lower level.

4. Intubation methods. Cervical instability may be an indication for awake fibreoptic intubation with the application of a collar or Crutchfield tongs, to maintain rigidity during surgery. Since spinal instability is usually in flexion, some authors believe that safe tracheal intubation can be achieved under general anaesthesia by careful extension of the head, except in the rare instances of posterior atlantoaxial subluxation when fibreoptic intubation is indicated (Heywood et al 1988). However, after a retrospective analysis of 78 patients with rheumatoid arthritis, Hakala and Randell (1998) concluded that the use of fibreoptic intubation in their department had increased the safety of intubation. Wattenmaker et al (1994) came to similar conclusions. Emergency control of the airway has been described using a laryngeal mask airway in a patient who developed acute pulmonary oedema following occipitocervical fusion (Calder et al 1990).

5. Deviation of the larynx may make fibreoptic laryngoscopy more difficult in some patients (Keenan et al 1983). Examination of the orientation of the larynx by indirect laryngoscopy at preoperative assessment may be helpful. If there is cricoarytenoid involvement, care should be taken with the choice of tracheal tube size and tube insertion. Cricoarytenoid arthritis may occasionally necessitate permanent tracheostomy (Absalom et al 1998). Acute arytenoid arthritis in a 4 year old was treated by 48 h of tracheal intubation, IPPV, and high-dose steroids (Vetter 1994).

6. Although the use of the laryngeal mask airway is increasingly common, as mentioned above, it cannot always be relied on in patients with severe flexion deformities of the neck.

7. Assessment of pulmonary function and reserve.

8. Examination for other significant complications, such as valvular disease, or pericardial effusion.

9. Extreme caution should be observed if epidural or caudal anaesthesia is to be undertaken in patients in whom intubation difficulties are anticipated. Even after a test dose to exclude an accidental spinal, or vascular penetration, the block should only be established very gradually.

10. The use of cervical epidural analgesia for treatment of digital vasculitis has been reported (Green & de Rosayro 1997).

Bibliography

Absalom AR, Watts R, Kong A 1998 Airway obstruction caused by rheumatoid cricoarytenoid arthritis. Lancet 351: 1099–100.

Bellamy MC, Natarajan V, Lenz RJ 1990 An unusual presentation of cardiac tamponade. Anaesthesia 45: 135–6.

Bollensen E, Schonle PW, Braun U et al 1991 [An unnoticed dislocation of the dens axis in a patient with primary chronic polyarthritis undergoing intensive therapy. English abstract.] Anaesthetist 40: 294–7.

Calder I, Ordman AJ, Jackowski A et al 1990 The Brain laryngeal mask airway. An alternative to emergency tracheal intubation. Anaesthesia 45: 137–9.

Camilleri JP, Douglas-Jones AG, Pritchard MH 1991 Rapidly progressive aortic valve incompetence in a patient with rheumatoid arthritis. British Journal of Rheumatology 30: 379–81.

Collins DN, Barnes CL, FitzRandolph RL 1991 Cervical spine instability in rheumatoid patients having total hip or knee arthroplasty. Clinical Orthopaedics 272: 127–35.

Dvorak J, Grob D, Baumgartner H et al 1989 Functional evaluation of the spinal cord by magnetic resonance imaging in patients with rheumatoid arthritis and instability of the upper cervical spine. Spine 14: 1057–64.

Geterud A, Bake B, Berthelsen B et al 1991a Laryngeal involvement in rheumatoid arthritis. Acta Otolaryngologie (Stockholm) 111: 990–8.

Geterud A, Bake B, Bjelle A et al 1991b Swallowing problems in rheumatoid arthritis. Acta Otolaryngologie (Stockholm) 111: 1153–61.

Green CR, de Rosayro AM 1997 Cervical epidural analgesia for management of pain associated with digital vasculitis secondary to rheumatoid arthritis. Regional Anesthesia 22: 188–91.

Hakala P, Randell T 1998 Intubation difficulties in patients with rheumatoid arthritis. A retrospective analysis. Acta Anaesthesiologica Scandinavica 42: 195–8.

Heywood AWB, Learmonth ID, Thomas M 1988 Cervical spine instability in rheumatoid arthritis. Journal of Bone & Joint Surgery 70B: 702–7.

Hodgkinson R 1981 Anesthetic management of a parturient with severe juvenile rheumatoid arthritis. Anesthesia & Analgesia 60: 611–12.

Howard RS, Henderson F, Hirsch NP et al 1994 Respiratory abnormality due to craniovertebral junction compression in rheumatoid disease. Annals of the Rheumatic Diseases 53: 134–6.

Ishimura H, Minami K, Sata T et al 1995 Impossible insertion of the laryngeal mask airway and oropharyngeal axis. Anesthesiology 83: 867–9.

Kauppi M, Neva MH 1998 Sensitivity of lateral view cervical spine radiography taken in the neutral position in atlantoaxial subluxation in rheumatic diseases. Clinical Rheumatology 17: 511–14.

Keenan MA, Stiles CM, Kaufman RL 1983 Acquired laryngeal deviation associated with cervical spine disease in erosive polyarticular arthritis. Anesthesiology 58: 441–9.

Kraus DR, Peppelman WC, Agarwal AK et al 1991 Incidence of subaxial subluxation in patients with generalized rheumatoid arthritis who have had previous occipital cervical fusions. Spine 16: S486–9.

Kwek TK, Lew TW, Thoo FL 1998 The role of preoperative cervical spine X-rays in rheumatoid arthritis. Anaesthesia & Intensive Care 26: 636–41.

Lehmann T, Nek W, Stalder B et al 1997 Fatal postoperative airway obstruction in a patient with rheumatoid arthritis. Annals of Rheumatic Diseases 56: 512–13.

Louthrenoo W, Ruttanaumpawan P, Aramrattana A et al 1999 Cardiovascular autonomic nervous system dysfunction in patients with rheumatoid arthritis and systemic lupus erythematosus. Quarterly Journal of Medicine 92: 97–102.

McConkey B 1982 Rheumatoid cervical myelopathy. British Medical Journal 284: 1731–2.

Marks JS, Sharp J 1981 Rheumatoid cervical myelopathy. Quarterly Journal of Medicine 199: 307–19.

Norton ML, Ghanma MA 1982 Atlanto-axial instability revisited; an alert for endoscopists. Annals of Otology, Rhinology & Laryngology 91: 567–70.

Salvarani C, Lasagni D, Casali B et al 1991 Recombinant human erythropoietin therapy in patients with rheumatoid arthritis with the anaemia of chronic disease. Journal of Rheumatology 18: 1168–71.

Vetter TR 1994 Acute airway obstruction due to arytenoid arthritis in a child with juvenile rheumatoid arthritis. Anesthesia & Analgesia 79: 1198–1200.

Wattenmaker I, Concepcion M, Hibberd P et al 1994 Upper-airway obstruction and perioperative management of the airway in patients managed with posterior operations on the cervical spine for rheumatoid arthritis. Journal of Bone & Joint Surgery 76A: 360–5.

Sarcoidosis

A multisystem, granulomatous disorder, of variable natural history and prognosis, most frequently presenting in young adults with bilateral hilar lymphadenopathy, pulmonary infiltration, cutaneous and ocular lesions. In some, an acute onset may resolve spontaneously; in others, slow onset may herald progressive disease with serious complications, such as pulmonary fibrosis, blindness, cardiac involvement, nephrocalcinosis, and renal failure. Heart and lung involvement are the most significant contributors to a fatal outcome. Cardiac sarcoid is difficult to diagnose and is reported to run a treacherous course (Mitchell et al 1997).

Preoperative abnormalities

1. The patient may be asymptomatic, and about one-third of cases present because of an abnormality found on CXR. With more advanced disease there may be variable degrees of respiratory impairment. CXR usually shows bilateral hilar lymphadenopathy with increased reticular shadowing in the lung fields. Lung function tests may be impaired. Restrictive gas transfer and obstructive defects may all occur at different stages of the disease. In advanced disease, pulmonary hypertension may develop.

2. Other more commonly involved organs are the skin, eyes, liver, spleen, and the bones of the hands and feet.

3. Hypercalcaemia may occur, which is secondary to the production of excess 1,25-dihydroxycholecalciferol. Nephrocalcinosis and renal failure may result.

4. Cardiac disease, though rare, is more common than was previously thought (Fleming 1986), and carries a poor prognosis. Its diagnosis is of anaesthetic importance.

The pathological lesions can be diffuse or focal. Localised granulomas and fibrous scarring most commonly occur in the basal portion of the ventricular septum and left ventricular wall.

These lesions will be asymptomatic unless they happen to involve the conducting system, in which case arrhythmias or conduction defects occur. Less commonly, the distribution of granulomas may be widespread, and they may coalesce to produce diffuse interstitial fibrosis. The resulting hypokinesia and subsequent heart failure is clinically indistinguishable from other cardiomyopathies (Fleming 1986).

Pericardial effusions may also occur. About 20% of 81 consecutive patients with proven sarcoid, but without clinical evidence of heart disease, were found to have pericardial effusions (Angomachalelis et al 1994). Myocardial imaging showed that the majority of these had an infiltrative cardiomyopathy. At autopsy on 84 patients with sarcoidosis, 27% were found to have myocardial granulomas, one-third of which had been unsuspected (Silverman et al 1978). In those patients diagnosed as having cardiac involvement, the signs in order of frequency of presentation were: complete heart block, ventricular ectopics or ventricular tachycardia, myocardial disease causing heart failure, sudden death, and first-degree heart block or bundle branch block. A further analysis of 57 patients with complete heart block and sarcoid revealed that in 72%, the heart block was the first sign of the disease (Pehrsson & Tornling 1985). Sudden death had occurred in two-thirds of patients in an autopsy study of cardiac sarcoid (Roberts et al 1977). In approximately 18% of these, death was the initial manifestation of cardiac involvement, and in the majority, death occurred during a period of exercise.

5. Central nervous system sarcoid also carries a poor prognosis. Presentation can vary widely and includes cranial nerve palsies, peripheral neuropathy, epilepsy, and cerebellar ataxia (Zajicek et al 1999).

6. Laryngeal sarcoidosis may occur. The commonest lesion reported is an oedematous, pale, diffuse enlargement of the supraglottic structures (Fortune & Courey 1998).

7. The diagnosis can be made on biopsy of a skin lesion, or lung and bronchial biopsy via a

fibreoptic bronchoscope. The Kveim test has a high positivity in the active stages, but is lower in the chronic disease. Serum angiotensin-converting enzyme (ACE) level is an indicator of sarcoid activity, and serum calcium and 24-h urinary calcium levels may also be increased in active sarcoid.

8. Treatment of active disease may include corticosteroids, immunosuppressants, methotrexate, NSAIDS, and calcium chelating agents.

Anaesthetic problems

1. In advanced disease, respiratory function may be profoundly impaired.

2. Although rare, cardiac disease may be unexpected, and can occur in young, previously asymptomatic patients. The sudden onset of complete heart block during anaesthesia in an athletic young man with sarcoid was described (Thomas & Mason 1988). Permanent pacing was required after surgery. Difficulties with pacemaker management can be a feature of cardiac sarcoidosis (Lie et al 1974). Patients with advanced disease may have automatic implantable cardioverter defibrillators inserted (Paz et al 1994) (see also Automatic implantable cardioverter defibrillator).

3. Infiltration of the airway may cause obstructive sleep apnoea (Shah et al 1998), and a case of upper airway obstruction secondary to laryngeal sarcoid has been described (Wills & Harris 1987).

Management

1. If there is widespread pulmonary involvement and the patient is symptomatic, lung function tests, including blood gases, should be performed.

2. A preoperative ECG is essential, even in young patients. If there is evidence of a conduction defect, a temporary pacemaker should be inserted before anaesthesia.

3. Assessment and management of laryngeal sarcoid.

4. Treatment of hypercalcaemia. Corticosteroids may improve symptoms and signs of cardiac and pulmonary sarcoidosis (Schaedel et al 1991).

5. Epidural anaesthesia for Caesarean section has been reported in a patient with advanced sarcoid, pulmonary hypertension, and restrictive lung disease (Euliano et al 1997). Pulmonary artery pressures were measured and dobutamine was required.

Bibliography

Angomachalelis N, Hourzamanis A, Salem N et al 1994 Pericardial effusion concomitant with specific heart muscle disease in systemic sarcoidosis. Postgraduate Medical Journal 70 (suppl 1): S8–12.

Euliano TY, White SE, Aleixo L 1997 Sarcoidosis in a pregnant woman. Journal of Clinical Anesthesia 9: 78–86.

Fleming HA 1986 Sarcoid heart disease. British Medical Journal 292: 1095–6.

Fortune S, Courey MS 1998 Isolated laryngeal sarcoidosis. Otolaryngology—Head & Neck Surgery 118: 868–70.

Lie JT, Hunt D, Valentine PA 1974 Sudden death from cardiac sarcoidosis with involvement of the conduction system. American Journal of the Medical Sciences 267: 123–8.

Mitchell DN, du Bois RM, Oldershaw P 1997 Cardiac sarcoidosis. British Medical Journal 314: 320–1.

Paz HL, McCormick DJ, Kutalek SP et al 1994 The automatic implantable cardioverter defibrillator. Prophylaxis in cardiac sarcoidosis. Chest 106: 1603–7.

Pehrsson SK, Tornling G 1985 Sarcoidosis associated with complete heart block. Sarcoidosis 2: 135–41.

Roberts WC, McAllister HA, Ferrans VJ 1977 Sarcoidosis of the heart. American Journal of Medicine 63: 86–108.

Schaedel H, Kirsten D, Schmidt A et al 1991 Sarcoid heart—results of follow-up investigations. European Heart Journal 12: 26–7.

Shah RN, Mills PR, George PJ et al 1998 Upper airways sarcoidosis presenting as obstructive sleep apnoea. Thorax 53: 232–3.

Silverman KJ, Hutchins GM, Bulkley BH 1978 Cardiac sarcoid: a clinicopathologic study of 84 unselected patients with systemic sarcoidosis. Circulation 58: 1204–11.

Thomas DW, Mason RA 1988 Complete heart block during anaesthesia in a patient with sarcoidosis. Anaesthesia 43: 578–80.

Wills MH, Harris MM 1987 An unusual airway complication with sarcoidosis. Anesthesiology 66: 554–5.

Zajicek JP, Scolding NJ, Foster O et al 1999 Central nervous system sarcoidosis—diagnosis and management. Quarterly Journal of Medicine 92: 103–17.

Schwartz–Jampel syndrome

One of the osteochondrodysplasias, an autosomal recessive disease in which myotonia and skeletal abnormalities feature. The diagnosis is made on the combination of clinical features and an abnormal EMG. A sodium channel defect has been suggested.

Preoperative abnormalities

1.   Features include generalised myotonia, with muscles that are stiff and firm, short stature, pinched face and small mouth, low-set ears, and blepharospasm. Feeding difficulties, choking fits and feeding apnoeas are common. There is a characteristic gait, with bowing of long bones together with contractures.

2.   Ocular abnormalities.

3.   Thermoregulatory dysfunction.

4.   EMG shows high-frequency discharges in facial muscles and distal muscles of hands and legs (Ishpekova et al 1996).

Anaesthetic problems

1.   Intubation problems (Theroux et al 1995).

2.   Obstructive sleep apnoea may result from a combination of a small oropharynx, a rigid, hypertrophied tongue base, and neuromuscular abnormalities (Cook & Borkowski 1997).

3.   Thermoregulatory problems have been reported. Although an association with MH was suggested after a temperature increase of 1.5°C developed over 10 min in a 23-month-old child, the CK was only 216 mU ml^{-1}, and no other corroborative evidence was produced (Seay & Ziter 1978).

Management

1.   Preparations should be made in the event of difficult intubation. Theroux et al (1995) described an infant in whom intubation and fibreoptic endoscopy had failed, but passage of a size 1 laryngeal mask airway was successful. A fibrescope was loaded with two size 3 tubes without adaptors and, after intubation through the laryngeal mask airway, the proximal tube was used to stabilise the distal one, whilst the laryngeal mask airway was removed.

2.   CPAP may be required for obstructive sleep apnoea.

3.   Care should be taken in monitoring both core temperature and neuromuscular function.

4.   The use of caudal anaesthesia has been described in an 8 year old having orthopaedic surgery (Ray & Rubin 1994).

Bibliography

Cook SP, Borkowski WJ 1997 Obstructive sleep apnea in Schwartz–Jampel syndrome. Archives of Otolaryngology—Head & Neck Surgery 123: 1348–50.

Ishpekova B, Rasheva M, Moskov M 1996 Schwartz–Jampel syndrome: clinical electromyographic and genetic studies. Electromyography & Clinical Neurophysiology 36: 91–7.

Ray S, Rubin AP 1994 Anaesthesia in a child with Schwartz–Jampel syndrome. Anaesthesia 49: 600–2.

Seay AR, Ziter FA 1978 Malignant hyperpyrexia in a patient with Schwartz–Jampel syndrome. Journal of Pediatrics 93: 83–4.

Theroux MC, Kettrick RG, Khine HH 1995 Laryngeal mask airway and fiberoptic endoscopy in an infant with Schwartz–Jampel syndrome. Anesthesiology 82: 605.

Scleroderma

A spectrum of diseases involving abnormal collagen deposition and microvascular changes in the skin and other organs. There is synthesis and deposition of excessive extracellular matrix and the presence of vascular anti-GBM (glomerular basement membrane) antibodies (McHugh 1994). Autoantibodies define subsets of the disease. These include anti-centromere antibody (ACA) and anti-topoisomerase-1 antibody (ATA).

Limited cutaneous scleroderma, previously known as CREST syndrome (Calcinosis, Raynaud's, (o)Esophageal problems, Sclerodactyly, and Telangiectasia), has a high prevalence of ACA.

Diffuse cutaneous scleroderma has ATA present in about 30% of patients. This is a more diffuse form with early onset of pulmonary, renal, gastrointestinal or myocardial disease. A third form has a high frequency of neurological disease.

Scleroderma occurs more commonly in women, often in the 30–50-year age group. Pregnancy may worsen the disease, and there is a high incidence of fetal loss. Pulmonary hypertension was found to be the most frequent cause of death, and renal, cardiac and pulmonary involvement were features associated with reduced survival (Lee et al 1992).

Preoperative abnormalities

1. The skin becomes taut, shiny and waxy looking. Skin folds are lost and there is a nonpitting oedema. Contractures of the joints and the mouth may develop. Multiple telangiectasia may occur. Sweating is reduced.

2. Disease of the peripheral vessels is predominant and Raynaud's phenomenon of the hands and feet is the presenting feature in 90% of cases.

3. Oesophageal involvement has been reported in up to 80% of patients, and may produce dysphagia, reflux oesophagitis, and strictures. It has been suggested that the basis of the dysphagia lies in disturbances of motility, rather than structural changes in the oesophagus. Telangiectasia can occur throughout the gastrointestinal tract. Gut involvement may cause malabsorption, and occasionally vitamin C deficiency. Intestinal obstruction can occur.

4. The lungs are commonly involved. Pulmonary vascular disease, progressing to pulmonary hypertension, and interstitial lung disease are the two main lesions, and pulmonary haemorrhage may occur (Arroliga et al 1992). Weakness of the respiratory muscles and diaphragm may develop.

5. Cardiac lesions occur in 50–90% of cases of systemic disease. A study of 46 patients with systemic disease showed that 56% had arrhythmias or conduction defects, and 28% had a pericardial effusion demonstrated by echocardiography (Clements et al 1981), some of which may be massive. Hypokinetic left ventricular wall abnormalities have been shown on echocardiography in a high proportion of patients, even in those with limited cutaneous scleroderma. Cardiac and pulmonary artery enlargement secondary to pulmonary vascular disease may be seen on CXR. In some individuals, skeletal myopathies and cardiac muscle disease coexist, and in this group sudden death may occur from arrhythmias (Follansbee et al 1993).

6. Renal disease and hypertension are common in the systemic form of the disease with progression to renal insufficiency. Scleroderma renal crisis is a rare and devastating syndrome, in which acute renal failure is associated with widespread microvascular disease. Treatment is with ACE inhibitors.

7. Antinuclear antibodies are present in 40–90% of cases. Catastrophic antiphospholipid syndrome has been described in a patient with scleroderma, who presented with digital gangrene and multiorgan failure, and died within 19 h (Kane et al 1998).

8. Patients may be receiving steroids or immunosuppressants.

Anaesthetic problems

1. Skin changes result in difficulties with venous access. The contractures of the mouth are susceptible to damage, and may give poor access to the oral cavity. Bleeding can occur from telangiectasia in the mouth. Several problems were encountered during dental extraction. Injection into a peripheral cannula produced local complications in the patient's hand, and insertion of the mouth prop caused a tear of the angle of the mouth (Davidson-Lamb & Finlayson 1977). Selective narrowing of the ulnar arteries, caused by smooth thickening along their whole length, has been found in a study of 20 patients (Stafford et al 1998).

2. Patients with oesophageal involvement may be more prone to acid reflux and regurgitation. Abnormalities of oesophageal function can occur even in asymptomatic individuals, and there is an inability of the oesophagus to empty without the aid of gravity. Mallory–Weiss syndrome has been reported to complicate pregnancy (Chin et al 1995). Severe bleeding can occur from gastrointestinal telangiectasia.

3. There is evidence that impaired nerve conduction occurs in scleroderma, affecting most sensory modalities (Schady et al 1991). In addition, complications have been described in association with local anaesthetic techniques. Prolonged sensory loss, which may be due to reduced blood flow, has been reported (Eisele & Reitan 1971, Lewis 1974). Injection of a large volume of solution can produce a degree of tension in the skin sufficient to interfere with local blood supply. Sclerotic skin may conceal landmarks.

4. Tracheal intubation may be more difficult than usual if there are mouth and neck contractures. Telangiectasia in the mouth or nose may bleed. Involvement of the larynx has been described (Rapp et al 1991).

5. Problems associated with systemic or pulmonary hypertension. Left ventricular failure, arrhythmias or pericardial effusions may occur. A 71-year-old patient with a 20-year history of scleroderma, undergoing surgery for gastric cancer, developed sinus arrest. A temporary pacemaker was inserted, but pacemaker dependence necessitated the insertion of a permanent device (Kihira et al 1995).

6. The combination of pulmonary abnormalities and contraction of the skin of the chest wall may contribute to postoperative respiratory inadequacy. Inflammatory alveolitis occurs in up to 50% of patients, and it is possible that interstitial fibrosis is an end result of this process (Silver et al 1990).

7. Pregnancy in diffuse scleroderma may be associated with increased skin thickening, and occasionally serious cardiovascular and renal problems. A maternal death was reported associated with the development of pulmonary oedema and pulmonary hypertension following Caesarean section (Younker & Harrison 1985). Severe hypertension and pulmonary oedema causing a maternal death in the 32nd week of pregnancy has also been noted (personal observation). Severe respiratory distress and pulmonary oedema occurred 24 h after Caesarean section in a patient with severe preeclampsia and thrombocytopenia (D'Angelo & Miller 1997). IPPV and renal dialysis were required for 2 and 3 months respectively. Secondary antiphospholipid antibody syndrome may occur (Kane et al 1998).

Oesophageal reflux worsens during pregnancy (Steen 1999).

Management

1. Assessment of respiratory function, including lung function tests and blood gases, if there is pulmonary involvement. There is a suggestion that bronchoalveolar lavage may help to identify patients with active alveolitis.

2. Adequate venous access may require the use of a central vein or a venous cutdown. Vasoconstriction can be reduced by keeping the theatre temperature high and by warming intravenous fluids.

3. If arterial cannulation is considered, Allen's test should be performed to assess the adequacy of the ulnar blood supply (Stafford et al 1998).

4. Precautions should be taken against acid aspiration.

5. Potential difficulties posed by tracheal intubation should be assessed preoperatively. Under certain circumstances, the possibility of an awake intubation, or tracheostomy under local anaesthesia will need to be considered.

6. Problems in measuring the blood pressure may be overcome by the use of an ultrasonic blood pressure device. If direct monitoring is essential, and Allen's test suggests that the ulnar circulation is impaired, a larger artery should be chosen.

7. Pregnancy requires careful antenatal evaluation and discussion of potential problems, particularly cardiovascular and renal disease. Renal crisis should be treated aggressively with ACE inhibitors. For Caesarean section, the choice between a general or regional technique may be difficult. Successful epidural anaesthesia was reported in a patient with advanced systemic sclerosis and the CREST syndrome (Thompson & Conklin 1983). Spinal anaesthesia has also been reported (Bailey et al 1999). A coagulation screen should be performed, and care taken with the dose of local anaesthetic used. Oesophageal reflux should be treated.

Bibliography

Arroliga AC, Podell DN, Matthay RA 1992 Pulmonary manifestations of scleroderma. Journal of Thoracic Imaging 7: 30–45.

Bailey AR, Wolmarans M, Rhodes S 1999 Spinal anaesthesia for Caesarean section in a patient with systemic sclerosis. Anaesthesia 54: 355–8.

Chin KA, Kaseba CM, Weaver JB 1995 Mallory-Weiss syndrome complicating pregnancy in a patient with scleroderma: diagnosis and management. British Journal of Obstetrics & Gynaecology 102: 498–500.

Clements PJ, Furst DE, Cabeen W et al 1981 The relationship of arrhythmias and conduction disturbances to other manifestations of cardiopulmonary disease in progressive systemic sclerosis. American Journal of Medicine 71: 38–46.

D'Angelo R, Miller R 1997 Pregnancy complicated by severe pre-eclampsia and thrombocytopenia in a patient with scleroderma. Anesthesia & Analgesia 85: 839–41.

Davidson-Lamb RW, Finlayson MCK 1977 Scleroderma: complications encountered during dental anaesthesia. Anaesthesia 32: 893–5.

Eisele JH, Reitan JA 1971 Scleroderma, Raynaud's phenomenon, and local anesthesics. Anesthesiology 34: 386–7.

Follansbee WP, Zerbe TR, Medsger TA Jr 1993 Cardiac and skeletal muscle disease in systemic sclerosis (scleroderma): a high risk association. American Heart Journal 125: 194–203.

Kane D, McSweeney F, Swan N et al 1998 Catastrophic antiphospholipid syndrome in primary systemic sclerosis. Journal of Rheumatology 25: 810–12.

Kihira C, Mizutani H, Shimizu M 1995 Sinus arrest during gastric cancer operation in a progressive systemic sclerosis patient. Journal of Dermatology 22: 357–9.

Lee P, Langevitz P, Alderdice CA et al 1992 Mortality in systemic sclerosis (scleroderma). Quarterly Journal of Medicine 82: 139–48.

Lewis GB 1974 Prolonged regional analgesia in scleroderma. Canadian Anaesthetists' Society Journal 21: 495–7.

McHugh NJ 1994 Systemic sclerosis: HLA antigens, autoantibodies and the brain. British Journal of Rheumatology 33: 323–6.

Rapp MF, Guram M, Konrad HR et al 1991 Laryngeal involvement in scleroderma. Otolaryngology—Head & Neck Surgery 104: 362–5.

Schady W, Sheard A, Hassell A et al 1991 Peripheral nerve dysfunction in scleroderma. Quarterly Journal of Medicine 80: 661–75.

Silver RM, Miller KS, Kinsella MB et al 1990 Evaluation and management of scleroderma lung disease using bronchiolar lavage. American Journal of Medicine 88: 470–6.

Stafford L, Englert H, Gover J et al 1998 Distribution of macrovascular disease in scleroderma. Annals of the Rheumatic Diseases 57: 476–9.

Steen VD 1999 Pregnancy in women with systemic sclerosis. Obstetrics & Gynecology 94: 15–20.

Thompson J, Conklin KA 1983 Anesthetic management of a pregnant patient with scleroderma. Anesthesiology 59: 69–71.

Younker D, Harrison B 1985 Scleroderma and pregnancy. Anaesthetic considerations. British Journal of Anaesthesia 57: 1136–9.

Scoliosis

A lateral curvature of the spine occurring in association with actual rotation of the vertebral body and spine, in the direction of the concavity of the curve. There is wedging of the vertebral body and discs. The resulting prominence of the posterior part of the ribs on the side of the convexity may give a false impression of kyphosis.

Scoliosis can be broadly divided into three categories, the commonest of which is the idiopathic form. Otherwise, scoliosis may be congenital, or may develop as a secondary feature of a variety of neuromuscular or connective tissue disorders. Causes of secondary scoliosis include poliomyelitis, syringomyelia, Friedreich's ataxia, muscular dystrophy, neurofibromatosis, Marfan's syndrome, and rheumatoid arthritis.

Scoliosis is described in terms of its angle (Cobb angle). The greater the angle, the more severe the respiratory and subsequent cardiovascular impairment. Surgery is indicated when angulation exceeds 50 degrees in the thoracic spine and 40 degrees in the lumbar spine.

Preoperative abnormalities

1. *Respiratory changes.* Respiratory impairment in scoliosis results from a number of factors. These include abnormalities in the development of the rib cage, the muscles of respiration, and in the distribution of the pulmonary vascular bed in relation to the alveoli. Respiratory impairment is usually restrictive, the vital capacity, total lung capacity, and functional residual capacity being 60–80% of that predicted. As the severity of the scoliosis increases, airway closure encroaches on the functional residual capacity. The greater the angle of scoliosis, the greater the abnormalities in lung function. Gas exchange is impaired as a result of ventilation/blood flow inequalities, and it has been suggested that the greater maldistribution is on the side of the concavity. A Pao_2 reduction occurs initially, and may deteriorate further with

increasing age. The respiratory response to CO_2 is abnormal, and pulmonary vascular resistance may be elevated. Subsequently, hypercapnoea may develop. Initially, the abnormalities may occur only during sleep, and studies have shown a decreased vital capacity, hypoxia and respiratory failure in some patients at night.

2. *Cardiovascular changes.* In the more severe cases, increased pulmonary vascular resistance is secondary to a combination of structural changes in the pulmonary vascular bed and the effects of hypoxia. An increased pulmonary vascular pressure results. In the later stages, the ECG will show signs of right atrial dilatation (P wave >2.5 mm in height), and right ventricular hypertrophy (R > S in leads V1 and V2). Right ventricular failure secondary to pulmonary disease may finally ensue.

3. *Associated problems.*

a) Neuropathic: poliomyelitis, Friedreich's ataxia, syringomyelia.

b) Myopathic: muscular dystrophy, spinal muscular atrophy.

c) Miscellaneous: neurofibromatosis, Marfan's syndrome, rheumatoid arthritis.

Anaesthetic problems

Surgery may be incidental, or for correction of the scoliosis. In general, the prognosis for patients with secondary scoliosis is less good than for the idiopathic form. Death from cardiac failure occurred in the seventh hour of a scoliosis correction in a 13-year-old patient with DMD (Sethna et al 1988). Another death was reported in a retrospective review of nine cases of DMD and one of Becker's muscle dystrophy, undergoing spinal fusion. The particular patient had a VC of only 12% of that predicted and could not be weaned from the ventilator (Milne & Rosales 1982).

Surgery in general

1. Problems attributable to the underlying cause, if the scoliosis is not idiopathic.

2. Respiratory problems depend upon the degree of existing impairment. An already decreased respiratory response to CO_2 may be made worse by the anaesthetic. Whilst mild hypoxia is common, the onset of hypercarbia, unless precipitated by an acute infection, is a bad prognostic sign. A biphasic CO_2 excretion waveform was demonstrated in a severe kyphoscoliotic during IPPV. This was thought to result from the patient having two lungs with entirely different mechanics. The early peak represented the appearance of exhaled gas from well-ventilated regions of the lung with low airway resistance having a relatively low CO_2 concentration, followed by that from poorly ventilated areas with high airway resistance having high CO_2 concentrations (Nichols & Benumof 1989).

3. As a result of the anatomical changes, the respiratory muscles function at a mechanical disadvantage, so that postoperative respiratory inadequacy and retention of secretions is common.

4. In advanced cases, there may be the problems of pulmonary hypertension and right ventricular failure. Cardiac abnormalities, including hypertrophic cardiomyopathy and conduction defects, occur in 90% of patients with Friedreich's ataxia.

5. In DMD there may be hypertrophic cardiomyopathy and diastolic failure. Some patients develop mitral valve prolapse. Marfan's syndrome can be associated with mitral or aortic regurgitation, dissecting aortic aneurysm, aortic or pulmonary dilatation, or coronary artery disease.

6. Hyperkalaemia following the use of suxamethonium has been reported in patients with neuromuscular problems, particularly in conditions in which there is a motor deficit.

7. Rhabdomyolysis and myoglobinuria may occur after suxamethonium or halothane in patients with myopathies.

8. Serious arrhythmias and cardiac arrest have been described following the use of halothane and suxamethonium in DMD (see also Duchenne muscular dystrophy).

9. Satisfactory regional anaesthesia, which is particularly indicated during labour, may be difficult to achieve because of anatomical distortion of the spinal column, and uneven spread of local anaesthetic (Moran & Johnson 1990).

Surgery for scoliosis

1. Inadequate preoperative respiratory reserve has resulted in deaths in patients subjected to surgery for scoliosis.

2. Evaluation of spinal cord function may be required after spinal distraction with Harrington rods. It may be necessary to waken the patient during the procedure, so that motor deficits can be detected and the spinal distraction decreased. The use of evoked cortical responses is also undertaken, although these have not always been reliable. Complications of monitoring the transcervical motor evoked potentials have been reported. Severe hypotension occurred during stimulation for motor evoked potentials, but stopped after the transcervical needle electrodes were repositioned. It was thought that the electrodes had been displaced when the position of the patient had been changed, such that they were stimulating sympathetic pathways (Hays & Schwengel 1999). In another, an artefact appeared on the ECG, which was treated as an SVT with adenosine (Chowdry et al 1998).

3. Blood loss may be substantial. Losses of up to 92% of the patient's blood volume have been recorded (Abott & Bentley 1980). Patients with DMD appear to bleed more than those with other conditions (Noordeen et al 1999).

4. Deliberate hypotensive techniques have been associated with a decrease in blood supply to the spinal cord and subsequent paraplegia.

5. The problems of surgery performed in the prone position. In patients with severe kyphoscoliosis, compression of the trachea, both at its midpoint (Mesrobian & Epps 1986), and at

the thoracic inlet (Bagshaw & Jardine 1995), has occurred in the prone position. Rittoo and Morris (1995) also reported complete tracheal obstruction and bronchoscopy confirmed a slit-like narrowing of the lower trachea distal to the tube, thought to be secondary to compression against the vertebral bodies. Aggressive manipulation of, or downward pressure upon, the thoracic spine by the surgeon may cause hypotension secondary to compression of the heart and great vessels (Bagshaw & Jardine 1995). Should cardiac arrest occur, resuscitation is difficult (Irwin & Henderson 1995, Reid & Appleton 1999).

6. Hypothermia may occur in prolonged procedures and when extensive blood loss has been replaced.

7. Haemopneumothorax.

8. Two fatal cases of air embolism have been reported during posterior spinal fusion and instrumentation (McCarthy et al 1990).

Management

Surgery in general

1. Respiratory assessment should include the VC measured in both seated and supine positions, FEV with and without bronchodilators, CXR, and blood gases.

2. Cardiovascular assessment. ECG and echocardiography may be needed. If the PVR and PAP are increased, and there are ECG changes and signs of RVH, then the prognosis is poor. Right ventricular failure must be treated.

3. In severe disease, a decision must be made as to whether or not elective surgery should be undertaken. A VC <50% predicted suggests a need for postoperative ventilation, should major surgery be required.

4. If possible, regional or local anaesthesia should be utilised.

5. Monitoring should include ECG, core temperature, $ETCO_2$, and blood pressure,

directly or indirectly. When indicated, urine output, central venous pressure, blood gases, and occasionally PAP monitoring may be required.

6. Regional anaesthesia should be considered (Sethna & Berde 1991), although technical difficulties may be encountered. Continuous spinal anaesthesia using combined hyperbaric and hypobaric bupivacaine was used after failed epidural anaesthesia during labour (Moran & Johnson 1990).

Surgery for scoliosis

1. A VC of at least $20\,ml\,kg^{-1}$ or 30% of predicted, and an inspiratory capacity of $15\,ml\,kg^{-1}$, have been suggested as being essential for scoliosis surgery (Milne & Rosales 1982). If respiratory reserve is <50% predicted, postoperative ventilation will be required. A VC >70% suggests that respiratory reserve is adequate (Winkler et al 1998).

2. The tracheal tube must be firmly secured.

3. A wake-up test, the earliest form of spinal cord monitoring, can be performed, provided the patient is a suitable subject and the matter has been discussed in advance.

4. More recently, the sensory-evoked potentials (SEP) and motor-evoked potentials (MEP) have been used both alone, and in conjunction with the wake-up test, to detect neurological damage (Loughnan & Fennelly 1995, Padberg et al 1998).

5. Theatre temperature should be maintained at a higher than usual level, and a warming blanket and blood warmer used.

6. A variety of techniques have been used when blood loss is predicted to be high. These include predonation, acute normovolaemic haemodilution, and intraoperative cell salvage (Anand et al 1998).

7. The use of deliberate hypotension should be carefully considered.

8. If the anterior approach through the

diaphragm is used, postoperative IPPV may be required.

Bibliography

Abott TR, Bentley G 1980 Intra-operative awakening during scoliosis surgery. Anaesthesia 35: 298–302.

Anand N, Idio FG Jr, Remer S et al 1998 The effects of perioperative blood salvage and autologous blood donation on transfusion requirements in scoliosis surgery. Journal of Spinal Disorders 11: 532–4.

Bagshaw ONT, Jardine A 1995 Cardiopulmonary complications during anaesthesia and surgery for severe thoracic lordoscoliosis. Anaesthesia 50: 890–2.

Chamberlain ME, Bradshaw EG 1985 The 'wake-up test'. Anaesthesia 40: 780–2.

Chowdry DK, Stayer SA, Rehman MA et al 1998 Electrocardiographic artefact with SSEP monitoring unit during scoliosis surgery. Paediatric Anaesthesia 8: 341–3.

Hays SR, Schwengel DA 1999 Transient hypotension as a complication of monitoring transcervical motor evoked potentials. Anesthesiology 90: 314–17.

Irwin MG, Henderson M 1995 Cardiac arrest during major spinal surgery in a patient with Duchenne's muscular dystrophy undergoing intravenous anaesthesia. Anaesthesia & Intensive Care 23: 626–9.

Loughnan BA, Fennelly ME 1995 Spinal cord monitoring. Anaesthesia 50: 101–2.

McCarthy RE, Lonstein JE, Mertz JD et al 1990 Air embolism in spinal surgery. Journal of Spinal Disorders 3: 1–5.

Mesrobian RB, Epps JL 1986 Midtracheal obstruction after Harrington rod placement in a patient with Marfan's syndrome. Anesthesia & Analgesia 65: 411–13.

Milne B, Rosales JK 1982 Anaesthetic considerations in patients with muscular dystrophy undergoing spinal fusion and Harrington rod insertion. Canadian Anaesthetists' Society Journal 29: 250–4.

Moran DH, Johnson MD 1990 Continuous spinal anesthesia with combined hyperbaric and hypobaric bupivacaine in a patient with scoliosis. Anesthesia & Analgesia 70: 445–7.

Nichols KP, Benumof JL 1989 Biphasic carbon dioxide excretion waveform from a patient with severe kyphoscoliosis. Anesthesiology 71: 986–7.

Noordeen MH, Haddad FS, Muntoni F et al 1999 Blood loss in Duchenne muscular dystrophy:

vascular smooth muscle dysfunction. Journal of Pediatric Orthopedics. Part B 8: 212–15.

Padberg AM, Wilson-Holden TJ, Lenke LG et al 1998 Somatosensory- and motor-evoked potential monitoring without a wake-up test during idiopathic scoliosis surgery. Spine 23: 1392–400.

Reid JM, Appleton PJ 1999 A case of ventricular fibrillation in the prone position during back stabilisation surgery in a boy with Duchenne's muscular dystrophy. Anaesthesia 54: 364–7.

Rittoo DB, Morris P 1995 Tracheal occlusion in the prone position in an intubated patient with Duchenne muscular dystrophy. Anaesthesia 50: 719–21.

Sethna NF, Berde CB 1991 Continuous subarachnoid analgesia in two adolescents with severe scoliosis and impaired pulmonary function. Regional Anesthesia 16: 333–6.

Sethna NF, Rockoff MA, Worthen HM et al 1988 Anesthesia related complications in children with Duchenne muscular dystrophy. Anesthesiology 68: 462–5.

Winkler M, Marker E, Hetz H 1998 The perioperative management of major orthopaedic procedures. Anaesthesia 53 (suppl 2): 37–41.

461

Shy–Drager syndrome (see Multiple system atrophy and Autonomic failure)

Sick sinus syndrome

(bradycardia/tachycardia syndrome)

A general term for various disorders of sino-atrial node function which usually present in the elderly, but can sometimes occur in young people. There is ECG evidence of sinus node dysfunction in combination with symptoms of cerebral or coronary insufficiency. Patients may have a sinus bradycardia and periods of sinus arrest with escape rhythms, and sometimes intermittent episodes of tachyarrhythmias (the bradycardia/tachycardia syndrome). The sino-atrial node is under autonomic control and is a small area of specialised muscle situated at the junction of the superior vena cava and the base of the right atrial appendage. Its arterial supply is variable, arising from the right coronary artery in 65%, and the left circumflex artery in 35%, of individuals. Dysfunction of the node most commonly results from its replacement by fibrous tissue. Other causes include coronary artery disease, drugs, and postcardiac surgery. For symptomatic patients, the use of atrial rather than dual pacing is now established as best practice (Marshall et al 1998). Ventricular pacing has been shown to be associated with a higher incidence of heart failure, consumption of diuretics, atrial fibrillation, and thromboembolism, than atrial pacing (Andersen et al 1994).

Preoperative abnormalities

1. A typical patient is commonly older than 60 years, and may complain of episodes of syncope, dizziness or palpitations, and extreme tiredness. A 24-h ambulatory ECG may show episodes of brady- or tachyarrhythmias which may be asymptomatic, but may coincide with the symptoms. Occasionally young people are affected, and this form may be familial. A group of nine people below the age of 25 with sino-atrial disease has been studied (Mackintosh 1981). They were all male, taller than average, and ambulatory monitoring of close relatives revealed an increased incidence of conducting system disorders.

2. Episodes of arrhythmia may cause fatigue, syncope, or precipitate angina or cardiac failure.

3. There is an inappropriate heart rate in response to stress or drugs. Patients cannot increase their rate in response to exercise. Often there is a sinus bradycardia of <60 beat min^{-1} during the awake state.

4. ECG may show alternate brady- and tachyarrhythmias. In sino-atrial block, P waves are dropped intermittently and the RR intervals are multiples of cycle length.

5. Electrophysiological tests may occasionally be required if the diagnosis is in doubt. Recently, an adenosine challenge test has been described (Sorrentino 1999).

6. There is an increased risk of atrial fibrillation and thromboembolism.

Anaesthetic problems

1. The occurrence of brady- or tachyarrhythmias during anaesthesia may reduce cardiac output and compromise cerebral or coronary artery circulation. A number of such episodes have been described during both spinal and general anaesthesia. Sinus bradycardias unresponsive to repeated doses of atropine or glycopyrronium (Pratila & Pratilas 1976, Levy 1990), recurrent episodes of sinus arrest with nodal escape (Burt 1982), and severe bradycardias (Levy 1990), have been reported. Sinus arrest occurred during gastrectomy in a 70 year old with scleroderma. A temporary pacemaker was inserted, after which she became pacemaker dependent (Kihira et al 1995). Asystole, which responded to cardiopulmonary resuscitation and atropine, occurred 10 min after administration of a spinal anaesthetic for prostatectomy in a patient with sinus bradycardia and RBBB (Cohen 1988). Several periods of asystole were reported in a 46-year-old woman, some hours after spinal anaesthesia for varicose vein surgery (Underwood & Glynn 1988). Sick sinus syndrome was diagnosed and a pacemaker inserted. Subsequent questioning revealed that the patient had a history of blackouts, usually related to vomiting.

2. A high incidence (15.3%) of systemic embolism has been reported in this syndrome. For this reason, the patient may already be anticoagulated.

3. Bradycardias associated with sick sinus syndrome, that do not respond to anticholinergics, should be distinguished from those that are secondary to drugs given during general anaesthesia, or which sometimes occur during regional block (Corr & Thomas 1989). These bradycardias are often precipitated by the use of drugs such as fentanyl and vecuronium, and they will respond to normal doses of atropine or glycopyrronium.

Management

1. Twenty-four-hour ambulatory monitoring

may be required to confirm the diagnosis. If there is inadequate time, and the diagnosis is in doubt, then the response of the patient to atropine may be tested. In a normal subject, atropine iv $0.02\,\mathrm{mg\,kg^{-1}}$ should increase the heart rate by more than 14 beat $\mathrm{min^{-1}}$.

2. If sick sinus syndrome is diagnosed, a temporary pacemaker should be inserted before anaesthesia. Halothane and enflurane may prolong conduction, and impair the ability of the myocardium to maintain cardiac output by increasing stroke volume. Under these circumstances there is no guarantee that cerebral or coronary perfusion will be adequate. Patients who are symptomatic are given a permanent atrial pacemaker rather than a dual chamber one.

3. Anticoagulation may be required after surgery.

Bibliography

Andersen HR, Thuesen L, Bagger JP et al 1994 Prospective randomised trial of atrial versus ventricular pacing in sick-sinus syndrome. Lancet 344: 1523–8.

Burt DER 1982 The sick sinus syndrome. A complication during anaesthesia. Anaesthesia 37: 1108–11.

Cohen LI 1988 Asystole during spinal anesthesia in a patient with sick sinus syndrome. Anesthesiology 68: 787–8.

Corr CS, Thomas DA 1989 Sick sinus syndrome manifest after spinal anaesthesia. Anaesthesia 44: 179.

Kihara C, Mizutani H, Shimizu M 1995 Sinus arrest during gastric cancer operation in a progressive systemic sclerosis patient. Journal of Dermatology 22: 357–9.

Levy DM 1990 Recurrent bradycardia due to latent sick sinus syndrome. Anaesthesia 45: 488–9.

Mackintosh AF 1981 Sinuatrial disease in young people. British Heart Journal 45: 62–6.

Marshall HJ, Gammage MD, Griffith MJ 1998 AAI pacing for sick sinus syndrome: first choice on all counts. Heart 80: 315–16.

Pratila MG, Pratilas V 1976 Sick-sinus syndrome manifest during anesthesia. Anesthesiology 44: 433–6.

Shaw DB, Holman RR, Gowers JI 1980 Survival in sinoatrial disorders (sick-sinus syndrome). British Medical Journal 280: 139–41.

Sorrentino RA 1999 Is an adenosine challenge a useful test for diagnosing sick sinus syndrome? American Heart Journal 137: 435–8.

Underwood SM, Glynn CJ 1988 Sick sinus syndrome manifest after spinal anaesthesia. Anaesthesia 43: 307–9.

Sipple's syndrome (MEN 2a) (see also Multiple endocrine neoplasia)

One of a group of dominantly inherited cancer syndromes associated with mutations of tumour suppressor genes. MEN is defined as the occurrence of tumours in two or more endocrine glands (Thakker 1998). In MEN 2a, medullary carcinoma of the thyroid is frequently associated with phaeochromocytoma, and, less commonly, with a parathyroid adenoma. It is caused by mutations of the receptor tyrosine kinase (RET) proto-oncogene on chromosome 10. First degree relatives have a 50% risk of developing the disease. There are three variants, of which MEN 2a is the most common.

Preoperative abnormalities

1. A thyroid mass may be associated with symptoms of hoarseness, dysphagia, cough, and cervical lymphadenopathy. Can present any time between the ages of 20 and 70 (Heath 1998).

2. The tumour may secrete a number of hormones including calcitonin, serotonin, prostaglandins and ACTH/MSH, or insulin. Symptoms depend upon the hormone secreted.

3. Fifty percent of cases have a phaeochromocytoma and 70% of these are bilateral. Regular screening of urinary metanephrines is required.

4. A parathyroid adenoma is present in 20% of cases.

5. Metastases may occur to the liver, lungs, and bone.

6. In many cases, a family history is present, but not elicited, or the significance is not recognised (Nishikawa et al 1993).

Anaesthetic problems

1. Those of a phaeochromocytoma crisis. Adult respiratory distress syndrome was the initial presentation in a 43-year-old woman. Asystole, from which she could not be resuscitated, occurred soon after tracheal intubation. Postmortem showed thyroid carcinoma, phaeochromocytoma, and a hypertrophied left ventricle (Van der Kleij 1999). A 65-year-old woman presented with multiple organ failure, pulmonary oedema and coma; a hypertensive crisis, with VT and VF, occurred on day 8. After successful removal of a phaeochromocytoma, a thyroid carcinoma was detected (Lorz et al 1993). Treatment of thyrotoxic symptoms with propranolol precipitated a hypertensive crisis in a patient who was found to have a phaeochromocytoma (Blodgett & Reasner 1990). The family history was later elicited. Extreme levels of catecholamines were thought to have been responsible for the increased levels of thyroid hormones.

2. Pregnancy may occur in patients with, or without, phaeochromocytoma (Van Der Vaart et al 1993, Wax et al 1997). A hypertensive crisis, precipitated by attempts at pharmacological manipulation of severe hypertension (phentolamine followed by norepinephrine (noradrenaline)) at 16 weeks' gestation, resulted in intrauterine death and a coagulopathy. There was a strong family history (Nishikawa et al 1993). In a pregnant patient with known Sipple's syndrome, elective Caesarean section was combined with removal of phaeochromocytoma, whilst thyroidectomy with block dissection of the neck was carried out 3 weeks later (Palot et al 1991).

3. Cardiovascular complications, if hormones such as serotonin or prostaglandins are secreted.

Management

1. Exclude the presence of a phaeochromocytoma. If present, preoperative preparation will be required (see Phaeochromocytoma).

Bibliography

Blodgett J, Reasner CA 1990 Transient thyrotoxicosis associated with a pheochromocytoma in a patient with multiple endocrine neoplasia type IIa. American Journal of Medicine 88: 302–3.

Heath D 1998 Multiple endocrine neoplasia. Journal of the Royal Society of Physicians of London 32: 98–101.

Lorz W, Cottier Chr, Imhof E et al 1993 Multiple organ failure and coma as initial presentation of pheochromocytoma in a patient with multiple endocrine neoplasia (MEN) type II A. Intensive Care Medicine 19: 235–8.

Nishikawa K, Yukioka H, Tatekawa S et al 1993 Phaeochromocytoma crisis in Sipple's syndrome with intrauterine death and disseminated intravascular coagulation. International Journal of Obstetric Anesthesia 2: 45–8.

Palot M, Burde A, Quereux C et al 1991 [Anesthesia for cesarean section and excision of pheochromocytoma caused by Sipple's syndrome. English abstract.] Annales Francaises d'Anesthesie et de Reanimation 10: 84–7.

Thakker RV 1998 Multiple endocrine neoplasia—syndromes of the twentieth century. Journal of Clinical Endocrinology & Metabolism 83: 2617–20.

Van der Kleij FGH 1999 Adult respiratory distress syndrome due to phaeochromocytoma as the initial presentation of multiple endocrine neoplasia type IIA syndrome. American Journal of Medicine 107: 401.

Van Der Vaart CH, Heronga MP, Dullaart RPF et al 1993 Multiple endocrine neoplasia presenting as phaeochromocytoma during pregnancy. British Journal of Obstetrics & Gynaecology 100: 1144–5.

Wax JR, Eggleston MK Jr, Teague KE 1997 Pregnancy complicated by multiple endocrine neoplasia type IIa (Sipple's syndrome). American Journal of Obstetrics & Gynecology 177: 461–2.

Sjögren's syndrome

A chronic inflammatory autoimmune disease, which results in drying of secretions, and involves a number of exocrine organs, in particular the lacrimal and salivary glands. There is intense lymphocytic infiltration of the tissues. Sjögren's may be primary or secondary. About 75% of cases are secondary to a connective tissue disorder, of which the commonest is rheumatoid arthritis. In the secondary form the glandular element is relatively mild, but in the primary disease, infiltration of the salivary and lacrimal glands predominates, and there may be considerable swelling, accompanied by extreme dryness of the eyes and mouth. Occasionally, in association with lymphadenopathy, this type may proceed to malignant lymphoma.

Preoperative abnormalities

1. Symptoms of the sicca syndrome include dryness of the eyes, mouth, vagina, and skin.

2. Conditions associated with the secondary form include rheumatoid arthritis, systemic lupus, scleroderma, the polymyositis/dermatomyositis complex, polyarteritis nodosa, chronic active hepatitis, and Grave's disease.

3. Swelling of the salivary and lacrimal glands may be prominent.

4. Lung complications are being detected more often, because of the greater sensitivity of tests of pulmonary disease (Cain et al 1998). Dessication of the nose and bronchial tree, obstructive airways disease particularly affecting the small airways (Papiris et al 1999), and interstitial lung disease, are the most common (Gardiner 1993). Lymphomas may develop.

5. Kidney, liver, pancreas and lymphoid tissue are other major organs at risk.

6. Either a sensory or motor neuropathy may occur and CNS lesions have been described.

7. The patient may be taking corticosteroids or occasionally immunosuppressive agents.

Anaesthetic problems

1. Occasionally, gross swelling of the salivary glands may make mask anaesthesia difficult.

2. Those of the primary disease (see Section 1, Rheumatoid arthritis, Scleroderma and Systemic lupus erythematosus).

3. The problems of pulmonary disease, if present.

4. The dry eyes are susceptible to damage during anaesthesia.

5. Allergy to antimicrobial agents, particularly penicillin, cephalosporins and trimethoprim, was found to be more common in patients with Sjögren's disease than in a group of osteoarthritis patients (Antonen et al 1999).

Management

1. If the patient's Sjögren's syndrome is secondary to another disorder, there should be careful assessment of the primary disease, and of any pulmonary involvement.

2. Drying agents should be avoided if possible.

3. The eyes should be protected with pads.

4. Anaesthetic gases should be humidified.

5. Steroid supplements may be required.

6. Care should be taken when prescribing antimicrobial agents.

Bibliography
Antonen JA, Markula KP, Pertovaara MI et al 1999 Adverse drug reactions in Sjögren's syndrome. Scandinavian Journal of Rheumatology 28: 157–9.
Cain HC, Noble PW, Matthay RA 1998 Pulmonary manifestations of Sjögren's syndrome. Clinics in Chest Medicine 19: 687–9.
Gardiner P 1993 Primary Sjögren's syndrome. Bailliere's Clinical Rheumatology 7: 59–71.
Papiris SA, Maniati M, Constantopoulos SH et al 1999 Lung involvement in primary Sjögren's syndrome is mainly related to the small airway disease. Annals of the Rheumatic Diseases 58: 61–4.

Solvent and volatile substance abuse

Volatile substances can be divided into two groups, according to their state at room temperature. Those that are liquid at room temperature include toluene-containing adhesives, cleaning agents and typewriter correction fluids, whereas pressurised aerosols and butane cigarette lighter refills are classified as 'gaseous'. The incidence of solvent abuse was common in Britain in the 1980s but peaked in 1990, probably as a result of education (Esmail et al 1992). An epidemiological study reported 282 deaths in the period 1971–83, and 80 deaths in 1983 (Anderson et al 1985). The latter represented 2% of all deaths in males between the ages of 10 and 19 years. Fifty-one percent of the deaths were attributed to direct toxic effects, 21% to plastic bag asphyxia, 18% to inhaled gastric contents, and 11% to trauma. However, in the late 1980s, deaths from solvents started to decrease, but those from butane refills/aerosols ('gaseous') agents continued to increase (Esmail et al 1992). In 1997, butane inhalation was the cause of death in 56% of cases (Edwards & Wenstone 2000).

Sudden death during 'sniffing' or 'huffing' is thought to result from arrhythmias associated with the sensitisation of the heart to the effect of endogenous catecholamines, by the inhaled volatile hydrocarbon (Cunningham et al 1987). Death is likely to occur more commonly, therefore, during periods of intense cardiac stimulation such as exercise. Animal studies with inhaled hydrocarbons would seem to confirm this. Serious ventricular arrhythmias can be provoked by both exogenous and endogenous catecholamines. Once an arrhythmia develops, the victim's heart becomes more resistant to resuscitation and the risk of a sudden arrhythmia remains for some hours after inhalation has taken place (Ashton 1990, Adgey et al 1995, Williams & Cole 1998, Edwards & Wenstone 2000). Conventional advanced CPR may therefore not be appropriate if an arrest is known to be secondary to volatile substance abuse, because the use of high doses of epinephrine (adrenaline) may worsen the situation (Adgey et al 1995).

Volatile hydrocarbons also have chronic effects on the liver, kidney, lung, and brain. Chronic cardiotoxicity may also occur (Boon 1987, Marjot 1989).

It has been suggested that interactions can occur with halothane, whose chemical structure closely resembles that of 1,1,1-trichloroethane (McLeod et al 1987).

Typical products inhaled include glues, dry cleaning agents, nail polish, paint thinners, antifreeze, lighter fuel, aerosol propellants for spray cans, and degreasing agents.

Preoperative abnormalities

1. Agents most frequently encountered:

a) Toluene ($C_6H_5CH_3$). A solvent in cements and glues. Cardiac arrhythmias are common during inhalation, and the most frequent cause of death is cardiac arrest precipitated by exercise.

b) 1,1,1-Trichloroethane. An industrial cleaning solvent and paint remover. Is present in Tippex fluid thinner, audiovisual equipment cleaners, glues, adhesive plaster removers, and degreasing agents used in steel welding. Sudden deaths can occur either with solvent abuse or following industrial accidents. Cardiac arrhythmias can occur at the time of abuse, but may also persist for up to 2 weeks after the exposure. It has now been shown that this agent can cause chronic cardiac damage, and that there may be provocation of symptoms of cardiac toxicity when re-exposure to the agent, or to chemically similar substances, occurs.

c) Butane from lighter fuel.

d) Fluorocarbons used as propellants in spray cans.

2. The abuser is most likely to be a teenager, 13–15 years being the peak age. There is a high incidence from social class V, and from the armed forces (Anderson et al 1985). Perioral eczema, erythematous spots around the nose and chronic inflammation of the upper respiratory tract may suggest repeated contact with a solvent or indicate the use of a plastic bag.

3. Cardiac arrhythmias may be noticed preoperatively; the risk of sudden arrhythmias lasts for some hours after the episode of abuse. A patient with severe hypertension, recurrent non-Q-wave myocardial infarction, and an ion gap acidosis with hypokalaemia (K^+ 2.8 mmol^{-1}) was found to be secretly sniffing an industrial solvent containing toluene (Hussain et al 1996).

4. There is evidence that long-term abuse may result in damage to a number of organs including the kidney, liver, heart, and lung (Marjot & McLeod 1989).

5. Toluene abuse is also associated with a variety of neurological effects including cognitive and behavioural changes, chronic pyschosis, temporal lobe epilepsy, a decreased IQ, and peripheral neuropathy (Byrne et al 1991, White & Proctor 1997).

Anaesthetic and resuscitative problems

1. *Cardiac arrhythmias during anaesthesia.* Cardiac problems in two patients chronically exposed to 1,1,1-trichloroethane were attributed to an interaction with halothane during anaesthesia (McLeod et al 1987). The first, a 14-year-old boy, developed multiple ventricular extrasystoles and ventricular tachycardia during tonsillectomy. The arrhythmias persisted postoperatively and needed treatment with a number of antiarrhythmic drugs. At one stage a pacemaker was required. Evidence of 1,1,1-trichloroethane abuse was subsequently found. The second was a 55-year-old man who had previously developed AF and cardiac failure. This was diagnosed as secondary to industrial exposure to 1,1,1-trichloroethane in the steel industry. He was removed from exposure and his condition did not worsen. Two years later, and following an anaesthetic (halothane, but no details), he became symptomatic. Echocardiography and myocardial biopsy indicated a deterioration in cardiac function of recent onset. Since halothane is similar in structure to 1,1,1-trichloroethane, it was postulated that this was reponsible for the cardiac problems encountered in both cases.

2. *Difficulties in resuscitation from the arrested state.* In most individuals, sudden death occurs because of the absence of resuscitation facilities. In those reached before death, VF seems to be the commonest arrest arrhythmia, although asystolic cardiac arrest has also been documented after butane inhalation (Roberts et al 1990). Out of hospital defibrillation was performed in a 15-year-old girl, but she had a severe residual neurological deficit (Williams & Cole 1998). It has been suggested that the use of high-dose epinephrine (adrenaline) for resuscitation from VF caused by volatile substance abuse may be harmful (Adgey et al 1995). A 17 year old man, after collapse following the use of butane lighter fuel, had recurrent episodes of VF for which he required 27 DC shocks. Circulation returned 10 min after receiving amiodarone 300 mg iv (Edwards & Wenstone 2000). After a stormy ITU course, with a myocardial infarction, recurrent pulmonary oedema and renal failure, he recovered without neurological deficit, but with an apical cardiac aneurysm.

3. *Chronic cardiac damage.* A cardiomyopathy developed in a 15-year-old boy, who had a 2-year history of solvent abuse with toluene-containing substances. He subsequently required cardiac transplantation (Wiseman & Banim 1987).

4. One patient presented with acute upper respiratory tract obstruction after inhalation of a propellant (Kuhn & Lassen 1999).

5. Intractable vomiting occurs in about 25% of butane gas overdoses and may result in pulmonary aspiration (Roberts et al 1990).

6. Acute psychosis may occur in the recovery period after resuscitation following toxicity associated with cardiopulmonary arrest (Roberts et al 1990).

7. Fatal cerebral oedema and tonsillar herniation has been reported after trichloroethane abuse (D'Costa & Gunasekera 1990).

8. Rhabdomyolysis, hyperchloraemic metabolic acidosis and quadriplegia occurred in a chronic glue sniffer (Hong et al 1996).

9. Toluene vapour abuse during pregnancy is associated with morbidity in both mother and child (Wilkins-Haug & Gabow 1991). Renal tubular acidosis, hypokalaemia, arrhythmias and rhabdomyolysis occurred in the women, and prematurity, growth retardation, craniofacial abnormalities and sometimes death amongst the infants (Jones & Balster 1998).

Management

1. The occurrence of unexpected arrhythmias in a teenager, particularly in the presence of spots around the mouth and nose, should alert the anaesthetist to the possibility of volatile agent abuse.

2. Continuous ECG monitoring during anaesthesia. These case reports underline the importance of ECG monitoring from the start of the anaesthetic, even in apparently fit young patients.

3. If arrest occurs, and is known to be secondary to volatile agent abuse, the resuscitation sequence should be modified. Adgey et al (1995) suggested that sympathomimetics should not be used, but beta adrenergic blockers given to protect the sensitised myocardium. They also advised avoiding early tracheal intubation in butane inhalation because of the danger of laryngospasm. However, since vomiting is a common problem, the lungs need to be protected from aspiration of gastric contents. Edwards and Wenstone (2000) have used iv amiodarone to stop recurrent VF. Treatment may be required for metabolic acidosis and hypokalaemia.

4. If gross cerebral oedema is suspected, hyperventilation and treatment with dexamethasone and mannitol should be instituted (D'Costa & Gunasekera 1990).

5. The possibility of abuse of other substances should be considered. In a US population, volatile agent abusers were 5–10 times more likely to abuse opioids, stimulants, depressants, and hallucinogens (Dinwiddie et al 1991).

Bibliography

Adgey AAJ, Johnston PW, McMechan S 1995 Current problems in resuscitation. Sudden cardiac death and substance abuse. Resuscitation 29: 219–21.

Anderson HR, Macnair RS, Ramsey JD 1985 Deaths from abuse of volatile substances: a national epidemiological study. British Medical Journal 290: 304–7.

Ashton CH 1990 Solvent abuse. Little progress after 20 years. British Medical Journal 300: 135–6.

Boon NA 1987 Solvent abuse and the heart. British Medical Journal 294: 722.

Byrne A, Kirby B, Zibin T, Ensminger S 1991 Psychiatric and neurological effects of chronic solvent abuse. Canadian Journal of Psychiatry 36: 735–8.

Cunningham SR. Dalzell GWN, McGirr P et al 1987 Myocardial infarction and primary ventricular fibrillation after glue sniffing. British Medical Journal 294: 739–40.

D'Costa DF, Gunasekera NPR 1990 Fatal cerebral oedema following trichloroethane abuse. Journal of the Royal Society of Medicine 83: 533–4.

Dinwiddie SH, Reich T, Cloniger CR 1991 The relationship of solvent to other substance abuse. American Journal of Drug & Alcohol Abuse 17: 173–86.

Edwards KE, Wenstone R 2000 Successful resuscitation from recurrent ventricular fibrillation secondary to butane inhalation. British Journal of Anaesthesia 84: 803–5.

Esmail A, Anderson HR, Ramsey JD et al 1992 Controlling deaths from volatile substance abuse in under 18s: the effects of legislation. British Medical Journal 305: 692.

Hong JJ, Lin JL, Wu MS et al 1996 A chronic glue sniffer with hyperchloraemia, metabolic acidosis, rhabdomyolysis, irreversible quadriplegia, central pontine myelinosis, and hypothyroidism. Nephrology, Dialysis, Transplantation 11: 1848–9.

Hussain TF, Heidenreich PA, Benowitz N 1996 Recurrent non-Q-wave myocardial infarction associated with toluene abuse. American Heart Journal 131: 615–16.

Jones HE, Balster RL 1998 Inhalant abuse in pregnancy. Obstetrics & Gynecology Clinics of North America 25: 153–67.

Kuhn JJ, Lassen LF 1999 Acute upper airway obstruction after recreational inhalation of a hydrofluorocarbon propellant. Otolaryngology—Head & Neck Surgery 120: 587–90.

McLeod AA, Marjot R, Monaghan MJ et al 1987 Chronic cardiac toxicity after inhalation of 1,1,1-trichloroethane. British Medical Journal 294: 727–9.

Marjot R 1989 The relevance of volatile substance abuse to anaesthetists. Anaesthesia 44: 162–3.

Marjot R, McLeod AA 1989 Chronic non-neurological toxicity from volatile substance abuse. Human Toxicology 8: 301–6.

Roberts MJD, McIvor RA, Adgey AAJ 1990 Asystole following butane gas inhalation. British Journal of Hospital Medicine 44: 294.

White RF, Proctor SP 1997 Solvents and neurotoxicity. Lancet 349: 1239–43.

Wilkins-Haug L, Gabow PA 1991 Toluene abuse during pregnancy: obstetric complications and perinatal outcomes. Obstetrics and Gynecology 77: 504–9.

Williams DR, Cole SJ 1998 Ventricular fibrillation following butane gas inhalation. Resuscitation 37: 43–5.

Wiseman MN, Banim S 1987 'Glue sniffer's' heart. British Medical Journal 294: 739.

Spinal muscular atrophy (see also Werdnig–Hoffmann disease)

A group of diseases affecting peripheral motor neurones, usually hereditary, and associated with anterior horn degeneration. Type I is a rapidly progressive disease of infants (see Werdnig–Hoffmann disease). In type II the course is similar, but death occurs more slowly. The onset of type III is later in childhood and it runs a slower course. Type IV presents in the adult and gradually evolves (Editorial 1990, Donaghy 1999). The genes involved have been mapped, but the underlying defect is unknown.

Preoperative abnormalities

1. The proximal muscles are involved more than the distal, and lower limbs more than upper. In mild disease, there is no arm involvement. Tongue fasciculation may be present. Function deteriorates with time (Russman et al 1996).

However, in a study of 11 patients with type II spinal muscular atrophy, although all became wheelchair bound, none required ventilation (Lyager et al 1995).

2. Scoliosis occurs in all but the mildest cases and is progressive, resulting in a slow deterioration in pulmonary reserve. Its onset is before puberty, at average age 8.8 years (Phillips et al 1990). Surgical correction may be required, and this is associated with reversal of the decline in lung function.

3. A study of respiratory function in 273 patients showed difficulty in coughing, and asynchronous movements of the abdomen and chest. There were no spontaneous periods of deep breathing, and some areas of lung were perfused but not ventilated (Barois & Estournet-Mathiaud 1997).

4. One patient presented with cricoarytenoid arthritis (Thaler & Weinstein 1997).

Anaesthetic problems

1. Suxamethonium may be hazardous in these patients. Massive rhabdomyolysis (CK 252 000 u l⁻¹) and myoglobinuria in a 13-year-old boy following suxamethonium, given during dental surgery, has been encountered by the author. A diagnosis of MH was assumed, but investigation 4 years later showed the patient to be MHN. Electron microscopy suggested a subclinical spinal muscular atrophy.

2. Increased sensitivity to nondepolarising neuromuscular blockers may occur.

3. If there is bulbar muscle involvement, the risk of aspiration exists.

4. Surgery for scoliosis will halt the progression of the deformity and improve sitting, but if respiratory reserve is poor, prolonged postoperative IPPV may be required (Phillips et al 1990).

5. Weakness may worsen in pregnancy and respiration may be compromised in the third

trimester (Dahl et al 1995). In one patient, vocal cord palsy added to the problems (Weston & DiFazio 1996).

Management

1. If major surgery is undertaken, careful respiratory assessment is crucial. Neuromuscular monitoring is essential and postoperative respiratory support may be required.

2. When there is bulbar involvement, precautions should be taken to prevent postoperative aspiration.

3. The use of suxamethonium is contraindicated.

4. Pregnancy should be monitored carefully for deterioration in lung function. Anaesthetists and neurologists should be involved at an early stage and a plan for delivery documented. Regional anaesthesia has been used for labour. Two parturients with type III spinal muscular atrophy received epidural anaesthesia, one for Caesarean section, the other for vaginal delivery (Wilson & Williams 1992). Another patient with type III disease, who had severe kyphoscoliosis and was wheelchair bound, had Caesarean section under spinal anaesthesia (Coker et al 1997). In one patient with a VC of 600 ml, Caesarean section was carried out under general anaesthesia (Dahl et al 1995).

Bibliography

Barois A, Estournet-Mathiaud B 1997 Respiratory problems in spinal muscular atrophies. Pediatric Pulmonology 24 (suppl 16): 140–1.

Coker A, Scott W, McCune G 1997 Antenatal care and delivery of a patient with spinal muscular atrophy complicated with severe kyphoscoliosis. Journal of Obstetrics & Gynaecology 17: 154–5.

Dahl B, Norregaard FO, Juhl B 1995 [Pregnancy and delivery in a woman with neuromuscular disease. Spinal muscular atrophy and severely reduced pulmonary function. Danish.] Ugeskrift for Laeger 157: 750–1.

Donaghy M 1999 Classification and clinical features of motor neurone diseases and motor neuropathies. Journal of Neurology 246: 331–3.

Editorial 1990 Spinal muscular atrophies. Lancet i: 280–1.

Harpey JP, Charpentier C, Paturneu-Jouas M et al 1990 Secondary metabolic defects in spinal muscular atrophy type II. Lancet 336: 629.

Lyager S, Steffensen B, Juhl B 1995 Indicators of need for mechanical ventilation in Duchenne muscular dystrophy and spinal muscular atrophy. Chest 108: 779–85.

Phillips DP, Roye DP Jr, Farcy J-P C et al 1990 Surgical treatment of scoliosis in a spinal muscular atrophy population. Spine 15: 942–5.

Russman BS, Buncher CR, White M et al 1996 Function changes in spinal muscular atrophy. II and III. Neurology 47: 973–6.

Thaler ER, Weinstein GS 1997 Interesting presentation of spinal muscular atrophy: cricoarytenoid joint fixation. Otolaryngology—Head & Neck Surgery 117: S128–30.

Weston LA, DiFazio CA 1996 Labor analgesia in a patient with spinal muscular atrophy and vocal cord palsy. Regional Anesthesia 21: 350–4.

Wilson RD, Williams KP 1992 Spinal muscular atrophy and pregnancy. British Journal of Obstetrics & Gynaecology 99: 516–17.

Spondyloepiphyseal dysplasia

One of the osteochondrodysplasias, a group of conditions that includes most of the numerous forms of dwarfism. The congenita form is detected at birth, the tarda one later. There is developmental disturbance in endochondral bone formation, degeneration of discs, and destruction of spinal facet joints. The congenita form produces more problems for the anaesthetist than tarda.

Preoperative abnormalities

1. Skeletal abnormalities include flattened vertebrae and pectus carinatus. Kyphosis and scoliosis develop in later childhood.

2. Cyanosis which occurs after crying and feeding, respiratory difficulties, poor head control and decreased exercise tolerance, may herald the onset of problems.

3. Neurological deficits from atlantoaxial

instability, secondary to odontoid peg hypoplasia and laxity of ligaments. In one series of the congenita form, six out of 16 patients had myelopathy and the critical space available for the spinal cord at the level of the atlas was 10 mm or less (Nakamura et al 1998).

4. May subsequently develop respiratory insufficiency.

5. Surgery may be required for the treatment of scoliosis.

Anaesthetic problems

1. Tracheal intubation may be difficult (Mogera & Muralidhar 1996). The small xiphisternum to symphysis pubis distance may be associated with a short trachea of 15 rings or less, so that accidental bronchial intubation is more likely (Wells et al 1989).

2. Two cases of laryngeal stenosis have been reported. In one there was circumferential stenosis from the cricoid cartilage to the third tracheal ring. The second had gradually increasing respiratory difficulty, followed by acute stridor requiring emergency tracheostomy (Myer & Cotton 1985).

3. Dysplastic odontoid peg and delayed ossification increases the risk of atlantoaxial instability. An 18 year old sustained spastic tetraparesis after intubation that had required moderate neck flexion and use of a guidewire (Redl 1998). Massive cord compression to a diameter of 6 cm led to an eventual fatal outcome.

4. In pregnancy, restricted lung function from skeletal deformities may be further compromised by the growing uterus. Caesarean section under spinal anaesthesia was performed at 33 weeks' gestation because of respiratory failure (Yoshimura et al 1998).

5. Deformities may increase the technical difficulties of regional anaesthesia. A shallow epidural space, located at 2.5 cm from the skin, was reported in one patient (Rodney et al 1991).

Management

1. Lateral cervical spine views and screening should be undertaken in flexion and extension.

2. If atlantoaxial instability is present when general anaesthesia is required, tracheal intubation should be achieved either by manual in-line stabilisation, or by an awake fibreoptic technique (Auden 1999).

3. Extreme care should be taken to check the position of the tube, so as to avoid one lung ventilation.

4. Regional anaesthesia may be appropriate, if technically feasible. Caesarean section was performed under epidural anaesthesia in a patient with C3–4 subluxation (Rodney et al 1991).

Bibliography

Auden SM 1999 Cervical spine instability and dwarfism: fiberoptic intubation for all. Anesthesiology 91: 580.

Mogera C, Muralidhar V 1996 Spondyloepiphyseal dysplasia congenita syndrome: anesthetic implications. Anesthesia & Analgesia 83: 433–4.

Myer CM, Cotton RT 1985 Laryngotracheal stenosis in spondyloepiphyseal dysplasia. Laryngoscope 95: 3–5.

Nakamura K, Miyoshi K, Haga N et al 1998 Risk factors of myelopathy at the atlantoaxial level in spondyloepiphyseal dysplasia congenita. Archives of Orthopaedic & Trauma Surgery 117: 468–70.

Redl G 1997 The pediatric high-risk patient in orthopedic surgery. Acta Anaesthesiologica Scandinavica Supplementum 111: 211–14.

Redl G 1998 Massive pyramidal tract signs after endotracheal intubation: a case report of spondyloepiphyseal dysplasia. Anesthesiology 89: 1262–4.

Rodney GE, Callander CC, Harmer M 1991 Spondyloepiphyseal dysplasia congenita. Caesarean section under epidural anaesthesia. Anaesthesia 46: 648–50.

Wells AL, Wells TR, Landing BH et al 1989 Short trachea, a hazard in tracheal intubation of infants and neonates. Anesthesiology 71: 367–73.

Yoshimura T, Nakamura T, Ito M et al 1998 Respiratory difficulty necessitated early delivery in a woman with spondyloepiphyseal dysplasia. Journal of Maternal–Fetal Investigation 8: 145–6.

Sturge–Weber syndrome (see also Klippel–Trenaunay–Weber syndrome)

A congenital syndrome of unknown aetiology, in which a cavernous haemangioma of one side of the face is associated with an intracranial angioma. The angiomas, which become increasingly calcified, are usually surgically untreatable, although subtotal hemispherectomy has been performed to control intractable epilepsy. The syndrome is associated with progressive neurological deterioration. General anaesthesia may be required for the management of glaucoma, which is difficult to treat (Ceyhan et al 1999). Sturge–Weber may be associated with Klippel–Trenaunay syndrome. In this condition, haemangiomas on the trunk or limbs are associated with spinal cord malformations that may bleed and result in paraplegia. Vascular occlusive therapy may be required to obliterate haemangiomas (Caiazzo et al 1998).

Preoperative abnormalities

1. A naevus (port wine stain) of one side of the face, which may involve one or more divisions of the trigeminal nerve. It is often associated with progressive mental retardation, which is present in 60%, and severe in 32%.

2. Skin haemangiomas can occur at other sites. Glaucoma and buphthalmos may occur. Massive involvement of the paranasal sinuses and facial distortion has been reported (Ku et al 1999).

3. Epilepsy, and a hemiparesis involving the contralateral side may occur. Uncontrolled status epilepticus may result in permanent cerebral damage. Fits may be refractory to drug control. Gum hypertrophy may be secondary to phenytoin therapy.

4. Stroke-like episodes. Decreased blood flow may affect neurological function by interfering with glucose metabolism.

5. There are variations in the full clinical picture. One side of the vault and the hemiparetic half of the body may be smaller than the other. There may be unilateral glaucoma, increased scalp vascularity, and unilateral hypertrophy of the carotid artery.

6. A venous haemangioma usually involves the meninges of the occipitoparietal surface of the brain. The adjacent cortex is gradually destroyed, possibly as a result of pressure. Deeper arteriovenous malformations, which occur only rarely, may be fed by large arteries and increasingly large veins. If this happens, a considerable arteriovenous shunt may result in cardiac hypertrophy and failure.

7. Skull X-ray shows linear calcification of the underlying brain tissue.

8. Arteriography or DVI will demonstrate the extent of the lesion.

Anaesthetic problems

1. The patient may be severely retarded and uncooperative. Seizure disorders are usual.

2. Mask anaesthesia is often difficult because of gross vascular hypertrophy of the lips, buccal mucosa, gums and tongue. In addition, if there is a significant AV shunt causing increased cardiac output, inhalational induction will be delayed. Airway obstruction occurred during gaseous induction in one patient (Aldridge 1987), but laryngoscopy and intubation were considered not to be difficult once induction is achieved (de Leon-Casasola & Lema 1991). However, two children with features of both the Klippel–Trenaunay–Weber and the Sturge–Weber syndromes presented with severe upper airway obstruction (Reich & Wiatrak 1995). The 10 year old required tracheostomy under local anaesthesia for an enlarging mass that had expanded to replace the hard palate and maxilla. The 9 year old, who had recurrent attacks of pneumonia and difficulty in breathing, was found to have a high arched palate, narrowed choanae, and a hypoplastic and hypotonic pharynx. A tracheostomy under general anaesthesia relieved his obstruction.

3. Straining and coughing increases

intraocular pressure, which may be hazardous in the presence of buphthalmos or glaucoma (Batra et al 1994). Increases in intracranial pressure can cause intracerebral haemorrhage and bleeding into haemangiomas. Patients are susceptible to uncontrolled venous hypertension, which can interfere with venous outflow.

4. The cerebral lesion is usually too large for operative surgery. However, should neurosurgery be required, it may be associated with massive bleeding.

5. In patients with large cavernous haemangiomas, hypovolaemia may precipitate thrombocytopenia and hypofibrinogenaemia which can progress to a coagulopathy.

6. Protracted status epilepticus may produce permanent cerebral damage (Coley et al 1998).

Management

1. Assessment of the degree of significance of the AV shunt.

2. Management of the retarded patient with epilepsy. Optimal seizure control is needed to prevent venous hypertension and brain damage (Coley et al 1998).

3. Prevent increases in intracerebral and intraocular pressure.

4. Extreme hyperventilation should be avoided. Preservation of venous outflow.

5. Assessment of possible airway difficulties. Early laryngoscopy and intubation has been advised because of difficulties with mask anaesthesia.

6. A hypotensive technique may be required for neurosurgical procedures.

Bibliography
Aldridge LM 1987 An unusual case of upper airway obstruction. Anaesthesia 42: 1239–40.

Batra RK, Gulaya V, Madan R et al 1994 Anaesthesia and the Sturge–Weber syndrome. Canadian Journal of Anaesthesia 41: 133–6.

Caiazzo A, Mehra P, Papageorge MB 1998 The use of preoperative percutaneous transcatheter vascular occlusive therapy in the management of Sturge–Weber syndrome: report of a case. Journal of Oral & Maxillofacial Surgery 56: 775 8.

Ceyhan A, Cakan T, Basar H et al 1999 Anaesthesia for Sturge–Weber syndrome. European Journal of Anaesthesiology 16: 339–41.

Coley SC, Britton J, Clarke A 1998 Status epilepticus and venous infarction in Sturge–Weber syndrome. Childs Nervous System 14: 693–6.

de Leon-Casasola OA, Lema MJ 1991 Anesthesia for patients with Sturge–Weber disease and Klippel–Trenaunay syndrome. Journal of Clinical Anesthesia 3: 409–13.

Ku PKM, Kew J, Rad FF et al 1999 Paranasal sinus enlargement in Sturge–Weber syndrome. Journal of Laryngology & Otology 113: 177–8.

Reich DS, Wiatrak BJ 1995 Upper airway obstruction in Sturge–Weber syndrome and Klippel–Trenaunay–Weber syndrome. Annals of Otology, Rhinology & Laryngology 104: 363–8.

473

Systemic lupus erythematosus (SLE) (see also Antiphospholipid syndrome)

An autoimmune connective tissue disorder, predominantly occurring in females between the ages of 20 and 50, and which involves formation of autoantibodies and immune complexes against nucleic acid antigens and phospholipids (Mills 1994). Anaesthetists may be involved in the management of pregnant patients with SLE. Secondary antiphospholipid syndrome, which has no major differences from the primary disease, may occur. In a multicentre study of 1000 patients, death was more commonly associated with active SLE, infections, and thromboses (Cervera et al 1999). Survival was reduced in those who had a nephropathy at the start of the study.

Preoperative abnormalities

1. Arthritis and cutaneous lesions are the commonest presenting features, and occur in 86–100% of patients. Skin lesions include the well-known, but often transient, butterfly facial rash, vasculitis, alopecia, and a photosensitivity

dermatitis. Other common features are inflammatory arthritis of the hands, renal involvement (40–75% of patients), and central nervous system lesions (60%).

2. Cardiac disease in SLE is common (Moder et al 1999). A literature analysis showed clinical or echocardiography prevalence to be 28%, and autopsy prevalence to be 65%. ECG may show PR depression and ST elevation. Conduction abnormalities occur in about 10%. Libman–Sacks endocarditis (13–74%), with noninfective verrucous vegetations, most commonly affects the mitral valve, although it can involve any valve. Myocarditis (10–40%) may cause dyspnoea, tachycardia, and sometimes congestive heart failure. Coronary artery disease (25–45%) is now known to occur and the risk of myocardial infarction is considerably greater than in the normal population.

3. SLE can affect virtually all components of the respiratory system. Pulmonary atelectasis is common and may be associated with lupus pneumonitis and occasionally fibrosing alveolitis. Pulmonary function tests may show a restrictive defect. The diaphragm may be elevated, and a diaphragmatic myopathy has been suggested as a cause of the 'vanishing lung' syndrome.

4. There may be anaemia, leucopenia, and occasionally thrombocytopenia. Laboratory tests show a variety of antibodies to nuclear and cytoplasmic components. Anti-cardiolipin antibodies in SLE were found to be associated with venous thrombosis, autoimmune thrombocytopenia, recurrent fetal loss, leg ulcers, transverse myelitis, and pulmonary hypertension (Alarcon-Segovia et al 1989). Lupus antibody, as assessed by diluted APTT, is strongly associated with thrombosis.

5. There can be exacerbations and remissions. The condition may be made worse by stress, drugs, infection, and pregnancy. A significant proportion of the patients develop atherosclerotic disease in late life.

6. Circulating lupus anticoagulant occurs in up to 37% of patients with SLE (Malinow et al

1987). Paradoxically, this is an autoantibody associated with systemic vascular thromboses, which actually causes prolongation of some coagulation tests. Fetal survival has improved with low-dose heparin treatment (Lockshin 1998).

7. Life-threatening complications can occur. In a study of 50 patients with catastrophic antiphospholipid syndrome, 15 had SLE. Microangiopathy and multiorgan failure were common features and the death rate was 50% (Asherson et al 1998).

8. Pregnancy. Although exacerbation of the disease may occur in pregnancy (Wong et al 1991), and activity in the early stages is associated with relapses, it is thought to be uncommon (Lockshin 1989). Adverse fetal outcomes have been reported (Editorial 1991), but were not shown in all series (Wong et al 1991). Pregnancies in the presence of a high titre of antiphospholipid antibodies usually result in fetal loss. The outcome of pregnancy has been substantially improved recently by treatment. The incidence of fetal loss may be reduced by therapy with low-dose aspirin or heparin (Backos et al 1999). A small proportion of infants of patients with anti-Ro antibodies develop neonatal lupus syndrome, which is associated with congenital heart block (Editorial 1991).

9. Medication may include corticosteroids, antimalarials, and pulsed cyclophosphamide. Experimental therapy in severe cases includes plasmapheresis or immunoglobulins.

Anaesthetic problems

1. Pulmonary involvement may result in a restrictive lung defect. The presence of either acute lupus pneumonitis or pulmonary hypertension is associated with an increased mortality.

2. Thrombotic problems. There is an association between SLE and the antiphospholipid syndrome. Up to 28% of patients with lupus anticoagulant may have

arterial or venous thrombotic episodes. Sudden massive, fatal pulmonary embolism occurred in a 71 year old after induction of anaesthesia for emergency cholecystectomy. A large thrombus was found in the main pulmonary trunk and small emboli were thought to have occurred in the few days before admission (Greilich et al 1998).

3. Coagulation tests in patients with lupus anticoagulant may show a prolonged PT, APTT or KCCT, or thrombocytopenia and platelet dysfunction. In addition, the patient may be receiving aspirin or low-dose heparin.

4. Pregnancy complications. Although fetal loss has been improved by treatment, pregnancy may exacerbate the disease and increase the morbidity and mortality from lung or cardiac complications. Pulmonary hypertension and pulmonary oedema occurred in a 31-week-pregnant patient. Caesarean section was performed under GA and IPPV was required overnight (Cuenco et al 1999). Fatalities may occur around the 30-week period. Death occurred from ARDS 19 days after Caesarean section (Katz et al 1996), from severe pulmonary hypertension 4 days postpartum (Ray & Sermer 1996), and from preeclampsia and pulmonary hypertension with vasculitis (Rubin et al 1995). Severe laryngeal oedema presented 20 min after Caesarean section in a patient with preeclampsia who had received a renal transplant 6 months before conception (O'Connor & Thorburn 1993).

5. Antiphospholipid antibodies and the antiphospholipid syndrome. The incidence of lupus anticoagulant and anticardiolipin antibodies is 37% in women with SLE, compared with 5.3% in the normal obstetric population (Kutteh 1997). Their presence can be associated with slow, progressive thrombosis and infarction in the placenta, and a high incidence of fetal loss and maternal morbidity. They can also be associated with a devastating clinical course. One 36-year-old female, admitted acutely with a pelvic mass, developed a coagulopathy and ARDS following laparoscopy. Initially, the patient's previous history of

thromboses and SLE was not known, because the notes were unavailable and she did not speak English. Subsequent laparotomy led to cardiorespiratory and renal failure, with death at 10 days (Menon and Allt-Graham 1993).

Management

1. Assessment of pulmonary, cardiac and renal function. Anaesthetic management will depend upon the affected organs (Davies 1991).

2. In labour, coagulation studies, including PT, APTT, platelets and bleeding time, should be performed. If these are prolonged, epidural anaesthesia is contraindicated, except when there is isolated elevation of PTT in association with lupus anticoagulant (Davies 1991).

3. There should be a multidisciplinary approach to the patient in pregnancy (Davies 1991). The problems posed by the presence of lupus anticoagulant in the pregnant patient who is on aspirin therapy have been discussed (Malinow et al 1987). Both authors suggest that the benefits of epidural anaesthesia must be weighed against the possibility (but very low risk) of an epidural haematoma developing. Increased fetal survival has been achieved with low-dose heparin.

4. For management, see also Antiphospholipid syndrome.

5. In the case of pulmonary hypertension and pulmonary oedema occurring in pregnancy, Cuenco et al (1999) suggest optimising pulmonary blood flow, by regulating the RV preload and PAP in a narrow range sufficient to overcome a high PVR without exacerbating pulmonary oedema.

6. If valvular lesions are present, antibiotic prophylaxis should be given, when appropriate. Treatment of cardiac failure with afterload-reducing agents, diuretics, and inotropic agents.

Bibliography
Alarcon-Segovia D, Deleze M, Oria CV et al 1989 Antiphospholipid antibodies and the antiphospholipid syndrome in systemic lupus erythematosus. Medicine 68: 353–65.

Asherson RA, Cervera R, Piette J-C et al 1998 Catastrophic antiphospholipid syndrome: clinical and laboratory features of 50 patients. Medicine 77: 195–207.

Backos M, Rai R, Baxter N et al 1999 Pregnancy complications in women with recurrent miscarriage associated with antiphospholipid antibodies treated with low dose aspirin and heparin. British Journal of Obstetrics & Gynaecology 106: 102–7.

Cervera R, Khamashta MA, Font J et al 1999 Morbidity and mortality in systemic lupus erythematosus during a 5-year period: a multicenter prospective study of 1000 patients. Medicine 78: 167–75.

Cuenco J, Tzeng G, Wittels B 1999 Anesthetic management of the parturient with systemic lupus erythematosus, pulmonary hypertension, and pulmonary edema. Anesthesiology 91: 568–70.

Davies SR 1991 Systemic lupus erythematosus and the obstetrical patient—implications for the anaesthetist. Canadian Journal of Anaesthesia 38: 790–6.

Editorial 1991 Systemic lupus erythematosus in pregnancy. Lancet 338: 87–8.

Greilich PE, Randle DW, Froelich EG et al 1998 Massive intraoperative pulmonary embolism coincident with the administration of succinylcholine. Anesthesia & Analgesia 87: 491–3.

Katz VL, Kuller JA, McCoy MC et al 1996 Fatal lupus pleuritis presenting in pregnancy. A case report. Journal of Reproductive Medicine 41: 537–40.

Kutteh WH 1997 Antiphospholipid antibodies and reproduction. Journal of Reproductive Immunology 35: 151–71.

Lockshin MD 1989 Pregnancy does not cause systemic lupus erythematosus to worsen. Arthritis & Rheumatism 32: 665–70.

Malinow AM, Rickford WJK, Mokriski BLK et al 1987 Lupus anticoagulant. Implication for obstetric anaesthetists. Anaesthesia 42: 1291–3.

Menon G, Allt-Graham J 1993 Anaesthetic implications of the anticardiolipin syndrome. British Journal of Anaesthesia 70: 587–90.

Mills JA 1994 Systemic lupus erythematosus. New England Journal of Medicine 330: 1871–9.

Moder KG, Miller TD, Tazelaar HD 1999 Cardiac involvement in systemic lupus erythematosus. Mayo Clinic Proceedings 74: 275–84.

O'Connor R, Thorburn J 1993 Acute pharyngolaryngeal oedema in a pre-eclamptic parturient with systemic lupus erythematosus and a recent renal transplant. International Journal of Obstetric Anesthesia 2: 53–4.

Ray J, Sermer M 1996 Systemic lupus erythematosus and pulmonary hypertension during pregnancy: report of a case fatality. Canadian Journal of Cardiology 12: 753–6.

Rubin LA, Geran A, Rose TH et al 1995 A fatal pulmonary complication of lupus in pregnancy. Arthritis & Rheumatism 38: 710–14.

Wong KL, Chan FY, Lee CP 1991 Outcome of pregnancy in patients with systemic lupus erythematosus. A prospective study. Archives of Internal Medicine 151: 269–73.

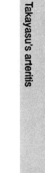

Takayasu's arteritis

A nonspecific chronic panarteritis, usually occurring in young women, and originally described in the Far East. In the early stages there is an inflammatory process in the large arteries that progresses to chronic arterial occlusion (Hall et al 1985). It is also known as 'pulseless disease', since there are usually reduced or absent pulses in the affected arteries. In a study of 60 patients, followed up for 6 months to 20 years, 97% were female, and the mean age at presentation was 25 years (Kerr et al 1994). Sixty-eight percent had extensive vascular disease, and stenotic lesions were more common than aneurysms (98% vv 27%). Treatment includes angioplasty or arterial bypass, or immunosuppressive therapy, but re-stenosis may occur. Criteria for disease activity include systemic features such as fever and muscular pains, increased ESR, and vascular ischaemia (Kerr et al 1994).

Type 1: involves the aortic arch and its branches.

Type 2: involves the descending thoracic and abdominal aorta, without arch involvement.

Type 3: is a mixed picture of types 1 and 2.

Type 4: can consist of any of the above features in association with pulmonary artery involvement.

Preoperative abnormalities

1. There may be pulse deficits, depending upon the stage of the disease and the arteries involved in the condition. Bruits may be heard over stenosed arteries. There are also ectatic lesions of the aorta with aneurysm formation, but these are much less common than stenoses.

2. Possible cerebrovascular or retinal insufficiency.

3. Renal involvement occurs in 63% of patients.

4. Hypertension, which is most often associated with renal artery stenosis.

5. In type 4 (45%) there may be moderate pulmonary hypertension.

6. Cardiac manifestations have been reported. Whilst cardiac failure can occur as a consequence of either systemic or pulmonary hypertension, valvular disease, most frequently aortic insufficiency, may also occur.

7. The ESR is related to the stage of the disease and is high in 78% of cases, notably in early inflammatory disease. There are ECG abnormalities in 40% and hypergamma-globulinaemia in 37%.

8. The patient may be taking corticosteroids, alone or with immunosuppressive agents.

9. Pregnancy can occur, but tends to be in those with the least severe disease.

Anaesthetic problems

1. There may be difficulties in haemodynamic monitoring because of an absence of palpable pulses (Ramanathan et al 1979, Warner et al 1983).

2. Pressure recording from one vessel does not necessarily reflect the pressure in another vessel. A 26 year old with type 3 disease had extreme differences in arterial pressures in the four limbs (Meikle & Milne 1997). The systolic varied from 90 mmHg in an arm, to 322 mmHg in a leg. In view of her previous stroke, there was concern about cerebral hypoxia, should the pressure be reduced.

3. Hypertension or pulmonary hypertension may be present, with or without heart failure. In a study of 54 patients, hypertension was found in 35 and congestive heart failure in 24; myocardial biopsy suggested that many patients had an inflammatory myocarditis that might account for the development of heart failure (Talwar et al 1991).

4. The myocardium may be sensitive to drugs with negative inotropic effects (Thorburn & James 1986).

5. In the presence of pulmonary hypertension, high lung inflation pressures may be required.

6. Hyperextension of the neck during laryngoscopy and intubation may reduce carotid artery blood flow.

7. Postoperative cerebral infarction has been described in a 53 year old. Initially no cause was identified, but on investigation the diagnosis of Takayasu's disease was made (Fawcett et al 1993).

8. Pregnancy may be associated with a worsening of hypertension, cerebral haemorrhage, and a hypercoagulable state. One patient had massive haemoptysis (Rocha et al 1994). Anaesthesia may be required for termination of pregnancy (Gaida et al 1991), labour (Crofts & Wilson 1991), or tubal ligation (McKay & Dillard 1991). Epidural anaesthesia was used for Caesarean section in a patient with multiple aortic aneurysms (Beilin & Bernstein 1993).

Management

1. The nature and degree of organ involvement must be assessed. Particular evidence of cardiac, respiratory, cerebral and renal insufficiency should be sought.

2. Hypertension or heart failure should be treated, if present.

3. For the purposes of blood pressure monitoring, the arteries involved in the disease process must be fully assessed.

4. The extent of monitoring depends upon the state of the patient, the accessibility of the arteries, and the magnitude of the surgery.

a) Care must be taken to monitor an artery representative of true arterial pressure (Thorburn & James 1986).

b) The use of a Doppler ultrasonic probe and a sphygmomanometer cuff, which permitted blood pressure recording despite an impalpable pulse, has been suggested (Warner et al 1983). The flow from a Doppler flow probe can also be displayed on an oscilloscope and recorded on a multichannel recorder (Ramanathan et al 1979).

c) The use of oximetry in combination with a mercury manometer to assess arterial blood pressure has been described (Chawla et al 1992), and the technique was successfully employed in two patients without arm pulses (Chawla et al 1990). The oximeter can still show a pulsatile plethysmographic waveform in clinically nonpulsatile arteries (Ramanathan et al 1979).

d) A cutdown onto the dorsalis pedis or superficial temporal arteries may be required for direct arterial monitoring. The appropriateness of these techniques will depend on the degree and distribution of the underlying ischaemia and the nature of the surgery being performed. If necessary, the surgeon can be requested to place a cannula in the aorta during surgery.

e) If pulmonary hypertension is present, a pulmonary artery catheter may be needed to measure PAP (Ramanathan et al 1979, Warner et al 1983). However, it must be remembered that pulmonary artery wedge pressures may be unreliable.

f) Measurement of cardiac stroke volume using an impedance cardiograph has been described (Ramanathan et al 1979).

g) Urine output may need careful monitoring.

5. In a patient with pulmonary hypertension, invasive haemodynamic monitoring demonstrated that epidural anaesthesia had a more beneficial effect on blood pressure and afterload control than vasodilators (Thorburn & James 1986).

6. Before anaesthesia is induced, the head should be fixed in a position that does not

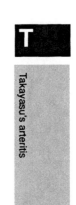

produce symptoms of cerebral blood flow impairment. A transcranial Doppler and continuous measurements of jugular venous oxygen saturation have been used to evaluate changes in cerebral perfusion (Nakajima et al 1992, Kawaguchi et al 1993).

7. Epidural anaesthesia for labour and postpartum tubal ligation (Crofts & Wilson 1991, McKay & Dillard 1991), combined general/epidural anaesthesia for abdominal hysterectomy in a patient with type 1 disease (Gozal et al 1995), and general anaesthesia for Caesarean section in type 2 (Herrema 1992, Mahmood et al 1997), have been described. Therapeutic abortion was performed under spinal anaesthesia (Hampl et al 1994). A patient with severe bilateral carotid artery stenoses demanded general anaesthesia for Caesarean section because she had experienced an unsatisfactory previous epidural. Processed EEG was used to monitor the adequacy of cerebral blood flow (Clark & al-Qatari 1998). A patient with a previous intrapartum cerebral haemorrhage had central pressure monitoring of the thoracic aorta during anaesthesia for elective Caesarean section (Tomioka et al 1998). Uneventful epidural anaesthesia was described for elective Caesarean section in a woman with hypertension, a pulseless left arm, extensive aortic disease, and needle phobia (Henderson & Fludder 1999).

Bibliography

Beilin Y, Bernstein H 1993 Successful epidural anesthesia for a patient with Takayasu's disease. Canadian Journal of Anaesthesia 40: 64–6.

Chawla R, Kumarvel V, Girdhar KK et al 1990 Oximetry in pulseless disease. Anaesthesia 45: 922–3.

Chawla R, Kumarvel V, Girdhar KK et al 1992 Can pulse oximetry be used to measure systolic blood pressure? Anesthesia & Analgesia 74: 196–200.

Clark AG, al-Qatari M 1998 Anaesthesia for Caesarean section in Takayasu's disease. Canadian Journal of Anaesthesia 45: 377–9.

Crofts SL, Wilson E 1991 Epidural analgesia for labour in Takayasu's arteritis. Case report. British Journal of Obstetrics & Gynaecology 98: 408–9.

Fawcett WJ, Razis PA, Berwick EP 1993 Post-operative cerebral infarction and Takayasu's disease. European Journal of Anaesthesiology 10: 33–5.

Gaida BJ, Gervais HW, Mauer D et al 1991 [Anesthesiology problems in Takayasu's syndrome. English abstract.] Anaesthesia 40: 1–6.

Gozal Y, Ginosar Y, Gozal D 1995 Combined general and epidural anesthesia for a patient with Takayasu's arteritis. Regional Anesthesia 20: 246–8.

Hall S, Barr W, Lie JT et al 1985 Takayasu arteritis. Medicine 64: 89–99.

Hampl KF, Klocke RK, Stoll M et al 1994 Spinal anaesthesia in a patient with Takayasu's disease. British Journal of Anaesthesia 72: 129–32.

Henderson K, Fludder P 1999 Epidural anaesthesia for Caesarean section in a patient with severe Takayasu's disease. British Journal of Anaesthesia 83: 956–9.

Herrema I 1992 Takayasu's disease and caesarean section. International Journal of Obstetric Anesthesia 1: 117–19.

Kawaguchi M, Ohsumi H, Nakajima T et al 1993 Intraoperative monitoring of cerebral haemodynamics in a patient with Takayasu's arteritis. Anaesthesia 48: 496–8.

Kerr GS, Hallahan CW, Giordano J et al 1994 Takayasu arteritis. Annals of Internal Medicine 120: 919–29.

McKay RSF, Dillard SR 1992 Management of epidural anesthesia in a patient with Takayasu's disease. Anesthesia & Analgesia 74: 297–9.

Mahmood T, Dewart PJ, Ralston AJ et al 1997 Three successive pregnancies in a patient with Takayasu's arteritis. Journal of Obstetrics & Gynaecology 17: 52–4.

Meikle A, Milne B 1997 Extreme arterial blood pressure differences in a patient with Takayasu's arteritis. Canadian Journal of Anaesthesia 44: 868–71.

Nakajima T, Kuro M, Hayashi Y et al 1992 Continuous monitoring of cerebral oxygen balance during cardiopulmonary bypass: on-line continuous monitoring of jugular venous oxyhemoglobin saturation. Anesthesia & Analgesia 74: 630–5.

Ramanathan S, Gupta U, Chalon J et al 1979 Anesthetic considerations in Takayasu arteritis. Anesthesia & Analgesia 58: 247–9.

Rocha MP, Guntupalli KK, Moise KJ Jr et al 1994 Massive haemoptysis in Takayasu's arteritis during pregnancy. Chest 106: 1619–22.

Talwar KK, Kumar K, Chopra P et al 1991 Cardiac involvement in nonspecific aortoarteritis (Takayasu's arteritis). American Heart Journal 122: 1666–70.

Thorburn JR, James MFM 1986 Anaesthetic management of Takayasu's arteritis. Anaesthesia 41: 734–8.

Tomioka N, Hirose K, Abe E et al 1998 Indications for peripartum aortic pressure monitoring in Takayasu's disease. A patient with a past history of intrapartum cerebral haemorrhage. Japanese Heart Journal 39: 255–60.

Warner MA, Hughes DR, Messick JM 1983 Anesthetic management of a patient with pulseless disease. Anesthesia & Analgesia 62: 532–5.

Tetanus

An infection caused by *Clostridium tetani*, an anaerobic bacillus present in soil and gut. It is able to survive for long periods outside the body. Under anaerobic conditions it multiplies and produces two potent, high molecular weight exotoxins, tetanolysin and tetanospasmin, which proteolyse some of the protein membranes involved in exocytosis (Ahnert-Hilger & Bilgalke 1995). Tetanospasmin is responsible for the acute clinical condition of tetanus and can travel up nerves into the spinal cord and medulla. The primary effect is on the spinal cord, with a lesser effect on the peripheral nerves. Tetanus neurotoxin is a high molecular weight protein, so its long half-life allows time for neural penetration. Tetanospasmin prevents transmission at inhibitory synapses in CNS, and therefore causes disinhibition of the motor system. The incubation period of the disease is 3–21 days. In about 60–65% of patients there is a history of a wound, but it is often trivial. Several cases have occurred following surgery, the commonest operation reported being cholecystectomy (Crokaert et al 1984, Lennard et al 1984, Farling et al 1989).

Cases may be classified (Edmondson & Flowers 1979) as:

Grade 1	Mild
Grade 2	Moderate
Grade 3a	Severe
Grade 3b	Very severe

In Edmondson and Flowers' report of 100 cases treated in Leeds, the mortality was 10%.

There is an increased risk of tetanus in heroin addicts (Sun et al 1994), in part due to additives such as quinine, which provide anaerobic conditions for multiplication of the bacilli. In fact, a high incidence of tetanus which was rapidly fatal has been seen following the use of im quinine for treatment of severe malaria (Yen et al 1994). Mortality is highest in severe disease, the elderly, and in drug addicts.

Presentation

1. General muscle hypertonicity.

2. Muscle spasm resulting in trismus (lockjaw), rigidity of the facial muscles (risus sardonicus), neck stiffness, or opisthotonos. Intermittent muscle spasms are superimposed on hypertonicity. Breathing difficulties can result from spasms of the laryngeal or intercostal muscles, and respiratory failure may ensue. Dysphagia may sometimes be the major symptom, with pooling of saliva and episodes of pharyngeal spasms (Kasanew et al 1989).

3. Occasionally, wounds in the head and neck may produce cephalic tetanus, which can result in a variety of cranial nerve palsies (Yanagi et al 1996).

4. A small number of patients have localised tetanus only.

5. Sympathetic disturbances occur in 23–60% of severe cases, probably as a result of the action of tetanospasmin on brainstem and autonomic interneurones causing increased circulating catecholamine levels. These consist of episodes of hypertension, tachycardia, arrhythmias, vasoconstriction, sweating, salivation, and pyrexia.

6. Episodes of hypotension and bradycardia have been reported, particularly after tracheal suction. These may be secondary to parasympathetic autonomic dysfunction.

Diagnosis

1. Is generally made on clinical grounds.

2. Tetanus is not an immunising disease, therefore it is possible to contract it on more than one occasion. This is probably because the toxin travels up the nerves and may not come into contact with gamma globulin. The blood level of tetanus antibody cannot be used as a diagnostic test for the disease (Stoddart 1979a).

3. Differentiation must be made from other conditions that mimic tetanus. These include hysteria, and treatment with drugs, such as the phenothiazines and butyrophenones, which can produce dyskinetic symptoms (Stoddart 1979b).

Anaesthetic (or intensive care) problems

1. Any strong external stimulus can precipitate severe muscle spasms. Death may occur because ventilatory impairment coincides with a greatly increased oxygen consumption by the muscles. In one patient, the diagnosis was only made when severe, recurrent pharyngeal spasms occurred after removal of the tracheal tube, following oesophagoscopy for dysphagia (Baronia et al 1991).

2. Cardiovascular instability, with episodes of hypertension and tachycardia, is often associated with increased circulating catecholamine levels (Domenighetti et al 1984).

3. Hypotension and bradycardia may occur, particularly after tracheal suction. There are several reports which suggest that treatment with beta blockers may predispose to bradycardias, and in one case, cardiac arrest occurred (Buchanan et al 1978).

4. Reduced plasma cholinesterase levels have been reported, the level often correlating with the severity of the disease. In one report, there was no enzymic activity for the first 3 days after admission (Porath et al 1977).

5. The use of suxamethonium in the later stages of the disease may cause cardiac arrest from hyperkalaemia.

6. Hypovolaemia occurs readily, from a combination of sweating, excess salivation, and gastrointestinal losses. Inappropriate ADH secretion may produce hyponatraemia.

7. Gastrointestinal stasis is a problem and gastrointestinal haemorrhage can occur.

8. Long-term ventilation and heavy sedation is associated with a high incidence of pulmonary complications and death.

9. Pyrexia may be secondary to infection, or it sometimes occurs as a result of autonomic dysfunction.

10. One patient is reported who required surgery during active tetanus (Farling et al 1989).

11. In patients who need IPPV for long periods, there is an increased risk of deep venous thrombosis and pulmonary embolism. In the Leeds series of 100 cases, nine venous thromboses, three pulmonary emboli, and one death occurred (Edmondson & Flowers 1979). Another embolic death has been reported, despite the use of low-dose heparin (Jenkins & Keep 1976).

Management

1. Initial management:

    a) Antitetanus immunoglobulin $30\,mg\,kg^{-1}$ im.

    b) Antibiotic: metronidazole 500 mg iv 6 hrly.

    c) Tetanus toxoid course is started.

    d) The wound should be excised and cleaned, and tissue sent for microscopy and bacterial culture. It has been suggested that this should be delayed for several hours after the immunoglobulin has been given, so that any neurotoxin released can be neutralised. Mutilating surgery is not justified.

2. Management of spasm and hypertonus.

Grade 1 Usually diazepam only.

Grade 2 Diazepam, tracheostomy, and nasogastric tube.

Grade 3a and 3b IPPV, sedatives, neuromuscular blockers, and analgesics.

More recently, other drugs have been reported for sedation and spasm. These include:

a) Propofol (Borgeat et al 1991), or midazolam and propofol (Orko et al 1988).

b) Inhaled isoflurane (Stevens et al 1993). The prolonged use of isoflurane was associated with potentially toxic concentrations of serum inorganic fluoride, although serum urea and creatinine levels remained within normal limits.

c) Intrathecal baclofen (Muller et al 1987, Brock et al 1995, Dressnandt et al 1997) for tetanus-induced spinal and supraspinal spasticity. Baclofen, a GABA agonist, may produce central depression, hypotonia, sedation, and coma. The central effects have been reversed using iv flumazenil followed by an infusion, thus preserving its spinal action (Saissy et al 1992).

d) Magnesium sulphate. Attygalle and Rodrigo (1997) used magnesium sulphate given iv as a 5-g loading dose, followed by an infusion of $2-3\,g\,h^{-1}$, increasing it to control spasms whilst retaining the patella reflex intact. Magnesium concentrations were kept within the therapeutic range of $2-4\,mmol\,l^{-1}$. Loss of reflexes occurs at magnesium levels in excess of $4\,mmol\,l^{-1}$. The authors found that this reduced the need for IPPV and sedation in patients with severe tetanus. If clinical signs of hypocalcaemia occurred, 10 ml 10% calcium gluconate was given.

3. Fluid replacement is required for sweating, salivation, and gastrointestinal losses. The latter depends on measured loss, but may amount to as much as $6-8\,l\,day^{-1}$. Nutrition is also needed,

either via a nasogastric tube or feeding gastrostomy, or parenterally if there is gastrointestinal failure.

4. Sympathetic overactivity has been treated in a number of ways. These have included:

a) Beta adrenoceptor blockade. However, the use of beta adrenoceptor blockers is controversial, since profound bradycardia may occur. Extremely high catecholamine levels, equivalent to those encountered in a phaeochromocytoma, were reported in one patient (Domenighetti et al 1984). During convalescence, these levels returned to normal. In this case, labetalol was used to treat sympathetic overactivity. The use of labetalol in 15 cases was reported to produce great variability of response and poor control of blood pressure (Wesley et al 1983). This is not surprising, since the beta blockade produced by labetalol is at least three to seven times greater than the alpha blockade. In addition, five of the treated patients had episodes of cardiac standstill. The death of a 4-year-old child was associated with the use of propranolol (Buchanan et al 1978). In the Leeds series (Edmondson & Flowers 1979), only two of the patients were treated with propanolol. Both had severe bradycardias and cardiac standstill after tracheal suction. More recently an infusion of esmolol, a short-acting beta blocker, has been tried (King & Cave 1991). This produced stability, but with less hypotension than that produced by propranolol.

b) Magnesium sulphate and clonidine (Sutton et al 1990).

c) Epidural anaesthesia. Bhagwanjee et al (1999) have reported the use of epidural bupivacaine and sufentanil to control sympathetic activity. Midazolam iv was used as the principle adjunctive sedative.

d) Morphine (5–30 mg in an infusion over 30 min every 2–8 h) for hypertension and/or tachycardia or hypotension (Wright et al 1989).

e) Atropine infusion 72–2756 mg day^{-1} (Dolar 1992).

f) Sodium valproate.

g) ACE inhibitors.

5. Patients should be pre-oxygenated prior to tracheal suction, to avoid hypoxia.

6. Low-dose heparin should be administered to prevent venous thrombosis. A fatal embolism occurred in an obese lady, despite low-dose heparin. The use of full anticoagulation has been suggested (Jenkins & Keep 1976).

7. General measures such as chest and limb physiotherapy, skin and mouth care, and treatment of depression.

Bibliography

Ahnert-Hilger G, Bigalke H 1995 Molecular aspects of tetanus and botulinum neurotoxin poisoning. Progress in Neurobiology 46: 83–96.

Attygalle D, Rodrigo N 1997 Magnesium sulphate for control of spasms in severe tetanus. Can we avoid sedation and artificial ventilation? Anaesthesia 52: 956–62.

Baronia AK, Singh PK, Dhiman RK 1991 Intractable pharyngeal spasm following tracheal extubation in a patient with undiagnosed tetanus. Anesthesiology 75: 1111.

Bhagwanjee S, Bosenberg AT, Muckart DJ 1999 Management of sympathetic overactivity in tetanus with epidural bupivacaine and sufentanil: experience with 11 patients. Critical Care Medicine 27: 1721–5.

Borgeat A, Popovic V, Schwander D 1991 Efficiency of a continuous infusion of propofol in a patient with tetanus. Critical Care Medicine 19: 295–7.

Brock H, Moosbauerk W, Gabriel C 1995 Treatment of severe tetanus by continuous intrathecal infusion of baclofen. Journal of Neurology, Neurosurgery & Psychiatry 59: 192–9.

Buchanan N, Smit L, Cane RD et al 1978 Death of a child with tetanus due to propranolol. British Medical Journal 2: 254–5.

Crokaert F, Glupczynski Y, Fastrez R et al 1984 Postoperative tetanus. Lancet i: 1466.

Dolar D 1992 The use of a continuous atropine infusion in the management of severe tetanus. Intensive Care Medicine 18: 26–31.

Domenighetti GM, Savary G, Stricker H 1984 Hyperadrenergic syndrome in severe tetanus; extreme rise in catecholamines responsive to labetolol. British Medical Journal 288: 1483–4.

Dressnandt J, Konstanzer A, Weinzierl FX et al 1997 Intrathecal baclofen in tetanus: four cases and a review of the literature. Intensive Care Medicine 23: 896–902.

Edmondson RS, Flowers MW 1979 Intensive care in tetanus: management, complications, and mortality in 100 cases. British Medical Journal 1: 1401–4.

Farling PA, Sharpe TD, Gray RC 1989 Major thoracic surgery during active tetanus. Anaesthesia 44: 125–7.

Jenkins J, Keep P 1976 Fatal embolism despite low dose heparin. Lancet i: 541.

Kasanew M, Browne B, Dawes P 1989 Tetanus presenting as dysphagia. Journal of Laryngology & Otology 103: 229–30.

King WW, Cave DR 1991 Use of esmolol to control autonomic instability of tetanus. American Journal of Medicine 91: 425–8.

Lennard JW, Gunn A, Sellars J et al 1984 Tetanus after elective cholecystectomy and exploration of the common bile duct. Lancet i: 1466–7.

Muller H, Borner U, Zierski J et al 1987 Intrathecal baclofen for treatment of tetanus-induced spasticity. Anesthesiology 66: 76–9.

Orko R, Rosenberg PH, Himberg J-J 1988 Intravenous infusion of midazolam, propofol and vecuronium in a patient with severe tetanus. Acta Anaesthesiologica Scandinavica 32: 590–2.

Porath A, Acker M, Perel A 1977 Serum cholinesterase in tetanus. Anaesthesia 32: 1009–11.

Saissy JM, Vitris M, Demaziere J et al 1992 Flumazenil counteracts intrathecal baclofen-induced CNS depression in tetanus. Anesthesiology 76: 1051–3.

Stevens JJWM, Griffin RM, Stow PJ 1993 Prolonged use of isoflurane in a patient with tetanus. British Journal of Anaesthesia 70: 107–9.

Stoddart JC 1979a The immunology of tetanus. Anaesthesia 34: 863–5.

Stoddart JC 1979b Pseudotetanus. Anaesthesia 34: 887–91.

Sun KO, Chan YW, Cheung RT et al 1994 Management of tetanus: a review of 18 cases. Journal of the Royal Society of Medicine 87: 135–7.

Sutton DN, Tremlett MR, Woodcock TE et al 1990 Management of autonomic dysfunction in severe tetanus: the use of magnesium sulphate and clonidine. Intensive Care Medicine 16: 75–80.

Wesley AG, Hariparsad D, Pather M et al 1983 Labetalol in tetanus. Anaesthesia 38: 243–9.

Wright DK, Lalloo UG, Nayiager S et al 1989 Autonomic nervous system dysfunction in severe tetanus: current perpectives. Critical Care Medicine 17: 371–5.

Yanagi F, Sawada N, Nishi M et al 1996 Cephalic tetanus in a non traumatized patient with left facial palsy. Anesthesia & Analgesia 83: 423–4.

Yen LM, Dao LM, Day NP et al 1994 Role of quinine in the high mortality of intramuscular injection tetanus. Lancet 344: 786–7.

Thalassaemia

An abnormality of haemoglobin resulting from an imbalance of globin chain synthesis, affecting the population in a wide geographical band from the Mediterranean area, through the Middle East, and into India and China.

In beta thalassaemia major (homozygous state) there is an absence, or a reduced production of beta chains, and therefore an increased production of alpha chains. The alpha chains precipitate in the red cell precursors, leading to ineffective erythropoiesis and shortened red cell survival. The haemolytic anaemia leads to tissue hypoxia and excess erythropoietin production, with marrow expansion and extramedullary erythropoiesis. Iron overload secondary to increased iron absorption and recurrent transfusion is another major clinical problem. When the capacity of ferritin is exceeded, plasma iron generates free radicals, and tissue damage occurs because of the inability of antioxidant systems to cope. Thalassaemia is a quantitative haemoglobinopathy, as opposed to sickle cell anaemia, in which the defect is qualitative.

In alpha thalassaemia there is absent or deficient alpha chain synthesis. Excess beta chains produce HbH, which has a high affinity for oxygen, but will not release it. Excess gamma chains in fetal haemoglobin produce HbBarts. Both HbH and HbBarts are physiologically useless.

The prognosis in thalassaemia major has improved since more aggressive treatment has been undertaken. Multiple blood transfusions to maintain the Hb at $10–12\,g\,dl^{-1}$ help to suppress erythropoiesis and reduce bone deformity. Simultaneous iron chelation with desferrioxamine decreases iron deposition in the body. The effects of starting treatment at an earlier age are being tried. Bone marrow transplantation to patients under 16 years of age can correct this disorder (Lucarelli et al 1990). The classical changes of the untreated disease are now rarely seen in the western world and survival is good in the treated patient (Olivieri 1999).

Patients with thalassaemia minor (heterozygous state) are normally symptom free, except when exposed to stresses such as pregnancy, when they may become anaemic, usually as a result of folic acid deficiency.

Anaesthesia may be required for splenectomy, maxillofacial surgery (Drew & Sachs 1997), cholecystectomy or bone marrow transplantation.

Preoperative abnormalities

Homozygous disease

1. Beta thalassaemia presents in the first year of life.

2. Haemolysis leads to gross anaemia.

3. Treatment with multiple transfusions to maintain the Hb between $10–12\,g\,dl^{-1}$ and chelation to reduce the iron load improves the prognosis.

4. In untreated disease, bony changes occur as a result of marrow hyperplasia. The marrow can expand to up to 30 times normal and increased erythropoietin synthesis may stimulate the formation of extramedullary tissue, leading to facial and skull deformities. Osteopenia and focal defects in bone mineralisation occur.

5. Iron deposition takes place, particularly in the liver, myocardium, and endocrine organs.

The commonest complications are those associated with iron overload. These include cardiac hypertrophy and dilatation, pulmonary hypertension, cirrhosis, and hypogonadism.

6. Hypothyroidism is seen in >17% of patients, diabetes mellitus in 8–15%, and hypocalcaemia in 7%.

7. There is gross hepatosplenomegaly.

8. A hyperdynamic circulation results from an increase in the circulating blood volume secondary to shunting through expanded marrow.

9. Neutropenia, and occasionally thrombcytopenia, secondary to hypersplenism or folate deficiency, may be seen.

10. There is an increased incidence of gallstones.

11. Patients treated with desferrioxamine commonly develop infection with *Yersinia* spp., which may result in abdominal complaints.

12. Recurrent transfusions increase the risk of blood-transmitted infections, such as hepatitis C and HIV.

Heterozygous beta thalassaemia

1. The haemoglobin level is normal, or there is only a mild anaemia, except during pregnancy.

2. The red cells are hypochromic and microcytic, therefore there is a low mean corpuscular haemoglobin and a low mean cellular volume.

3. The HbA_2 may be elevated to 4–6%. Fifty percent of subjects have HbF levels of 1–5%.

Anaesthetic problems of homozygous disease

There are few case reports of anaesthesia in thalassaemia major. The management of open heart surgery in patients with haemoglobinopathies was described (de Laval et al 1974). No complications were experienced in the three patients with thalassaemia.

1. Anaemia, associated with a hyperdynamic circulation.

2. Cardiac failure, pulmonary hypertension (Du et al 1997) and restrictive lung disease (Factor et al 1994) may occur, even in treated patients.

3. Intubation difficulties have been reported. In untreated patients, frontal bossing and maxillary bone enlargement may occur secondary to bone marrow hyperplasia. Intubation problems in an 11-year-old child were due to massive forward protrusion of the maxilla (Orr 1967). Marrow hyperplasia is now reduced by starting transfusion therapy at an earlier age.

4. An increased risk of transfusion reactions and the presence of irregular red-cell antibodies.

5. Increased risk of overwhelming infection in splenectomised patients, particularly those receiving desferrioxamine.

6. Now that patients are intensively treated, pregnancy does occur. In a study of 25 pregnancies, nine were by induction of ovulation. Of the two patients with cardiac disease, one died 9 months after delivery and the other developed atrial flutter and LVF (Tuck et al 1998). It is recommended that fertility treatment should only be undertaken in those without significant cardiomyopathy (Jensen et al 1995).

Management

1. Patients with homozygous disease will be having regular transfusions at 2–4-week intervals to maintain the Hb at about $12\,g\,dl^{-1}$, and desferrioxamine iv or sc to chelate iron. Those whose blood requirements exceeds 1.5 times the standard requirement of splenectomised patients may undergo splenectomy (Rebulla & Modell 1991).

2. Transfusion reactions are reduced by the routine use of white-cell filters.

3.   In untreated patients, the possible potential intubation difficulties should be considered.

4.   Serum ferritin levels will indicate the iron status in patients with thalassaemia minor.

5.   Bone marrow transplantation in suitable patients improves survival.

6.   Pregnancy may be safe, provided patients have had long-term treatment with chelation, vigorous transfusion regimens, and there is echocardiographic evidence of good left ventricular function (Aessopos et al 1999).

7.   Prophylaxis before and after splenectomy. Three vaccines should be given, preferably 2 weeks before splenectomy.

   a)   Pneumovax 0.5 ml sc or im and repeat once between 5 and 10 years later.

   b)   HIB vaccine 0.5 ml sc or im once only.

   c)   Mengivac (A + C) 0.5 ml sc or im and repeat every 2 years.

Antibiotic prophylaxis; benzylpenicillin 600 mg 12 hrly iv or oral penicillin V 250 mg 12 hrly. If penicillin allergic, erythromycin 500 mg 12 hrly iv or oral 250 mg 12 hrly.

Bibliography

Aessopos A, Karabatsos F, Farmakis A et al 1999 Pregnancy in patients with well-treated beta-thalassemia: outcome for mothers and newborn infants. American Journal of Obstetrics & Gynecology 180: 360–5.

de Laval MR, Taswell HF, Bowie EJW et al 1974 Open heart surgery in patients with inherited hemoglobinopathies, red cell dyscrasias and coagulopathies. Archives of Surgery 109: 618–22.

Drew SJ, Sachs SA 1997 Management of the thalassemia-induced skeletal facial deformity: case reports and review of the literature. Journal of Oral & Maxillofacial Surgery 55: 1331–9.

Du ZD, Roguin N, Milgram E et al 1997 Pulmonary hypertension in patients with thalassemia major. American Heart Journal 134: 532–7.

Factor JM, Pottipati SR, Rappoport I et al 1994 Pulmonary function abnormalities in thalassemia major and the role of iron overload. American Review of Respiratory & Critical Care Medicine 149: 1570–4.

Jensen CE, Tuck SM, Wonke B 1995 Fertility in beta thalassaemia major: a report of 16 pregnancies, preconceptual evaluation and a review of the literature. British Journal of Obstetrics & Gynaecology 102: 625–9.

Lucarelli G, Galimberti M, Polchi P et al 1990 Bone marrow transplantation in patients with thalassaemia. New England Journal of Medicine 322: 417–21.

Olivieri NF 1999 The beta-thalassemias. New England Journal of Medicine 341: 99–109

Orr D 1967 Difficult intubation: a hazard in thalassaemia. British Journal of Anaesthesia 39: 585–7.

Rebulla P, Modell B 1991 Transfusion requirements and effects in patients with thalassaemia major. Lancet 337: 277–80.

Tuck SM, Jensen CE, Wonke B et al 1998 Pregnancy management and outcomes in women with thalassaemia major. Journal of Pediatric Endocrinology 11 (suppl 3): 923–8.

Thalidomide-related deformities and other phocomelias

An association between the ingestion of thalidomide in early pregnancy and limb defects was suspected and subsequently confirmed in 1961 (Editorial 1981). About 450 individuals in the UK were affected and they are therefore now in their forties. A number of the abnormalities have required surgery (Fletcher 1980).

Preoperative abnormalities

1.   A range of defects, from absence of a limb to minor anomalies of thumbs or toes. The upper limb is more commonly involved. Hands and feet, which are deformed and rotated, may grow out directly of shoulders or trunk. The head and trunk size is normal.

2.   Other anomalies described include a depressed nasal bridge, ocular and facial palsies, coloboma, spinal abnormalities, congenital heart defects, profuse sweating, absence of ears, or small ears, with deafness, bowel, urological and gynaecological defects (Quibell 1981).

Anaesthetic problems

1. Potential sites for venous access are limited and femoral or subclavian veins may be poorly developed. There may be difficulties in obtaining blood for pathological investigations. Internal jugular cannulation failed in a pregnant patient with tetra-amelia who required LSCS, but a right subclavian catheter was eventually sited (Williams & Bailey 1999).

2. Arterial blood pressure measurement may be extremely difficult.

3. The reduction in total body skeletal muscle mass of about 75% resulted in rapid induction of anaesthesia followed by fluctuations in depth of anaesthesia in a patient having inhalational anaesthesia for minor gynaecological surgery (McCrory 1988).

4. Spinal abnormalities appear to be more common than was first thought, and they particularly involve fusion of vertebrae in the dorsolumbar region.

5. Patients may present for obstetric interventions, particularly since uterine and vaginal abnormalities have been described. A high Caesarean section rate has been found in women with major malformations (Maouris & Hirsch 1988). Epidural anaesthesia for Caesarean section has been described (Grayling & Young 1989). Another patient refused to have an epidural, but eventually required an emergency LSCS (Williams & Bailey 1999).

6. In those who are deaf and have speech impairment, there may be communication difficulties.

Management

1. May required jugular venous cannulation. A cannula of suitable length must be chosen.

2. The use of a paediatric sphygmomanometer cuff with a carbon microphone pulse meter on a rudimentary hand to measure blood pressure was described by Grayling and Young (1989).

Bibliography

Editorial 1981 Thalidomide: 20 years on. Lancet ii: 510–11.

Fletcher I 1980 Review of the treatment of thalidomide children with limb deficiency in Great Britain. Clinical Orthopaedics and Related Research 148: 18–25.

Grayling GW, Young PN 1989 Anaesthesia and thalidomide-related deformities. Anaesthesia 44: 69.

Maouris PG, Hirsch PJ 1988 Pregnancy in women with thalidomide-induced disabilities. Case report and a questionnaire. British Journal of Obstetrics & Gynaecology 95: 717–19.

McCrory JW 1988 Anaesthesia and thalidomide-related deformities. Anaesthesia 43: 613–14.

Quibell EP 1981 The thalidomide embryopathy. An analysis from the UK. Practitioner 225: 721–6.

Williams AR, Bailey MK 1999 Anesthetic management of a patient with tetra-amelia. Southern Medical Journal 92: 325–7.

Thyrotoxicosis (see also Section 2, Thyrotoxic crisis)

A state of thyroid overactivity, which should be controlled before elective surgery, to avoid precipitating a thyroid crisis (Pronovost & Parris 1995). If antithyroid drugs are used, preparation for thyroid surgery may take up to 2 months. With beta adrenoceptor blockers and potassium iodide alone, control can be achieved within 2 weeks, but not all are agreed on the adequacy of this method for patients who need surgery. Beta blockers only block the peripheral effects of the hormones. They do not affect their synthesis or release, and may obscure a crisis (Eriksson et al 1977). Since they are short acting, their omission in the perioperative period may lead to an unexpected crisis. Occasionally a thyrotoxic patient requires urgent surgery. Alternatively, surgery may be unwittingly undertaken in a thyrotoxic patient, because the diagnosis is obscured by other pathology. Thyrotoxicosis may also be precipitated by infections, labour, trauma, acute medical illness, and stress (Smallridge 1992). The diagnosis is most frequently missed in elderly patients, or during pregnancy, when it is difficult to distinguish it from physiological increases in metabolic rate.

Preoperative abnormalities

1. A history of weight loss, heat intolerance, tremor, sweating, palpitations, fatigue, diarrhoea, and anxiety.

2. Tachycardia, in particular an increased sleeping pulse rate, atrial fibrillation in the elderly, and occasionally heart failure.

3. There may be thyroid swelling, exophthalmos, and lid lag. Rarely, a goitre may cause tracheal compression.

4. The diagnosis is made on an increased serum T_4, free thyroxine index and T_3 concentrations with an undetectable TSH. The TRH test may be needed in difficult cases.

5. Clinically obvious myopathy is infrequent, but there is some degree of EMG abnormality in 90% of thyrotoxic patients.

Anaesthetic problems

1. Tachyarrhythmias are common during anaesthesia. High thyroid hormone concentrations may result in beta adrenoceptor up-regulation, so that larger doses of propranolol than normal may be needed to control tachycardias, because the clearance is increased in the disease. In fact, control with propranolol may be unsuccessful (Isley et al 1990, Knighton & Crosse 1997).

2. A hypermetabolic state may occur that can resemble malignant hyperthermia (Peters et al 1981, Stevens 1983). Atrial fibrillation was precipitated by induction of anaesthesia in one patient (Bennett & Wainwright 1989). Factitious thyrotoxicosis has occurred in a patient who was subsequently found to have taken 14 thyroxine 0.1-mg tablets on the morning of surgery, because she had not taken any for 2 weeks (Ambus et al 1994). Tachycardia and increased CO_2 was associated with a serum thyroxine level of $27 \mu g dl^{-1}$ (normal range $4.5-12 \mu g dl^{-1}$).

3. Pulmonary oedema may develop intraoperatively. This can present as cyanosis, tachycardia, and respiratory distress. It is caused by a combination of hypertension, tachycardia, and increased blood volume. An undiagnosed thyrotoxic patient with a fractured hip developed pulmonary oedema, pyrexia and tachycardia during surgery (Stevens 1983). This hypermetabolic state was diagnosed and treated as malignant hyperthermia. The true diagnosis was only revealed during postoperative investigations.

4. Rarely, a thyroid crisis, or storm, may develop after surgery and present with agitation, pyrexia, sweating, tachycardia, hypertension, and cardiac failure (Jamison & Dove 1979, Knighton & Crosse 1997). Similarly this may occur during labour or Caesarean section (Halpern 1989).

5. The crisis can be masked by beta blockers, which do not block the output of thyroid hormones (Jones & Solomon 1981). In addition, the negative inotropic effect may be disadvantageous. Circulatory collapse has been reported during the use of propranolol to control severe thyrotoxicosis in an elderly patient (Vijayakumar et al 1989).

6. Thyrotoxic myopathy occasionally results in delayed recovery from neuromuscular blocking agents. In one patient beta blockers masked the signs of thyrotoxicosis, but not the thyrotoxic myopathy (Uusitupa et al 1980).

7. When proptosis is present the eyes are more vulnerable to damage than normal.

8. In pregnancy, thyrotoxicosis is difficult to diagnose, because the two states share common features. Cardiac dysfunction may accompany thyrotoxicosis, and has been reported with both Caesarean section (Clark et al 1985) and septic abortion (Hankins et al 1984). Intraoperative tachycardia, followed by deterioration in conscious level, occurred in an anxious patient after general anaesthesia for Caesarean section. She was acidotic (base excess -13.2) and hyperkalaemic ($8.1 \text{ mmol } l^{-1}$). Propranolol and cardioversion failed to control the pulse rate and eventually thyrotoxicosis was diagnosed (Pugh et al 1994).

9. A functioning metastatic thyroid

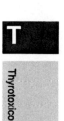

carcinoma caused a thyroid storm on the 19th day after severe burns, in a patient who had previously undergone thyroidectomy for malignancy (Naito et al 1997). A major increase in free hormone level was demonstrated after each new surgical procedure and attributed to transient decreases in hormone binding protein levels.

10. Deterioration in conscious level. One patient presented to the emergency department in coma (Gilbert et al 1992), and one failed to recover consciousness after emergency Caesarean section (Pugh et al 1994).

11. Thyrotoxic periodic paralysis is a type of hypokalaemic periodic paralysis that occurs in thyrotoxic patients. Hypophosphataemia and mild hypomagnesaemia are common accompanying features. In a study of 24 episodes of paralysis in 19 patients, the serum potassium ranged from 1.1 to 3.4 mmol l⁻¹ (Manoukian et al 1999).

Management

1. A euthyroid state should be achieved before surgery.

a) Antithyroid drugs inhibit thyroid hormone synthesis and block T_3 and T_4, but will take 6–8 weeks to become fully effective. The physical size of the thyroid gland may significantly increase during this therapy.

b) Potassium iodide will reduce the concentration of circulating hormone to well within the normal range, but its action only lasts for 10 days.

c) Beta adrenoceptor blockers will block the peripheral effects of the hormones, but will not block hormone release. Thyroid hormone will therefore still be present, as will the catabolic state. For those with a small gland, beta blockers are effective in combination with potassium iodide, but this is not so for the more toxic patients.

i) Propanolol 40–120 mg daily in divided doses for 2–3 weeks, with the addition of potassium iodide for the last 10 days. However, the systemic clearance of propranolol is increased by thyrotoxicosis, and, since the thyroxine already in the circulation has a long half-life, therapy needs to be continued for a week after operation. Propranolol may also produce hypoglycaemia in the perioperative period. If it cannot be given orally, an infusion will be required. The dose required to maintain therapeutic blood levels has been suggested to be 1 mg h⁻¹ (Prys-Roberts 1984) and 3 mg h⁻¹ (Smulyan et al 1982).

ii) Nadolol is more slowly metabolised by the liver, more slowly eliminated, and its clearance not altered by thyrotoxicosis. It can be given in a single daily dose of 160 mg, which gives prolonged beta blockade and more satisfactory blood levels than propranolol (Peden et al 1982). Preoperative potassium iodide is added in the usual manner. Bradycardias have been noticed more frequently than with propranolol, and atropine has been recommended as a premedication.

iii) The use of esmolol to control the tachycardia in severe thyrotoxicosis that was refractory to treatment has been described (Thorne & Bedford 1989). Surgery was urgent because of airway compromise. An infusion was started in the anaesthetic room and continued for 10 h after the end of surgery. On one occasion, a dose of 351 μg kg⁻¹ min⁻¹ was required, which exceeds the dose recommended by the manufacturer. In two adults, esmolol was used when propranolol had failed to work, or had caused problems. In a pregnant patient for laparotomy, a total of propranolol 27 mg failed to control the tachycardia, whereas an esmolol infusion was successful (Isley et al 1990). In a second patient, the use of propranolol had resulted in cardiovascular collapse (Vijayakumar et al 1989). Esmolol was used under similar circumstances in a 14-month-old infant after thyroidectomy for uncontrolled nonautoimmune hyperthyroidism (Knighton & Crosse 1997). The success of esmolol infusion is attributed to its more selective beta-1 adrenoceptor blocking action, its ease of titration, and the lowered systemic vascular resistance.

2.   Atrial fibrillation, heart failure or hypertension should be treated preoperatively.

3.   The eyes should be carefully protected.

4.   Treatment of a thyrotoxic crisis (see Section 2, Thyrotoxic crisis or storm).

5.   Management of thyrotoxicosis in pregnant or possibly pregnant women produces the potential problem of effects on the fetus (Drake & Wood 1998, O'Doherty et al 1999). At present, treatment is based on propylthiouracil.

6.   Regional anaesthesia, with cervical plexus block and local infiltration, has been used for thyroidectomy in two patients with amiodarone-induced thyrotoxicosis. This was refractory to treatment, and they were unfit for general anaesthesia (Klein et al 1997).

Bibliography

Ambus T, Evans S, Smith NT 1994 Thyrotoxicosis factitia in the anesthetized patient. Anesthesiology 81: 254–6.

Bennett MH, Wainwright AP 1989 Acute thyroid crisis on induction of anaesthesia. Anaesthesia 44: 28–30.

Burger AG, Philippe J 1992 Thyroid emergencies. Bailliere's Clinical Endocrinology & Metabolism 6: 77–93.

Clark SL, Phelan JP, Montoro M et al 1985 Transient ventricular dysfunction associated with cesarean section in a patient with hyperthyroidism. American Journal of Obstetrics & Gynecology 151: 384–6.

Drake WM, Wood DF 1998 Thyroid disease in pregnancy. Postgraduate Medical Journal 74: 583–6.

Eriksson M, Rubenfeld S, Garber AJ et al 1977 Propranolol does not prevent thyroid storm. New England Journal of Medicine 296: 263–4.

Gilbert RE, Thomas GW, Hope RN 1992 Coma and thyroid dysfunction. Anaesthesia & Intensive Care 20: 86–7.

Halpern S 1989 Anaesthesia for Caesarean section in patients with uncontrolled hyperthyroidism. Canadian Journal of Anaesthesia 36: 454–9.

Hankins GDV, Lowe TW, Cunningham FG 1984 Dilated cardiomyopathy and thyrotoxicosis complicated by septic abortion. American Journal of Obstetrics & Gynecology 149: 85–6.

Isley WL, Dahl S, Gibbs H 1990 Use of esmolol in managing a thyrotoxic patient needing emergency surgery. American Journal of Medicine 89: 122–3.

Jamison MH, Dove HJ 1979 Postoperative thyrotoxic crisis in a patient prepared for thyroidectomy with propranolol. British Journal of Clinical Practice 32: 82–3.

Jones DK, Solomon S 1981 Thyrotoxic crisis masked by treatment with beta blockers. British Medical Journal 283: 659.

Klein SM, Greengrass RA, Knudsen N et al 1997 Regional anesthesia for thyroidectomy in two patients with amiodarone-induced hyperthyroidism. Anesthesia & Analgesia 85: 222–4.

Knighton JD, Crosse MM 1997 Anaesthetic management of childhood thyrotoxicosis and the use of esmolol. Anaesthesia 52: 67–70.

Manoukian MA, Foote JA, Crapo LM 1999 Clinical and metabolic features of thyrotoxic periodic paralysis in 24 episodes. Archives of Internal Medicine 159: 601–6.

Naito Y, Sone T, Kataoka K et al 1997 Thyroid storm due to functioning metastatic thyroid carcinoma in a burn patient. Anesthesiology 87: 433–5.

O'Doherty MJ, McElhatton PR, Thomas SH 1999 Treating thyrotoxicosis in pregnant or potentially pregnant women. British Medical Journal 318: 5–6.

Peden NR, Gunn A, Browning MCK et al 1982 Nadolol and potassium iodide in combination in the surgical patient. British Journal of Surgery 69: 638–40.

Peters KR, Nance P, Wingard DW 1981 Malignant hyperthyroidism or malignant hyperthermia. Anesthesia & Analgesia 60: 613–15.

Pronovost PH, Parris KH 1995 Perioperative management of thyroid disease. Prevention of complications related to hyperthyroidism and hypothyroidism. Postgraduate Medicine 98: 83–6, 96–8.

Prys-Roberts C 1984 Kinetics and dynamics of beta adrenoceptor antagonists. In: Pharmacokinetics of anaesthesia. Blackwell Scientific Publications, Oxford.

Pugh S, Lalwani K, Awal A 1994 Thyroid storm as a cause of loss of consciousness following anaesthesia for emergency Caesarean section. Anaesthesia 49: 35–7.

Smallridge RC 1992 Metabolic and anatomic thyroid emergencies: a review. Critical Care Medicine 20: 276–91.

Smulyan H, Weinberg SE, Howanitz PJ 1982 Continuous propranolol infusion following abdominal surgery. Journal of the American Medical Association 247: 2539–42.

Stevens JJ 1983 A case of thyrotoxic crisis that mimicked malignant hyperthermia. Anesthesiology 59: 263.

Thorne AC, Bedford RF 1989 Esmolol for perioperative management of thyrotoxic goiter. Anesthesiology 71: 291–4.

Uusitupa M, Aro A, Korhon ENT et al 1980 Beta blockade, myopathy and thyrotoxicosis. British Medical Journal 1: 183.

Vijayakumar HR, Thomas WO, Ferrara JJ 1989 Perioperative management of severe thyrotoxicosis with esmolol. Anaesthesia 44: 406–8.

Torsade de pointes (atypical ventricular tachycardia)

An atypical, paroxysmal VT associated with delayed repolarisation of the ventricle. It is frequently drug induced, but may also occur with metabolic abnormalities and the familial long QT syndromes (see also QT syndromes). It is now known that, in addition to antiarrhythmic drugs, there are a number of noncardiac drugs that provoke torsade de pointes (T de P) VT. They share a common feature in that they block one component of a particular type of potassium channel, resulting in lengthening of the QT interval (Yap & Camm 2000). Drugs include terfenadine, astemizole, some macrolide antibiotics, tricyclic antidepressants, neuroleptics such as haloperidol and thioridazine, cisapride and pimozide.

Presentation

1. The patient may collapse, or complain of episodes of palpitations, faintness, or fatigue.

2. As an unusual type of VT. Instead of a rapid succession of extrasystoles of identical configuration, the axis of the QRS complex appears to rotate around the baseline. Before the event there is a characteristic 'long–short' sequence in which a premature ectopic beat is followed by a long pause, then another premature ectopic initiates the torsade de pointes.

3. The VT is not resolved by conventional antiarrhythmic treatment.

4. Factors that predispose to the development of torsade de pointes include:

   a) Drug therapy.

      i) Prenylamine.

      ii) Disopyramide. Intraoperative T de P was attributed to sevoflurane, but was much more likely to have been due to disopyramide given on induction of anaesthesia to treat atrial fibrillation (Abe et al 1998).

      iii) Quinidine.

      iv) Tricyclic antidepressants.

      v) Haloperidol. T de P occurred following cardiac bypass grafting in a patient who had been given large doses of haloperidol (Perrault et al 2000).

      vi) Sotalol.

      vii) Cisapride

      viii) Terfenadine and astemizole.

   b) Conduction problems.

      i) Sick sinus syndrome.

      ii) Congenital long QT interval syndromes.

      iii) Atrioventricular block.

c) Electrolyte imbalance.

i) Hypokalaemia. A combination of hypokalaemia, hypocalcaemia and alkalosis prolonged the QT_c interval in two patients undergoing surgery (Soroker et al 1995). Isolated hypokalaemia in a 4 year old secondary to high-dose frusemide has also been reported (Chvilicek et al 1995). A combination of erythromycin and mechanical bowel preparation caused a long QT_c interval and T de P (Vogt & Zollo 1997).

ii) Hypomagnesaemia. T de P has been reported after massive blood transfusion for severe postpartum haemorrhage (Kulkarni et al 1992). Magnesium infusion restored the QT interval to normal and temporary ventricular pacing prevented further ventricular arrhythmias.

iii) Hypocalcaemia.

d) Right radical neck dissection (Otteni et al 1983). Prolongation of the QT interval occurred in association with right-sided neck surgery, but not with left, and persisted in more than one-third of 32 patients studied. Three patients had episodes of T de P in the postoperative period.

e) Coronary artery spasm occurring during abdominal surgery was thought to be responsible for two episodes of T de P (Mizutani et al 1996).

Diagnosis

1. Is best made on a 12-lead ECG. A VT is shown with the QRS axis undulating over 5–6 beats and with a change in direction. The 'long–short' initiating sequence may be seen.

2. In between episodes of T de P the corrected QT interval (QT_c) may be prolonged.

Management

1. The underlying cause is corrected.

a) Any potentially causative drug is stopped. A recurrent VT appeared 6 h after pleurectomy in a patient with severe lung disease (Alexander & Potgieter 1983). A further 20 h of treatment with a number of drugs including lidocaine (lignocaine), disopyramide, digoxin, procainamide and propranolol, and DC shock, was unsuccessful. A 12-lead ECG showed an undulating QRS axis and the QT_c in between episodes of tachycardia was 0.863 s. A diagnosis of atypical VT was made. All drugs were stopped and the hypokalaemia corrected. Review of earlier ECGs also showed a prolonged QT_c.

b) Metabolic causes such as hypokalaemia, hypocalcaemia or hypomagnesaemia are corrected.

c) Patients with the long QT syndrome should remain permanently on beta adrenoceptor blocking drugs. The use of labetalol in a patient with recurrent T de P, refractory to treatment, has been described (Grubb 1991).

2. Avoid the use of class I antiarrhythmics, and those drugs already mentioned.

3. In cases in which the tachycardia persists, atrial pacing may be required.

4. If VF occurs, defibrillation will be necessary.

5. Isoprenaline may increase the heart rate and therefore shorten the QT interval. A dose of $1–2\,\mu g\,kg^{-1}$ has been recommended, but extreme caution is required. Contraindications include myocardial ischaemia and hypertensive heart disease.

6. Bretylium, lidocaine (lignocaine) and magnesium sulphate have on occasions been successful.

7. Nicorandil, a potassium channel activator, abolished intraoperative T de P (Saitoh et al 1998).

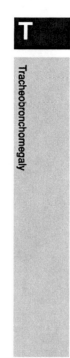

Bibliography

Abe K, Takada K, Yoshiya I 1998 Intraoperative torsade de pointes ventricular tachycardia and ventricular fibrillation during sevoflurane anesthesia. Anesthesia & Analgesia 86: 701–2.

Alexander MG, Potgieter PD 1983 Atypical ventricular tachycardia (torsade de pointes). Anaesthesia 38: 269–74.

Chvilicek JP, Hurlbert BJ, Hill GE 1995 Diuretic-induced hypokalaemia inducing torsades de pointes. Canadian Journal of Anaesthesia 42: 1137–9.

Grubb BP 1991 The use of oral labetalol in the treatment of arrhythmias associated with the long QT syndrome. Chest 100: 1724–5.

Kulkarni P, Bhattacharya S, Petros AJ 1992 Torsade de pointes and long QT syndrome following major blood transfusion. Anaesthesia 47: 125–7.

Lusyik SJ, Eichelberger JP, Chhibber AK et al 1998 Torsade de pointes during orthotopic liver transplantation. Anesthesia & Analgesia 87: 300–3.

Mizutani K, Toyoda Y, Kubota H 1996 Torsade de pointes ventricular tachycardia following coronary artery spasm during general anaesthesia. Anaesthesia 51: 858–60.

Otteni JC, Pottecher RT, Bronner G et al 1983 Prolongation of the Q–T interval and sudden cardiac arrest following right radical neck dissection. Anesthesiology 59: 358–61.

Perrault LP, Denault AY, Carrier M et al 2000 Torsades de pointes secondary to haloperidol after cardiac bypass graft. Canadian Journal of Anaesthesia 47: 251–4.

Saitoh K, Suzuki H, Hirabayashi Y et al 1998 Nicorandil successfully abolished intraoperative torsade de pointes. Anesthesiology 88: 1669–71.

Soroker D, Ezri T, Szmuk P et al 1995 Perioperative torsade de pointes ventricular tachycardia induced by hypocalcemia and hypokalemia. Anesthesia & Analgesia 80: 630–3.

Vogt AW, Zollo RA 1997 Long Q–T syndrome associated with oral erythromycin used in preoperative bowel preparation. Anesthesia & Analgesia 85: 1011–13.

Yap YG, Camm J 2000 Risk of torsade de pointes with non-cardiac drugs. British Medical Journal 320: 1158–9.

Tracheobronchomegaly

A congenital condition in which atrophy and thinning of the elastic fibres of the membraneous and cartilaginous parts of the trachea results in significant tracheal and bronchial dilatation, sometimes with diverticulum formation. Stenosis may subsequently occur.

Preoperative abnormalities

1. Presents in the third to fourth decade, usually in males. Symptoms include a loud, ineffective cough, dyspnoea, episodes of choking, recurrent, nonproductive chest infections, respiratory insufficiency, and cor pulmonale.

2. The trachea is abnormally dilated (>30 mm); weakness occurs in the membraneous and cartilaginous parts, which can easily collapse. Sometimes the trachea becomes stenosed secondary to fibrous tissue formation around it.

3. A flow–volume loop reveals extrathoracic narrowing.

4. Bronchoscopy shows gross dilatation of the trachea or bronchi, and collapse on expiration or coughing. There may be large tracheal diverticuli.

5. The diagnostic criteria on CT scan have been defined (Woodring et al 1991). In women, it is diagnosed if the transverse and sagittal diameters exceed 21 mm and 23 mm respectively; in men, when the transverse and sagittal diameters exceed 25 mm and 27 mm respectively. On plain X-ray, which magnifies the tracheal size, a diameter in a male in excess of 30 mm, is diagnostic. There may be an abrupt transition between the normal and the dilated segments.

Anaesthetic problems

1. A 22-year-old male receiving IPPV after a head injury was noticed on day 2 to have tracheal dilatation to 29 mm at the site of the cuff. The patient was extubated on day 15, by which time the trachea was no longer dilated. Progressive stenosis followed rapidly and, after

failed bougie dilatation, resection of the stenosed segment was undertaken at 2 months (Messahel 1989).

2.   The tracheal wall can easily collapse during respiration, resulting in partial or complete obstruction. This gives conflicting results on investigation. In a 66-year-old male, videofluoroscopy showed the extrathoracic A–P diameter to be 30 mm, collapsing down to 22 mm (Bourne et al 1995). During anaesthesia, 18 ml air in the tube cuff was required to produce a seal.

3.   Secretions may pool in the redundant mucosa or diverticulae, and result in chronic suppurative lung disease, emphysema, and pulmonary fibrosis. Patients are more prone to postoperative atelectasis. One patient, with respiratory failure secondary to bronchiectasis, was found to have large airways filled with copious thick secretions (Schwartz & Rossoff 1994).

Management

1.   There is some disagreement about the best way to avoid complications. Using an uncuffed tube with packing has been suggested to result in aspiration, whereas prolonged damage from a tracheal tube cuff may produce stenosis (Messahel 1989, Bourne et al 1995).

2.   The collapsed airways may be maintained open with CPAP.

3.   Treatment may be by resection or stenting. However, since the disease is widespread, the role of surgery is limited (Sane et al 1992).

Bibliography

Bourne TM, Raphael JH, Tordoff SG 1995 Anaesthesia for a patient with tracheobronchomegaly (Mounier–Kuhn syndrome). Anaesthesia 50: 545–7.

Collard P, Freitag L, Reynaert MS et al 1996 Respiratory failure due to tracheobronchomalacia. Thorax 51: 224–6.

Messahel FM 1989 Tracheal dilatation followed by stenosis in Mounier–Kuhn syndrome. Anaesthesia: 44: 227–9.

Sane AC, Effmann EL, Brown SD 1992 Tracheobronchomegaly. The Mounier–Kuhn syndrome in a patient with the Kenney–Caffey syndrome. Chest 102: 618–19.

Schwartz M, Rossoff L 1994 Tracheobronchomegaly. Chest 106: 1589–90.

Smith DL, Withers N, Holloway et al 1994 Tracheobronchomegaly: an unusual presentation of a rare condition. Thorax 49: 840–1.

Woodring JH, Howard RS 2nd, Rehm SR 1991 Congenital tracheobronchomegaly (Mounier–Kuhn syndrome): a report of 10 cases and review of the literature. Journal of Thoracic Imaging 6: 1–10.

Treacher Collins syndrome (see also Pierre Robin syndrome)

A craniofacial defect associated with developmental anomalies of the first arch. Abnormalities vary from minimal, to the complete syndrome. Patients may require anaesthesia for manoeuvres to improve upper airway obstruction temporarily, or for correction of some of the congenital defects. Obstruction and a requirement for multiple operations increases the need for tracheostomy (Posnick 1997). In a retrospective review of Treacher Collins and Nager syndromes, 28 out of 59 patients required tracheostomy at some stage (Sculerati et al 1998).

Preoperative abnormalities

1.   Features may include mandibular and malar hypoplasia, antimongoloid palpebral fissure, a large mouth and irregular maloccluded teeth, microphthalmia, lower lid defects, cleft palate, macroglossia, and auricular deformities.

2.   Associated abnormalities include mental retardation, deafness, dwarfism, cardiac defects, and skeletal deformities.

3.   The predominant problem is one of chronic upper respiratory tract obstruction, which in its severest form leads to retarded growth and occasionally cor pulmonale. If the child is failing to compensate for his/her airway

dysfunction, growth will be well below the average percentile (Mallory & Paradise 1979).

4. Sleep apnoea has been described.

Anaesthetic problems

1. Airway obstruction. In the small baby this may require urgent temporary corrective manoeuvres, such as stitching the tongue to the lower lip.

2. Excess secretions may hamper induction of anaesthesia.

3. Gaseous induction may be difficult.

4. Tracheal intubation. A number of papers have described difficult or failed intubation (Sklar & King 1976, Miyabe et al 1985, Rasch et al 1986). One resulted in a near fatality (Ross 1963).

5. Obstructive sleep apnoea may occur postoperatively (Roa & Moss 1984).

6. Pulmonary oedema. Respiratory arrest and pulmonary oedema were reported in a 15-year-old boy 40 min after a N_2O/O_2/halothane anaesthetic (Roa & Moss 1984).

Management

1. Respiratory depressant agents should be avoided, both for premedication, and postoperatively.

2. Drying agents should always be used.

3. A muscle relaxant must never be given until the airway has been secured.

4. Awake intubation or awake direct laryngoscopy to visualise the vocal cords should be considered. A successful direct laryngoscopy, performed with the patient in the sitting position, and using a 5-G feeding tube taped to the side of the laryngoscope to give oxygen, has been described (Rasch et al 1986). The use of the fibreoptic bronchoscope or tracheostomy under local anaesthetic has been recommended in order to avoid the hazards of gaseous

induction and failed intubation. In older children, some of whom are retarded, this may not be possible.

5. If general anaesthesia is essential, a number of techniques have been described to assist intubation.

a) The use of an anterior commissure laryngoscope, which prevents the tongue from falling in on the laryngoscope, has been described (Handler & Keon 1983, see Pierre Robin syndrome for a full description).

b) A tactile nasal intubation technique was used in a 4-year-old boy (Sklar & King 1976). Induction was with halothane followed by ether, and the tongue was pulled downwards and forwards. The tube was initially used as a nasal airway, whilst the index and middle finger were used to palpate the epiglottis, through which the tube was then passed.

c) The use of an assistant to pull out the tongue with forceps, and at the same time to apply cricoid pressure, was found to assist laryngoscopy (Miyabe et al 1985).

d) A 14-year-old boy was anaesthetised with incremental ketamine. A gum elastic bougie was inserted into the larynx and the tube was threaded over the top (MacLennan & Roberts 1981).

e) A laryngeal mask airway instead of a tracheal tube was used in a patient undergoing tympanoplasty (Ebata et al 1991). A laryngeal mask airway has also been inserted under propofol anaesthesia (Bahk et al 1999). It has been suggested as a conduit for the passage of a bougie or a fibreoptic bronchoscope. However, Inada et al (1995) showed that only the fibrescope was of use in Treacher Collins, because the posteriorly placed tongue tended to displace the glottis anteriorly.

f) The Bullard intubating laryngoscope has been used to achieve nasotracheal intubation in a 17-month-old child with tongue tie (Brown et al 1993).

g) The Augustine guide was used for nasotracheal intubation in an awake, sedated patient having multiple operations for facial reconstruction (Kovac 1992).

6. The tracheal tube should remain in place until the patient is fully awake. There have been a number of reports of airway obstruction occurring during the recovery period. These have necessitated reintubation and, in one case, a tracheostomy.

7. Patients should be nursed in a high-dependency area postoperatively. The combination of sleep apnoea and drugs with CNS-depressant effects may make them particularly susceptible to respiratory arrest.

Bibliography

Bahk J-H, Han S-M, Kim S-D 1999 Management of difficult airways with a laryngeal mask airway under propofol anaesthesia. Paediatric Anaesthesia 9: 163–6.

Brown RE Jr, Vollers JM, Rader GR et al 1993 Nasotracheal intubation in a child with Treacher Collins syndrome using the Bullard intubating laryngoscope. Journal of Clinical Anesthesia 5: 492–3.

Ebata T, Nishiki S, Masuda A et al 1991 Anaesthesia for Treacher Collins syndrome using a laryngeal mask airway. Canadian Journal of Anaesthesia 38: 1043–5.

Handler SD, Keon TP 1983 Difficult laryngoscopy/intubation: the child with mandibular hypoplasia. Annals of Otology, Rhinology & Laryngology 92: 401–4.

Inada T, Fujise K, Tachibana K et al 1995 Orotracheal intubation through the laryngeal mask airway in paediatric patients with Treacher Collins syndrome. Paediatric Anaesthesia 5: 129–32.

Kovac AL 1992 Use of the Augustine stylet anticipating difficult tracheal intubation in Treacher Collins syndrome. Journal of Clinical Anesthesia 4: 409–12.

MacLennan F, Robertson GS 1981 Ketamine for induction and intubation in Treacher Collins syndrome. Anaesthesia 36: 196–8.

Mallory SB, Paradise JL 1979 Glossoptosis revisited: on the development and resolution of airway obstruction in the Pierre Robin syndrome. Pediatrics 64: 946–8.

Miyabe M, Dohi S, Homma E 1985 Tracheal intubation in an infant with Treacher Collins syndrome—pulling out the tongue by a forceps. Anesthesiology 62: 213–14.

Posnick JC 1997 Treacher Collins syndrome: perspectives in evaluation and treatment. Journal of Oral & Maxillofacial Surgery 55: 1120–33.

Rasch DJ, Browder F, Barr M et al 1986 Anaesthesia for Treacher Collins and Pierre Robin syndromes: a report of three cases. Canadian Anaesthetists' Society Journal 33: 364–70.

Roa NL, Moss KS 1984 Treacher Collins syndrome with sleep apnea: anesthetic considerations. Anesthesiology 60: 71–3.

Ross ED 1963 Treacher Collins syndrome. An anaesthetic hazard. Anaesthesia 18: 350–4.

Sculerati N, Gottlieb MD, Zimbler MS et al 1998 Airway management in children with major craniofacial abnormalities. Laryngoscope 108: 1806–12.

Sklar GS, King BD 1976 Endotracheal intubation and Treacher Collins syndrome. Anesthesiology 44: 247–9.

Tuberous sclerosis

A neurocutaneous disease associated with hamartomas in multiple organ systems, skin lesions, and learning difficulties. Skeletal muscle is not involved. It is an autosomal dominant condition and recent genetic linkage studies have implicated abnormalities of the 9q34 protein encoded by the tuberin and hamartin genes. Both are tumour suppressor genes on chromosomes 9 and 16 (O'Callaghan 1999). For full diagnostic criteria, see Webb and Osbourne (1995).

Preoperative abnormalities

1. Cutaneous. Facial and ungual angiofibroma.

2. Neurological. Mental retardation in 60%, and seizures in 80–90%. Giant cell astrocytomas, obstruction of the third ventricle, and retinal astrocytomas.

3. Cardiovascular. Cardiac rhabdomyomas may cause outlet obstruction. The presence of a cardiomyoma increases the risk of pre-excitation and arrhythmias, in particular WPW syndrome (O'Callaghan et al 1998). Cardiomyomas regress with the passage of time and surgery may be

required only occasionally in neonates, if the tumour causes obstructive heart failure.

4. Renal angiomyolipoma, which may bleed, and renal cysts.

5. Occasionally, pulmonary lymphangiomatosis occurs.

6. In a series of 355 patients at the Mayo Clinic, 49 died. The main causes of death were cardiac failure, renal disease, brain tumours, and lymphangiomatosis of the lung (Shepherd et al 1991).

Anaesthetic problems

1. Cardiac arrhythmias associated with WPW syndrome.

2. Rupture of a renal angiomyolipoma and placental abruption occurred in a 37-week-pregnant woman. A right nephrectomy was performed (Forsnes et al 1996). Severe haemorrhage can occur in those renal angiomyolipomas that exceed 8 cm in diameter. Laparotomy was required for bleeding into a tumour that resulted in an Hb of 5 g dl⁻¹ (Ong & Koay 2000).

3. Anaesthesia has been reported for repair of an 8-cm-diameter aortic aneurysm in a 4-year-old child (Tsukui et al 1995).

4. The problems of anaesthesia for a patient with epilepsy (Nott & Halfacre 1996).

Management

1. Careful examination and investigation for involvement of different organ systems, in particular pulmonary involvement (Lee et al 1994).

2. Management of the patient with seizures.

3. ECG and echocardiography if cardiac rhabdomyoma is suspected.

Bibliography
Forsnes EV, Eggelston MK, Burtman M 1996 Placental abruption and spontaneous rupture of renal angiomyolipoma in a pregnant woman with tuberous sclerosis. Obstetrics & Gynecology 88: 725.
Lee JJ, Imrie M, Taylor V 1994 Anaesthesia and tuberous sclerosis. British Journal of Anaesthesia 73: 421–5.
Nott MR, Halfacre J 1996 Anaesthesia for dental conservation in a patient with tuberous sclerosis. European Journal of Anaesthesiology 13: 413–15.
O'Callaghan FJ 1999 Tuberous sclerosis. British Medical Journal 318: 1019–20.
O'Callaghan FJ, Clarke AC, Joffe H et al 1998 Tuberous sclerosis complex and Wolff–Parkinson–White syndrome. Archives of Disease in Childhood 78: 159–62.
Ong EL, Koay CK 2000 Tuberous sclerosis presenting for laparotomy. Anaesthesia & Intensive Care 28: 94–6.
Shepherd CW, Gomez MR, Lie JT et al 1991 Causes of death in patients with tuberous sclerosis. Mayo Clinic Proceedings 66: 792–6.
Tsukui A, Noguchi R, Honda T et al 1995 Aortic aneurysm in a four-year-old child with tuberous sclerosis. Paediatric Anaesthesia 5: 67–70.
Webb DW, Osbourne JP 1995 Tuberous sclerosis. Archives of Disease in Childhood 72: 471–4.

Turner's syndrome

A syndrome associated with a sex chromosome abnormality, it includes gonadal dysgenesis, primary amenorrhoea, skeletal, renal, cardiovascular and other anomalies. Cardiovascular complications are the single source of increased mortality and may be associated with aortic wall weakness. Those with the 45,X karyotype were particularly susceptible (Gotzsche et al 1994). There is a high incidence of sternal abnormalities, insulin resistance, and neoplastic conditions (Saenger 1996).

Preoperative abnormalities

1. Skeletal abnormalities may include short stature, a short, webbed neck, with fusion of cervical vertebrae, a low hairline, cubitus valgus, a high arched palate, micrognathia, a shield chest, scoliosis, inverted, widely spaced nipples, and a short fourth metacarpal. Nail dysplasia and dental defects may occur. There is an increased incidence of fractures and osteoporosis.

2. In a survey of patients, or families of patients, 52% had cardiovascular malformations (Lin et al 1998). Left-sided obstructive lesions, namely bicuspid aortic valve, aortic stenosis and coarctation, were most common, although aortic dilatation and dissection may occur. Other cardiac defects include partial anomalous pulmonary venous drainage and pulmonary valve anomalies (Moore et al 1990, Gotzsche et al 1995). Hypertension is common.

3. Associated anomalies such as renal dysgenesis, peripheral lymphoedema, and ocular and aural defects.

4. Metabolic abnormalities are more common than normal. There is an increased incidence of diabetes and autoimmune thyroid disease.

Anaesthetic problems

1. Intubation difficulties may result from the short neck and fused cervical vertebrae.

2. The distance between the vocal cords and carina may be reduced. A patient developed left lung collapse following accidental one lung anaesthesia during laparoscopy (Divekar et al 1983). Subsequent X-rays showed that the bifurcation of the trachea was in an abnormally high position, at the level of the sternoclavicular joint.

3. Problems of renal disease.

4. Natural pregnancies in Turner's syndrome are rare. However, assisted conception is becoming more common, although pregnancy carries high risks. Two deaths from aortic dissection have been reported in the third trimester of assisted pregnancy (Lin et al 1998). A further patient collapsed at 24 weeks' gestation with a myocardial infarction secondary to aortic dissection (Garvey et al 1998). At surgery she was found to have severe aortic regurgitation, and mild coarctation in addition. Although she survived surgery under cardiopulmonary bypass

and her child was delivered at 27 weeks, she died 88 days later.

Management

1. It has been recommended that patients with Turner's syndrome have 5-yearly echocardiography and regular monitoring of blood pressure and aortic root diameter, particularly the 45,X karyotype individuals with bicuspid aortic valves. However, it has been suggested that this is unnecessary in the absence of structural cardiac malformations at the first cardiological screening (Sybert 1998). Thus, the extent of preoperative cardiac assessment will depend on how recently investigations have been undertaken.

2. Potential intubation difficulties must be anticipated and the risk of inadvertent one lung anaesthesia borne in mind.

3. Full medical evaluation and counselling should be undertaken before assisted pregnancy is attempted.

Bibliography

Divekar VM, Kothari MD, Kamdar BM 1983 Anaesthesia in Turner's syndrome. Canadian Anaesthetists' Society Journal 1983; 30: 417–18.

Garvey P, Elovitz M, Landsberger EJ 1998 Aortic dissection and myocardial infarction in a pregnant patient with Turner syndrome. Obstetrics & Gynecology 91: 864.

Gotzsche CO, Krag-Olsen B, Nielsen J et al 1995 Prevalence of cardiovascular malformations and association with karyotypes in Turner's syndrome. Archives of Disease in Childhood 71: 433–6.

Lin AE, Lippe B, Rosenfeld RG 1998 Further delineation of aortic dilatation, dissection, and rupture in patients with Turner syndrome. Pediatrics 102: e12.

Moore JW, Kirby WC, Rogers WM et al 1990 Partial anomalous pulmonary venous drainage associated with 45,X Turner's syndrome. Pediatrics 86: 273–6.

Saenger P 1996 Turner's syndrome. New England Journal of Medicine 335: 1749–54.

Sybert VP 1998 Cardiovascular malformations and complication in Turner syndrome. Pediatrics 101: E11.

Varicella

A common infectious disease of childhood caused by the DNA varicella zoster virus, although the introduction of varicella virus vaccine has reduced the incidence. In adults, the disease may run a more severe course than in children, and anaesthetists may be involved in the treatment of patients with varicella pneumonia and other complications. Herpes zoster may follow, possibly as a result of reactivation of the virus within the spinal sensory ganglia. Severe disease is most common in the immunocompromised patient.

Preoperative abnormalities

1. The incubation period is about 15–18 days. In children the rash starts immediately, whereas in adults there is a prodromal illness. Lesions begin in the mouth, hard palate, fauces, and uvula. Those on the trunk spread from the back to the front, then onto the face and limbs. Hollows and protected parts may be particularly affected. There is cropping of the rash, in contrast to smallpox, in which lesions tend to be of the same age. Thus in chickenpox macule, papule, vesicle, pustule and scab may be seen at any one time.

2. Complications, which particularly affect adults, include encephalitis, pneumonia, sepsis, hepatitis (Patti et al 1990), and thrombocytopenia. Musculoskeletal complications such as osteomyelitis, septic arthritis and necrotising fasciitis may necessitate surgery and sometimes amputation (Schreck et al 1996, Burke & Chambers 1997).

3. In children, cerebral vasculitis and stroke may occur in the recovery period.

4. Varicella pneumonia is more common in adults (almost exclusively affecting those who are smokers), in the immunologically compromised, and during pregnancy. It carries a significant morbidity and mortality. Cough and breathlessness usually starts 2–5 days after the rash appears, but occasionally before. CXR initially shows diffuse fine nodular shadowing, followed by an increase in nodular size, finally progressing to patchy consolidation. Patients may deteriorate rapidly, and the onset of hypoxia that is unresponsive to treatment is associated with a poor prognosis. Hyponatraemia is a common finding.

Anaesthetic problems

1. Anaesthetists are predominantly involved in the management of varicella pneumonia, in patients who develop progressive hypoxia that is refractory to treatment (Clark et al 1991). Varicella pneumonia tends to be more common, and more severe, in pregnancy (Esmonde et al 1989). Bacterial superinfection, endotoxic shock and ARDS may ensue (Chandra et al 1998).

2. It has been suggested that, if IPPV is required, there is an increased risk of laryngeal oedema following prolonged tracheal intubation. Laryngeal oedema has been reported after extubation in three adults (Boyd & Grounds 1991). In two, difficulties in reintubation resulted in cardiac arrest.

3. One HIV-infected patient developed ARDS, septic shock and a coagulopathy, and died at 1 month (Mofredj et al 1996).

Management

1. In cases of varicella pneumonia, close observation for hypoxia, and early admission to the ITU in the face of deterioration, is essential (Potgieter & Hammond 1997).

2. Antiviral agents. There have been no really satisfactory studies to define the place of acyclovir in the management of varicella. There is some evidence that oral acyclovir 4 g day^{-1} reduces the severity of the illness in adults, provided that it is given within 24 h of the rash appearing (Feder 1990, Brody & Moyer 1997). A retrospective study of varicella pneumonia in previously healthy adults suggested that iv cyclovir given within 36 h of hospital admission

was associated with a reduction in fever and tachypnoea, and an improvement in oxygenation (Haake et al 1990). Varicella-zoster immune globulin may be effective in exposed individuals who are at risk (Brody & Moyer 1997).

3. Treatment of hypoxia, initially by mask. Assisted nasal breathing with inspiratory pressure support of 35 cmH$_2$O was used to improve oxygenation in a 44-year-old woman (Jankowski & Petros 1991). However, this technique requires patient cooperation and, in the event of severe hypoxia, IPPV and PEEP usually will be required. In one pregnant patient, the use of ECMO was reported to be life-saving (Clark et al 1991). In severe cases it has been suggested that early institution of extracorporeal life support (ECLS) improves survival rate (Lee et al 1998).

4. In view of the possibility of laryngeal oedema, it is important to inspect the larynx before extubation. If, in the presence of laryngeal oedema, the tube needs to be changed, the use of a bougie or tube exchange catheter will be of assistance. It has been suggested that tracheal intubation be avoided, if possible. If not, tracheostomy should be considered at an earlier stage than normal, but at least 7 days after the last lesion has appeared.

5. In the third trimester of pregnancy, delivery may have to be expedited and the decision made whether or not to give varicella-zoster immune globulin to the neonate (Chandra et al 1998).

Bibliography

Boyd OF, Grounds RM 1991 Life threatening laryngeal oedema after prolonged intubation for chickenpox pneumonia. British Medical Journal 302: 516–17.

Brody MB, Moyer D 1997 Varicella-zoster virus infection. Postgraduate Medicine 102: 187–94.

Burke GA, Chambers TL 1997 Musculoskeletal side-effects of varicella. Lancet 349: 818–19.

Chandra PC, Patel H, Schiavello HJ et al 1998 Successful pregnancy outcome after complicated varicella pneumonia. Obstetrics & Gynecology 92 (4 II suppl): 680–2.

Clark GPM, Dobson PM, Thickett A et al 1991 Chickenpox pneumonia, its complications and management. Anaesthesia 46: 376–80.

Esmonde TF, Herdman G, Anderson G 1989 Chickenpox pneumonia: an association with pregnancy. Thorax 44: 812–15.

Feder HM Jr 1990 Treatment of adult chickenpox with oral acyclovir. Archives of Internal Medicine 150: 2061–5.

Haake DA, Zakowski PC, Haake DL et al 1990 Early treatment with acyclovir for varicella pneumonia in otherwise healthy adults: retrospective controlled study and review. Review of Infectious Diseases 12: 788–98.

Jankowski S, Petros AJ 1991 Chickenpox pneumonia: NAB before IPPV? Anaesthesia 46: 993–4.

Lee WA, Kolla S, Schreiner RJ Jr et al 1998 Prolonged extracorporeal life support (ECLS) for varicella pneumonia. Critical Care Medicine 26: 1138–9.

Mofredj A, Guerin JM, Madec Y et al 1996 Respiratory distress syndrome and septic shock due to varicella in an HIV-infected adult. Intensive Care Medicine 22: 835–6.

Patti ME, Selvaggi KJ, Kroboth FJ 1990 Varicella hepatitis in the immunocompromised adult: a case report and review of the literature. American Journal of Medicine 88: 77–80.

Potgieter PD, Hammond JM 1997 Intensive care management of varicella pneumonia. Respiratory Medicine 91: 207–12.

Schreck P, Schreck P, Bradley J et al 1996 Musculoskeletal complications of varicella. Journal of Bone & Joint Surgery 78A: 1713–19.

Vipoma

One of the APUDomas (Amine Precursor Uptake and Decarboxylation) that secretes vasoactive intestinal polypeptide (VIP), but may also produce other hormones. Tumours in adults are most commonly of pancreatic endocrine origin, whereas in children they are usually ganglioneuroblastomas arising from the sympathetic chain. Vipomas can also occur as a manifestation of the MEN 1 syndrome (Thakker 1998). VIP is one of a number of hormones that can be secreted by bronchial carcinomas, neuroblastomas, and paraganglionomas. Neurogenic tumours almost all produce the syndrome, whereas in vipomas of pancreatic origin, only about 85% are associated with it.

Tumours greater than 20 mm in size are more likely to produce symptoms. Intravenous administration of VIP causes hypotension secondary to vasodilatation, hyperglycaemia, diarrhoea, inhibition of gastric acid output, and respiratory stimulation. Vipomas are malignant and about 50% of patients have metastatic spread at the time of diagnosis (Krejs 1987). Although surgery is the first line of treatment, the introduction of somatostatin has resulted in dramatic improvement of symptoms (Philippe 1992), and in some cases, long-term remission has been reported (Brunani et al 1991).

Preoperative abnormalities

1. The syndrome, as it was originally described, consisted of Watery Diarrhoea, Hypokalaemia and Achlorhydria or hypochlorhydria (WDHA syndrome). The diarrhoea is secretory and continues even when fasting (Perry & Vinik 1995). It is accompanied by weight loss and dehydration, and a history of abdominal colic and cutaneous flushing.

2. The picture may be complicated by the effects of additional hormones.

3. Biochemical changes include hypokalaemia, acidosis, hypercalcaemia, increased blood urea, diabetic glucose tolerance, increased plasma VIP, and increased plasma pancreatic polypeptide (Park et al 1996).

4. Tumour location may be by CT scan and arteriography.

5. If the tumour can be located and is large, excision is necessary. If not, or if it cannot be localised, symptomatic therapy includes somatostatin, corticosteroids, indometacin, and lithium (Perry & Vinik 1995).

Anaesthetic problems

1. Gross fluid and electrolyte imbalance can be a major problem, since losses of up to 8 l day^{-1}

may occur (Bouloux 1987). One patient, whose serum potassium was only 1.3 mmol l^{-1}, presented with a quadriparesis. This resolved completely after potassium infusion (Taylor et al 1977).

2. Secretion of VIP during handling of the tumour may produce profound hypotension. The patient mentioned above had an adrenal ganglioneuroblastoma that secreted both VIP and norepinephrine (noradrenaline). Before removal of the tumour, these had mutually antagonistic effects. However, following its removal there was severe hypotension, probably as a result of the more prolonged action of VIP.

3. There may be associated hypercalcaemia (Venkatesh et al 1989).

Management

1. Correction of fluid and electrolyte imbalance before surgical removal is a priority. In particular, total body potassium losses may be appreciable.

2. Treatment with somatostatin by sc injection or infusion (50–150 μg 8 hrly). Somatostatin treatment has been associated with complete relief of diarrhoea, return of serum potassium to normal, and a decrease in plasma levels of VIP. Diarrhoea is reduced within 12–24 h from 20–22 l day^{-1} and electrolyte imbalance resolves within 48 h (Wynick & Bloom 1991). However, there is no evidence that somatostatin arrests the progression of the tumour (Brunani et al 1991).

3. Correction of hypercalcaemia, if present.

Bibliography

Bouloux P-M 1987 Multiple endocrine neoplasia. Surgery 1: 1180–5.

Brunani A, Crespi C, De Martin M et al 1991 Four year treatment with a long acting somatostatin analogue in a patient with Verner–Morrison syndrome. Journal of Endocrinological Investigation 14: 685–9.

Krejs GJ 1987 VIPoma syndrome. American Journal of Medicine 82 (suppl 5B): 37–48.

Park SK, O'Dorisio MS, O'Dorisio TM 1996 Vasoactive intestinal polypeptide-secreting tumours: biology and therapy. Baillieres Clinical Gastroenterology 10: 673–96.

Perry RR, Vinik AI 1995 Clinical review 72: diagnosis and management of functioning islet cell tumours. Journal of Clinical Endocrinology & Metabolism 80: 2273–8.

Philippe J 1992 APUDomas: acute complications and their medical management. Baillieres Clinical Endocrinology & Metabolism 6: 217–28.

Taylor AR, Chulajata D, Jones DH et al 1977 Adrenal tumour secreting vasoactive intestinal peptide and noradrenaline. Anaesthesia 32: 1012–16.

Thakker RV 1998 Multiple endocrine neoplasia— syndromes of the twentieth century. Journal of Clinical Endocrinology & Metabolism 83: 2617–20.

Venkatesh S, Vassilopoulou-Sellin R, Samaan NA 1989 Somatostatin analogue: use in the treatment of vipoma with hypercalcaemia. American Journal of Medicine 87: 356–7.

Wynick D, Bloom SR 1991 Clinical review 23. The use of long-acting somatostatin analog octreotide in the treatment of gut neuroendocrine tumours. Journal of Clinical Endocrinology & Metabolism 73: 1–3.

Von Gierke's disease and type 1b

glycogenolysis

An autosomal recessive, inherited glycogen storage disease (Cori type Ia) in which there is an absence, or reduction in levels, of glucose-6-phosphatase. Glycogen is a polymer made up of straight and branching chains of glucose monomer units. Blood glucose is normally maintained by the breakdown of glycogen.

Glucose-6-phosphatase is present in the liver, kidney, gut, and platelets. It is the enzyme involved in the final step in the conversion of glycogen to free glucose. An absence, or a reduction in levels of the enzyme, results in severe hypoglycaemia, multiple metabolic abnormalities and accumulation of glycogen within the liver and kidney. Patients require a regular intake of glucose 2–3 hrly and limitation of fructose and lactose. Some patients have been helped by a portacaval shunt (Casson 1975), which improves most aspects of the disease apart from fasting hypoglycaemia, and by liver transplantation.

In type 1b glycogenolysis, there is a deficiency of glucose-6-phosphate microsomal translocase, which is required for glucose-6-phosphate to be transported to the inner surface of the microsome. This results an inability to hydrolyse glycogen in hepatocytes and other cells. The signs and symptoms of type 1a and 1b are similar. There is also a type 1c involving another transporter, but this is rare and will not be considered further (Wolfsdorf et al 1999).

Preoperative abnormalities

1. Presents in infancy with gross hepatomegaly that results from accumulation of glycogen and fat in the liver.

2. Severe hypoglycaemia, occurring 3–4 h after a meal, is secondary to impaired glycogenolysis and gluconeogenesis. This does not respond to glucagon, fructose, or epinephrine (adrenaline), and may lead to fits and failure to thrive. In spite of this, patients tend to be obese, secondary to deposition of subcutaneous fat.

3. The kidneys are also enlarged and renal disease (chronic proteinuria, renal stones, nephrocalcinosis), and renal failure, are common (Chen et al 1988).

4. A chronic lactic acidosis results from free conversion of pyruvate to lactate, and increased pyruvate levels.

5. Hypertriglyceridaemia and high levels of free fatty acids occur as a result of increased synthesis, and stimulation of their release from fat.

6. Hyperuricaemia and gout, and gouty nephropathy.

7. Platelet dysfunction, secondary to biochemical derangements, may produce coagulation problems. These are reversed when treatment is instituted. Neutrophil dysfunction may also occur.

8. Hepatic adenomas are common (Wolfsdorf et al 1999), and an increased incidence of cirrhosis and hepatocellular carcinoma has been reported (Conti & Kemeny 1992).

9. Diagnosis can be confirmed by liver biopsy, and histochemistry.

10. Dietary management is now well established. Uncooked cornstarch provides an accessible source of glucose (Chen et al 1984, Wolfsdorf et al 1999). Management can include measures such as continuous intragastric, nasogastric or parenteral feeding, and portacaval shunt, all of which improve metabolic control and ameliorate the signs and symptoms of the disease.

Anaesthetic problems

1. Starvation produces severe hypoglycaemia and lactic acidosis. In a review of 12 patients, one 17-year-old boy developed a pH of 7.08 during surgery after 7 h of starvation (Cox 1968). Death occurred in another child, who had a cardiac arrest at the end of a tonsillectomy, but no details were given.

2. The present, successful, continuous metabolic management of these children reduces the tolerance to low blood glucose levels that normally occurs in the untreated child.

3. In untreated patients, there may be recurrent hypoglycaemia resulting in convulsions and brain damage (Shenkman et al 1996).

4. There may be spontaneous epistaxes or bruising, or bleeding may occur after dental or other surgery. The metabolic disturbances are probably responsible for a reduction in adhesiveness and impaired aggregation of platelets, because the defects can be reversed by strict metabolic control.

5. Muscle development is poor and may result in postoperative respiratory insufficiency.

6. Although there is a delay in sexual development and reproductive capacity is low,

pregnancy has been reported (Chen et al 1984, Johnson et al 1990).

Management

1. To prevent an acidosis occurring at the beginning of surgery, a dextrose infusion should be given during the period of preoperative starvation (Shenkman et al 1996). In one case, intragastric feeding was maintained until 3 h preoperatively, and replaced by an infusion of glucose to give $0.4\,g\,kg^{-1}h^{-1}$ (Bevan 1980).

2. If major surgery, such as a portacaval shunt or liver transplantation, is contemplated, preoperative parenteral nutrition is advisable (Casson 1975). Liver size is decreased and platelet function improved.

3. Plasma glucose and acid–base status should be monitored regularly throughout the perioperative period (Bevan 1980). Acidaemia can occur without ketonuria, therefore testing for urinary ketones alone may be an unreliable predictor of acidosis.

4. Lactate-containing solutions are absolutely contraindicated. Fructose should not be given because it induces hyperuricaemia.

5. Platelet function can be assessed by performing a bleeding time. If this is significantly prolonged, regional anaesthesia is inadvisable.

6. Neuromuscular monitoring.

7. Careful postoperative observation is required, to detect respiratory insufficiency.

8. The management of pregnancy and labour involving the use of 3-hrly cornstarch feeds has been described (Chen et al 1984). As much as 325 g cornstarch may be needed to meet the requirements of both mother and fetus. Protein loss secondary to severe preeclampsia necessitated the use of parenteral nutrition in one patient (Johnson et al 1990).

Bibliography
Bevan JC 1980 Anaesthesia in Von Gierke's disease. Current approach to management. Anaesthesia 35: 699–702.

Casson H 1975 Anaesthesia for portacaval bypass in patients with metabolic diseases. British Journal of Anaesthesia 47: 969–75.

Chen YT, Cornblath M, Sidbury JB 1984 Cornstarch therapy in type I glycogen-storage disease. New England Journal of Medicine 310: 171–5.

Chen YT, Coleman RA, Scheinman JI et al 1988 Renal disease in type I glycogen storage disease. New England Journal of Medicine 318: 7–11.

Conti JA, Kemeny N 1992 Type Ia glycogenolysis associated with hepatocellular carcinoma. Cancer 69: 1320–2.

Cox JM 1968 Anesthesia and glycogen storage disease. Anesthesiology 29: 1221–5.

Johnson MP, Compton A, Drugan A et al 1990 Metabolic control of von Gierke disease (glycogen storage disease type IA) in pregnancy: maintenance of euglycemia with cornstarch. Obstetrics & Gynecology 75: 507–10.

Shenkman Z, Golub Y, Meretyk S et al 1996 Anaesthetic management of a patient with glycogen storage disease type 1b. Canadian Journal of Anaesthesia 43: 467–70.

Wolfsdorf JI, Holm IA, Weinstein DA 1999 Glycogen storage diseases. Phenotypic, genetic, and biochemical characteristics, and therapy. Endocrine & Metabolism Clinics of North America 28: 801–23.

Von Hippel–Lindau disease (vHLD)

A rare, autosomal dominant, inherited neuroectodermal disorder, that involves mutations of the vHL tumour suppressor gene on the short arm of chromosome 3 (Maher & Kaelin 1997). It usually presents in young adults with one or more of a variety of manifestations. Amongst the most serious of these are cerebellar, medullary or spinal haemangioblastomas, retinal angiomatosis, renal cell carcinoma and phaeochromocytoma. A high incidence of pancreatic lesions has recently been found (Neumann et al 1991). Genetic studies suggest familial clustering of the features (Neumann & Wiestler 1991).

Preoperative abnormalities

1. The predominant and earliest features are retinal angiomatosis and cerebellar haemangioblastomas, both of which occur in about 60% of affected individuals (Maher & Kaelin 1997). Lesions usually present separately, and, unless there is a known family history, the diagnosis of vHLD may only be made in retrospect. Tumours may recur, or new tumours appear. The frequency of phaeochromocytomas is 7–20%. A 14-year-old boy initially presented with a phaeochromocytoma and subsequently developed a cerebral angioblastoma, retinal angiomatosis, and a second phaeochromocytoma (personal observation).

2. Other associated conditions include renal and pancreatic cysts, islet cell tumours, angiomas of the liver and kidneys, epididymal cystadenoma, and spinal cord haemangioblastomas. About 25% of patients with CNS haemangioblastomas subsequently turn out to have vHLD.

3. Erythrocytosis and a high haematocrit are common.

Anaesthetic problems

1. Surgery for one manifestation of the disease may be complicated by the presence of an undiagnosed phaeochromocytoma.

2. The problems of management of a phaeochromocytoma, if present. Pharmacological control of phaeochromocytoma becomes the priority and surgery may have to be carried out in two stages (Mugawar et al 1998).

3. Spinal anaesthesia may be hazardous in the presence of an undiagnosed cerebral or spinal tumour, and spinal cord haemangioblastomas can occur at more than one level. However, epidural anaesthesia has been performed for Caesarean section in a patient with a known, small haemangioblastoma (Wang & Sinatra 1999). Following MRI of the spine, the needle was sited distal to the lesion.

4. Patients with known disease may become pregnant; others may present during pregnancy. In one patient, laminectomy was

performed at 35 weeks for acute paraplegia resulting from a bleed into a spinal haemangioblastoma. Elective Caesarean section under epidural anaesthesia was subsequently undertaken at 37 weeks (Ogasawara et al 1995). Occasionally, Caesarean section and phaeochromocytoma removal may be combined (Joffe et al 1993). The safe management of the pregnant patient with a previously resected cerebral tumour has been reported (Matthews & Halshaw 1986). There is some suggestion that pregnancy may worsen the disease, by increasing the vascularity of tumours. One week after delivery, a patient with vHLD developed an oppressive headache and was found to have severe papilloedema. Urgent MRI showed hydrocephalus and cerebellar tonsillar herniation, secondary to a cyst from a haemangioblastoma, that had not been present on a previous scan. Neurosurgical intervention was lifesaving (Othmane et al 1999). A retrospective analysis of 56 unselected pregnancies in vHLD showed that although maternal morbidity was 5.4%, the survival rate of the fetus was 96.4% (Grimbert et al 1999).

5. Surgery may be required for more than one lesion at the same time. Ercan et al (1996) describe the combined removal of bilateral phaeochromocytoma and spinal cord haemangioblastoma.

Management

1. Careful assessment should be made for lesions other than the one for which anaesthesia is required, and in particular for any symptoms and signs of cerebral, cerebellar or spinal cord tumours. Patients with CNS haemangioblastomas have a 23% incidence of vHLD.

2. In the situation in which two lesions are present, decisions may have to be made as to whether to operate simultaneously or separately (Ercan et al 1996). During pregnancy the management of the delivery must be carefully planned in advance.

3. Although 24-h urinary screening for catecholamines can be performed, plasma normetanephrines and metanephrines are the most sensitive tests for detecting phaeochromocytomas in patients with family predisposition (Eisenhofer et al 1999).

4. In the presence of phaeochromocytoma, the pharmacological control of this becomes a priority. For preparation for phaeochromocytoma surgery (see Phaeochromocytoma).

Bibliography

Eisenhofer G, Lenders JWM, Linehan WM et al 1999 Plasma normetanephrine and metanephrine for detecting phaeochromocytoma in von Hippel–Lindau disease and multiple endocrine neoplasia type 2. New England Journal of Medicine 340: 1872–9.

Ercan M, Kahraman S, Basgul E et al 1996 Anaesthetic management of a patient with von Hippel–Lindau disease: a combination of bilateral phaeochromocytoma and spinal cord haemangioblastoma. European Journal of Anaesthesiology 13: 81–3.

Grimbert P, Chaveau D, Remy SRP et al 1999 Pregnancy in von Hippel–Lindau disease. American Journal of Obstetrics & Gynecology 180: 110–11.

Joffe D, Robbins R, Benjamin A 1993 Caesarean section and phaeochromocytoma resection in a patient with von Hippel–Lindau disease. Canadian Journal of Anaesthesia 40: 870–4.

Maher ER, Kaelin WG Jr 1997 von Hippel–Lindau disease. Medicine 76: 381–91.

Matthews AJ, Halshaw J 1986 Epidural anaesthesia in von Hippel–Lindau disease. Anaesthesia 41: 853–5.

Mugawar M, Rajender Y, Purohit AK et al 1998 Anesthetic management of von Hippel–Lindau syndrome for excision of cerebellar hemangioma and pheochromocytoma surgery. Anesthesia & Analgesia 86: 673–4.

Neumann HP, Wiestler OD 1991 Clustering of features of von Hippel–Lindau syndrome: evidence for a complex genetic locus. Lancet 337: 1052–4.

Neumann HP, Dinkel E, Brambs H et al 1991 Pancreatic lesions in the von Hippel–Lindau syndrome. Gastroenterology 101: 465–71.

Ogasawara KK, Ogasawara EM, Hirata G 1995 Pregnancy complicated by von Hippel–Lindau disease. Obstetrics & Gynecology 85: 829–31.

Othmane IS, Shields C, Singh A et al 1999 Postpartum
cerebellar herniation in von Hippel–Lindau
syndrome. American Journal of Ophthalmology
128: 387–9.

Wang A, Sinatra RS 1999 Epidural anesthesia for
Cesarean section in a patient with von
Hippel–Lindau disease and multiple sclerosis.
Anesthesia & Analgesia 88: 1083–4.

Von Recklinghausen's disease (see
Neurofibromatosis type 1 and 2)

Von Willebrand's disease

A group of autosomal dominant inherited
haemorrhagic diseases associated with reduced,
abnormal or absent von Willebrand factor
(vWF : Ag). In plasma, vWF : Ag forms a
complex with factor VIII (VIII/vWF : Ag),
although the two proteins are controlled by
genes on different chromosomes. During
coagulation the complexes are dissociated.

Since the formation of a complex with
vWF : Ag protects Factor VIII from premature
destruction, Factor VIII clotting activity levels
are also reduced in most cases of von
Willebrand's disease (vWD). However, levels
usually remain above 5% and, on occasions, may
even be normal.

vWF : Ag has been demonstrated to be
present in endothelial cells, platelets and
megakaryocytes, and is involved in the link
between platelets and damaged endothelium.
Von Willebrand's disease is therefore associated
with defects in platelet adhesiveness and
aggregation, and a prolonged bleeding time. Von
Willebrand factor is also found in plasma and
intact subendothelium. Electrophoretic
techniques have allowed laboratory classification
of three major types, and further subtypes, of
vWD (Cameron & Kobrinsky 1990). The
different types of the disease vary in their clinical
severity, the mode of inheritance, laboratory
abnormalities, and in their response to different
therapies and to pregnancy. Mild disease is

common and may occur in up to 3% of the
population.

1. Type I is the commonest form and is
responsible for about 90% of cases; all vWF (von
Willebrand factor) multimers are decreased
quantitatively, and the haemophilic part (VIII C)
may also be decreased. The PT and PTT (partial
thromboplastin time) are usually normal; the
bleeding time may be prolonged, but can be
normal despite a history of bleeding. In addition,
results may vary on different occasions; for
example, pregnancy and oestrogens may result in
an increase in vWF, and the menopause may be
associated with excessive menstrual bleeding.

2. Type IIa (9%) in which large and
intermediate vWF multimers are absent from
plasma and platelets, and Factor VIII C levels
may be normal or reduced. Bleeding time is
prolonged. There is usually no improvement in
the disease in pregnancy.

3. Type IIb (1%) in which vWF multimers are
reduced in the plasma, but increased on the
platelet surface. There is decreased platelet survival
and a mild to moderate thrombocytopenia.
Bleeding time is prolonged. Pregnancy may be
associated with worsening thrombocytopenia.
Infusions of desmopressin may further reduce the
platelet count and should be avoided.

4. Type III, an autosomal recessive form, is
the severest type, in which no vWF or Factor
VIII C is detectable. The PTT will always be
abnormal in this form. Bleeding time is
prolonged.

There have been recent changes in the treatment
of bleeding problems in vWD. New virus-
inactivated products, Factor VIII concentrates
rich in vWF, are now being produced and they
carry less risk of virus transmission than
cryoprecipitate. These are now preferred to
cryoprecipitate.

Preoperative abnormalities

1. Clinically, the bleeding in vWD differs
from that seen in haemophilia. Bruising occurs

easily, and bleeding tends to be mucosal in type, from the nose, mouth, gastrointestinal tract, lungs, and uterus. Immediate bleeding tends to follow trauma and surgery in vWD, whereas in haemophilia it is usually delayed. In the homozygous form, cutaneous and deep tissue bleeding may also occur.

2. The bleeding time is usually prolonged, and platelet aggregation and adhesion reduced. Factor VIII clotting activity may be reduced or normal, and therefore the partial thromboplastin time may or may not be abnormal. There are a number of laboratory tests for vWF : Ag activity, which remain in the province of the haematologist. The Ristocetin cofactor activity is the most reliable in clinical terms.

3. Acquired vWD may suddenly develop, particularly in association with monoclonal gammopathies and lympho- or myelo-proliferative disorders (Mohri et al 1998, van Genderen & Michiels 1998).

Anaesthetic problems

1. Bleeding after trauma or surgery may occur, the degree being dependent upon the severity of the disease. Although bleeding is not usually as severe as in haemophilia, major anaesthetic problems may arise from time to time. Massive tonsillar haemorrhage was reported in a patient with severe vWD, despite cooperation with the haematologists (Alusi et al 1995). Examination of 150 women with menorrhagia and normal pelvic examination showed that 17% had an inherited bleeding disorder, of which vWD was the most common (Kadir et al 1998b).

2. Pregnancy and delivery may be complicated (Kadir et al 1998a). Whilst many patients with type I disease show improvement in clotting factors during pregnancy, other types do not. A proportion of infants will be affected. Vaginal delivery may cause trauma and haemorrhage in infants of severely affected mothers, and in these patients Caesarean section is required. In such cases, blood loss at Caesarean section may be considerable. There is an increased incidence of miscarriage, postabortion bleeding, and primary and secondary postpartum haemorrhage, particularly when factor levels are <50 iu dl⁻¹. Bleeding associated with surgical delivery or perineal damage usually occurs postpartum because of the rapid decline in Factor VIII and vWF levels after delivery (Walker et al 1994).

3. Desmopressin may cause water retention. Two patients were described in whom desmopressin, given in labour, produced water retention. In one hyponatraemic fits occurred (Chediak et al 1986). Another undergoing vaginal hysterectomy, who had four doses of desmopressin $0.3 \mu g\,kg^{-1}$, had a reduction in plasma sodium from 134 to 108 mmol⁻¹ and fitted at 48 h (Bertholini & Butler 2000). In 67 patients given desmopressin before adenotonsillectomy, three had significant postoperative hyponatraemia, and one had a fit (Allen et al 1999). Those with hyponatraemia had received significantly more iv fluids than those without.

4. Menorrhagia may increase in menopausal women with vWD, because of the decrease in oestrogen levels. Oestrogens generally increase vWF levels in the commonest type of vWD, therefore care should be taken to exclude a history of other bleeding in women requiring hysterectomy (Kadir et al 1998b).

Management

1. Careful clinical and haematological assessment of the type and severity of the disease is required. Advice is obtained from a haematologist as to the appropriate therapy to cover the proposed surgery, or for pregnancy. Blood samples for coagulation studies should be taken with care. Stasis, or damage to blood by difficult aspiration, may produce unreliable results with some tests.

2. Avoid all antiplatelet drugs (particularly salicylates, which may worsen the defect), im

injections, and rectal medication (Shah et al 1998).

3. Treatment depends on the severity and type of vWD. In the less severe forms of the disease (type I or IIa), clinical and laboratory improvement is associated with both pregnancy and the administration of oestrogens or desmopressin (DDAVP). These have the benefits of avoiding the use of blood products. For adenotonsillectomy, in patients shown to respond, desmopressin $0.3\,\mu g\,kg^{-1}$ was given 20–30 min preoperatively (Allen et al 1999). It has been suggested that better haemostasis is obtained by using laser for surgery (Shah et al 1998). Serum sodium levels should be checked for hyponatraemia. Similar preparations should take place before dental surgery (Wilde & Cook 1998).

This treatment should not be given to patients with type IIb, for which desmopressin is contraindicated (Lethargen et al 1997).

4. In more severe cases, or in the event of bleeding in milder ones, virally inactivated select Factor VIII concentrates may be required in addition. These are safer and more effective in replacing vWF than cryoprecipitate, which used to be given. However, there are considerable variations in AHF-vWF products and hopefully vWF depleted of Factor VIII will soon be available. Haemate P Factor VIII concentrate (Centeon Limited, Eastbourne, Sussex, UK) contains vWF : Ag and activity sufficient for correction of coagulation in most cases of vWD. The aim should be to increase the factor concentrations $>50\,iu\,dl^{-1}$. Platelets alone do not correct the bleeding time, but may occasionally be required in addition, when blood loss occurs during surgery or trauma and results in thrombocytopenia. Desmopressin is contraindicated in type II disease because it may exacerbate the thrombocytopenia by increasing platelet/vWF binding.

5. Pregnancy requires collaboration between obstetricians, haematologists, anaesthetists, and paediatricians; a management plan should be in place. Haematological advice should be sought early, so that coagulation factors can be monitored through pregnancy. Regular review at least every 8–12 weeks is required, and at 34–36 weeks the delivery should be finally planned. If problems are anticipated, it might be advisable to plan an actual date (Watanabe et al 1997). There are guidelines for pregnancy produced by the Working Party of the Haemostasis and Thrombosis Taskforce (Walker et al 1994).

6. On admission, blood should be sent for full blood and platelet count, coagulation screen, appropriate factor or vWF assays, blood grouping, and antibody screening.

7. Type III will need blood products and prophylaxis for 3–5 days. Types IIa and IIb may require them, but type I only rarely.

8. Intramuscular drugs should be avoided.

9. Opinion is divided as to whether regional anaesthesia should be performed. In normal pregnancy, Factor VIII levels increase, and it has been suggested that regional anaesthesia is feasible in patients with mild vWD, provided the APTT and the bleeding time are close to normal. Caesarean section under epidural anaesthesia has been reported in a patient with vWD who fulfilled these criteria (Milaskiewicz et al 1990). As pregnancy had progressed, the patient's bleeding time had decreased from 15 min to 6 min and the Factor VIII C level had increased from 42% to 108%. It has been suggested that women should not be denied the benefits of regional anaesthesia, provided clotting factors are $>50\,iu\,dl^{-1}$ in the third trimester, and the coagulation screen normal at presentation in labour (Kadir et al 1998a). However, once the patient is delivered, the coagulation factors return rapidly to the pre-pregnant state, therefore early removal of the epidural catheter is advisable unless concentrates are continued. In one patient with type IIa vWD, severe preeclampsia and low Ristocetin cofactor activity (RCF), Haemate P was given to correct the RCF before the epidural was sited (Jones et al 1999). A further dose was give at 8.5 h when RCF decreased, then 12 hrly for 48 h and daily until day 6.

10.   The clinical courses of pregnancies in 31 patients with vWd have been reviewed (Kadir et al 1998a). Caesarean section will be required unless the defect is mild, because the trauma of delivery may cause haemorrhage in a susceptible infant. If both desmopressin and oxytocin are required, only small volumes of saline 0.9% should be used as the diluent, and the plasma sodium levels should be estimated regularly during treatment. Fluid retention may require treatment with furosemide (frusemide) $0.25–0.5\,\mathrm{mg\,kg^{-1}}$.

Bibliography

Allen GC, Armfield DR, Bontempo FA et al 1999 Adenotonsillectomy in children with von Willebrand disease. Archives of Otolaryngology—Head & Neck Surgery 125: 547–51.

Alusi GH, Grant WE, Lee CA et al 1995 Bleeding after tonsillectomy in severe von Willebrand's disease. Journal of Laryngology & Otology 109: 437–9.

Bertholini DM, Butler CS 2000 Severe hyponatraemia secondary to desmopressin therapy in von Willebrand's disease. Anaesthesia & Intensive Care 28: 199–201.

Cameron CB, Kobrinsky N 1990 Perioperative management of patients with von Willebrand's disease. Canadian Journal of Anaesthesia 37: 341–7.

Chediak JR, Alban GM, Maxey B 1986 von Willebrand's disease and pregnancy: management during delivery and outcome of offspring. American Journal of Obstetrics & Gynecology 155: 618–24.

Jones BP, Bell EA, Maroof M 1999 Epidural labor analgesia in a parturient with von Willebrand's disease type IIA and severe preeclampsia. Anesthesiology 90: 1219–20.

Kadir RA, Lee CA, Sabin CA et al 1998a Pregnancy in women with von Willebrand's disease or factor XI deficiency. British Journal of Obstetrics & Gynaecology 105: 314–21.

Kadir RA, Economides DL, Sabin CA et al 1998b Frequency of inherited bleeding disorders in women with menorrhagia. Lancet 351: 485–9.

Lethagen S, Flordal P, Van Aken H et al 1997 The UK guidelines for the use of desmopressin in patients with von Willebrand's disease. Von Willebrand Working Party of the United Kingdom Haemophilia Centre Director's Organization. European Journal of Anaesthesiology Supplement 14: 19–22.

Milaskiewicz RM, Holdcroft A, Letsky E 1990 Epidural anaesthesia and von Willebrand's disease. Anaesthesia 45: 462–4.

Mohri H, Motomura S, Kanamori H et al 1998 Clinical significance of inhibitors in acquired von Willebrand syndrome. Blood 91: 3623–9.

Shah SB, Lalwani AK, Koerper MA 1998 Perioperative management of von Willebrand's disease in otolaryngologic surgery. Laryngoscope 108: 32–6.

van Genderen PJ, Michiels JJ 1998 Acquired von Willebrand disease. Baillières Clinical Haematology 11: 319–30.

Walker ID, Walker JJ, Colvin BT et al 1994 Investigation and management of haemorhagic disorders of pregnancy. Journal of Clinical Pathology 47: 100–8.

Watanabe T, Minakami H, Sakata Y 1997 Successful management of pregnancy in a patient with von Willebrand disease Normandy. American Journal of Obstetrics & Gynecology 89: 859.

Wilde JT, Cook RJ 1998 von Willebrand disease and its management in oral and maxillofacial surgery. British Journal of Oral & Maxillofacial Surgery 36: 112–18.

Wegener's granulomatosis

A systemic granulomatous vasculitis, usually affecting the age group 20–40 years, in which granulomas of the upper and lower respiratory tract are associated with a focal necrotising glomerulonephritis, and a widespread vasculitis involving other organs. The clinical features overlap with microscopic polyarteritis, and the antineutrophil cytoplasmic antibody is positive in both. A survey of 85 cases showed that all patients had either upper or lower respiratory tract involvement, and 85% had documented renal disease (Fauci et al 1983). In the past, without treatment, the condition was almost universally fatal, and up to 90% of deaths were associated with renal failure. Treatment with cyclophosphamide and corticosteroids has improved the prognosis. In early cases, some response to sulfamethoxazole has been shown (Valeriano-Marcet & Spiera 1991). A limited form of the disease may occur in which there are mucosal lesions. Patients may require anaesthesia for oral or ENT procedures, or for biopsy of airway lesions, before the diagnosis has been made.

Preoperative abnormalities

1. Head and neck problems include nasal discharge, crusting, bleeding and ulceration, sometimes progressing to septal perforation and nasal collapse. Infection or ulceration may occur in the sinuses, palate, and pharynx. Granulomas, ulceration and stenosis may involve the larynx. Subglottic stenosis occurs in 20% of adults (O'Devaney et al 1998), but the condition is more common in childhood-onset, than in adult-onset, disease (Rottem et al 1993). Ophthalmic and aural complications were reported in 58% and 61% of cases respectively.

2. More than 90% of patients have pulmonary involvement (Langford & Hoffman 1999). Symptoms include cough, haemoptysis, chest pain and breathlessness. Chest X-ray shows changing, nodular pulmonary opacities, that are often multiple and bilateral. Some of these cavitate and simulate lung carcinoma. In one series, fibreoptic bronchoscopy was found to be abnormal in 55% of patients, the main lesions being inflammation, haemorrhage, and ulceration (Cordier et al 1990). Partial bronchial stenosis was less common and occurred in 17.5%.

3. Renal disease may present with haematuria, proteinuria or red cell casts. Untreated, patients progress to kidney failure.

4. Cardiac involvement occurs in up to 44% of patients and includes pericarditis, arrhythmias, myocarditis, valvular and coronary disease (Goodfield et al 1995).

5. Other systems that may be involved in a diffuse vasculitis include the skin (45%), nervous (22%) and cardiovascular systems (12%). Severe intestinal lesions occur rarely.

6. General symptoms include joint pains, malaise and fever.

7. Patients may be taking cyclophosphamide and steroids.

8. There may be anaemia, high ESR, hypergammaglobulinaemia and leucocytosis (unless cyclophosphamide has caused a leucopenia), eosinophilia, and thrombocytosis. The test for antineutrophil cytoplasmic antibody is usually positive in systemic disease, but not necessarily in the local form.

9. Plasmapheresis may have a place for those in renal failure.

Anaesthetic problems

1. Patients may present insidiously with ear, nose or throat problems, some time before the diagnosis has been made (D'Cruz et al 1989). Granulomas of the upper airway may cause bleeding, or result in obstruction (Cohen et al 1978, Lake 1978).

2. Subglottic stenoses, tracheal granulomas and tracheo-oesophageal fistulae have all been described. Subglottic stenosis is usually circumferential, most frequently affects females,

and usually requires permanent tracheostomy (Arauz & Fonseca 1982, McDonald et al 1982). A 17 year old with a saddle nose had a biopsy under general anaesthesia as a day case. The following day he developed acute respiratory distress and died 1 h later. At autopsy there was a large mass of polypoid tissue in the subglottis and upper trachea and, in retrospect, subglottic irregularity could be seen on the sinus X-rays (Matt 1996). It is an unusual cause of stridor in children (Passey & Walker 2000), although childhood-onset disease is five times more likely to be complicated by subglottic stenosis than adult-onset (Rottem et al 1993). Recurrent subglottic stenosis may occur (Hoare et al 1989). Bronchoscopy shows endobronchial abnormalities in almost 60% (Daum et al 1995). Rarely, proximal bronchial stenosis has been reported, which in this case responded to cyclophosphamide and cotrimoxazole (Hirsch et al 1992).

3. Nasal intubation may dislodge tissue or cause bleeding.

4. Oral lesions that may ulcerate and resemble malignancies have been reported (Allen et al 1991).

5. Renal failure is common.

6. A peripheral arteritis may result in digital ischaemia. In such cases arterial cannulation is hazardous.

7. Pulmonary lesions may lead to consolidation, cavitation, bleeding, and arterial hypoxia.

8. Cardiac lesions can cause heart failure, conduction defects or coronary insufficiency, although this is rare.

9. Pregnancy may be associated with worsening of the disease, or with its initial presentation (Milford & Bellini 1986, Pauzner et al 1994, Dayoan et al 1998). One patient presented with the disease at 18 weeks' gestation and had termination of pregnancy so that treatment could be started, whilst another had an uneventful delivery but developed a lower lobe opacity 3 weeks later (Habib et al 1996). Another developed acute pulmonary haemorrhage in the first trimester and required aggressive, life-saving treatment (Palit & Clague 1990). However, sometimes regression can occur following delivery.

10. Treatment for the disease may cause immunosuppression. Cyclophosphamide most commonly causes leucopenia, hair loss, and haemorrhagic cystitis (Fauci et al 1983). Cholinesterase activity may be reduced.

Management

1. A careful assessment of the systems that may be affected by the disease must be undertaken. If there are signs that the airway is involved, indirect laryngoscopy and airway tomography may be indicated.

2. Investigations required may include Hb, WCC, platelet count, ESR, CXR, arterial blood gases, and tests of renal and liver function.

3. Corticosteroid supplements may be needed.

4. If airway obstruction is diagnosed, laryngoscopy, or intubation under local anaesthesia, or occasionally tracheostomy, may be necessary (D'Cruz et al 1989). Otherwise, examination of the palate, pharynx and larynx for lesions should be carried out during laryngoscopy. Patients may require tracheal dilatation, laser treatment, or insertion of stents (Daum et al 1995). In a review of 20 patients with subglottic stenosis treated with intratracheal dilatation and glucocorticoid injection therapy, none required tracheostomy and six with existing tracheostomies could be decannulated (Langford et al 1996).

5. The management of renal failure.

6. If the patient has both airway lesions and renal failure, local anaesthesia should be considered. However, any neurological lesions secondary to the disease should be accurately documented prior to anaesthesia.

7. If pregnancy occurs, the risks and benefits of continuing the pregnancy with or without drug treatment must be discussed (Harber et al 1999). However, cyclophosphamide has been given beyond the first trimester without harm to the fetus (Dayoan et al 1998).

Bibliography

Allen CM, Camisa C, Salewski C et al 1991 Wegener's granulomatosis: report of three cases with oral lesions. Journal of Oral & Maxillofacial Surgery 49: 294–8.

Arauz JC, Fonseca R 1982 Wegener's granulomatosis appearing initially in the trachea. Annals of Otology, Rhinology & Laryngology 91: 593–4.

Cohen SR, Landing BH, King KK et al 1978 Wegener's granulomatosis causing laryngeal and tracheobronchial obstruction in an adolescent girl. Annals of Otology, Rhinology & Laryngology 87 (S52): 15–19.

Cordier JF, Valeyre D, Guillevin L et al 1990 Pulmonary Wegener's granulomatosis. A clinical and imaging study of 77 cases. Chest 97: 906–12.

Daum TE, Specks U, Colby TV et al 1995 Tracheobronchial involvement in Wegener's granulomatosis. American Journal of Respiratory & Critical Care Medicine 151: 522–6.

Dayoan ES, Dimen LL, Boylen CT 1998 Successful treatment of Wegener's granulomatosis during pregnancy: a case report and review of the medical literature. Chest 113: 836–8.

D'Cruz DP, Baguley E, Asherson RA et al 1989 Ear, nose and throat symptoms in subacute Wegener's granulomatosis. British Medical Journal 299: 419–22.

Fauci AS, Haynes BF, Katz P et al 1983 Wegener's granulomatosis: prospective clinical and therapeutic experiences. Annals of Internal Medicine 98: 76–85.

Goodfield NE, Bhandari S, Plant WD et al 1995 Cardiac involvement in Wegener's granulomatosis. British Heart Journal 73: 110–15.

Habib A, MacKay K, Abrons HL 1996 Wegener's granulomatosis complicating pregnancy. Clinical Nephrology 46: 332–6.

Harber MA, Tso A, Taheri S et al 1999 Wegener's granulomatosis in pregnancy—the therapeutic dilemma. Nephrology, Dialysis & Transplantation 14: 1789–91.

Hirsch MM, Houssiau FA, Collard P et al 1992 A rare case of bronchial stenosis in Wegener's granulomatosis. Dramatic response to intravenous cyclophosphamide and oral cotrimoxazole. Journal of Rheumatology 19: 821–4.

Hoare TJ, Jayne D, Rhys Evans P et al 1989 Wegener's granulomatosis, subglottic stenosis and antineutrophil cytoplasm antibodies. Journal of Laryngology & Otology 103: 1187–91.

Lake CL 1978 Anesthesia and Wegener's granulomatosis: case report and review of the literature. Anesthesia & Analgesia 57: 353–9.

Langford CA, Hoffman GS 1999 Rare diseases. 3: Wegener's granulomatosis. Thorax 54: 629–37.

Langford CA, Sneller MC, Hallahan CW et al 1996 Clinical features and therapeutic management of subglottic stenosis in patients with Wegener's granulomatosis. Arthritis & Rheumatism 39: 1754–60.

McDonald TJ, Neel HB, DeRemee RA 1982 Wegener's granulomatosis of the subglottis and the upper portion of the trachea. Annals of Otology, Rhinology & Laryngology 91: 588–92.

Matt BH 1996 Wegener's granulomatosis, acute laryngotracheal airway obstruction and death in a 17-year-old female: case report and review of the literature. International Journal of Pediatric Otorhinolaryngology 37: 163–72.

Milford CA, Bellini M 1986 Wegener's granulomatosis arising in pregnancy. Journal of Laryngology & Otology 100: 475–6.

O'Devaney K, Ferlito A, Hunter BC et al 1998 Wegener's granulomatosis of the head and neck. Annals of Otology, Rhinology & Laryngology 107: 439–45.

Palit J, Clague RB 1990 Wegener's granulomatosis presenting during first trimester of pregnancy. British Journal of Rheumatology 29: 389–90.

Passey J, Walker R 2000 Wegener's granulomatosis in a child. An unusual cause of upper airway obstruction. Anaesthesia 55: 682–4.

Pauzner H, Mayan H, Hershko E et al 1994 Exacerbation of Wegener's granulomatosis during pregnancy. Report of a case with tracheal stenosis and literature review. Journal of Rheumatology 21: 1153–6.

Rottem M, Fauci AS, Hallahan CW et al 1993 Wegener's granulomatosis in children and adolescents: clinical presentation and outcome. Journal of Pediatrics 122: 26–31.

Valeriano-Marcet J, Spiera H 1991 Treatment of Wegener's granulomatosis with sulfamethoxazole-trimethoprim. Archives of Internal Medicine 151: 1649–52.

Werdnig–Hoffmann disease (see also Spinal muscular atrophy)

One of a group of inherited diseases, the spinal muscular atrophies, in which there is neuronal degeneration and loss of neurones in the anterior horn cells. Werdnig–Hoffmann (Type I or infantile spinal muscular atrophy or floppy infant syndrome) is the most severe, with onset of symptoms before age 6 months. Type II disease has an onset between 6 and 18 months, and type III an onset after 18 months. It is an autosomal recessive disease with an incidence of 1 in 10 000. Usually the onset of type I is at birth, or in the early weeks of life, and death occurs by the age of 3 years. Genetic mapping has recently shown the gene to be located on chromosome 5q (Editorial 1990).

Preoperative abnormalities

1. A floppy infant, with muscle weakness and wasting which begins in the back, pelvic, and shoulder girdles. There are depressed tendon reflexes. There is tongue fasciculation and loss of sucking ability.

2. Intercostal and accessory muscles may be involved, resulting in increasing respiratory difficulty. Since the diaphragm is spared until late in the disease, lower rib indrawing may occur on inspiration. Respiratory failure, usually in association with pneumonia, is responsible for the early death.

3. Diagnosis by muscle biopsy, and this is the most common reason for anaesthesia.

Anaesthetic problems

1. Increasing muscle weakness and respiratory compromise, particularly in the later stages of the disease.

2. The possibility that suxamethonium may precipitate hyperkalaemia or rhabdomyolysis should be considered.

Management

1. Nondepolarising neuromuscular blockers and respiratory depressants should be avoided because of the risks of hypoventilation and respiratory failure.

2. Suxamethonium should not be used.

3. Ketamine has been given for diagnostic muscle biopsy (Ramachandra et al 1990). Thirty-two children from 3 months to 12 years were given diazepam 0.2 mg kg^{-1} im as premedication followed by either ketamine 2 mg kg^{-1} iv or ketamine 10 mg kg^{-1} im as an anaesthetic.

4. For longer procedures, controlled ventilation and postoperative respiratory support may be required.

Bibliography
Editorial 1990 Spinal muscle atrophies. Lancet 336: 629–30.
Ramachandra PS, Anisya V, Gourie-Devi M 1990 Ketamine monoanaesthesia for diagnostic muscle biopsy in neuromuscular disorders in infancy and childhood: floppy infant syndrome. Canadian Journal of Anaesthesia 37: 474–6.
Thaler ER, Weinstein GS 1997 Interesting presentation of spinal muscular atrophy: cricoarytenoid joint fixation. Otolaryngology—Head & Neck Surgery 117: 154–7.

Williams syndrome (Williams–Beuren syndrome)

An autosomal dominant condition in which cardiovascular abnormalities, in particular severe biventricular outflow tract obstruction and coronary artery stenosis, are associated with an elfin face, growth retardation, learning difficulties, gregarious personality, and hypercalcaemia. The cardiovascular elements of the disease are progressive (Greenberg 1989). The disease is associated with abnormalities of elastin production and in most cases there is a correlation with elastin gene deletion on chromosome 7 (Metcalfe 1999). The wide spectrum of the disease is attributed to the elastin defects and the term 'elastin arteriopathy' has been suggested as a more appropriate name.

Preoperative abnormalities

1. A characteristic 'elfin' face, with mandibular and dental hypoplasia, hoarse voice, hypotonia, mental and physical retardation, but a gregarious personality.

2. Cardiovascular anomalies include supravalvular aortic stenosis, supravalvular and valvular pulmonary stenosis, and carotid artery stenoses. In one echocardiographic and Doppler study, a high incidence of mitral or tricuspid valve prolapse was found (Brand et al 1989). Premature coronary artery disease has been described in these children, possibly secondary to abnormal haemodynamics around the coronary ostia and limited diastolic coronary filling (Terhune et al 1985, Conway et al 1990). Sudden deaths are often associated with evidence of myocardial infarction.

3. Systemic hypertension and a wide range of peripheral vascular anomalies may be present.

4. Idiopathic hypercalcaemia.

5. A spectrum of renal abnormalities, such as renal artery stenosis, nephrocalcinosis, urethral stenosis, reflux, kidney anomalies and systemic hypertension, have been described (Ingelfinger & Newburger 1991).

6. Bowel and joint problems.

7. Reports of adults with Williams syndrome are rare and the small number of studies have shown progressive multisystem problems. However, correction of aortic stenosis was found to be worthwhile (Morris et al 1990, Kececioglu et al 1993).

Anaesthetic problems

1. Intubation difficulties may occur because of mandibular hypoplasia. In adults, progressive joint limitation may exacerbate this.

2. Masseter muscle spasm after halothane and suxamethonium has been reported (Patel & Harrison 1991). However, this might have been a normal response to suxamethonium given in standard (Leary & Ellis 1990) or low dosages (Matthews & Vernon 1991), particularly since halothane had been given before the suxamethonium (Carroll 1987). A suspected case of malignant hyperthermia was reported (Mammi et al 1996).

3. Cardiovascular disease is a prominent feature and may add to the risks of anaesthesia. Apart from the congenital cardiac lesions and left ventricular hypertrophy, myocardial insufficiency has been reported. A 16-month-old child with supravalvular aortic stenosis was admitted with episodes of cyanosis that were associated with ECG changes suggestive of subendocardial ischaemia (Terhune et al 1985). She was given morphine, but inadvertently in an overdose of 8 mg. The error was immediately recognised, naloxone was given, and a tracheal tube inserted. Ninety minutes later the child had a cardiac arrest and resuscitation failed. At postmortem, 80% occlusion of the lumen of the left anterior descending coronary artery was found, together with an area of recent myocardial infarction. Although the death was attributed to the child's cardiac state, rather than the morphine, the problems sometimes associated with the use of naloxone in cardiac disease cannot be ignored.

The risk of sudden death during or after cardiac catheterisation is well known to paediatric cardiologists. In 19 cases of Williams syndrome in which sudden death occurred, 11 died in association with anaesthesia for cardiac catheterisation (Conway et al 1990, Bird et al 1996). Most of the deaths occurred during manipulation of the catheter, but two took place immediately afterwards, and a third at 72 h. In most cases, death was preceded by bradycardia and hypotension, which was resistant to treatment. The majority of postmortem reports showed recent or remote myocardial infarctive changes, in addition to supravalvular pulmonary or aortic stenosis. However, there was no mention of the anaesthetic techniques used.

A 3 year old with a dilated cardiomyopathy having bilateral inguinal hernia repair had a postoperative cardiac arrest (Bonnet et al 1997). Occlusion of the left main coronary artery trunk was found, together with a long QT interval.

4.   The problems of managing anaesthesia for MRI angiographic investigations of the vascular tree (Andrzejowski & Mundy 2000).

Management

1.   Cardiovascular assessment is particularly important in view of the range of anomalies described. Management of the patient must be based on this knowledge. The reports of myocardial ischaemia and sudden deaths associated with cardiac catheterisation mean that these children should be treated with particular caution throughout the whole perioperative period. It has been suggested that, in a patient suspected of having Williams syndrome, blood pressure should be measured at least once in all four limbs. When supravalvular aortic stenosis is present, the systolic and mean blood pressures may be higher in the right arm than in the other three extremities.

2.   Management of difficult intubation, if applicable.

3.   The problems of anaesthesia for surgical correction of supravalvular aortic stenosis under deep hypothermia, in a child who additionally had left carotid artery stenosis, have been described (Larson & Warner 1990). The use of transoesophageal echocardiography has been reported in a 15 year old undergoing aortoplasty (Kawahito et al 1998). Anaesthesia for MRI angiographic investigation has been reported (Andrzejowski & Mundy 2000).

Bibliography

Andrzejowski J, Mundy J 2000 Anaesthesia for MRI angiography in a patient with Williams syndrome. Anaesthesia 55: 97–8.

Bird LM, Billman GF, Lacro RV et al 1996 Sudden death in Williams syndrome; report of ten cases. Journal of Pediatrics 129: 926–31.

Bonnet D, Cormier V, Villain E et al 1997 Progressive left main coronary artery obstruction leading to myocardial infarction in a child with Williams syndrome. European Journal of Pediatrics 156: 751–3.

Brand A, Keren A, Reifen RM et al 1989 Echocardiographic and Doppler findings in the Williams syndrome. American Journal of Cardiology 63: 633–5.

Carroll JB 1987 Increased incidence of masseter spasm in children with strabismus anaesthetised with halothane and succinyl choline. Anesthesiology 67: 559–61.

Conway EE Jr, Noonnan J, Marion RW et al 1990 Myocardial infarction leading to sudden death in the Williams syndrome: report of three cases. Journal of Pediatrics 117: 593–5.

Greenberg F 1989 Williams syndrome. Pediatrics 84: 922–3.

Ingelfinger JR, Newburger JW 1991 Spectrum of renal anomalies in patients with Williams syndrome. Journal of Pediatrics 119: 771–3.

Kawahito S, Kitahata H, Kimura H et al 1998 Anaesthetic management of a patient with Williams syndrome undergoing aortoplasty for supravalvular stenosis. Canadian Journal of Anaesthesia 45: 1203–6.

Kececioglu D, Kotthoff S, Vogt J 1993 Williams–Beuren syndrome: a 30-year follow-up of natural and postoperative course. European Heart Journal 14: 1458–64.

Larson JS, Warner MA 1989 Williams syndrome: an uncommon cause of supravalvular aortic stenosis in a child. Journal of Cardiothoracic Anesthesia 3: 337–40.

Leary NP, Ellis FR 1990 Masseteric muscle spasm as a normal response to suxamethonium. British Journal of Anaesthesia 64: 488–92.

Mammi I, Iles DE, Smeetes D et al 1996 Anesthesiologic problems in Williams syndrome: the CACNL2A locus is not involved. Human Genetics 98: 317–20.

Matthews AJ, Vernon JM 1991 Masseter spasm in Williams syndrome. Anaesthesia 46: 706.

Metcalfe K 1999 Williams syndrome: an update on clinical and molecular aspects. Archives of Disease in Childhood 81: 198–200.

Morris CA, Leonard CO, Dilts C et al 1990 Adults with Williams syndrome. American Journal of Medical Genetics Supplement 6: 102–7.

Patel J, Harrison MJ 1991 Williams syndrome: masseter spasm during anaesthesia. Anaesthesia 46: 115–16.

Sadler LS, Gingell R, Martin DJ 1998 Carotid ultrasound examination in Williams syndrome. Journal of Pediatrics 132: 354–6.

Terhune PE, Buchino JJ, Rees AH 1985 Myocardial infarction associated with supravalvular aortic stenosis. Journal of Pediatrics 106: 251–4.

Wolff–Parkinson–White syndrome

A congenital pre-excitation syndrome in which an accessory pathway, an anomalous band of conducting tissue, occurs between the atrial and ventricular myocardium (the bundle of Kent). This permits the initiation of excitation and contraction of the ventricles, before the normal atrial impulse has crossed the AV node to the bundle of His. The different excitation recovery times of the two pathways allow repeated circulation of impulses between the atria and ventricles. Subjects are thus liable to develop episodes of supraventricular tachycardia, and sometimes rapid atrial fibrillation. The myocardium is usually normal, but prolonged periods of tachycardia may cause hypotension, and occasionally heart failure. Aborted sudden death has been reported in 2.2% of a population of 690 patients, predominantly in men, and usually involving a septal accessory pathway (Timmermans et al 1995). For more detailed explanations of the electrophysiology, see Ganz and Friedman (1995).

WPW may occur in up to 0.3% of the general population, and the incidence can be even higher in close relatives of affected individuals.

In patients who are refractory to treatment, surgical division of the relevant accessory pathway may be required. This may be particularly appropriate to avoid long-term drug therapy in the young (Hood et al 1991). However, it is probably unnecessary to subject asymptomatic individuals, who are incidentally found to have the WPW pattern on ECG, to electrophysiological studies (Fisch 1990).

Preoperative abnormalities

1. The PR interval is short, usually less than 0.12 s. This is best seen in lead V1.

2. The QRS interval is broader than normal (>0.12 s, best seen in leads II, V5 and V6), and the initial QRS deflection is slow rising and slurred, and is known as the delta wave. Early depolarisation occurs via the accessory pathway, but further spread is slow, since it does not involve specialised conducting tissue. It therefore merges into the normal QRS complex. In some patients the ECG may be entirely normal.

3. WPW was originally classified into two types: type A, in which the ventricular complex was predominantly positive in V1, and type B, in which it was predominantly negative. Classification is now known to be more complex than this, since the pathway may be in any segment of the myocardium (Ganz & Friedman 1995).

4. The clinical history is of episodes of 'palpitations' which are precipitated by exercise, stress, or excitement. During an attack the patient may complain of faintness, chest pain, breathlessness, or polyuria. If the arrhythmia persists, cardiac failure may occur.

5. The ECG during attacks may show an AV re-entrant tachycardia (120–140 beat min^{-1}), atrial fibrillation, or atrial flutter. Ventricular rates of up to 300 beat min^{-1} may occur, and ventricular fibrillation has been reported. Death occasionally occurs (Brechenmacher et al 1977). During the re-entrant tachycardia there will be narrow, regular ventricular complexes. If the P wave can be seen, it will occur midway between ventricular complexes. Atrial fibrillation will, in general, be faster than normal; most of the impulses will show delta waves, although some will not.

6. Routine drug therapy includes procainamide, flecainide, and bretylium.

Anaesthetic problems

1. Since pre-excitation may be intermittent, WPW may present during anaesthesia, despite the patient having had a normal preoperative ECG. One case was unmasked by the development of glycine absorption syndrome

during prostatectomy (Lubarsky & Wilkinson 1989). Another presented with tachyarrhythmias during spinal anaesthesia (Nishikawa et al 1993).

2. Tachyarrhythmias may be precipitated by anxiety, surgical stimulation, induction of anaesthesia, intubation, or hypotension. Rapid AF with a wide QRS complex occurred after administration of neostigmine without atropine to reverse a patient with intermittent WPW syndrome following surgery. Two synchronised cardioversions of 100 J and 200 J restored sinus rhythm (Kadoya et al 1999).

3. During an attack, hypotension and a significant decrease in cardiac output may occur. Recurrent episodes of SVT were reported in a patient in late pregnancy. Failure to respond to drug therapy on one occasion, and the occurrence of hypotension and fetal distress from the practolol therapy on the second, necessitated the use of direct current cardioversion on both occasions (Klepper 1981).

4. ECG abnormalities may be misinterpreted. Tachycardia, chest pain and large inferior Q waves on ECG in a young cocaine user led to the incorrect diagnosis of myocardial infarction (Lustik et al 1999). Successful ablation of the accessory pathway was accompanied by return to normal of the short PR interval and disappearance of the Q wave.

5. Anaesthesia for surgical ablation of the accessory pathway. Sympathetic stimulation may precipitate tachyarrhythmias, whilst anaesthetic agents that significantly alter conduction in the normal or accessory pathways might hinder identification of the pathway. Halothane, enflurane and isoflurane all depress conduction in normal and accessory pathways and may be unsuitable in these particular circumstances (Dobkowski et al 1990, Sharpe et al 1990). Sevoflurane had no significant effect on electrophysiology of the AV or accessory pathways or SA node activity (Sharpe et al 1999).

6. In patients with WPW undergoing nonablative procedures, agents that increase the refractory period are most suitable.

7. Patients with asymptomatic WPW may become symptomatic during pregnancy (Afridi et al 1992, Kounis et al 1995).

Management

1. If the patient with WPW is already receiving drug treatment, this should be maintained.

2. Sympathetic stimulants, such as atropine and pancuronium, should be avoided.

3. For nonablative surgical procedures, drugs producing tachycardia, or techniques of light anaesthesia resulting in sympathetic stimulation, should be avoided. It is probably better to choose anaesthetics that increase the refractory period of the accessory pathway. Droperidol, in doses of $0.2–0.6\,mg\,kg^{-1}$, was found to increase the antegrade and retrograde effective refractory period of the action potential (Gomez-Arnau et al 1983). Enflurane, isoflurane and halothane (in decreasing order of effect) all increase accessory and atrial pathway refractory periods (Sharpe et al 1994, Chang et al 1996). Although propofol was reported to have no effect on cardiac electrophysiology, abolition of WPW changes was reported in one patient (see below).

4. For ablative procedures, agents are required that have no effects on the refractory period of the accessory pathway. The development of catheter ablation techniques in patients with accessory pathways has given the opportunity to perform electrophysiological studies on the effects of a wide variety of anaesthetic agents before surgical section. Alfentanil–midazolam anaesthesia was studied on eight patients during accessory pathway ablation (Dobkowski et al 1991, Sharpe et al 1992). No effect was found on conduction in either the normal or the accessory pathway and there were no tachyarrhythmias. The authors concluded that this was a suitable technique for surgical ablation. Propofol (Sharpe et al 1995) and sevoflurane (Sharpe et al 1999), studied under similar circumstances, have both been suggested as being suitable for patients undergoing ablative

surgery because of their lack of significant effect on cardiac electrophysiology. However, a single patient, whose delta wave disappeared after the start of a propofol infusion, only to reappear 5 min after its cessation, has been reported (Seki et al 1999).

5. If an acute attack occurs, vagal stimulation by carotid sinus massage, a Valsalva manoeuvre or squatting, can be tried. To be effective, these need to be instituted as soon as possible after the beginning of the tachycardia (Wellens et al 1987). If they fail, then drug or other methods of treatment will be needed. Individual patients may respond differently to different drugs. In addition, if atrial fibrillation is present, it can be made worse by verapamil and digoxin.

a) For supraventricular tachycardias (Ganz & Friedman 1995):

i) Adenosine, an A_1 receptor agonist, is first choice in emergency treatment of supraventricular tachycardias associated with WPW, but should not be used in AF. Give rapid iv injection into a large peripheral or central vein, 3 mg over 2 s, if necessary followed by 6 mg after 1–2 min and 12 mg after a further 1–2 min. Ninety per cent will be terminated, but its effect is shortlived. Adenosine was used successfully in a pregnant patient during labour (Afridi et al 1992).

ii) Verapamil 5–10 mg over 1 min (but should not be used if the patient is receiving beta blockers, or is in pre-excitation atrial fibrillation or atrial flutter).

iii) Other drugs that prolong the refractory period of either the aberrant pathway, or the AV node, can be tried. These include flecainide, disopyramide, diltiazem, beta blockers, procainamide, or amiodarone.

iv) Drugs producing reflex bradycardia may occasionally be successful. Phenylephrine 200 μg, and a subsequent phenylephrine infusion, finally terminated a refractory tachycardia in a patient having squint surgery, when other drugs had failed (Jacobsen et al 1985).

b) For atrial fibrillation:

i) In the case of AF with an anterogradely conducting pathway, iv procainamide will slow the ventricular rate by blocking conduction over the accessory pathway. Other drugs which act in this way include disopyramide, amiodarone, and flecainide.

c) Direct current cardioversion should be considered early in AF, particularly if there is haemodynamic compromise. It can also be used if tachycardias fail to respond to drug treatment. Recurrent attacks of SVT in a patient in late pregnancy which produced serious maternal hypotension required cardioversion (Klepper 1981).

d) Atrial pacing may be used as a last resort.

e) Surgical transection may be considered for patients with recurrent arrhythmias or intolerance to drug therapy.

6. For prophylaxis, or long-term medical treatment, little difference is reported between verapamil, digoxin, and propranolol (Ganz & Friedman 1995).

Bibliography

Afridi I, Moise Jr KJ, Rokey R 1992 Termination of supraventricular tachycardia with intravenous adenosine in a pregnant woman with Wolff–Parkinson–White syndrome. Obstetrics & Gynecology 80: 481–2.

Brechenmacher R, Coumel PH, Fauchier J-P et al 1977 Intractable paroxysmal tachycardia which proved fatal in type A Wolff–Parkinson–White syndrome. Circulation 43: 408–17.

Chang RK, Stevenson WG, Wetzel GT et al 1996 Effects of isoflurane on electrophysiological measurements in children with Wolff–Parkinson–White syndrome. Pacing & Clinical Electrophysiology 19: 1082–8.

Dobkowski WB, Murkin JM, Sharpe MD et al 1990

The effect of isoflurane (1 MAC) on the normal AV conduction system and accessory pathways. Anesthesia & Analgesia 70: S86.

Dobkowski WB, Murkin JM, Sharpe MD et al 1991 The effect of combined alfentanil and midazolam anaesthesia on the normal AV conduction system and accessory pathways in patients with Wolff–Parkinson–White syndrome. Canadian Journal of Anaesthesia 38: A168.

Fisch C 1990 Clinical electrophysiological studies and the Wolff–Parkinson–White pattern. Circulation 82: 1872–3.

Ganz LI, Friedman PL 1995 Supraventricular tachycardia. New England Journal of Medicine 332: 162–71.

Gomez-Arnau J, Marquez-Montes J, Avello F 1983 Fentanyl and droperidol effects on the refractoriness of the accessory pathway in the Wolff–Parkinson–White syndrome. Anesthesiology 58: 307–13.

Hood MA, Smith WM, Robinson MC et al 1991 Operations for Wolff–Parkinson–White syndrome. Journal of Thoracic & Cardiovascular Surgery 101: 998–1003.

Jacobsen L, Turnquist K, Masley S 1985 Wolff–Parkinson–White syndrome. Anaesthesia 40: 657–60.

Kadoya T, Seto A, Aoyama K et al 1999 Development of rapid atrial fibrillation with a wide QRS complex after neostigmine in a patient with intermittent Wolff–Parkinson–White syndrome. British Journal of Anaesthesia 83: 815–18.

Klepper I 1981 Cardioversion in late pregnancy. Anaesthesia 36: 611–16.

Kounis NG, Zavras GM, Papadaki PJ et al 1995 Pregnancy-induced increase of supraventricular arrhythmias in Wolff–Parkinson–White syndrome. Clinical Cardiology 18: 137–40.

Lubarsky D, Wilkinson K 1989 Anesthesia unmasking benign Wolff–Parkinson–White syndrome. Anesthesia & Analgesia 68: 172–4.

Lustik SJ, Wojtczak J, Chhibber AK 1999 Wolff–Parkinson–White syndrome simulating inferior myocardial infarction in a cocaine abuser for urgent dilatation and evacuation of the uterus. Anesthesia & Analgesia 89: 609–12.

Nishikawa K, Mizoguchu M, Yukioka H et al 1993 Concealed Wolff–Parkinson–White syndrome detected during spinal anaesthesia. Anaesthesia 48: 1061–4.

Seki S, Ichimiya T, Tschida H et al 1999 A case of normalization Wolff–Parkinson–White syndrome conduction during propofol anesthesia. Anesthesiology 90: 1779–81.

Sharpe MD, Murkin JM, Dobkowski WB et al 1990 Halothane depresses conduction of normal and accessory pathways during surgery for Wolff–Parkinson–White syndrome. Anesthesia & Analgesia 70: S365.

Sharpe MD, Dobkowski WB, Murkin JM et al 1992 Alfentanil–midazolam anaesthesia has no electrophysiological effects upon the normal conduction system or accessory pathways in patients with Wolff–Parkinson–White syndrome. Canadian Journal of Anaesthesia 39: 816–21.

Sharpe MD, Dobkowski WB, Murkin JM et al 1994 The electrophysiological effects of volatile anesthetics and sufentanil on the normal atrioventricular conduction system and accessory pathways in Wolff–Parkinson–White syndrome. Anesthesiology 80: 63–70.

Sharpe MD, Dobkowski WB, Murkin JM et al 1995 Propofol has no direct effect on sinoatrial node function or on normal atrioventricular and accessory pathway conduction in Wolff–Parkinson–White syndrome during alfentanil/midazolam anaesthesia. Anesthesiology 82: 888–95.

Sharpe MD, Cuillerier DJ, Lee JK et al 1999 Sevoflurane has no effect on sinoatrial node function or on normal atrioventricular and accessory pathway conduction in Wolff–Parkinson–White syndrome during alfentanil/midazolam anaesthesia. Anesthesiology 90: 60–5.

Timmermans C, Smeets JL, Rodriguez LM et al 1995 Aborted sudden death in the Wolff–Parkinson–White syndrome. American Journal of Cardiology 76: 492–4.

Wellens HJJ, Brugada P, Penn OC 1987 The management of the preexcitation syndromes. Journal of the American Medical Association 257: 2325–33.

Zenker's diverticulum

A pharyngeal pouch, which is formed by an outpouching of pharyngeal mucosa in the posterior wall of the hypopharynx at its junction with the oesophagus through Killian's dehiscence. At this site there is an area of weakness that lies between the cricopharyngeus and the inferior pharyngeal constrictor muscles. There may be a functional component to the condition, because neuromuscular dysfunction, particularly in the relaxation of cricopharyngeus, has been found.

Preoperative abnormalities

1. The main complaints are of food sticking in throat and dysphagia, bouts of coughing, swelling in the neck, and regurgitation.

2. Aspiration pneumonitis occurs in about 25% of patients and results in bronchitis or recurrent pneumonia (Aggerholm & Illum 1990).

3. Weight loss and poor nutrition.

4. It has been suggested that reflux oesophagitis and hiatus hernia occur more frequently than in the normal population, but this has been disputed (Gage-White 1988).

Anaesthetic problems

1. Problems of aspiration and leakage around the tracheal tube.

2. The use of oral medication may be ineffective, because the tablets lodge within the pouch and absorption may be delayed.

3. Postoperative complications are most often associated with inhalation of food or debris from the pouch.

Management

1. The pouch should be emptied pre-operatively.

2. Induction with a head-up tilt has been recommended.

3. There is argument about the method of induction. Awake fibreoptic intubation has been recommended by some authors, and a smooth general anaesthetic by others (Cope & Spargo 1990, Thiagarajah et al 1990). Cricoid pressure is ineffective.

4. The use of endoscopic stapling is now considered to be superior to the open approach, in terms of reduced complications, shorter hospital stay and more rapid resumption of feeding (von Doersten & Byl 1997, Narne et al 1999, van Eeden et al 1999).

5. Treatment with antibiotics after pouch surgery reduces the number of local infective complications, and possibly the incidence of pouch recurrence.

Bibliography

Aggerholm K, Illum P 1990 Surgical treatment of Zenker's diverticulum. Journal of Laryngology & Otology 104: 312–14.

Cope R, Spargo P 1990 Anesthesia for Zenker's diverticulum. Anesthesia & Analgesia 71: 312.

Gage-White L 1988 Incidence of Zenker's diverticulum with hiatus hernia. Laryngoscope 98: 527–30.

Narne S, Cutrone C, Bonavina L et al 1999 Endoscopic diverticulotomy for the treatment of Zenker's diverticulum: results in 102 patients with staple-assisted endoscopy. Annals of Otology, Rhinology & Laryngology 108: 810–15.

Thiagarajah S, Lean E, Keh M 1990 Anesthetic implications of Zenker's diverticulum. Anesthesia & Analgesia 70: 109–11.

van Eeden S, Lloyd RV, Tranter RM 1999 Comparison of the endoscopic stapling technique with more established procedures for pharyngeal pouch. Journal of Laryngology & Otology 113: 237–40.

Von Doersten PG, Byl FM 1997 Endoscopic Zenker's diverticulectomy (Dohlman procedure): forty cases reviewed. Otolaryngology—Head & Neck Surgery 116: 209–12.

SECTION 2

EMERGENCY CONDITIONS ARISING DURING ANAESTHESIA OR IN THE IMMEDIATE PERIOPERATIVE PERIOD

Addisonian crisis or acute adrenocortical insufficiency (see

also Section 1, Addison's disease)

An extremely rare cause of perioperative cardiovascular collapse. May result from primary adrenocortical disease, in which case all three zones of the adrenal cortex will be affected, or secondary, which manifests itself as pure glucocorticoid deficiency associated with atrophy of the zona fasciculata.

Although rare, it must not be overlooked. An unrecognised and untreated Addisonian crisis can be fatal. The preoperative diagnosis is difficult to make in patients with mild clinical disease, yet these are the individuals in whom the adrenocortical responses to the stresses of anaesthesia and surgery may be inadequate. In patients with adenocarcinomas, adrenal metastases are not uncommon (Ihde et al 1990), but clinically apparent disease occurs only after a 90% loss of adrenocortical tissue.

Presentation

1. Acute cardiovascular collapse can occur under a wide variety of circumstances. (Occasional individuals may be apparently normotensive, if they were hypertensive before the crisis.)

   a) Cardiac arrest during appendicectomy in a 15-year-old girl responded to cardiac massage, saline, and bicarbonate (Salam & Davies 1974). She was subsequently found to have a normal resting blood cortisol, but no response to adrenal stimulation.

   b) An acute Addisonian crisis associated with a serum sodium of 106 mmol l^{-1} was deliberately provoked by a patient who stopped his own steroid therapy, then cut his neck and wrists (Smith & Byrne 1981). Another patient with chronic insufficiency developed a crisis after cardiac surgery, despite adequate preoperative replacement (Serrano et al 2000).

   c) Severe perioperative hypotension, despite the administration of fluids and inotropic agents, occurred in a young man with an acute abdominal emergency (Hertzberg & Schulman 1985). An improvement in his condition only took place when steroids were given. His postoperative complications included myocardial infarction and pericarditis. A subsequent adrenal stimulation test indicated Addison's disease.

   d) A patient with a previous history of TB, who was undergoing preoperative workup for head and neck cancer surgery, collapsed on the fifth day. His admission serum sodium of 124 mmol l^{-1} had decreased to 118 mmol l^{-1} and he was hypoglycaemic (Aono et al 1999).

   e) Patients with adrenocortical insufficiency may be subfertile. Cardiovascular collapse occurred in a young woman undergoing infertility investigations under general anaesthesia (personal observation). Sudden death occurred a week later, in a period of steroid withdrawal, during adrenocortical investigations.

   f) A patient with severe diarrhoea and vomiting presented with hypotension, tachycardia, and fever (Frederick et al 1991). Despite rehydration and inotropic support on the ITU, he developed acute respiratory distress with hypoxia and died 10 h later. It was later discovered that his brother had primary Addison's disease, and the patient's own plasma cortisol level before death was 2 μg dl^{-1} (normal 6–25 μg dl^{-1}).

   g) Should pregnancy occur, which is rare because these patients are subfertile, a crisis may present during pregnancy (Seaward et al 1989). One woman, admitted with apparent hyperemesis gravidarum, was found to have a plasma sodium level 115 mmol l^{-1} (Abu et al 1997).

h) Adrenocortical insufficiency has been reported after the removal of apparently nonfunctioning adrenal adenomas (Huiras et al 1989). Although there were no stigmata of adrenal hyperactivity, it was suggested that there was sufficient secretion from the adenoma to produce basal cortisol levels, whilst suppressing the other gland.

i) Two patients with high-output circulatory failure and negative blood cultures were found to have primary adrenal insufficiency (Dorin & Kearns 1988).

j) In patients with cancer, adrenocortical insufficiency is particularly difficult to diagnose, since anorexia, nausea, orthostatic hypotension and confusion may be attributed to the disease itself (Kung et al 1990).

2. A patient receiving anticoagulants who became hypotensive and confused after CABG surgery, developed a serum sodium of $118 \, \text{mmol} \, \text{l}^{-1}$ on day 14. An enlarged right adrenal was seen and adrenal failure secondary to adrenal haemorrhage was diagnosed (Hardy et al 1992).

3. Other symptoms and signs include abdominal pain, vomiting, diarrhoea, orthostatic hypotension, syncope, confusion, stupor, and mucosal hyperpigmentation. If Addison's disease is present, other endocrine abnormalities (hypothyroidism or panhypopituitarism) should be sought (Frederick et al 1991).

4. There may be a history of steroid therapy within the previous 12 months. Adrenocortical atrophy is detectable 5 days after the onset of glucocorticoid therapy of the equivalent of prednisone $20–30 \, \text{mg} \, \text{day}^{-1}$, HPA axis suppression can occur after the equivalent of $20–30 \, \text{mg} \, \text{day}^{-1}$, and a return to completely normal homeostasis was suggested to take up to 1 year (Axelrod 1976). However, recent studies indicate that the problem has been overexaggerated (Nicholson et al 1998). Current recommendations for treatment in the perioperative period are given in Section 1 (Addison's disease).

5. The cardiac effects of adrenal insufficiency have recently been recognised. Seven patients with newly diagnosed disease underwent echocardiographic and Doppler studies before treatment, and 4–8 months after. A reduction in cardiac dimensions seen in all patients, and mitral valve prolapse in four, regressed after treatment (Fallo et al 1999). One child undergoing treatment for an acute crisis developed congestive heart failure, which was found to be secondary to a cardiomyopathy (Derish et al 1996).

Management

1. Hydrocortisone hemisuccinate iv 200 mg, followed by an infusion of hydrocortisone 400 mg in saline 0.9%, to be given over 24 h.

2. Saline 0.9% iv, 1 litre rapidly initially, then more slowly.

3. Dextrose 10% iv to correct hypoglycaemia.

4. Subsequently, the presumptive diagnosis must be confirmed or refuted with plasma cortisol estimations and adrenal stimulation tests. Before these, hydrocortisone should be changed to dexamethasone, which does not register in plasma cortisol assays.

Bibliography

Abu MAE, Sinha P, Totoe I 1997 Addison's disease in pregnancy presenting as hyperemesis gravidarum. Journal of Obstetrics & Gynaecology 17: 278–9.

Aono J, Mamiya K, Ueda W 1999 Abrupt onset of adrenal crisis during routine preoperative examination in a patient with unknown Addison's disease. Anesthesiology 90: 313–14.

Axelrod L 1976 Glucocorticoid therapy. Medicine 55: 39–65.

Derish M, Eckert K, Chin C 1996 Reversible cardiomyopathy in a child with Addison's disease. Intensive Care Medicine 22: 460–3.

Dorin RI, Kearns PJ 1988 High output circulatory failure in acute adrenal insufficiency. Critical Care Medicine 16: 296–7.

Fallo F, Betterle C, Budano S et al 1999 Regression of cardiac abnormalities after replacement therapy in Addison's disease. European Journal of Endocrinology 140: 425–8.

Frederick R, Brown C, Renusch J et al 1991 Addisonian crisis: emergency presentation of primary adrenal insufficiency [clinical conference]. Annals of Emergency Medicine 20: 802–6.

Hardy K, Mead B, Gill G 1992 Adrenal apoplexy after coronary artery bypass surgery leading to Addisonian crisis. Journal of the Royal Society of Medicine 85: 577–8.

Hertzberg LB, Schulman MS 1985 Acute adrenal insufficiency in a patient with appendicitis during anesthesia. Anesthesiology 62: 517–19.

Huiras CM, Pehling GB, Caplan RH 1989 Adrenal insufficiency after operative removal of apparently nonfunctioning adrenal adenoma. Journal of the American Medical Association 261: 894–9.

Ihde JK, Turnbull AD, Bajorunas DR 1990 Adrenal insufficiency in the cancer patient: implications for the surgeon. British Journal of Surgery 77: 1335–7.

Kung AWC, Pun KK, Lam K et al 1990 Addisonian crisis as presenting feature in malignancies. Cancer 65: 177–9.

Nicholson G, Burrin JM, Hall GM 1998 Peroperative steroid supplementation. Anaesthesia 53: 1091–4.

Salam AA, Davies DM 1974 Acute adrenal insufficiency during surgery. British Journal of Anaesthesia 46: 619–22.

Seaward PG, Guidozzi F, Sonnendecker EW 1989 Addisonian crisis in pregnancy. Case report. British Journal of Obstetrics & Gynaecology 96: 1348–50.

Serrano N, Jiminez JJ, Brouard MT et al 2000 Acute adrenal insufficiency after cardiac surgery. Critical Care Medicine 28: 569–70.

Smith MG, Byrne AJ 1981 An Addisonian crisis complicating anaesthesia. Anaesthesia 56: 681–4.

Air embolism

Air embolism can occur in any situation in which there is an open vein and a subatmospheric pressure. When a patient is in an upright position, air inadvertently entering the venous system will normally be carried to the right side of the heart, where it localises initially at the junction of the right atrium and the superior vena cava. Some air may remain in the upper part of the right atrium, while the rest is carried through the tricuspid valve and into the pulmonary artery. There is experimental evidence to suggest that small venous air emboli are eliminated primarily in the pulmonary arterioles (Presson et al 1989), and that this elimination depends on diffusion of gas across the arteriolar walls into the alveolar spaces. Larger amounts of air may cause pulmonary outflow obstruction and a reduction in cardiac output. However, new work on dogs has suggested that adoption of the head-down position during resuscitation confers no haemodynamic benefit (Geissler 1997).

Many studies using transoesophageal echocardiography have now shown the presence of gas bubbles in the right side of the heart during a variety of different surgical procedures. Derouin et al (1996) showed gas bubbles in 11 out of 16 patients having laparoscopic cholecystectomy. In five, the entry occurred during peritoneal insufflation, and in six, during gall bladder dissection. In this series, however, there were no associated cardiovascular events.

Particular concern has focused on the subject of 'paradoxical' air embolism (Clayton et al 1985, Black et al 1989). At postmortem, 20–35% of all patients have a 'probe patent' foramen ovale, and several transoesophageal echocardiographic studies have demonstrated passage of contrast across the interatrial septum in 22% of 50 patients (Konstadt et al 1991). In a patient with a patent foramen ovale, if the RAP were to exceed the LAP, venous air could theoretically enter the systemic circulation. Haemodynamic studies have shown that, in the sitting position, the interatrial pressure gradient can become reversed (Perkins-Pearson et al 1982). It has been suggested that, if the incidence of air embolism in the sitting position is 30–40%, and that of patent foramen ovale is 20–35%, one in ten patients operated on in this position could have conditions that predispose to the entry of air into the systemic circulation (Gronert et al 1979). This 'paradoxical' air embolism can account for a number of cases of air embolism in which Doppler changes occurred without ETCO$_2$ changes, when ST segment or QRS changes suggested entry of air into the coronary arteries, or where there were postoperative clinical signs of cerebral air embolism. The possibility of a transpulmonary route for access of venous air to the systemic circulation has also been suggested.

Haemodynamic studies have shown that, in the sitting position, the interatrial pressure gradient can be reversed transiently (Perkins-Pearson et al 1982), particularly during sustained application of PEEP (Jaffe et al 1992), or at sudden release of positive airway pressure. However, work on preoperative identification of flow-patent foramen ovale is still in its early stages, interpretation is difficult, and sometimes results are conflicting (Rafferty 1992).

Systemic air embolism, although a rare event, can occur after blunt and penetrating injuries, induction of artificial pneumothorax, and during laser surgery to bronchial carcinoma. There are pathognomonic antemortem signs, but the diagnosis may easily be missed at postmortem.

Presentation and origin

1. *Type of surgery.* The incidence of air embolism reported depends on the monitoring techniques employed. The Doppler method is particularly sensitive and capable of detecting extremely small emboli.

a) Neurosurgery in the sitting position. Using Doppler detection, an incidence of up to 58% has been reported in patients having posterior fossa or cervical disc surgery in the sitting position.

b) Several patients had air emboli whilst undergoing stereotactic surgery for Parkinson's disease, when sedated and in the sitting position (Suarez et al 1999). Symptomatic emboli usually occur soon after dural puncture, when the cerebral venous channels are open to atmosphere. Cough and hyperventilation are associated with hypotension, decreases in $ETCO_2$, and hypoxia (Stone et al 1997).

c) Craniectomy (Faberowski et al 2000). Using echocardiographic techniques, 66% of infants undergoing craniectomy in the supine position show evidence of venous air embolism (Harris et al 1987).

d) Head and neck surgery. Emboli can also occur when large veins are opened in head and neck operations if there is a head-up tilt.

e) Hip surgery. In hip arthoplasty, Doppler evidence of air embolism was seen in 30% of patients, immediately following the insertion of the femoral cement, but an associated decrease in blood pressure occurred in only 4% (Michel 1980).

f) Caesarean section. Air may also enter the uterine sinuses in up to 40% of Caesarean deliveries. However, massive emboli are rare, and are most likely to occur in hypovolaemic patients, bleeding from placenta praevia or placental abruption (Younker et al 1986).

g) Central venous catheter insertion or removal. The increasing use of CVP lines has been associated with a number of incidents of accidental introduction of air (Seidelin et al 1987, Ely et al 1999). Disconnection of a three-way tap in a patient receiving chemotherapy at home resulted in a nonfatal paradoxical embolism (Jensen & Hansen 1989). Air embolism occurred after removal of central venous catheters (Turnage & Harper 1991), presumably secondary to air entrainment through the track formed by the device.

h) In association with the administration of Haemaccel using a pressure bag (Gray & Glover 1999). Warming the infusion, and the use of certain pumps, can potentially increase the volume of air infused.

i) In association with perioperative blood salvage. Five fatal cases were described in which blood was being reinfused under pressure (Linden et al 1997).

j) Lumbar disc surgery. Three patients undergoing lumbar laminectomy in the prone position developed sudden air embolism (Albin et al 1991). This is a rare occurrence, but in each case a frame was used to retain the patient in a 'four-poster' position. In this posture, the pressure in the inferior vena cava is low and there is a gravitational gradient between the right side of the heart and the operative site.

k) Transurethral resection of prostate. Fatal massive air embolism occurred after TURP (Vacanti & Lodhia 1991). At the end of surgery, there was no drainage from the Foley catheter, so repeated attempts to unblock it were made with a 60-ml syringe containing fluid and air. The patient collapsed after he was moved from the lithotomy position and, at postmortem, air was found throughout the venous side of the circulation. The air was probably contained within the femoral veins until the patient was moved.

l) Epidural injection. A suspected air embolism has been described during insertion of a Tuohy needle in the C7/T1 space for injection of epidural steroids in a seated patient (Jackson & Rauck 1991).

m) Laparoscopic procedures. A sudden decrease in end-tidal CO_2 with oxygen desaturation, which occurred just after accidental penetration of the liver by the sapphire tip of an Nd : YAG laser, was the first sign of air embolism during laparoscopic cholecystectomy (Greville et al 1991). The surgeon was unaware that the laser was cooled with air flowing at $0.5\,l\,min^{-1}$ from ports proximal to the tip, and this air must have entered the hepatic venous system during the 15 s of inadvertent penetration. Fatal CO_2 embolism and haemorrhage has also occurred during laparoscopic salpingectomy (Beck & McQuillan 1994).

n) Transcervical resection of endometrium. Similar accidents again resulted in two deaths during laser endometrial ablation using artificial sapphire tips with gaseous cooling systems (Baggish & Daniel 1989). Another patient developed venous air embolism (VAE) 40 min into TCRE surgery secondary to the use of a roller pump for delivering fluid (Babita et al 2000).

o) During hysteroscopy, undertaken with and without anaesthesia (Nishiyama & Hanaoka 1999). An unmonitored, awake patient developed convulsions and cardiac arrest just after hysteroscopy, in which CO_2 was used as the inflating gas. She died 25 h after the event.

p) During irrigation of a wound with hydrogen peroxide (Neff et al 1996, Schwab & Dilworth 1999).

q) Laser application to bronchial tumours. A massive, fatal, systemic air embolism, a rare event, resulted from a fistula produced between the right main bronchus and a branch of the pulmonary vein during Nd : YAG laser of an obstructing bronchial carcinoma (Peachey et al 1988). The emergence of bright red froth from the arterial cannula, palpation of crepitus in the brachial, femoral and carotid arteries, and observation of air in the retinal vessels on ophthalmoscopy, confirmed the diagnosis. Three patients were described in whom gas embolism occurred as a result of jet ventilation during bronchial laser surgery. On ECG, ST segment elevation accompanied cardiovascular collapse in two, and all three initially developed left hemipareses. Air was seen in the brain on CT scan.

r) During endoscopically assisted varicose vein surgery (Vidovich & Lojeski 1999).

2. *Factors affecting clinical signs.* The effects of air embolism depend on the rate of entry and quantity of air, the differences between the venous and atmospheric pressures, and the percentage of nitrous oxide being administered. Animal studies show that a rate of

$0.5 \, ml \, kg^{-1} \, min^{-1}$ can produce symptoms. The entry of large boluses of air has been associated with the insertion of CVP lines, especially when the head-down position was not used and if the CVP was low. Experiments have shown that with a pressure difference of $5 \, cmH_2O$, as much as $100 \, ml \, air \, s^{-1}$ can be drawn through a 2-mm needle. The concomitant administration of N_2O effectively increases the volume of air drawn into the bloodstream. A concentration of 50% N_2O produces an effective increase of 200%, and 75% N_2O one of 400%.

3. *Source or timing of entry.* In neurosurgical procedures, air enters most frequently via veins held open by the neck muscles, or those in the dura, venous sinuses, or bone. In sterotactic procedures under local anaesthesia the event often occurred immediately after opening the dura (Stone et al 1997).

a) During spinal fusion and instrumentation for scoliosis, four fatal cases have occurred (McCarthy et al 1990, Sutherland & Winter 1997).

b) In hip surgery, emboli can occur when cement is inserted into the femoral shaft.

c) Of 79 cases of air embolism associated with central venous lines, the majority involved technical problems (Seidelin et al 1987). One-third happened during catheter insertion, and death occurred in 32% of the cases reported.

d) During Caesarean section, there is evidence of entry of gas bubbles in 37–50% of patients, sometimes associated with chest pain and dyspnoea, in the period between uterine incision and delivery (Malinow et al 1987, Matthews & Greer 1990).

4. *Clinical signs of venous air embolism.* These may include a hissing sound from the wound, hypotension, arrhythmias, cyanosis, or changes in respiratory pattern in a spontaneously breathing patient. However, with adequate monitoring, subclinical air entry should be detected before many of these signs occur.

5. *Clinical signs of systemic air embolism.*

a) Circulatory collapse, followed by pupillary dilatation. Although brief, there may be a preceding period of hypertension; this may be missed without direct arterial monitoring.

b) Other signs include marbling of the skin, secondary to gas bubbles in the subcutaneous tissues causing venous stasis (Dullye et al 1998), air bleeding from arteries, bubbles of air in the retinal vessels, and pallor of part of the tongue.

c) Although the mill wheel murmur is said to be absent, it may be heard if large amounts of gas pass through the left ventricle from a pulmonary vein (Peachey et al 1988).

d) Systemic air embolism may be missed at postmortem, if the diagnosis is not suspected, because air disappears within a few hours of death.

Diagnosis

1. A precordial Doppler produces the earliest signs of air embolism, but is very sensitive. The use of an oesphageal Doppler has been described. The diagnosis can sometimes be confirmed by aspiration through a right heart catheter, if it has been placed high in the right atrium.

2. A decrease in $ETCO_2$ occurs before clinical signs, but will not necessarily change as quickly, or as much, if a paradoxical air embolus has also occurred.

3. Later signs of significant emboli include a 'mill wheel' murmur, arrhythmias, hypotension, a decrease in oxygen saturation, and increases in CVP or in PAWP.

4. The occurrence of paradoxical air embolism is difficult to prove, unless a neurosurgeon observes air in small cerebral arteries. However, it may be inferred if ECG changes of ST elevation or depression or cardiac

arrest occur. Monitored changes of cerebral function have been attributed to cerebral emboli. Localisation of air in the cardiac chambers has been seen using two-dimensional TOE. Out of 21 patients, paradoxical embolism occurred in three, only after the most severe venous air embolism and within 20–30 s of it (Mammoto et al 1998). Fatal paradoxical air embolus occurred in a 26 year old during hepatic dissection in a liver transplantation. At autopsy there was a 2-cm patent foramen ovale and evidence of myocardial ischaemic changes, assumed to be secondary to air within the coronary arteries (Olmedilla et al 2000).

Management

1. Individual.

a) *In neurosurgery.* Identify the site of access, and prevent further entry. Cover or flood the wound. Compress the neck to show open veins. Deal surgically with the open vein or apply bone wax, if appropriate. Although aspiration of air from a right heart catheter may have a diagnostic role, its therapeutic value is doubtful.

b) *Central venous catheter.* To prevent air embolism during insertion of a central venous line, it is important to have the patient in a head-down position. Occlusion of the catheter after insertion, and use of a three-way tap when disconnecting infusion sets, will reduce the risks. The catheter should be removed in the supine position and the site covered with an occlusive dressing. It has been suggested that patients remain supine for 1 h afterwards (Turnage & Harper 1991).

c) *Total hip replacement.* Insertion of cement into the femoral shaft using a cement gun is less likely to produce air embolism than when the cement is inserted by hand (Evans et al 1989).

d) *Hysteroscopy using CO_2 without anaesthesia* should not be undertaken unless the patient is being monitored.

e) In *blood salvage techniques*, avoid infusing direct from the recovery chamber. Limit the use of reinfusion under pressure, and, if essential, watch carefully or use air detection devices. If only small volumes are salvaged, consider whether or not reinfusion is worthwhile (Linden et al 1997).

f) During *laser treatment of endobronchial carcinoma*, if bleeding occurs, the airway pressure should be minimised and the bronchoscope withdrawn to above the carina (Dullye et al 1998).

2. If the entry of a large amount of air occurs, CPR may be required. Although it has traditionally been taught that assumption of the left head-down position will relocate the air and reduce pulmonary outflow obstruction, experimental work on dogs has suggested that positional changes do not confer haemodynamic benefit. Arterial hypotension, increased RV afterload and possible ischaemia, appear to be the major causes of cardiac dysfunction (Geissler et al 1997).

3. It has been suggested that morbidity and mortality is such that the sitting position should no longer be used for neurosurgical procedures. However, an analysis of 554 cases showed that with careful patient selection, monitoring, and anaesthetic and surgical skills, emboli can be minimised (Matjasko et al 1985). Increasing work is being done on the recognition of the flow-patent foramen ovale by TOE (Rafferty 1992, Fuchs et al 1998), although techniques for identification are dependent on the skill of the operator. If a right-to-left shunt is demonstrated, the sitting position should not be used. Since reversal of pressure gradients can be caused by the sudden release of positive airway pressure, positive airway pressures should be avoided in the seated patient.

4. An inflatable neck tourniquet, which could be used to identify venous bleeding points during the incision through muscle and bone, has been described (Sale 1984).

Bibliography

Albin MS, Ritter RR, Pruett CE et al 1991 Venous air embolism during lumbar laminectomy in the prone position: report of three cases. Anesthesia & Analgesia 73: 346–9.

Babita G, Jayalakshmi TS, Amit S 2000 Air embolism: a complication during TCRE. Anesthesiology 90: 763–4.

Baggish MS, Daniell JF 1989 Death caused by air embolism associated with neodymium:yttrium–aluminium–garnet laser surgery and artificial sapphire tips. American Journal of Obstetrics & Gynecology 161: 877–80.

Beck DH, McQuillan PJ 1994 Fatal carbon dioxide embolism and severe haemorrhage during laparoscopic salpingectomy. British Journal of Anaesthesia 72: 243–5.

Black S, Cucchiara RF, Nishimura RA et al 1989 Parameters affecting occurrence of paradoxical air embolus. Anesthesiology 71: 235–41.

Clayton DG, Evans P, Williams C et al 1985 Paradoxical air embolism during neurosurgery. Anaesthesia 40: 981–9.

Derouin M, Couture P, Boudreault D 1996 Detection of gas embolism by transesophageal echocardiography during laparoscopic cholecystectomy. Anesthesia & Analgesia 82: 119–24.

Dullye KK, Kaspar MD, Ramsay MA et al 1998 Laser treatment of endobronchial lesions. Anesthesiology 86: 1387–90.

Ely EW, Hite RD, Baker AM et al 1999 Venous air embolism from central venous catheterization: a need for increased physician awareness. Critical Care Medicine 27: 2113–17.

Evans RD, Palazzo MGA, Ackers JWL 1989 Air embolism during total hip replacement: comparison of two surgical techniques. British Journal of Anaesthesia 62: 243–7.

Faberowski LW, Black S, Mickle JP 2000 Incidence of venous air embolism during craniectomy for craniosynostosis. Anesthesiology 92: 20–7.

Fuchs G, Schwarz G, Stein J et al 1998 Doppler color-flow imaging: screening of a patent foramen ovale in children scheduled for neurosurgery in the sitting position. Journal of Neurosurgical Anesthesiology 10: 5–9.

Geissler HJ, Allen SJ, Mehlhorn U et al 1997 Effect of body repositioning after venous air embolism. An echocardiographic study. Anesthesiology 86: 710–17.

Gray AJ, Glover P 1999 Air emboli with Haemaccel. Anaesthesia 54: 790–2.

Greville AC, Clements EAF, Erwin DC et al 1991 Pulmonary air embolism during laparoscopic laser cholecystectomy. Anaesthesia 46: 113–14.

Gronert GA, Messick JM Jr, Cucchiara RF et al 1979 Paradoxical air embolism from a patent foramen ovale. Anesthesiology 50: 548–9.

Harris MM, Yemen TA, Davidson A et al 1987 Venous air embolism during craniectomy in supine infants. Anesthesiology 67: 816–19.

Jackson KE, Rauck RL 1991 Suspected venous air embolism during epidural anesthesia. Anesthesiology 74: 190–1.

Jaffe RA, Pinto FJ, Schnittger I et al 1992 Aspects of mechanical ventilation affecting interatrial shunt flow during general anesthesia. Anesthesia & Analgesia 75: 484–8.

Jensen AG, Hansen PA 1989 Non-fatal paradoxical air embolism. British Journal of Anaesthesia 63: 244.

Konstadt SN, Louie EK, Black S et al 1991 Intraoperative detection of patent foramen ovale by transesophageal echocardiography. Anesthesiology 74: 212–16.

Linden JV, Kaplan HS, Murphy MT 1997 Fatal air embolism due to perioperative blood recovery. Anesthesia & Analgesia 84: 422–6.

McCarthy RE, Lonstein JE, Mertz JD et al 1990 Air embolism in spinal surgery. Journal of Spinal Disorders 3: 1–5.

Malinow AM, Naulty JS, Hunt CO et al 1987 Precordial ultrasonic monitoring during Cesarean delivery. Anesthesiology 66: 816–19.

Mammoto T, Hayashi Y, Ohnishi Y et al 1998 Incidence of venous and paradoxical air embolism in neurosurgical patients in the sitting position: detection by transesophageal echocardiography. Acta Anaesthesiologica Scandinavica 42: 643–7.

Matjasko J, Petrozza P, Cohen M et al 1985 Anesthesia and surgery in the seated position: analysis of 554 cases. Neurosurgery 17: 695–702.

Matthews NC, Greer G 1990 Embolism during Caesarean section. Anaesthesia 45: 964–5.

Michel R 1980 Air embolism in hip surgery. Anaesthesia 35: 858–62.

Neff SPW, Zululeta L, Miller R 1996 Hydrogen peroxide: an unusual cause of arterial and venous gas embolism. Anaesthesia 51: 683–4.

Nishiyama T, Hanaoka K 1999 Gas embolism during hysteroscopy. Canadian Journal of Anaesthesia 46: 379–81.

Olmedilla L, Garutti I, Perez-Pena J et al 2000 Fatal paradoxical air embolism during liver transplantation. British Journal of Anaesthesia 84: 112–14.

Peachey T, Eason J, Moxham J et al 1988 Systemic air embolism during laser bronchoscopy. Anaesthesia 43. 872–5.

Perkins-Pearson N, Marshall W, Bedford R 1982 Atrial pressures in the seated position. Anesthesiology 57: 493–7.

Presson RG, Kirk KR, Haselby KA et al 1989 The fate of air emboli in the pulmonary circulation of the dog. Anesthesia & Analgesia 68: S227.

Rafferty TD 1992 Intraoperative transesophageal saline-contrast imaging of flow-patent foramen ovale. Anesthesia & Analgesia 475–80.

Sale JP 1984 Prevention of air embolism during sitting neurosurgery. Anaesthesia 39: 795–9.

Schwab C, Dilworth K 1999 Gas embolism produced by hydrogen peroxide abscess irrigation in an infant. Anaesthesia & Intensive Care 27: 418–20.

Seidelin PH, Stolarek IH, Thompson AM 1987 Central venous catheterisation and fatal air embolism. British Journal of Hospital Medicine 38: 438–9.

Stone JG, Schwartz AE, Berman MF et al 1997 Air embolization in seated, sedated, spontaneously breathing, neurosurgical patients. Anesthesiology 87: 1244–7.

Suarez S, Ornaque I, Fabregas N et al 1999 Venous air embolism during Parkinson surgery in patients with spontaneous ventilation. Anesthesia & Analgesia 88: 793–4.

Sutherland RW, Winter RJ 1997 Two cases of fatal air embolism in children undergoing scoliosis surgery. Acta Anaesthesiologica Scandinavica 41: 1073–6.

Turnage WS, Harper JV 1991 Venous air embolism occurring after removal of central venous catheter. Anesthesia & Analgesia 72: 559–60.

Vacanti CA, Lodhia KL 1991 Fatal massive air embolism during transurethral resection of the prostate. Anesthesiology 74: 186–7.

Vidovich MI, Lojeski EW 1999 Probable carbon monoxide embolism during endoscopically assisted varicose vein stripping. Anesthesiology 91: 1527–9.

Younker D, Rodriguez V, Kavanagh J 1986 Massive air embolism during Cesarean section. Anesthesiology 65: 77–9.

Amniotic fluid embolism

This term refers to a rare and potentially devastating syndrome of the peripartum period, in which acute hypoxia, haemodynamic changes and coagulopathy coexist. There is an increase in the number of maternal deaths associated with the condition (May 1999). Amniotic fluid embolism (AFE) is a clinical diagnosis, and there is no specific or consistent confirmatory test. It has been described in association with normal labour (or immediately postpartum), Caesarean section, therapeutic abortion, amniocentesis, and artificial rupture of the membranes. The exact aetiology is unknown, but it appears to be associated with exposure of maternal blood vessels to fetal tissue. Whilst amniotic fluid, which contains electrolytes, nitrogenous compounds, lipids, prostaglandins and fetal elements such as squames, hairs, vernix and meconium, has been found in the lungs, it is probably not an embolus according to the strict definition of the term. The syndrome has been said to resemble both anaphylaxis and septic shock, and Clark et al (1995) believe that a more appropriate term would be 'anaphylactoid syndrome of pregnancy'.

Earlier papers suggested that pulmonary hypertension was the principal haemodynamic feature of the condition, and that treatment should be with pulmonary vasodilators. More recently, invasive haemodynamic monitoring has been undertaken in several patients in the acute stage of the disease. An initial period of pulmonary hypertension, hypoxia and increased right heart pressures is succeeded by left ventricular failure secondary to impaired left ventricular function (Clark et al 1988, Clark 1991, Vanmaele et al 1991). The haemodynamic findings would therefore vary, according to the stage at which monitoring was first undertaken. This would account for the high incidence (70%) of pulmonary oedema seen on the CXR of survivors, and the variety of features described in the few patients in whom invasive monitoring has been undertaken. These features include pulmonary hypertension (Shah et al 1986), left heart failure (Girard et al 1986, Vanmaele et al 1990, Choi & Duffy 1995), and left and right heart failure (Moore et al 1982).

There is increasing evidence that the pathophysiology involves a two-stage response to the release of vasoactive metabolites of arachidonic acid (prostaglandins and leukotrienes), that directly or indirectly damage the myocardium, leading to left ventricular failure. Expression of endothelin-1, which has vasoconstrictor and bronchoconstrictor effects, has been found in two cases of AFE (Khong 1998). In addition, circulating amniotic fluid has thromboplastic activity and the entry of a significant amount is usually associated with a coagulopathy. Abnormal fibrinolysis often occurs as well. Immunoassays and functional assays suggest that coagulation changes are caused by tissue factors contained in amniotic fluid (Lockwood et al 1991). There is increasing evidence that some form of anaphylactoid reaction takes place. Immunohistochemical studies in fatalities from amniotic fluid embolism, anaphylaxis and trauma, showed an increase in numbers of pulmonary mast cells in the first two groups, compared with those who died from trauma (Fineschi et al 1998).

The mortality rates reported vary according to the series, and may reflect differences in selection methods. The National Registry analysed 41 cases (which fulfilled their strict criteria) in which the maternal mortality was 61% (Clark et al 1995). A later study of 53 cases occurring in California, in a 2-year period, reported a maternal mortality rate of 26.4% (Gilbert & Danielsen 1999). It was suggested that the former represented 'worst cases', and the latter, 'population frequency'. The condition is largely nonpreventable, but with better understanding of the pathophysiology, and an increasing use of ITU facilities for haemodynamic monitoring, a continuing improvement in mortality rate might be expected in the future.

Presentation

1. Reviews of 272 cases (Morgan 1979), 46 cases (Clark et al 1995) and 53 cases (Gilbert & Danielsen 1999) have shown similar presenting symptoms. In Clark's series there was hypotension in 100%, fetal distress in 100%, pulmonary oedema or ARDS in 93%,

cardiopulmonary arrest in 87%, coagulopathy in 83%, and cyanosis in 83%. Seizures (or seizure-like activity) were also common. Patients were often multiparous. A high incidence (41%) of patients had a history of atopy or allergy. Bronchospasm is rare.

2. The onset is often dramatic. In an analysis of 46 cases, it occurred during labour in 70% of women, after vaginal delivery in 11%, and during Caesarean section after delivery of the infant in 19% (Clark et al 1995). Most patients had ruptured membranes. Sometimes it occurs in association with the use of oxytocin (Alon & Atanassoff 1992). Those who collapsed after vaginal delivery, did so within 5 min.

3. One fatal case presented with an asymptomatic decrease in oxygen saturation, as measured by pulse oximetry, during Caesarean section under epidural anaesthesia (Quance 1988).

4. At Caesarean section, collapse has been reported after delivery of the placenta (McDougall & Duke 1995). However, delayed embolism occurred 60 min following Caesarean section under spinal anaesthesia. Over the next 60 min a severe coagulopathy developed (Margarson 1995). It was suggested that a combination of the offset of spinal anaesthesia, and return of venous tone, might have mobilised amniotic fluid lodged in a uterine vessel.

5. In some patients there has been a temporal association between artificial rupture of the membranes or placement of a uterine pressure catheter, and collapse (Clark et al 1995). One patient in whom a uterine catheter was inserted developed a coagulopathy before delivery, uterine hypotonia and massive haemorrhage afterwards, and became disorientated and unresponsive. She died despite all attempts at resuscitation. It was suggested that a small tear in the posterior cervix had allowed a slow, but steady leakage of amniotic fluid into the maternal circulation (Bastien et al 1998).

6. A proportion of those who survive suffer permanent neurological damage (Noble & St-Amand 1993, Clark et al 1995).

7. Coagulopathy results in decreased fibrinogen levels, increased fibrinogen degradation products, and increased APTT. Thrombocytopenia is not a prominent feature initially. In the National Registry series, only six out of 46 patients had a platelet count $<50 \times 10^9\,l^{-1}$. In some patients there may be a delay in development of coagulopathy of up to 3 h, and presentation is with sudden massive haemorrhage. However, there has often been some preceding event involving hypotension, or decrease in SpO_2, during Caesarean section (Quinn & Barrett 1993).

Diagnosis

This is made on clinical grounds alone. The primary concern is that of resuscitation of the collapsed patient.

Treatment

1. Cardiovascular collapse, or even cardiac arrest, may be the initial event. CPR is instituted and, if the fetus is still in utero, the uterus should be displaced laterally, or the Cardiff wedge should be used, to prevent aortocaval compression. Hypoxia is treated with high flow oxygen and, if necessary, IPPV and PEEP. Emergency Caesarean section may be appropriate during resuscitation (Alon & Atanassoff 1992).

2. Hypotension requires careful management on an ITU, such as is given to any patient with cardiogenic shock. In the situation in which the obstetric unit is geographically isolated from such facilities, a decision must be made about the optimum time for transfer. Clark (1991) suggests initial treatment with fluids, followed by circulatory support with an inotropic agent such as dopamine. Monitoring with a pulmonary artery catheter may sometimes be necessary. Once the blood pressure improves, fluid restriction may be required to prevent or treat pulmonary oedema. Inhaled aerosolised prostacyclin has been used as a selective pulmonary vasodilator (Van Heerden et al 1996).

3. On the basis that the syndrome resembles that of anaphylaxis, the use of epinephrine (adrenaline) and steroids (hydrocortisone 100 mg) has been suggested (Clark et al 1995). To test this hypothesis, blood should be taken for plasma tryptase levels (Benson & Lindberg 1996).

4. Replacement of blood volume may be needed if there is significant haemorrhage. Treatment of any bleeding diathesis will require repeated coagulation tests and specialist haematological advice. In general, packed red cells are followed by fresh frozen plasma and the tests repeated. There is not sufficient evidence to support the use of heparin, which has sometimes been recommended.

5. Continuous arteriovenous haemofiltration was used in a patient with an AFE syndrome that occurred in association with premature labour and Caesarean delivery (Weksler et al 1994).

Bibliography

Alon E, Atanassoff PG 1992 Successful cardiopulmonary resuscitation of a parturient with amniotic fluid embolism. International Journal of Obstetric Anesthesia 1: 205–7.

Bastien JL, Graves JR, Bailey S 1998 Atypical presentation of amniotic fluid embolism. Anesthesia & Analgesia 87: 124–6.

Benson MD, Lindberg RE 1996 Amniotic fluid embolism, anaphylaxis, and tryptase. American Journal of Obstetrics & Gynecology 175: 737.

Choi DM, Duffy BL 1995 Amniotic fluid embolism. Anaesthesia & Intensive Care 23: 741–3.

Clark SL 1991 Amniotic fluid embolism. Critical Care Clinics 7: 877–82.

Clark SL, Cotton DB, Gonik B et al 1988 Central hemodynamic alterations in amniotic fluid embolism. American Journal of Obstetrics & Gynecology 158: 1124–6.

Clark SL, Hankins GD, Dudley DA et al 1995 Amniotic fluid embolism: analysis of the national registry. American Journal of Obstetrics & Gynecology 172: 1158–67.

Fineschi V, Gambassi R, Gherardi M et al 1998 The diagnosis of amniotic fluid embolism: an immunohistochemical study for the quantification of pulmonary mast cell tryptase. International Journal of Legal Medicine 111: 238–43.

Gilbert WM, Danielsen B 1999 Amniotic fluid embolism: decreased mortality in a population-based study. Obstetrics & Gynecology 93: 973–7.

Girard P, Mal H, Laine J-F et al 1986 Left heart failure in amniotic fluid embolism. Anesthesiology 64: 262–5.

Khong TY 1998 Expression of endothelin-1 in amniotic fluid embolism and possible pathophysiological mechanism. British Journal of Obstetrics & Gynaecology 105: 802–4.

Lockwood CJ, Bach R, Guha A et al 1991 Amniotic fluid contains tissue factor, a potent initiator of coagulation. American Journal of Obstetrics & Gynecology 5: 1335–41.

McDougall RJ, Duke GJ 1995 Amniotic fluid embolism: case report and review. Anaesthesia & Intensive Care 23: 735–40.

Margarson MP 1995 Delayed amniotic fluid embolism following Caesarean section under spinal anaesthesia. Anaesthesia 50: 804–6.

May AE 1999 The Confidential Enquiry into Maternal Deaths 1994–1996. International Journal of Obstetric Anesthesia 8: 77–8.

Moore PG, James OF, Saltos N 1982 Severe amniotic fluid embolism: case report with haemodynamic findings. Anaesthesia & Intensive Care 10: 40–4.

Morgan M 1979 Amniotic fluid embolism. Anaesthesia 34: 20–32.

Noble WH, St-Amand J 1993 Amniotic fluid embolus. Canadian Journal of Anaesthesia 40: 971–80.

Quance D 1988 Amniotic fluid embolism: detection by pulse oximetry. Anesthesiology 68: 951–2.

Quinn A, Barrett T 1993 Delayed onset of coagulopathy following amniotic fluid embolism: two case reports. International Journal of Obstetric Anesthesia 2: 177–80.

Shah K, Karlman R, Heller J 1986 Ventricular tachycardia and hypotension with amniotic fluid embolism during Cesarean section. Anesthesia and Analgesia 65: 533–5.

Van Heerden PV, Webb SA, Hee G et al 1996 Inhaled aerosolized prostacyclin as a selective pulmonary vasodilator for the treatment of severe hypoxaemia. Anaesthesia & Intensive Care 24: 87–90.

Vanmaele L, Noppen M, Vincken W et al 1990 Transient left heart failure in amniotic fluid embolism. Intensive Care Medicine 16: 269–71.

Weksler N, Ovadia L, Stav A et al 1994 Continuous arteriovenous hemofiltration in the treatment of amniotic fluid embolism. International Journal of Obstetric Anesthesia 3: 92–6.

Anaphylactoid/anaphylactic reactions to intravenous agents

A general term for a drug-related clinical event that either threatens life or disrupts the course of an operation. It is a multisystem response to a drug, or drug combination, to which the patient may or may not have been previously exposed. The term anaphylactoid does not explain the mechanism. Usually, the type of reaction may only be elucidated subsequently, by evaluation of history, immunology and, if appropriate, skin testing. Unfortunately more than one drug may have been given immediately before the reaction.

Epinephrine (adrenaline) has been recommended as the key drug for treatment for some years, and a report in which anaphylaxis occurred when transcranial Doppler monitoring was in place confirmed its effectiveness in restoring cerebral blood flow (Fox et al 1999). The collection of blood samples for immunological studies should start as soon as possible after the event. Understanding the mechanism of the reaction is important for the subsequent management of the patient. Both intradermal and skin prick testing have been used to determine the drug responsible. In a prospective non-randomised study, there was no evidence that one test was superior. However, since there are no data on the safety of subsequent anaesthesia based on the results of prick testing alone, in cases of doubt, both tests should be performed (Fisher & Bowey 1997).

There appears to be an increase in the number of these reactions and they occur more frequently in women than in men. An analysis of 154 serious cases in France showed that 70% occurred in women (Laxenaire et al 1985). In a later study of 1585 patients, 813 were recognised as having an immunological basis to their reactions. Substances involved were muscle relaxants (70%), latex (12.6%), colloids (4.7%), hypnotics (3.6%), antibiotics (2.6%), benzodiazepines (2%), and opioids (1.7%) (Laxenaire et al 1993). The female predominance remained consistent (3:1).

1. Drugs producing reactions.

a) *Induction agents.* Thiopental causes more reactions than either methohexitone or etomidate. Etomidate has caused a low incidence of anaphylactoid reactions. There have been a few reports of reactions to propofol (de Leon-Casasola et al 1992, Laxenaire et al 1992).

b) *Neuromuscular blocking agents.* These produce a surprising number of anaphylactoid responses and may be involved in up to 50% of reactions during anaesthesia. In 1985, Watkins showed that those involved in anaphylactoid reactions, in decreasing order of frequency, were: suxamethonium, alcuronium, atracurium, tubocurarine, pancuronium, vecuronium, and gallamine. At the time of Watkins' study, pancuronium was in very common use, yet rarely involved. In a later survey of 590 clinically severe reactions (Watkins 1994b), suxamethonium still predominated (48%), with atracurium 18% and vecuronium 12%. Anaphylactic reactions to cisatracurium have been reported (Clendenen et al 1997), and in one, high levels of serum tryptase and urinary methylhistamine were demonstrated (Toh et al 1999). Results of skin testing to atracurium and its stereoisomer cisatracurium appear to be identical, therefore only one may be needed when testing (Fisher 1999). Anaphylaxis to mivacurium (Baird & Futter 1996) and rocuronium (Yee & Fernandez 1996), have also been described. Sometimes, a family history has been elicited (Duvaldestin et al 1999).

Skin testing does not always accurately predict responses to neuromuscular blockers. Fisher et al (1999) reported three patients in whom false-negative skin tests led to a second severe reaction to another neuromuscular blocker.

c) *Neostigmine.* Only one case of anaphylaxis to neostigmine has been confirmed by testing (Seed & Ewan 2000). In addition, skin prick test to neostigmine was strongly positive, whereas that to edrophonium was negative, so an alternative drug would be available.

d) *Plasma expanders.* Anaphylactoid reactions to colloid volume substitutes were studied in 1977 (Ring & Messmer), and at that time were shown to occur most commonly with the dextrans. A study of 50 dextran-induced reactions identified a metabolic acidosis as having occurred in all the severe reactions, and also frequently in the less severe ones (Ljungstrom and Renck 1987). Although a technique of hapten administration (dextran 1) prior to the use of dextran was shown to be effective (Ljungstrom et al 1988), serious reactions still occurred despite immunoprophylaxis (Berg et al 1991). Dextrans are now rarely used. Although a severe reaction to hydroxyethyl starch has been reported (Cullen & Singer 1990), antigenicity appears to be low, and reactions to starches are rare compared with other plasma expanders (Dieterich et al 1998). A number of adverse reactions to gelatin products have been reported. Although some of these are severe, in 43 patients reported to the Sheffield Unit over 5 years, histamine release was a feature, but there was little evidence of an IgE-mediated reaction (Watkins 1994a).

e) *X-ray contrast media.* Adverse systemic reactions to the older types of contrast media occurred in 5% of patients (Goldberg 1984). The majority receiving these had an increased serum osmolality, a decreased haematocrit, and a subsequent osmotic diuresis. In addition, some patients will develop an actual anaphylactoid response, usually within 2 min of the injection. Nausea and vomiting, cardiovascular collapse, upper airway obstruction, bronchospasm, and hypoxia could occur. The newer contrast media are much safer from this point of view.

f) *Local anaesthetic agents.* The differentiation between anaphylactoid and toxic reactions is difficult. However, the incidence of true allergy is probably very low (Incaudo et al 1978). Proven cases have, however, been reported. Lidocaine (lignocaine) mixed with propofol for induction resulted in cardiovascular collapse and a widespread rash. Skin prick testing to lidocaine produced a skin wheal 28 mm in diameter (Ismail & Simpson 1997).

g) *Antibiotics.* Penicillin produces a high incidence of anaphylactic reactions, a proportion of which are fatal. IgE is frequently involved (Sogn 1984). Up to 8% of patients allergic to penicillin are said to react to cephalosporins. All intraoperative antibiotics should be given slowly and well diluted. Requests that they be given at induction of anaesthesia should be resisted. If a reaction occurs, there may be major difficulty in identifying the drug responsible.

h) *Latex* (see Sections 1 & 2, Latex allergy). This has increasingly been reported, but only in the last 15 years (Leynadier et al 1989). Extracted from the sap of *Hevea brasiliensis*, latex is used in the manufacture of rubber gloves, balloons, catheters, and elastic adhesives. Reactions, which have included rash, wheezing, urticaria, and hypotension, are of delayed onset, the earliest time usually being 40 min from induction of anaesthesia (Gold et al 1991), but may occur much later because elution of the protein from the rubber gloves is required (Hirshman 1992). Exceptions to this may be in high-risk children, and in adults having catheterisation, when it may occur considerably earlier. Strategies for latex allergies have been described (Dakin & Yentis 1998).

2. *Types of reactions.* Most immunologists now believe that nonspecific anaphylactoid reactions are more common than immune-mediated ones, although they may still be severe.

a) *Type I hypersensitivity response.* A true anaphylactic or allergic response which depends upon previous exposure to the drug. On the first occasion, lymphocytes produce specific IgE antibodies which become attached to the membrane of mast cells and basophils. A second exposure results in cross-linkages between these primed cells, changes in the cell membrane, and mast cell and basophil degranulation. Mediators such as histamine and leukotriene C are released from mast cells, causing some or all of the pharmacological effects associated with anaphylactic reactions. Complement is not involved. IgE involvement is most common, IgG may be concerned, and C4 is consumed. Disappearance of basophils is said to be highly indicative of a type I reaction (Watkins 1987). This type of reaction may occur after multiple exposures to thiopentone, and although uncommon, can be fatal.

b) *Complement-mediated reaction.* This classical reaction can occur on initial exposure to the drug. Activation of C1–C9, the complement cascade, occurs, and C4 and C3 are consumed. C3a and C5a (anaphylatoxins) are mast cell degranulators. Once again chemical mediators are released.

c) *Alternate complement pathway.* Activation of this results in direct conversion of C3, C3a once again being released. A previous exposure is not necessary. Reactions to cremophor-containing drugs were frequently of this type.

d) *Non-immune anaphylactoid responses.* They are common and it may be difficult to identify the responsible drug. Chemical mediators are released as a result of a direct or an indirect effect on mast cells and basophils. The diagnosis is generally one of exclusion. No IgE changes occur, and complement C3 and C4 are not consumed. It has been suggested that this reaction may occur on exposure to a particular group of drugs, such as muscle relaxants, when they share common molecular characteristics (Baldo 1986). There may be predisposing factors such as chronic atopy, complement abnormalities, or a history of regular exposure to the particular drug. The greater the amount of drug and the more rapid its administration, the more severe the reaction is likely to be.

e) *Miscellaneous.* In some cases a similar response may be due to drug interactions, or drug overdose. Rarely, it is secondary to an unexpected pathology, such as a hormone-secreting tumour.

Presentation

Life-threatening effects include cardiovascular collapse (90%), bronchospasm (30%), angio-oedema (25%), and pulmonary oedema (49%) (Fisher 1992). Hypotension alone occurs in only about 10% of cases.

1. *Cutaneous lesions.* Include flushing and urticaria and may cause significant fluid depletion. The development of a 1-mm layer of subcutaneous fluid over the whole body is approximately equivalent to a loss of 1.5 litres of extracellular volume.

2. *Cardiovascular symptoms.* Feature most commonly and vary in severity from moderate hypotension to cardiovascular collapse. Hypotension is secondary to release of histamine (and other vasoactive peptides), which causes widespread capillary vasodilatation and increased capillary permeability. Changes in heart rate or rhythm accompany the hypotension. ECG changes were analysed in 186 cases (Fisher 1986). A supraventricular tachycardia developed in 153 (82%), and this was accompanied by ST elevation in a further eight patients. The remaining arrhythmias included asystole, rapid AF, and VF. Arrhythmias other than SVT tended to be associated with pre-existing cardiac disease. This was so in 24 out of 26 patients with heart

disease, whereas 151 out of the 160 patients without cardiac disease had SVT alone. The four episodes of VF came from both groups, and were usually associated with the administration of epinephrine (adrenaline) in the presence of halothane.

3. *Bronchospasm.* This was noted to have occurred in 39% of cases studied in France (Laxenaire et al 1985). It is serious and can be responsible for deaths, secondary to cerebral hypoxia.

4. *Glottic oedema.* May occur occasionally.

5. *Gastrointestinal.* Immediately after recovery from the reaction, the patient may complain of abdominal pain, diarrhoea, or vomiting. This may be secondary to hyperperistalsis and oedema of the gut.

6. *Miscellaneous.* Other effects include AV conduction defects, leucopenia, and coagulation disorders. Widespread fibrin deposition and haemorrhage found at postmortem examination suggested a coagulopathy in a patient who had died on induction of anaesthesia with thiopentone and suxamethonium (Wright et al 1989). The formation of colloid aggregates was suggested to be the cause.

Management

1. *Initial cardiopulmonary resuscitation.*

a) Stop administration of the suspected drug and turn off all volatile agents. There is no place for these in the treatment of anaphylactoid bronchospasm.

b) Administer 100% oxygen and maintain the airway.

c) Give epinephrine (adrenaline) iv, 0.1–0.5 mg (0.1–0.5 ml of 1 : 1000 solution, or 5 μg kg^{-1}) for cardiovascular collapse. For less severe reactions dilute to 1 : 10 000 and give 0.5–1 ml and repeat as required.

Epinephrine (adrenaline) is the drug of first choice in anaphylactoid reactions and should be given early. The route of administration has been the subject of debate; there is evidence that any route (iv, im, sc, or via the airway) is better than none (Fisher 1992). In view of its brevity of action, in severe reactions, an epinephrine (adrenaline) infusion may be required subsequently. Additional to its cardiovascular effects, epinephrine inhibits further degranulation of mast cells and basophils, by increasing levels of intracellular AMP. There is also evidence from incidental transcranial Doppler monitoring that it is associated with increases in cerebral blood flow that are independent of arterial blood pressure (Fox et al 1999). Occasionally, norepinephrine (noradrenaline) may be required (McKinnon & Wildsmith 1995).

In six out of seven fatal reactions, epinephrine (adrenaline) had been given late in the treatment (Fisher 1986). For patients taking beta blockers, the hypotension does not respond well to epinephrine (Laxenaire et al 1985), and isoprenaline may have to be given in higher than normal doses. In less severe reactions the epinephrine can be diluted and given more slowly. Its effects require close monitoring, and caution is essential if halothane has been in use, since VF may be precipitated.

d) Give crystalloid or colloid iv to expand the vascular volume. Following analysis of treatment given to 203 cases, it was concluded that colloid was preferable (Fisher 1986). Whilst colloid is important for the replacement of intravascular losses, it should not be relied upon solely. It cannot be given at a sufficient speed to counteract hypotension in the severe case and does not have the additional benefits of epinephrine (adrenaline) in stopping the progress of the reaction and worsening of oedema, and treatment of bronchospasm.

e) Manage the airway. In the presence of severe laryngeal oedema and failure to intubate, tracheostomy or cricothyroidotomy may be required.

f) Measure pH and blood gases. Severe acidosis may occur and require treatment with sodium bicarbonate (Ljungstrom & Renck 1987).

2. *Second line treatment.*

a) Antihistamines. Chlorpheniramine iv 10–20 mg can be given slowly over 1 min. Antihistamines occupy cellular H_1-receptor sites and are competitive inhibitors of histamine binding. However, they only partially reverse anaphylactoid responses, because chemicals other than histamine are involved. Also, it may not be possible to achieve complete block of certain histamine receptor sites.

b) Aminophylline. A dose of 250–500 mg ($5 \, mg \, kg^{-1}$) given slowly over 20 min may be required if bronchospasm persists. Aminophylline prevents degradation of 3,5-cyclic AMP, and reduces the release of histamine and arachnidonic acid metabolites. Its effect on respiratory function is not solely that of bronchodilatation.

c) Corticosteroids. There is little place for corticosteroids in the immediate treatment, since their onset of action at a cellular level may take several hours. However, they may be used where the reaction does not resolve quickly and hypotension persists.

3. *Investigations.*

a) Immediate.

   i) As soon as possible, blood samples should be taken for subsequent assessment of the mechanisms of the reaction.

   ii) Additional advice can be obtained from specialist centres.

iii) Take two sets of venous blood samples in two EDTA tubes as soon as possible after the start of the reaction (EDTA stabilises plasma complement proteins). Further duplicated samples should be taken at 3 h, 6 h, 12 h, and 24 h.

iv) The first set should go to the local haematology department for Hb, WCC (total and differential), platelet count, and haematocrit.

v) Plasma should be separated from the second set. This should be stored at −20 to −25°C until ready for despatch (without ice) by first class post to an Immunology Laboratory (such as the Protein Reference Unit, Sheffield), as soon as the 24-h collection is complete. Some hospitals may have their own facilities for performing complement and immunoglobulin levels.

vi) Detailed documentation should accompany the samples. This will include a full record of the incident, the agents and batch numbers, details of previous administration of these substances and relevant history, such as allergies and atopy.

vii) Other similar, but more complex protocols exist, arising from recommendations by a joint European workshop in Nancy (Laxenaire et al 1983).

viii) Plasma histamine levels are increased but they are difficult to measure. Histamine has a short half-life and studies suggest that plasma levels should be measured between 10 min and 1 h after the reaction and samples should not be haemolysed (Laroche et al 1991).

ix) Measurement of plasma tryptase concentrations plays an important role in investigation of reactions (Fisher & Baldo 1998). Plasma tryptase, a protease in mast cell granules, has a longer half-life (approximately 2 h) than histamine. Thus, increases may be documented 1–2 h after the reaction, but in any case, not more than 6 h (Laroche et al 1991). Increased levels are a valuable indicator of anaphylactic reactions, but they do not always distinguish between the two. However, skin testing is still required even in the absence of increased levels (Fisher & Baldo 1998).

If, as more frequently happens, the reaction involves neither IgE nor complement, then the offending drug may be more difficult to identify.

b) Subsequent.

i) Skin prick testing with clinical concentrations of drugs (Pepys et al 1994).

ii) Intradermal skin testing with drugs at low dilutions, 6 weeks after the initial reaction. A regimen for intradermal testing has been described, with recommendations on drug dilutions (Fisher 1984). This should preferably be undertaken by someone experienced in the technique.

iii) RAST test. This radioallergosorbent test involves the use of commercially prepared antigen to detect drug-specific IgE antibodies. At present the usefulness of this test is limited, both by the availability of preparations, and by the occurrence of false-positive and false-negative results. The suxamethonium test proved to be reliable and the thiopentone test may be so (Assem 1990).

4. *Communication of information.*

a) Report the reaction to the Committee on Safety of Medicines via the Yellow Card system.

b) Inform the patient of the results of investigations. Issue a warning card or suggest a Medic Alert bracelet.

c) Document the results clearly in the patient's notes.

d) Inform the patient's general practitioner.

5. *Management of subsequent anaesthetics.*

a) If the reaction is shown to be immune-mediated and the drug is identified by skin testing, then this drug should not be used again. In an immune-mediated reaction, there is no place for the use of iv test doses, since even minute amounts of a drug may prove fatal.

b) If the reaction is nonspecific, then future anaesthetics should be conducted using drugs considered to be relatively safe, whilst avoiding those known to more readily produce reactions. Currently, drugs with the fewest reports of serious problems are fentanyl, etomidate, vecuronium, pancuronium, and atracurium. If closely repeated anaesthetics are required in the same patient, consideration should be given to varying the techniques and drugs used. All drugs should be given slowly.

c) Pretreatment with H_1 and H_2 antagonists has been recommended by some authors. However, since other mediators are also involved, this does not guarantee freedom from a response.

6. *Fatal reactions.* Since there are no specific postmortem changes in death associated with anaphylaxis, there may be medicolegal pressures to establish a diagnosis. Sera, taken both before and after death, can help to resolve the diagnosis (Fisher et al 1991). Radioimmunoassay for drug-specific IgE antibodies was performed on blood taken for preoperative laboratory tests in two cases, and resulted in revision of the preliminary postmortem diagnosis to one of anaphylaxis. In a further two fatal cases, mast cell tryptase levels were also shown to be valuable, even when the blood is taken after death (Fisher & Baldo 1993).

Bibliography

Assem ESK 1990 Anaphylactic anaesthetic reactions. The value of paper radioallergosorbent tests for IgE antibodies to muscle relaxants and thiopentone. Anaesthesia 45: 1032–8.

Baird MB, Futter M 1996 Anaphylaxis to mivacurium. Anaesthesia & Intensive Care 24: 486–8.

Baldo BA 1986 Cross-reactions of neuromuscular blocking drugs and anaphylactoid reactions. Anaesthesia 41: 550–1.

Baldo B, Fisher MMcD 1983 Detection of serum IgE antibodies that react with alcuronium and tubocurarine after life-threatening reactions to muscle relaxants. Anaesthesia & Intensive Care 11: 194–7.

Berg EM, Fasting S, Sellevold OFM 1991 Serious complications with dextran-70 despite hapten prophylaxis. Is it best avoided prior to delivery? Anaesthesia 46: 1033–5.

Clendenen SR, Harper JV, Wharen RE et al 1997 Anaphylactic reaction after cisatracurium. Anesthesiology 87: 690–2.

Cullen MJ, Singer M 1990 Severe anaphylactoid reaction to hydroxyethyl starch. Anaesthesia 45: 1041–2.

Dakin MJ, Yentis SM 1998 Latex allergy: a strategy for management. Anaesthesia 53: 774–81.

de Leon-Casasola OA, Weiss A, Lema MJ 1992 Anaphylaxis due to propofol. Anesthesiology 77: 384–6.

Dieterich H-J, Kraft D, Sirtl C et al 1998 Hydroxyethyl starch antibodies in humans: incidence and clinical relevance. Anesthesia & Analgesia 86: 1123–6.

Duvaldestin P, Wigdorowicz C, Gabriel I 1999 Anaphylactic shock to neuromuscular blocking agents: a family history. Anesthesiology 90: 1211–12.

Fisher MM 1984 Intradermal testing after anaphylactoid reactions to anaesthetic drugs. Practical aspects of performance and interpretation. Anaesthesia & Intensive Care 12: 115–20.

Fisher MMcD 1986 Clinical observations on the pathophysiology and treatment of anaphylactic cardiovascular collapse. Anaesthesia & Intensive Care 14: 17–21.

Fisher M 1992 Treating anaphylaxis with sympathomimetic drugs. In severe anaphylaxis adrenaline by any route is better than none. British Medical Journal 305: 1107–8.

Fisher MM 1999 Cisatracurium and atracurium as antigens. Anaesthesia & Intensive Care 27: 369–70.

Fisher MM, Baldo BA 1992 Persistence of allergy to anaesthetic drugs. Anaesthesia & Intensive Care 20: 143–6.

Fisher MM, Baldo B 1993 The diagnosis of fatal anaphylactic reactions during anaesthesia: employment of immunoassays for mast cell tryptase and drug-reactive IgE antibodies. Anaesthesia & Intensive Care 21: 353–7.

Fisher MM, Baldo BA 1998 Mast cell tryptase in anaesthetic anaphylactoid reactions. British Journal of Anaesthesia 80: 26–9.

Fisher MMcD, Bowey CJ 1997 Intradermal compared with prick testing in the diagnosis of anaesthetic allergy. British Journal of Anaesthesia 79: 56–63.

Fisher MMcD, Baldo BA, Silbert BS 1991 Anaphylaxis during anesthesia: use of radioimmunoassay to determine etiology and drugs responsible in fatal cases. Anesthesiology 75: 1112–15.

Fisher MM, Merefield D, Baldo B 1999 Failure to prevent an anaphylactic reaction to a second neuromuscular blocking drug during anaesthesia. British Journal of Anaesthesia 82: 770–3.

Fox AJ, McLaren IM, Naylor AR 1999 Cerebral perfusion monitored using transcranial Doppler during acute anaphylaxis. Anaesthesia 57: 678–82.

Gold M, Swartz JS, Braude BM et al 1991 Intraoperative anaphylaxis: an association with latex sensitivity. Journal of Allergy & Clinical Immunology 87: 662–6.

Goldberg M 1984 Systemic reactions to intravascular contrast media. Anesthesiology 60: 46–56.

Hirshman CA 1992 Latex anaphylaxis. Anesthesiology 77: 223–5.

Incaudo G, Schatz M, Patterson R et al 1978 Administration of local anesthetics to patients with a history of prior adverse reaction. Journal of Allergy & Clinical Immunology 61: 339–45.

Ismail K, Simpson PJ 1997 Anaphylactic shock following intravenous administration of lignocaine. Acta Anaesthesiologica Scandinavica 41: 1071–2.

Laroche D, Vergnaud M-C, Sillard B et al 1991 Biochemical markers of anaphylactoid reactions to drugs. Anesthesiology 75: 945–9.

Laxenaire M-C, Moneret-Vautrin DA, Watkins J 1983 Diagnosis of the causes of anaphylactoid anaesthetic reactions. A report of the recommendations of the joint Anaesthetic and Immuno-allergological Workshop, Nancy, France: 19 March 1982. Anaesthesia 38: 147–8.

Laxenaire M-C, Moneret-Vautrin DA, Vervloet D 1985 The French experience of anaphylactoid

reactions. International Anesthesiology Clinics 23: 145–60.

Laxenaire M-C, Mata-Bermejo E, Moneret-Vautrin DA et al 1992 Life-threatening anaphylactoid reactions to propofol (Diprivan). Anesthesiology 77: 275–80.

Laxenaire M-C, Mouton C, Moneret-Vautrin DA et al 1993 Drugs and other agents involved in anaphylactic shock occurring during anaesthesia. A French multicenter epidemiological study. Annales Francaises d'Anesthesie et de Reanimation 21: 91–6.

Leynadier F, Pecquet C, Dry J 1989 Anaphylaxis to latex during surgery. Anaesthesia 44: 547–50.

Ljungstrom K-G, Renck H 1987 Metabolic acidosis in dextran-induced anaphylactic reactions. Acta Anaesthesiologica Scandinavica 31: 157–60.

Ljungstrom K-G, Renck H, Hedin H et al 1988 Hapten inhibition and dextran anaphylaxis. Anaesthesia 43: 729–32.

McKinnon RP, Wildsmith JAW 1995 Histaminoid reactions in anaesthesia. British Journal of Anaesthesia 74: 217–28.

Pepys J, Pepys EO, Baldo BA et al 1994 Anaphylactic/anaphylactoid reactions to anaesthetic and associated agents. Skin prick tests. Anaesthesia 49: 470–5.

Ring J, Messmer K 1977 Incidence and severity of anaphylactoid reactions to colloid volume substitutes. Lancet i: 466–9.

Seed MJ, Ewan PW 2000 Anaphylaxis to neostigmine. Anaesthesia 55: 574–5.

Sogn DD 1984 Penicillin allergy. Journal of Allergy & Clinical Immunology 74: 589–93.

Toh KW, Deacock S, Fawcett WJ 1999 Severe anaphylactic reaction to cisatracurium. Anesthesia & Analgesia 88: 462–4.

Watkins J 1985 Adverse anaesthetic reactions. An update from a proposed national reporting and advisory service. Anaesthesia 40: 797–800.

Watkins J 1987 Investigation of allergic and hypersensitivity reactions to anaesthetic agents. British Journal of Anaesthesia 59: 104–11.

Watkins J 1994a Reactions to gelatin plasma expanders. Lancet 344: 328–9.

Watkins J 1994b Adverse reaction to neuromuscular blockers: frequency, investigation, and epidemiology. Acta Anaesthesiologica Scandinavica 38(suppl 102): 6–10.

Watkins J, Nimmo WS 1985 'Allergic' drug reactions during anaesthesia. Anaesthesia 40: 813–14.

Wright PJ, Shortland JR, Stevens JD et al 1989 Fatal

haemopathological consequences of general anaesthesia. British Journal of Anaesthesia 62: 104–7.

Yee R, Fernandez JA 1996 Anaphylactic reaction to rocuronium bromide. Anaesthesia & Intensive Care 24: 601–4.

Angioneurotic oedema

A general term applied to the development of acute oedema in the subcutaneous or submucous tissues. Anaesthetic help may be sought during an attack, when oedema of the lips, tongue or larynx may cause respiratory problems. Angioedema may be secondary to release of histamine, or a number of other vasoactive substances such as the bradykinins, prostaglandins or leukotrienes. It is thought that paediatric and adult angioedemas differ. Children are less likely to required intubation or tracheostomy than adults (Ishoo et al 1999, Shah & Jacobs 1999). Recent work in adults has shown substantial increases in plasma bradykinin during attacks of hereditary, acquired or captopril-induced angioedema (Nussberger et al 1998). The development of oedema may be:

1. Part of a general anaphylactoid or anaphylactic reaction to a drug, bite, sting or the ingestion of a substance (see Anaphylactoid/ anaphylactic reactions to intravenous agents).

2. A manifestation of hereditary angioneurotic oedema, a condition caused by a deficiency of C1 esterase inhibitor (see Section 1, Hereditary angioneurotic oedema).

3. A result of an acquired form of C1 esterase inhibitor deficiency which usually occurs in association with a B-lymphocyte malignancy (see Section 1, C1 esterase inhibitor deficiency).

4. A known side effect of a drug. Recently, there have been a number of cases of angioedema reported, usually involving the tongue, floor of the mouth, epiglottis and aryepiglottic folds, secondary to treatment with ACE inhibitors (Gannon & Eby 1990, Rodgers

et al 1991). Most occur in the first week of treatment, but may be delayed for up to a year (Ogbureke et al 1996). Can be associated with elevated serum bradykinin levels (Nussberger et al 1998). In a profile of cases, 22% were considered to be life threatening, and fatalities have occurred (Slater et al 1988). The presence of painful dysphagia and tongue oedema were found to be associated with the need for laryngoscopy (Agah et al 1997). At present, it is impossible to predict which patients will develop the complication.

Presentation

1. There may be a history of a predisposing factor. This can be ingestion of food or a drug, an infection, bite or sting, a family history of angioedema, or a B-lymphocytic malignancy.

2. Oedema of subcutaneous tissue may occur alone, or be accompanied by hypotension.

3. Patients taking ACE inhibitors have developed problems in the perioperative period. Angioedema of the tongue occurred 15 min after tracheal tube removal (Kharasch 1992). A man who had taken ACE inhibitors for 13 months developed severe facial oedema, airway obstruction and respiratory arrest 5 h after a spinal anaesthetic and sedation for transurethral resection of a bladder tumour. He was successfully resuscitated with cricothyroidotomy, followed by tracheostomy (Mchaourab et al 1999).

4. A patient with acquired C1 esterase inhibitor deficiency undergoing cardiopulmonary bypass had massive activation of the common pathway, coagulopathy, pulmonary oedema and circulatory collapse (Bonser et al 1991).

Management

1. Assessment of severity of airway obstruction.

2. If the angioedema is part of an

anaphylactic or anaphylactoid reaction, see appropriate section.

a) Give epinephrine (adrenaline) iv or im, 0.1–0.5 mg depending on the severity.

b) If the condition is severe and involves the glottis, an airway should be established, either by tracheal intubation, cricothyroidotomy, or tracheostomy. In a series of 93 episodes in 80 patients, intervention was required in nine patients. A predictive system was suggested, based on the site of presentation (Ishoo et al 1999). Those with tongue and laryngeal oedema usually required ITU admission.

c) Second-line treatment includes iv fluids, chlorpheniramine iv 10–20 mg, and steroids.

3. Hereditary angioneurotic oedema, or acquired C1 esterase inhibitor deficiency. These do not respond to epinephrine (adrenaline) or antihistamines, but to replacement of the deficient inhibitor by either:

a) An infusion of fresh frozen plasma. There is a risk that the additional presence of C2 and C4 may initially cause a deterioration, but this objection appears to be largely theoretical.

b) Purified C1 esterase inhibitor can be obtained from Immuno Ltd (Rye Lane, Dunton Green, Sevenoaks, Kent TN14 5HB. UK, tel 01732 458101).

Bibliography

Agah R, Bandi V, Guntupalli KK 1997 Angioedema: the role of ACE inhibitors and factors associated with poor clinical outcome. Intensive Care Medicine 23: 793–6.

Bonser RS, Dave J, Morgan J et al 1991 Complement activation during bypass in acquired C1 esterase inhibitor deficiency. Annals of Thoracic Surgery 52: 541–3.

Gannon TH, Eby TL 1990 Angioedema from angiotensin converting inhibitors: a cause of upper airway obstruction. Laryngoscope 100: 1156–60.

Ishoo E, Shah UK, Grillone GA et al 1999 Predicting airway risk in angioedema: staging system based on presentation. Otolaryngology—Head & Neck Surgery 121: 263–8.

Kharasch ED 1992 Angiotensin-converting enzyme inhibitor-induced angioedema associated with endotracheal intubation. Anesthesia & Analgesia 74: 602–4.

Mchaourab A, Sarantopoulos C, Stowe DF 1999 Airway obstruction due to late-onset angioneurotic edema from angiotensin-converting enzyme inhibitors. Canadian Journal of Anaesthesia 46: 975–8.

Nussberger J, Cugno M, Amstutz C et al 1998 Plasma bradykinin in angio-oedema. Lancet 351: 1693–7.

Ogbureke KU, Cruz C, Johnson JV et al 1996 Perioperative angioedema in a patient on long-term angiotensin-converting enzyme inhibitors. Journal of Oral & Maxillofacial Surgery 54: 917–20.

Rodgers GK, Galos RS, Johnson JT 1991 Hereditary angioedema: case report and review of management. Otolaryngology—Head & Neck Surgery 104: 394–8.

Shah UK, Jacobs IN 1999 Pediatric angioedema: ten years' experience. Archives of Otolaryngology—Head & Neck Surgery 125: 791–5.

Slater EE, Merrill DD, Guess HA et al 1988 Clinical profile of angioedema associated with angiotensin converting-enzyme inhibitor. Journal of the American Medical Association 260: 967–70.

Aortocaval fistula

Rare, but most commonly the result of rupture of an atheromatous abdominal aortic aneurysm. It can result from trauma (vehicular or gunshot), or as a complication of surgery for lumbar discectomy (Fruhwirth et al 1996). Occasionally the aneurysm may be syphilitic, or associated with a connective tissue disease such as Marfan and Ehler–Danlos syndrome. Aortocaval fistulae may present pre-, intra- or postoperatively. In a study of 18 patients, 78% had abdominal pain, 61% had a bruit, and 56% had a pulsatile abdominal mass (Davis et al 1998). A significant proportion of the cardiac output may flow into the inferior vena cava: this steal phenomenon reduces arterial pressure and flow to the coronary circulation. In these circumstances, vasopressors are ineffective and will simply increase the shunt of blood through the fistula.

If the fistula is associated with an aneurysm, the signs and symptoms will depend upon the presence or absence of external rupture of the aneurysm, and whether or not there is compression of the IVC by the aneurysm (Phipps 1988). If there is significant compression, the increased venous pressure is directed distally; if there is not, the pressure is transmitted in both directions. The diagnosis is easily missed and, even if it is made, the condition carries a mortality of up to 50%.

Presentation

1. Abdominal signs and symptoms. Lower abdominal or back pain radiating into testes or legs. There is a pulsatile, tender mass, an abdominal bruit and a thrill.

2. Cardiac signs. Inappropriate jugular venous distension and a hyperdynamic circulation, despite hypotension and shock. High-output cardiac failure, hepatomegaly, and signs of myocardial insufficiency or decompensation.

3. Systemic signs. Shock and poor perfusion if the aortic aneurysm is ruptured. Anuria, increased blood urea and renal failure may ensue.

4. Venous signs in the lower part of the body with truncal dusky cyanosis. Limb discoloration and oedema, haematuria, rectal bleeding, or priapism.

5. Paradoxical embolism of aneurysmal debris or a mural thrombus (Hecker & Lynch 1983, Davis et al 1998).

6. Unexpected presentation during aortic aneurysm surgery (Bodenham 1990, Tsolakis et al 1999), sometimes with massive venous haemorrhage after cross clamping of the aorta.

7. Signs of blood loss during or after lumbar disc surgery.

8. In an analysis of seven cases without aortic rupture, the median Hb level was within normal limits, but the PCV was low. This is because no blood has actually been lost from the vascular compartment. An absolute lymphocytopenia was also found, probably associated with cardiac failure (Burke & Jamieson 1983).

9. If invasive monitoring is undertaken, there is a high mixed venous oxygen saturation and a discrepancy between right and left heart pressures.

Diagnosis

Diagnosis can be made in a variety of ways. It may be demonstrated on a CT scan, DVI, MRI, or an aortogram. A femoral catheter can be passed into the IVC to show increased pressure, oxygen content or saturation. Fibreoptic oximetry was used to confirm the diagnosis in a patient following resection of an unruptured aneurysm (Khan et al 1992). An oximetric flotation catheter was passed up the femoral vein. A damped arterial waveform was identified, that was maximal at 15 cm, and increasing oxygen saturations were recorded as the fistula was approached.

Management

1. When the diagnosis is suspected preoperatively, the morbidity and mortality is considerably lower than when it is unexpected. The use of intraoperative cell salvage may reduce complications (Davis et al 1998).

2. Attempts at resuscitation are fruitless and will simply overload the circulation. Surgery must be undertaken expeditiously. Control of the IVC above and below the fistula is most important (Delaney & Brady 1998). Preliminary control of the fistula with a balloon catheter has been reported, but this may risk venous damage or thrombosis (Ingoldby et al 1990).

3. Agents should be used that minimise changes in arterial pressure. Vasopressor drugs that will increase the shunt should be avoided. Although vasodilators may reduce blood flow through fistulae, they may worsen the haemodynamics.

Bibliography

Alexander JJ, Imbembo AL 1989 Aorto-vena cava fistula. Surgery 105: 1–12.

Bodenham A 1990 Anaesthetic hazards of aortocaval fistula. British Journal of Anaesthesia 65: 723–5.

Burke AM, Jamieson GG 1983 Aorto-caval fistula associated with ruptured aortic aneurysm. British Journal of Surgery 70: 431–3.

Davis PM, Gloviczki P, Cherry KJ Jr et al 1998 Aorto-caval and ilio-iliac arteriovenous fistulae. American Journal of Surgery 176: 115–18.

Delaney CP, Brady MP 1998 Ruptured aortic aneurysm with aortocaval fistula. Journal of the Royal Society of Medicine 91: 645–6.

Editorial 1991 Aortocaval fistula. Lancet 338: 415–16.

Fruhwirth J, Koch G, Amann W et al 1996 Vascular complications of lumbar disc surgery. Acta Chirurgica 138: 912–16.

Hecker BR, Lynch C 1983 Intraoperative diagnosis and treatment of massive pulmonary embolism complicating surgery of the abdominal aorta. British Journal of Anaesthesia 55: 689–91.

Ingoldby CJ, Case WG, Primrose JN 1990 Aortocaval fistulas and the use of transvenous balloon tamponade. Annals of the Royal College Surgeons of England 72: 335–8.

Khan KJ, Tsnag GMK, Fielding JWL et al 1992 Fibreoptic oximetry in the diagnosis of aortocaval fistula. A case study and review of the literature. Anaesthesia 47: 237–9.

Phipps RF 1988 Spontaneous aortocaval fistulas. British Journal of Hospital Medicine 39: 306–7.

Tsolakis JA, Papadouplas S, Kakkos SK 1999 Aortocaval fistula in ruptured aneurysms. European Journal of Vascular & Endovascular Surgery 17: 390–3.

Arrhythmias (see also under Automatic implantable cardioverter defibrillators, QT interval syndrome (long), Torsade de pointes ventricular tachycardia, Wolff–Parkinson–White syndrome)

Arrhythmias may occur unexpectedly in the perioperative period; alternatively, anaesthetists may be involved in anaesthesia for one of a number of therapeutic antiarrhythmic procedures. Some knowledge of recent advances is therefore important. As a result of several large, randomised controlled trials, there have been significant changes in the management of some arrhythmias (Hammill & Hubmayr 2000). Anaesthetists may now be involved in anaesthesia for automatic implantable cardioverter defibrillator (AICD) insertion in patients with ventricular arrhythmias; for incidental surgery in patients who already have AICDs; for catheter ablation techniques in supraventricular tachycardias (and some cases of AF); and for cardioversion (Stoneham 1996).

The diagnosis and treatment of certain cardiac arrhythmias in the perioperative period can on occasions be complex and may require cardiological expertise. However, during anaesthesia a cardiologist may not be available immediately, therefore the anaesthetist needs a basic working knowledge of the common abnormalities and their likely causes. There is often a correctable surgical or anaesthetic precipitating factor, so the need for complex antiarrhythmic therapy in the operating theatre is unusual.

If the use of an antiarrhythmic is contemplated, careful thought should be given to possible interactions. In the presence of anaesthetic agents, or preoperative drug therapy, the iv administration of potent cardiac drugs can precipitate serious side effects. The anaesthetist must be aware of these and be prepared to treat complications should they arise. However, on occasions, the urgent treatment of a life-threatening arrhythmia may be essential.

Particular care must taken if the patient has an AICD, when the minimum energy requirements to deliver an effective shock may be altered by certain drugs. This is more likely to be a problem shortly after insertion of the AICD (Jones et al 1991, Zaidan 1999).

In general, if rhythm disturbances appear for the first time in the perioperative period, the initial search should be for a precipitating cause, associated with either the surgery or anaesthesia.

Predisposing factors

1. General problems. Hypoxia, hypercarbia, metabolic and electrolyte abnormalities, light anaesthesia, or manoeuvres that stimulate the output of endogenous catecholamines. Bowel cleansing with sodium picosulphate and magnesium citrate (picolax) or sodium phosphate preparations (Fleet) may occasionally precipitate AF (personal observation).

2. Drug causes. Accidental overdose with local anaesthetics, absorption of epinephrine (adrenaline) during surgical infiltration, or pre-existing medication with drugs such as digoxin.

3. Pre-existing cardiac disease. Ischaemic heart disease, congenital heart disease, cardiomyopathy, WPW syndrome, mitral valve prolapse, or one of the long QT syndromes.

4. Rare causes. Undiagnosed thyrotoxicosis, phaeochromocytoma, carcinoid syndrome, 'athlete's heart', malignant hyperthermia, and drug or solvent abuse (see under individual entries).

Presentation

1. *Atrial fibrillation.* Fast chaotic atrial activity, irregular fibrillation waves of 350–600 beat min^{-1}, best seen in V1. An irregular ventricular response of 100–200 beat min^{-1} and varying AV conduction. Only if AF is associated with AV block is the ventricular rate regular. Causes include ischaemic, hypertensive and rheumatic heart disease, thyrotoxicosis, sick sinus syndrome, alcohol abuse, and atrial septal defect. Transient AF may occur during an acute toxic illness. Patients are at risk from systemic embolism.

2. *Atrial flutter.* Regular atrial rate of 250–350 beat min^{-1} with saw-toothed flutter waves, which are best seen in leads II, III, AVF and V1. There may be a 2 : 1 or 3 : 1 AV block. The ventricular rate is also regular, varying from 125 to 350 min^{-1}. Causes are similar to those for AF.

3. *Atrial tachycardia with AV block.* P waves are visible but often inverted in leads II, III, and AVF.

The atrial rate is regular at 120–250 beat min^{-1}, with a fixed or varying degree of AV block. Ventricular activity is usually normal, but occasionally bundle branch block occurs. Most often associated with digitalis toxicity, but can be due to ischaemic heart disease, cardiomyopathy, or sick sinus syndrome.

4. *Paroxysmal supraventricular tachycardia (AV nodal re-entrant tachycardia).* Ventricular rate regular at 130–250 beat min^{-1}. No normal P waves seen, but inverted ones follow the QRS complex. Normal ventricular activity, sometimes with BBB. Often occurs in the absence of cardiac disease, but can be associated with WPW syndrome or Ebstein's anomaly. An abrupt onset of palpitations may cause hypotension, syncope, chest pain, polyuria and, if it persists, occasionally heart failure occurs.

5. *Atrial ectopic beats.* A premature, abnormal-shaped or sometimes inverted, P wave, best shown in V1. The QRS is usually normal and there is no compensatory pause after the ectopic. The next beat occurs exactly one sinus cycle after the ectopic, thus resetting the cycle. Atrial ectopics are frequently benign, but if they occur with heart disease, they may presage AF.

6. *Ventricular ectopic beats.* A widened bizarre-shaped QRS, without a preceding ectopic P wave. There is a short interval between a normal beat and the ectopic, followed by a compensatory pause before the next normal beat. If the ectopic falls early onto the T wave of the previous contraction (R on T), then ventricular tachycardia or fibrillation may be precipitated. Causes include ischaemic heart disease, cardiomyopathies, digoxin toxicity, and valvular disease. However, the cause may not be obvious.

7. *Ventricular fibrillation.* An incoordinate contraction of ventricular myocardial fibres associated with loss of consciousness and an absence of cardiac output.

8. *Ventricular tachycardia.* A rapid ventricular rhythm of 120–250 beats min^{-1}, lasting for at least three or more beats, with abnormal-shaped complexes. Evidence of separate atrial activity

occurring at a slower rate, with P waves dissociated from ventricular complexes, helps to distinguish it from supraventricular tachycardia. If in doubt, the distance between any visible P waves may be shown to be mathematically related. R waves occur only in V1 and the QRS width is >140 ms.

9. *Torsade de pointes ventricular tachycardia.* This is an atypical ventricular tachycardia in which the QRS complexes vary in form and amplitude, and the axis of the complexes twists around the baseline (see Section 2, Torsade de pointes).

Problems

1. The presenting arrhythmia may result in hypotension and a reduction in cardiac output. Atrial fibrillation causes a rapid ventricular rate and the loss of the atrial component to diastole. Ventricular fibrillation, and occasionally ventricular tachycardia, cause circulatory arrest.

2. Myocardial ischaemia may be provoked.

3. If there is pre-existing left-sided heart disease, there may be cardiac decompensation and pulmonary oedema.

4. The arrhythmia may precipitate a more serious or fatal one, such as ventricular tachycardia or ventricular fibrillation.

5. A risk of systemic thromboembolism or stroke. In the presence of AF there are a number of clinical risk factors that greatly increase the chance of developing emboli. These include hypertension, a history of CHF or previous embolus, diabetes, woman >75 years of age, left ventricular dysfunction with an EF <40%, and a left atrial size >2.5 cm m^{-2} (Hammill & Hubmayr 2000). It has been shown that patients with one or more risk factors should be anticoagulated with warfarin to an INR of 2–3 (Ezekowitz 1999).

Management

1. *Atrial fibrillation.* Digoxin slows the ventricular response rate to atrial activity.

Verapamil will slow the ventricular rate. In AF of acute onset, particularly when the patient is already anaesthetised, direct current cardioversion may be the best treatment and should result in sinus rhythm. For management of cardioversion, see Stoneham (1996).

2. *Atrial flutter.* Verapamil and digoxin may not control the ventricular rate. Cardioversion may be successful in reverting flutter to sinus rhythm. Atrial pacing can be tried.

3. *Atrial tachycardia with AV block.* Stop digoxin, correct any hypokalaemia and give lidocaine (lignocaine) iv 1 mg kg^{-1}. Should this fail, direct current cardioversion or rapid atrial pacing may be tried. If the patient is not already taking digoxin, treatment with this may control the ventricular rate.

4. *Paroxysmal supraventricular tachycardia.* Carotid sinus massage or a Valsalva manoeuvre to increase vagal tone (for details see Section 1, Autonomic failure). Pressure should be exerted by two fingers over the carotid artery at the level of the thyroid cartilage. Verapamil iv 5–10 mg is usually successful, but should not be given if the patient is taking beta blockers. Digoxin, propranolol, quinidine, procainamide, disopyramide and cardioversion can also be used.

5. *Atrial ectopic beats.* No treatment is usually necessary, unless they are very frequent, or are associated with cardiac disease. In such a case digoxin may help.

6. *Ventricular ectopic beats.* In general no treatment is needed, unless they are frequent, or of the early R on T type. A lidocaine infusion or a beta blocker may then be needed.

7. *Ventricular fibrillation.* A single precordial blow can be tried, otherwise defibrillation and full CPR is required. If the heart is resistant to defibrillation then prior treatment with bretylium tosylate iv 400 mg may increase the fibrillation threshold. Recurrent VF may be an indication for AICD implantation (see Section 1, Automatic implantable cardioverter defibrillator).

8. *Ventricular tachycardia (see also Section 1, Torsade de pointes).* The urgency and method of

Emergency conditions arising during anaesthesia

treatment depends upon the degree of haemodynamic impairment. In the presence of severe hypotension, direct current cardioversion is required. If hypotension is not a major problem, or for short episodes of VT, drug treatment can be used. Lidocaine (lignocaine) is the first choice. If this fails, disopyramide, flecainide or mexiletine can be used.

Bibliography

Ezekowitz MD 1999 Preventing stroke in patients with atrial fibrillation. Journal of the American Medical Association 281: 1830–5.

Hammill SC, Hubmayr RD 2000 The rapidly changing management of cardiac arrhythmias. American Journal of Respiratory and Critical Care Medicine 161: 1070–3.

Jones DL, Klein GJ, Guiraudon GM et al 1991 Effects of lidocaine and verapamil on defibrillation in humans. Journal of Electrocardiography 24: 299–305.

Moss AJ, Hall HJ, Cannom DS et al 1996 Improved survival with an implanted defibrillator in patients with coronary disease at high risk for ventricular arrhythmia: multicenter Automatic Defibrillator Implantation Trial Investigation. New England Journal of Medicine 335: 1933–40.

Nathanson MH, Gajraj NM 1998 The peri-operative management of atrial fibrillation. Anaesthesia 53: 665–76.

Stoneham MD 1996 Anaesthesia for cardioversion. Anaesthesia 51: 565–70.

Zaidan JR 1999 Implantable cardioverter-defibrillators. Journal of Cardiothoracic & Vascular Anesthesia 13: 475–83.

Bronchospasm (see also Section 1, Asthma)

An incidence of bronchospasm of 0.17% was reported in a large study of anaesthetic complications. It was usually triggered in susceptible patients by mechanical stimuli (Olsson 1987). Other causes include anaphylactoid reactions, inhalation of gastric contents, and rarely, certain hormone-secreting tumours.

Presentation

1. Predisposing factors to intraoperative bronchospasm include asthma, obstructive airways disease, respiratory infection, and tracheal intubation. Reversible bronchoconstriction has been shown in association with tracheal intubation, but not with laryngeal mask airway insertion (Kim & Bishop 1999). Bronchospasm is most likely to occur during airway manipulation in a patient who has previously exhibited a capacity for airway constriction.

2. Bronchospasm may be one manifestation of an anaphylactoid reaction. Other signs, such as flushing, urticaria, hypotension, and tachycardia, should be sought.

3. It may result from silent aspiration of gastric contents. This may have been associated with difficulties in tracheal intubation.

4. In rare hormone-secreting tumours, such as carcinoids, flushing and hypotension may additionally occur.

Management

1. Bronchospasm is frequently associated with tracheal intubation or airway manipulation, in a patient with a history of bronchitis, asthma, or wheezing. Its incidence can be significantly reduced by preoperative preparation, avoidance of intubation during light anaesthesia, and the use of iv lidocaine (lignocaine) (Kingston & Hirshman 1984, Hirshman & Bergman 1990, Hirshman 1991). If it occurs in spite of these measures, an attempt should be made to deepen the anaesthetic, using a volatile agent and oxygen. Halothane, enflurane, isoflurane and sevoflurane are all effective at reversing antigen-induced bronchospasm. An inhalational induction with sevoflurane was given for emergency Caesarean section in a patient with status asthmaticus (Que & Lusaya 1999). Halothane sensitises the heart to the effect of exogenous and endogenous catecholamines. In addition, it interacts with aminophylline to produce arrhythmias. Isoflurane or sevoflurane, therefore, are probably the best choices.

2. A bronchodilator, such as a salbutamol infusion 5–20 μ g min^{-1} or aminophylline 5 mg kg^{-1} over 10–15 min can be given.

3. If the clinical situation suggests an anaphylactoid reaction, or the bronchospasm is severe enough, then epinephrine (adrenaline) 1–10 ml 1 : 10 000 iv is the treatment of choice (see also Anaphylactoid/anaphylactic reactions to intravenous agents).

4. If there is evidence of pulmonary aspiration, appropriate treatment should be instituted.

Bibliography

Hirshman CA 1991 Perioperative management of the asthmatic patient. Canadian Journal of Anaesthesia 38: R26–32.

Hirshman CA, Bergman NA 1990 Factors influencing intrapulmonary airway calibre during anaesthesia. British Journal of Anaesthesia 65: 30–42.

Kim ES, Bishop MI 1999 Endotracheal intubation, but not LMA insertion, produces reversible bronchoconstriction. Anesthesiology 90: 391–4.

Kingston HGG, Hirshman CA 1984 Perioperative management of the patient with asthma. Anesthesia and Analgesia 63: 844–55.

Olsson GL 1987 Bronchospasm during anaesthesia. A computer-aided incidence study of 136 929 patients. Acta Anaesthesiologica Scandinavica 31: 244–52.

Que JC, Lusaya VO 1999 Sevoflurane induction for emergency cesarean section in a parturient in status asthmaticus. Anesthesiology 90: 1475–6.

Carcinoid syndrome (see also Section 1, Carcinoid syndrome)

Less than 25% of patients with carcinoid tumours have carcinoid syndrome. The majority with the syndrome have liver metastases. Exceptions are the tumours whose venous drainage bypasses the liver. Flushing and hypertension have occurred rarely during anaesthesia in the absence of metastases (Jones & Knight 1982), and these were attributed to release of hormones resulting from manipulation of the tumour itself. Preoperative features include flushing, diarrhoea, wheezing and valvular lesions of the heart. The patient may present unexpectedly, during anaesthesia or investigative procedures, with cardiovascular or respiratory complications from secretion of vasoactive chemical mediators such as serotonin, bradykinins, tachykinins, prostaglandins, or histamine. Octreotide, a somatostatin analogue, is now the most important antagonist for prophylaxis, or the treatment of complications of carcinoid syndrome. A new longer-acting somatostatin analogue, lanreotide, has recently been introduced (Ruszniewski et al 1996).

Presentation

1. Release of hormones from carcinoid tissue may occur as a result of certain stimuli during anaesthesia, surgery, or investigative procedures. These include tracheal intubation, biopsy, tumour handling, hypotension, and catecholamine release.

2. Serotonin is known to cause hyperkinetic states of hypertension, tachycardia, and certain sorts of flushing. Bradykinins and tachykinins may produce hypotension, increased capillary permeability, oedema, flushing, and bronchospasm. Other vasoactive peptides such as histamine and prostaglandins may be involved, but their part in the syndrome has not, as yet, been elucidated.

3. Serious reactions during anaesthesia have included the following: severe hypertension that responded to ketanserin (Casthely et al 1986), and to ketanserin and octreotide (Hughes & Hodkinson 1989), cardiovascular collapse which responded to octreotide (Marsh et al 1987, Quinlivan & Roberts 1994, Veall et al 1994), severe bronchospasm (Miller et al 1980), and facial oedema.

4. General anaesthesia is not always a requirement; a fatal acute crisis has occurred immediately after fine needle liver biopsy of liver metastases (Bissonnette et al 1990), and a nonfatal one after bronchial biopsy (Sukamaran et al 1982), both of which procedures were performed under local anaesthesia.

Management

1. Somatostatin analogues, which inhibit the release of active mediators from carcinoid tumours, now form the basis of therapy for acute carcinoid crises, as well as in the preoperative management of patients with known carcinoid syndrome. Although octreotide (Sandostatin, Sandoz SMS 201–995) is not licensed for iv use, the authors of several case reports have suggested that, in the situation of an acute crisis, it has been lifesaving. Octreotide (in doses of 25–100μg iv) was used for intraoperative treatment during excision of metastatic carcinoid tumours (Roy et al 1987), and in one case in which cardiovascular collapse occurred the beneficial effect was dramatic (Marsh et al 1987).

2. A number of different antiserotoninergic drugs have been used in attempts to treat complications arising during anaesthesia. These include methotrimeprazine iv 2.5 mg (Mason & Steane 1976), cyproheptadine iv 1 mg (Solares et al 1987), ketanserin iv 10 mg over 3 min and an infusion of 3 mg h⁻¹ (Fischler et al 1983, Casthely et al 1986). The choice is often governed by availability of the drug.

3. Antibradykinin drugs include aprotinin (infusion of 200 000 kiu in 250 ml saline), and corticosteroids. However, there have been variable reports of their effectiveness in treating complications.

4. The role of histamine is uncertain. Flushing was successfully blocked in a patient with a gastric carcinoid using a combination of H_1 and H_2 antagonists (Roberts et al 1979).

5. It should be remembered that acute events during surgery are not always the result of tumour hormone secretion. Intractable hypotension without flushing or bronchospasm occurred following cardiopulmonary bypass in a patient undergoing valve replacement. This was thought to be of cardiac origin and the cautious use of epinephrine (adrenaline) resulted in an improvement in the patient's condition (Hamid & Harris 1992). Cardiovascular collapse occurred in a patient who had an atypical carcinoid tumour (Bachelor & Conacher 1992),

and the authors discussed the problems of differentiating a carcinoid crisis from an anaphylactoid reaction.

Bibliography

Bachelor AM, Conacher ID 1992 Anaphylactoid or carcinoid? British Journal of Anaesthesia 69: 325–7.

Bissonnette RT, Gibney RG, Berry BR et al 1990 Fatal carcinoid crisis after percutaneous fine-needle biopsy of hepatic metastasis: case report and review of the literature. Radiology 174: 751–2.

Casthely PA, Jablons M, Griepp RB et al 1986 Ketanserin in the preoperative and intraoperative management of a patient with carcinoid tumour undergoing tricuspid valve replacement. Anesthesia & Analgesia 65: 809–11.

Fischler M, Dentan M, Westerman MN et al 1983 Prophylactic use of ketanserin in a patient with carcinoid syndrome. British Journal of Anaesthesia 55: 920.

Hamid SK, Harris DNF 1992 Hypotension following valve replacement surgery in carcinoid heart disease. Anaesthesia 47: 490–2.

Hughes EW, Hodkinson BP 1989 Carcinoid syndrome: the combined use of ketanserin and octreotide in the management of an acute crisis during anaesthesia. Anaesthesia & Intensive Care 17: 367–70.

Jones RM, Knight D 1982 Severe hypertension and flushing in a patient with a non-metastatic carcinoid tumour. Anaesthesia 37: 57–9.

Marsh HM, Martin JK, Kvols LK et al 1987 Carcinoid crisis during anaesthesia: successful treatment with a somatostatin analogue. Anesthesiology 66: 89–91.

Mason RA, Steane PA 1976 Carcinoid syndrome: its relevance to the anaesthetist. Anaesthesia 31: 228–42.

Miller R, Boulukos PA, Warner RRP 1980 Failure of halothane and ketamine to alleviate carcinoid syndrome-induced bronchospasm during anesthesia. Anesthesia & Analgesia 59: 621–3.

Quinlivan JK, Roberts WA 1994 Intraoperative octreotide for refractory carcinoid-induced bronchospasm. Anesthesia & Analgesia 78: 400–2.

Roberts LJ II, Marney SR Jr, Oates JA 1979 Blockade of the flush associated with metastatic gastric carcinoid by combined histamine H_1 and H_2 receptor antagonists. New England Journal of Medicine 300: 236–8.

Roy RC, Carter RF, Wright PD 1987 Somatostatin, anaesthesia, and the carcinoid syndrome. Anaesthesia 42: 627–32.

Ruszniewski P, Ducreux M, Chayvialle JA et al 1996 Treatment of the carcinoid syndrome with the long acting somatostatin analogue lanreotide: a prospective study in 39 patients. Gut 39: 279–83.

Solares G, Blanco E, Pulgar S et al 1987 Carcinoid syndrome and intravenous cyproheptadine. Anaesthesia 42: 989–92.

Sukamaran M, Wilkinson ZS, Christianson L 1982 Acute carcinoid syndrome: a complication of flexible fibreoptic bronchoscopy. Annals of Thoracic Surgery 34: 702–5.

Veall GRQ, Peacock JE, Bax NDS et al 1994 Review of the anaesthetic management of 21 patients undergoing laparotomy for carcinoid syndrome. British Journal of Anaesthesia 72: 335–41.

Cardiac tamponade (see also Section 1, Cardiac tamponade)

Can occur when a pericardial effusion, or a collection of blood within the pericardial cavity, restricts cardiac filling during diastole, by the effect of external pressure. At the point at which the pericardium becomes no longer distensible, a small volume increase results in a rapid rise in intrapericardial pressure. There is a fixed, decreased diastolic volume of both ventricles. Induction of anaesthesia may cause cardiovascular collapse, although in the case of aortic dissection, problems are more likely to occur after relief of tamponade. When perforation results from CVP insertion, cardiovascular collapse may occur some time into surgery. Tamponade secondary to aortic dissection is frequently fatal and requires special management if the patient is to survive (Norman & Mycyk 1989).

Presentation

1. Causes include:

a) Malignancy, which may present as a large mediastinal mass on CXR (Keon 1981).

b) Recent cardiac surgery (Skacel et al 1991).

c) Blunt or sharp chest trauma, especially in the presence of sternal tenderness, chest bruising, wedge fractures of the thoracic or upper lumbar vertebrae (Cyna et al 1990, Breen & MacVay 1996, Jain 1998).

d) Closed cardiac massage.

e) Intracardiac injection.

f) CVP (Jiha et al 1996, Leech et al 1999) or pacemaker insertion.

g) Anticoagulant therapy.

h) Aortic dissection (Bond et al 1987, Norman & Mycyk 1989).

i) Systemic disease such as rheumatoid arthritis (Bellamy et al 1990).

2. In the presence of one of the predisposing factors, a high venous pressure, rapid low volume pulse, hypotension (Beck's triad), and reflex peripheral arterial and venous vasoconstriction, may arouse suspicions of tamponade, particularly if respiratory distress is accentuated in the supine position, or if there is a history of 'fainting' attacks.

3. Pulsus paradoxicus. Normally on inspiration there is a slight decrease in systolic pressure. In cardiac tamponade this decrease is accentuated, usually to >10 mmHg, and sometimes even to >20 mmHg. Pulsus paradoxicus is easily detected by palpation, but may be detected by an auscultation method (Lake 1983). Using a sphygmomanometer, the cuff pressure should first be reduced until the sound is intermittent, then deflation continued until all beats are heard. The difference between the two pressures is then measured.

4. Tamponade presented as cardiovascular collapse on induction of anaesthesia in two children with mediastinal masses (Keon 1981, Halpern et al 1983). At postmortem, both were found to have lymphomas enveloping the heart and infiltrating the pericardium.

5. Intraoperative tamponade has occurred secondary to central venous cannulation (Jiha et al 1996, Leech et al 1999). In the first patient, a 51-year-old man, it occurred 90 min after insertion of a subclavian catheter. In the second,

a 7-month-old infant, signs appeared 2 h into orthotopic liver transplantation.

6. Cardiac tamponade may complicate aortic dissection, in which case median sternotomy may relieve the tamponade. However, under these circumstances exsanguination may occur because of the sudden increase in arterial pressure in a patient under light anaesthesia (Norman & Mycyk 1989).

Diagnosis

1. Initially, the diagnosis must be considered, either from the history or on clinical examination. If cardiac arrest occurs, it is one cause of pulseless electrical activity ((EMD) electromechanical dissociation).

If the fluid collection is >250 ml, the CXR may show an enlarged, globular cardiac outline, the border of which may be straight or even convex. The right cardiophrenic angle is less than 90 degrees. The lung fields are clear. Reduced cardiac pulsation may be detected on fluoroscopy. Echocardiography is the most reliable method of diagnosis.

2. In the case of aortic dissection, the diagnosis may also be made during angiography.

Management

1. Monitor direct arterial and central venous pressures.

2. Minimise factors that worsen the haemodynamic situation. These include:

a) An increase in intrathoracic pressure. If artificial ventilation is already being undertaken, for example after cardiac surgery, then PEEP should be avoided since it further reduces cardiac output, especially at slow rates of ventilation (Mattila et al 1984).

b) A low intravascular volume. Maintain the blood volume with iv fluids, according to the haemodynamic responses.

c) A decreased myocardial contractility. Dopamine may have a favourable effect on haemodynamics, even in the presence of severe tamponade (Mattila et al 1984).

3. Urgent relief of tamponade. If possible, needle pericardiocentesis, with or without catheter insertion, should be performed under local anaesthesia. If time allows, ECG, radiological screening and facilities for emergency thoracotomy should be available. A subxiphoid approach can be used. Local anaesthesia is infiltrated between the xiphisternum and the left costal margin. With the patient at 30–45 degrees head up, a long, 16- or 18-G needle is directed towards the left shoulder. Safety may be increased by the use of a sterile ECG lead attached to the needle. When the epicardium is located, there is elevation of the ST segment. Continuous gentle aspiration assists identification of the pericardial sac. A sample of blood is injected onto a gauze swab; defibrinated pericardial blood does not clot. A Seldinger technique with insertion of a soft catheter should be used. More recently a technique of percutaneous balloon pericardiotomy has been described. This involves passage of a guidewire into the pericardium via a subxiphoid approach, draining the effusion with a pigtail catheter, then dilating the pericardium with a balloon dilating catheter. The pigtail catheter can be left in place for 24 h. A maximum drainage rate of 50 ml min $^{-1}$ has been suggested (Hamaya et al 1993). Since symptomatic improvement occurs with the removal of the first 50–200 ml of fluid withdrawn, there is no urgency to fully decompress the heart.

4. Sudden drainage of a chronic cardiac tamponade may cause acute haemodynamic changes and pulmonary oedema (Vandyke et al 1983, Downey et al 1991, Hamaya et al 1993). This gradually resolves over 24 h. In one patient, a volume of 500 ml of pericardial fluid had been removed. Full haemodynamic monitoring was being undertaken and there was a sudden increase in pulmonary artery pressure after pericardiocentesis. In cardiac tamponade it is the

right, rather than the left, ventricle that is being compressed. After release of the tamponade there is sudden overload of the left ventricle, while the PVR is still high. Acute dilatation of the thinner walled right ventricle and temporary mismatch between the output of the two ventricles was thought to have been responsible for the pulmonary oedema in these cases.

5. In the case of aortic dissection, the management may have to be modified. Norman and Mycyk described two patients: the first, who was managed conventionally, exsanguinated when sudden relief of tamponade restored cardiac output; in the second patient, who survived, femorofemoral bypass was instituted before sternotomy, and propranolol and vasodilators were given to control systemic arterial pressure.

Bibliography

Bellamy MC, Natarajan V, Lenz RJ 1990 An unusual presentation of cardiac tamponade. Anaesthesia 45: 135–6.

Bond DM, Milne B, Pym J et al 1987 Cardiac tamponade following anaesthetic induction for repair of ascending aorta dissection. Canadian Journal of Anaesthesia 34: 291–3.

Breen PH, MacVay MA 1996 Pericardial tamponade: a case for awake endotracheal intubation. Anesthesia & Analgesia 83: 658.

Cyna AM, Rodgers RC, McFarlane H 1990 Hypotension due to unexpected cardiac tamponade. Anaesthesia 45: 140–2.

Downey RJ, Bessler M, Weissman C 1991 Acute pulmonary oedema following pericardiocentesis for chronic cardiac tamponade secondary to trauma. Critical Care Medicine 19: 1323–5.

Halpern S, Chatten J, Meadows AT et al 1983 Anterior mediastinal masses: anesthesia hazards and other problems. Journal of Pediatrics 102: 407–10.

Hamaya Y, Dohi S, Ueda N et al 1993 Severe circulatory collapse immediately after pericardiocentesis in a patient with chronic cardiac tamponade. Anesthesia & Analgesia 78: 169–71.

Jain AK 1998 Survival after cardiac tamponade and arrest in a paediatric patient with penetrating trauma to pulmonary artery. Paediatric Anaesthesia 8: 345–8.

Jiha JG, Weinberg GL, Laurito CE 1996 Intraoperative cardiac tamponade after central venous cannulation. Anesthesia & Analgesia 82: 664–5.

Keon TP 1981 Death on induction of anesthesia for cervical node biopsy. Anesthesiology 55: 471–2.

Lake CL 1983 Anesthesia and pericardial disease. Anesthesia & Analgesia 62: 431–43.

Leech RC, Watts ADJ, Heaton ND et al 1999 Intraoperative cardiac tamponade after central venous cannulation in an infant during orthotopic liver transplantation. Anesthesia & Analgesia 89: 342–3.

Mattila I, Takkunen O, Mattila P et al 1984 Cardiac tamponade and different modes of ventilation. Acta Anaesthesiologica Scandinavica 28: 236–40.

Norman PH, Mycyk T 1989 Dissection of ascending thoracic aorta complicated by cardiac tamponade. Canadian Journal of Anaesthesia 36: 470–2.

Skacel M, Harrison GA, Verdi IS 1991 A case of isolated right atrial compression following cardiac surgery. Anaesthesia & Intensive Care 19: 114–15.

Vandyke WH, Cure J, Chakko CS et al 1983 Pulmonary oedema after pericardiocentesis for cardiac tamponade. New England Journal of Medicine 309: 595–6.

Central anticholinergic syndrome

A term given to a syndrome of blockade of central cholinergic neurotransmission, probably involving muscarinic receptors, which produces a clinical picture similar to that of atropine intoxication (Schneck & Rupreht 1989). It may be caused by any drug that has central anticholinergic actions, sometimes even after normal doses. It occurs most commonly following general anaesthesia, but also after acute intoxication from self poisoning, in association with sedation on the ITU, or during acute withdrawal states. The conscious level is usually impaired, or the patient may exhibit unpredictable behaviour. It has been described in association with a wide variety of drugs including atropine, hyoscine, benzodiazepines, tricyclic antidepressants, phenothiazines, butyrophenones (especially droperidol), cimetidine, phenobarbitone, opiates, and datura stramonium. Patients can vary considerably in their sensitivity to the anticholinergic effects.

It is a difficult condition to diagnose with absolute certainty, since nothing is measurable. However, a dramatic improvement in conscious

C

level after a small dose of physostigmine, a cholinesterase inhibitor that crosses the blood–brain barrier and increases brain acetylcholine levels, is suggestive of the diagnosis.

It has been observed that central anticholinergic syndrome is reported far more often in Europe than in the UK (Cook & Spence 1997). This was attributed to the different profile of drugs used on the continent. In a report from Germany of 18 cases of central anticholinergic syndrome out of 962 patients, eight had been given droperidol, in doses from 2.5 to 25 mg, nine had received either diazepam or phenobarbitone, and all had had promethazine and atropine (Link et al 1997). In the UK, in the past, it was frequently linked to the use of hyoscine, a drug that is now rarely used (personal observation).

Presentation

1. Unexpected delayed recovery from anaesthesia, stupor, restlessness, agitation, amnesia, hallucinations, respiratory depression, confusion, or seizures. In the perioperative period, after premedication with morphine 10 mg and hyoscine 0.4 mg, a young man developed hyperthermia (39.3°C increasing to 42°C), tachycardia, and confusion which resolved immediately after physostigmine 3 mg (Torline 1992). A young woman given glycopyrrolate 0.2 mg became hot and dry and developed headache, tachycardia, widely dilated pupils; this responded to physostigmine (Grum & Osborne 1991). This is a surprising reaction, since glycopyrrolate has limited passage across the blood–brain barrier, and it was subsequently suggested that ranitidine might have potentiated the effects of glycopyrrolate (Wingard 1991). Two patients had been given hyoscine as premedication. One was deeply unconscious in the recovery room, the other developed agitation and confusion (Martin & Howell 1997). In one patient, dramatic extrapyramidal symptoms after anaesthesia responded to physostigmine; in this case fentanyl was thought to have been responsible, but naloxone had failed

to reverse the symptoms (Dehring et al 1991). Hyoscine 0.4 mg given iv before awake fibreoptic intubation for an obstructing thyroid, resulted in sedation and apnoea, followed by agitation and lack of cooperation 3 h later (Ezri et al 1996).

2. After overdoses involving psychoactive drugs that have anticholinergic effects. After anaesthesia for colonic surgery, a 40-kg, 73 year old had delayed recovery and facial flushing, that responded dramatically to physostigmine 0.5 mg. It was initially thought to have been a sensitivity to atropine 0.3 mg, given for intraoperative bradycardia. However, relapse into unconsciousness occurred 2 h later and it transpired that, because of her anxiety about surgery, her regular daily dose of chlordiazepoxide 10 mg had been increased to 40 mg daily for the previous 5 days! The patient had IPPV overnight (without need for sedation) and eventually emerged the following day with little memory for events (personal observation).

3. On the ITU after a prolonged period of sedation.

4. A dramatic response to a small dose of physostigmine was the common features in all patients.

Differential diagnosis

Disturbances of glucose and electrolytes, endocrine disorders (myxoedema and thyrotoxicosis), hypoxia and hypercarbia, neuropsychiatric disorders, stroke, neuroleptic malignant syndrome, and drug dependence.

Management

1. Increase the levels of acetylcholine in the brain by the use of a drug such as phyostigmine, a cholinesterase inhibitor, that crosses the blood–brain barrier, and which possesses minimal muscarinic effects. A small dose of physostigmine (increments of 0.5 mg) can be

used as a diagnostic test and for treatment of the more serious symptoms (arrhythmias, seizures, autonomic side effects, or delirium) of drug overdose. In the case of overdoses, it should not be used simply to arouse the patient. Physostigmine has a relatively brief duration of action; most is eliminated within 2 h, therefore repeated doses may be needed.

2. Ensure oxygenation and respiratory adequacy. If in doubt, tracheal intubation should be performed and IPPV instituted.

Bibliography

Cook B, Spence AA 1997 Post-operative central anticholinergic syndrome. European Journal of Anaesthesiology 14: 1–2.

Dehring DJ, Gupta B, Peruzzi WT 1991 Postoperative opisthotonos and torticollis after fentanyl, enflurane and nitrous oxide. Canadian Journal of Anaesthesia 38: 919–25.

Ezri T, Szmuk P, Konichezsky S et al 1996 Central anticholinergic syndrome complicating management of a difficult airway. Canadian Journal of Anaesthesia 43: 1079–80.

Grum DF, Osborne LR 1991 Central anticholinergic syndrome following glycopyrrolate. Anesthesiology 74: 191–3.

Link J, Papadopoulos G, Dopjans D et al 1997 Distinct central anticholinergic syndrome following general anaesthesia. European Journal of Anaesthesiology 14: 15–23.

Martin B, Howell PR 1997 Physostigmine: going..going..gone? Two cases of central anticholinergic syndrome following anaesthesia and its treatment. European Journal of Anaesthesiology 14: 467–70.

Schneck HJ, Rupreht J 1989 Central anticholinergic syndrome in anaesthesia and intensive care. Acta Anaesthesiologica Belgica 40: 219–28.

Torline RL 1992 Extreme hyperpyrexia associated with central anticholinergic syndrome. Anesthesiology 76: 470–1.

Wingard DW 1991 Glycopyrrolate and the central anticholinergic syndrome. Anesthesiology 75: 1125–6.

Glycine absorption (see TURP syndrome)

Latex allergy

Reports of intraoperative reactions began in the late 1980s in the USA, although it is possible that they had occurred previously, but latex was not recognised as the cause. In one patient, anaphylaxis to latex was only diagnosed at the end of a long history of multiple anaesthetic drug reactions (Sethna et al 1992). Factors that may account for the recent appearance of the problem include the increasing use of latex gloves by hospital workers, and changes in the manufacturing processes and chemicals used, necessitated by the sudden great demand for latex products (Hirshman 1992).

Reactions can be either delayed type IV or immediate type 1. The majority of anaphylactic reactions in children are due to latex allergy (Holzman 1997). Spina bifida is one risk factor (D'Astous et al 1992, Meehan et al 1992). In a study of 80 children, those with spina bifida and those who had undergone multiple operations had similar incidences of latex sensitisation (Porri et al 1997). Whilst most of those affected do have predisposing factors, the occasional, otherwise fit child has been reported (Zestos & Creighton 1997). Patients often forget to mention rubber allergies. Fisher (1997) reported two patients who denied any allergy until prompted by a positive skin prick test. A parturient, known by her dentist to be latex sensitive, developed anaphylaxis that was initially attributed to epidural bupivacaine. In retrospect, it had coincided with the insertion of a latex catheter (Rae et al 1997).

Presentation

1. The patient may fall into one of the categories of high risk for latex allergy. These include: patients who require repeated bladder catheterisation; those with spina bifida and congenital urogenital abnormalities, such as bladder and cloacal exstrophy; individuals who have multiple surgical procedures; occupational exposure, in particular, healthcare workers; and those with a history of atopy, drugs allergies, and

food allergies for bananas, kiwi fruit, and avocados.

2. Reactions are usually associated with exposure to the surgeon's latex gloves, from which the latex leaches out and enters the patient's circulation. In adults, reactions have been observed 45 min (Swartz et al 1990), 25 min (McKinstry et al 1992) and 40 min (Hodgson & Andersen 1994) after induction. However, in a report of 21 children, whose average number of operations was 11, the onset was earlier, often only minutes after the induction of anaesthesia, and rarely beyond 30 min (Dormans et al 1994). Extensive visceral exposure to latex may accelerate the onset and severity of the reaction. A parturient developed dyspnoea, bronchospasm, cyanosis and cardiovascular collapse, only 5 min after insertion of a Foley catheter, before Caesarean section for preeclampsia (Stewart & Bogod 1995).

3. Reaction. Generalised urticaria, periorbital oedema, bronchospasm (Zestos & Creighton 1997) and profound cardiorespiratory collapse have been reported.

4. Source of reaction. Usually the surgeon's rubber gloves. Other sources, have included a latex urethral catheter (Stewart & Bogod 1995), the stopper of a medication vial (Vassallo et al 1995), and a pulmonary artery catheter balloon (Gosgnach et al 1995).

Treatment

1. As for anaphylaxis (see also Association of Anaesthetists 1995):

   a) For hypotension, epinephrine (adrenaline) 50–100μg iv over 1 min (0.5–1 ml 1 : 10 000), with further doses as required.

   b) For cardiovascular collapse epinephrine (adrenaline) 0.5–1 mg (5–10 ml 1 : 10 000).

2. Intravascular volume expansion with colloid or crystalloid.

3. Secondary treatment; antihistamines (chlorpheniramine 10–20 mg); corticosteroids;

hydrocortisone 100–300 mg.

4. Epinephrine (adrenaline) infusion 4–8μg min^{-1} (0.05–0.1μg kg^{-1} min^{-1})); norepinephrine (noradrenaline) infusion 4–8μg min^{-1} (0.05–1μg kg^{-1} min^{-1}); isoprenaline 0.05–1μg min^{-1}.

5. Bronchodilators for bronchospasm (salbutamol, aminophylline).

6. Observe for airway oedema on extubation. If necessary use an airway exchanger, which can stay in place until the security of the airway has been ascertained.

Subsequent diagnosis

1. Made by skin prick test, performed after saline has been pressed into a piece of rubber glove (Pepys et al 1994). A drop of the test agent is placed on the volar surface of the forearm and the tip of an orange needle, bevel upwards, is introduced into the epidermis with a gentle, lifting motion. Saline solution can be used as control. Positive reactions show a wheal plus flare, often with itching, and can be graded according to diameter. Since a number of different antigenic latex proteins have been described, samples of the actual suspect articles should be retained for dermatological testing (Dakin & Yentis 1998).

2. The presence of IgE antibodies to latex.

3. Increases in plasma tryptase have been reported, which subsequently returned to normal (Volcheck & Li 1994, Fisher 1997).

4. There is now a latex allergy website: http://www.latexallergy.com/

Subsequent management

1. Inform the patient and general practitioner, as for anaphylaxis.

2. For management of further surgery, see Latex allergy (Section 1).

Bibliography

Association of Anaesthetists 1995 Suspected anaphylactic reactions associated with anaesthesia, Revised edn. Association of Anaesthetists of Great Britain & Ireland and The British Association of Clinical Immunology, London.

Ballantine JC, Brown E 1995 Latex anaphylaxis: another case, another cause. Anesthesia & Analgesia 81: 1303–4.

D'Astous J, Drouin MA, Rhine E 1992 Intraoperative anaphylaxis secondary to allergy to latex in children who have spina bifida. Report of two cases. Journal of Bone & Joint Surgery 74: 1084–6.

Dakin MJ, Yentis SM 1998 Latex allergy: a strategy for management. Anaesthesia 53: 774–81.

Dormans JP, Templeton JJ, Edmonds C et al 1994 Intraoperative anaphylaxis due to exposure to latex (natural rubber) in children. Journal of Bone & Joint Surgery 76A: 1688–91.

Fisher MMcD 1997 Latex allergy during anaesthesia: cautionary tales. Anaesthesia & Intensive Care 25: 302–3.

Gosgnach M, Bourel LM, Ducart A et al 1995 Pulmonary artery catheter balloon: an unusual cause of severe anaphylactic reaction. Anesthesiology 83: 220–1.

Hirshman CA 1992 Latex anaphylaxis. Anesthesiology 77: 223–5.

Hodgson CA, Andersen BD 1994 Latex allergy: an unfamiliar cause of intra-operative cardiovascular collapse. Anaesthesia 49: 507–8.

Holzman RS 1997 Clinical management of latex-allergic children. Anesthesia & Analgesia 85: 529–33.

McKinstry LJ, Fenton WJ, Barrett P 1992 Anaesthesia in the patient with latex allergy. Canadian Journal of Anaesthesia 39: 587–9.

Meehan PL, Galina MP, Daftari T 1992 Intraoperative anaphylaxis due to allergy to latex. Report of two cases. Journal of Bone & Joint Surgery 74A: 1087–9.

Pepys J, Pepys EO, Baldo BA et al 1994 Anaphylactic/anaphylactoid reactions to anaesthetic and associated agents. Skin prick tests in aetiological diagnosis. Anaesthesia 49: 470–5.

Porri F, Pradal M, Lemiere C et al 1997 Association between latex sensitization and repeated latex exposure in children. Anesthesiology 86: 599–602.

Rae SM, Milne MK, Wildsmith JAW 1997 Anaphylaxis associated with, but not caused by, extradural bupivacaine. British Journal of Anaesthesia 78: 224–6.

Sethna NF, Sockin SM, Holzman RS et al 1992 Latex allergy in a child with a history of multiple anesthetic drug allergies. Anesthesiology 77: 372–5.

Stewart PD, Bogod D 1995 Latex anaphylaxis during late pregnancy. International Journal of Obstetric Anesthesia 4: 48–50.

Swartz J, Braude BM, Gilmour RF et al 1990 Intraoperative anaphylaxis to latex. Canadian Journal of Anaesthesia 37: 589–92.

Vassallo SA, Thurston TA, Kim SH et al 1995 Allergic reaction to latex stopper of a medication vial. Anesthesia & Analgesia 80: 1057–8.

Volcheck GW, Li JTC 1994 Elevated serum tryptase level in a case of intraoperative anaphylaxis caused by latex allergy. Archives of Internal Medicine 154: 2243–5.

Zestos MM, Creighton R 1997 Latex anaphylaxis during tissue expander insertion in a healthy child. Canadian Journal of Anaesthesia 44: 1275–7.

Local anaesthetic toxicity

557

Local anaesthetic toxicity may occur if the maximum safe dose is exceeded, or if transient high blood levels are achieved by accidental intravenous injection, or rapid absorption from an inflamed or vascular area. However, maximum safe doses are extremely difficult to define, since they depend upon a number of factors, including the concentration of the local anaesthetic, and the site of administration (Scott 1986). When continuous infusion techniques are employed, additional factors, in particular those that affect the rate of absorption, drug metabolism and excretion, become important.

There has been increasing use of local anaesthetics combined with opiates for epidural anaesthesia following surgery. This decreases the amount of local anaesthetic required, which in turn reduces sympathetic vasodilatation, the degree of muscular paralysis, and risk of systemic local anaesthetic toxicity. However, in the USA in particular, techniques of continuous caudal or lumbar epidural anaesthesia in children using local anaesthesia alone have become more popular. Sometimes these are continued for several days and there have been reports of seizures, and in some cases, cardiotoxicity occurred without warning (Berde 1992).

Now that bupivacaine is no longer recommended for intravenous regional anaesthesia, the safety of this technique seems to have increased. However, the lessons learned from deaths which occurred in accident and emergency units, where the technique was used by nonanaesthetic staff, must not be forgotten (Heath 1982). In unfamiliar hands, accidental deflation of an automatic tourniquet can occur before the local anaesthetic has become fixed. Inappropriately high doses of the drug may be given. Resuscitation procedures in casualty for unexpected convulsions may be inadequate.

Other problems with bupivacaine also led to revisions in the clinical indications in the USA and the UK. A series of reports of deaths, chiefly associated with obstetric anaesthesia, and the subsequent evidence presented to the FDA (Albright 1979, Reiz & Nath 1986), resulted in the withdrawal of bupivacaine 0.75% for obstetric use in the USA. Following this, in the UK, the manufacturers' literature stated that the 0.75% solution was contraindicated in obstetric anaesthesia, and that bupivacaine should not be used for intravenous regional anaesthesia.

These problems led to a search for less toxic drugs. However, CNS toxicity still occurs with all of the local anaesthetics given for a wide variety of regional blocks. Complications result from injection directly into a vessel, administration of a drug at its upper limit of safety, and the use of continuous infusions over several days. The narrower margin of safety for bupivacaine and etidocaine, and their potential for cardiotoxicity, are well known. Convulsions with ropivacaine seem to occur equally readily, but so far, there has been only one report of cardiac complications (Ruetsch et al 1999). Three patients with CNS toxicity from ropivacaine became anxious and vocalised during injection (Klein & Benveniste 1999). The authors attributed this unexpected behaviour to disinhibition of select neural pathways. Interestingly, an almost identical sequence was described with levobupivacaine (Kopacz & Allen 1999). Levobupivacaine also produces convulsions, but again at a higher threshold than with bupivacaine (toxic threshold levobupivacaine 2–4 μg ml^{-1}, bupivacaine >1.5 μg ml^{-1}).

Presentation

1. Contributory factors include administration of a local anaesthetic in doses exceeding the toxic levels, the sudden release of a normal dose into the circulation, or the injection of small amounts into an artery supplying the brain. The arterial concentration, and in particular the proportion of blood going to the brain, is important in acute toxicity. Toxicity is therefore likely to be most serious in a hypovolaemic or shocked patient (Scott 1986). The threshold for CNS toxicity with lidocaine (lignocaine) is 5 μg ml^{-1}, which is close to the therapeutic dose for treatment of ventricular extrasystoles. Respiratory depression, coma and circulatory collapse occur at levels in excess of 10 μg ml^{-1} (Dawling et al 1989).

a) *Interscalene block.* Accidental injection into the vertebral artery during interscalene brachial plexus block resulted in transient, reversible 'locked-in' syndrome (Durrani & Winnie 1991), probably as a result of a direct toxic effect of mepivacaine and tetracaine on the brainstem. Unconsciousness, apnoea and hypotension occurred after interscalene injection of 20 ml 0.75% bupivacaine and epinephrine (adrenaline) (Tuominen et al 1991); this was also attributed to accidental entry into the vertebral artery. Convulsions, but no arrhythmias, occurred when 18 ml 0.75% ropivacaine was used for an interscalene block (Korman & Riley 1997).

b) The presence of volatile anaesthetics delays the onset of convulsions. A child was anaesthetised for abdominal surgery using sevoflurane and epidural analgesia. Convulsions occurred immediately on recovery and were associated with high

plasma mepivacaine concentrations (Saitoh et al 1996). Accidental iv injection of lidocaine (lignocaine) 20 mg kg^{-1} instead of 2 mg kg^{-1} in an anaesthetised patient before tracheal intubation resulted in cardiovascular collapse and tachyarrhythmias. Convulsions only appeared 10 min later, after discontinuance of anaesthesia (Yukioka et al 1990). In both cases, the convulsions were presumably suppressed by the anaesthetic agent.

c) *Stellate ganglion block* (Wulf et al 1991). In a study of plasma bupivacaine concentrations after stellate ganglion block, three out of 11 exceeded the threshold for CNS toxicity of 1.5–2 μg ml^{-1}. Maximum values were reached in 5 min. Intra-arterial injection may still occur, even after negative aspiration tests (Romanoff & Ellis 1991).

d) *Intrapleural block.* Continuous intrapleural block with bupivacaine resulted in convulsions in a child 21 h after the start (Agarwal et al 1992). The blood bupivacaine level was 5.6 μg ml^{-1}.

e) *Lumbar epidural anaesthesia.* A continuous lumbar epidural block in a child was associated with convulsions at 56 h and a blood bupivacaine level of 5.4 μg ml^{-1} (Agarwal et al 1992). A similar technique in a 4 year old, using 0.57 mg kg^{-1} h^{-1}, resulted in a convulsion at 40 h (Peutrell & Hughes 1995). The plasma bupivacaine concentration was 4.5 mg l^{-1} (toxic concentration >1.5–2 mg l^{-1}). Epidural injection of levobupivacaine 17 ml 0.75% caused CNS signs, despite negative aspiration and a test dose. The patient was given thiopentone before the onset of convulsions could occur and a blood level at 14 min was 2.5 μg ml^{-1}. The level at convulsions was presumably much higher than this. The patient was haemodynamically stable (Kopacz & Allen 1999). A total of 120 mg of ropivacaine was injected in divided doses over 11 min

into a patient with an epidural catheter having postpartum sterilisation. A complaint of nervousness was followed by a convulsion lasting 1 min. She recovered spontaneously (Abouleish et al 1998). Accidental iv injection of ropivacaine 20 mg during an epidural given for chronic pain resulted in a convulsion in a 44-kg patient (Plowman et al 1998).

f) *Caudal epidural anaesthesia.* Three cases of bupivacaine toxicity with continuous caudal anaesthesia were reported (McCloskey et al 1992). A neonate developed bradycardia, hypotension and ventricular tachycardia, then seizures 2 h later; an 8-year-old child had convulsions at 25 h, and a 4 year old had convulsions at 34 h. The blood bupivacaine levels taken at the time of the event were 5.6 μg ml^{-1}, 6.6 μg ml^{-1}, and 10.2 μg ml^{-1} respectively. In none of the children had warning signs of toxicity been evident.

g) *Sciatic nerve block.* Injection of 30 ml 0.75% ropivacaine into the sciatic nerve and psoas compartment resulted in a convulsion within 90 s. This was accompanied by bradycardia and increasing QRS interval (Ruetsch et al 1999). The threshold for toxicity is 3–4 μg ml^{-1} (see 4 below).

2. Symptoms of toxicity include lightheadedness, circumoral tingling, numbness of the tongue, a metallic taste, tinnitus, visual disturbances, anxiety, and restlessness. Convulsions and apnoea may follow.

3. The combination of apnoea and convulsions can lead to hypoxia, respiratory and metabolic (in particular lactic) acidosis. With drugs such as lidocaine (lignocaine), it had been accepted that a wide margin existed between CNS and cardiovascular toxicity. However, the situation with bupivacaine was different, in that following convulsions, hypotension, serious ventricular arrhythmias or cardiac arrest were reported. Resuscitation proved to be particularly difficult or impossible (Albright 1979, Prentiss

1979). Successful resuscitation has however been reported on occasions (Davis & de Jong 1982, Mallampati et al 1984). In late pregnancy the associated problems of aortocaval occlusion and supine resuscitation cannot be ignored.

4. The newer drugs, ropivacaine and levobupivacaine, seem to have a wider margin between CNS and cardiac toxicity than do bupivacaine and etidocaine (Knudsen et al 1997). The cardiac effects of bupivacaine, of which depression of cardiac function is the chief one, was not attributable solely to hypoxia and acidosis, and is probably in part related to differences in myocardial uptake of the drug (Morishima et al 1985). An inhibition of energy metabolism was suggested as one explanation for bupivacaine-induced cardiotoxicity (Eledjam et al 1989). Acute toxicity studies of ropivacaine in fit volunteers suggest that it causes fewer CNS symptoms and is at least 25% less toxic than bupivacaine (Scott et al 1989). So far, there has only been one patient in whom cardiac problems occurred in association with convulsions (Ruetsch et al 1999). These consisted of bradycardias, lengthening QRS intervals, followed by SVT and transient AF. Based on total ropivacaine concentrations in blood taken 7 and 12 min after the event, and extrapolated back to the time of the arrhythmia, a level of $7.5 \, mg \, l^{-1}$ was estimated (threshold for appearance of CNS symptoms in volunteers $1–2 \, mg \, l^{-1}$, toxic levels $>4 \, mg \, l^{-1}$). This seems to confirm the wide margin between CNS and cardiovascular toxicity.

5. There is clinical and experimental evidence to suggest that pregnant patients are particularly vulnerable to bupivacaine toxicity (Morishima et al 1983). Severe ventricular arrhythmias occurred with bupivacaine in pregnant sheep, even when the acidosis was rapidly corrected (Marx 1984). A pregnancy-associated increase in availability of free bupivacaine, which does not occur with mepivacaine, was suggested to account for the differences (Santos et al 1989). Studies with ropivacaine suggest that ovine pregnancy, at least, is not associated with a gestational-related

increase in the availability of free drug (Santos et al 1991).

6. Methaemoglobinaemia is associated with toxic doses of prilocaine. A brachial plexus block with 35 ml 1.5% prilocaine resulted in a pulse oximetry reading of 88% despite a Pao_2 of 48.6 kPa (Bardoczky et al 1990). There have been several reports of toxicity in infants and children given EMLA cream, a eutectic mixture of prilocaine and lidocaine (lignocaine) (Jakobsen & Nilsson 1985, Frayling et al 1990), and ointments containing benzocaine (Adachi et al 1999).

7. Physical injury may sometimes result from local anaesthetic toxicity. Convulsions caused posterior dislocation of the shoulder in two patients, after bupivacaine injection during sacral and epidural anaesthesia respectively (Pagden et al 1986).

Prophylaxis

1. A benzodiazepine premedication may suppress some of the manifestations of local anaesthetic toxicity. In pigs, however, although convulsions were suppressed, the threshold for cardiovascular toxicity was unaltered (Bernards et al 1989).

2. Do not exceed the maximum safe dose for the particular local anaesthetic being used. When continuous infusions are used for prolonged periods, this requires particular care. It has been suggested that doses for prolonged caudal or lumbar epidural analgesia should not exceed $0.2–0.4 \, mg \, kg^{-1} h^{-1}$ in infants, and $0.2–0.75 \, mg \, kg^{-1} h^{-1}$ in children, and that caudal analgesia should be limited to 48 h (Berde 1992). Additional risk factors, such as fever or reduced clearance, should be taken into account (Peutrell & Hughes 1995).

3. With epidural anaesthesia there is no foolproof method of ensuring that intravascular or subarachnoid injection has not occurred.

4. All injections should be given slowly and the dose should be fractionated. Where a large

volume of local anaesthetic is required, a rate not exceeding 1 ml s^{-1} and the use of a 10-ml rather than a 30-ml syringe has been recommended.

5. Aspiration for blood and CSF should always be performed. However, a negative test does not ensure safe placement of the epidural catheter.

6. The use of a test dose is controversial and remains so (Birnbach & Chestnut 1999). It has been suggested that, for a single test dose of local anaesthetic to be of value in signalling the possibility of an iv or subarachnoid injection, it must contain a dose of local anaesthetic sufficient to rapidly produce evidence of spinal anaesthesia plus 0.015 mg epinephrine (adrenaline). Thus a systemic tachycardia will give warning of an accidental intravascular injection (Moore & Batra 1981). This means the use of 3 ml of local anaesthetic containing 1 : 200 000 epinephrine. However, there are doubts about the safety of using epinephrine in obstetric patients. It was found to decrease uterine blood flow in up to 50% of pregnant ewes, sometimes with signs of fetal distress (Hood et al 1986). The heart rate in the pregnant patient is so variable that its reliability has also been called into question (Leighton et al 1987). In addition the use of epinephrine does not guarantee identity of inadvertent subarachnoid or iv injection (Blomberg & Lofstrom et al 1991). The test dose will not consistently identify misplaced catheters. Failure to identify subdural placement has been reported (Crosby & Halpern 1989). Extensive sensory neural blockade followed injection of 13 ml lidocaine (lignocaine) 1.5%, into a catheter, thought to be positioned epidurally (Crosby & Halpern 1989). Response to the test dose had not led to suspicions of misplacement.

7. The patient's mental state should be continuously assessed throughout the injection, usually by engaging him/her in active conversation. Each subsequent dose of local anaesthetic should be administered as if it were a test dose. Pulse oximetry should be used if the patient is sedated.

8. The immediate availability of resuscitation equipment and experienced personnel.

Management

The method by which the convulsions are controlled is arguable and depends partly upon the experience of the attendant and partly on the choice of drugs immediately available. All of the following have been reported.

1. Oxygenation and control of convulsions.

a) Thiopentone 150–200 mg.

b) Suxamethonium will immediately control the muscular activity (but not the cerebral activity), and allow oxygen to be given by bag and mask ventilation, before intubation. During local anaesthetic-induced convulsions, severe hypoxia, hypercarbia and lactic acidosis occur simultaneously. Lactic acid production stops immediately after administration of suxamethonium. Rapid intubation is permitted, no myocardial depression occurs, and its effects wear off rapidly.

c) Diazepam 2–10 mg has also been recommended. However it takes several minutes to become effective, during which time the convulsions continue and acidosis progresses. It is a long-acting drug, and it has respiratory-depressant properties.

d) Propofol, in a dose of 50 mg, has also been reported to stop ropivacaine-induced convulsions (Ruetsch et al 1999).

2. Cardiac resuscitation. May be required with a massive local anaesthetic overdose or if bupivacaine has been used. ECG monitoring may show bradycardia, asystole, ventricular tachycardia, or ventricular fibrillation.

a) External cardiac massage must be sustained and effective, because bupivacaine remains longer in the myocardium than lidocaine (lignocaine).

b) Hypoxia and acidosis must be corrected rapidly.

c) If ventricular fibrillation occurs, defibrillation may not be successful on the first occasion.

d) Ventricular tachycardia is treated. The ventricular tachycardia threshold has been tested during bupivacaine toxicity in dogs (Kasten & Martin 1985). Bretylium raised the ventricular tachycardia threshold, whereas lidocaine (lignocaine) was either ineffective or further lowered it. It was noted that bupivacaine prolonged the QT interval and produced a ventricular tachycardia similar to that of a torsade de pointes atypical VT. Bretylium tosylate 5–10 mg kg^{-1} (diluted to 10 mg ml^{-1} with 5% dextrose or 0.9% saline) can be given slowly over 8–10 min, with ECG observation.

e) Hypotension may need to be treated with inotropes or vasopressors.

f) Cardiopulmonary bypass was successful in treating bupivacaine-induced cardiac arrest (Long et al 1989).

Bibliography

Abouleish EI, Elias M, Nelson C 1998 Ropivacaine-induced seizure after extradural anaesthesia. British Journal of Anaesthesia 80: 843–4.

Adachi T, Fukumoto M, Uetsuki N et al 1999 Suspected severe methemoglobinemia caused by topical application of an ointment containing benzocaine around the enterostomy. Anesthesia & Analgesia 88: 1190–1.

Agarwal R, Gutlove DP, Lockhart CH 1992 Seizures occurring in pediatric patients receiving continuous infusions of bupivacaine. Anesthesia & Analgesia 75: 284–6.

Albright GA 1979 Cardiac arrest following regional anesthesia with etidocaine or bupivacaine. Anesthesiology 51: 285–7.

Bardoczky GI, Wathieu M, D'Hollander A 1990 Prilocaine-induced methaemoglobinaemia evidenced by pulse oximetry. Acta Anaesthesiologica Scandinavica 34: 162–4.

Berde CB 1992 Convulsions associated with pediatric regional anesthesia. Anesthesia & Analgesia 75: 164–6.

Bernards CM, Carpenter RL, Rupp SM et al 1989 Effect of midazolam and diazepam premedication on central nervous system toxicity and cardiovascular toxicity of bupivacaine in pigs. Anesthesiology 70: 318–23.

Birnbach DJ, Chestnut DH 1999 The epidural test dose in obstetric patients: has it outlived its usefulness? Anesthesia & Analgesia 88: 1073–6.

Blomberg RG, Lofstrom JB 1991 The test dose in regional anaesthesia. Acta Anaesthesiologica Scandinavica 35: 465–8.

Crosby ET, Halpern S 1989 Failure of a lidocaine test dose to identify subdural placement of an epidural catheter. Canadian Journal of Anaesthesia 36: 445–7.

Davis NL, de Jong RH 1982 Successful resuscitation following massive bupivacaine overdose. Anesthesia & Analgesia 61: 62–4.

Dawling S, Flanagan RJ, Widdop B 1989 Fatal lignocaine poisoning: report of two cases and review of the literature. Human Toxicology 8: 389.

Durrani Z, Winnie AP 1991 Brainstem toxicity with reversible locked-in syndrome after intrascalene brachial plexus block. Anesthesia & Analgesia 72: 249–52.

Eledjam JJ, de la Coussaye JE, Brugada J et al 1989 In vitro study on bupivacaine-induced depression of myocardial contractility. Anesthesia & Analgesia 69: 732–5.

Frayling IM, Addison GM, Chattergee K et al 1990 Methaemoglobinaemia in children treated with prilocaine-lignocaine cream. British Medical Journal 301: 153–4.

Heath M 1982 Deaths after intravenous regional anaesthesia. British Medical Journal 285: 913–14.

Hood DD, Dewan DM, James FM 1986 Maternal and fetal effects of epinephrine in gravid ewes. Anesthesiology 64: 610–13.

Jakobson B, Nilsson A 1985 Methaemoglobinaemia associated with a prilocaine-lidocaine cream and trimethoprim-sulphamethazole. Acta Anaesthesiologica Scandinavica 29: 453–5.

Kasten GW, Martin ST 1985 Bupivacaine cardiovascular toxicity. Comparison of treatment with bretylium and lignocaine. Anesthesia & Analgesia 64: 911–16.

Klein SM, Benveniste H 1999 Anxiety, vocalization, and agitation following peripheral nerve block with ropivacaine. Regional Anesthesia & Pain Medicine 24: 175–8.

Knudsen K, Beckman Suurkula M, Blomberg S et al 1997 Central nervous and cardiovascular effects of i.v. infusions of ropivacaine, bupivacaine and placebo in volunteers. British Journal of Anaesthesia 78: 507–14.

Kopacz DJ, Allen HW 1999 Accidental intravenous levobupivacaine. Anesthesia & Analgesia 89: 1027–9.

Korman B, Riley RH 1997 Convulsions induced by ropivacaine during interscalene brachial plexus block. Anesthesia & Analgesia 85: 1128–9.

Leighton B, Norris M, Sosis M et al 1987 Limitations of ephedrine as a marker of intravascular injection in laboring women. Anesthesiology 66: 688–91.

Long WB, Rosenblum S, Grady IP 1989 Successful resuscitation of bupivacaine-induced cardiac arrest using cardiopulmonary bypass. Anesthesia & Analgesia 69: 403–6.

McCloskey JJ, Haun SE, Deshpande JK 1992 Bupivacaine toxicity secondary to continuous caudal epidural infusion in children. Anesthesia & Analgesia 75: 287–90.

Mallampati SR, Liu PL, Knap RM 1984 Convulsions and ventricular tachycardia from bupivacaine with epinephrine: successful resuscitation. Anaesthesia & Analgesia 63: 856–9.

Marx GF 1984 Cardiotoxicity of local anesthetics— the plot thickens. Anesthesiology 60: 3–5.

Moore DC, Batra MS 1981 The components of an effective test dose prior to epidural block. Anesthesiology 55: 693–6.

Morishima HO, Pedersen H, Finster M et al 1983 Is bupivacaine more cardiotoxic than lignocaine? Anesthesiology 59S: A409.

Morishima HO, Pedersen H, Finster M et al 1985 Bupivacaine toxicity in pregnant and non-pregnant ewes. Anesthesiology 63: 134–9.

Pagden D, Halaburt AS, Wirpszor R et al 1986 Posterior dislocation of the shoulder complicating regional anaesthesia. Anesthesia & Analgesia 65: 1063–5.

Peutrell JM, Hughes DG 1995 A grand mal convulsion in a child in association with a continuous epidural infusion of bupivacaine. Anaesthesia 50: 563–4.

Plowman AN, Bolsin S, Mather LE 1998 Central nervous system toxicity attributable to epidural ropivacaine hydrochloride. Anaesthesia & Intensive Care 26: 204–6.

Prentiss JE 1979 Cardiac arrest following regional anaesthesia with etidocaine or bupivacaine. Anesthesiology 51: 285–7.

Reiz S, Nath S 1986 Cardiotoxicity of local anaesthetic agents. British Journal of Anaesthesia 58: 736–46.

Reiz S, Haggmark S, Johansson G et al 1989 Cardiotoxicity of ropivacaine—a new amide local anaesthetic agent. Acta Anaesthesiologica Scandinavica 33: 93–8.

Romanoff ME, Ellis JS 1991 Bupivacaine toxicity after stellate ganglion block. Anesthesia & Analgesia 73: 505–6.

Ruetsch YA, Fattinger KE, Borgeat A 1999 Ropivacaine-induced convulsions and severe cardiac dysrhythmia after sciatic block. Anesthesiology 90: 1784–6.

Saitoh K, Tsukamoto N, Mitsuhata H et al 1996 Convulsions associated with epidural analgesia during sevoflurane anaesthesia. Paediatric Anaesthesia 6: 495–7.

Santos AC, Pedersen H, Harmon TW et al 1989 Does pregnancy alter the systemic toxicity of local anesthetic? Anesthesiology 70: 991–5.

Santos AC, Arthur GR, Pedersen H et al 1991 Systemic toxicity of ropivacaine during ovine pregnancy. Anesthesiology 75: 137–41.

Scott DB 1986 Toxic effects of local anaesthetic agents on the central nervous system. British Journal of Anaesthesia 58: 732–5.

Scott DB, Lee A, Fagan D et al 1989 Acute toxicity of ropivacaine compared with that of bupivacaine. Anesthesia & Analgesia 69: 563–9.

Tuominen MK, Pere P, Rosenberg PH 1991 Unintentional arterial catheterization and bupivacaine toxicity associated with continuous interscalene brachial plexus block. Anesthesiology 75: 356–8.

Wulf H, Maier C, Schele HH-A et al 1991 Plasma concentrations of bupivacaine after stellate ganglion blockade. Anesthesia & Analgesia 72: 546–8.

Yukioka H, Hayashi IM, Fujimori M 1990 Lidocaine toxicity during general anesthesia. Anesthesia & Analgesia 71: 200–12.

Malignant hyperthermia (see also

Section 1, Malignant hyperthermia)

Nowadays, fulminant MH crisis, which was so common in the early days, will be unusual. The widespread use of monitoring means that the signs of MH are likely to be identified at an early stage. However, many of these signs are nonspecific, so that the problem arises as to how seriously they should be taken, particularly since a decreasing percentage of cases referred to the Leeds Unit for investigation subsequently turn out to be MHS (Ellis et al 1990).

The anaesthetist must be aware, therefore, of the spectrum of signs associated with MH. Should the possibility of MH be entertained during surgery, certain investigations must be undertaken at the time of the event. There is nothing worse for a family (or for subsequent anaesthetists) to be told that an individual could possibly be MH susceptible, when no effort was made at the time to seek evidence of muscle involvement.

Presentation

1. The clinical signs and symptoms of MH can be broadly divided into two:

a) Signs of metabolic stimulation.

b) Signs of abnormal muscle activity.

  However, it should be remembered that there are conditions other than MH that can cause either, or both, of these signs. A combination of metabolic and muscle signs under anaesthesia may occur with Duchenne or Becker muscular dystrophy, spinal muscle atrophy, myotonia congenita, McArdle's disease, and carnitine palmitoyl transferase deficiency.

2. Signs of metabolic stimulation.

a) Hypercarbia. Tachypnoea occurs in a spontaneously breathing patient, whilst in the paralysed patient there is an apparently increased requirement for neuromuscular blockers. Both states initially result from stimulation of respiration by an increasing alveolar CO_2. An increase in $ETCO_2$ is the earliest sign of MH.

b) Metabolic acidosis. In early reports of fulminating cases, an arterial pH of less than 7.0 was not uncommon. Severe acidosis may have been responsible for the

cases in which sudden death occurred unexpectedly in the operating theatre.

c) Arrhythmias.

d) Increase in core temperature; this is a late sign.

e) Hypoxaemia. In the later stages of an MH crisis, cyanosis occurs secondary to the combination of a massive increase in oxygen consumption, and ventilation perfusion defects.

3. Signs of abnormal muscle activity.

a) Failure of the jaw to relax after suxamethonium. An increase in tone in the masseter muscle is a normal response to suxamethonium and in some patients the tension developed may be very marked (Leary & Ellis 1990, Saddler et al 1990). However, it may also be an early sign of MH. Susceptibility to MH was found in about half of a series of 77 patients who developed masseter muscle rigidity (MMR) (Rosenberg & Fletcher 1986). In view of this, it was suggested that any patient who developed MMR after suxamethonium should be assumed to be MHS and anaesthesia terminated. However, a 1% incidence of MMR was found in children receiving halothane and suxamethonium (Carroll 1987) and it soon became apparent that MMR, although occurring frequently in MH, was not exclusive to it. (See also Masseter muscle rigidity.)

b) Rigidity of certain, but not necessarily all, groups of muscles. Although a nonrigid group has been described, it is not yet known whether this is a different biochemical process, or an earlier stage of the same process. A contracture of the muscle actually takes place and, if the process is not aborted, oedema of the muscle, and subsequently ischaemia can develop.

c) Hyperkalaemia, with or without cardiac arrest; potassium may be released in large quantities, particularly after the use of suxamethonium. However, this complication is not exclusive to MH, and can occur with other muscle diseases, particularly the muscular dystrophies. In addition, hyperkalaemia can occur even when suxamethonium has not been given. Hyperkalaemia and cardiac arrest has been reported after inhalation anaesthesia alone in both Duchenne (Chalkiadis & Branch 1990) and Becker muscular dystrophies (Bush & Dubovitz 1991).

d) Myoglobin and potassium may be released in large quantities, sometimes resulting in massive myoglobinuria and renal failure. Myoglobin may be detected in the blood and urine almost immediately, but its transient appearance means that its presence is frequently missed.

e) A greatly elevated serum CK; this may be in excess of $100\,000\,\text{iu}\,\text{l}^{-1}$. Unlike myoglobin, which can be detected almost immediately and is transient in its appearance, the serum CK takes several hours to increase. Often, the maximum blood concentration will not be seen until the following day, and levels will remain elevated for several days after this.

4. Later complications.

a) A coagulopathy may occur in advanced cases, possibly secondary to thromboplastin release.

b) Cerebral and pulmonary oedema may develop.

Management

1. Nowadays, the increased quality of monitoring means that the fulminant case is rarely seen. However, it also means that there is an increase in the number of aborted or doubtful cases. Since the early signs of MH are nonspecific, it is the responsibility of the anaesthetist, should MH be suspected, to gain as much information as possible at the time of the event.

2. What should be done if intraoperative signs occur which are not specific to MH, and are not life-threatening, but raise the suspicion of MH? Under these circumstances, Ellis et al (1990) recommended that attention is paid to the following features.

a) Good record keeping of the time sequence of clinical events:

  i) MMR (duration and degree).

  ii) Presence or absence of generalised rigidity.

  iii) Arrhythmias.

  iv) Tachypnoea with signs of CO_2 production.

  v) Cyanosis.

  vi) Increase in core temperature.

b) Laboratory tests:

  i) Arterial blood gases.

  ii) Serum potassium.

  iii) Initial, 12- and 24-h CK. Serial CK levels taken under these circumstances are very important. Whilst the CK is normally of little diagnostic help in MH, if an anaesthetic has been given which is associated with evidence of hypermetabolism, the serum CK is of considerable value. If the CK is very high, it is likely that the event that occurred was of significance. It may not necessarily be MH, but could be associated with one or another of a variety of myopathies, as mentioned above.

  iv) Evidence of myoglobinuria.

3. If a tentative intraoperative diagnosis of MH is made, the treatment required will depend upon the severity of the reaction at the time of diagnosis. The patient's susceptibility, the promptness of the diagnosis and hence the dose of the triggering agent received, are important factors. With a short exposure and a rapid

diagnosis the syndrome will be aborted by the first measure in 4 (below).

4.   Treatment of established MH.

a)   Stop the use of all MH trigger agents. Terminate surgery if possible. Observe ECG and capnograph. Estimate blood gases.

b)   Delegate one person to prepare dantrolene sodium, 1 mg kg^{-1}.

c)   Record core temperature, pulse rate and blood pressure every 5 min.

d)   Hypercarbia should be treated with hyperventilation.

e)   Treat acidosis with sodium bicarbonate 2–4 mmol kg^{-1}, and oxygenation maintained.

f)   Send venous samples for electrolytes, calcium, and CK.

g)   Give dantrolene sodium iv 1 mg kg^{-1} and repeat, up to 10 mg kg^{-1}.

h)   If the syndrome is severe, treat symptomatically. Institute cooling and treat hyperkalaemia if necessary. Give calcium chloride 10% 10 ml. Give glucose 50% 50 ml with 20 u actrapid insulin. If necessary, follow with an infusion of glucose 20% 1 litre, with insulin 100 u, and infuse at 2 ml kg^{-1}h^{-1}.

i)   Save the first urine sample for myoglobin estimation. Measure urine output. If there is obvious myoglobinuria, give iv fluids, with mannitol or furosemide (frusemide) to reduce the possibility of renal failure.

j)   The use of steroids is debatable. They may be indicated in the severe case, particularly if there is cerebral oedema.

k)   Repeat the serum CK at 24 h.

l)   Treat coagulopathy, if necessary.

m)   The half-life of dantrolene is only 5 h; therefore if retriggering occurs in the first 24 h, it may need to be repeated.

Bibliography

Bush A, Dubowitz V 1991 Fatal rhabdomyolysis complicating general anaesthesia in a child with Becker muscular dystrophy. Neuromuscular Disorders 1: 204–10.

Carroll JB 1987 Increased incidence of masseter spasm in children with strabismus anesthetised with halothane and succinylcholine. Anesthesiology 67: 559–61.

Chalkiadis GA, Branch KG 1990 Cardiac arrest after isoflurane anaesthesia in a patient with Duchenne's muscular dystrophy. Anaesthesia 45: 22–5.

Ellis FR, Halsall PJ 1984 Suxamethonium spasm. British Journal of Anaesthesia 56: 381–4.

Ellis FR, Halsall PJ, Christian AS 1990 Clinical presentation of suspected malignant hyperthermia during anaesthesia in 402 probands. Anaesthesia 45: 838–41.

Leary NP, Ellis FR 1990 Masseteric muscle spasm as a normal response to suxamethonium. British Journal of Anaesthesia 64: 488–92.

Rosenberg H, Fletcher JE 1986 Masseter muscle rigidity and malignant hyperthermia susceptibility. Anaesthesia & Analgesia 65: 161–4.

Saddler JM, Bevan JC, Plumley MH et al 1990 Jaw muscle tension after succinylcholine in children undergoing strabismus surgery. Canadian Journal of Anaesthesia 37: 21–5.

Masseter muscle rigidity (MMR)

Masseter muscle spasm is a clinical diagnosis; it has been defined as jaw tightness to a degree that it interferes with tracheal intubation, and occurs despite usually adequate doses of suxamethonium (Saddler et al 1990). Since MMR occurs in 50% of patients who are MHS, it was assumed to be an exclusive sign presaging an MH crisis. However, it is now known that an increase in masseter muscle tone may be a normal response to suxamethonium.

In a study of 50 healthy patients, the majority showed myotonia which lasted for less than 100 s (Leary & Ellis 1990). In about 40%, the maximum tone was greater than 500 g, and in 1% it was greater than 1 kg. On occasions, the rigidity can last several minutes, and may be such that the jaw can barely be opened. Intubation may temporarily be impossible, although ventilation on a mask is usually feasible. A similar situation was found in studies on eight patients having squint surgery (Saddler et al 1990). At the same time, an increase in tension, but to a lesser degree, was found in the adductor pollicis muscles. This hypertonus is more likely to occur in young patients, particularly if a volatile agent has been given before the suxamethonium. Most of these individuals will have a minor degree of rhabdomyolysis, as evidenced by an increase in serum CK level. The masseter spasm may be associated with ventricular arrhythmias and myoglobinuria.

Thus, although MMR is certainly one sign of MH, and features in a high proportion of patients subsequently found to be MHS, transient MMR commonly occurs in normal patients, and is severe in about 1% of the population. As a result, the significance of MMR, and its subsequent management if it occurs, has been a controversial subject.

Previously, it was assumed that since a proportion of cases would be associated with MH, anaesthesia should be stopped, or the drugs used should be changed to nontriggering agents. The masseter muscle is known to contain a unique form of myosin. This may explain the localisation of the spasm to the jaw muscles (Fletcher 1987).

The controversies

1. *MMR as normal response to suxamethonium.* Two studies claim that masseter spasm occurs in as many as 1% of children after halothane induction followed by suxamethonium administration (Schwartz et al 1984, Carroll 1987). Littleford et al (1991), in a study of 42 000 anaesthetics over a 10-year period, found that it occurred in 0.3% of inhalational anaesthetics in which suxamethonium was given. They found no morbidity or mortality in 57 children who developed isolated MMR and suggested that anaesthesia can continue in the presence of this sign. However, this is controversial. The discrepancy between these figures, and the 50% incidence of MHS with MMR, was difficult to

explain. A difference in definition of MMR may have contributed (Rosenberg 1987). MMR is a situation in which the jaw can hardly be opened, even with considerable effort by the anaesthetist. This situation, which is rare, must be differentiated from a mere increase in muscle tone, which is common among children (van der Spek et al 1987) and passes off fairly rapidly. In addition, those referred to a centre for screening are likely to have been a selected group of patients who had additional signs of MH.

2. *MMR associated with malignant hyperthermia.* The exact percentage of patients with MMR found subsequently to be MH susceptible (MHS) varies with the studies reported. One claimed an incidence of 100% in 15 patients (Schwartz et al 1984). However the diagnosis of MH was made on the basis of a sarcoplasmic reticulum calcium uptake test. This had not been accepted as diagnostic by a number of workers in the field, and an incidence as high as this was therefore disputed (Ellis & Halsall 1986).

Using caffeine and halothane contracture tests, other workers have found the incidence to be between 40% and 60%. Nearly 50% of 77 patients who had developed MMR after suxamethonium were found to be MHS using these tests (Rosenberg & Fletcher 1986). Another study reported four out of six boys with isolated MMR to be MHS (Flewellen & Nelson 1984).

Muscle rigidity, not necessarily of the masseter alone, is a common feature in MH episodes. It appeared in about 80% of MHS patients studied by Britt and Kalow (1970). In 31 out of 75 patients, MH episodes with muscle rigidity occurred after the use of suxamethonium. In another study of 147 patients found to be MHS after referral for investigation (Ellis & Halsall 1984), 65% had responded to suxamethonium with muscle spasm. In 5% of these MHS patients, the suxamethonium spasm was the only sign of MHS.

3. *MMR not associated with malignant hyperthermia but with other muscle disorders.* Further investigations of the group of patients with

MMR who were shown not to be susceptible to malignant hyperthermia (MHN) revealed a small number who had some other myopathy. These included Duchenne and Becker muscle dystrophies and myotonia congenita. The remainder must be assumed to have had abnormal reactions to suxamethonium.

Presentation

1. Administration of suxamethonium is associated with a degree of rigidity of the jaw muscles, such that the patient's mouth can hardly be opened. It may last anywhere between 90 s and several minutes. Sometimes it results in intubation difficulty. A 25 year old involved in major trauma developed masseter muscle spasm after suxamethonium, when tracheal intubation was performed for resuscitation. He was transferred to the operating theatre, and isoflurane was given 2.5 h after suxamethonium, following which an episode of MH was triggered (Ramirez-R et al 1998).

2. Peripheral muscles are usually flaccid, and there is no response to nerve stimulation.

3. The episode may be accompanied by tachycardia or ventricular arrhythmias.

4. Pyrexia can develop subsequently, or the patient may be apyrexial.

5. Myoglobinuria may occur and the serum CK level may be increased and myoglobinuria may occur, within the first 24 h after anaesthesia.

6. Muscle pains, stiffness, and occasionally weakness may last for several days.

7. A small number of patients may proceed to MH, although this may not be immediately clinically obvious.

Management

1. If a patient develops increased masseter muscle tone after suxamethonium, it should be remembered that in the majority of cases, this is a normal reaction. However, rarely, it is an early sign of MH and this should be borne in mind. At present there is no way of distinguishing the types of MMR, except that the 'normal' myotonia usually returns to baseline after 60–90 s (Leary & Ellis 1990), and the patient's lungs can be ventilated with oxygen by mask during this time. Anaesthetists should be wary if the rigidity is particularly severe or prolonged.

2. In the mid-1980s, the profession was divided as to whether or not surgery should be continued if masseter spasm occurred. This author believes that surgery should be continued, with close metabolic and acid–base monitoring, and should only be stopped if signs suggest an abnormal metabolic response, or other signs of muscular involvement occur. If in doubt, an experienced anaesthetist should be consulted.

3. In all cases, heart rate, core temperature, end-tidal CO_2 and blood gas tensions must be measured. At the same time blood should be taken for serum CK and the urine examined for myoglobin.

4. If there is no evidence of hyper-metabolism, it is safe to continue surgery.

5. If there is evidence of hypermetabolism, if the MMR is very severe and prolonged, or if the patient has generalised rigidity, MH should be suspected and elective surgery stopped. If surgery is urgent, a nontriggering technique should be used (propofol/narcotic analgesic/nondepolarising relaxant), and CO_2, temperature and biochemistry closely monitored. If necessary, dantrolene 2.5 mg kg^{-1} may be administered.

6. Postoperative serum CK levels should always be measured. In all patients with MMR, the serum CK is likely to be elevated to some degree. However, in one study, levels above 20 000 iu l^{-1} occurred only in patients found to be MHS, or patients with muscle dystrophy (Rosenberg & Fletcher 1986). The peak serum CK level does not usually occur until the following day.

7. If there is frank myoglobinuria,

intravenous fluids and an osmotic diuretic should be given. Renal function requires monitoring. Myoglobin is present in the blood and urine almost immediately and its appearance may be missed.

8. If any patient shows evidence of both hypermetabolism and muscle signs, they should subsequently be referred for investigation of possible MH. If there is doubt, discussion with an investigating unit is suggested. Ellis et al (1990) have outlined the important information required to elucidate the diagnosis of an event during anaesthesia suspected as being MH. Good record keeping of the clinical events is necessary, including.

a) Duration and degree of MMR.

b) Generalised rigidity.

c) Arrhythmias.

d) Tachypnoea and/or signs of increased CO_2 production.

e) Cyanosis.

f) Increase in core temperature.

g) Arterial blood gases.

h) Serum potassium.

i) Initial, 12- and 24-h serum CK level.

j) Evidence of myoglobinuria.

9. The results of investigations should be clearly conveyed to the patient and recorded in the notes.

Bibliography

Britt BA, Kalow W 1970 Malignant hyperthermia: a statistical review. Canadian Anaesthetists' Society Journal 17: 293–315.

Carroll JB 1987 Increased incidence of masseter spasm in children with strabismus anaesthetised with halothane and succinyl choline. Anesthesiology 67: 559–61.

Ellis FR, Halsall PJ 1984 Suxamethonium spasm. A differential diagnostic conundrum. British Journal of Anaesthesia 56: 381–4.

Ellis FR, Halsall PJ 1986 Improper diagnostic test may account for high incidence of malignant hyperthermia associated with masseter spasm. Anesthesiology 64: 291.

Ellis FR, Halsall PJ, Christian AS 1990 Clinical presentation of suspected malignant hyperthermia during anaesthesia of 402 probands. Anaesthesia 45: 838–41.

Fletcher R 1987 4th International Hyperpyrexia Workshop. Report of a meeting. Anaesthesia 42: 206.

Flewellen EH, Nelson TE 1982 Masseter spasm induced by succinylcholine in children: contracture testing for malignant hyperthermia: report of 6 cases. Canadian Anaesthetists' Society Journal 29: 42–9.

Flewellen EH, Nelson TE 1984 Halothane–succinylcholine induced masseter spasm: indicative of malignant hyperthermia susceptibility? Anesthesia & Analgesia 63: 693–7.

Leary NP, Ellis FR 1990 Masseteric muscle spasm as a normal response to suxamethonium. British Journal of Anaesthesia 64: 488–92.

Littleford JA, Patel LR, Bose D et al 1991 Masseter muscle spasm in children: implications of continuing the triggering anesthetic. Anesthesia & Analgesia 72: 151–60.

Ramirez-R JA, Cheetham ED, Laurence AS et al 1998 Suxamethonium, masseter spasm and later malignant hyperthermia. Anaesthesia 53: 1111–16.

Rosenberg H 1987 Trismus is not trivial. Anesthesiology 67: 453–5.

Rosenberg H, Fletcher JE 1986 Masseter muscle rigidity and malignant hyperthermia susceptibility. Anesthesia & Analgesia 65: 161–4.

Saddler JM, Bevan JC, Plumley MH et al 1990 Jaw muscle tension after succinylcholine in children undergoing strabismus surgery. Canadian Journal of Anaesthesia 37: 21–5.

Schwartz L, Rockoff MA, Koka BV 1984 Masseter spasm and anesthesia: incidence and implications. Anesthesiology 61: 772–5.

van der Spek AFL, Fang WB, Ashton-Miller JA et al 1987 The effect of suxamethonium on mouth opening. Anesthesiology 67: 459–65.

Methaemoglobinaemia

Methaemoglobin is produced when the iron in the haem group of the haemoglobin molecule is oxidised from the ferrous to the ferric form. Methaemoglobin is continuously formed during red cell metabolism, but it is then converted back to reduced Hb. Under normal circumstances, its concentration never exceeds 1%. However, sometimes the capacity of the enzyme system is exceeded. Methaemoglobinaemia is a clinical condition in which more than 1% of the blood has been oxidised to the ferric form. It can arise from:

1. Congenital methaemoglobinaemia due to NADH-diaphorase deficiency. The inheritance is autosomal recessive.

2. Toxic methaemoglobinaemia, which occurs when various drugs or toxic substances oxidise haemoglobin, e.g. aniline and nitrobenzene.

3. Haemoglobin M disease, a form of haemoglobinopathy.

Cyanosis is seen when the level of methaemoglobin exceeds 1.5 g dl^{-1}. In congenital methaemoglobinaemia, the level of methaemoglobin varies between 8% and 40%. In general, 20% of methaemoglobin is required before symptoms occur. Higher levels can be tolerated without symptoms in the congenital condition, as compared with the acute toxic form.

Presentation

1. *Signs and symptoms.* The patient looks cyanosed, his/her actual appearance often being described as a 'slatey grey'. Arterial blood takes on an unusual chocolate brown colour. About 1.5 g dl^{-1} of methaemoglobin causes cyanosis, compared with the 5 g dl^{-1} required for reduced Hb. The diagnosis may also be suspected when unexpectedly low oxygen saturation readings are recorded using a pulse oximeter, in the presence of a normal Pa_{O_2} on a blood gas sample. However, the effect of methaemoglobin on the oximeter reading is complex (Ralston et al 1991). For technical reasons, the presence of MetHb will bias the saturation reading towards 85%, so that either over- or underestimation may occur (Bardoczky et al 1990). Very high MetHb levels will therefore mask profound desaturation (Rieder et al 1989). Carboxyhaemoglobin, and

dyes such as methylene blue, have also caused spurious oximeter readings (Eisenkraft 1988).

2. *Causes in normal subjects.* Methaemoglobinaemia has been reported to have been caused by a variety of substances.

a) Ingestion of aniline or nitrobenzene compounds (Harrison 1977).

b) Prilocaine in doses exceeding 600–900 mg (8 mg kg^{-1}), due to a metabolite, orthotoluidine (Duncan & Kobrinsky 1983, Bardoczky et al 1990). Methaemoglobin levels peak at 60–90 min after administration of prilocaine, but may sometimes be delayed for 6 h.

c) Benzocaine in toxic doses (O'Donohue et al 1980). One adult had a 1-s spray of benzocaine (200 mg) for bronchoscopy. This was repeated 2 h later, after which he became blue and the SpO$_2$ decreased to 84%. The methaemoglobin level was 22.5% (Nguyen et al 2000). Infants and children are particularly susceptible to benzocaine because fetal haemoglobin is more easily oxidised, and they have lower levels of NADH-methaemoglobin reductase, catalase, and glutathione peroxidase (Severinghaus et al 1991).

d) Methylene blue, in doses of >7 mg kg^{-1}, from oxidation of haemoglobin.

e) Treatment with antimalarials.

f) Antileprosy drugs (Mayo et al 1987). One 14 year old took an overdose of 8–9 g dapsone and presented with confusion, agitation, and convulsions. The first MetHb level was in excess of 55% (Ferguson & Lavery 1997).

g) A combination of EMLA cream (prilocaine and lidocaine (lignocaine) and a sulphonamide in a baby (Jakobsen & Nilsson 1985).

3. *Techniques.*

a) 'Three-in-one-block' using prilocaine (Bellamy et al 1992).

b) Brachial plexus block using prilocaine (Marks & Desgrand 1991).

c) During methylene blue infusion for parathyroid location.

d) Axillary block (Schroeder et al 1999).

4. *Metabolic defects with risk of methaemoglobinaemia.*

a) A woman undergoing tubal patency tests with methylene blue developed cyanosis and a SpO_2 reading of 86%, 30 min after injection of the dye. She was subsequently found to have glucose-6-phosphate dehydrogenase deficiency (Bilgin et al 1998).

b) A 17 year old, noted to have an SpO_2 of 92% during anaesthesia, even with 100% oxygen, was found to have congenital methaemoglobinaemia secondary to low levels of the enzyme NADH-diaphorase (Sugahara et al 1998).

Anaesthetic or resuscitative problems

1. The oxygen carrying capacity is reduced, and the oxygen dissociation curve is shifted to the left.

a) 20% MetHb is required before symptoms occur.

b) 20–50% produces tachycardia, giddiness, headache, and dyspnoea.

c) 60–70% or more may be associated with confusion, coma, convulsions, cardiovascular collapse, and death.

d) Unexplained cyanosis may occur. Cyanosis during appendicectomy in a child was subsequently found to be due to dapsone 200 mg, administered to him by his father (Mayo et al 1987). Although methylene blue 1–2 mg kg^{-1} is used in the treatment of methaemoglobinaemia, higher doses may oxidise haemoglobin to methaemoglobin. Thus, a rapid infusion of methylene blue can itself produce transient cyanosis. An infusion of methylene blue 5 mg kg^{-1} is frequently used to assist identification of the parathyroid glands during parathyroid surgery. Studies of the resulting methaemoglobin levels have shown a peak of 7.1% (Whitwam et al 1979) in one, and a range from 4.5% to 17.4% (Lamont et al 1986) in another. The first authors thought that such levels might be dangerous in a patient with haemoglobin M disease, or where there was an abnormality of the hexose monophosphate pathway. The second paper concluded that with normal doses, problems were unlikely.

e) High levels of MetHb may be followed by haemolysis, starting 3–5 days after the event (Ferguson & Lavery 1997).

Management

1. Ascorbic acid 300–600 mg daily can be used for chronic methaemoglobinaemia.

2. If acute symptomatic methaemoglobinaemia occurs, methylene blue 1–2 mg kg^{-1} should be given. This stimulates the relevant reducing enzymes.

Excess methylene blue (>7 mg kg^{-1}) can itself cause methaemoglobinaemia.

3. In cases of severe poisoning with a drug such as dapsone, activated charcoal can be given to bind unabsorbed drug and break its enterohepatic circulation (Ferguson & Lavery 1997). Exchange transfusion may sometimes be required (Harrison 1977).

Bibliography

Bardoczky GI, Wathieu M, D'Hollander A 1990 Prilocaine-induced methemoglobinemia evidenced by pulse oximetry. Acta Anaesthesiologica Scandinavica 34: 162–4.

Bellamy MC, Hopkins PM, Halsall PJ et al 1992 A study into the incidence of methaemoglobinaemia after 'three-in-one' block with prilocaine. Anaesthesia 47: 1084–5.

Bilgin H, Oczam B, Bilgin T 1998
Methemoglobinemia induced by methylene blue
perturbation during laparoscopy. Acta
Anaesthesiologica Scandinavica 42: 594–5.

Duncan P, Kobrinsky N 1983 Prilocaine-induced
methemoglobinemia in a newborn infant.
Anesthesiology 59: 75–6.

Eisenkraft JB 1988 Pulse oximeter desaturation due
to methemoglobinemia. Anesthesiology 68:
279–80.

Ferguson AJ, Lavery GG 1997 Deliberate self-
poisoning with dapsone. A case report and
summary of relevant pharmacology and treatment.
Anaesthesia 52: 359–63.

Harrison MR 1977 Toxic methaemoglobinaemia.
Anaesthesia 32: 270–2.

Jakobsen B, Nilsson A 1985 Methaemoglobinaemia
associated with a prilocaine–lidocaine cream and
trimethoprim–sulphamethazole. Acta
Anaesthesiologica Scandinavica 29: 453–5.

Lamont ASM, Roberts MS, Holdsworth DG et al
1986 Relationship between methaemoglobin
production and methylene blue plasma
concentrations under general anaesthesia.
Anaesthesia & Intensive Care 14: 360–4.

Marks LF, Desgrand D 1991 Prilocaine associated
methaemoglobinaemia and the pulse oximeter.
Anaesthesia 41: 703.

Mayo W, Leighton K, Robertson B et al 1987
Intraoperative cyanosis: a case of dapsone-induced
methaemoglobinaemia. Canadian Journal of
Anaesthesia 34: 79–82.

Nguyen ST, Cabrales RE, Bashour CA 2000
Benzocaine-induced methemoglobinemia.
Anesthesia & Analgesia 90: 369–71.

O'Donohue WJ, Moss LM, Angelillo VA 1980 Acute
methemoglobinemia induced by topical
benzocaine and lidocaine. Archives of Internal
Medicine 1980; 140: 1508–9.

Ralston AC, Webb RK, Runciman WB 1991 Potential
errors in pulse oximetry. III: Effects of interference,
dyes, dyshaemoglobins and other pigments.
Anaesthesia 46: 291–5.

Rieder HU, Frei FJ, Zbinden AM, Thomson DA 1989
Pulse oximetry in methaemoglobinaemia.
Anaesthesia 44: 326–7.

Schroeder TH, Dieterich HJ, Muhlbauer B 1999
Methemoglobinemia after axillary block with
bupivacaine and additional injection of lidocaine in
the operative field. Acta Anaesthesiologica
Scandinavica 43: 480–2.

Severinghaus JW, Xu F-D, Spellman MJ 1991

Benzocaine and methemoglobinemia:
recommended actions. Anesthesiology 74: 385–6.

Sugahara K, Sadohara T, Kawaguchi T et al 1998
NADH-diaphorase deficiency identified in a
patient with congenital methemoglobinaemia
detected by pulse oximetry. Intensive Care
Medicine 24: 706–8.

Whitwam JG, Taylor AR, White JM 1979 Potential
hazard of methylene blue. Anaesthesia 34: 181–2.

Phaeochromocytoma

Patients with unsuspected phaeochromocytoma may undergo anaesthesia for surgical, investigative or obstetric procedures. The danger of this situation is underlined by the results of a study of 54 patients in whom tumours were shown at autopsy. These had been clinically unsuspected prior to the event leading to death, or were only diagnosed postmortem (Sutton et al 1981). One-third of these patients had died suddenly during, or immediately after, minor operations for unrelated conditions. Death was associated with either hypotensive or hypertensive crises. With the passage of years, the situation has changed little. A retrospective survey of 62 death certificates registering phaeochromocytoma as a cause of death between 1981 and 1989, showed that in only 17 patients was the diagnosis made before death, and 16 had undergone surgery in the previous week (Platts et al 1995).

Severe complications may occur with remarkable rapidity. If disaster is to be averted, the anaesthetist must be aware of the possibility of the diagnosis, the detailed pharmacology of the condition, and the correct method of treatment. Tachycardia treated blindly with beta blockers may result in extreme hypertension (Ambesh 1999). Patients are at risk from cerebral haemorrhage, encephalopathy, pulmonary oedema, myocardial infarction, ventricular fibrillation, or renal failure. Phaeochromocytoma during pregnancy carries a particularly bad prognosis. A maternal mortality of 48% and a fetal mortality of 55% have been reported (Mitchell et al 1987). Crises may also occur after drugs, chemotherapy, tumour embolisation (Quezado et al 1992) and angiography (Brueckel & Boehm 1998).

The most frequent preoperative clinical features are episodes of headache, pallor, palpitations, and sweating. In the series of autopsies reported by Platts et al (1995), typical symptoms of phaeochromocytoma had been present for more than 3 months prior to death in 61%. Patients may have an unusually labile blood pressure and a pressor response to the induction of anaesthesia. One patient, who developed major cardiovascular complications during surgery for cerebral arteriovenous malformation, was found to have had a series of potentially life-threatening events over a 20-year period (Jones et al 1999).

Beware of surgery for apparently asymptomatic 'nonfunctioning' adrenal tumours (adrenalomas) diagnosed incidentally on CT scan. A patient with negative VMA screening and a normal mIBG scan developed a systolic arterial pressure in excess of 250 mmHg during creation of the pneumoperitoneum. High levels of plasma catecholamines confirmed an active tumour (Harioka et al 1999). In a series of 57 patients with adrenalomas, four turned out to be phaeochromocytomas (Linos et al 1996).

Presentation

1. *Blood pressure changes.* Severe hypertension or severe hypotension during the perioperative period (Bittar 1979, 1982, Jones & Hill 1981, Sutton et al 1981, Wooster & Mitchell 1981, Voros et al 1996). However, the classical signs are not always present and sometimes they are masked by other pathology. Several cases have been reported following cardiopulmonary bypass (Brown & Caplan 1986, Fenje et al 1989). An unexpected bladder tumour revealed itself as intermittent hypertension and bradycardia during cystoscopy (Takimoto & Ueda 1995).

2. *Tachyarrhythmias.* A patient with an abdominal mass, high output left ventricular failure and hypertension underwent laparotomy.

Severe cardiovascular instability was treated with practolol and phentolamine. Massive blood loss was reduced by means of sodium nitroprusside. Direct arterial and pulmonary artery pressure monitoring helped cardiovascular control. Subsequent histology confirmed a phaeochromocytoma (Darby & Prys-Roberts 1976).

3. *Acute pulmonary oedema.* This has been described in several cases (Greaves & Barrow 1989, Jones et al 1999). A 43-year-old man, with a history of attacks of sweating and palpitations, was admitted to ITU with pulmonary oedema and shock (Blom et al 1987). He was treated with IPPV and cardiovascular monitoring. Biochemistry indicated a predominantly epinephrine- (adrenaline-) secreting phaeochromocytoma. A 39-year-old woman developed abdominal pain, hypertension, tachycardia and pulmonary oedema immediately after vaginal hysterectomy (Fahmy et al 1997).

4. *Myocardial depression and cardiogenic shock.* Segmental ST changes after massive catecholamine release in two patients with metastatic phaeochromocytoma have been described (Quezado et al 1992). In both, high levels of all three catecholamines were found, and, as levels decreased, haemodynamic function improved. In one, the episode had been precipitated by an injection of metoclopramide, whilst the second occurred 24 h after embolisation of the right superior gluteal artery. Both had large tumours. Cardiac arrest and multiorgan failure occurred in a male following knee arthroscopy (Cooper & Mihm 1999). Myocardial infarction and death followed Caesarean section in a patient with both phaeochromocytoma and protein S deficiency (Zangrillo et al 1999).

5. *Events during pregnancy.* Phaeochromocytomas presenting in pregnancy are associated with a high mortality. The condition may be forgotten, or misdiagnosed as preeclampsia. One actually presented with a convulsion and the diagnosis was only made at autopsy (Harper et al 1989). Intra- or postoperative tachycardia, hypotension,

pulmonary oedema and death are the commonest modes of presentation (Sardesai et al 1990). Tachycardia and gross pulmonary oedema occurred on extubation at the end of a Caesarean section, in a patient with preeclampsia. Death occurred 3 days later, and the diagnosis was only made at autopsy (personal communication). Severe neck and facial oedema accompanied by hypertension occurred after Caesarean section under epidural anaesthesia for 'preeclampsia' (Botchan et al 1995).

6. *An acute abdominal emergency.* Haemorrhagic necrosis of the tumour mimicked an acute abdominal emergency in two cases (Jones & Durning 1985). One patient developed pulmonary oedema after induction, and surgery was abandoned. The second developed a tachycardia of 180 beat min^{-1} and an unrecordable BP during surgery. Both died postoperatively. Acute abdominal pain and severe respiratory distress was the presenting feature in a patient with a ruptured haemorrhagic phaeochromocytoma (Spencer et al 1993).

7. *As a mimic of malignant hyperthermia.* Hypertension, tachycardia, pyrexia, acidosis, hypoxaemia and cardiac arrest occurred perioperatively in a patient undergoing cholecystectomy. The patient survived and subsequently underwent surgical removal of the tumour (Crowley et al 1988, Allen & Rosenberg 1990).

8. *As a mimic of a thyroid crisis.* A 29 year old presented with clinical hyperthyroidism, which was treated with carbimazole and atenolol. Thyroidectomy was planned when she became euthyroid, but hypertension and tachycardia occurred after induction of anaesthesia. Propranolol 2 mg precipitated a pressure of 240/148 and severe systemic vasconstriction, so surgery was postponed. The pressures were only finally controlled using nitroprusside and glyceryl trinitrate infusions. Plasma catecholamine levels and a CT scan confirmed a right adrenal tumour (Ambesh 1999).

9. *Multiorgan failure.* Rarely, phaeochromocytoma presents as a crisis with

multiple system organ failure, hyperthermia, encephalopathy, and hyper- or hypotension (Newell et al 1988).

10. *Crisis after beta blockers.* This has occurred when beta blockers have been given alone, sometimes despite the diagnosis having been made (Sheaves et al 1995). The first patient, who had been given a slow-release preparation of propranol in outpatients after confirmation of the tumour, was admitted to hospital cold, clammy and delirious, with extreme blood pressure lability. During treatment she developed a dense hemiplegia and never regained consciousness. A second patient had palpitations, anxiety and headaches whilst receiving atenolol and nifedipine for hypertension. He developed chest pain, and whilst on the CCU was given a labetalol infusion. Severe hypertension developed 5 min later and he had a seizure.

11. *Other presentations.* Bilateral dilated, nonreactive pupils, accompanied by only moderate cardiovascular changes, were the only signs of a phaeochromocytoma in a patient undergoing nephrectomy for renal cell carcinoma (Larson & Herman 1992). The possibility of phaeochromocytoma was suspected (and later confirmed), therefore appropriate management was instituted.

Management

1. Incidental surgery in a patient with an undiagnosed phaeochromoytoma carries a high mortality. The patient's best chance of survival lies in the early recognition of the condition, cessation of the proceedings, and admission to an ITU for haemodynamic monitoring (Smith et al 1978).

2. Phentolamine, phenoxybenzamine and sodium nitroprusside have all been used to control hypertension. Magnesium sulphate has been used in a pregnant patient (James et al 1988). Magnesium is known to inhibit catecholamine release from the adrenal medulla, to decrease the sensitivity of the alpha adrenoceptors to catecholamines, and to cause

vasodilatation. A bolus of magnesium sulphate iv 4 g over 15 min was used, followed by an infusion of $1.5\,g\,h^{-1}$.

3. If hypotension occurs, phenylephrine or dopamine have been suggested as the most appropriate agents to use (Roizen et al 1982). Aggressive ITU support, invasive monitoring, and treatment with alpha and beta adrenoceptor antagonists for cardiogenic shock, are required.

4. Beta blockers should only be used to treat a tachycardia after alpha blockers have been given.

Bibliography

Allen GC, Rosenberg H 1990 Phaeochromocytoma presenting as acute malignant hyperthermia—a diagnostic challenge. Canadian Journal of Anaesthesia 37: 593–5.

Ambesh SP 1993 Occult pheochromocytoma in association with hyperthyroidism presenting under general anesthesia. Anesthesia & Analgesia 77: 1074–6.

Bittar DA 1979 Innovar-induced hypertensive crises in patients with pheochromocytoma. Anesthesiology 50: 366–9.

Bittar DA 1982 Unsuspected phaeochromocytoma. Canadian Anaesthetists' Society Journal 29: 183–4.

Blom HJ, Karsdop V, Birnie R et al 1987 Phaeochromocytoma as a cause of pulmonary oedema. Anaesthesia 42: 646–50.

Botchan A, Hauser R, Kupfermine M et al 1995 Pheochromocytoma in pregnancy: case report and review of the literature. Obstetrical & Gynecological Survey 50: 321–7.

Brown P, Caplan RA 1986 Recognition of an unsuspected phaeochromocytoma during elective coronary artery bypass surgery. Canadian Anaesthetists' Society Journal 33: 785–9.

Brueckel J, Boehm BO 1998 Crisis after angiography. Lancet 352: 1940.

Cooper ZA, Mihm FG 1999 Blood pressure control with fenoldopam during excision of a pheochromocytoma. Anesthesiology 91: 558–60.

Crowley KJ, Cunningham AJ, Conroy B et al 1988 Phaeochromocytoma—a presentation mimicking malignant hyperthermia. Anaesthesia 43: 1031–2.

Darby E, Prys-Roberts C 1976 Unusual presentation of phaeochromocytoma. Management of anaesthesia and cardiovascular monitoring. Anaesthesia 31: 913–16.

Fahmy N, Assaad M, Bathija P et al 1997 Postoperative pulmonary edema: a rare presentation of pheochromocytoma. Clinical Nephrology 48: 122–4.

Fenje N, Lee LW, Jamieson WRE et al 1989 Phaeochromocytoma and mitral valve replacement. Canadian Journal of Anaesthesia 36: 198–9.

Greaves DJ, Barrow PM 1989 Emergency resection of phaeochromocytoma presenting with hyperamylasaemia and pulmonary oedema. Anaesthesia 44: 841–2.

Harioka T, Nomura K, Hosoi S et al 1999 Laparoscopic resection of unsuspected pheochromocytoma. Anesthesia & Analgesia 89: 1068.

Harper MA, Murnaghan GA, Kennedy L et al 1989 Phaeochromocytoma in pregnancy. Five cases and a review of the literature. British Journal of Obstetrics & Gynaecology 96: 594–606.

James MFM, Huddle KRL, Owen AD et al 1988 Use of magnesium sulphate in the anaesthetic management of phaeochromocytoma in pregnancy. Canadian Journal of Anaesthesia 35: 178–82.

Jones DJ, Durning P 1985 Phaeochromocytoma presenting as an acute abdomen: report of two cases. British Medical Journal 291: 1267–9.

Jones RM, Hill AB 1981 Severe hypertension associated with pancuronium in a patient with a phaeochromocytoma. Canadian Anaesthetists' Society Journal 28: 394–6.

Jones SE, Redfern N, Shaw IH et al 1999 Exaggerated cardiovascular response to anaesthesia—a case for investigation. Anaesthesia 54: 882–4.

Larson MD, Herman WC 1992 Bilateral dilated nonreactive pupils during surgery in a patient with undiagnosed pheochromocytoma. Anesthesiology 77: 200–2.

Linos DA, Stylopoulos N, Raptis SA 1996 Adrenaloma: a call for more aggressive treatment. World Journal of Surgery 20: 788–93.

Mitchell SZ, Freilich JD, Brant D et al 1987 Anesthetic management of pheochromocytoma resection during pregnancy. Anesthesia & Analgesia 66: 478–80.

Newell KA, Prinz RA, Pickleman J et al 1988 Pheochromocytoma multisystem crisis. Archives of Surgery 123: 956–9.

Platts JK, Drew PJ, Harvey JN 1995 Death from phaeochromocytoma: lessons from a post-mortem survey. Journal of the Royal College of Physicians 29: 299–306.

Quezado ZN, Keiser HR, Parker MM 1992

Reversible myocardial depression after massive catecholamine release from pheochromocytoma. Critical Care Medicine 20: 549–51.

Roizen MF, Horrigan RW, Koike M et al 1982 A prospective randomised trial of 4 anaesthetic techniques for resection of pheochromocytoma. Anesthesiology 57: A43.

Sardesai SH, Mourant AJ, Sivathandon Y et al 1990 Phaeochromocytoma and catecholamine-induced cardiomyopathy presenting as heart failure. British Heart Journal 63: 234–7.

Sheaves R, Chew SL, Grossman AB 1995 The dangers of unopposed beta-adrenergic blockade in phaeochromocytoma. Postgraduate Medical Journal 71: 58–9.

Smith DS, Aukberg SM, Levit JD 1978 Induction of anesthesia in a patient with undiagnosed pheochromocytoma. Anesthesiology 49: 368–9.

Spencer E, Pycock C, Lytle J 1993 Phaeochromocytoma presenting as acute circulatory collapse and abdominal pain. Intensive Care Medicine 19: 356–7.

Sutton MStJ, Sheps SG, Lie JT 1981 Prevalence of clinically unsuspected pheochromocytoma. Mayo Clinic Proceedings 56: 354–60.

Takimoto E, Udea W 1995 Unsuspected pheochromocytoma of the urinary bladder. Anesthesia & Analgesia 80: 1243–4.

Voros DC, Smyrniotis B, Argyra E et al 1996 Undiagnosed phaeochromocytoma in the perioperative period. European Journal of Surgery 162: 985–7.

Wooster L, Mitchell RI 1981 Unsuspected phaeochromocytoma presenting during surgery. Canadian Anaesthetists' Society Journal 28: 471–4.

Zangrillo A, Valentini G, Casati A et al 1999 Myocardial infarction and death after cesarean section in a woman with protein S deficiency and undiagnosed pheochromocytoma. European Journal of Anaesthesiology 16: 268–70.

Pituitary apoplexy (see also Section 1 for detailed review)

A complication of a previously undiagnosed pituitary adenoma caused by its sudden enlargement, usually as a result of spontaneous haemorrhage into the adenoma, or tumour infarction (Editorial 1986, Lewin et al 1988). Pituitary adenomas may be susceptible to infarction because of compromised blood supply of abnormal tumour vessels, and the nature of the pituitary blood supply. Symptoms may be related to compression of optic chiasma and other structures around the sella, or can be associated with hormonal disturbances. A number of precipitating factors have been identified, of which anaesthesia and surgery are two.

Presentation

1. Headache, visual disturbances, ophthalmoplegias, and impaired conscious level. May present with meningism and blood in the CSF and can be difficult to distinguish from subarachnoid haemorrhage. The majority of perioperative cases have occurred after coronary artery bypass surgery (Shapiro 1990), possibly because of the nonpulsatile flow and decreased perfusion pressure on bypass. However, pituitary apoplexy has been reported after cholecystectomy under combined GA and epidural anaesthesia (Yahagi et al 1992), and total hip replacement under spinal anaesthesia (Lennon et al 1998).

2. Onset of symptoms have varied from immediately (Meek et al 1998) to 3 weeks after surgery (Wiesmann et al 1999).

3. Endocrine disturbances, usually mild, either due to the adenoma, or secondary to pituitary or hypothalamic damage. Multiple pituitary hormone deficiencies may occur.

4. Diagnosis by CT scan or MRI.

5. The differential diagnosis includes SAH (subarachnoid haemorrhage), brain abscess, and cavernous sinus thrombosis.

Management

1. Suspicion of pituitary apoplexy should be aroused if, in the perioperative period, a patient develops unusual symptoms and signs, referable to the cranial nerves.

2. A neurological opinion should be sought; CT scan, or MRI will confirm the diagnosis.

3. Early diagnosis and urgent surgical decompression may be needed, although conservative management has been described.

4. Check endocrine function; disturbances may be mild. Treat any hypopituitarism.

Bibliography

Editorial 1986 Pituitary tumours and the empty sella syndrome. Lancet ii: 1371–2.

Lennon M, Seigne P, Cunningham AJ 1998 Pituitary apoplexy after spinal anaesthesia. British Journal of Anaesthesia 81: 616–18.

Lewin IG, Mohan J, Norman PF et al 1988 Pituitary apoplexy. British Medical Journal 297: 1526–7.

Meek EN, Butterworth J, Kon ND et al 1998 Pituitary apoplexy following mitral valve repair. Anesthesiology 89: 1580–2.

Shapiro LM 1990 Pituitary apoplexy following coronary artery bypass surgery. Journal of Surgical Oncology 44: 66–8.

Wiesmann M, Gliemroth J, Kehler U et al 1999 Pituitary apoplexy after cardiac surgery presenting as deep coma with dilated pupils. Acta Anaesthesiologica Scandinavica 43: 236–8.

Yahagi N, Nishikawa A, Matsui S et al 1992 Pituitary apoplexy following cholecystectomy. Anaesthesia 47: 234–6.

Pulmonary oedema (see Section 1)

Subdural block (accidental)

The subdural space is a potential space, between the arachnoid mater and the dura mater, which contains minimal amounts of serous lubricating fluid. It extends from L2 into the cranial cavity, and runs for a short distance along the spinal and cranial nerves. Autopsy studies have confirmed the fact that it is possible to open up the subdural space with saline, using either a Tuohy needle or an epidural catheter (Blomberg 1987). During myelography an incidence of subdural injection as high as 13% has been reported, occasionally with extensive spread of contrast material the whole length of the subdural space. The spread is extensive presumably because the space has a limited capacity and the injected fluid cannot escape. Accidental subdural injection may therefore be associated with either spinal or epidural anaesthesia.

The incidence after spinal anaesthesia is about 7%, and subdural injection may account for the so-called 'failed spinal'.

During epidural anaesthesia, the incidence of penetration of the subdural space is much lower, and is estimated to be 0.05–1.125%. In a study of 2182 patients having epidural analgesia, 0.82% of patients met the criteria for subdural block (Lubenow et al 1988). The signs and symptoms produced can vary widely, although the chief features are those of a more extensive block than would normally be expected for the dose of local anaesthetic given, but in the presence of a negative aspiration test. The presentation presumably depends upon the site of the catheter, the precise distribution of the local anaesthetic, its volume and concentration, and the force with which the anaesthetic has been injected.

Several papers have included X-rays, CT or MRI scans, to show the distribution of contrast injected through misplaced catheters (Ralph & Williams 1996). Since there is potentially more capacity posteriorly and laterally in the subdural space, a sensory block is more likely to occur, and significant motor and sympathetic blockade is rare. However, the subsequent positioning of the patient may influence the symptoms and signs (McMenemin et al 1992). Clinical signs of mixed blocks may occur, and CT scans have also shown evidence of spread within both the epidural and subdural spaces. If motor blockade does occur, it seems either to be associated with the use of larger volumes, or more concentrated solutions, or a mixed block.

Reynolds and Speedy (1991) suggest that there are nine possible sequelae when a catheter is passed through a needle that has penetrated the dura. They believe that this may account not only for the typical delayed onset and the profound and extensive conduction blockade, but also for a series of other unexplained features. Radio-opaque dye introduced into 100 catheters thought to be in the epidural space showed that 17 were just outside the spinal canal, or only partly in the space (Mehta & Salmon 1985).

Presentation

1. Extensive segmental spread of local anaesthetic following an epidural block in the presence of a negative aspiration test. Slow, progressive ascent of signs from 15 min for up to 1.5 h. There is less of a reduction in systemic blood pressure than would be expected with spinal anaesthesia, and the hypotension is easy to control. The sensory block extends high, but sacral sensation is retained (Morgan 1990). Occasionally a motor block occurs (Soni & Holland 1981), but this is relatively unusual. Progressive respiratory depression may occur. There is usually complete recovery in 2 h, although one patient who received 20 ml of a 1.5% lidocaine (lignocaine) and 0.5% bupivacaine mixture developed a rapid, extensive bilateral motor block up to C2 and required IPPV for 3 h. Dye spread into both epidural and subdural spaces (Chauhan et al 1995).

2. The volume of local anaesthetic in the subdural space may lead to compression of the dural contents (Reynolds & Speedy 1991, McMenemin et al 1992, Tripathi et al 1997). This second paper reported a patient in whom frontal headache occurred on injection of local anaesthetic, and this was followed by the development of atypical signs. A subsequent CT scan with contrast showed the catheter lying anteriorly within the spinal canal, and a long posterior fluid level, clearly influenced by gravity, with pooling at the most dependent level. An axial scan at T7 showed anterior displacement of the spinal cord within the subarachnoid space by the contrast. The authors considered that such displacement could potentially produce direct spinal cord damage, or indirect damage from ischaemia resulting from pressure on a vessel. They suggested that subdural injection might account for the occasional reports of permanent nerve damage following epidural analgesia.

3. A predominantly unilateral block occurs in some patients (Brindle-Smith et al 1984). Total unilateral (left-sided) analgesia occurred in one patient, and injection of 2 ml of a contrast material showed it ascending within the left lateral subdural space, with minimal spread to the right side, or caudal to the site of entry of the catheter (Manchanda et al 1983).

4. Although the aspiration test is usually negative, if the bevel of the needle straddles the subdural and subarachnoid spaces, CSF may be obtained (Stevens & Stanton-Hicks 1985).

5. The incidence of subdural block may be increased by dural tears (caused by a preceding lumbar puncture, a spinal anaesthetic, or dural puncture), rotation of the needle, catheter stiffness, or intermittent advancement of the needle using loss of resistance to air.

6. Often there has been a failure to use a test dose, or to fractionate the local anaesthetic (Collier 1992), although one paper showed that test doses of local anaesthetic do not consistently identify misplaced catheters (Crosby & Halpern 1989).

7. It is possible to perform surgery successfully with a subdural block. One patient had an adequate sensory level after epidural blockade, but no demonstrable motor block. Subsequently, injection of radio-opaque dye showed a typical subdural distribution (Gershon 1996). Injection of morphine 2–3 mg has been reported in three gravid patients in whom subdural placement of the catheter was subsequently confirmed radiologically (Chadwick et al 1992). Although there were atypical signs during the development of the block, anaesthesia for Caesarean section and postoperative opiate analgesia were successful in each case. In no patient did signs of opiate respiratory depression occur.

8. Occasionally, if the local anaesthetic reaches the cranial nerves, pupillary dilatation, trigeminal nerve block and respiratory depression occurs.

9. Following successful epidural blockade, migration of the catheter into the subdural space can occur (Abouleish & Goldstein 1986).

10. Multihole epidural catheters may straddle the epidural and subdural spaces, resulting in spread of local anaesthetic to both, thus giving a multicompartmental block (Sala-Blanch et al 1996).

11. Catheters placed accidentally within the subdural space can enter the subarachnoid space. One patient who had an initial apparently normal response to a therapeutic epidural injection developed dyspnoea, drowsiness, hand and facial numbness, and nystagmus after a second dose. The remainder of labour was managed using only small doses of bupivacaine (2 ml 0.25%) at each top-up. A CT scan with contrast subsequently showed the dye only within the subdural and subarachnoid spaces, whilst the epidural space was contrast free. It was assumed the catheter had originally been sited subdurally, and only later had arachnoid rupture occurred (Elliott et al 1996).

Diagnosis

1. Accidental subdural placement should be suspected if abnormal symptoms and signs follow epidural analgesia, particularly if a more extensive block than expected is obtained.

2. The emergence of free fluid dribbling from the catheter may suggest subdural injection. This occurred in one patient who developed high neurological signs following a second dose. The pressure was 36 mmHg and slow aspiration of 7 ml fluid (shown not to be CSF by the absence of glucose) promptly reversed the excessive blockade (Tripathi et al 1997). The authors suggested a mechanical rather than a pharmacological cause for the neurological signs.

3. Injection of contrast medium into the catheter will show a characteristic 'string of beads' dorsally and laterally around the nerve roots, with a 'railroad track' appearance on the anteroposterior view.

4. A range of findings on CT scan have been shown (Dake et al 1986, McMenemin et al 1992).

Management

1. Inadvertent subdural block is difficult to detect; however, the incidence may be reduced by the application of constant pressure to the plunger of a saline-filled syringe, so that the dura is pushed away.

2. Appropriately trained staff, who can recognise the signs of abnormal placement of an epidural catheter and treat the resulting complications, must be present at all times.

3. Symptomatic treatment for hypotension or respiratory depression. Oxygen, tracheal intubation and IPPV may sometimes be required (Abouleish & Goldstein 1986).

4. Alternative forms of analgesia must be given, although satisfactory anaesthesia is produced on occasions (Chadwick et al 1992, Gershon 1996).

5. The catheter should be removed, with or without performing an X-ray to confirm misplacement. Although some authors have left the catheter in place for further analgesia, this strategy is potentially hazardous, because complications may be unpredictable (Bell & Taylor 1994), and rupture can occur through the arachnoid. In such circumstances, total spinal blockade may occur and there is the likelihood of developing postdural puncture headache (Scrutton et al 1996).

Bibliography

Abouleish E, Goldstein M 1986 Migration of an extradural catheter into the subdural space. A case report. British Journal of Anaesthesia 58: 1194–7.

Bell GT, Taylor JC 1994 Subdural block—further points. Anaesthesia 49: 794–5.

Blomberg RG 1987 The lumbar subdural extra-arachnoid space of humans; an anatomical study using spinaloscopy in autopsy cases. Anesthesia & Analgesia 66: 177–80.

Brindle-Smith G, Barton FL, Watt JH 1984 Extensive spread of local anaesthetic solution following subdural insertion of an epidural catheter during labour. Anaesthesia 39: 355–8.

Chadwick HS, Bernards CM, Kovarik DW et al 1992 Subdural injection of morphine for analgesia for Cesarean section: a report of three cases. Anesthesiology 77: 590–4.

Chauhan S, Gaur A, Tripathi M et al 1995 Unintentional combined epidural and subdural block: case report. Regional Anesthesia 20: 249–51.

Collier CB 1992 Accidental subdural block: four more cases and a radiographic review. Anaesthesia & Intensive Care 20: 215–32.

Crosby ET, Halpern S 1989 Failure of a lidocaine test dose to identify subdural placement of an epidural catheter. Canadian Journal of Anaesthesia 36: 445–7.

Dake MD, Dillon WP, Dowart RH 1986 CT of extraarachnoid metrizamide installation. American Journal of Roentgenology 147: 583–6.

Elliott DW, Voyvodic F, Brownridge P 1996 Sudden onset of subarachnoid block after subdural catheterization: a case of arachnoid rupture? British Journal of Anaesthesia 76: 322–4.

Gershon RY 1996 Surgical anaesthesia for Caesarean section with a subdural catheter. Canadian Journal of Anaesthesia 43: 1068–71.

Lee A, Dodd KW 1986 Accidental subdural catheterisation. Anaesthesia 41: 847–9.

Lubenow T, Keh-Wong E, Kristof K et al 1988 Inadvertent subdural injection: a complication of an epidural block. Anesthesia & Analgesia 67: 175–9.

McMenemin IM, Sissons GRJ, Brownridge P 1992 Accidental subdural catheterization: radiological evidence of a possible mechanism for spinal cord damage. British Journal of Anaesthesia 69: 417–19.

Manchanda VN, Murad SHN, Shilyansky G et al 1983 Unusual clinical course of accidental subdural local anesthetic injection. Anesthesia & Analgesia 62: 1124–6.

Mehta M, Salmon N 1985 Extradural block, confirmation of the injection site by X-ray monitoring. Anaesthesia 40: 1009–12.

Morgan B 1990 Unexpectedly extensive conduction blocks in obstetric analgesia. Anaesthesia 45: 148–52.

Ralph CJ, Williams MP 1996 Subdural or epidural? Confirmation with magnetic resonance imaging. Anaesthesia 51: 175–7.

Reynolds F, Speedy HM 1991 The subdural space: the third place to go astray. Anaesthesia 45: 120–3.

Sala-Blanch X, Martinez-Palli G, Agusti-Lasus M et al 1996 Misplacement of multihole epidural catheters—a report of two cases. Anaesthesia 51: 386–8.

Scrutton M, Porter J, Russell R et al 1995 Subdural or epidural? Anaesthesia 51: 708–9.

Soni N, Holland R 1981 An extensive lumbar epidural block. Anaesthesia & Intensive Care 9: 150–3.

Stevens RA, Stanton-Hicks MA 1985 Subdural injection of local anesthetic: a complication of epidural anesthesia. Anesthesiology 63: 323–6.

Tripathi M, Babo N, Gaur A et al 1997 Accidental subdural injection of local anaesthetic: diagnosis by pressure measurement and response to aspiration of injectate. European Journal of Anaesthesiology 14: 455–7.

Suxamethonium apnoea (see also Section 1, Plasma cholinesterase abnormalities)

Prolonged apnoea and neuromuscular blockade may occur following the administration of suxamethonium or mivacurium, either from the presence of a genetic variant of plasma cholinesterase, or as a result of low levels of the normal enzyme. Plasma cholinesterase levels decrease during pregnancy and do not return to normal until 6 weeks postpartum (Davis et al 1997). Since cocaine is metabolised by plasma cholinesterase, the individual with a deficiency is more susceptible to the toxic effects of cocaine.

Presentation

1. During anaesthesia, spontaneous respiration fails to return after suxamethonium or mivacurium have been given in normal clinical doses. Mivacurium, a synthetic, nondepolarising blocker, is metabolised by plasma cholinesterase, and the rate of hydrolysis is about 70–88% that of suxamethonium. Duration of action is therefore increased in those with reduced plasma cholinesterase activity. Doses as low as 0.03 mg kg^{-1} have caused prolonged response in patients homozygous for the atypical gene (Ostergaard et al 1995). Lengths of apnoea recorded with doses of 0.12–0.2 mg kg^{-1} vary from 3 h in a heterozygous patient to 8 h in a homozygous patient.

2. During pregnancy, there is a decrease in plasma cholinesterase activity of about 20% in the first trimester, and values do not return to normal until about 6 weeks after delivery (Davis et al 1997). Thus, pregnancy may result in prolonged apnoea following suxamethonium or mivacurium in heterozygous individuals. A parturient requiring manual removal of placenta was given both suxamethonium and mivacurium. Inadequate respirations, and reduced TOF without fade, necessitated IPPV overnight with sedation. A low plasma cholinesterase level, which returned to normal 1 month postpartum, was found (Davies & Landy 1998).

3. A family history of plasma cholinesterase abnormalities.

4. Toxicity of cocaine. Plasma cholinesterase is essential for the metabolism of cocaine. Individuals with enzyme abnormality or deficiency are therefore at risk from sudden death (Cregler & Mark 1986). There is now definite evidence that those with cocaine-induced complications have significantly lower levels of plasma cholinesterase than those without complications (Om et al 1993).

5. Low levels of normal enzyme may result from a number of pathological causes, including severe liver disease, tetanus, malnutrition, renal failure, malignancy, collagen disorders, and Huntington's disease.

6. Iatrogenic causes include radiotherapy, renal dialysis, plasmapheresis, following cardiac bypass, cytotoxic drugs, ecothiopate eye drops, oral contraceptives, propanidid, neostigmine, chlorpromazine, pancuronium, tacrine, and exposure to organophosphorus compounds (Whittaker 1980, Davis et al 1997).

Diagnosis

Confirm complete neuromuscular blockade with a peripheral nerve stimulator. During the return of neuromuscular function there will be signs of a phase II block, with fade in response to train-of-four stimulation.

Management

1. Continue IPPV until adequate respiration is re-established. Maintain light anaesthesia to reduce distress.

2. After full recovery, a detailed anaesthetic, family and drug history should be taken from the patient.

3. A clotted blood sample should be taken for plasma cholinesterase activity, dibucaine and fluoride numbers.

4. The results should be given to the patient and the general practitioner, and a warning card issued, if applicable. The investigation of other close relatives may be suggested.

Bibliography

Cregler LL, Mark H 1986 Medical complications of cocaine abuse. New England Journal of Medicine 315: 1495–500.

Davies P, Landy M 1998 Suxamethonium and mivacurium sensitivity from pregnancy-induced plasma cholinesterase deficiency. Anaesthesia 53: 1109–11.

Davis L, Britten JJ, Morgan M 1997 Cholinesterase: its significance in anaesthetic practice. Anaesthesia 52: 244–60.

Om A, Ellahham S, Ornato JP et al 1993 Medical complications of cocaine: possible relationship to low plasma cholinesterase enzyme. American Journal of Cardiology 125: 1114–17.

Ostergaard D, Jensen FS, Viby-Mogensen J 1995 Reversal of intense mivacurium block with human plasma cholinesterase in patients with atypical plasma cholinesterase. Anesthesiology 82: 1295–8.

Whittaker M 1980 Plasma cholinesterase variants and the anaesthetist. Anaesthesia 35: 174–97.

Whittaker M, Britten JJ 1987 Phenotyping of individuals sensitive to suxamethonium. British Journal of Anaesthesia 59: 1052–5.

Thyrotoxic crisis or storm (see also Thyrotoxicosis)

The abrupt onset of symptoms of a severe hypermetabolic state, associated with the output of thyroxine, in a patient with pre-existing thyroid disease. This is a clinical, not a bichemical, diagnosis, and biochemically it is difficult to distinguish between the two. However, serum free T_4 concentrations are significantly higher in a thyroid crisis compared with thyrotoxicosis. It may occur in a patient with occult thyroid disease, in whom a crisis may be precipitated by an acute medical, traumatic or surgical event. It can also occur in treated thyrotoxic patients following thyroidectomy, either if there is inadequate preoperative control (Jamison & Done 1979, Knighton & Crosse 1997), or if antithyroid therapy has been discontinued too early in the postoperative period. Thyrotoxicosis may be difficult to diagnose during pregnancy, and a thyroid crisis may be precipitated by delivery or Caesarean section (Clark et al 1985, Halpern 1989).

Although the onset of the crisis is most likely to occur in the postoperative period, intraoperative problems have also been described. A thyroid crisis can also be concealed by the use of beta adrenoceptor blockers (Jones & Solomon 1981). Beta blockers only affect the peripheral effects on beta adrenoceptors, not the output of thyroid hormone or the thyroid hormone tests.

Presentation

1. Intraoperative tachycardia or atrial fibrillation (Robson 1985, Bennett & Wainwright 1989), ventricular tachycardia, and cardiac arrest (Peters et al 1981).

2. A hypermetabolic state which may resemble malignant hyperthermia (Murray 1978, Peters et al 1981, Stevens 1983, Bennett & Wainwright 1989). Respiratory and metabolic acidosis occurs, with increased oxygen consumption.

3. Intraoperative pulmonary oedema. This may present as cyanosis, tachycardia, and respiratory distress. It is secondary to a combination of increased cardiac output, tachycardia or atrial fibrillation, mild hypertension, increased red cell mass, and increased blood volume. An undiagnosed thyrotoxic patient with a fractured hip developed pulmonary oedema, pyrexia and tachycardia during surgery (Stevens 1983). This state was diagnosed and treated as malignant hyperthermia. The true diagnosis was only made during postoperative investigations.

4. Depression of myocardial function. A dilated cardiomyopathy complicated by a septic abortion (Hankins et al 1984) and ventricular dysfunction during Caesarean section (Clark et al 1985), have been described. In pregnant patients with untreated disease, thyroid crisis is most likely to occur during labour, surgery, infection, or with preeclampsia. Heart failure is common. The stillbirth rate is high.

5. The sudden onset of confusion or mania in the perioperative period; alternatively, patients may occasionally present to the emergency department in coma (Gilbert et al 1992). Deterioration in conscious level occurred in an anxious patient after Caesarean section under general anaesthesia. She had a tachycardia of 180 beat min^{-1}, a BE (base excess) of -13.2, and a serum potassium of 8.1 mmol l^{-1}. Although a phaeochromocytoma was suspected, urgent thyroid screening showed thyrotoxicosis (Pugh et al 1994).

6. Postoperatively, it can present with hyperthermia, tachycardia, agitation, nausea, vomiting, abdominal pain, diarrhoea, jaundice, hepatomegaly, dehydration, and infection. A 14-month-old infant with nonautoimmune hyperthyroidism, that was difficult to control medically, developed pyrexia, agitation and tachycardia 3 h following surgery (Knighton & Crosse 1997).

7. Crisis may be precipitated by trauma. A 26-year-old male with multiple trauma had a persistent tachycardia and pyrexia of 39.4°C 6 h following surgery. The cardiac index was high and SVR low. High T_3 and T_4 levels, with low TSH, confirmed the diagnosis (Fitz-Henry & Riley 1996). Subsequent discussion with his relatives revealed that he had recently been to his GP for investigation of weight loss, palpitations, and anxiety. The importance of adequate history taking was emphasised.

8. A thyrotoxic crisis may also occur in an adequately prepared toxic patient in whom therapy is stopped too soon after surgery, or when the thyrotoxicosis is being treated with propranolol alone (Eriksson et al 1977).

9. As an acute abdominal event. A 61-year-old female presented with vomiting and colicky abdominal pain, tachycardia, hyperthermia, and neutrophilia. After negative laparotomy and one episode of AF, she was found to have a very low TSH and high free plasma T_4, but normal total T_4 levels (Bhattacharyya & Wiles 1997). Thyroid storm may also be precipitated by a genuine acute abdominal emergency (Yeung et al 1995).

10. Thyroid crisis has also occurred from functioning metastases from a thyroid carcinoma, that had already been completely excised (Naito et al 1997). This revealed itself on day 18 following 60% burns, with pyrexia, hypertension, and confusion. It became apparent that a major increase in free thyroid hormone levels occurred after each surgical procedure. It was suggested that levels were increased by transient decreases in hormone binding protein.

11. Factitious thyrotoxicosis occurred in a patient who was subsequently found to have taken 14 thyroxine 0.1-mg tablets on the morning of surgery, because she had not taken any for 2 weeks (Ambus et al 1994). Tachycardia and increased CO_2 was associated with a serum thyroxine level of $27 \mu g\,dl^{-1}$ (normal range $4.5–12 \mu g\,dl^{-1}$).

Management

1. Antithyroid drugs.

a) Carbimazole 60–120 mg or propylthiouracil 600–1200 mg, given orally or, if necessary, by nasogastric tube. This usually starts to act within 1 h of administration.

b) Potassium or sodium iodide acts immediately to inhibit further release of thyroid hormone; this should not be given until 1 h after the antithyroid drug (Smallridge 1992).

2. Beta adrenoceptor antagonists:

a) Propranolol oral 20–80 mg 6-hrly, or iv 1–5 mg 6-hrly.

b) Esmolol infusion can be used for short-term control, in an emergency, particularly if propranolol fails to work (Thorne & Bedford 1989, Vijaykumar et al 1989, Isley et al 1990, Knighton & Crosse 1997). Dilute two ampoules of 2.5 g concentrate in 500 ml saline to give $10\,mg\,ml^{-1}$. Give a loading dose of $500 \mu g\,kg^{-1}$ over 1 min followed by $50–200 \mu g\,kg^{-1}\,min^{-1}$.

3. Active cooling to reduce metabolic demands.

4. IPPV and muscle paralysis if necessary.

5. Steroids. Hydrocortisone iv 100 mg 6-hourly.

6. In the presence of atrial fibrillation, digoxin may be required, in which case beta blockers should be given with caution.

7. Fluid iv (including dextrose) to replace insensible losses and vitamins. In the elderly, haemodynamic monitoring may be required.

8. Sources of infection should be sought, and some authors recommend the empirical use of antibiotics.

9. Dantrolene was given to a child with thyroid storm who failed to respond to conventional treatment (Christensen & Nissen 1987). Although dantrolene successfully controlled the hypermetabolic state, the patient subsequently died from respiratory and renal failure. Dantrolene was also used in a young man who developed a hypermetabolic state on induction of anaesthesia. It was thought to be MH, but subsequent investigation showed thyrotoxicosis (Bennett & Wainwright 1989).

Bibliography

Ambus T, Evans S, Smith NT 1994 Thyrotoxicosis factitia in the anesthetized patient. Anesthesiology 81: 254–6.
Bennett MH, Wainwright AP 1989 Acute thyroid crisis on induction of anaesthesia. Anaesthesia 44: 28–30.

T

584

Bhattacharyya A, Wiles PG 1997 Thyrotoxicosis presenting as acute abdomen. Journal of the Royal Society of Medicine 90: 681–2.

Christensen PA, Nissen LR 1987 Treatment of thyroid storm in a child with dantrolene. British Journal of Anaesthesia 59: 522–6.

Clark SL, Phelan JP, Montoro M et al 1985 Transient ventricular dysfunction associated with cesarean section in a patient with hyperthyroidism. American Journal of Obstetrics & Gynecology 151: 384–6.

Eriksson M, Rubenfeld S, Garber AJ et al 1977 Propranolol does not prevent thyroid storm. New England Journal of Medicine 296: 263–4.

Fitz-Henry J, Riley B 1996 Thyrotoxicosis in a patient with multiple trauma: value of 'AMPLE' history taking. British Medical Journal 313: 997–8.

Gilbert RE, Thomas GW, Hope RN 1992 Coma and thyroid dysfunction. Anaesthesia & Intensive Care 20: 86–7.

Halpern SH 1989 Anaesthesia for Caesarean section in patients with uncontrolled hyperthyroidism. Canadian Journal of Anaesthesia 36: 454–9.

Hankins GDV, Lowe TW, Cunningham FG 1984 Dilated cardiomyopathy and thyrotoxicosis complicated by septic abortion. American Journal of Obstetrics & Gynecology 149: 85–6.

Isley WL, Dahl S, Gibbs H 1990 Use of esmolol in managing a thyrotoxic patient needing emergency surgery. American Journal of Medicine 89: 122–3.

Jamison MH, Done HJ 1979 Postoperative thyrotoxic crisis in a patient prepared for thyroidectomy with propranolol. British Journal of Clinical Practice 32: 82–3.

Jones DK, Solomon S 1981 Thyrotoxic crisis masked by treatment with beta blockers. British Medical Journal 283: 659.

Knighton JD, Crosse MM 1997 Anaesthetic management of childhood thyrotoxicosis and the use of esmolol. Anaesthesia 52: 67–70.

Murray JF 1978 Hyperpyrexia of unknown origin. British Journal of Anaesthesia 50: 387–8.

Naito Y, Sone T, Kataoka K et al 1997 Thyroid storm due to functioning metastatic thyroid carcinoma in a burn patient. Anesthesiology 87: 433–5.

Peters KR, Nance P, Wingard DW 1981 Malignant hyperthyroidism or malignant hyperthermia? Anesthesia & Analgesia 60: 613–15.

Pugh S, Lalwani K, Awal A 1994 Thyroid storm as a cause of loss of consciousness following anaesthesia for Caesarean section. Anaesthesia 49: 35–7.

Robson NJ 1985 Emergency surgery complicated by thyrotoxicosis and thyroid periodic paralysis. Anaesthesia 40: 27–31.

Stevens JJ 1983 A case of thyrotoxic crisis that mimicked malignant hyperthermia. Anesthesiology 59: 263.

Thorne AC, Bedford RF 1989 Esmolol for perioperative management of thyrotoxic goiter. Anesthesiology 71: 291–4.

Vijayakumar HR, Thomas WO, Ferrara JJ 1989 Perioperative management of severe thyrotoxicosis with esmolol. Anaesthesia 44: 406–8.

Yeung SC, Go R, Balasubramanyam A 1995 Rectal administration of iodide and propylthiouracil in the treatment of thyroid storm. Thyroid 5: 403–5.

Torsade de pointes (T de P) (see also Section 1 and QT interval syndromes)

An atypical, paroxysmal ventricular tachycardia associated with delayed repolarisation of the ventricles. It is frequently drug induced, but may also occur with metabolic abnormalities and the congenital long QT syndromes.

It is now known that, in addition to anti-arrhythmic drugs, there are a number of noncardiac drugs that provoke T de P. They share a common feature in that they block one component of a particular type of potassium channel, resulting in lengthening of the QT interval (Yap & Camm 2000). These noncardiac drugs include terfenadine, astemizole, some macrolide antibiotics, tricyclic antidepressants, neuroleptics such as haloperidol and thioridazine, cisapride, and pimozide.

Presentation

1. The patient may complain of episodes of palpitations, faintness, or fatigue. Sudden death may occur.

2. ECG shows paroxysms of an atypical ventricular tachycardia in which the QRS complexes vary in form and amplitude, and the axis of the complexes twists around the baseline. During periods of ordinary sinus rhythm there is a prolonged QT_c of >0.44 s or an uncorrected

QT interval of >0.5 s. Immediately before the onset of the event there is a characteristic 'long–short' sequence (Raehl et al 1985) in which a premature ectopic is followed by a long pause, then a second premature ectopic initiates the torsade de pointes.

3. Predisposing factors.

a) Any disease that causes prolongation of the QT interval. There are at least six familial mutations that include Romano–Ward, Jervell and Lange–Nielsen syndromes, and familial ventricular tachycardia.

b) Metabolic abnormalities. These include hypokalaemia, hypomagnesaemia, and hypocalcaemia. Hypomagnesaemia should be considered in any patient with a combination of gastrointestinal losses and T de P. Torsades de pointes occurred following massive blood transfusion and hypomagnesaemia (Kulkarni et al 1992). A combination of hypokalaemia and hypocalcaemia and alkalosis prolonged the QT_c interval in two patients undergoing surgery (Soroker et al 1995). Isolated hypokalaemia in a 4 year old secondary to high-dose furosemide (frusemide) has also been reported (Chvilicek et al 1995). A combination of erythromycin and mechanical bowel preparation caused a long QT_c interval and T de P (Vogt & Zollo 1997).

c) Drug induced. A number of cardiac drugs, some of which prolong myocardial repolarisation, have been reported to precipitate T de P. These include amiodarone, disopyramide, lidoflazine, prenylamine, procainamide, propranolol, quinidine, and sotalol. Others include terfenadine, astemizole, some macrolide antibiotics, tricyclic antidepressants (amitriptyline, imipramine), neuroleptics (haloperidol and thioridazine), maprotiline, cisapride, pimozide, trifluoperazine, vasopressin, and diuretics.

d) T de P occurred following cardiac bypass grafting in a patient who had been given large doses of haloperidol for acute mania (Perrault et al 2000).

e) In a patient undergoing sigmoid colectomy, intraoperative T de P was attributed to sevoflurane, but was much more likely to have been due to disopyramide, given on induction of anaesthesia to treat atrial fibrillation (Abe et al 1998).

f) Following surgery which involved a block dissection of the right side of the neck (Otteni et al 1983).

Diagnosis

Torsade de pointes can be differentiated from polymorphous ventricular tachycardia by the long QT_c and the 'long–short' initiating sequence.

Management

1. Stop any potentially causative drug.

2. Avoid the use of class I antiarrhythmics, or any of those already mentioned.

3. Correct potential metabolic causes such as hypokalaemia, hypocalcaemia, or hypomagnesaemia. Magnesium therapy is often given empirically.

4. Defibrillation, if VF occurs.

5. Atrial or ventricular pacing may be required until the QT_c is normal. The duration of pacing required will depend upon the half-life of the precipitating drug.

6. Treatment can either be directed towards shortening the action potential durations with beta agonists or vagolytic agents, or suppressing early after-depolarisation (Rosen & Schwartz 1991).

7. Thus, isoprenaline may increase the heart rate and therefore shorten the QT interval. A

dose of $1–2\,\mu g\,min^{-1}$ has been recommended. However, this is a potentially dangerous treatment and should be used with caution. Contraindications to its use include myocardial ischaemia and hypertensive heart disease (Raehl et al 1985).

8. Early after-depolarisation can be suppressed with calcium channel blockers, magnesium sulphate (Ramee et al 1985, Martinez 1987), or beta adrenoceptor blockers.

9. Occasionally bretylium (Raehl et al 1985) and lidocaine (lignocaine) have been reported to be effective.

Bibliography

Abe K, Takada K, Yoshiya I 1998 Intraoperative torsade de pointes ventricular tachycardia and ventricular fibrillation during sevoflurane anesthesia. Anesthesia & Analgesia 86: 701–2.

Chvilicek JP, Hurlbert BJ, Hill GE 1995 Diuretic-induced hypokalaemia inducing torsades de pointes. Canadian Journal of Anaesthesia 42: 1137–9.

Kulkarni P, Bhattacharyra S, Petros AJ 1992 Torsade de pointes and long QT syndrome following major blood transfusion. Anaesthesia 47: 125–7.

Martinez R 1987 Torsade de pointes: atypical rhythm, atypical treatment. Annals of Emergency Medicine 16: 878–84.

Otteni JC, Pottecher RT, Bronner G et al 1983 Prolongation of the Q-T interval and sudden cardiac arrest following right radical neck dissection. Anesthesiology 59: 358–61.

Perrault LP, Denault AY, Carrier M et al 2000 Torsades de pointes secondary to haloperidol after cardiac bypass graft. Canadian Journal of Anaesthesia 47: 251–4.

Raehl CL, Patel AK, LeRoy M 1985 Drug-induced torsade de pointes. Clinical Pharmacology 4: 675–90.

Ramee SR, White CJ, Svinarich JT et al 1985 Torsade de pointes and magnesium deficiency. American Heart Journal 109: 164–7.

Rosen MR, Schwartz DJ 1991 The 'Sicilian Gambit'. A new approach to the classification of antiarrhythmic drugs based on their actions on arrhythmogenic mechanisms. Taskforce of the Working Group on Arrhythmias of the European Society of Cardiology. European Heart Journal 12: 1112–13.

Soroker D, Ezri T, Szmuk P et al 1995 Perioperative torsade de pointes ventricular tachycardia induced by hypocalcemia and hypokalemia. Anesthesia & Analgesia 80: 630–3.

Vogt AW, Zollo RA 1997 Long Q-T syndrome associated with oral erythromycin used in preoperative bowel preparation. Anesthesia & Analgesia 85: 1011–13.

Yap YG, Camm J 2000 Risk of torsade de pointes with non-cardiac drugs. British Medical Journal 320: 1158–9.

Total spinal anaesthesia

A syndrome of central neurological blockade. It occurs when a volume of local anaesthetic solution, intended for epidural anaesthesia, enters the subarachnoid space and ascends to the cervical region. This results in cardiovascular collapse, phrenic nerve paralysis, and unconsciousness. Deaths have occasionally been reported.

Accidental total spinal analgesia may occur in association with the original epidural, or subsequently following a top-up dose, as a result of accidental puncture of the dura by the epidural catheter.

Presentation

1. The circumstances:

a) After a known dural tap. Cardiovascular collapse usually takes place immediately after the epidural injection, although delays of up to 45 min have been reported (Woerth et al 1977). Three cases of total spinal anaesthesia occurred when epidural injections of local anaesthetic were given into the interspace adjacent to an inadvertent dural perforation (Hodgkinson 1981). In all three incidents, the patients were in active labour. It was suggested that frequent uterine contractions can result in some of the local anaesthetic solution being forced through a puncture hole into the subarachnoid space.

In a 68-year-old man, having an epidural sited before colonic surgery, ropivacaine 1% 20 ml was injected over 4 min, after a negative aspiration, but without a test dose. Loss of leg power was immediately followed by asystole, loss of consciousness, and respiratory arrest. After stabilisation, surgery was undertaken, and the patient recovered full power 8 h after the ropivacaine injection. Subsequent aspiration showed that the catheter had entered the subarachnoid space, but the original needle had not (Esteban et al 2000).

b) After epidural top-ups. High spinal anaesthesia has occurred after top-ups of epidural catheters (Philip & Brown 1976). This is unlikely to result from catheter migration, but may happen if part of the catheter lies within the epidural space and part within the subarachnoid. With a slow injection, the solution will emerge from the proximal holes, and with a rapid one from the more distal (Morgan 1990). Cardiovascular collapse usually takes place immediately after the injection, although delays of up to 45 min have been reported (Woerth et al 1977). There is severe hypotension secondary to blockade of the sympathetic outflow. Occasionally cardiac arrest occurs.

In one patient, attempted epidural resulted in two accidental dural punctures. Seven hours later the patient needed Caesarean section, so 1.5 ml 0.75% bupivacaine was injected into the subarachnoid space. Within 2 min the patient experienced hand weakness and respiratory difficulty. It was suggested that leakage of CSF into the epidural space and the lower CSF pressure resulted in compression of the dural sac (Wagner 1994).

A delayed block, resulting in prolonged coma and quadriparesis, occurred 1.5 h following injection of 10 ml bupivacaine 0.25% with 100 μg fentanyl through an epidural catheter during labour. It was thought that the solution

had passed through a hole made at a first unsuccessful attempt at an epidural and this was supported by finding air bubbles in the subarachnoid space of the brain. The patient finally recovered and was extubated about 28 h later (Evron et al 2000). Severe respiratory depression occurred within 4 min of injection of diamorphine 4 mg in 8 ml 0.125% bupivacaine into an epidural catheter following combined spinal–epidural anaesthesia for Caesarean section. This was 5 h after uneventful injection down the catheter. It was assumed that the catheter had migrated through the hole in the dura made by the spinal needle (Ferguson et al 1997).

2. Rapidly increasing paralysis involves the respiratory muscles, resulting in apnoea and hypoxia.

3. The pupils become dilated and consciousness is lost.

4. Apnoea may vary from 20 min to 6 h, unconsciousness from 25 min to 4 h, while full recovery of sensation may take up to 9 h (Gillies & Morgan 1973). The lengths of time vary with the agent, the dose and volume of local anaesthetic given. Bupivacaine lasts longer than lidocaine (lignocaine).

Management

1. Precautions should be taken to prevent the occurrence of total spinal anaesthesia. A test dose of local anaesthetic is recommended. The injection of 3 ml of the local anaesthetic containing epinephrine (adrenaline) 1 : 200 000, followed by an adequate pause to assess the effects, has been suggested (Moore & Batra 1980). The use of this during labour is controversial (see Local anaesthetic toxicity). It has been recommended that, if dural puncture occurs during active labour when a Caesarean section is required, then further attempts should not be made. Either a spinal or a general anaesthetic should be employed as an alternative (Hodgkinson 1981). Others claim never to have seen this complication, and challenge the advice (Crawford 1983).

2. If a total spinal does occur, a nonpregnant patient should be turned supine, tilted head down, and the legs elevated to encourage venous return. The pregnant patient should be tilted in the lateral position to prevent aortocaval compression (Rees & Willis 1988).

3. The lungs should be inflated with oxygen.

4. A pressor agent such as ephedrine i.v. in 5–10-mg increments up to 30 mg is recommended. Epinephrine (adrenaline) 0.1–0.5 mg may occasionally be required but should preferably be avoided in patients in labour.

5. Intravenous fluids should be infused rapidly.

6. A tracheal tube can then be inserted. IPPV may have to be continued for up to 2 h, depending upon the local anaesthetic and the volume used.

Bibliography

Crawford JS 1983 Collapse after epidural injection following inadvertent dural perforation. Anesthesiology 59: 78–9.

Esteban JL, Gomez A, Gonzalez-Miranda F 2000 Unintended total spinal anaesthesia with ropivacaine. British Journal of Anaesthesia 84: 697–8.

Evron S, Krumholtz S, Wiener Y et al 2000 Prolonged coma and quadriplegia after accidental subarachnoid injection of a local anesthetic with an opiate. Anesthesia & Analgesia 90: 116–18.

Ferguson S, Brighouse D, Valentine S 1997 An unusual complication following combined spinal-epidural anaesthesia for caesarean section. International Journal of Obstetric Anesthesia 6: 190–3.

Gillies IDS, Morgan M 1973 Accidental total spinal analgesia. Anaesthesia 28: 441–5.

Hodgkinson R 1981 Total spinal block after epidural injection into an interspace adjacent to an inadvertent dural perforation. Anesthesiology 55: 593–5.

Moore DC, Batra MS 1981 The components of an effective test dose prior to epidural block. Anesthesiology 55: 693–6.

Morgan B 1990 Unexpectedly extensive conduction blocks in obstetric analgesia. Anaesthesia 45: 148–52.

Philip JH, Brown WV 1976 Total spinal late in the course of obstetric bupivacaine epidural block. Anesthesiology 44: 340–1.

Rees GAD, Willis BA 1988 Resuscitation in late pregnancy. Anaesthesia 43: 347–9.

Wagner DL 1994 Total spinal anesthesia during cesarean section hours after previous unintentional dural puncture. Anesthesiology 81: 260–1.

Woerth SD, Bullard JR, Alpert CC 1977 Total spinal anesthesia. A late complication of epidural anesthesia. Anesthesiology 47: 380–1.

TURP syndrome

A syndrome which may occur during transurethral resection of the prostate, in which large quantities of glycine 1.5% irrigating fluid are absorbed into the circulation through open veins in the prostatic bed, although some is also absorbed more slowly from the retroperitoneal or perivesical spaces. Glycine 1.5% is a nonelectrolytic, slightly hypotonic solution (2.1% would be isotonic), which on absorption is mainly confined to the ECF. Plasma sodium levels are decreased by more than would be caused by an equivalent volume of water alone. Large intravascular volume expansion results in significant patient weight gain (Gravenstein 1997).

In general, the amount absorbed depends upon the number and size of prostatic venous sinuses opened, the hydrostatic pressure of the irrigating fluid, and the length of exposure (although this has been disputed, since development of the syndrome has been reported after quite brief resection times). Absorption studies suggest an average rate of 20 ml min^{-1}, although as much as 87 ml min^{-1} has been reported (Alexander et al 1986). Risk factors for the development of a severe syndrome may include a large prostate, profuse bleeding from open prostatic veins, perforation of the prostatic capsule, and pre-existing hyponatraemia. Several deaths from the syndrome have been reported (Aasheim 1973, Osborn et al 1980, Rhymer et al 1985). In patients undergoing regional anaesthesia it has been found that the smallest volume absorbed which gives rise to symptoms is 1000 ml, and more severe symptoms occur when it exceeds 2000 ml (Hahn 1989, 1990).

In some centres, isotonic dextrose was used as the irrigating fluid. In a study of 22 patients, dextrose was found to give a significantly greater decrease in plasma sodium than glycine, and some patients developed severe hyperglycaemia (Allen et al 1981).

A decrease in body temperature usually accompanies significant absorption of glycine, and surgery is associated with increased systemic vascular resistance, decreased stroke volume, and decreased cardiac output (Evans et al 1992). Haemodynamic stresses have been suggested to contribute to the higher long-term mortality found following TURP compared with open prostatectomy (Roos et al 1989, Editorial 1991).

Presentation

1. The patient is usually undergoing a TURP, and glycine 1.5% (or sorbitol 3%) is being used as an irrigating fluid. Glycine absorption has also been described during percutaneous ultrasonic lithotripsy (Sinclair et al 1985), and transcervical resection of the endometrium (Van Boven et al 1989, Rosenberg 1995).

2. The time of onset is variable. In one case, a convulsion occurred during spinal anaesthesia after only 15 min of resection (Hurlbert & Wingard 1979). There were no warning signs, despite the plasma sodium having decreased to 104 mmol l^{-1}. Absorption of glycine may continue beyond the resection time into the postoperative period.

3. Initially, there is an increase in systolic blood pressure and a widening of pulse pressure. This is followed by bradycardia, hypotension, and occasionally cardiac arrest (Charlton 1980). Other ECG abnormalities, including nodal rhythm and U waves, have been reported. Blood loss may mask the initial hypertensive phase.

4. The syndrome is likely to present earlier in a conscious patient undergoing spinal anaesthesia than in one having a general anaesthetic. Facial warmth, visual disturbances, restlessness, confusion, headache, nausea and retching may herald its onset. Convulsions have been reported. During general anaesthesia, detection may be delayed, particularly if the initial hypertensive phase is masked by blood loss.

5. Pulmonary oedema may occur (Aasheim 1973, Allen et al 1981). The patient can present with respiratory distress and cyanosis in the postoperative period (Rhymer et al 1985).

6. Cerebral oedema may result in mental confusion and seizures. Several cases of visual disturbances (Ovassapian et al 1982) and transient blindness (Russell 1990) have been described. These are attributed to the effects of high glycine levels on the retinal synapses, although oedema of the occipital cortex has also been suggested as a cause (Ovassapian et al 1982). Wang et al (1989) studied four patients with visual aberrations following TURP and found that increased serum glycine levels correlated significantly with a decrease in serum sodium levels. Blindness has also occurred following hysteroscopy, in which glycine was infused at a pressure of 150 mmHg. A serum ammonia level seven times the upper limit of normal was recorded (Levin & Ben-David 1995). Return of sight occurred at 36 h. Delayed awakening from anaesthesia has been reported (Roesch et al 1983).

7. Profound hyponatraemia can occur, plasma sodium levels of 102–105 mmol l^{-1} often being reported. In one fatal case, the plasma sodium, after more than 5 h resection, was 83 mmol l^{-1}. The sodium level does not necessarily correlate with the amount of fluid absorbed, since the presence of glycine enhances the hyponatraemia. In a study of 372 prostatectomies, 15% of patients had plasma sodium levels below 125 mmol l^{-1}. All had clinical evidence of hyponatraemia (Shearer & Standfield 1981). By contrast, other authors claimed to have seen patients with levels of 104 mmol l^{-1}, without clinical signs (Allen et al 1981).

8. Decreased serum osmolality usually occurs, but the degree is very variable.

9. The extent to which high levels of glycine and its metabolites contribute to the CNS effects of the syndrome is the subject of continuing debate. Products of glycine metabolism include serine, ammonia, oxalate, and glycolate. Glycine (and to a lesser extent serine) is known to be an inhibitory neurotransmitter in the brain, spinal cord and retina, with a similar action to GABA on chloride channels.

Although early reports suggested that ammonia accumulation was not a problem, in one case, delayed recovery from anaesthesia was associated with a serum ammonia level of $500\,\mu\,mol\,l^{-1}$ (Roesch et al 1983). It was suggested that some patients may be more susceptible to ammonia production and toxicity than others.

Twenty-four-hour urinary oxalate and glycolate levels were studied in three patients, who were selected from a total of 34 patients, on the basis of hyponatraemia the morning after surgery (Fitzpatrick et al 1981). Urinary levels of oxalate and glycolate were high in all three patients and oxalate continued to be excreted for up to 2 weeks.

Diagnosis

1. Plasma sodium. Values as low as $83\,mmol\,l^{-1}$ have been reported.

2. Plasma osmolality may be reduced.

3. Hb and haematocrit levels are decreased.

4. The use of irrigating fluid tagged with 1% ethanol. Absorption in litres has been calculated to equal to 3.6 EB-ethanol (max) divided by the ethanol concentration in % in the irrigating fluid (Hulten et al 1991).

5. Plasma glycine levels are high ($n = 176{-}332\,\mu mol\,l^{-1}$). The results of glycine estimations may take several days to return, and are therefore not of immediate use. Levels as high as $8000\mu\,mol\,l^{-1}$ have been reported.

6. Blood ammonia may be increased ($n = 11{-}35\,\mu mol\,l^{-1}$). In the patient with delayed recovery from anaesthesia, the blood ammonia was $500\,\mu mol\,l^{-1}$.

7. When isotonic dextrose was used as the irrigating fluid, one patient developed a blood glucose of $61.8\,mmol\,l^{-1}$ (Allen et al 1981).

8. Urinary oxalate ($n = 0.1{-}0.5\,mmol\,24\,h^{-1}$) and glycolate levels ($n = 0.10{-}0.35\,mmol\,24\,h^{-1}$) may be elevated.

Management

1. Prophylaxis and anticipation.

a) Prostatic resection time should, in general, be limited to 1 h. However, in one patient, convulsions and a sodium of $104\,mmol\,l^{-1}$ developed after only 15 min (Hurlbert & Wingard 1979).

b) Irrigating pressure should be kept to about $60{-}70\,cmH_2O$, and certainly should never be allowed to exceed $100\,cmH_20$.

c) Sodium-free iv solutions should not be used during prostatic resection.

d) Postoperatively, the bladder irrigation fluid should be changed from glycine to saline.

2. Early detection of absorption of glycine and prompt cessation of surgery, if the amount suspected approaches 2000 ml. Methods of detecting this include the use of an ethanol 'marker' in the glycine. Hahn (1990) reported the use of glycine 1.5% with ethanol 1% in 100 consecutive patients having TURP under epidural anaesthesia, and subsequently the technique was found to be applicable to anaesthetised patients (Hulten et al 1991, Stalberg et al 1992). An alcohol meter (Alcolmeter, Lions Laboratories Ltd, Barry, Wales) was used each 10 min (or each 5 min if absorption was detected), and irrigant absorption was calculated according to a formula determined in a previous study (Hahn 1989), where EBV is the expired breath volume:

Absorption of glycine in litres = 3.6 EBV – ethanol (max) divided by the ethanol concentration in % in the irrigating fluid

The use of 1% alcohol allowed the absorption of 100–150 ml per 10-min period to be detected, and if 2% alcohol was used, as little as 50 ml per 10-min period could be detected.

3. Treatment of hyponatraemia. This is controversial. Recommendations range from no treatment at all, to saline 0.9%, hypertonic saline, mannitol, loop diuretics, and peritoneal dialysis. Mannitol was found to be an effective alternative to furosemide (frusemide) to promoting diuresis after TURP (Crowley et al 1990).

Those who have reservations about the use of active therapy observed that some patients with a sodium of 104 mmol l⁻¹ were asymptomatic, and that spontaneous correction of hyponatraemia normally occurred within 12–24 h. However, a number of deaths associated with the syndrome have been reported, and in the elderly patient cardiac arrhythmias, convulsions, and pulmonary and cerebral oedema, are dangerous complications. A study of 13 men undergoing TURP, and five women having TCRE, showed that 14 patients treated with hypertonic saline survived, whereas the four who were not thus treated suffered respiratory arrest and died (Ayus & Arieff 1997).

a) Each case must be dealt with individually, with a knowledge of the patient's clinical state, his/her cardiovascular and respiratory status, and the biochemical results.

b) If active therapeutic correction of the hyponatraemia is required, it should be carried out with extreme caution. Saline 0.9% is usually sufficient, perhaps with the addition of a loop diuretic. However, a loop diuretic is less effective in dilutional hyponatraemia, and has the disadvantage of causing the loss of sodium in addition to water. If the serum osmolality is very low, hypertonic saline may be required. A plasma sodium correction rate to achieve an increase in serum sodium of 1–2 mmol l⁻¹ h⁻¹ has been proposed, until symptoms improve (Fraser & Arieff 1999), stopping at a level of 133 mmol l⁻¹. Others recommend a lower rate of 6–8 mmol l⁻¹ day⁻¹ (Sterns 1992). It is important not to overcorrect.

c) Prophylactic IPPV and ITU monitoring are essential, at least until the plasma sodium and hypervolaemia are corrected, if the hyponatraemia is severe. This will prevent hypoxia, minimise the effects of cerebral oedema or convulsions, and allow detection and treatment of cardiac arrhythmias.

4. Calcium and inotropic agents may be required. The routine use of calcium gluconate 10% 10 ml, has been recommended, particularly if cardiovascular collapse has occurred.

5. Coagulation studies should be performed if there is persistent bleeding and hyponatraemia. Dilutional abnormalities are the most frequent, although a coagulopathy may also occur. Deficiencies should be treated appropriately.

6. Should blindness occur, ophthalmological advice should be sought; however, in those cases reported, sight has always been restored within 12–36 h.

7. Urinary volumes should be maintained postoperatively, to prevent the deposition of calcium oxalate in the urinary tract.

Bibliography

Aasheim GM 1973 Hyponatraemia during transurethral surgery. Canadian Anaesthetists' Society Journal 20: 274–80.

Alexander JP, Polland A, Gillespie IA 1986 Glycine and transurethral resection. Anaesthesia 41: 1189–95.

Allen PR, Hughes RG, Goldie DJ et al 1981 Fluid absorption during transurethral resection. British Medical Journal 282: 740.

Ayus JC, Arieff AI 1997 Glycine-induced hypo-osmolar hyponatremia. Archives of Internal Medicine 157: 223–6.

Charlton AJ 1980 Cardiac arrest during transurethral prostatectomy after absorption of 1.5% glycine. Anaesthesia 35: 804–6.

Crowley K, Clarkson K, Hannon V et al 1990 Diuretics after transurethral prostatectomy: a double-blind controlled trial comparing frusemide and mannitol. British Journal of Anaesthesia 65: 337–41.

Editorial 1991 Monitoring TURP. Lancet 338: 606–7.

Evans JWH, Singer M, Chapple CR et al 1992 Haemodynamic evidence for cardiac stress during transurethral resection of the prostate. British Medical Journal 304: 666–71.

Fitzpatrick JM, Kasidas GP, Rose GA 1981 Hyperoxaluria following glycine irrigation for transurethral prostatectomy. British Journal of Urology 53: 250–2.

Fraser CL, Arieff AI 1997 Epidemiology, pathophysiology, and management of hyponatremic encephalopathy. American Journal of Medicine 102: 67–77.

Gravenstein D 1997 Transurethral resection of the prostate (TURP) syndrome: a review of the pathophysiology and management. Anesthesia & Analgesia 84: 438–46.

Hahn RG 1989 Early detection of the TUR syndrome by marking the irrigating fluid with 1% ethanol. Acta Anaesthesiologica Scandinavica 33: 146–51.

Hahn RG 1990 Prevention of TUR syndrome by detection of trace ethanol in the expired breath. Anaesthesia 45: 577–81.

Hahn RG 1991 The transurethral resection syndrome. Acta Anaesthesiologica Scandinavica 35: 557–67.

Hulten J, Sarma VJ, Hjertberg H et al 1991 Monitoring of irrigating fluid absorption during transurethral prostatectomy. A study in anaesthetised patients using a 1% ethanol solution. Anaesthesia 46: 349–53.

Hurlbert BJ, Wingard DW 1979 Water intoxication after 15 minutes of transurethral resection of the prostate. Anesthesiology 50: 355–6.

Levin H, Ben-David B 1995 Transient blindness during hysteroscopy: a rare complication. Anesthesia & Analgesia 81: 880–1.

Osborn DE, Rao PN, Greene MJ et al 1980 Fluid absorption during transurethral resection. British Medical Journal 281: 1549–50.

Ovassapian A, Joshi CW, Brunner EA 1982 Visual disturbances: an unusual symptom of transurethral prostate resection reaction. Anesthesiology 57: 332–4.

Rhymer JC, Bell TJ, Perry KC et al 1985 Hyponatraemia following transurethral resection of the prostate. British Journal of Urology 57: 450–2.

Roesch RP, Stoelting RK, Lingeman JE et al 1983 Ammonia toxicity resulting from glycine absorption during a transurethral resection of the prostate. Anesthesiology 58: 577–9.

Roos NP, Wennberg JE, Malenka DJ et al 1989 Mortality and reoperation after open and transurethral resection of the prostate for benign hyperplasia. New England Journal of Medicine 320: 1120–4.

Rosenberg MK 1995 Hyponatremic encephalopathy after rollerball endometrial ablation. Anesthesia & Analgesia 80: 1046–8.

Russell D 1990 Painless loss of vision after transurethral resection of the prostate. Anaesthesia 45: 218–21.

Shearer RJ, Standfield NJ 1981 Fluid absorption during transurethral resection. British Medical Journal 282: 740.

Sinclair JF, Hutchison A, Baraza R et al 1985 Absorption of 1.5% glycine after percutaneous ultrasonic lithotripsy for renal stone disease. British Medical Journal 291: 691–2.

Stalberg HP, Hahn RG, Jones AW 1992 Ethanol monitoring of transurethral resection of the prostate during inhaled anesthesia. Anesthesia & Analgesia 75: 983–8.

Sterns RH 1992 Severe hyponatraemia: the case for conservative management. Critical Care Medicine 20: 534–9.

Van Boven MJ, Singelyn F, Donnez J et al 1989 Dilutional hyponatremia associated with intrauterine endoscopic laser surgery. Anesthesiology 71: 449–50.

Wang JM, Creel DJ, Wong KC 1989 TURP, serum glycine levels and ocular evoked potential. Anesthesiology 70: 36–41.

APPENDIX

USEFUL ADDRESSES,
TELEPHONE NUMBERS
AND WEBSITES

Association of Anaesthetists
9 Bedford Square
London WC1B 3RA
020 7631 1650
www.aagbi.org
Anaesthesia online:
www.blackwell-science.com/ana

British Medical Association
BMA House
Tavistock Square
London WC1H 9JP
020 7387 4499
www.bma.org.uk

British Journal of Anaesthesia
BJA online: www.bja.oupjournals.org

Cholinesterase Research Unit
Hammersmith Hospital
Du Cane Road
London W12 0HS
020 8383 1000

**Committee on Safety of Medicines/
Medicine Control Agency**
1 Nine Elms Lane
London SW8 5NQ
020 7273 0574 (9am–5pm)
020 7210 3000 (other times)

Department of Health
Quarry House
Quarry Hill
Leeds LS2 7UE
0113 254 5715

General Medical Council
178 Great Portland Street
London W1N 6JE
020 7580 7642
www.gmc-uk.org

Malignant Hyperthermia Unit
St James's University Hospital
Beckett Street
Leeds LS9 7TF
0113 206 5274

Medical Defence Union
230 Blackfriars Road
London SE1 8PJ
020 7202 1500
0800 716 376
www.the-mdu.com

Medical Devices Agency
Hannibal House
Elephant & Castle
London SE1 6TQ
020 7972 8080/8100
www.medical-devices.gov.uk

Medical Protection Society
33 Cavendish Square
London W1
020 7399 1300

Medical Research Council
20 Park Crescent
London W1N 4AL
020 7636 5422

Medicine Control Agency (Adverse reactions
to drugs)
CSM Freepost
London SW8 5BR
0800 731 6789 (24-hour)

Regional Centres

CSM Mersey
Freepost
Liverpool L3 3AB
0151 794 8113

CSM Northern
Freepost 1085
Newcastle upon Tyne NE1 1BR
0191 232 1525

CSM Wales
Freepost
Cardiff CF4 1ZZ
029 2074 4181

CSM West Midlands
Freepost SW2991
Birmingham B18 7BR
No telephone number

National Assembly for Wales
Cathays Park
Cardiff CF10 3NQ
029 2082 5111

National Confidential Enquiry into Perioperative Deaths
35-43 Lincoln's Inn Fields
London WC2A 3PN
020 7831 6430
www.ncepod.org.uk

POISONS CENTRES

Belfast 028 9024 0503

Birmingham 0121 507 5588/9

Cardiff 029 2070 9901

Dublin 00 353 1 837 9964/9966

Edinburgh 0131 536 2300

London 020 7635 9191

Newcastle 0191 282 0300

Porphyria
Supplies of Haem arginate from on call pharmacist:

University Hospital of Wales, Cardiff
029 2074 7747

St James's University Hospital, Leeds
0113 243 3144 or 0113 283 7010

St Thomas's Hospital London
020 7928 9292

Royal College of Anaesthetists
48 Russell Square
London WC1B 4JP
020 7813 1900
www.rcoa.ac.uk

Royal College of Surgeons of England
35 Lincolns Inn Fields
London WC2A 3PN
020 7405 3474
www.rcseng.ac.uk

Royal College of Surgeons of Edinburgh
Nicholson Street
Edinburgh EH8 9DW
0131 527 1600
www.rcsed.ac.uk

Royal Society of Medicine
1 Wimpole Street
London W1G 0AE
020 7290 2900

Index

A

acetanilid 208
acetazolamide 151, 189
acetylcholine receptors 340
achalasia of oesophagus 3–4, 313
achondroplasia 5–8
acid maltase deficiency
   adult onset 405, 406, 407
   Pompe's disease 405–7
acromegaly 8–11
acyclovir 499
addiction 12–13
   see also alcoholism
Addisonian crisis 16, 336, 337, 523–4
Addison's disease 14–16, 263
adenosine 518
adrenocortical deficiency 368
   acute 523–4
   steroid therapy withdrawal 14, 16
      surgical cover 16
   see also Addison's disease
AIDS (acquired immunodeficiency syndrome) *see*
HIV infection/AIDS
air embolism 525–9
   management 529
   'paradoxical' 525
albendazole 256
albuterol 167
alcohol abuse 23–6, 546
alcohol withdrawal 23, 24, 25
alcuronium 536
aldosterone 107
aldosteronism, primary *see* Conn's syndrome
alendronate 375
alfentanil 28, 87, 160, 517
   adverse reactions 144, 378
      perioperative excitatory events 178
alimemazine (trimeprazine) 442
alkalosis
   Conn's syndrome 107
   Cushing's disease 112
alkaptonuria 26–7

alpha methylparatyrosine 388
alveolar proteinosis 27–9
amiloride 115
aminocaproic acid 244
aminoglycosides, safety in porphyria 411
aminophylline 57, 538, 549
   halothane interaction 55, 57
4-aminopyridine 153, 154
amiodarone 63, 83, 85, 389, 518
   adverse reactions
      thyrotoxicosis 490
      torsade de pointes 585
amitryptiline 182, 585
amniotic fluid embolism 531–3
   treatment 533
amphetamine abuse 12–13, 29–32, 179
   rhabdomyolysis 443, 446
ampicillin 175
   Haemophilus influenzae resistance 174, 175
amyloidosis 32–5
   autonomic dysfunction 66
   heart disease 33–4, 35, 83
amyotrophic lateral sclerosis (motor neurone disease)
330–2
anaemia
   Gaucher's disease 203
   hypothyroidism 263
   myeloma 344
   relapsing polychondritis 439
   systemic lupus erythematosus 474
   Wegener's granulomatosis 510
anaphylactic/anaphylactoid reactions 309
   drug-related 309, 310, 535–6
   hydatid disease 255, 256
   intravenous agents 534–40
   latex allergy 555, 556
   management 537–40
   subsequent anaesthetics 540
   types of reaction 536–7
angioneurotic oedema 542–3
   acquired C1 esterase inhibitor deficiency 93–4,
     542, 543

hereditary 93, 94, 238–40, 542, 543
angiotensin converting enzyme (ACE) inhibitors 326, 455, 457
    adverse reactions 93
        angioneurotic oedema 542
    dilated (congestive) cardiomyopathy 83
aniline, toxic methaemoglobinaemia 570
ankylosing spondylitis 36–9
antibiotic prophylaxis 329
    aortic regurgitation 45
    Down's syndrome 138
    Ebstein's anomaly 156
    Ehlers–Danlos syndrome 164
    Eisenmenger's syndrome 168
    Fallot's tetralogy 184
    hereditary haemorrhagic telangiectasia 244
    Klippel–Feil syndrome 283
    mitral valve disease 322, 324, 327
    sickle cell anaemia 220, 222
    splenectomy 486
    systemic lupus erythematosus 475
antibiotics
    adverse reactions
        anaphylactic/anaphylactoid 465, 534, 536
        torsade de pointes 491, 584, 585
    Ludwig's angina 293
anticholinergic bronchodilators 54
anticonvulsants 179
    drug interactions 177, 179
antihistamines (H1 and H2 antagonists) 94, 291, 309, 538, 550
    premedication 56
antioestrogen therapy 344
antiphospholipid syndrome 40–2, 73, 455
    systemic lupus erythematosus 473, 474, 475
antiretroviral agents 18, 19, 20
antitetanus immunoglobulin 481
antithrombin III deficiency 74
antithyroid drugs 489, 583
aortic dilatation/dissection
    cardiac tamponade 551, 552, 553
    Ehlers–Danlos syndrome type IV 163, 164
    Marfan syndrome 303, 304, 305, 306
    Turner's syndrome 498
aortic regurgitation (incompetence) 43–5, 439
    rheumatoid arthritis 449–50
aortic stenosis 46–8
aortocaval fistula 543–4
aprotinin 276, 550
APUDomas 500
Arnold–Chiari malformation 49–51
arthrogryposis multiplex congenita 51–3

aspiration of gastric contents
    achalasia of oesophagus 3, 4
    arthrogryposis multiplex congenita 52, 53
    CHARGE association 97
    Cockayne syndrome 107
    cri du chat syndrome 111
    dermatomyositis/polymyositis complex 126
    dystrophia myotonica 150
    epidermolysis bullosa 171
    Fabry's disease 182
    Gaucher's disease 203
    Huntington's disease 250
    motor neurone disease 331
    nemaline myopathy 350
    obese patients 362
    Opitz–Frias syndrome 370
    Prader–Willi syndrome 414
    preeclampsia/eclampsia 158, 160
    Riley–Day syndrome 186, 187
    scleroderma 457
    Zenker's diverticulum 520
aspirin 41, 42, 74, 208, 209, 227, 279, 475
    safety in porphyria 411
astemizole 491, 584, 585
asthma 54–8, 99
    bronchospasm 55, 56, 57, 548
    drug treatment 54–5
athletic heart syndrome 59–61, 546
atlantoaxial instability
    alkaptonuria 27
    diffuse idiopathic skeletal hyperostosis 135
    Down's syndrome 136, 137–8
    Ehlers–Danlos syndrome type IV 163
    Lesch–Nyhan disease 292
    Morquio's syndrome 328–9
    Paget's disease 376
    rheumatoid arthritis 448–9, 450
    spondyloepiphyseal dysplasia 470–1
atlanto-occipital instability, mucopolysaccharidoses 253
atracurium 25, 57, 96, 124, 149, 154, 180, 190, 299, 312, 319
    anaphylactic/anaphylactoid reactions 536
    anticonvulsant interactions 179
    myasthenia gravis 342
    safety in porphyria 411
atrial ectopic beats 546, 547
atrial fibrillation 546, 547
atrial flutter 546, 547
atrial pacing 547
    sick sinus syndrome 462, 463
    Wolff–Parkinson–White syndrome 518

atrial tachycardia with atrioventricular block 546, 547
atrioventricular-nodal re-entrant (paroxysmal
    supraventricular) tachycardia 546
atropine 48, 56, 60, 84, 91, 187, 233, 299, 315, 341,
    343, 350, 395, 483
    central anticholinergic syndrome 553, 554
    contraindications
        mitral valve disease 324, 326
        phaeochromocytoma 388
        Wolff–Parkinson–White syndrome 517
    safety in porphyria 411
    sick sinus syndrome 462, 463
automatic implantable cardioverter defibrillator
    (AICD) 62–5, 83, 545
    anaesthesia for insertion/testing 63, 64
    antiarrhythmic drug interactions 64
    device 62
    insertion indications 62–3
    long QT syndrome 433, 434, 436
autonomic dysfunction 66–8
    alcoholic patients 24
    Creutzfeldt–Jakob disease 110
    diabetes mellitus 129, 130, 131
    Down's syndrome 136
    Eaton–Lambert syndrome 153, 154
    Fabry's disease 182
    familial dysautonomia 186, 187
    Guillain–Barré syndrome 214, 215
    HIV infection/AIDS 18, 19
    motor neurone disease 331
    multiple system atrophy 337
    Parkinson's disease 378, 379
    Prader–Willi syndrome 414
    rheumatoid arthritis 448
    tetanus 480
awake intubation
    acromegaly 11
    ankylosing spondylitis 38, 39
    cardiac tamponade 81
    cherubism 98
    cri du chat syndrome 112
    Cushing's disease 113
    diabetes mellitus 131
    diffuse idiopathic skeletal hyperostosis 135
    fibrodysplasia ossificans progressiva 197
    juvenile hyaline fibromatosis 278
    Ludwig's angina 293
    Morquio's syndrome 329
    mucopolysaccharidoses 253
    obesity 361
    obstructive sleep apnoea 366
    Pierre Robin syndrome 395

rheumatoid arthritis 450
spondyloepiphyseal dysplasia 471
Treacher Collins syndrome 495
Zenker's diverticulum 520
axillary block
    epidermolysis bullosa 171
    hypokalaemic periodic paralysis 190
azathioprine 341, 383
azlocillin 117

B
baclofen 124
    intrathecal 482
bacterial endocarditis 43, 48, 101, 103, 166, 167, 183,
    184, 368
    Ebstein's anomaly 155, 156
    mitral valve disease 322, 324, 325, 327
    Morquio's syndrome 329
barbiturates
    adverse reactions 148
    porphyria 410
basilar impression
    osteogenesis imperfecta 371
    Paget's disease 375
Becker muscular dystrophy 70–1, 142, 144, 298, 339,
    445
    hyperkalaemic cardiac arrest 70, 71
    malignant hyperthermia-like reactions 297, 564
    masseter muscle rigidity 568
    rhabdomyolysis 443, 444
Becker's myotonia 151–2
Beck's triad 79, 80, 551
Beckwith–Wiedemann syndrome 71–2
beclometasone 54, 55
benserazide 377
benzhexol 209
benzocaine
    methaemoglobinaemia 570
    toxicity 560
benzodiazepines 25, 31, 86, 105, 295, 299, 310, 427,
    560
    adverse reactions 148
        anaphylactic 534
        central anticholinergic syndrome 553
        rhabdomyolysis 443
    contraindication in opiate addicts 369
    premedication 56
benzylpenicillin 246, 486
beta-2-adrenoceptor agonists 54, 55
    pulmonary oedema 429–31
    rhabdomyolysis 443
beta-adrenoceptor blockers 25

599

cardiac arrhythmias 547
cocaine-related cardiotoxicity 104
hypertension 109
hypertrophic cardiomyopathy 83, 86
long QT syndrome 433, 434, 435, 436, 492
Marfan syndrome 303, 304, 305, 306
mitral stenosis 323, 324–5
  pulmonary oedema 425
mitral valve prolapse 326
phaeochromocytoma 387, 389, 574, 575
porphyria 411
tetanus 482
thyroid crisis (thyroid storm) 583
thyrotoxicosis 487, 489
torsade de pointes 492, 586
Wolff–Parkinson–White syndrome 518
beta-interferon 124
betamethasone 16, 237
biguanides, safety in porphyria 411
biphosphonates 344
bradycardia/tachycardia syndrome *see* sick sinus
  syndrome
bradykinins 76, 77
bretylium 433, 492, 516, 586
bromocriptine 9, 337, 355, 356, 377
bronchial cysts 313
bronchoalveolar lavage (BAL) 27–8
bronchodilators
  asthma 54, 56
  cystic fibrosis 117
bronchospasm 548–9
  anaphylactic/anaphylactoid reactions 537
  asthma 55, 56, 57
  carcinoid syndrome 76
  latex allergy 556
Budd–Chiari syndrome 73–4, 380, 381, 404
budesonide 54, 55
Buerger's disease 74–5
bupivacaine 8, 38, 53, 78, 135, 156, 192, 342, 421,
  482, 587
  accidental subdural block 578
  safety in porphyria 411, 412
  toxicity 558, 559, 560, 561
buprenorphine 227
  methadone equivalent dosage 369
  safety in porphyria 411
busulphan 403
butane abuse 466, 467
butyrophenones 249, 250, 378
  adverse reactions 481
    central anticholinergic syndrome 553
  contraindications 379

C
C1 esterase inhibitor deficiency
  acquired 93–4
  hereditary form (angioneurotic oedema) 93, 94,
    238–40, 542, 543
C1 esterase inhibitor therapy 239, 240, 543
Caesarean section
  achondroplasia 7
  air embolism 526, 528
  amniotic fluid embolism 532, 533
  amphetamine abuse 31
  amyloidosis 35
  aortic stenosis 47, 48
  arthrogryposis multiplex congenita 52–3
  Budd–Chiari syndrome 73
  Charcot–Marie–Tooth disease 96
  Chiari malformations 50, 51
  coarctation of aorta 101
  cocaine abuse 102, 103, 104
  demyelinating disease/multiple sclerosis 125
  dilated cardiomyopathy 86
  dystrophia myotonica 149, 150
  Ebstein's anomaly 156
  Ehlers–Danlos syndrome 163, 164, 165
  Eisenmenger's syndrome 167
  familial dysautonomia 187
  Friedreich's ataxia 201
  haemophilia A carriers 227
  HELLP syndrome 235, 237
  HIV infection/AIDS 19, 20
  hypertrophic cardiomyopathy 87
  hypokalaemic periodic paralysis 190
  Kawasaki disease 279, 280
  Klippel–Feil syndrome 283
  Klippel–Trenaunay–Weber syndrome 285
  Marfan syndrome 305, 306
  mitochondrial encephalopathies 319
  mitral prolapse 326
  mitral regurgitation 323
  mitral stenosis 324, 325
  nemaline myopathy 350
  neurofibromatosis 352, 353
  Noonan's syndrome 358
  obese patients 362
  osteogenesis imperfecta 373
  paramyotonia 192
  pemphigus vulgaris 383
  porphyria 412
  preeclampsia/eclampsia 160
  protein S deficiency 418
  pulmonary hypertension 421–2
  sarcoidosis 453

scleroderma 456, 457
sickle cell trait 221
spondyloepiphyseal dysplasia 471
status asthmaticus 57
systemic lupus erythematosus 475
Takayasu's arteritis 479
thalidomide-related deformities/phocomelias 487
von Hippel–Lindau disease 505
von Willebrand's disease 508, 509
CAGE assessment 23
calcitonin 197, 214, 257, 375, 376
calcium channel blockers 107, 586
  cocaine-related cardiotoxicity 105
  mitral stenosis 323
  phaeochromocytoma 388
  pulmonary hypertension 420
calcium channel disorders 188, 189
Caplan's syndrome 447
captopril 93
carbamazepine
  drug interactions 179
  porphyria 410
carbidopa 377, 378, 379
carbimazole 583
carbromal 410
carcinoid syndrome 76–8, 546, 549–50
  bronchospasm 76, 548, 549
cardiac arrest
  aortic stenosis 47
  cardiac tamponade 79, 80, 552
  Guillain–Barré syndrome 215, 216
  hypothyroidism 263–4
  infectious mononucleosis 267, 268
  long QT syndrome 434, 435
  phaeochromocytoma 573
  solvent abuse 467, 468
  see also cardiorespiratory arrest; cardiovascular
    collapse
cardiac arrhythmias 545–8
  asthma 55
  athletic heart syndrome 60, 61
  automatic implantable cardioverter defibrillators
    (AICD) 62
  autonomic dysfunction 68
  Becker muscular dystrophy 70
  carcinoid syndrome 549
  cardiac myxoma 347, 348
  dilated cardiomyopathy 84
  dystrophia myotonica 148, 149
  Ebstein's anomaly 155
  Ehlers–Danlos syndrome 163–4
  Eisenmenger's syndrome 166–7

Emery–Dreifuss muscular dystrophy 169
  Fallot's tetralogy, corrected 183–4
  Friedreich's ataxia 201
  Guillain–Barré syndrome 215, 216
  hypercalcaemia 257
  hypokalaemic periodic paralysis 189
  levodopa-related 377
  local anaesthetic toxicity 559, 560, 561–2
  long QT syndrome *see* QT syndrome, prolonged
  malignant hyperthermia 298, 564
  management 547–8
  Marcus Gunn jaw winking phenomenon 303
  mediastinal masses 314–15
  mitral valve prolapse 325, 326
  obstructive sleep apnoea 364
  phaeochromocytoma 572, 573
  Prader–Willi syndrome 414
  solvent abuse 466, 467, 468
  tetanus 480, 481
  thyroid crisis 582, 583
  thyrotoxicosis 488, 489–90
  tuberous sclerosis 496, 497
  TURP syndrome 589, 591
  Wolff–Parkinson–White syndrome 516, 517
cardiac disease, congenital
  cardiac arrhythmias 546
  CHARGE association 96, 97
  cri du chat syndrome 111
  Dandy–Walker syndrome 122
  Down's syndrome 136, 137, 138
  Goldenhar's syndrome 211
  Klippel–Feil syndrome 282, 283
  Miller's syndrome 317
cardiac myxoma 346–8
cardiac tamponade 79–81, 551–3
  mediastinal masses 314, 315
cardiogenic pulmonary oedema 424–6
cardiomyopathy 82–7, 546
  phaeochromocytoma 384, 385, 389
cardiopulmonary resuscitation
  air embolism 529
  amniotic fluid embolism 533
  anaphylactic/anaphylactoid reactions 537–8
  ankylosing spondylitis 38
  aortic stenosis 47, 48
  local anaesthetic toxicity 561–2
  near drowning 139
  ventricular fibrillation 547
cardiorespiratory arrest
  cardiac myxoma 347
  CHARGE association 97
  epiglottitis 173

cardiovascular collapse
  Addison's disease 14–15, 523
  air embolism 528
  amniotic fluid embolism 533
  carcinoid syndrome 549, 550
  cardiac tamponade 551
  carotid body tumour 90, 91
  latex allergy 556
  local anaesthetic toxic reactions 559
  total spinal anaesthesia 586, 587
  see also cardiac arrest; cardiorespiratory arrest
cardiovascular disorders
  acromegaly 9, 10
  adrenocortical deficiency 524
  alcoholic patients 24, 25
  alkaptonuria 26, 27
  alveolar proteinosis 28
  amyloid disease 33–4, 35
  anaphylactic/anaphylactoid reactions 537
  ankylosing spondylitis 36–7, 38, 39
  antiphospholipid syndrome 40–1
  aortic regurgitation 43–5
  aortic stenosis 46–8
  autonomic dysfunction 67
  Becker muscular dystrophy 70, 71
  Beckwith–Wiedemann syndrome 71
  carcinoid syndrome 76, 77
  coarctation of aorta 100–1
  cocaine abuse 102, 103, 104
  Cushing's disease 112, 113
  dermatomyositis/polymyositis complex 126
  diabetes mellitus 129, 130, 131
  Duchenne muscular dystrophy 142, 143, 144, 145
  Ehlers–Danlos syndrome 163
  Emery–Dreifuss muscular dystrophy 169
  Fabry's disease 182
  familial dysautonomia 186, 187
  Friedreich's ataxia 200–1
  hypothyroidism 263
  Kawasaki disease 279, 280
  Kearns–Sayre syndrome 281
  Marfan syndrome 303, 304
  Maroteaux–Lamy syndrome 307
  mitochondrial encephalopathies 319
  Morquio's syndrome 328, 329
  mucopolysaccharidoses 251, 253
  myeloma 344
  nemaline myopathy 350
  Noonan's syndrome 357, 358
  obesity 360, 361
  osteogenesis imperfecta 371
  Paget's disease 375

  phaeochromocytoma 384, 389
  Pompe's disease 405, 406
  pulmonary hypertension 420
  pulmonary oedema 424–6
  relapsing polychondritis 439
  rheumatoid arthritis 448, 449
  sarcoidosis 452, 453
  scleroderma 455
  scoliosis 458
  Sturge–Weber syndrome 472, 473
  systemic lupus erythematosus 474, 475
  Takayasu's arteritis 477, 478
  thalassaemia 485
  thyrotoxicosis 488, 489–90
  tuberous sclerosis 496
  Turner's syndrome 497, 498
  Wegener's granulomatosis 510, 511
  Williams syndrome 513, 514, 515
carnitine palmitoyl transferase 89
carnitine palmitoyl transferase deficiency 88–9, 443, 444
carotid body tumour 90–1, 384
caudal anaesthesia, local anaesthetic toxic reactions 559, 560
central anticholinergic syndrome 553–5
central core disease 91–3
centronuclear (myotubular) myopathy 345–6
cephalosporins
  anaphylactic/anaphylactoid reactions 536
  epiglottitis 174, 175
  safety in porphyria 411
cerebral berry aneurysm 100
cerebral oedema
  preeclampsia 157, 158, 161
  TURP syndrome 589
cerebral protection 206
cervical spine abnormalities
  ankylosing spondylitis 36, 37, 39
  fibrodysplasia ossificans progressiva 196, 197
  Goldenhar's syndrome 211
  Klippel–Feil syndrome 282, 283
  Maroteaux–Lamy syndrome 307
  neurofibromatosis 352–3
  Paget's disease 375–6
  rheumatoid arthritis 448–9, 450
  Turner's syndrome 497, 498
  see also atlantoaxial instability
Charcot–Marie–Tooth disease (peroneal muscular atrophy) 95–6
CHARGE association 96–7
cherubism 98
Chiari malformations 49–51

chloramphenicol 208
  porphyria 410
chlordiazepoxide 554
  porphyria 410
chlormethiazole 25
chloroprocaine 31
chloroquine 209
chlorphenamine *see* chlorpheniramine
chlorpheniramine 309, 538, 543, 556
  safety in porphyria 411
chlorpromazine 31, 295, 400, 411, 427
  adverse reactions
    neuroleptic malignant syndrome 355
    suxamethonium apnoea 581
  safety in porphyria 411
choanal atresia 96, 97
Christmas disease (haemophilia B) 224, 227–8
Churg–Strauss syndrome 56, 99, 400
cimetidine 188, 309
  anticonvulsant interactions 177
  central anticholinergic syndrome 553
  porphyria 410
cisapride 107
  torsade de pointes 491, 584, 585
cisatracurium 536
cleft lip/palate
  arthrogryposis multiplex congenita 52
  Dandy–Walker syndrome 122
  Miller's syndrome 317
  Pierre Robin syndrome 393
  Treacher Collins syndrome 494
clodronate 257
clonidine 25, 91, 482
coagulation abnormalities
  alcoholic patients 24, 25
  amniotic fluid embolism 533
  amyloidosis 34, 35
  antiphospholipid syndrome 40, 41
  Factor IX deficiency 227
  Fallot's tetralogy 184
  Gaucher's disease 203
  haemophilia A 224–5
  HELLP syndrome 236
  malignant hyperthermia 299
  Noonan's syndrome 358
  preeclampsia 158
  TURP syndrome 591
  von Gierke's disease 502, 503
  von Willebrand's disease 506, 507
  see also haemostatic defects
coarctation of aorta 100–1
cocaine

abuse 12–13, 102–5, 179
  anaesthetic interactions 103
  cardiotoxicity 102, 103, 104
  plasma cholinesterase deficiency-related toxicity
    401, 580, 581
  rhabdomyolysis 443
Cockayne syndrome 106–7
codeine, safety in porphyria 411
collagen vascular disease 420
compartment syndrome 445, 446
congestive (dilated) cardiomyopathy 82, 83
Conn's syndrome (primary aldosteronism) 107–9
consent
  AIDS dementia 19
  Jehovah's witnesses 274
contractures, congenital 51
contrast media, anaphylactic/anaphylactoid reactions
    536
convulsions *see* seizures/convulsions
cortisone 16
co-trimoxazole 18
coumarins, safety in porphyria 411
craniocarpotarsal dysplasia (Freeman–Sheldon
    syndrome; distal arthrogryposis type 2) 199–200
CREST syndrome (limited cutaneous scleroderma)
    455, 457
Creutzfeldt–Jakob disease (CJD) 109–11
cri du chat syndrome 111–12
Cushing's disease 112–13
Cushing's syndrome 112–13
cutaneous mastocytosis 308, 309
cyclophosphamide 99, 420, 474, 510, 511
cyclosporin 420
cyproheptadine 77, 78, 550
cystic fibrosis 114–18
  chest infections 115, 116–17
cystic hygroma (lymphangioma) 119–20

D

danazol 94, 239, 240
Dandy–Walker syndrome 122
dantrolene sodium 31, 92, 150, 229, 296, 299, 300,
    301, 355, 356, 372, 446, 566, 583
dapsone 571
datura stramonium 553
delerium tremens 24, 25
demyelinating disease 123–5
dermatomyositis/polymyositis complex 125–6, 465
desferrioxamine 484, 485
desflurane 388
  adverse reactions 92
    malignant hyperthermia 299

desipramine 355
desmogleins 382
desmopressin 226, 244, 276, 507, 508, 509
  adverse reactions 225
dexamethasone 15, 16, 113, 222, 237, 398, 427
dexamethasone test 112
dextromoramide 369
diabetes insipidus 127–8
  acromegaly 9
diabetes mellitus 129–33
  acromegaly 9
  autonomic dysfunction 66, 67, 68
  Cushing's disease 112, 113
  Friedreich's ataxia 201
  glucagonoma 207
  glycaemic control
    assessment 131–2
    elective surgery 132
    glucose/insulin/potassium (GIK) technique 132
  hypothyroidism association 263
  infection susceptibility 129, 130
  insulin resistance 133
  insulin-dependent (type I) 129, 130, 132
  ketoacidosis 133
  noninsulin-dependent (type II) 129, 132
  obesity association 360
3,4-diaminopyridine 153, 154
diathermy
  automatic implantable cardioverter defibrillators
    (AICD) 64
  pacemaker complications 230–1, 233
diazepam 25, 81, 160, 187, 188, 383, 561
  adverse reactions 204
    central anticholinergic syndrome 554
  porphyria 410
diazoxide 269, 270
  safety in porphyria 411
dibucaine number 399, 401
difficult intubation
  achondroplasia 5, 7
  acromegaly 10, 11
  amyloidosis 33, 35
  ankylosing spondylitis 37, 38–9
  arthrogryposis multiplex congenita 52, 53
  CHARGE association 97
  cherubism 98
  Cockayne syndrome 107
  cri du chat syndrome 111
  diabetes mellitus 131
  diffuse idiopathic skeletal hyperostosis 135
  Down's syndrome 137
  fibrodysplasia ossificans progressiva 197

Fraser syndrome 198
Freeman–Sheldon syndrome 199–200
Gaucher's disease 203, 204
Goldenhar's syndrome 211
Gorham's syndrome 214
juvenile hyaline fibromatosis 277, 278
Klippel–Feil syndrome 282, 283
laryngeal papillomatosis 287, 288
Ludwig's angina 293
Maroteaux–Lamy syndrome 307
Miller's syndrome 317
Morquio's syndrome 329
mucopolysaccharidoses 252
nemaline myopathy 350
Noonan's syndrome 357, 358
obesity 360, 361
obstructive sleep apnoea 365
Opitz–Frias syndrome 370
osteogenesis imperfecta 372
Pierre Robin syndrome 393, 394–5
Pompe's disease 407
Prader–Willi syndrome 414
relapsing polychondritis 440
Schwartz–Jampel syndrome 454
scleroderma 456, 457
spondyloepiphyseal dysplasia 471
thalassaemia 485
Treacher Collins syndrome 495–6
Turner's syndrome 498
Williams syndrome 514, 515
diffuse idiopathic skeletal hyperostosis 134–5
digitalis toxicity 546
digoxin 85, 322, 323, 324, 326, 425, 492, 518, 547, 583
  safety in porphyria 411
dihydrocodeine 227
dilated (congestive) cardiomyopathy 82, 83, 84–5, 86
diltiazem 83, 419, 420, 518
diphenhydramine 379
dipipanone 369
disopyramide 83, 492, 518, 547, 548
  torsade de pointes 491, 585
distal arthrogryposis type 2 (Freeman–Sheldon
    syndrome; craniocarpotarsal dysplasia) 199–200
distal muscular dystrophy 340
diuretics 83, 192
  neurogenic pulmonary oedema 427
  pulmonary hypertension 421
  torsade de pointes 585
  TURP syndrome 591
dobutamine 45, 86, 324, 425, 427
dopamine 81, 86, 575

Down's syndrome 136–8
droperidol 299, 427, 517
    adverse reactions 346, 355
        central anticholinergic syndrome 553, 554
        neuroleptic malignant syndrome 355
    aortic regurgitation 45
    contraindication in phaeochromocytoma 388
    safety in porphyria 411
drowning *see* near drowning
drug abuse 12–13, 173, 546
    seizures 179
Duchenne muscular dystrophy 142–6, 298, 339, 445,
    459
        malignant hyperthermia-like reactions 143, 144,
            297, 564
        masseter muscle rigidity 568
        rhabdomyolysis 443, 444, 445
dwarfism *see* spondyloepiphyseal dysplasia
dystrophia myotonica 147–50
dystrophin 70, 142

E
Eaton–Lambert (Lambert–Eaton; myasthenic)
    syndrome 153–4
Ebstein–Barr virus 267
Ebstein's anomaly 155–6, 546
eclampsia 156–61
    convulsions management 160–1
    postpartum fits 161
ecstasy (MDMA) 13, 30, 31
    acute hyponatraemia 259
    rhabdomyolysis 443, 446
edrophonium 340
Ehlers–Danlos syndrome 43, 162–5, 325, 543
    ecchymotic form (type IV) 162–3, 164–5
Eisenmenger's syndrome 166–8
electroconvulsive therapy (ECT) 63, 64–5
emerin 169
Emery–Dreifuss muscular dystrophy 169, 339
EMLA cream
    methaemoglobinaemia 570
    toxicity 560
enalapril 93
endoglin 241
enflurane 48, 56, 57, 87, 362, 548
    contraindications 70, 86
        Wolff–Parkinson–White syndrome 517
    perioperative excitatory events 178
    porphyria 410, 411
ephedrine 588
epidermolysis bullosa 170–2
    junctional 170

    recessive dystrophic 170
    simplex 170
epidural anaesthesia
    accidental subdural block 577, 579
    accidental total spinal anaesthesia 586–8
    achondroplasia 7–8
    amphetamine abuse 31, 32
    amyloidosis 35
    ankylosing spondylitis 38, 39
    aortic regurgitation 45
    aortic stenosis 48
    carcinoid syndrome 78
    Charcot–Marie–Tooth disease 96
    Chiari malformations 50, 51
    cystic fibrosis 118
    demyelinating disease/multiple sclerosis 124–5
    dilated cardiomyopathy 86
    dystrophia myotonica 149
    Ebstein's anomaly 156
    Ehlers–Danlos syndrome 163, 164
    epidermolysis bullosa 172
    Friedreich's ataxia 201–2
    Guillain–Barré syndrome 216
    haemophilia A carriers 227
    hereditary haemorrhagic telangiectasia 243
    HIV infection/AIDS 19, 20
    hypertrophic cardiomyopathy 86
    hypokalaemic periodic paralysis 190, 191
    Kawasaki disease 279, 280
    Kearns–Sayre syndrome 281
    local anaesthetic toxic reactions 559, 560
    Marfan syndrome 305
    mitral valve prolapse 326
    motor neurone disease 331
    myasthenia gravis 342
    nemaline myopathy 350
    Noonan's syndrome 358
    obesity 361
    obstructive sleep apnoea 365
    paramyotonia 192
    pemphigus vulgaris 383
    phaeochromocytoma 388
    preeclampsia/eclampsia 159
    pulmonary hypertension 421–2
    Rett syndrome 442
    rheumatoid arthritis 450
    sarcoidosis 453
    spondyloepiphyseal dysplasia 471
    Takayasu's arteritis 479
    test dose 561, 587
    tetanus 482
    thalidomide-related deformities/phocomelias 487

605

von Hippel–Lindau disease 505
von Willebrand's disease 508
epidural blood patch, HIV infection/AIDS patients
    19, 20
epiglottitis 172–5
    intubation 174, 175
epilepsy 176–80
    generalised seizures 176
    partial seizures 176
epinephrine (adrenaline) 57, 94, 175, 233, 256, 310,
    533, 534, 543, 549
    adverse reactions
        cardiac arrhythmias 546
        long QT syndrome 435–6
    anaphylactic/anaphylactoid reactions 537–8
    cardiovascular collapse 556
    latex allergy 556
    phaeochromocytoma 384, 385
    safety in porphyria 411
epsilon aminocaproic acid 240, 285
ergometrine 87, 425, 430
ergot alkaloids 410
erythromycin 133, 246, 486
    porphyria 410, 411
erythropoietin 274–5
esmolol 86, 105, 389, 426, 431, 436, 482, 489, 490, 583
etidronate 197, 375
etomidate 15, 28, 56, 76, 78, 113
    adverse reactions
        anaphylactic/anaphylactoid 536
        perioperative excitatory events 177–8
    porphyria 410
eve (MDEA) 13, 30, 446
extracorporeal shock wave lithotripsy (ESWL)
    automatic implantable cardioverter defibrillators
        (AICD) 63, 65
    pacemaker problems 231, 234

F
Fabry's disease 83, 182
Factor IX deficiency 224, 227
Factor IX therapy 226, 227, 228
Factor V Leiden 73, 74, 418
Factor VIII deficiency 224
Factor VIII inhibitors (acquired haemophilia) 224,
    225–6, 227
Factor VIII therapy 225, 226, 508
    intraoperative 226
    pregnancy management 227
Fallot's tetralogy 183–5
familial dysautonomia (Riley–Day syndrome) 66,
    186–8

familial periodic paralyses 188–93
familial ventricular tachycardia 585
    see also QT syndrome, prolonged
famotidine 309
facioscapulohumeral (Landouzy–Dejerine) muscular
    dystrophy 340
fat embolism 193–5
felypressin 103
fenoterol 429, 430
fentanyl 8, 27, 76, 78, 81, 87, 112, 156, 185, 207, 333,
    334, 342, 362, 414, 421, 587
    adverse reactions 148, 253, 346
        central anticholinergic syndrome 554
        perioperative excitatory events 178
    porphyria 410, 411
    regional anaesthesia 86, 117
        myasthenia gravis 342
fetal haemoglobin 218
    sickle cell disease 219, 220
fetal loss 40, 42
fibrillin 303
fibrodysplasia (myositis) ossificans progressiva 196–7
flecainide 516, 518, 548
fludrocortisone 16, 337, 338
flumazenil 482
flunitrazepam 410
fluoride number 399, 401
fluorocarbons abuse 466
fluphenazine 355
fluticasone cromoglycate 55
fosphenytoin 180
fracture susceptibility
    osteogenesis imperfecta 370, 371, 372
    Paget's disease 375, 376
    Turner's syndrome 497
Fraser syndrome 198
frataxin 200
Freeman–Sheldon syndrome (distal arthrogryposis
    type 2; craniocarpotarsal dysplasia) 199–200
Friedreich's ataxia 200–2, 458, 459
frusemide 261, 301, 425, 591
    porphyria 410

G
gabapentin 124, 331
gallamine 536
gastro-oesophageal reflux
    cystic fibrosis 116, 117
    Noonan's syndrome 357
    Pierre Robin syndrome 393, 394
    scleroderma 456
gastroparesis 67

Gaucher's disease 203–4
Gerstmann–Straussler–Schenker disease 109
giant axonal neuropathy 204
Gilbert's disease (idiopathic unconjugated
  hyperbilirubinaemia) 205
glomus jugulare tumour 205–7
glucagon 207
glucagonoma 207–8
glucose-6-phosphate dehydrogenase deficiency
  208–9, 570
glucose/insulin/potassium (GIK) technique 132
glutethimide 410
glyceryl trinitrate 45, 101, 306, 388, 389, 422, 425,
  430
  safety in porphyria 411
glycine irrigation fluid 588, 589
glycogen storage diseases 209–10
  classification 210
  type Ia (von Gierke's disease) 502–3
  type IIa (Pompe's disease) 405–7
  type V (myophosphorylase deficiency; McArdle's
    syndrome) 298, 311–12, 443, 444, 445, 564
  type VI (Hers' disease) 246–7
glycogen synthase deficiency 210
glycopyrrolate 299
  central anticholinergic syndrome 554
  ranitidine interaction 554
Goldenhar's syndrome (oculo-auriculo-vertebral
  dysplasia) 210–11
Goodpasture's syndrome 212
Gorham's syndrome 213–14
Graves' disease 465
griseofulvin 410
growth hormone 8, 9
guanidine 153
Guillain–Barré syndrome 214–16, 267, 445
  autonomic dysfunction 66
  rhabdomyolysis 443, 444

H

H1 antagonists *see* antihistamines
H2 antagonists 24, 107, 117, 291, 309, 362, 550
haem metabolism 407, 408
haemoglobin 218
haemoglobin Barts 484
haemoglobin H 484
haemoglobin M disease 570
haemoglobinopathies 218
haemolytic anaemia
  glucose-6-phosphate dehydrogenase deficiency
    208, 209
  hereditary spherocytosis 245, 246

paroxysmal nocturnal haemoglobinuria 380
sickle cell anaemia 219
haemophilia A 224–7
  acquired 224, 225–6, 227
haemophilia B (Christmas disease) 224, 227–8
haemostatic defects
  Ehlers–Danlos syndrome 162, 163
  polycythaemia vera 403, 404, 405
  see also coagulation abnormalities
Hallervorden–Spatz disease (neuronal dystrophy)
  228–9, 354
haloperidol 25
  adverse reactions 92
    neuroleptic malignant syndrome 355
    torsade de pointes 491, 584, 585
halothane 30, 31, 48, 56–7, 58, 80, 87, 174, 358, 362,
  548
  adverse reactions 355, 442
    Freeman–Sheldon syndrome 199
    Williams syndrome 514
  contraindications 25, 32, 70, 86
    Duchenne muscular dystrophy 143, 145–6, 459
    pacemakers 231
    phaeochromocytoma 388
    Pompe's disease 407
    Wolff–Parkinson–White syndrome 517
  drug interactions
    aminophylline 55, 57
    anticonvulsants 177
  myasthenia gravis 342
  porphyria 410, 411
  rhabdomyolysis 459
heart block 229–34
  acquired 230
  classification 230
  congenital 229–30
  Kearns–Sayre syndrome 281
  obstructive sleep apnoea 364, 365
  pacemakers *see* pacemakers
  sarcoidosis 452, 453
  torsade de pointes 491
heat stroke 298
HELLP syndrome 157, 158, 235–7
heparin 41, 42, 74, 168, 248, 417, 418, 420, 474, 475,
  483
  safety in porphyria 411
hepatitis A 225
hepatitis B 13, 103, 136
  opiate addicts 368, 369
  transmission in blood products 225
hepatitis C 225, 485
hepatitis, chronic active 465

607

hereditary angioneurotic oedema 93, 94, 238–40, 542, 543
hereditary coproporphyria 409
hereditary haemorrhagic telangiectasia (Osler–Weber–Rendu disease) 241–4
hereditary spherocytosis 245–6
heroin abuse 179, 480
    abstinence syndrome 369
    methadone equivalent dosage 369
Hers' disease (Cori type VI glycogen storage disease) 246–7
histamine
    asthma 54
    carcinoid syndrome 76, 77, 549, 550
    mastocytosis 308, 309, 310
HIV infection/AIDS 13, 17–21, 103, 173
    autonomic dysfunction 66
    occupational post-exposure prophylaxis 20, 21
    opiate addicts 368, 369
    transmission 485
        blood products 225
        occupational 17–18, 19–20, 21
homocystinuria 247–8
Hughes' syndrome *see* antiphospholipid syndrome
human papillomavirus 287, 288
Hunter syndrome 250, 251–2, 253, 335
Huntington's disease 249–50, 400
Hurler syndrome 250, 251, 252, 253, 335
Hurler–Scheie syndrome 250, 251, 254, 335
hydantoins 410
hydatid disease 255–6
hydralazine 159, 237, 306
    porphyria 410
hydrocephalus
    achondroplasia 5, 7
    Chiari malformations 50
    Dandy–Walker syndrome 122
    neurofibromatosis 353
    osteogenesis imperfecta 371
hydrocortisone 16, 524, 556, 583
hydroxyurea 220, 222, 403, 405
hyoscine
    central anticholinergic syndrome 553, 554
    safety in porphyria 411
hypercalcaemia 256–7, 336
    acromegaly 9
    Addison's disease 14
    myeloma 344, 345
    sarcoidosis 452, 453
    vipoma 501
    Williams syndrome 514
hyperemesis gravidarum 14, 257, 523

hyperglycaemia
    Cushing's disease 112
    diabetes mellitus 129, 130, 133
    hyponatraemia 261
hyperglycaemic hyperosmolar nonketotic coma 133
hyperkalaemia
    Addison's disease 14
    amphetamine abuse 30
    Becker muscular dystrophy 70, 71
    Duchenne muscular dystrophy 142, 143
    malignant hyperthermia 299, 301, 564–5
    periodic paralysis 188, 191–3
    rhabdomyolysis 444
    suxamethonium-related 445, 459
hypermetabolic reactions
    arthrogryposis multiplex congenita 52, 53
    dystrophia myotonica 149
    myotonia congenita 149, 151
    osteogenesis imperfecta 371, 372
    thyroid crisis (thyroid storm) 582
    thyrotoxicosis 488
    see also malignant hyperthermia-like reactions
hypertension 546
    acromegaly 9, 10
    amphetamine abuse 30, 32
    carcinoid syndrome 76, 77, 78, 549
    carotid body tumour 90, 91
    coarctation of aorta 100, 101
    cocaine abuse 104
    Conn's syndrome (primary aldosteronism) 107, 108, 109
    Cushing's disease 112, 113
    HELLP syndrome 235, 237
    intubation response 157–8
        drug modification 160
    Marfan syndrome 305–6
    neurofibromatosis 352
    obesity 360
    obstructive sleep apnoea 364, 365
    phaeochromocytoma 159, 384, 385, 386, 387, 572, 573
        intraoperative management 389
    preeclampsia 156, 157, 159, 160
    scleroderma 455, 456
    Takayasu's arteritis 477
    tetanus 480, 481, 482
    Turner's syndrome 498
    Williams syndrome 514
hyperthermia, amphetamine abuse 30, 31
hypertrophic cardiomyopathy 82–3, 84, 85, 86–7, 142, 459
    Friedreich's ataxia 201

Noonan's syndrome 357, 358
hyperviscosity
  myeloma 344, 345
  polycythaemia vera 403
hypocalcaemia, torsade de pointes 492, 585
hypoglycaemia
  Addison's disease 14, 16, 524
  alcoholic patients 24, 25
  Beckwith–Wiedemann syndrome 72
  diabetes mellitus 129, 130, 133
  Hers' disease 246, 247
  homocystinuria 248
  insulinoma 269, 270
  phaeochromocytoma surgery 386
  Prader–Willi syndrome 413, 414
  propranolol-related 489
  status epilepticus 180
  von Gierke's disease 502, 503
hypokalaemia
  alcoholic patients 24, 25
  Conn's syndrome 107, 108, 109
  Cushing's disease 112, 113
  periodic paralysis 188, 189–91
  torsade de pointes 492, 585
  vipoma 501
hypomagnesaemia, torsade de pointes 492, 585
hyponatraemia 258–62
  active treatment 260, 261
  Addison's disease 14
  dilutional 258, 259, 261
    prevention 261
  encephalopathy 260
  Guillain–Barré syndrome 215
  neuroleptic malignant syndrome 355
  pulmonary oedema 260
  solute losses 259–60, 261
  syndrome of inappropriate ADH secretion 259, 261
  tetanus 481
  TURP syndrome 589, 591
  varicella pneumonia 499
hypotension
  Addisonian crisis 523, 524
  amniotic fluid embolism 533
  aortic stenosis 47
  autonomic dysfunction 67, 68
  carcinoid syndrome 549, 550
  cardiac arrhythmias 547
  cardiac myxoma 347
  cardiac tamponade 79, 80
  familial dysautonomia 186, 187
  hypothyroidism 263–4
  latex allergy 556

mastocytosis 309, 310
mitral valve prolapse 326
multiple system atrophy 337, 338
opiate addicts 369
Parkinson's disease 377
phaeochromocytoma 572, 573, 575
  surgery 386, 389
tetanus 480, 483
TURP syndrome 589
hypotensive anaesthesia, glomus jugulare tumour
  surgery 206
hypothermia
  glomus jugulare tumour surgery 206
  near drowning 139, 140, 141
hypothyroidism 262–5
hypoxaemia
  alveolar proteinosis 28, 29
  cardiac myxoma 347
  Duchenne muscular dystrophy 142
  Fallot's tetralogy 184
  Goodpasture's syndrome 212
  hereditary haemorrhagic telangiectasia 243
  malignant hyperthermia 298, 564
  pulmonary hypertension 420, 421
  secondary polycythaemia 402

idiopathic unconjugated hyperbilirubinaemia
  (Gilbert's disease) 205
imipramine
  porphyria 410
  torsade de pointes 585
immunoglobulin, intravenous
  Eaton–Lambert syndrome 154
  Guillain–Barré syndrome 216
  Kawasaki disease 279
  pemphigus vulgaris 383
  systemic lupus erythematosus 474
immunosuppressive therapy
  scleroderma 455
  Takayasu's arteritis 477
indinavar 21
indomethacin 309
infectious mononucleosis 267–8
insulin therapy 129, 130
  diabetic ketoacidosis 133
  elective surgery 132
  glucose/insulin/potassium (GIK) technique 132
  safety in porphyria 411
insulin-like growth factor (somatomedin) 8–9
insulinoma 207, 269–70
intercostal block, hypokalaemic periodic paralysis 190

609

interferon therapy 289, 344
intermittent porphyria, acute 407, 408, 409
interscalene block, local anaesthetic toxic reactions
    558
intracranial haemorrhage
    haemophilia A 225
    hereditary haemorrhagic telangiectasia 242
    pregnancy 157, 161
    Sturge–Weber syndrome 473
intrapleural block, local anaesthetic toxic reactions
    559
ion channelopathies 147
iron overload 484, 485
ischaemic heart disease 546
    cardiac arrhythmias 546
    pulmonary oedema 424, 425
isoflurane 25, 56, 57, 64, 81, 87, 207, 310, 333, 334,
    362, 482, 548
    adverse reactions
        Duchenne muscular dystrophy 143
        long QT syndrome 435
    contraindications 87
        Wolff–Parkinson–White syndrome 517
    drug interactions 103
    myasthenia gravis 342, 343
    perioperative excitatory event suppression 178
isoprenaline 86, 109, 233, 256, 422, 427, 492, 556, 585
isosorbide dinitrate 425
isoxuprine 429

J
jaundice
    Gilbert's disease 205
    glucose-6-phosphate dehydrogenase deficiency
        209
    HELLP syndrome 236
    paroxysmal nocturnal haemoglobinuria 380
Jehovah's witnesses 272–6
    acceptable products 273, 274
    autologous intraoperative transfusion 273, 274,
        275–6
    blood loss minimization 275
    blood loss treatment 275–6
    children 272, 274
    discussion/agreement with patients 272, 274
    legal issues 272–3
        informed consent 274
    plasma expanders 273–4
    preoperative erythropoietin therapy 274–5
Jervell and Lange–Nielsen syndrome 436, 585
    see also QT syndrome, prolonged
juvenile hyaline fibromatosis 277–8

K
Kasabach–Merritt syndrome 285
Kawasaki disease (mucocutaneous lymph node
    syndrome) 279–80
Kearns–Sayre syndrome 280–1, 318
ketamine 53, 56, 57, 171, 185, 197, 315, 372, 379, 383,
    395, 407, 442, 495, 513
    drug interactions 103
    malignant hyperthermia 299
    perioperative excitatory events 179
    porphyria 410, 411
ketanserin 77, 78, 549, 550
Klippel–Feil syndrome 282–3
Klippel–Trenaunay–Weber syndrome 284–6, 472
knee–elbow position 444
Korsakoff's psychosis 24
kuru 109
kyphoscoliosis
    achondroplasia 5
    acromegaly 9
    cystic fibrosis 115
    Ehlers–Danlos syndrome type VI 163
    fibrodysplasia ossificans progressiva 196
    Freeman–Sheldon syndrome 199
    homocystinuria 247
    Klippel–Feil syndrome 283
    Maroteaux–Lamy syndrome 307
    Morquio's syndrome 328
    neurofibromatosis 1 351, 352
    Noonan's syndrome 357
    osteogenesis imperfecta 371
kyphosis
    Prader–Willi syndrome 413
    spondyloepiphyseal dysplasia 470

L
labetalol 104, 105, 159, 306, 387, 482, 492
    safety in porphyria 411
lactic acidosis 133
    local anaesthetic toxic reactions 559
    mitochondrial encephalopathies 319, 320
    von Gierke's disease 503
Lambert–Eaton (Eaton–Lambert; myasthenic)
    syndrome 153–4
lamivudine 21
Landouzy–Dejerine (facioscapulohumeral) muscular
    dystrophy 340
lanreotide 77
laryngeal mask airway
    ankylosing spondylitis 37, 39
    asthma 55, 56

Cockayne syndrome 107
cri du chat syndrome 112
diffuse idiopathic skeletal hyperostosis 135
epidermolysis bullosa 170, 171
Freeman–Sheldon syndrome 200
Gaucher's disease 203
juvenile hyaline fibromatosis 278
mucopolysaccharidoses 252, 253
osteogenesis imperfecta 373
Pierre Robin syndrome 395–6
rheumatoid arthritis 449, 450
Treacher Collins syndrome 495
laryngeal oedema
 HELLP syndrome 236
 hereditary angioneurotic oedema 239
 preeclampsia/eclampsia 158–9
 varicella pneumonia 500
laryngeal papillomatosis 287–9
laryngeal sarcoidosis 452, 453
lateral decubitus position 444
latex allergy 290–1, 534, 536, 555–6
 preoperative prophylaxis 290, 291
Leber's hereditary optic neuropathy 318
Lesch–Nyhan disease 291–2
leukotriene receptor antagonists 54, 55, 56
leukotrienes 54
levobupivacaine toxicity 558, 560
levodopa 209, 337, 377, 378, 379, 385
 drug interactions 378
 withdrawal-related neuroleptic malignant
  syndrome 354, 355
levomepromazine (methotrimeprazine) 78, 550
Libman–Sacks endocarditis 474
lidocaine (lignocaine) 31, 56, 63, 64, 76, 84, 91, 160,
 395, 492, 547, 548, 586
 accidental subdural block 578
 anaphylactic/anaphylactoid reactions 536
 porphyria 410, 411
 toxicity 558, 559, 560
lidoflazine 585
limited cutaneous scleroderma (CREST syndrome)
 455, 457
lisuride 377
lithium 127
lithotomy position 443–4, 445
liver dysfunction
 alcoholic patients 24, 25
 Budd–Chiari syndrome 73, 74
 cystic fibrosis 114, 115, 116
 HELLP syndrome 236, 237
 hereditary haemorrhagic telangiectasia 242
 infectious mononucleosis 267

 mastocytosis 308
 mitochondrial encephalopathies 319
 opiate addiction 368
 plasma cholinesterase abnormalities 400
 von Gierke's disease 503
local anaesthesia
 anaphylactic/anaphylactoid reactions 536
 demyelinating disease/multiple sclerosis 124
 diabetes mellitus 131
 Duchenne muscular dystrophy 145
 dystrophia myotonica 149
 Ehlers–Danlos syndrome 164
 familial dysautonomia 187
 mucopolysaccharidoses 254
 Pompe's disease 407
 safety in porphyria 411
 toxicity 557–62
long QT syndrome *see* QT syndrome, prolonged
lorazepam 176
 safety in porphyria 411
low-molecular-weight heparin 42, 419
Ludwig's angina 292–4
lung function tests
 alveolar proteinosis 27
 asthma 55
 dystrophia myotonica 149
 Goodpasture's syndrome 212
 Gorham's syndrome 214
 sarcoidosis 453
 sickle cell disease 222
 systemic lupus erythematosus 474
lung transplantation, cystic fibrosis 117–18
lupus anticoagulant 474
 thromboembolic complications 474–5
lupus pneumonitis 474
lupus syndrome 40
lymphangioma (cystic hygroma) 119–20
lysergic acid diethylamide (LSD) abuse 12, 294–5

M

macroglossia
 amyloidosis 33, 34, 35
 Beckwith–Wiedemann syndrome 71, 72
 Dandy–Walker syndrome 122
 Maroteaux–Lamy syndrome 307
 Pompe's disease 406, 407
 Treacher Collins syndrome 494
magnesium sulphate 58, 157, 160, 388, 389, 482, 492,
 574, 586
 preeclampsia/eclampsia 159, 160
magnetic resonance imaging, automatic implantable
 cardioverter defibrillators (AICD) 64

MAGPIE trial 157, 160
malignant hyperthermia 52, 53, 143, 144, 209,
 296–301, 445, 546, 563–6, 574
 associated conditions 297–8
 central core disease 92–3
 neuroleptic malignant syndrome 354–5, 356
 postoperative pyrexia 301
 diagnostic criteria 297, 298, 299, 301
 hyperkalaemia 564–5
 management 296, 565–6
 fulminant syndrome 300–1
 intraoperative 300
 masseter muscle rigidity 564, 567
 nontriggering anaesthetics 299–300, 301
 presentation 564–5
 prophylaxis 296
 rhabdomyolysis 443, 444, 445
 trigger agents 296, 299
malignant hyperthermia-like reactions 564
 hyperkalaemic periodic paralysis/paramyotonia
 191–2
 hypokalaemic periodic paralysis 190
 osteogenesis imperfecta 372
 Schwartz–Jampel syndrome 454
 see also hypermetabolic reactions
Mallory–Weiss syndrome 456
mannitol 261, 301, 591
maprotiline 585
Marcus Gunn jaw winking phenomenon 303
Marfan's syndrome 43, 44, 303–6, 325, 458, 459, 543
Maroteaux–Lamy syndrome 251, 252, 307
mask ventilation problems
 achondroplasia 5
 acromegaly 10
masseter muscle rigidity 444, 564, 566–9
massive pulmonary fibrosis 447
mast-cell leukaemia 308
mastocytosis 308–10
McArdle's syndrome (myophosphorylase deficiency)
 298, 311–12, 443, 444, 445
 malignant hyperthermia-like reactions 564
mebendazole 256
mediastinal masses 313–16
 airway obstruction 313–14, 315, 316
 anaesthetic hazards 313, 314–15
 myocardial/pericardial involvement 314–15
 pulmonary artery obstruction 314
 superior vena cava obstruction 313, 314, 315
MEN 336
mepivacaine 559
meprobamate 410
metaraminol 256, 326

metformin 131
methadone 369
methaemoglobinaemia 569–71
methohexitone 177
methotrexate
 pulmonary hypertension with collagen vascular
 disease 420
 sarcoidosis 453
methotrimeprazine (levomepromazine) 78, 550
methoxamine 87, 167
methyldopa 159, 385
 porphyria 410
methylene blue 208, 209
 methaemoglobinaemia 570, 571
methylprednisolone 16
metoclopramide 182, 299
 contraindications 379
 neuroleptic malignant syndrome 355
 plasma cholinesterase inhibition 400
 porphyria 410
metocurine 179
metoprolol 295, 389
metronidazole 481
metyrapone 113
mexilitene 151, 192, 548
micrognathia/microstomia
 arthrogryposis multiplex congenita 52
 CHARGE association 97
 cri du chat syndrome 111
 Dandy–Walker syndrome 122
 Freeman–Sheldon syndrome 199
 Goldenhar's syndrome 211
 Miller's syndrome 317
 Noonan's syndrome 357
 Opitz–Frias syndrome 370
 Pierre Robin syndrome 393
 Prader–Willi syndrome 414
 Turner's syndrome 497
midazolam 25, 250, 315, 482, 517
 safety in porphyria 411
Miller's syndrome 317–18
mithramycin 375
mitochondrial encephalopathies 318–20
mitochondrial encephalopathy with lactic acidosis
 and stroke-like episodes (MELAS) 318, 320
mitral stenosis 323–5
 pulmonary oedema 425
mitral valve disease 321–7
 pulmonary oedema 424
mitral valve prolapse 325–7, 434, 546
mitral valve regurgitation 321–3, 325, 326, 439
mivacurium 96, 319

adverse reactions
   anaphylactic/anaphylactoid 536
   apnoea 580–1
  myasthenia gravis 342
  plasma cholinesterase hydrolysis 399, 400
montelukast 55
morphine 87, 182, 222, 332, 366, 425, 482
  abstinence syndrome 369
  accidental subdural block 578
  adverse reactions 205
   central anticholinergic syndrome 554
  contraindication in phaeochromocytoma 388
  intrathecal 342
  methadone equivalent dosage 369
  safety in porphyria 411
  spinal 167
  tolerance 368, 369
Morquio's syndrome 328–9
motor neurone disease (amyotrophic lateral sclerosis) 330–2
moyamoya disease 332–4
mucocutaneous lymph node syndrome (Kawasaki disease) 279–80
mucopolysaccharidoses 250–4, 335
multiple endocrine neoplasia 336–7
  phaeochromocytoma 384
multiple endocrine neoplasia (MEN) 1 336
  insulinoma 269
  vipoma 500
multiple endocrine neoplasia (MEN) 2A (Sipple's syndrome) 336, 463–4
multiple endocrine neoplasia (MEN) 2B 336
multiple sclerosis 123, 124
multiple system atrophy 66, 68, 337–9
muscle relaxants
  anaphylactic/anaphylactoid reactions 536
  Duchenne muscular dystrophy 143, 144, 145
  dystrophia myotonica 148
  Eaton–Lambert syndrome 153, 154
  familial dysautonomia 187
  Friedreich's ataxia 201
  Huntington's disease 240, 250
  hyperkalaemic periodic paralysis/paramyotonia 192, 193
  hypokalaemic periodic paralysis 190
  Kearns–Sayre syndrome 281
  mitochondrial encephalopathies 319
  motor neurone disease 331
  myasthenia gravis 341, 342
   reversal 343
  myotonia congenita 151
  myotubular myopathy 346

nemaline myopathy 350
neurofibromatosis 353
safety in porphyria 411
tetanus 182
thyrotoxicosis 488
Werdnig–Hoffman disease 513
muscular dystrophies 339–40
  malignant hyperthermia 297
  scoliosis 458
muscular weakness
  acromegaly 9
  Charcot–Marie–Tooth disease 95
  Conn's syndrome 107
  Cushing's disease 112, 113
  dermatomyositis/polymyositis complex 125
  Duchenne muscular dystrophy 142, 143
  dystrophia myotonica 147
  Eaton–Lambert syndrome 153
  Emery–Dreifuss muscular dystrophy 169
  giant axonal neuropathy 204
  Guillain–Barré syndrome 215, 216
  Kearns–Sayre syndrome 281
  motor neurone disease 330
  myasthenia gravis 340, 341, 342
  myotubular myopathy 346
  nemaline myopathy 350
  Pompe's disease/adult onset acid maltase deficiency 405, 406
  Werdnig–Hoffman disease 513
myasthenia gravis 340–3
  muscle relaxants 341, 342
   reversal 343
myasthenic (Eaton–Lambert; Lambert–Eaton) syndrome 153–4
myeloma/multiple myeloma 344–5
myeloproliferative disorders 73, 74
myoclonic epilepsy with red-ragged fibres (MERRF) 318
myophosphorylase deficiency *see* McArdle's syndrome
myositis (fibrodysplasia) ossificans progressiva 196–7
myotonia congenita (Thomsen's disease) 147, 151–2, 298
  malignant hyperthermia-like reactions 564
  masseter muscle rigidity 568
  rhabdomyolysis 443, 444
myotonic syndromes 147
  malignant hyperthermia 297
myotubular (centronuclear) myopathy 345–6
myxoma 346–8, 424

N

NADH-diaphorase deficiency 570, 571

613

nadolol 489
nalidixic acid 208
    porphyria 410
naloxone 369, 425, 554
    adverse reactions 431
near drowning 139–41, 434, 435
    hypothermia 139, 140, 141
nedocromil sodium 54, 55
nemaline myopathy 350
neostigmine 149, 153, 299, 341, 343, 400
    anaphylactic/anaphylactoid reactions 536
    safety in porphyria 411
    suxamethonium apnoea 581
neuroblastoma 72
neurofibromatosis 351–3, 384, 458
neurofibromatosis 1 (von Recklinghausen's disease)
    351–2
neurofibromatosis 2 351, 352, 353
neurogenic pulmonary oedema 426–7
neuroleptic malignant syndrome 354–6, 446
    associated drugs 355
    Hallervorden–Spatz disease 229
    malignant hyperthermia relationship 297, 354–5,
        356
    Parkinson's disease-related susceptibility 378
    rhabdomyolysis 443
neuronal dystrophy (Hallervorden–Spatz disease)
    228–9, 354
neuropathy, ataxia and retinitis pigmentosa (NARP)
    318
new variant Creutzfeldt–Jakob disease (CJD) 109, 110
nicardipine 388, 389
nicorandil 492
nifedipine 4, 43, 105, 107, 159, 295, 306, 419, 420,
    422
nikethimide 410
nimodipine 334
nitrazepam 410
nitric oxide 419, 422
nitrobenzene, toxic methaemoglobinaemia 570
nitrofurantoin 208
nitroprusside 45, 86, 91, 209, 389, 422, 425, 427, 574
    safety in porphyria 411
nitrous oxide 86, 174, 185, 299, 324, 414, 421
    contraindication in phenylketonuria 391, 392
    safety in porphyria 411
Noonan's syndrome 83, 357–8
norepinephrine (noradrenaline) 338, 422
    phaeochromocytoma 384, 385

O

obesity 360–2

Cushing's disease 112, 113
    Prader–Willi syndrome 413, 414
    sleep apnoea 364, 366, 367
    von Gierke's disease 502
occupational transmission
    HIV infection/AIDS 17–18, 19–20, 21
    human papillomavirus 288, 289
octreotide 9, 11, 76, 77, 78, 208, 269, 336, 549, 550
ocular muscular dystrophy 340
oculo-auriculo-vertebral dysplasia (Goldenhar's
    syndrome) 210–11
oculopharyngeal muscular dystrophy 340
oesophageal duplication 313
oesophageal varices 24, 26, 115
ondansetron 76
opiates
    addiction 12, 368–9
        abstinence syndromes 368, 369
        methadone equivalent dosages 369
    adverse reactions 148
        anaphylactic reactions 534
        central anticholinergic syndrome 553
        long QT syndrome 435
        perioperative excitatory events 178–9
    Guillain–Barré syndrome 216
    haemophilia A postoperative care 227
    motor neurone disease 331, 332
    reversal-related pulmonary oedema 431
    tolerance 368, 369
Opitz–Frias syndrome 370
organophosphates exposure 400, 581
Osler–Weber–Rendu disease (hereditary
    haemorrhagic telangiectasia) 241–4
osmotic demyelination syndrome 258, 260
osteogenesis imperfecta 325, 370–3
    type I 371
    type II 371
    type III 371, 372
    type IV 371, 372
osteoporosis
    Cushing's disease 112, 113
    cystic fibrosis 115
oxidative phosphorylation diseases 280, 318

P

pacemakers 229, 281
    defibrillation 234
    diathermy complications 230–1, 233
    dysfunction detection 233
    extracorporeal shock wave lithotripsy 231, 234
    failure during anaesthesia/surgery 231, 233–4
    hypertrophic cardiomyopathy 83

long QT syndrome 433
markings 232
mitochondrial encephalopathies 319
MRI contraindications 232
scleroderma 456
sick sinus syndrome 462, 463
threshold 233
type/function 232–3
see also atrial pacing; temporary pacing
Paget's disease 375–6
pain relief
carcinoid syndrome 78
cystic fibrosis postoperative care 117
demyelinating disease/multiple sclerosis 125
Fabry's disease 182
Guillain–Barré syndrome 215, 216
haemophilia A postoperative care 227
HIV infection/AIDS 19, 21
motor neurone disease 331–2
obese patients 362
obstructive sleep apnoea 366
opiate addicts 369
Paget's disease 375
pulmonary hypertension 422
safe drugs in porphyria 411
sickle cell crises 219, 221, 222
palm sign 131
palmitoyl transferase deficiency 564
pamidronate 214, 257, 372, 375
pancuronium 45, 53, 78, 281, 333, 414
adverse reactions 400
anaphylactic/anaphylactoid 536
suxamethonium apnoea 581
contraindications
phaeochromocytoma 388
Wolff–Parkinson–White syndrome 517
drug interactions 179
myasthenia gravis 341
porphyria 410, 411
papaveretum 205
paracetamol 209, 227
adverse reactions 205
safety in porphyria 411
paraganglionomas 90
paraldehyde 410
paramyotonia 147, 188, 191–3
paraproteinaemias 344
pargyline 410
Parkinson's disease 376–9
autonomic dysfunction 66
neuroleptic malignant syndrome 354, 355
paroxysmal nocturnal haemoglobinuria 73, 74, 380–2

paroxysmal supraventricular (AV nodal re-entrant) tachycardia 546, 547
Pearson's syndrome 318
pemphigus foliaceous 382, 383
pemphigus vulgaris 382–3
penicillin 220, 222, 246, 486
anaphylactic/anaphylactoid reactions 536
safety in porphyria 411
pentamidine 18
pentazocine 227, 369
methadone equivalent dosage 369
perioperative excitatory events 178
porphyria 410
pergolide 377
pericardiocentesis 80, 81
periodic paralysis 147
malignant hyperthermia 297
peripheral neuropathy
alcoholic patients 24, 26
diabetes mellitus 129
familial dysautonomia 186
myeloma 344
rheumatoid arthritis 448
sarcoidosis 452
pernicious anaemia 263
peroneal muscular atrophy (Charcot–Marie–Tooth disease) 95–6
pethidine
abstinence syndrome 369
contraindication in phaeochromocytoma 388
drug interactions 378
methadone equivalent dosage 369
perioperative excitatory events 179
porphyria 410, 411
phaeochromocytoma 90, 91, 159, 207, 336, 337, 384–9, 418, 430, 431, 463, 464, 546, 572–5
hypertensive crisis 384, 385, 464
neurofibromatosis association 351, 352, 353
preoperative stabilization 386–8
von Hippel–Lindau disease 504, 505
phenacetin 208, 209
phencyclidine abuse 179
phenobarbitone 179
central anticholinergic syndrome 553, 554
drug interactions 177
phenothiazines 105, 378
adverse reactions 481
central anticholinergic syndrome 553
malignant hyperthermia 299
contraindications 379
phenoxybenzamine 91, 249, 385, 386, 387, 427, 574
porphyria 410

615

phentolamine 104, 295, 387, 389, 427, 574
phenylbutazone 209
phenylephrine 48, 87, 105, 167, 184, 185, 326, 334,
    518, 575
    drug interactions 103
phenylketonuria 391–2
phenytoin 148, 151, 170, 179, 209, 433
    drug interactions 177, 179
phocomelias 486–7
physostigmine 554, 555
Pierre Robin syndrome 393–6
pimozide 491, 584, 585
pituitary adenoma 9, 11
pituitary apoplexy 397–8, 576–7
plasma cholinesterase abnormalities 104, 399–401
    disease states 399–400
    genetic variants 399
    iatrogenic causes 400
    pregnancy 400
    suxamethonium apnoea 580, 581
plasma expanders, anaphylactic/anaphylactoid
    reactions 536
Pneumocystis carinii pneumonia 18, 19
pneumothorax
    cystic fibrosis 115, 116, 117
    Ehlers–Danlos syndrome type IV 164
    epiglottitis 173
poliomyelitis 458
polyarteritis nodosa 465
polycythaemia 73, 402
    Fallot's tetralogy 183, 184, 185
    secondary 402, 404
polycythaemia vera 402–5
polymyositis *see* dermatomyositis/polymyositis
    complex
polyneuropathy
    Churg–Strauss syndrome 99
    HIV infection/AIDS 19
    rhabdomyolysis 443
Pompe's disease 405–7
porphyria 407–12
    acute crises 409, 410, 411
        treatment 411–12
    drug-related attacks 408, 409–10, 411
    haem metabolism 407, 408
    safe drugs 411
potassium iodide 487, 489, 583
Prader–Willi syndrome 413–14
pranlukast 55
prayer sign 129
prazosin 387
prednisolone 16, 175, 382

prednisone 16
preeclampsia 156–61, 235
    see also HELLP syndrome
pregnancy
    achondroplasia 8
    Addison's disease 14, 523
    alveolar proteinosis 29
    amphetamine abuse 30, 31
    ankylosing spondylitis 39
    antiphospholipid syndrome 40, 41, 42
    aortic stenosis 47, 48
    arthrogryposis multiplex congenita 52–3
    asthma 57
    Budd–Chiari syndrome 73, 74
    Charcot–Marie–Tooth disease 95
    coarctation of aorta 101
    cocaine abuse 104, 105
    Conn's syndrome 107, 109
    Cushing's disease 112, 113
    cystic fibrosis 114, 116, 118
    demyelinating disease/multiple sclerosis 123, 124,
        125
    dermatomyositis/polymyositis complex 126
    diabetes insipidus 127, 128
    drug abuse 13
    dystrophia myotonica 149
    Ebstein's anomaly 156
    Ehlers–Danlos syndrome type IV 163, 164–5
    Eisenmenger's syndrome 167, 168
    Fallot's tetralogy, corrected 184, 185
    fibrodysplasia ossificans progressiva 197
    Friedreich's ataxia 201
    Gaucher's disease 203, 204
    Goodpasture's syndrome 212
    Gorham's syndrome 214
    Guillain–Barré syndrome 216
    haemophilia A
        acquired 227
        carriers 225, 227
    hereditary angioneurotic oedema 240
    hereditary haemorrhagic telangiectasia 243
    hereditary spherocytosis 245–6
    HIV infection/AIDS 19, 20
    homocystinuria 248
    hypercalcaemia 257
    hypertrophic cardiomyopathy 85
    hypokalaemic periodic paralysis 191
    hypothyroidism 263
    insulinoma 269
    Kawasaki disease 279, 280
    Kearns–Sayre syndrome 281
    Klippel–Feil syndrome 283

Klippel–Trenaunay–Weber syndrome 285
local anaesthetic toxic reactions 560, 561
long QT syndrome 436
Marfan syndrome 304, 305
mitochondrial encephalopathies 320
mitral stenosis 324, 325
mitral valve regurgitation 322
motor neurone disease 331
moyamoya disease 333, 334
neurofibromatosis 352, 353
Noonan's syndrome 358
obesity 361
opiate addicts 368, 369
paroxysmal nocturnal haemoglobinuria 381
pemphigus vulgaris 383
peripartum cardiomyopathy 84–5
phaeochromocytoma 159, 385, 386, 389, 572,
    573–4
phenylketonuria 392
plasma cholinesterase abnormalities 400
    suxamethonium apnoea 580, 581
preeclampsia/eclampsia 156–61
protein C deficiency 416, 417
protein S deficiency 418, 419
pulmonary hypertension 420, 421
relapsing polychondritis 439, 440
scleroderma 455, 456, 457
sickle cell disease 221, 222–3
Sipple's syndrome 464
spinal muscular atrophy 469–70
spondyloepiphyseal dysplasia 471
systemic lupus erythematosus 474, 475
Takayasu's arteritis 477, 478, 479
thalassaemia 485, 486
thalidomide-related deformities/phocomelias 487
thyrotoxicosis 488, 490
toluene abuse 468
Turner's syndrome 498
varicella 500
von Gierke's disease 503
von Hippel–Lindau disease 504–5
von Willebrand's disease 507, 508, 509
Wegener's granulomatosis 511, 512
Wolff–Parkinson–White syndrome 517
premature labour 429
prenylamine 491, 585
prilocaine 209
    methaemoglobinaemia 570, 571
    toxicity 560
primaquine 208
primidone 433
    drug interactions 177

prion diseases 109–10
    iatrogenic transmission 110
procainamide 148, 151, 192, 492, 516, 518, 547
    torsade de pointes 585
procaine 411
prochloperazine 411
promazine 411
promethazine
    central anticholinergic syndrome 554
    safety in porphyria 411
propanidid 581
propantheline 341
propofol 28, 52, 56, 58, 63, 64, 78, 87, 117, 149, 200,
    250, 299, 306, 320, 334, 342, 366, 373, 435, 482,
    561
    adverse reactions 144, 148, 149
        anaphylactic/anaphylactoid 536
        perioperative excitatory events 177, 178
    contraindication in epilepsy 177, 179
    porphyria 410, 411
propranolol 104, 185, 295, 326, 387, 416, 435, 482,
    488, 489, 490, 492, 518, 547, 553, 583
    safety in porphyria 411
    torsade de pointes 585
propylthiouracil 490, 517, 583
prostacyclin 101
prostaglandins 76, 77
protein C deficiency 73, 74, 415–17
    homozygous infants 415, 416–17
protein S deficiency 74, 418–19
proton pump inhibitors 107
pseudohyponatraemia 260, 261, 262
pseudostatus epilepticus (psychogenic seizures) 179,
    180
pseudoxanthoma elasticum 325
psychogenic seizures (pseudostatus epilepticus) 179,
    180
pulmonary arteriovenous malformations 242, 243
pulmonary hypertension 419–22
    amniotic fluid embolism 531
    cardiac myxoma 347
    cystic fibrosis 114, 115
    Eisenmenger's syndrome 166, 167
    Gaucher's disease 203
    mitral stenosis 323
    obstructive sleep apnoea 364
    opiate addiction 368
    primary 419, 420, 421
    scleroderma 455, 456
    scoliosis 459
    systemic lupus erythematosus 475
    Takayasu's arteritis 477, 478

thalassaemia 485
pulmonary oedema 423–31
    aortic regurgitation 45
    aortic stenosis 47
    beta-2-sympathomimetics-related 429–31
    cardiac arrhythmias 547
    cardiac tamponade drainage complication 80
    cardiogenic 424–6
    causes 423–4
    cocaine abuse 103
    epiglottitis 173–4, 175
    hyponatraemia 260
    ischaemic heart disease 424, 425
    McArdle's syndrome 312
    mediastinal masses 314
    mitral stenosis 323, 324–5, 425
    mitral valve disease 322, 424
    mucopolysaccharidoses 253
    myxoma 424
    naloxone-related 431
    near drowning 139
    neurogenic 426–7
    opiate addiction 368
    pericardiocentesis complication 552–3
    permeability 424
    phaeochromocytoma 384–5, 386, 573
    Pierre Robin syndrome 394
    preeclampsia 158
    systemic lupus erythematosus 475
    thyroid crisis 582
    thyrotoxicosis 488
    Treacher Collins syndrome 495
    TURP syndrome 589
    upper airway obstruction 427–8
pulsus paradoxus 79, 551
pyridostigmine 153, 341, 343, 400

Q
QT syndrome, prolonged 63, 433–6, 442, 546
    ECG abnormalities 434
    genetic studies 433, 435
    surgery-related arrhythmias 435
    torsade de pointes 491, 492, 584, 585
quinidine 208, 322, 547
    torsade de pointes 491, 585
quinine 151, 208, 480

R
radial artery cannulation
    acromegaly 10
    scleroderma 457

radiotherapy, automatic implantable cardioverter
    defibrillators (AICD) 64
ranitidine 291, 309
    glycopyrrolate interaction 554
Raynaud's disease 420
receptor tyrosine kinase (RET) proto-oncogene 336,
    463
regional anaesthesia
    achondroplasia 6
    antiphospholipid syndrome 42
    aortic stenosis 48
    arthrogryposis multiplex congenita 53
    asthma 57
    athletic heart syndrome 60
    contraindications
        haemophilia A 225
        homocystinuria 248
    dilated cardiomyopathy 86
    Ehlers–Danlos syndrome 163, 164
    epidermolysis bullosa 172
    familial dysautonomia 187
    hypertrophic cardiomyopathy 86
    Klippel–Trenaunay–Weber syndrome 285
    local anaesthetic toxic reactions 557–62
    multiple system atrophy 338
    neurofibromatosis 352
    obesity 360, 361
    osteogenesis imperfecta 373
    Parkinson's disease 379
    porphyria 412
    pulmonary hypertension 421–2
    rheumatoid arthritis 450
    scoliosis 459, 460
    spondyloepiphyseal dysplasia 471
    thyrotoxicosis 490
    von Willebrand's disease 508
relapsing polychondritis 439–41
remifentanil 25, 87, 101, 117, 323, 342
renal function impairment
    diabetes mellitus 129, 131
    Goodpasture's syndrome 212
    HELLP syndrome 236, 237
    myeloma 344, 345
    plasma cholinesterase abnormalities 400
    preeclampsia 158
    rhabdomyolysis 443, 444, 446
    rheumatoid arthritis 448
    sarcoidosis 452
    scleroderma 455
    sickle cell disease 219, 221
    tuberous sclerosis 497
    Turner's syndrome 498

von Gierke's disease 502
Wegener's granulomatosis 510, 511
Williams syndrome 514
renin-angiotensin system 107
reperfusion-related rhabdomyolysis 444
respiratory dysfunction
  achondroplasia 5, 6
  Addison's disease 15
  ankylosing spondylitis 37, 38
  cardiac tamponade 79, 80
  Charcot–Marie–Tooth disease 95, 96
  cocaine abuse 103–4
  cystic fibrosis 114, 115, 116
  demyelinating disease/multiple sclerosis 123
  dermatomyositis/polymyositis complex 125, 126
  diabetes mellitus 130
  Duchenne muscular dystrophy 143, 144, 145, 146
  dystrophia myotonica 148, 149
  familial dysautonomia 186
  fat embolism 195
  fibrodysplasia ossificans progressiva 196–7
  Fraser syndrome 198
  Friedreich's ataxia 201
  Goodpasture's syndrome 212
  Guillain–Barré syndrome 214, 215, 216
  hydatid disease 255
  Marfan syndrome 305
  Morquio's syndrome 329
  motor neurone disease 330–1
  multiple system atrophy 337, 338
  myasthenia gravis 342, 343
  myotubular myopathy 346
  near drowning 139
  neurofibromatosis 351, 352
  Noonan's syndrome 357
  obesity 360, 361
  obstructive sleep apnoea 365
  Prader–Willi syndrome 413, 414
  pulmonary hypertension 420
  Rett syndrome 442
  rheumatoid arthritis 447–8, 450
  sarcoidosis 452, 453
  scleroderma 455, 456
  scoliosis 458, 459
  sickle cell disease 220, 221
    acute chest syndrome 222
  spondyloepiphyseal dysplasia 470, 471
  systemic lupus erythematosus 474
  tetanus 480, 481
  tracheobronchomegaly 493, 494
  varicella pneumonia 499, 500
  Wegener's granulomatosis 510, 511

Werdnig–Hoffman disease 513
respiratory failure
  achalasia of oesophagus 3
  autonomic dysfunction 68
  Chiari malformations 50
  cystic fibrosis 114, 115, 116
restrictive cardiomyopathy 83, 84, 85, 87
Rett syndrome 441–2
rhabdomyolysis 442–6
  amphetamine abuse 30, 31
  Becker muscular dystrophy 70, 443, 444
  biochemical features 444–5
  carnitine palmitoyl transferase deficiency 89
  cocaine abuse 103, 105
  compartment syndrome 445, 446
  drug-related 443, 444
  Duchenne muscular dystrophy 144–5, 146, 443, 444, 445
  Emery–Dreifuss muscular dystrophy 169
  Guillain–Barré syndrome 443, 444
  halothane 459
  hyperkalaemia 444
  intraoperative factors 443–4
  malignant hyperthermia 443, 444, 445
  management 445–6
  McArdle's syndrome 312
  myotonia congenita 443, 444
  neuroleptic malignant syndrome 355, 443
  polyneuropathy 443
  predisposing factors 443
  spinal muscle atrophy 443, 444, 469
  status epilepticus 443
  suxamethonium 459, 469
  tourniquets 444, 446
rhabdomyosarcoma 72
rheumatic heart disease 43, 546
rheumatoid arthritis 447–50, 458, 465
  intubation methods 450
Riley–Day syndrome (familial dysautonomia) 66, 186–8
riluzole 331
ritodrine 429
Robin sequence 393
rocuronium 319
  anaphylactic/anaphylactoid reactions 536
Romano–Ward syndrome 585
  see also QT syndrome, prolonged
ropivacaine toxicity 558, 560
ryanodine receptors 296

S

salbutamol 57, 549, 556

adverse reactions 429
salicylates 309
salmetrol 55
Sanfilippo's syndrome 335
sarcoidosis 452–3
 heart disease 83, 452, 453
Scheie syndrome 250, 251, 335
Schwartz–Jampel syndrome 454
sciatic nerve block, local anaesthetic toxic reactions
 559
scleroderma 325, 455–7, 465
 diffuse cutaneous 455
 limited cutaneous (CREST syndrome) 455, 457
 pulmonary hypertension 419, 420, 455
scoliosis 458–61
 cardiovascular changes 458
 Duchenne muscular dystrophy 142, 143, 144, 145,
  458
 Friedreich's ataxia 201, 458
 Klippel–Feil syndrome 282
 Marfan syndrome 304, 305, 458
 nemaline myopathy 350
 osteogenesis imperfecta 371, 372
 Prader–Willi syndrome 413, 414
 pulmonary hypertension 459
 respiratory changes 458
 Rett syndrome 442
 spinal muscular atrophy 469
 spondyloepiphyseal dysplasia 470, 471
 surgical correction 143, 144, 145, 458, 459–61
 surgical problems 458–9
seizures/convulsions
 alcohol withdrawal 24
 anaesthetic drug-related perioperative excitatory
  events 177
 cocaine abuse 105
 eclampsia 157, 158, 160–1
 emergency department management 179
 local anaesthetic toxic reactions 558, 559, 560, 561
 mitochondrial encephalopathies 319
 moyamoya disease 333
 phenylketonuria 392
 Prader–Willi syndrome 414
 psychogenic 179, 180
 Rett syndrome 441
 Sturge–Weber syndrome 472
 tuberous sclerosis 496, 497
 TURP syndrome 589
 see also epilepsy
selegiline 377, 378
 drug interactions 378
serotonin 76, 77

sevoflurane 25, 50, 57, 174, 185, 270, 362, 517, 548
 adverse reactions 92
  long QT syndrome 435
  perioperative excitatory events 178
 malignant hyperthermia 299
short tetracosactrin test 15
Shy–Drager syndrome *see* multiple system atrophy
sick cell syndrome 259, 260, 261, 262
sick sinus syndrome 461–3, 491, 546
sickle cell disease 218–23
 haemoglobin electrophoresis 219
 red cell sickling 218, 219, 220
  intraoperative prevention 222
 screening 219, 221
 sickle cell anaemia 218, 219
  painful crises 219, 221
  pulmonary hypertension 419, 420
 sickle cell HbC disease 219
 sickle cell trait 218, 220–1
Sipple's syndrome (multiple endocrine neoplasia 2a)
 463–4
sitting position 525, 526
Sjögren's syndrome 464–5
sleep apnoea/obstructive sleep apnoea 363–7
 achondroplasia 5
 acromegaly 9, 10, 11
 adverse reactions 346
 Chiari malformations 50
 children 363, 364, 365
 contributing factors 363–4
 cri du chat syndrome 111
 diffuse idiopathic skeletal hyperostosis 135
 Down's syndrome 137
 Duchenne muscular dystrophy 142
 dystrophia myotonica 148
 Friedreich's ataxia 201
 Goldenhar's syndrome 211
 hypothyroidism 264
 Klippel–Feil syndrome 283
 laryngeal papillomatosis 287
 lymphangioma 120
 Marfan syndrome 304, 305
 Morquio's syndrome 329
 motor neurone disease 331
 mucopolysaccharidoses 253
 multiple system atrophy 337, 338
 obese patients 360–1, 364, 366, 367
 palatal surgery 366–7
 Pierre Robin syndrome 393
 Prader–Willi syndrome 414
 rheumatoid arthritis 449
 sarcoidosis 453

Schwartz–Jampel syndrome 454
Treacher Collins syndrome 495
sodium channel disorders 192
sodium cromoglycate 54, 309, 310
sodium iodide 583
sodium valproate 179, 483
  drug interactions 177, 179
solvents abuse 12, 465–8, 546
somatostatin therapy 501
sotalol
  contraindications 436
  torsade de pointes 491, 585
spinal anaesthesia
  accidental subdural block 577
  ankylosing spondylitis 38, 39
  aortic stenosis 48
  demyelinating disease/multiple sclerosis 124
  diabetes mellitus 130
  dystrophia myotonica 149
  Ehlers–Danlos syndrome 163, 164
  Friedreich's ataxia 201
  haemophilia A carriers 227
  hypokalaemic periodic paralysis 191
  Morquio's syndrome 329
  mucopolysaccharidoses 254
  multiple system atrophy 338
  Paget's disease 376
  pemphigus vulgaris 383
  von Hippel–Lindau disease 504
spinal muscular atrophy 298, 469–70
  malignant hyperthermia-like reactions 297, 564
  rhabdomyolysis 443, 444
  scoliosis 469
spironolactone 189
splenectomy
  antibiotic prophylaxis 246, 486
  hereditary spherocytosis 245
  infectious mononucleosis 267, 268
  prophylactic vaccination 246, 486
  thalassaemia 484, 485, 486
spondyloepiphyseal dysplasia 470–1
spongiform encephalopathy 50
stanozolol 94, 239, 240
status asthmaticus 548
status epilepticus 176
  rhabdomyolysis 443
  treatment 179–80
stellate ganglion block, local anaesthetic toxic
  reactions 559
steroid therapy 94
  anaphylactic/anaphylactoid reactions 256, 538
  asthma 54, 55, 56

carcinoid syndrome 550
Churg–Strauss syndrome 99
cystic fibrosis 117
Eaton–Lambert syndrome 153
epidermolysis bullosa 170
epiglottitis 175
equivalent dosages 16
fibrodysplasia ossificans progressiva 197
Goodpasture's syndrome 212
HELLP syndrome 235, 237
hypercalcaemia 257
hypothyroidism 265
laryngeal papillomatosis 289
malignant hyperthermia 301
mineralocorticoid effects 16
myasthenia gravis 341
myeloma 344
neurogenic pulmonary oedema 427
paroxysmal nocturnal haemoglobinuria 382
pemphigus vulgaris 382, 383
Pneumocystis carinii pneumonia 18
porphyria attacks 410
pulmonary hypertension with collagen vascular
  disease 420
relapsing polychondritis 439, 440
sarcoidosis 453
scleroderma 455
systemic lupus erythematosus 474
Takayasu's arteritis 477
thyroid crisis 583
Wegener's granulomatosis 510
withdrawal-related adrenocortical deficiency 14,
  523, 524
  surgical cover 16
stiff joint syndrome 129–30, 131
streptokinase 273
streptomycin 209
streptozotocin 269
Sturge–Weber syndrome 284, 285, 472–3
subdural block, accidental 577–9
substance abuse 173
sudden death
  Addisonian crisis 523
  aortic stenosis 47
  asthma 55
  autonomic dysfunction 68
  cardiac myxoma 347
  coarctation of aorta 100
  congenital heart block 230
  dilated cardiomyopathy 84
  dystrophia myotonica 148
  Emery–Dreifuss muscular dystrophy 169

epiglottitis 173
Fallot's tetralogy, corrected 184
familial dysautonomia 186, 187
Guillain–Barré syndrome 215, 216
hypertrophic cardiomyopathy 83
infectious mononucleosis 267
Kearns–Sayre syndrome 281
long QT syndrome 433, 434
mitral valve prolapse 325
phaeochromocytoma crisis 384
primary pulmonary hypertension 419
relapsing polychondritis 440
Rett syndrome 442
sickle cell trait 220
solvent abuse 466
torsade de pointes 584
Williams syndrome 514
Wolff–Parkinson–White syndrome 516
sufentanil 48, 388, 482
sulfamethoxazole 510
see also co-trimoxazole
sulfones 208
sulphonamides 177, 208
porphyria 410
sulphonylureas 410
superior vena cava obstruction, mediastinal masses 313, 314, 315
suxamethonium 31, 76, 95, 126, 257, 281, 561
adverse reactions 92, 277–8, 283, 297, 350, 378, 399, 400, 413
anaphylactic/anaphylactoid 536
apnoea 580–1
hyperkalaemia 445, 459
hypokalaemic periodic paralysis 190
malignant hyperthermia 299
masseter muscle rigidity 298, 444, 564, 567, 568
rhabdomyolysis 444, 459
contraindications 19, 70, 71, 78, 89, 92, 93, 445
Duchenne muscular dystrophy 143, 144, 145, 459
dystrophia myotonica 149
Freeman–Sheldon syndrome 200
Guillain–Barré syndrome 215, 216
Hallervorden–Spatz disease 229
hyperkalaemic periodic paralysis/paramyotonia 193
Lesch–Nyhan disease 292
McArdle's syndrome 312
motor neurone disease 331
myotonia congenita 151, 152
osteogenesis imperfecta 372
phaeochromocytoma 388

Pompe's disease/adult onset acid maltase deficiency 407
spinal muscular atrophy 469
tetanus 481
Werdnig–Hoffman disease 513
Williams syndrome 514
myasthenia gravis 341, 342
plasma cholinesterase hydrolysis 399
safety in porphyria 411
syndrome of inappropriate ADH secretion 259, 261
syringobulbia 50
syringomyelia 49, 50, 51
scoliosis 458
systemic lupus erythematosus 74, 465, 473–5
antiphospholipid syndrome 40, 473, 474, 475
pulmonary hypertension 419, 420
systemic mastocytosis 308, 309, 310
systemic sclerosis 40, 41

T
tachykinins 76, 77
tacrine 581
Takayasu's arteritis 477–9
Taurius' syndrome 443
temazepam 411
temporary pacing
sarcoidosis 453
sick sinus syndrome 463
temporomandibular joint disorders
ankylosing spondylitis 36, 38
arthrogryposis multiplex congenita 52
rheumatoid arthritis 449
terbutaline 429, 430, 443
terfenadine 309
torsade de pointes 491, 584, 585
tetanolysin 480
tetanospasmin 480
tetanus 66, 480–3
toxoid 481
tetrabenazine 249, 250
neuroleptic malignant syndrome 355
thalassaemia 218, 484–6
alpha 484
beta major (homozygous disease) 484–5
beta minor (heterozygous state) 484, 485
splenectomy 484, 485, 486
thalidomide-related deformities 486–7
theophylline 54, 55
porphyria 410
rhabdomyolysis 443, 446
thiapride 355
thiazide diuretics 258, 259

thiopentone 25, 31, 84, 95, 105, 180, 299, 334, 427, 561
  adverse reactions 409
    anaphylactic/anaphylactoid 536
    long QT syndrome 435
  contraindications 86
  drug interactions 270
  porphyria 410
thioridazine
  neuroleptic malignant syndrome 355
  torsade de pointes 491, 584, 585
Thomsen's disease *see* myotonia congenita
thrombocytopenia
  anticonvulsants-related 177
  cocaine abuse 104, 105
  Gaucher's disease 203
  HELLP syndrome 235, 236
  infectious mononucleosis 267, 268
  paroxysmal nocturnal haemoglobinuria 380
  systemic lupus erythematosus 474
thromboembolic complications
  antiphospholipid syndrome 40, 41
  cardiac arrhythmias 546, 547
  cardiac myxoma 347
  Cushing's disease 113
  Eisenmenger's syndrome 166, 167, 168
  Fabry's disease 182
  glucagonoma 207, 208
  homocystinuria 248
  Klippel–Trenaunay–Weber syndrome 284, 285
  lupus anticoagulant 474–5
  mitral stenosis 323
  obesity 361, 362
  paroxysmal nocturnal haemoglobinuria 380, 381
  polycythaemia vera 403
  protein C deficiency 415, 416
  protein S deficiency 418
  sick sinus syndrome 462
  systemic lupus erythematosus 474
  tetanus 481
thrombotic thrombocytopenic purpura 73
thyroid crisis (thyroid storm) 488, 489, 574, 581–3
thyroid medullary carcinoma 463
thyrotoxic periodic paralysis 188–9, 489
thyrotoxicosis 487–90, 546
thyroxine therapy 263, 264, 265, 488, 583
  safety in porphyria 411
tobramycin 117
tocainide 151
tolazoline 422
tolbutamide 208
toluene abuse 466, 467, 468

torsade de pointes 491–2, 547, 584–6
  drug-induced 491, 584
total spinal anaesthesia 586–8
tourniquet-induced rhabdomyolysis 444, 446
toxic methaemoglobinaemia 570
tracheobronchomegaly 493–4
tracheostomy
  angioneurotic oedema 543
  laryngeal papillomatosis 288
  lymphangioma 120
  multiple system atrophy 338
  myasthenia gravis 343
  Pierre Robin syndrome 393, 394
  relapsing polychondritis 440
  tetanus 482
  Treacher Collins syndrome 494
  Wegener's granulomatosis 511
tranexamic acid 94, 226, 227, 276
transcutaneous electrical nerve stimulation (TENS) 64
tranylcypromine 410
Treacher Collins syndrome 494–6
triamcinolone 16
triamterene 189
1,1,1,-trichloroethane abuse 466, 467
tricyclic antidepressants
  central anticholinergic syndrome 553
  torsade de pointes 491, 584, 585
trifluoperazine
  adverse reactions
    neuroleptic malignant syndrome 355
    torsade de pointes 585
  safety in porphyria 411
trimeprazine (alimemazine) 442
trimethoprim 209
  see also co-trimoxazole
trismus
  arthrogryposis multiplex congenita 52
  fibrodysplasia ossificans progressiva 196, 197
  Gaucher's disease 203
  Ludwig's angina 293, 294
  tetanus 480
tuberous sclerosis 496–7
tubocurarine 51
  anaphylactic/anaphylactoid reactions 536
  safety in porphyria 411
Turner's syndrome 43, 44, 497–8
TURP syndrome 588–91

U
upper airway obstruction
  achalasia of oesophagus 3, 4

623

achondroplasia 5, 7
acromegaly 9, 10, 11
amyloidosis 33, 35
arthrogryposis multiplex congenita 52
asthma 55, 56
Beckwith–Wiedemann syndrome 72
CHARGE association 97
Down's syndrome 137, 138
epiglottitis 173, 174
infectious mononucleosis 267
Klippel–Trenaunay–Weber syndrome 285
laryngeal papillomatosis 287
Ludwig's angina 293, 294
lymphangioma 119, 120
mediastinal masses 313–14, 315, 316
Miller's syndrome 317
Morquio's syndrome 329
motor neurone disease 331
mucopolysaccharidoses 251, 252
myasthenia gravis 340
neurofibromatosis 352
Parkinson's disease 377–8
Pierre Robin syndrome 393, 394, 395
pulmonary oedema 427–8
relapsing polychondritis 439, 440
Sturge–Weber syndrome 472
Treacher Collins syndrome 494–5
Wegener's granulomatosis 511

V
Valsalva manoeuvre 67
valvular heart disease 546
varicella 499–500
varicella-zoster immune globulin 500
variegate porphyria 407, 409
vasculitis
    rheumatoid arthritis 448
    Wegener's granulomatosis 510
vasopressin 127, 128
    torsade de pointes 585
vecuronium 78, 126, 144, 149, 180, 299, 312, 319,
    388, 407
    anaphylactic/anaphylactoid reactions 536
    drug interactions 179
    myasthenia gravis 341, 342
    safety in porphyria 411
venous access
    achondroplasia 5–6, 7
    arthrogryposis multiplex congenita 52
    Cushing's disease 113
    Ehlers–Danlos syndrome 163, 164

epidermolysis bullosa 171
haemophilia A 225
hereditary haemorrhagic telangiectasia 243
Miller's syndrome 317
mucopolysaccharidoses 253
obesity 360
opiate addicts 368
pemphigus vulgaris 383
scleroderma 456
thalidomide-related deformities/phocomelias 487
ventricular ectopic beats 546, 547
ventricular fibrillation 546, 547
ventricular tachycardia 546, 547–8
ventriculoperitoneal shunt 50
verapamil 63, 64, 83, 425, 433, 518, 547
vertebrobasilar insufficiency, ankylosing spondylitis
    36, 37, 39
vipoma 500–1
vitamin supplements 25, 170
volatile agents
    adverse reactions 148
        Duchenne muscular dystrophy 143, 144, 146
        malignant hyperthermia 299
    safety in porphyria 411
volatile substance abuse 465–8
von Gierke's disease 502–3
von Hippel–Lindau disease 125, 504–5
    phaeochromocytoma association 384
von Recklinghausen's disease *see* neurofibromatosis 1
von Willebrand's disease 506–9
    treatment 507, 508
    types 506

W
warfarin 41, 42, 197, 416, 417, 418, 420
water intoxication, acute 258–9, 261
    prevention 261
WDHA syndrome 501
Wegener's granulomatosis 510–12
Werdnig–Hoffman disease 513
Wernicke's encephalopathy 24, 25
Williams (Williams–Beuren) syndrome 46, 513–15
Wilm's tumour 72
Wolff–Parkinson–White syndrome 516–18, 546
    acute attack management 518
    tuberous sclerosis 496, 497

Z
zafirlukast 55
Zenker's diverticulum 520
zidovudine 18, 21

Printed in the United Kingdom by
Lightning Source UK Ltd., Milton Keynes
139555UK00002B/9/P